Nursing for Wellness in
Older Adults

Nursing *for Wellness in* Older Adults

SIXTH EDITION

Carol A. Miller, MSN, RN-BC, AHN-BC

Gerontological Clinical Nurse Specialist and Nurse Case Manager
Care & Counseling, Miller/Wetzler Associates
Cleveland, Ohio

Clinical Faculty
Frances Payne Bolton School of Nursing
Case Western Reserve University
Cleveland, Ohio

. Wolters Kluwer | Lippincott Williams & Wilkins
Health

Philadelphia · Baltimore · New York · London
Buenos Aires · Hong Kong · Sydney · Tokyo

Executive Acquisitions Editor: Elizabeth Nieginski
Product Managers: Helene T. Caprari and Betsy Gentzler
Design Coordinator: Holly Reid McLaughlin
Art Director, Illustration: Brett MacNaughton
Manufacturing Coordinator: Karin Duffield
Prepress Vendor: Aptara, Inc.

Sixth Edition

9 8 7 6 5 4 3 2 1

Printed in China

Library of Congress Cataloging-in-Publication Data
Miller, Carol A. (Carol Ann), 1945- author.
  Nursing for wellness in older adults / Carol A. Miller. — Sixth
edition.
     p. ; cm.
  Includes bibliographical references and index.
  ISBN 978-1-60547-777-0 (hardback : alkaline paper)
  1. Geriatric nursing.   I. Title.
     [DNLM: 1. Geriatric Nursing.   2. Aged—psychology.   3. Health Promotion.
  4. Nursing Theory. WY 152]
     RC954.M55 2011
     618.97′0231—dc22

                                              2010043818

    Care has been taken to confirm the accuracy of the information presented and to describe generally accepted practices. However, the author, editors, and publisher are not responsible for errors or omissions or for any consequences from application of the information in this book and make no warranty, expressed or implied, with respect to the currency, completeness, or accuracy of the contents of the publication. Application of this information in a particular situation remains the professional responsibility of the practitioner; the clinical treatments described and recommended may not be considered absolute and universal recommendations.

    The author, editors, and publisher have exerted every effort to ensure that drug selection and dosage set forth in this text are in accordance with the current recommendations and practice at the time of publication. However, in view of ongoing research, changes in government regulations, and the constant flow of information relating to drug therapy and drug reactions, the reader is urged to check the package insert for each drug for any change in indications and dosage and for added warnings and precautions. This is particularly important when the recommended agent is a new or infrequently employed drug.

    Some drugs and medical devices presented in this publication have Food and Drug Administration (FDA) clearance for limited use in restricted research settings. It is the responsibility of the health care providers to ascertain the FDA status of each drug or device planned for use in his or her clinical practice.

LWW.com

Associate Professor, Faculty of Community
Mount Royal College, School of Nursing
University of South Alabama, College of Nursing
Mobile, Alabama

Associate Professor
...

Clinical Assistant Professor
Betty Irene Moore School of Nursing
...

Snow Community College, School of Nursing
...

K... College of Nursing
... College of Nursing, Practice
Assistant Professor
Associate Professor of Nursing
...

CONTRIBUTORS

Georgia Anetzberger, PhD, ACSW
Assistant Professor, Health Care Administration
Cleveland State University and Case Western Reserve
   Unviersity
Cleveland, Ohio

Casey R. Shillam, RN, MSN, PhD
Post-doctoral fellow
Betty Irene Moore School of Nursing
University of California Davis
Sacramento, California

REVIEWERS

Alice Brnicky
Texas Woman's University
Irving, Texas

Virginia Burggraf
Radford University
Radford, Virginia

Nathania Bush, MSN, APRN, BC
Associate Professor of Nursing
Morehead State University
Clay City, Kentucky

Eunice Cleeland, MSN, RN
Contract Faculty
University of Alabama at Birmingham, School of Nursing
Birmingham, Alabama

Kimberly F. Craven, BSN, MSN
Instructor of Nursing
Jacksonville State University, School of Nursing and
   Health Sciences
Jacksonville, Alabama

Winifred Dolph
Mid-Plains Community College
North Platte, Nebraska

A Student's Perspective Contributors
*These features were contributed by students
from the following programs:*

Brigham Young University
Provo, Utah

Western Michigan University
Kalamazoo, Michigan

Angelo State University
San Angelo, Texas

Judith Draper, MSN, GNP, BC
University of Pennsylvania
Philadelphia, Pennsylvania

Marybeth K. Fischer, RN, MSN
Instructor
St. Luke's School of Nursing
Bethlehem, Pennsylvania

Patricia Fuehr, MSN, RN, FNP-BC
Faculty Specialist
Western Michigan University, Bronson School
   of Nursing
Kalamazoo, Michigan

Barbara A. Heise, PhD, APRN, BC
Assistant Professor
Brigham Young University, College of Nursing
Provo, Utah

Barbara Hulsman, RN, MN
Assistant Professor
Carson-Newman College, School of Nursing
   and Behavioral Health
Jefferson City, Tennessee

Kathy J. Keister, PhD, RN, CNE
Associate Professor
Wright State University, College of Nursing & Health
Dayton, Ohio

Norma Krumwiede, EdD, MEd, MN, RN
Professor
Minnesota State University
Mankato, Minnesota

Lisa A. Lacko, RN, MSN
Assistant Professor
Cedar Crest College
Allentown, Pennsylvania

Bonnie Launhardt
Grant MacEwan Community College
Edmonton, Alberta, Canada

Heidi McCoy, RN, MSN
University of Nebraska Medical Center, College of Nursing
Lincoln, Nebraska

Siobhan McMahon, MSN, MPH, GNP-BC
Assistant Professor of Nursing
The College of St. Scholastica, School of Nursing
Duluth, Minnesota

Elizabeth A. Peterson, DMin, RN
Associate Professor of Nursing
Bethel University
St. Paul, Minnesota

L. Sue Sprinkle, BSN, MSN, HFA, RN
Assistant Professor
Indiana Wesleyan University, Pre-Licensure Division
    School of Nursing
Marion, Indiana

Gregg Trueman, NP, PhD, CHPCN(c)
Associate Professor, Faculty of Community and
    Health Studies
Mount Royal College, School of Nursing
Calgary, Alberta, Canada

Joyce McCullers Varner, DNP, GNP-BC, GCNS
Associate Professor, Adult Health Nursing Department
University of South Alabama, College of Nursing
Mobile, Alabama

Gail Vitale, EdDc, RN, GCNS-BC
Associate Professor
Lewis University, College of Nursing and
    Health Professions
Romeoville, Illinois

Molly J. Walker, PhD, RN, CNS, CNE
Associate Professor, Graduate Advisor
Angelo State University
San Angelo, Texas

Judith Webb, DNP, ANP-BC
Clinical Assistant Professor
MGH Institute of Health Professions
Boston, Massachusetts

Donna Williams-Newman
Knox Community College, School of Nursing
Clarendon, Florida

Preface

When I began my nursing career in 1970, I chose to work in a visiting nurse program that addressed the unique needs of older adults in home settings. When asked why I would want to work full time with the "geriatric population," I enthusiastically responded that this presented a wide open opportunity to meet the needs of people who were neglected by most health care professionals. At that time, "geriatrics'" and "gerontology" were the newcomers in health care, and little was known about the unique nursing care needs of older adults. It would be 4 years before gerontological nursing would be an approved specialization and 5 years before the first gerontological nursing journal would be published. During the past four decades, the percentage of the U.S. population defined as "older adults" has been gradually increasing, with projections that by 2050, 20% of the U.S. population will be aged 65 years and older. Concomitantly, our knowledge about how to provide evidence-based care for older adults has been expanding at a rapid pace. Thus, it is imperative that nurses keep up-to-date on aging-related research and issues so that they can apply this knowledge to identify and address the unique needs of older adults.

In addition to the increasing focus on care of older adults, "wellness" has been emerging as a major focus of health care in recent years. The concept is usually associated with physical fitness and "preventing aging"; however, a major premise of this text is that there is no age limit to achieving wellness when it is holistically conceptualized in the context of one's body, mind, and spirit. Another major premise is that nurses have primary roles in promoting wellness for older adults because we holistically address the needs of our patients, which for older adults involves supporting their optimal level of functioning and quality of life. Thus, the intent of this text is to serve as a foundation for providing wellness-oriented nursing care for older adults in any health care setting.

This sixth edition of *Nursing for Wellness in Older Adults* has been extensively updated to incorporate recent evidence-based information that is pertinent to providing wellness-oriented care for older adults. In addition, a major focus is on the multitude of opportunities that nurses have for promoting health and improving quality of life for older adults. As in previous editions, this text focuses on the aspects of physiologic and psychosocial function that are most relevant to nursing care of older adults. The Functional Consequences Theory provides a framework for identifying the many interacting factors that affect the level of functioning and quality of life of older adults within the context of the nursing process. For each aspect of functioning, nurses can use the assessment and intervention guidelines to identify and address factors that affect the functioning and quality of life of older adults. Evidence-based boxes provide information about recent research that supports assessment of and interventions for conditions commonly addressed when caring for older adults. Nursing interventions focus on health promotion, and many of the intervention guides can be used as health education tools to teach older adults, their families, and their caregivers about actions they can take to promote wellness. Chapters also include information about applicable wellness nursing diagnoses and wellness outcomes. Theory illustrations at the beginning of chapters illustrate how the Functional Consequences Theory is integrated with the nursing process with regard to specific aspects of functioning.

ORGANIZATION

Nursing for Wellness in Older Adults has 29 chapters, organized into five parts. Chapters in Parts 1 and 2 introduce topics relevant to aging, wellness, older adults, and the role of nurses in promoting wellness in older adults. Chapters in Parts 3 and 4 are organized around the Functional Consequences Theory of Gerontological Nursing, so each facet of physiologic or psychosocial function is presented according to age-related changes, risk factors, functional consequences, nursing assessment, nursing diagnosis, wellness outcomes, nursing interventions, and evaluation of nursing care. The three chapters in Part 5 helps nurses provide holistic care for older adults during illness.

The intent of Part 1 (Chapters 1 through 4), *Older Adults and Wellness,* is to help nurses apply a wellness philosophy to their care of older adults. Chapters 1 and 2 integrate the concepts of wellness and aging and provide an overview of characteristics and diversity of older adults. Chapter 3 explicates the Functional Consequences Theory, which is applied throughout this text as a framework for wellness-oriented nursing care of older adults. Chapter 4 provides an overview of theories that are pertinent to aging well.

Part 2 (Chapters 5 through 10), *Nursing Considerations for Older Adults,* introduces gerontological nursing as a subspecialty within nursing and addresses the unique challenges of caring for older adults, with an extensive discussion of health promotion in relation to older adults. Roles for gerontological nurses are described in relation to diverse settings that comprise the continuum of care for older adults. This section also covers the complex topics of assessment, medications, and legal and ethical concerns because nurses address these aspects of care with the majority of the older adults for whom they provide care. Elder abuse and neglect also is addressed in this section because nurses need to be aware of this concern when caring for older adults.

Part 3 (Chapters 11 through 15), *Promoting Wellness in Psychosocial Function*, extensively reviews cognitive and psychosocial function and provides guidelines for a comprehensive nursing assessment of psychosocial function, with emphasis on healthy older adults. In addition, this part covers delirium, dementia, and depression, which are three of the most commonly occurring pathologic conditions that have serious psychosocial consequences for older adults.

Part 4 (Chapters 16 through 26), *Promoting Wellness in Physical Function*, includes chapters that address each of the following specific aspects of functioning in older adults: hearing, vision, digestion and nutrition, urinary function, cardiovascular function, respiratory function, mobility and safety, integument, sleep and rest, thermoregulation, and sexual function. Selected common pathologic conditions also are addressed in these chapters when these conditions affect a particular aspect of functioning in older adults.

Part 5 (Chapters 27 through 29), *Promoting Wellness in All Stages of Health and Illness*, has been added to address topics of caring for older adults during illness and when they are experiencing pain or are at the end of life.

NEW AND SPECIAL FEATURES

Special features from past editions have been retained in this edition, and several new features have been added.

Pedagogical Features

- **Learning Objectives** help the reader identify important chapter content and focus his or her reading.
- **Key Terms** listed at the beginning of the chapter and bolded in the text highlight important vocabulary.
- **Theory Illustrations** at the beginning of each chapter on specific aspects of functioning present an overview of the Functional Consequences Theory in the context of the nursing process.
- **Icons** identify the five major components of the Functional Consequences Theory:

 Age-related changes

 Risk factors

 Functional consequences

 Nursing assessment

 Nursing interventions

- **Progressive Case Studies** provide real-life examples of the effects of age-related changes and risk factors, beginning in young-old adulthood and continuing through all the stages of later adulthood. **Thinking Points** after each segment of the case assist the student in applying the content of the chapter to the case example. Many chapters include a concluding Case Study with a sample **Nursing Care Plan**.
- **Chapter Highlights** in an easy-to-read bulleted format facilitate review of the material.
- **Critical Thinking Exercises**, at the end of each chapter, help readers to gain insight and develop problem-solving skills through purposeful, goal-directed thinking.
- **References** give readers additional information about the most up-to-date research that supports evidence-based practice.

Practice-Oriented Features

- *NEW!* **Evidence-Based Practice** boxes are included in clinically oriented chapters to summarize guidelines for research-based care of older adults.
- **Wellness Opportunities** are sprinkled throughout the clinically oriented chapters to draw attention to ways in which nurses can promote wellness during the usual course of their care activities.
- **A Student's Perspective** provides reality-based stories written by nursing students that illustrate the application of wellness concepts in clinical practice.
- **Cultural Considerations** boxes help the reader to appreciate cultural differences that may influence his or her approach to a patient, resident, or client.
- **Diversity Notes** give brief information about differences among specific groups (e.g., men and women, whites and African Americans).
- **Assessment Boxes** provide the reader with specific approaches for nursing assessment. Commonly used assessment tools are described (and, in many cases, illustrated).
- **Interventions Boxes** provide succinct guides for nursing interventions, with a strong focus on health promotion. Guides for "best practices" in nursing interventions are given. Many of the interventions boxes can be used as tools for teaching older adults and their caregivers about how to improve functional abilities. Interventions boxes that double as teaching tools can be downloaded from thePoint at http://thepoint.lww.com/miller6e.
- **Resources** sections direct the reader to sources for clinical tools, evidence-based practice, and health education.

TEACHING AND LEARNING PACKAGE

Instructor Resources

Tools to assist you with teaching your course are available upon adoption of this text on thePoint at http://thePoint. lww.com/Miller6e. Many of these tools are also included on the Instructor's Resource DVD-ROM.

- An **E-Book** allows access to the book's full text and images online.
- The **Test Generator** lets you generate new tests from a bank of NCLEX-style questions to help you assess your students' understanding of the course material.
- **PowerPoint Presentations** provide an easy way for you to integrate the textbook with your students' classroom experience, either via slide shows or handouts. Multiple-choice and True/False questions are integrated into the presentations to promote class participation and allow you to use i-clicker technology.
- A sample **Syllabus** provides guidance for structuring your course.
- An **Image Bank** contains illustrations from the book in formats suitable for printing and incorporating into PowerPoint presentations and Internet sites.
- **Journal Articles**, corresponding to book chapters, offer access to current research available in Lippincott Williams & Wilkins journals.
- Access to all student resources.

Student Resources

Students can also visit thePoint at http://thePoint.lww.com/miller6e and access the following tools and resources using the codes printed in the front of their textbooks:

- An **E-Book** allows access to the book's full text and images online.
- **Journal Articles**, corresponding to book chapters to offer access to current research available in Lippincott Williams & Wilkins journals.
- **Internet Resources**, include links to clinical tools, evidence-based practice, and health education materials.
- Plus **NCLEX alternate-item format tutorial**, a **Spanish–English audio glossary, Learning Objectives**, and **Interventions Boxes** from the textbook.

SUMMARY

Providing wellness-oriented nursing care for older adults is an opportunity to care for people who are striving to meet the challenges of remaining healthy and functional as they cope with age-related changes and risk factors that affect their functioning and quality of life. The goal of *Nursing for Wellness in Older Adults* is to provide nurses and nursing students with a practical approach to assisting older adults in meeting the many challenges of older adulthood in positive and creative ways.

Carol A. Miller, MSN, RN-BC, AHN-BC

Acknowledgments

I am deeply grateful to my family, friends, and colleagues who have supported me on my journey as this book has grown from a dream to a reality and now into its sixth edition. Pat Rehm, in particular, has constantly supported and encouraged me to pursue my goals as a nurse and author. My work with older adults and their families provides valuable lessons that have become part of this text. These experiences, which cannot be learned in books, have taught me to care deeply about, and to care sensitively for, older adults. I thank these older adults and their families and appreciate their contributions to my life and my writings.

I appreciate and acknowledge the many people who have helped bring this text to fruition. I want to extend my deepest appreciation to the staff at Wolters Kluwer | Lippincott Williams & Wilkins who assisted with all phases of development and production. I thank all these people, and many unnamed people, for the advice, guidance, support, assistance, and encouragement on my journey through all six editions of *Nursing for Wellness in Older Adults*.

Contents

PART **1**

Older Adults and Wellness   1

CHAPTER **1**
Seeing Older Adults Through the Eyes of Wellness   1

IMAGES OF AGING 1

THE RELATIONSHIP BETWEEN WELLNESS AND AGING 2
Wellness and Older Adults 2
Wellness and Nursing Care of Older Adults 2
Definitions of Aging 3
Descriptions of Successful Aging 4

ATTITUDES TOWARD AGING 5
Shifting Trends 5
Ageism 5
Effects of Ageism 6
Addressing Attitudes of Nurses 8

DEBUNKING MYTHS: UNDERSTANDING REALITIES ABOUT OLDER ADULTS IN THE UNITED STATES 8
Demographics of Aging 9
Health Characteristics 11
Socioeconomic Characteristics 11
Living Arrangements of Older Adults 13

OLDER ADULTS IN FAMILIES 14
Trends in Caregiving 14
Older Adults as Recipients and Givers of Care 15
Grandparents Raising Grandchildren 16

OLDER ADULTS IN THE WORLD 16

CHAPTER **2**
Addressing Diversity of Older Adults   20

CULTURAL DIVERSITY IN THE UNITED STATES 20

CULTURAL COMPETENCE 21
Performing a Cultural Self-Assessment 21

Obtaining Information About Culturally Diverse Groups 22
Linguistic Competence in Care of Older Adults 23

CULTURAL PERSPECTIVES ON WELLNESS 23

HEALTH DISPARITIES 24

OVERVIEW OF CULTURAL GROUPS OF OLDER ADULTS IN THE UNITED STATES 26
African Americans 26
Hispanics or Latinos 27
Asians and Pacific Islanders in the United States 29
American Indians and Alaska Natives 30

OLDER ADULTS IN OTHER DIVERSE GROUPS 31
Older Adults in Rural Areas 32
Homeless Older Adults 32
Lesbian, Gay, Bisexual, and Transgender Older Adults 32

CHAPTER **3**
Applying a Nursing Model for Promoting Wellness in Older Adults   36

A NURSING THEORY FOR WELLNESS-FOCUSED CARE OF OLDER ADULTS 36

CONCEPTS UNDERLYING THE FUNCTIONAL CONSEQUENCES THEORY 37
Functional Consequences 37
Age-Related Changes and Risk Factors 39
Person 40
Nursing 41
Health 41
Environment 42

APPLYING THE THEORY TO PROMOTE WELLNESS IN OLDER ADULTS 42

CHAPTER **4**
Theoretical Perspectives on Aging Well   45

HOW CAN WE LIVE LONG AND WELL? 45
Life Span and Life Expectancy 46

Rectangularization of the Curve and
Compression of Morbidity 46
Active Life Expectancy 47
Relationships Among Aging, Disease,
and Death 48
Studies of Healthy Aging 48

HOW DO WE EXPLAIN BIOLOGIC AGING? 49
Wear-and-Tear Theories 49
Cross-Linkage Theory 49
Free Radical Theory 49
Neuroendocrine and Immunity Theories 49
Genetic Theories 50
Apoptosis Theory 50
Caloric Restriction Theories 50
Conclusions About Biologic Theories and
Relevance to Nurses 50

SOCIOCULTURAL PERSPECTIVES ON AGING 51
Disengagement Theory 52
Activity Theory 52
Subculture and Age Stratification Theories 52
Emerging Sociocultural Theories 53
Person–Environment Fit Theory 53
Relevance of Sociocultural Theories of
Aging to Nurses 53

PSYCHOLOGICAL PERSPECTIVES ON AGING 54
Human Needs Theory 54
Life-Course and Personality Development
Theories 54
Theory of Gerotranscendence 55
Theories About Gender and Aging 55
Relevance of Psychological Theories of
Aging to Nurses 55

**A HOLISTIC PERSPECTIVE ON AGING
AND WELLNESS 56**

PART 2

**Nursing Considerations for
Older Adults 59**

CHAPTER 5
**Gerontological Nursing and Health
Promotion 59**

GERONTOLOGY AND GERIATRICS 59
GERONTOLOGICAL NURSING 60
Gerontological Nursing Education and Practice 60
Roles for Gerontological Nurses 61

Evidence-Based Practice for Gerontological
Nursing 61
**HEALTH, WELLNESS, AND HEALTH
PROMOTION 63**
Health Promotion for Older Adults 64
Health Promotion Initiatives for Older Adults 64
Types and Examples of Health Promotion
Interventions for Older Adults 65
Promotion of Physical Activity as a Nursing
Intervention for Wellness 68

**THE TRANSTHEORETICAL MODEL OF HEALTH
PROMOTION 69**

CHAPTER 6
**Diverse Health Care Settings for
Older Adults 75**

**DEVELOPMENT OF A CONTINUUM OF
CARE FOR OLDER ADULTS 75**
ACUTE CARE SETTINGS 77
Specialized Geriatric Acute Care Units 77
Subacute Care Units 77
Hospital-at-Home Model 77
Transitional Care Models 78
Roles for Gerontological Nurses in
Acute Care Settings 78

NURSING HOME SETTINGS 78
Levels of Nursing Home Care 78
Admission to Long-Term Care 79
Trends in Nursing Home Care 79
Roles for Gerontological Nurses in
Nursing Home Settings 80

NEWER MODELS OF NURSING HOME CARE 80
The Culture Change Movement 80
Evidence for Positive Outcomes With
Culture Change 81
Pioneer Network 81
Assisted-Living Facilities 81
Roles for Nurses in Newer Models of Care 82

HOME CARE SERVICES 82
Trends in Home Care Services 82
Skilled Home Care 83
Long-Term Home Care 83
Sources of Home Care Services 83

**COMMUNITY-BASED SERVICES FOR
OLDER ADULTS 84**
Adult Day Centers 84
Respite Services 85
Parish Nursing Programs 85
Health Promotion Programs 85

Roles for Gerontological Nurses in Home and
Community Settings 85

**MODELS ADDRESSING COORDINATION
OF CARE 86**
Comprehensive Models 86
Chronic Care Models 87
Care and Case Management Services 87

**PAYING FOR HEALTH CARE SERVICES
FOR OLDER ADULTS 88**
Out-of-Pocket Expenses 88
Medicare 88
Medigap Insurance 88
Medicaid 89
Older Americans Act 90
Long-Term Care Insurance 90

CHAPTER **7**
**Assessment of Health and
Functioning 94**

ASSESSING HEALTH OF OLDER ADULTS 94

NURSING ASSESSMENT TOOLS 95

ASSESSING FUNCTION OF OLDER ADULTS 95
Using Functional Assessment Tools 95
Assessing Activities of Daily Living 99
Assessing Instrumental Activities of Daily
Living 101
Assessing Function in Cognitively Impaired
Older Adults 101
Assessing the Use or Potential Use of Adaptive
and Assistive Devices 105

COMPREHENSIVE GERIATRIC ASSESSMENTS 106

**ASSESSING OLDER ADULTS IN RELATION TO THEIR
ENVIRONMENTS 106**

**ASSESSING AND ADDRESSING DRIVING
SAFETY 108**
Identifying Risks and Consequences 108
Addressing Risk Factors 109
Referring to Community Resources 109
Working With Caregivers 110

CHAPTER **8**
**Medications and Other Bioactive
Substances 113**

INTRODUCTION TO BIOACTIVE SUBSTANCES 113
Considerations Regarding Medications 113
Considerations Regarding Herbs and
Homeopathy 115

**AGE-RELATED CHANGES THAT AFFECT BIOACTIVE
SUBSTANCES IN OLDER ADULTS 118**
Changes That Affect the Action of Bioactive
Substances in the Body 118
Changes That Affect Behaviors Related to
Taking Bioactive Substances 120

**RISK FACTORS THAT AFFECT BIOACTIVE
SUBSTANCES 120**
Pathologic Processes and Functional
Impairments 121
Behaviors Based on Myths and
Misunderstandings 121
Communication Barriers 122
Lack of Information 122
Inappropriate Prescribing Practices 122
Polypharmacy and Inadequate Monitoring of
Medications 124
Medication Nonadherence 124
Financial Concerns Related to Prescription
Drugs 124
Insufficient Recognition of Adverse Medication
Effects 125

MEDICATION INTERACTIONS 125
Medication–Medication Interactions 125
Medications and Herbs 126
Medications and Nutrients 127
Medications and Alcohol 128
Medications and Caffeine 128
Medications and Nicotine 128

**FUNCTIONAL CONSEQUENCES ASSOCIATED
WITH BIOACTIVE SUBSTANCES IN OLDER
ADULTS 129**
Altered Therapeutic Effects 129
Increased Potential for Adverse Effects 129
Anticholinergic Adverse Effects 130
Altered Mental Status 130
Tardive Dyskinesia and Drug-Induced
Parkinsonism 131
Antipsychotics in People With Dementia 131

**NURSING ASSESSMENT OF MEDICATION
USE AND EFFECTS 131**
Communication Techniques for Obtaining
Accurate Information 132
Scope of a Medication Assessment 132
Observing Patterns of Medication Use 134
Linking the Medication Assessment to the
Overall Assessment 135
Identifying Adverse Medication Effects 135

NURSING DIAGNOSIS 136

PLANNING FOR WELLNESS OUTCOMES 136

NURSING INTERVENTIONS TO PROMOTE HEALTHY MEDICATION-TAKING PATTERNS 136

Implementing Evidence-Based Interventions 136
Teaching About Medications 137
Teaching About Herbs and Other Bioactive Substances 138
Addressing Factors That Affect Adherence 139
Decreasing the Number of Medications 141

EVALUATING EFFECTIVENESS OF NURSING INTERVENTIONS 142

CHAPTER 9
Legal and Ethical Concerns 149

AUTONOMY AND RIGHTS 149
Competency 150
Decision-Making Capacity 150

ADVANCE DIRECTIVES 151
Living Wills and Do Not Resuscitate (DNR) Orders 152
Durable Power of Attorney for Health Care 152

LEGAL ISSUES SPECIFIC TO LONG-TERM CARE SETTINGS 153

ETHICAL ISSUES COMMONLY ADDRESSED IN GERONTOLOGICAL NURSING 153
Ethical Issues in Everyday Care of Older Adults 153
Ethical Issues Specific to Long-Term Care Settings 154
Ethical Issues Related to Artificial Nutrition and Hydration 154

CULTURAL ASPECTS OF LEGAL AND ETHICAL ISSUES 155

ROLE OF NURSES REGARDING LEGAL AND ETHICAL ISSUES 156
Implementing Advance Directives 156
Facilitating Decisions About Care 158

CHAPTER 10
Elder Abuse and Neglect 162

OVERVIEW OF ELDER ABUSE AND NEGLECT 162
Characteristics of Elder Abuse 162
Historical Recognition of a Social Problem 163
Prevalence and Causes 163
Cultural Considerations 164

RISK FACTORS FOR ELDER ABUSE AND NEGLECT 165
Invisibility and Vulnerability 165
Psychosocial Factors 165
Caregiver Factors 165

ELDER ABUSE AND NEGLECT IN NURSING HOMES 166

FUNCTIONAL CONSEQUENCES ASSOCIATED WITH ELDER ABUSE AND NEGLECT 167

NURSING ASSESSMENT OF ABUSED OR NEGLECTED OLDER ADULTS 168
Unique Aspects of Elder Abuse Assessment 168
Physical Health 169
Activities of Daily Living 171
Psychosocial Function 171
Support Resources 172
Environmental Influences 172
Threats to Life 173
Cultural Aspects 173

NURSING DIAGNOSIS 174

PLANNING FOR WELLNESS OUTCOMES 175

NURSING INTERVENTIONS TO ADDRESS ELDER ABUSE AND NEGLECT 175
Interventions in Institutional Settings 175
Interventions in Community Settings 176
Interventions in Multidisciplinary Teams 176
Referrals 177
Prevention and Treatment Interventions 177

LEGAL INTERVENTIONS 178
Adult Protective Services 179
Ethical Issues 181

EVALUATING EFFECTIVENESS OF NURSING INTERVENTIONS 182

PART 3

Promoting Wellness in Psychosocial Function 187

CHAPTER 11
Cognitive Function 187

AGE-RELATED CHANGES THAT AFFECT COGNITION 187
Central Nervous System 188
Fluid and Crystallized Intelligence 189
Memory 189
Adult Psychological Development 190

RISK FACTORS THAT AFFECT COGNITIVE WELLNESS 191
Personal, Social, and Attitudinal Influences 191
Physical and Mental Health Factors 192

Medication Effects 192
Smoking and Environmental Factors 192

FUNCTIONAL CONSEQUENCES AFFECTING
COGNITIVE FUNCTION 193

NURSING ASSESSMENT OF COGNITIVE
FUNCTION 193

NURSING DIAGNOSIS 194

PLANNING FOR WELLNESS OUTCOMES 194

NURSING INTERVENTIONS TO PROMOTE
COGNITIVE WELLNESS 194
Teaching About Memory and Cognition 195
Improving Concentration and Attention 195
Encouraging Participation in Mentally Stimulating
Activities 195
Adapting Health Education Materials 197

EVALUATING EFFECTIVENESS OF
NURSING INTERVENTIONS 198

CHAPTER **12**
Psychosocial Function   202

LIFE EVENTS: AGE-RELATED CHANGES
AFFECTING PSYCHOSOCIAL FUNCTION 202
Retirement 203
Relocation 204
Chronic Illness and Functional Impairments 204
Decisions About Driving a Vehicle 204
Widowhood 205
Death of Friends and Family 205
Ageist Attitudes 205

THEORIES ABOUT PSYCHOSOCIAL FUNCTION IN
OLDER ADULTS 206
Theories About Emotional Development During
Later Adulthood 206
Theories About Stress 206
Theories About Coping 207

FACTORS THAT INFLUENCE PSYCHOSOCIAL
FUNCTION IN OLDER ADULTS 208
Religion and Spirituality 208
Cultural Considerations 209

RISK FACTORS THAT AFFECT PSYCHOSOCIAL
FUNCTION 211

FUNCTIONAL CONSEQUENCES ASSOCIATED WITH
PSYCHOSOCIAL FUNCTION IN OLDER ADULTS 212

NURSING ASSESSMENT OF PSYCHOSOCIAL
FUNCTION 212

NURSING DIAGNOSIS 212

PLANNING FOR WELLNESS OUTCOMES 213

NURSING INTERVENTIONS TO PROMOTE HEALTHY
PSYCHOSOCIAL FUNCTION 213
Enhancing Self-Esteem 214
Promoting a Sense of Control 215
Involving Older Adults in Decision Making 215
Addressing Role Loss 216
Encouraging Life Review and Reminiscence 216
Fostering Social Supports 217
Addressing Spiritual Needs 217
Promoting Wellness Through Healthy
Aging Classes 218

EVALUATING THE EFFECTIVENESS OF NURSING
INTERVENTIONS 221

CHAPTER **13**
Psychosocial Assessment   226

OVERVIEW OF PSYCHOSOCIAL ASSESSMENT
OF OLDER ADULTS 226
Purposes of the Psychosocial Assessment
Process 227
Procedure for the Psychosocial Assessment 227
Scope of the Psychosocial Assessment 228

COMMUNICATION SKILLS FOR
PSYCHOSOCIAL ASSESSMENT 229
Identifying Communication Barriers 229
Enhancing Communication With Older Adults 230
Creating an Environment That Supports Good
Communication 231

MENTAL STATUS ASSESSMENT 233
Physical Appearance 234
Motor Function and Psychomotor Behaviors 234
Social Skills 235
Response to the Interview 235
Orientation 235
Alertness and Attention 236
Memory 236
Speech and Language Characteristics 237
Higher Language Skills 238

DECISION-MAKING AND EXECUTIVE FUNCTION 238

AFFECTIVE FUNCTION 240
Guidelines for Assessing Affective Function 240
Mood 241
Anxiety 241
Self-Esteem 242
Depression 243
Happiness and Well-Being 243

CONTACT WITH REALITY 244
Delusions 244
Hallucinations and Illusions 247

Special Considerations for Assessing Contact With
   Reality in Older Adults 249

SOCIAL SUPPORTS 249
   Social Network 250
   Barriers to Obtaining Social Supports 251
   Economic Resources 251

RELIGION AND SPIRITUALITY 251

CHAPTER 14
Impaired Cognitive Function: Delirium and Dementia 255

DELIRIUM 255
   Overview and Types 255
   Prevalence, Risk Factors, and Functional
      Consequences of Delirium 256
   Nursing Assessment of Delirium 256
   Nursing Diagnosis and Outcomes 257
   Nursing Interventions for Delirium 257

OVERVIEW OF DEMENTIA 259
   Terminology to Describe Dementia 259
   Theories to Explain Dementia 259
   Diagnosing Dementia 260

TYPES OF DEMENTIA 260
   Alzheimer's Disease 261
   Vascular Dementia 263
   Lewy Body Dementia 264
   Frontotemporal Dementia 264

FACTORS ASSOCIATED WITH DEMENTIA 264

FUNCTIONAL CONSEQUENCES ASSOCIATED
WITH DEMENTIA IN OLDER ADULTS 265
   Stages of Dementia 265
   Self-awareness of People With Dementia 266
   Personal Experiences of Dementia 266
   Behavioral and Psychological Symptoms of
      Dementia 268

NURSING ASSESSMENT OF DEMENTIA IN OLDER
ADULTS 269
   Factors That Interfere With the Assessment of
      Dementia 269
   Initial Assessment 269
   Ongoing Assessment of Consequences 269

NURSING DIAGNOSIS 270

PLANNING FOR WELLNESS OUTCOMES 271

NURSING INTERVENTIONS TO ADDRESS
DEMENTIA 271
   Promoting Wellness for People With Dementia 273
   Theoretical Frameworks for Nursing
      Interventions 273

General Principles of Nursing Interventions in
   Different Settings 273
Improving Safety and Function Through
   Environmental Modifications 275
Communicating With Older Adults With
   Dementia 276
Teaching About Pharmacologic Interventions 276

EVALUATING THE EFFECTIVENESS OF
NURSING INTERVENTIONS 279

CHAPTER 15
Impaired Affective Function: Depression 287

THEORIES ABOUT LATE-LIFE DEPRESSION 287
   Psychosocial Theories 287
   Cognitive Triad Theory 289
   Biologic and Genetic Theories 289
   Theories About Depression and Dementia 289

CLASSIFICATION OF DEPRESSION 290

RISK FACTORS FOR DEPRESSION IN OLDER
ADULTS 290
   Demographic Factors and Psychosocial Influences 290
   Medical Conditions and Functional
      Impairments 291
   Effects of Medications and Alcohol 292

FUNCTIONAL CONSEQUENCES ASSOCIATED
WITH DEPRESSION IN OLDER ADULTS 292
   Physical Health and Functioning 292
   Psychosocial Function and Quality of Life 293

NURSING ASSESSMENT OF DEPRESSION
IN OLDER ADULTS 294
   Identifying the Unique Manifestations of
      Depression 294
   Using Screening Tools 295

NURSING DIAGNOSIS 296

PLANNING FOR WELLNESS OUTCOMES 296

NURSING INTERVENTIONS TO
ADDRESS DEPRESSION 296
   Alleviating Risk Factors 297
   Improving Psychosocial Function 297
   Promoting Health Through Physical
      Activity and Nutrition 297
   Providing Education and Counseling 298
   Facilitating Referrals for Psychosocial Therapies 299
   Teaching About and Managing Antidepressant
      Medications 299
   Teaching About Electroconvulsive Therapy 301
   Teaching About Complementary and
      Alternative Interventions 302

EVALUATING THE EFFECTIVENESS OF NURSING
INTERVENTIONS 302

SUICIDE 302

   Assessing the Risks for Suicide 303

   Nursing Diagnosis and Outcomes 305

   Nursing Interventions for Preventing Suicide 305

   Evaluating the Effectiveness of Nursing
      Interventions 305

P A R T **4**

Promoting Wellness in Physical Function 311

CHAPTER **16**
Hearing 311

AGE-RELATED CHANGES THAT AFFECT
HEARING 311

   External Ear 311

   Middle Ear 312

   Inner Ear 313

   Auditory Nervous System 314

RISK FACTORS THAT AFFECT HEARING
WELLNESS 314

   Lifestyle and Environmental Factors 314

   Impacted Cerumen 315

   Medication Effects 315

   Disease Processes 316

FUNCTIONAL CONSEQUENCES AFFECTING
HEARING WELLNESS 316

   Effects on Communication 316

   Effects of Hearing Loss on Overall Wellness 317

PATHOLOGIC CONDITION AFFECTING
HEARING: TINNITUS 318

NURSING ASSESSMENT OF HEARING 318

   Interviewing About Hearing Changes 318

   Observing Behavioral Cues 320

   Using Hearing Assessment Tools 320

NURSING DIAGNOSIS 321

PLANNING FOR WELLNESS OUTCOMES 322

NURSING INTERVENTIONS FOR HEARING
WELLNESS 322

   Promoting Hearing Wellness for All Older
      Adults 322

   Preventing and Alleviating Impacted Cerumen 323

   Compensating for Hearing Deficits 323

   Communicating With Hearing-Impaired
      Older Adults 328

EVALUATING EFFECTIVENESS OF NURSING
INTERVENTIONS 329

CHAPTER **17**
Vision 333

AGE-RELATED CHANGES THAT AFFECT VISION 333

   Eye Appearance and Tear Ducts 333

   The Eye 335

   The Retinal–Neural Pathway 336

EFFECTS OF AGE-RELATED CHANGES ON VISION 336

   Loss of Accommodation 337

   Diminished Acuity 337

   Delayed Dark and Light Adaptation 337

   Increased Glare Sensitivity 337

   Reduced Visual Field 337

   Diminished Depth Perception 337

   Altered Color Vision 338

   Diminished Critical Flicker Fusion 338

   Slower Visual Information Processing 338

RISK FACTORS THAT AFFECT VISUAL
WELLNESS 338

FUNCTIONAL CONSEQUENCES AFFECTING VISUAL
WELLNESS 339

   Effects on Safety and Function 339

   Effects on Quality of Life 340

   Effects on Driving 340

PATHOLOGIC CONDITIONS AFFECTING VISION 341

   Cataracts 341

   Age-Related Macular Degeneration 343

   Glaucoma 343

NURSING ASSESSMENT OF VISION 345

   Interviewing About Vision Changes 345

   Identifying Opportunities for Health Promotion 345

   Observing Cues to Visual Function 346

   Using Standard Vision Tests 347

NURSING DIAGNOSIS 348

PLANNING FOR WELLNESS OUTCOMES 348

NURSING INTERVENTIONS FOR VISUAL
WELLNESS 348

   Health Promotion for Visual Wellness 348

   Comfort Measures for Dry Eyes 350

   Environmental Modifications 350

   Low-Vision Aids 350

   Maintaining and Improving the Quality of Life 351

EVALUATING EFFECTIVENESS OF NURSING
INTERVENTIONS 353

CHAPTER 18
Digestion and Nutrition   358

AGE-RELATED CHANGES THAT AFFECT
DIGESTION AND EATING PATTERNS 358
   Smell and Taste 358
   Oral Cavity 359
   Esophagus and Stomach 360
   Intestinal Tract 360
   Liver, Pancreas, and Gallbladder 360

AGE-RELATED CHANGES IN NUTRITIONAL
REQUIREMENTS 360
   Calories 361
   Protein 361
   Carbohydrates and Fiber 361
   Fats 361
   Water 361

RISK FACTORS THAT AFFECT DIGESTION
AND NUTRITION 362
   Conditions Related to Oral Care 363
   Functional Impairments and Disease Processes 363
   Medication Effects 364
   Lifestyle Factors 364
   Psychosocial Factors 365
   Cultural and Socioeconomic Factors 365
   Environmental Factors 366
   Behaviors Based on Myths and
     Misunderstandings 367

FUNCTIONAL CONSEQUENCES AFFECTING
DIGESTION AND NUTRITION 367
   Ability to Procure, Prepare, and Enjoy Food 367
   Changes in Oral Function 367
   Nutritional Status and Weight Changes 368
   Quality of Life 368

PATHOLOGIC CONDITIONS AFFECTING
DIGESTIVE WELLNESS: CONSTIPATION 369

NURSING ASSESSMENT OF DIGESTION
AND NUTRITION 369
   Interviewing About Digestion and Nutrition 369
   Observing Cues to Digestion and Nutrition 370
   Using Physical Assessment and Laboratory
     Information 370
   Using Assessment Tools 371

NURSING DIAGNOSIS 372

PLANNING FOR WELLNESS OUTCOMES 374

NURSING INTERVENTIONS TO PROMOTE
HEALTHY DIGESTION AND NUTRITION 374
   Addressing Risk Factors That Interfere With
     Digestion and Nutrition 374
   Promoting Oral and Dental Health 375

   Promoting Optimal Nutrition and
     Preventing Disease 376

EVALUATING EFFECTIVENESS OF NURSING
INTERVENTIONS 377

CHAPTER 19
Urinary Function   383

AGE-RELATED CHANGES THAT AFFECT
URINARY WELLNESS 383
   Changes in the Kidneys 383
   Changes in the Bladder and Urinary Tract 385
   Changes in Control Mechanisms 385
   Changes Affecting Control Over Socially
     Appropriate Urinary Elimination 386

RISK FACTORS THAT AFFECT URINARY
WELLNESS 386
   Behaviors Based on Myths and
     Misunderstandings 386
   Functional Impairments 387
   Pathologic Conditions 387
   Medication Effects 388
   Environmental Factors 388

FUNCTIONAL CONSEQUENCES AFFECTING
URINARY WELLNESS 389
   Effects on Homeostasis 389
   Effects on Voiding Patterns 389

PATHOLOGIC CONDITION AFFECTING URINARY
FUNCTION: URINARY INCONTINENCE 390

NURSING ASSESSMENT OF URINARY FUNCTION 391
   Talking With Older Adults About Urinary
     Function 391
   Identifying Opportunities for Health Promotion 392
   Using Laboratory Information 393

NURSING DIAGNOSIS 395

PLANNING FOR WELLNESS OUTCOMES 395

NURSING INTERVENTIONS TO PROMOTE
HEALTHY URINARY FUNCTION 395
   Teaching About Urinary Wellness 395
   Promoting Continence and Alleviating
     Incontinence 396
   Managing Incontinence 401

EVALUATING EFFECTIVENESS OF
NURSING INTERVENTIONS 402

CHAPTER 20
Cardiovascular Function   408

AGE-RELATED CHANGES THAT AFFECT
CARDIOVASCULAR FUNCTION 408

Myocardium and Neuroconduction
   Mechanisms 409
Vasculature 410
Baroreflex Mechanisms 410

RISK FACTORS THAT AFFECT
CARDIOVASCULAR FUNCTION 410
Atherosclerosis 411
Physical Inactivity 411
Tobacco Smoking 412
Dietary Habits 412
Obesity 412
Hypertension 412
Lipid Disorders 413
Metabolic Syndrome 414
Psychosocial Factors 414
Heredity and Socioeconomic Factors 415
Risk for Cardiovascular Disease in Women
   and Minority Groups 415

FUNCTIONAL CONSEQUENCES AFFECTING
CARDIOVASCULAR WELLNESS 416
Effects on Cardiac Function 416
Effects on Pulse and Blood Pressure 416
Effects on the Response to Exercise 416
Effects on Circulation 416

PATHOLOGIC CONDITIONS AFFECTING
CARDIOVASCULAR WELLNESS: ORTHOSTATIC
AND POSTPRANDIAL HYPOTENSION 417

NURSING ASSESSMENT OF CARDIOVASCULAR
FUNCTION 417
Assessing Baseline Cardiovascular Function 418
Assessing Blood Pressure 418
Identifying Risks for Cardiovascular Disease 418
Assessing Signs and Symptoms of Heart Disease 419
Assessing Knowledge About Heart Disease 422

NURSING DIAGNOSIS 422

PLANNING FOR WELLNESS OUTCOMES 423

NURSING INTERVENTIONS TO PROMOTE HEALTHY
CARDIOVASCULAR FUNCTION 423
Addressing Risks Through Nutrition and Lifestyle
   Interventions 423
Secondary Prevention 424
Addressing Risks Through Pharmacologic
   Interventions 425
Preventing and Managing Hypertension 425
Preventing and Managing Lipid Disorders 428
Preventing and Managing Orthostatic or
   Postprandial Hypotension 429

EVALUATING EFFECTIVENESS OF NURSING
INTERVENTIONS 429

CHAPTER 21
Respiratory Function 435

AGE-RELATED CHANGES THAT AFFECT
RESPIRATORY FUNCTION 435
Upper Respiratory Structures 435
Chest Wall and Musculoskeletal Structures 436
Lung Structure and Function 437

RISK FACTORS THAT AFFECT RESPIRATORY
WELLNESS 438
Tobacco Use 438
Secondhand Smoke and Other Environmental
   Factors 439
Additional Risk Factors for Compromised
   Respiratory Function 439

FUNCTIONAL CONSEQUENCES AFFECTING
RESPIRATORY WELLNESS 440

PATHOLOGIC CONDITION AFFECTING
RESPIRATORY FUNCTION: COPD 441

NURSING ASSESSMENT OF RESPIRATORY
FUNCTION 441
Identifying Opportunities for Health
   Promotion 441
Detecting Lower Respiratory Infections 442
Assessing Smoking Behaviors 443
Identifying Other Risk Factors 444
Physical Assessment Findings 444

NURSING DIAGNOSIS 445

PLANNING FOR WELLNESS OUTCOMES 445

NURSING INTERVENTIONS FOR RESPIRATORY
WELLNESS 445
Promoting Respiratory Wellness 445
Preventing Lower Respiratory Infections 446
Eliminating the Risk From Smoking 447

EVALUATING EFFECTIVENESS OF NURSING
INTERVENTIONS 448

CHAPTER 22
Mobility and Safety 452

AGE-RELATED CHANGES THAT AFFECT
MOBILITY AND SAFETY 452
Bones 452
Muscles 453
Joints and Connective Tissue 454
Nervous System 454
Osteopenia and Osteoporosis 454

RISK FACTORS THAT AFFECT MOBILITY
AND SAFETY 454

Risk Factors That Affect Overall Musculoskeletal
Function 455
Risk Factors for Osteoporosis and Osteoporotic
Fractures 455
Risk Factors for Falls 456

PATHOLOGIC CONDITION AFFECTING
MUSCULOSKELETAL FUNCTION:
OSTEOARTHRITIS 458

FUNCTIONAL CONSEQUENCES AFFECTING
MUSCULOSKELETAL WELLNESS 459
Effects on Musculoskeletal Function 459
Susceptibility to Falls and Fractures 459
Fear of Falling 460

NURSING ASSESSMENT OF MUSCULOSKELETAL
FUNCTION 460
Assessing Musculoskeletal Performance 460
Identifying Risks for Osteoporosis 461
Identifying Risks for Falls and Injury 462

NURSING DIAGNOSIS 464

PLANNING FOR WELLNESS OUTCOMES 464

NURSING INTERVENTIONS FOR
MUSCULOSKELETAL WELLNESS 464
Promoting Healthy Musculoskeletal Function and
Preventing Falls 464
Health Education About Osteoporosis 465
Preventing Falls and Fall-Related Injuries 467

EVALUATING EFFECTIVENESS OF NURSING
INTERVENTIONS 471

CHAPTER 23
Integument 477

AGE-RELATED CHANGES THAT AFFECT
THE SKIN 477
Epidermis 477
Dermis 479
Subcutaneous Tissue and Cutaneous Nerves 479
Sweat and Sebaceous Glands 479
Nails 479
Hair 479

RISK FACTORS THAT AFFECT SKIN WELLNESS 480
Genetic Influences 480
Lifestyle and Environmental Influences 480
Medication Effects 480

FUNCTIONAL CONSEQUENCES AFFECTING
SKIN WELLNESS 481
Susceptibility to Injury 481
Response to Ultraviolet Radiation 481
Comfort and Sensation 481
Cosmetic Effects 481

PATHOLOGIC CONDITIONS AFFECTING SKIN: SKIN
CANCER AND PRESSURE ULCERS 482
Skin Cancer 482
Pressure Ulcers 483

NURSING ASSESSMENT OF SKIN 487
Identifying Opportunities for Health Promotion 487
Observing Skin, Hair, and Nails 487

NURSING DIAGNOSIS 490

PLANNING FOR WELLNESS OUTCOMES 490

NURSING INTERVENTIONS FOR SKIN
WELLNESS 491
Promoting Healthy Skin 491
Preventing Skin Wrinkles 491
Preventing Dry Skin 492
Detecting and Treating Harmful Skin Lesions 492

EVALUATING EFFECTIVENESS OF NURSING
INTERVENTIONS 492

CHAPTER 24
Sleep and Rest 496

AGE-RELATED CHANGES THAT AFFECT
SLEEP AND REST PATTERNS 496
Sleep Quantity 497
Sleep Quality 498
Circadian Rhythm 498

RISK FACTORS THAT CAN AFFECT SLEEP 499
Psychosocial Factors 499
Environmental Factors 499
Pathophysiologic Factors 500
Effects of Bioactive Substances 500

FUNCTIONAL CONSEQUENCES AFFECTING
SLEEP WELLNESS 501

PATHOLOGIC CONDITION AFFECTING SLEEP:
OBSTRUCTIVE SLEEP APNEA 502

NURSING ASSESSMENT OF SLEEP 503
Identifying Opportunities for Health Promotion 503
Evidence-Based Assessment Tools 503

NURSING DIAGNOSIS 504

PLANNING FOR WELLNESS OUTCOMES 504

NURSING INTERVENTIONS FOR SLEEP
WELLNESS 504
Evidence-Based Interventions 504
Self-Care Actions to Promote Healthy
Sleep Patterns 505
Complementary and Alternative Care
Practices 505
Improving Sleep for Older Adults in
Institutional Settings 506

Modifying the Environment to Promote Sleep 507
Educating Older Adults About Medications
and Sleep 507
Teaching About Management of Sleep
Disorders 507

EVALUATING EFFECTIVENESS OF
NURSING INTERVENTIONS 509

CHAPTER 25
Thermoregulation 513

AGE-RELATED CHANGES THAT AFFECT
THERMOREGULATION 513
Response to Cold Temperatures 513
Response to Hot Temperatures 515
Normal Body Temperature and Febrile
Response to Illness 515

RISK FACTORS THAT AFFECT
THERMOREGULATION 515
Pathophysiologic Conditions That Alter
Thermoregulation 515
Environmental and Socioeconomic Influences 515
Behaviors Based on Lack of Knowledge 516

FUNCTIONAL CONSEQUENCES ASSOCIATED WITH
THERMOREGULATION IN OLDER ADULTS 516
Altered Response to Cold Environments 517
Altered Response to Hot Environments 517
Altered Thermoregulatory Response to Illness 517
Altered Perception of Environmental
Temperatures 517
Psychosocial Consequences of Altered
Thermoregulation 517

NURSING ASSESSMENT OF
THERMOREGULATION 518
Assessing Baseline Temperature 518
Identifying Risk Factors for Altered
Thermoregulation 518
Assessing for Hypothermia 519
Assessing for Hyperthermia 519
Assessing the Older Adult's Febrile
Response to Illness 520

NURSING DIAGNOSIS 520

PLANNING FOR WELLNESS OUTCOMES 520

NURSING INTERVENTIONS TO PROMOTE HEALTHY
THERMOREGULATION 520
Addressing Risk Factors 520
Promoting Healthy Thermoregulation 521

EVALUATING EFFECTIVENESS OF
NURSING INTERVENTIONS 521

CHAPTER 26
Sexual Function 525

AGE-RELATED CHANGES THAT AFFECT
SEXUAL FUNCTION 525
Changes Affecting Older Women 525
Changes Affecting Older Men 527

RISK FACTORS THAT AFFECT SEXUAL
FUNCTION 527
Societal Influences 527
Attitudes and Behaviors of Families and
Caregivers 528
Limited Opportunities for Sexual Activity 528
Adverse Effects of Medication, Alcohol,
and Nicotine 529
Chronic Conditions 529
Gender-Specific Conditions 530
Functional Impairments and Dementia 530

FUNCTIONAL CONSEQUENCES AFFECTING
SEXUAL WELLNESS 530
Reproductive Ability 531
Response to Sexual Stimulation 531
Sexual Interest and Activity 531
Male Sexual Dysfunction 532
Female Sexual Dysfunction 532

PATHOLOGIC CONDITION AFFECTING
SEXUAL WELLNESS: HUMAN
IMMUNODEFICIENCY VIRUS 533
Risk Factors for HIV 533
Role of Nurses in Assessment and
Interventions 534

NURSING ASSESSMENT OF SEXUAL
FUNCTION 534
Self-Assessment of Attitudes About
Sexual Function and Aging 534
Assessing Sexual Function in Older Adults 535

NURSING DIAGNOSIS 537

PLANNING FOR WELLNESS OUTCOMES 537

NURSING INTERVENTIONS TO PROMOTE
HEALTHY SEXUAL FUNCTION 537
Teaching Older Adults About
Sexual Wellness 537
Addressing Risk Factors 537
Promoting Sexual Wellness in Long-Term Care
Settings 539
Teaching Women About Interventions 539
Teaching Men About Interventions 540

EVALUATING EFFECTIVENESS OF NURSING
INTERVENTIONS 541

PART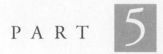

Promoting Wellness in All Stages of Health and Illness 547

CHAPTER **27**
Caring for Older Adults During Illness 547

CHARACTERISTICS OF ILLNESS IN OLDER ADULTS 547
CONNECTING THE CONCEPTS OF WELLNESS, AGING, AND ILLNESS 548
HOLISTICALLY CARING FOR OLDER ADULTS WHO ARE ILL: FOCUSING ON CARING AND COMFORTING 549
APPLYING WELLNESS CONCEPTS IN SPECIFIC PATHOLOGIC OR CHRONIC CONDITIONS 550
    Promoting Wellness for Older Adults With Cancer 550
    Promoting Wellness for Older Adults With Diabetes Mellitus 552
    Promoting Wellness for Older Adults With Heart Failure 553
ADDRESSING NEEDS OF FAMILIES AND CAREGIVERS 555

CHAPTER **28**
Caring for Older Adults Experiencing Pain 560

ACUTE VERSUS PERSISTENT PAIN 560
ANATOMY AND PHYSIOLOGY OF PAIN 561
TYPES OF PAIN 562
CAUSES OF PAIN IN OLDER ADULTS 562
AGE-RELATED CHANGES THAT AFFECT PAIN 563
BARRIERS TO PAIN MANAGEMENT 563
FUNCTIONAL CONSEQUENCES OF PAIN IN OLDER ADULTS 563

CULTURAL ASPECTS OF PAIN ASSESSMENT AND MANAGEMENT 563
NURSING ASSESSMENT OF PAIN IN OLDER ADULTS 565
    Collecting Pertinent Information 565
    Assessment of Pain Components 566
    Assessment in Cognitively Impaired Older Adults 568
PRINCIPLES OF ANALGESIC MEDICATION 568
    Classifications of Analgesics 569
    The World Health Organization's Three-Step Pain Relief Ladder for Pain Management 570
    Management of Side Effects and Risks of Tolerance, Dependence, and Addiction 571
    Developing a Wellness-Focused Pain Management Plan 571

CHAPTER **29**
Caring for Older Adults at the End of Life 575

THE DYING PROCESS AND DEATH 575
NURSING SKILLS FOR PALLIATIVE CARE 576
PERSPECTIVES ON DEATH AND DYING 576
    Sites of Death and Dying 576
    Views of Death and Dying in Western Culture 576
    Older Adults' Perspective on Death and Dying 577
    Health Care Professionals' Perspective on Death and Dying 577
    Culturally Diverse Perspectives on Death and Dying 578
QUALITY OF CARE AT THE END OF LIFE 578
    Promoting Wellness at the End of Life 579
    Hospice Care 580
NURSING INTERVENTIONS IN END-OF-LIFE CARE 581
    Promoting Communication 581
    Offering Spiritual Support 581
    Managing Symptoms 582

INDEX 589

Assessment, Intervention & Evidence-Based Practice Boxes

ASSESSMENT BOXES

Safety and Functioning

Box 7-1   Criteria for Assessing Activities of Daily Living (ADLs), 100

Box 7-2   Criteria for Assessing Instrumental Activities of Daily Living (IADLs), 101

Box 7-3   Guidelines for Assessing the Safety of the Environment, 107

Medications

Box 8-4   Guidelines for Medication Assessment, 133

Psychosocial Assessment

Box 13-1   Self-Assessment of Attitudes About Psychosocial Aspects of Aging, 228

Box 13-3   Guidelines for Assessing Physical Appearance, Motor Function, Social Skills, and Response to the Interview, 236

Box 13-4   Guidelines for Assessing Orientation, Alertness, and Memory, 237

Box 13-5   Guidelines for Assessing Speech Characteristics, and Calculation and Higher Language Skills, 238

Box 13-6   Guidelines for Assessing Affective Function, 244

Box 13-7   Guidelines for Assessing Contact With Reality, 249

Box 13-8   Guidelines for Assessing Social Supports, 250

Box 13-9   Guidelines for Assessing Spiritual Needs, 253

Impaired Cognitive Function

Box 14-3   Assessing Progressive Cognitive Impairment in Older Adults, 270

Impaired Affective Function

Box 15-6   Guidelines for Assessing Suicide Risk, 304

Hearing

Box 16-2   Guidelines for Assessing Hearing, 319

Box 16-3   Guidelines for Assessing Behavioral Cues Related to Hearing, 321

Box 16-4   Guidelines for Otoscopic and Tuning Fork Assessment, 321

Vision

Box 17-1   Guidelines for Assessing Vision, 346

Box 17-2   Guidelines for Assessing Behavioral and Environmental Cues Related to Visual Performance, 347

Box 17-3   Guidelines for Using Vision Screening Tests, 347

Digestion and Nutrition

Box 18-2   Guidelines for Assessing Digestion and Nutrition, 370

Box 18-3   Behavioral Cues to Nutrition and Digestion, 371

Box 18-4   Physical Assessment and Laboratory Data, 372

Urinary Function

Box 19-2   Guidelines for Assessing Urinary Elimination, 392

Box 19-3   Guidelines for Assessing Behavioral Cues to and Environmental Influences on Incontinence, 393

Cardiovascular Function

Box 20-2   Guidelines for Assessing Blood Pressure, 419

Box 20-3   Guidelines for Assessing Risks for Cardiovascular Disease in Older Adults, 422

Box 20-4   Guidelines for Assessing Cardiovascular Function in Older Adults, 422

Respiratory Function

Box 21-2   Guidelines for Assessing Respiratory Function, 443

Box 21-3   Guidelines for Nursing Assessment of Older Adults Who Smoke, 444

Mobility and Safety

Box 22-3   Guidelines for Assessing Overall Musculoskeletal Function and Risks for Falls and Osteoporosis, 461

Integument

Box 23-1   Interview Questions for Assessing the Integument, 488

Box 23-2   Observations Regarding the Integument, 490

Sleep and Rest

Box 24-1   Guidelines for Assessing Sleep and Rest, 503

Thermoregulation

Box 25-2   Guidelines for Assessing Thermoregulation, 519

Sexual Function

Box 26-3   Assessing Personal Attitudes Toward Sexuality and Aging, 535

Box 26-4   Guidelines for Assessing Sexual Function in Older Adults, 536

Illness

Box 27-2   Assessment Guidelines for Older Adults With Diabetes, 553
Box 27-3   Assessment Guidelines for Older Adults With Heart Failure, 554

Pain

Box 28-3   Sample Questions for Pain Assessment in Older Adults, 566

INTERVENTIONS BOXES

Health Promotion

Box 5-3   Guidelines for Prevention and Health Promotion Interventions for Older Adults, 67
Box 5-4   Health Education About Types of Exercise, 69

Medications

Box 8-5   Tips on Safe and Effective Medication Use, 138
Box 8-6   Tips on the Use of Herbs and Homeopathic Remedies, 139

Legal and Ethical Concerns

Box 9-3   Model for Facilitating Decisions About the Care of People With Dementia, 158

Cognitive Function

Box 11-2   Memory Training for Older Adults, 196
Box 11-3   Guidelines for Health Education for Older Adults, 197

Psychosocial Function

Box 12-1   Nursing Interventions to Promote Self-Esteem, 215
Box 12-2   Nursing Interventions to Promote Psychosocial Wellness, 218
Box 12-3   Nursing Interventions to Address Spiritual Needs, 219

Psychosocial Assessment

Box 13-2   Strategies to Enhance Communication With Older Adults, 234

Impaired Cognitive Function

Box 14-6   Nursing Interventions for People With Dementia Based on the Progressively Lowered Stress Threshold Model (PLST), 274
Box 14-9   Environmental Adaptations and Techniques for Improving Safety and Functioning in People With Dementia, 277
Box 14-10   Facilitating Communication With People Who Have Dementia, 277
Box 14-11   Guidelines for Decisions About Behavior-Modifying Medications for People With Dementia, 278

Impaired Affective Function

Box 15-4   Health Education About Antidepressant Medications, 301

Box 15-5   Interventions Commonly Used for Preventing or Alleviating Depression, 302
Box 15-7   Nursing Interventions for People Who Are Potentially Suicidal, 305

Hearing

Box 16-5   Health Promotion Teaching About Hearing, 322
Box 16-6   Use and Care of Hearing Aids, 327
Box 16-7   Techniques for Communicating With Hearing-Impaired People, 328

Vision

Box 17-4   Health Promotion Teaching About Visual Wellness, 349
Box 17-5   Eye Care Practitioners, 349
Box 17-6   Considerations for Optimal Illumination, 350
Box 17-7   Environmental Adaptations for Improving Visual Performance, 351
Box 17-8   Low-Vision Aids for Improving Visual Performance, 352
Box 17-9   Guidelines for Using Magnifying Aids, 353

Digestion and Nutrition

Box 18-5   Health Education Regarding Constipation, 375
Box 18-6   Health Education Regarding Oral and Dental Care, 376
Box 18-7   Guidelines for Daily Food Intake for Older Adults, 377

Urinary Function

Box 19-4   Health Education to Promote Urinary Wellness, 396
Box 19-5   Instructions for Performing Pelvic Muscle Exercises, 397
Box 19-6   Continence Training Programs, 399
Box 19-7   Environmental Modifications for Preventing Incontinence, 400
Box 19-8   Considerations Regarding Continence Aids and Equipment, 402

Cardiovascular Function

Box 20-5   Health Promotion Activities to Reduce the Risks for Cardiovascular Disease, 425
Box 20-6   Guidelines for Nursing Management of Hypertension, 426
Box 20-7   Nutritional Interventions for People With High Cholesterol, 428
Box 20-8   Education Regarding Orthostatic and Postprandial Hypotension, 429

Respiratory Function

Box 21-4   Health Promotion Teaching About Respiratory Problems, 446
Box 21-5   Health Promotion Teaching About Cigarette Smoking, 447

Mobility and Safety

Box 22-4   Health Promotion Teaching About Osteoporosis, 466
Box 22-5   A Fall-Prevention Program for Older Adults Being Cared for in Hospitals or Nursing Homes, 468

Integument

Box 23-3   Health Promotion Teaching About Skin Care for Older Adults, 491

Sleep and Rest

Box 24-2   Health Promotion Teaching About Sleep, 505
Box 24-3   Relaxation and Mental Imagery Techniques That Promote Sleep, 506
Box 24-4   Health Promotion Teaching About Medications and Sleep, 508

Thermoregulation

Box 25-3   Health Promotion Teaching About Hypothermia and Heat-Related Illness, 522

Sexual Function

Box 26-5   Health Education About Sexual Activity for Older People, 538
Box 26-6   Health Education About Sexual Activity for People With Arthritis, 538
Box 26-7   Health Education About Sexual Activity for People With Cardiovascular Disease, 539

Illness

Box 27-1   Health Promotion Interventions Related to Cancer and Older Adults, 552

Pain

Box 28-4   Recommendations for Maintaining Bowel Function in Patients Taking Opioid Medications, 571

End of Life

Box 29-3   Supportive Interventions for Relationship Building, 582
Box 29-4   Communicating With Dying Patients and Their Families, 582

EVIDENCE-BASED PRACTICE BOXES

Box 8-1   Reducing Adverse Drug Events, 137
Box 13-1   Detection and Assessment of Late-Life Anxiety, 242
Box 15-1   Depression in Older Adults, 303
Box 16-1   Impacted Cerumen, 324
Box 17-1   Vision Changes, 336
Box 18-1   Dysphagia, 364
Box 20-1   Evidence-Based Practice Related to Prevention of Cardiovascular Disease, 414
Box 21-1   Nursing Care of Dyspnea, 442
Box 22-1   Osteoporosis, 465
Box 22-2   Prevention of Falls, 471
Box 23-1   Pressure Ulcers, 484
Box 24-1   Excessive Sleepiness, 502
Box 27-1   Family Caregiving, 556

Older Adults and Wellness

CHAPTER 1

Seeing Older Adults Through the Eyes of Wellness

LEARNING OBJECTIVES

After reading this chapter, you will be able to:

1. Describe the relationship between aging and wellness.
2. Identify barriers to and opportunities for nurses to promote wellness in older adults.
3. Define aging from several perspectives.
4. Recognize the effects of ageism and attitudes about aging.
5. Identify myths that affect nursing care of older adults.
6. Describe demographic, health, and socioeconomic characteristics of older adults in the United States.
7. Discuss how population trends affect relationships of older adults and their families.
8. Describe living arrangements of older adults.

KEY POINTS

age attribution	comorbidities
age identity	functional age
ageism	high-level wellness
aging	informal caregiver
aging anxiety	perceived age
anti-aging	sandwich generation
baby boomers	skipped-generation
caregiver burden	households
chronologic age	successful aging

People in modern societies often associate being "old" or "elderly" with decline, disease, disability, decrepitude, and death. However, it is imperative to recognize that these images do not accurately reflect the realities of aging because they are rooted in myths and stereotypes that are based on a lack of knowledge.

IMAGES OF AGING

Many images of aging arise from long-term patterns of falsely attributing pathologic conditions and undesirable characteristics to normal aging. Unfortunately, these misperceptions have been reinforced by terms, such as *senility,* that equate aging with impaired functioning. In reality, studies confirm that most older adults function independently and report high levels of satisfaction with their health and quality of life, even with their high prevalence of chronic conditions. For example, 78% of a large cohort of 85-year olds rated their health as good to excellent despite the presence of significant levels of disease and 20% of the subjects were completely independent in their daily functioning (Collerton et al., 2009). Studies of nonagenarians indicate that loss of independence declines only slightly between the ages of 92 and 100 years (Christensen, Doblhammer, Rau, & Vaupel, 2009). It is widely recognized that adults at any age aspire to live a long, healthy, satisfying, and high-functioning life.

Because many challenges of older adulthood involve health and functioning, older adults need accurate information, not only about normal aging but also about interventions to promote wellness. Nurses are in ideal positions to teach older adults about health and aging and empower them to implement problem-solving strategies directed toward wellness, improved functioning, and quality of life. The intent of this gerontological nursing text is to provide comprehensive and research-based information so that nurses can distinguish between the changes associated with normal aging and those that result from risk factors. In addition, the text provides tools for nursing assessment, interventions, and health education in relation to all aspects of physical and psychosocial functioning. Nurses can use these tools to promote wellness—which includes improved health, functioning, and quality of life—for the older adults for whom they provide care.

This chapter provides an overview of concepts related to wellness and aging and reviews some myths about aging and older adults. To combat myths about aging, this chapter also presents information about older adults in the United States in terms of demographic, health, and socioeconomic characteristics. The chapter also presents information about aging worldwide to provide a broader perspective.

THE RELATIONSHIP BETWEEN WELLNESS AND AGING

If asked to define *wellness* and *aging*, most people associate wellness with peak achievement in younger adulthood and aging with declining health that eventually leads to death. Although somewhat accurate with regard to biologic aging, this description of wellness does not address well-being of the body, mind, and spirit. Similarly, many definitions of human aging focus narrowly on physical health and functioning rather than holistically—and accurately—on humans as complex bio-psycho-social-spiritual individuals. Thus, the apparent disconnect between definitions of wellness and aging results not only from misunderstandings about aging but also from a narrow focus on physical health and functioning.

Promoting wellness in older adults is an ideal; however, nurses may not believe it is achievable in practice because of barriers such as the following:

- Older adults may be pessimistic about their ability to improve their health and functioning.
- Survival needs and a multitude of health problems may take precedence over the "luxury" of being able to focus on wellness and quality of life.
- Despite the purported emphasis on wellness and health promotion, health care environments focus more on treating disease than on preventing illness and addressing whole-person needs.
- Older adults and health care providers often mistakenly attribute symptoms to aging rather than identify and address the contributing factors that are reversible and treatable.
- Health care providers may not believe that older adults are capable of learning and implementing health-promoting behaviors that are inherent in wellness-oriented care.
- Because many of these barriers arise from myths, misperceptions, and lack of knowledge, accurate information about older adults and the relationship between aging and wellness is an indispensable tool for addressing these barriers.

Wellness and Older Adults

The concept of wellness came to public attention in the early 1960s when Halbert L. Dunn, MD, PhD, retired from his formal public health career and became a "lecturer and consultant in high-level wellness work" (Dunn, 1961, p. 244). Dunn believed that education at all points in a person's life was the key to high-level wellness, and he developed a series of radio talks with the theme "High-Level Wellness for Man and Society." He defined **high-level wellness** as an "integrated method of functioning that is oriented toward maximizing each person's potential, while maintaining a continuum of balance and purposeful direction within the person's environment" (Dunn, 1961, pp. 4–5). In one radio program, Dunn addressed stereotypes about aging and emphasized that "healthy maturity" is characterized not only by physical decline but also by wisdom. Moreover, he discussed the relationship between mind, body, and spirit and stressed the importance of older adults having a purpose in life, communicating with others, maintaining personal dignity, and contributing to society (Dunn, 1961).

Even before addressing aging in his public education series, Dunn had published an article in *Geriatrics* while he was chief of the National Office of Vital Statistics. In the article, he advised all health care workers to foster a sense of value and dignity for older adults by directing interventions toward improved health and functioning (Dunn, 1958). Dunn described the role of health care professionals with regard to older adults as follows (1958, p. 51):

> The later years of life will come to be more widely regarded as years of opportunity for older people and for society if, in addition to prevention, care, and various health-related activities, direct attention is devoted to the promotion of high-level wellness. This will require a major reorientation.

Wellness and Nursing Care of Older Adults

Nurses have many opportunities to promote wellness for older adults through actions that are integral to holistic nursing. A major focus of a "wellness approach" to older adult health care is addressing the body–mind–spirit interconnectedness of each older adult as a unique and respected individual. This requires that nurses assess each older adult in the full context of his or her personal history and current situation. Based on this holistic assessment, nurses identify realistic wellness outcomes and plan interventions directed toward improved health, functioning, and quality of life. This approach may seem challenging—or even impossible—for older adults who are seriously or terminally ill or for those who have overwhelming chronic conditions. Even when there are serious physical challenges, however, nurses need to recognize that they can implement interventions directed toward improved physical comfort and psychological and spiritual growth. Some nursing actions that promote wellness for older adults are as follows:

- Addressing the body–mind–spirit interrelatedness of each older adult

- Identifying and challenging ageist attitudes (including their own), especially those that interfere with optimal health care
- Assessing each older adult from a whole-person perspective
- Incorporating wellness nursing diagnoses as a routine part of care
- Planning for wellness outcomes, which are directed toward improved health, functioning, and quality of life
- Using nursing interventions to address the factors that interfere with optimal functioning (including lack of accurate information about aging)
- Recognizing each older adult's potential for improved health and functioning as well as psychological and spiritual growth
- Teaching about self-care behaviors to improve health and functioning (or teaching caregivers of dependent older adults)
- Promoting wellness for caregivers and other people who provide care for older adults (including self-care for nurses).

Definitions of Aging

Gerontologists and lay people define aging from many perspectives. Objectively, **aging** is a universal process that begins at birth; in this context, it applies equally to young and old people. Subjectively, however, aging is typically associated with being "old" or reaching "older adulthood," and people define aging in terms of personal meaning and experience. Children usually do not view themselves as aging, but they delight in announcing how old they are and they anticipate birthdays with great enthusiasm. They view their birthdays as positive events that will permit them to enjoy additional opportunities and responsibilities. Adolescents, likewise, view aging as the mechanism that allows them to participate legally in important activities, such as driving and voting.

In contrast, adults tend to view "old age" as something to be avoided and they are likely to define the onset of older adulthood as a decade beyond their current age. The term **age identity** (also referred to as *feel* age or *subjective age*) is used to describe someone's perception of his or her age. Studies have found that older people judge the onset of both middle and older age as occurring at a later chronologic age than do younger people (Musaiger & D'Souza, 2009; Prevc & Doupona, 2009). Nurses often observe this phenomenon when they hear people whose chronologic age is 75 years, 80 years, or older refer to "old people" as if they were a group older than and distinct from themselves.

Since the 1980s, gerontologists have used the concept of **perceived age**, which is another person's estimated age of someone based on appearances, in many studies including several large longitudinal studies. These studies have confirmed that perceived age correlates very closely with health and is a strong predictor of survival, especially for people aged 70 years and older (Christensen, Thinggaard, et al., 2009).

Objectively, people define **chronologic age** as the length of time that has passed since birth. North American culture is particularly fascinated by numbers, quantities, and relative values that can be measured. Among the questions frequently asked and answered are *How much? How far? How often?* and *How old?* Our fascination with age is particularly evident in newspaper articles, which invariably state the age of the subjects, regardless of the relevance of age to the topic. In addition to being easily measured, another advantage of chronologic age is that it serves as an objective basis for social organization. For example, societies establish chronologic age criteria for certain activities, such as education, voting, driving, marriage, employment, alcohol consumption, military service, and the collection of retirement benefits. To participate legally in these activities, people must provide documentation of a certain chronologic age.

With the passage of the 1935 Social Security Act and the 1965 amendment that created Medicare, the age of 65 years was established as the standard age criterion for eligibility for retirement and health care benefits in the United States. This age-based determination for retirement was determined in part on the socioeconomic condition of the United States after the Depression. In recent years, the legal age for Social Security retirement benefits has been increasing gradually because of current socioeconomic trends, including increased longevity and improved health status. Even this chronologic age criterion, however, varies across different government-sponsored programs, such as the Older Americans Act (OAA). For example, the qualifying age for Native Americans' participation in OAA-funded programs is 45 years in Montana, but it is 55 years in all other states.

During the 1960s, gerontologists also viewed 65 years of age as an acceptable chronologic criterion for aging processes. In recent decades, however, gerontologists agree that aging is too complex to be defined only by one's birth date. From both scientific and humanistic perspectives, a person's chronologic age is relatively insignificant because there is no biologic measurement that applies to everyone at a specific age. Consequently, gerontologists have commonly divided older adulthood into subgroups, such as young-old, middle-old, old-old, and oldest-old. As one of the first gerontologists to challenge the original criterion stated:

> We have used sixty-five as the economic marker, then as the social and psychological marker, of old age. A set of stereotypes has grown up that older persons are sick, poor, enfeebled, isolated, and desolated. While these stereotypes have been greatly overdrawn even for the old-old, they have become uncritically attached to the whole group over sixty-five (Neugarten, 1978, pp. 47–48).

The trend in gerontology to divide old age into chronologic subcategories is an improvement over the categorization of all people older than 65 years as one homogeneous group, but it has the disadvantage of creating additional stereotypes and age biases. For example, if a chronologically old-old person needs a complicated or expensive medical treatment to maintain or potentially improve his or her health status, such treatment may be denied or withheld based on advanced age.

More recently, there is increasing recognition that decisions about treatment approaches should be based on broad evidence-based criteria, especially for those people who are chronologically categorized as old-old (Lerolle et al., 2010; Wilson, Thurston, & Lichlyter, 2010).

For health care providers whose practice focuses on older adults, as well as for most older adults, the important indicators of age are physiologic health, psychological well-being, socioeconomic factors, and the ability to function and participate in desirable activities. Based on this understanding of aging, gerontologists have used the term **functional age** for several decades. This concept is associated with a shift in emphasis from chronologic factors to such factors as whether individuals can contribute to society and benefit others and themselves. Functional age is a concept that is used worldwide, but its definition varies according to different cultural contexts. For example, industrialized societies may associate functional age with self-sufficiency and physiologic function, whereas other cultures might associate it more closely with social or psychological function than with physiologic function.

One advantage of functional definitions of age over chronologic definitions is that the former are associated with higher levels of well-being and with more positive attitudes about aging. From a holistic perspective, the concept of functional age provides a more rational basis for care than the measurement of how many years have passed since the person was born. Thus, the question *How functional?* is more relevant than *How old?* Even more relevant for promoting wellness in older adults are questions such as the following:

- How well do you feel?
- What goals do you have for improving your level of wellness?
- Is there anything that you would like to do that you cannot do?
- What goals do you have for improving your quality of life?

In this text, the term *older adult* applies to individuals experiencing the cumulative effects of age-related changes and risk factors that affect their health and functioning (refer to Chapter 3 for further definition and discussion). From a holistic perspective, this conceptualization addresses all aspects of bio-psycho-social-spiritual health and functioning, as discussed in the next section in relation to successful aging.

Descriptions of Successful Aging

For several decades, gerontologists have focused on identifying the most agreed-upon components of **successful aging** and determining how many older adults can be categorized as such. A widely recognized model, which is based on the large-scale longitudinal studies of the MacArthur Research Network on Successful Aging, identified three components of successful aging: an active engagement with life, high cognitive and physical function, and low probability of disease and disability (Rowe & Kahn, 1997). A review of 28 English-language studies of definitions of successful aging found that

A Student's Perspective

My interview with Mr. H. was an enlightening experience. I was able to learn a great deal about the time period in which this man grew up. Also, it was eye opening to see how healthy a man of 84 years could be. His health reinforced what we are learning. He does have a chronic illness, diabetes (like 80% of those aged 65+), but he still is independent and free of any noticeable cognitive impairments. He can still drive and get around, which also defeats a lot of ageist attitudes. Negative attitudes that I have heard about elders were defeated by this man. Reading about aging in a book is one thing, but actually interacting with elders and learning first hand is much more influential. Mr. H. really taught me not to hold ageist attitudes.

Jordan S.

the mean reported proportion of successful agers was 35.8% (Depp & Jeste, 2006).

Currently, there is emphasis on optimal physical, mental, and social well-being and function as essential components of successful aging. The federally funded Prevention Research Centers on Healthy Aging Research Network (PRC-HAN) is focusing on adopting and maintaining attitudes and behaviors that promote health and well-being of older adults, with emphasis on cognitive health (Logsdon, Hochhalter, & Sharkey, 2009). One PRC-HAN study of a diverse group of older adults found that all or most racial/ethnic groups identified longevity, leisure, spirituality, social involvement, continuous learning, and good physical and cognitive health as essential aspects of successful aging (Laditka et al., 2009). Studies also found that having a sense of purpose in life is an important aspect of successful aging (Boyle, Barnes, Buchman, & Bennett, 2009; Gruenewald, Karlamangla, Greendale, Singer, & Seeman, 2009). Studies of successful aging in Brazil and Britain found that leisure activities, psychosocial support, functional capacity, health and perceived well-being, and family and social relationships and engagement were important components of active or successful aging (Bowling, 2009; Chaves, Camozzato, Eizirik, & Kaye, 2009). A nursing study found that older adults in Brazil viewed old age as a time for experiencing new possibilities and felt that being healthy was essential for maintaining their autonomy (Silva & Boemer, 2009).

Gerontologists are also emphasizing that the concept of successful aging can be applied to people who have overcome disabilities and disease, in which case the term *aging successfully* is used (Morley, 2009). To illustrate this concept, Morley cited the following examples of well-known people who have aged successfully:

- Grandma Moses (Anna Maria Robertson) became a famous painter after arthritis interfered with her ability to make quilts.
- Monet developed the painting technique known as modern impressionism after his eyesight was clouded by cataracts.
- Renoir painted with a clenched fist after he developed arthritis.

- Pablo Casals played his cello each day in his 90s.
- Maurice Ravel composed the famous *Bolero* after he was affected with dementia.

The concept of aging successfully also has been applied to nonagenarians and centenarians, who are viewed as special subgroups of "healthy agers" (Engberg, Oksuzyan, Jeune, Vauper, & Christensen, 2009; Zikic et al., 2009).

ATTITUDES TOWARD AGING

Historically, societal attitudes toward aging have ranged from respect and veneration to fear of aging and idealization of youth. As indicated in Figure 1-1, the pendulum is slowly swinging again toward positive attitudes toward aging and older adulthood.

Shifting Trends

This shift is attributable to the increasing emphasis on successful aging and the emergence of accurate information about the difference between aging and disease. Fortunately, gerontologists and other health care professionals are now focusing on preventing and addressing the problems most commonly associated with older adulthood. Despite this focus on successful aging, however, care of older adults continues to be influenced by long-standing negative attitudes toward aging that are held by society as well as health care professionals. Thus, an important part of gerontological nursing is to recognize the effects of ageism and address attitudes that can interfere with holistic care of older adults.

Ageism

The term *ageism* was coined by Robert Butler in 1968 and was first used in a publication, *The Gerontologist*, the next year (Butler, 1969). With the publication of Butler's Pulitzer Prize-winning book *Why Survive? Being Old in America* (1975), *ageism* became an accepted new word in the English language. Butler defines **ageism** as "the prejudices and stereotypes that are applied to older people sheerly on the basis of their age. . . . Ageism, like racism and sexism, is a way of pigeonholing people and not allowing them to be individuals with unique ways of living their lives" (Butler, Lewis, & Sunderland, 1991, p. 243).

A review of ageism among younger and older adults proposed that younger adults develop ageist attitudes to protect themselves from death anxiety because they associate death with aging. In contrast, older adults develop ageist attitudes because of negative stereotypes about their own group (Bodner, 2009). Common manifestations of ageism include negative stereotypes of social isolation, psychological rigidity, asexual behavior, lack of creativity, physical and mental

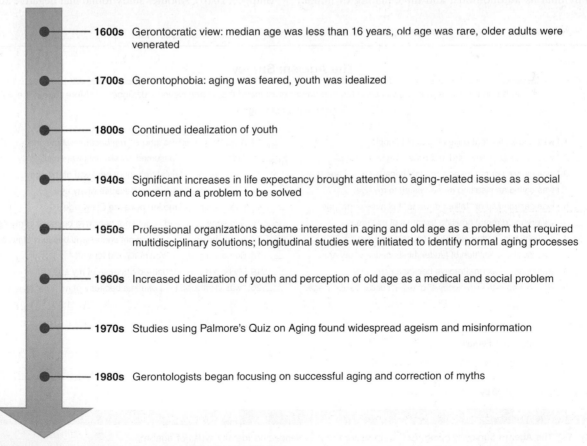

1600s Gerontocratic view: median age was less than 16 years, old age was rare, older adults were venerated

1700s Gerontophobia: aging was feared, youth was idealized

1800s Continued idealization of youth

1940s Significant increases in life expectancy brought attention to aging-related issues as a social concern and a problem to be solved

1950s Professional organizations became interested in aging and old age as a problem that required multidisciplinary solutions; longitudinal studies were initiated to identify normal aging processes

1960s Increased idealization of youth and perception of old age as a medical and social problem

1970s Studies using Palmore's Quiz on Aging found widespread ageism and misinformation

1980s Gerontologists began focusing on successful aging and correction of myths

FIGURE 1-1 Historic trends in views on aging in the United States.

decline, and economic and familial burden. For example, a review of 262 articles published in the *Economist* between 1997 and 2008 found that 64% portrayed an ageist view of older people being a burden on society (Martin, Williams, & O'Neill, 2009).

In the late 1960s, Erdman Palmore and other researchers concluded that between 1950 and 1970, the effects of ageism diminished more slowly than those of racism (Palmore, 2005). Based on his research, Palmore developed two versions of a 25-item Facts on Aging Quiz, as indirect measures of ageism. These quizzes have been used in hundreds of studies and classrooms and consistently show more negative bias than positive bias toward older adults (Palmore, 2005). Palmore later developed a 20-item Ageism Survey to directly measure older adults' experiences of ageism (Figure 1-2). Studies using this survey in Canada and the United States have found that most respondents in both countries frequently experienced ageism (Palmore, 2005). For example, one study of 247 community-dwelling adults between the ages of 60 and 92 years found that 84% of the participants said they had experienced at least one type of ageism, with the most common forms being jokes and greeting cards that poked fun at older people (McGuire, Klein, & Chen, 2008).

Although ageism is not unique to the United States, it does not exist in all cultures. In North America, ageism has developed and grown as a result of dominant cultural beliefs and trends, such as the glorification of youth, the perception of the individual as autonomous, and the equating of human worth with economic worth. Contrasting cultural perspectives on independence versus interdependence is another factor that can account for differences in attitudes about aging (Plath, 2009). For example, Levy and Leifhelt-Limson (2009) found that older adults in the United States and Japan were likely to make age attributions, but these were associated with worse functional health only among the Americans. This difference was attributed to the Japanese acceptance of interdependence, which is rooted in the Confucian precept that adult children should respect and support parents. A potentially positive outcome of the increasing cultural diversity in the United States is that the dominant cultural values that foster ageism may be challenged by cultural values of other groups. See Cultural Considerations 1-1 for a summary of various cultural perspectives on elders.

Effects of Ageism

In recent years, gerontologists have identified some of the specific effects of negative attitudes and stereotypes on older adults. Studies have found that members of stigmatized groups—which includes "the aged"—are more likely to become depressed, have less social interaction, have lower self-esteem, and have poorer function and self-confidence (Dobbs et al., 2008; Kang & Chasteen, 2009). One study found that women, but not men, associated older age identities with pessimistic outlooks about their own cognitive aging (Schafer & Shippee, 2010). Another study found that negative attitudes of

---

The Ageism Survey

Please put a number in the blank that shows how often you have experienced that event: Never = 0; Once = 1; More than once = 2.
("Age" means older age.)

_____ 1. I was told a joke that pokes fun at old people.

_____ 2. I was sent a birthday card that pokes fun at old people.

_____ 3. I was ignored or not taken seriously because of my age.

_____ 4. I was called an insulting name related to my age.

_____ 5. I was partronized or "talked down to" because of my age.

_____ 6. I was refused rental housing because of my age.

_____ 7. I had difficulty getting a loan because of my age.

_____ 8. I was denied a position of leadership because of my age.

_____ 9. I was rejected as unattractive because of my age.

_____ 10. I was treated with less dignity and respect because of my age.

_____ 11. A waiter or waitress ignored me because of my age.

_____ 12. A doctor or nurse assumed my ailments were caused by my age.

_____ 13. I was denied medical treatment because of my age.

_____ 14. I was denied employment because of my age.

_____ 15. I was denied promotion because of my age.

_____ 16. Someone assumed I could not hear well because of my age.

_____ 17. Someone assumed I could not understand because of my age.

_____ 18. Someone told me, "You're too old for that."

_____ 19. My house was vandalized because of my age.

_____ 20. I was victimized by a criminal because of my age.

Please write in your age: _____

Please check: Male _____ Female _____

What is the highest grade in school that you completed? _____

Survey © Copyright 2000 by Erdman Palmore.

FIGURE 1-2 The Ageism Survey is being used to measure the prevalence and identify types of ageism. (Used with permission from Palmore, E. [2000]. *The ageism survey.* Durham, NC: Duke Center for the Study of Aging.)

Cultural Perspectives on Elders and Family Caregiving Relationships

African Americans

- Elders are a source of wisdom and deserve respect.
- Grandparents are often involved with caring for grandchildren and may live in the same household.

American Indians/Alaskan Natives

- Elder status is characterized by health status and roles as counselors, teachers, or grandparents.
- Grandparents often care for grandchildren, who then are expected to care for the elders; grandmother may be called mother.

Chinese

- Traditional Chinese values place family and society above the individual.
- Elders are highly respected and honored.
- Multigenerational households are common.

Filipinos

- Respect for elders is a cornerstone of Filipino values, demonstrated by deference in verbal and nonverbal communication.
- Children (especially the oldest daughter) are expected to care for parents to repay their debt of gratitude (*utang na loob*).

Germans

- Close intergenerational relationships are maintained by first- and second-generation German Americans, but family mobility may affect this.
- Children are expected to help their parents stay in their own homes as long as possible.
- Because Amish and German Baptists view family relationships as reciprocal throughout life, grandparents usually live with their children or move from child to child.

Greeks

- Elderly women have higher status and more power within the family than younger women do and are expected to live with or near adult children, especially daughters.

Haitians

- Elders assume roles as family advisers, babysitters, historians, and consultants.
- Children are expected to care for elders at home.

Japanese

- Elders are highly respected and those who are able help in caring for children and grandchildren.
- Elders commonly maintain separate households; when they need help, the eldest son's family is expected to care for them at home.

Koreans

- Caring for elderly kin is a family duty that is associated with respect for elders and family bonds inherent in Confucianism.
- Grandparents frequently provide care for grandchildren; elders are welcome to live with family during times of need.

Mexican Americans

- Elders are revered, but acculturation reduces the sense of obligation to provide care.
- Obligation to care for an elder parent or relative does not preclude placement in long-term care facility.

Puerto Ricans

- *La abuela(o)* (elder or grandparent) is a figure of respect, wisdom, and admiration.
- Both men and women care for elders and share caregiving responsibilities with family members and a close family network.

Russians

- Elders are highly respected and remain close to their children.
- Even if elders do not live with their children, they are expected to help raise grandchildren and participate in decision making.

Vietnamese

- They believe that the more one respects the elderly, the greater one's chance is of reaching old age.
- Young adults are expected to assume full responsibility for caring for elders at home.

From Lipson, J. G., & Dibble, L. (2005). *Culture & clinical care.* San Francisco: UCSF Nursing Press.

younger generations, especially lack of respect for older generations, can affect well-being of older adults (Cheng, 2009).

Another outcome of ageism is **aging anxiety**, which is experienced by people of all ages as fears and worries about detrimental effects associated with older adulthood (e.g., social losses, financial insecurity, changes in appearance, and declines in health and functioning). One study found that aging anxiety about loss of attractiveness was higher among women who are younger, white, employed, heterosexual, separated or divorced, and less financially independent (Barrett & Robbins, 2008). Aging anxiety is reinforced by negative stereotypes of older adults and the associated fear that these problems are likely to occur in one's own later life. In contrast, people who have accurate information about aging and positive experiences with older adults are less likely to have aging anxiety.

One aspect of ageism that is particularly relevant to providing care for older adults is related to **age attribution**, which is the tendency to attribute problems to the aging process rather than to pathologic and potentially treatable conditions. For example, the phrase *senior moment* has been used since the mid-1990s to describe a lapse in memory. Because age attribution can have the effect of a self-fulfilling prophecy, health care professionals need to be cognizant of messages they give to older adults. Negative effects of age attribution include worse physical functioning, delayed treatment for health problems, and an increased risk of mortality (Levy, Ashman, & Slade, 2009). One study found that exposure to images associated with healthy aging had a more positive effect on older adults, as compared with younger adults (Lineweaver, Berger, & Hertzog, 2009).

When older adults or health care professionals falsely attribute symptoms of pathologic conditions to normal aging, they are likely to overlook treatable conditions, and significant harm can result from this negligence. An important responsibility of gerontological nurses is to be knowledgeable about the differences between age-related changes and pathologic conditions, so appropriate nursing interventions can be initiated. An essential first step in planning interventions, especially health-promotion interventions, is to identify those factors that are not inherent consequences of aging. Throughout this text, emphasis is placed on differentiating between age-related changes, which cannot be modified, and those factors that can be addressed through interventions. Chapter 3 describes a nursing model for this approach to promoting wellness for older adults.

Another consequence of ageism is the emergence of the **anti-aging** movement, which has been promoted by the American Academy of Anti-Aging Medicine since the early 1990s. The anti-aging movement views aging as a process that can be stopped and the lifespan as something that can be extended for up to 200 years. Anti-aging interventions include exercise and lifestyle modifications, but there also is strong emphasis on dietary supplements and other products that have not been proved effective. A main criticism is that the anti-aging movement is directed more toward selling products than toward the advancement of sound scientific evidence. One gerontologist concluded that anti-aging concepts are based on an understanding of aging as a bodily failure, which can be counteracted only when scientists no longer hold ageist preconceptions that are embedded in a wider ageist culture (Vincent, 2008).

Addressing Attitudes of Nurses

Negative attitudes about aging that are held by health care workers can negatively affect the care older adults receive. For example, a nursing study found that ageism was a major source of ethical issues for nurses for older adults (Rees, King, & Schmitz, 2009). Health care workers are likely to be influenced not only by ageism in society but also by their own experiences in health care, which often are with those older adults who are the most impaired and in need of interventions. It is important, therefore, that health care workers in all clinical settings recognize that most older adults are healthy and functional and strive toward improved levels of wellness and functioning.

Attitudes are changed through education, but changing attitudes requires first recognizing their existence. Because ageism is subtle but pervasive in American society, nurses first need to become aware of the attitudes they hold toward older adults. The first critical thinking exercise at the end of this chapter suggests ways of becoming aware of one's own attitudes about older adults.

Another way of addressing attitudes of nurses and other health care workers toward older adults is through experiential educational activities. For example, *Into Aging* is a simulation game developed by nurses in the late 1980s to challenge the myths of aging (available at www.slackbooks.com). This game has been used successfully to improve attitudes and staff behaviors toward care of older adults in a variety of settings (Dillon, Ailor, & Amato, 2009). A simpler method of addressing attitudes is to listen carefully to older adults as they talk about beliefs, values, hopes, and experiences that are integral to their self-identities. Nurses have daily opportunities to learn about aging and older adulthood simply by listening to the older adults for whom they provide care. In addition, nurses can equip themselves with accurate information about the older adult population. Accurate information may be the most effective antidote to negative attitudes resulting from misunderstandings or myths. The next sections address myths about aging by providing an accurate snapshot of older adults in the United States.

A Student's Perspective

I personally have aging anxiety. After working at an assisted living facility for the past year and a half, I have seen some pretty tragic and depressing events happen in the lives of these residents. Many of these residents tell me they do not know why God has kept them around this long. But listening to the stories of others has given me hope. I found it very encouraging to see the elderly people taking classes and enjoying the discussions they were a part of. I would imagine that it would be tempting to give up when the mental or physical functioning is not what it used to be, but some of the people gave me hope for aging. They make me want to be a stronger person even now at the age of 19 years. They seem to have so much passion and intensity to their lives. Not only can they serve to encourage people in their younger years to continually embrace life, but I hope other elderly people can be encouraged that they do not have to let go of their dreams just because they are aging. You can age successfully as these people have by living life to its fullest and persevering to keep your individuality and talents alive.

Jessica S.

DEBUNKING MYTHS: UNDERSTANDING REALITIES ABOUT OLDER ADULTS IN THE UNITED STATES

As a consequence of ageism and negative attitudes about aging, many myths and negative stereotypes about older adults have been perpetuated, especially with regard to aspects of health and functioning. These myths and stereotypes can be particularly detrimental when health care providers lack accurate information on which to base their decisions or actions about older adults because misconceptions lead to suboptimal goals for care. At best, older adults do not experience the benefits of wellness-focused care; at worst, they experience unnecessary decline.

This chapter provides information about characteristics of the older adult population, and Chapter 2 extends this overview by addressing cultural diversity of older adults. Chapters in Part 3 of this text address aspects of functioning that can be significantly affected by myths and misunderstandings about aging. Table 1-1 lists some of the myths and

TABLE 1-1 Myths and Realities of Aging

Myth	Reality
Older adulthood is something to be dreaded because it represents disability and death.	Most older adults live independently, have high levels of self-reported health, and are aging successfully. *(Chapter 1)*
People consider themselves "old" on their 65th birthday.	People usually feel old based on their health and function, rather than on their chronologic age. *(Chapter 1)*
Gerontologists have discovered that, by the age of 75 years, people are quite homogeneous as a group.	The more gerontologists learn about aging, the more they realize that, with increased age, people become more diverse, and individuals become less like their age peers. *(Chapters 1, 2, and 4)*
Ageism is a natural part of all societies.	Ageism is more common in industrialized societies and is highly influenced by stereotypes and cultural values. *(Chapter 1)*
Gerontologists have recently discovered a theory that explains biologic aging.	Theories about biologic aging continue to evolve, and there is little agreement on any one theory. *(Chapter 4)*
In today's society, families no longer care for older people.	In the United States, 80% of the care of older adults is provided by their families. *(Chapter 1)*
As people grow older, it is natural for them to want to withdraw from society.	Because older people are unique individuals, each of them responds differently to society. *(Chapter 4)*
By the age of 70 years, an individual's psychological growth is complete.	People never lose their capacity for psychological growth. *(Chapters 4 and 12)*
Increased disability in older people is attributable to age-related changes alone.	Although age-related changes increase one's vulnerability to functional impairments, the disabilities are attributable to risk factors, such as diseases and adverse medication effects. *(Chapter 3)*
Health-promotion efforts are not beneficial to older adults who have two or more chronic conditions.	Research has debunked the myths that prevention is not effective after onset of chronic illness. *(Chapter 5)*
About 20% of people aged 65 years and older live in nursing homes as long-term residents.	Between 4% and 5% of older adults live in a nursing home at any time. *(Chapters 1 and 6)*
Widowhood and other life events have been found to have a consistently negative impact on older people.	No one life event affects all older people negatively. The most important consideration governing the impact of an event is its unique meaning for the individual. *(Chapter 12)*
In old age, there is an inevitable decline in all intellectual abilities.	A few areas of cognitive ability decline in healthy older adults but other areas show improvement. *(Chapter 11)*
Older adults cannot learn complex new skills.	Older adults are capable of learning new things, but the speed with which they process information slows down with age. *(Chapter 11)*
Constipation develops primarily because of age-related changes.	Constipation is attributable primarily to risk factors, such as restricted activity and poor dietary habits. *(Chapter 18)*
Urinary incontinence is a normal consequence of aging that is best managed by using incontinence products.	In most cases, underlying causes of urinary incontinence can be addressed and a variety of self-care methods can be initiated. *(Chapter 19)*
Skin wrinkles can be prevented by using oils and lotions.	The best way to prevent skin wrinkles is to avoid exposure to ultraviolet light. *(Chapter 23)*
Older people are less sexually active primarily because they lose the ability to enjoy sex.	Declines in sexual activity in older people are primarily because of risk factors, such as diseases, adverse medication effects, and loss of partner. *(Chapter 26)*
Health care professionals readily recognize adverse medication effects in older adults.	Adverse medication effects are often overlooked in older adults because they are mistakenly attributed to aging or pathologic conditions. *(Chapter 8)*
Some degree of "senility" is normal in very old people.	"Senility" is an inaccurate term used to refer to dementing conditions, which are always caused by pathologic changes. *(Chapter 14)*
Most old people are depressed and should be allowed to withdraw from society.	About one-third of older people exhibit depressive symptoms; however, depression is a very treatable condition at any age. *(Chapter 15)*

misperceptions about aging that are commonly held by older adults and health care professionals. The related realities about each aspect of health and functioning also are identified, along with a reference to the chapter that provides accurate information to dispel the myths.

The characteristics of the older adult population in the United States summarized in this chapter are based on census data and other reliable sources; however, this information can only reflect trends and compilations. The intent is to provide an overview of population demographics and characteristics of older adults that are most pertinent to holistically caring for older adults. Nurses need to keep in mind that older adults are a highly diverse group and this general information does not necessarily apply to every older individual.

Demographics of Aging

Discussions of current demographic trends in the United States inevitably focus on the so-called **baby boomers**, which is the large group of people born between 1946 and 1964. This group, which comprised about 30% of the population in 1994, began turning 65 in 2011, and will bring about major demographic changes. The influence of this and other population trends, such as greater cultural diversity (see Chapter 2) and increased life expectancy (see Chapter 4), is reflected in the statistics summarized in Box 1-1 and Figures 1-3 and 1-4.

Statistics about anticipated trends are based on forecasts about a variety of factors that will affect morbidity and mortality of people who are baby boomers now as well as generations who are not yet born. The most commonly cited projections are

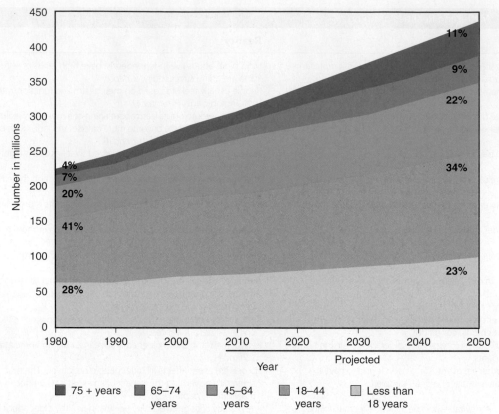

FIGURE 1-3 Actual and projected total population of the United States by age, 1980 to 2050. (*Source: U.S. Census Bureau, Population Estimates & Projections.*)

Box 1-1   Stats in Brief: Changing Demographics of Aging in the United States

Median Age
- 1900   23 years
- 2000   35 years
- 2035   39 years

Average Life Expectancy at Age 65 Years
- 1900   11.9 years
- 1960   14.4 years
- 2007   18.6 years (19.8 for women, 17.1 for men)

Actual and Projected Percentage of People Aged 65+ Years
- 1900   4.1%
- 2010   12.8%
- 2050   20.6%

Actual and Estimated Number and Percentage of People Aged 85+ Years
- 1900   100,000 (0.2%)
- 2006   5.3 million (1.8%)
- 2050   21 million (5%)

Approximate or Estimated Number of Centenarians
- 1990   37,300
- 2009   104,000
- 2050   1.5 million

Source: U.S. Census Bureau, American Fact Finder (2010).

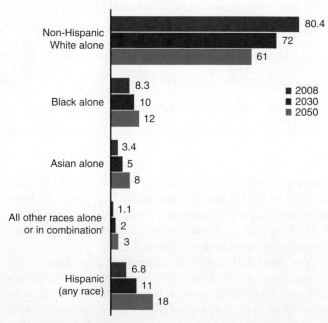

¹The race group "All other races alone or in combination" includes American Indian and Alaska Native alone, Native Hawaiian and Other Pacific Islander alone, and all people who reported two or more races.

FIGURE 1-4 Population age 65+, by race and Hispanic origin, 2008 and projected through 2050. (*Source: U.S. Census Bureau, Population Estimates & Projections.*)

based on government agency assumptions that the pace of improvements in mortality will be slowing down. However, the MacArthur Foundation Research Network on an Aging Society has concluded that a combination of control of behavioral risk factors and medical advances that slow down aging can result in as much as 7.9 additional years of life expectancy at birth in 2050 (Olshansky, Goldman, Zheng, & Rowe, 2009).

Health Characteristics

A major focus of health characteristics of older adults is on chronic conditions and levels of functioning. Many studies show that the prevalence of disability among older adults has decreased dramatically during the past few decades, despite the increasing in the prevalence of chronic conditions among middle-aged and older adults (Manton, 2008; Martin, Freedman, Schoeni, & Andreski, 2009). These improvements are attributed to advances in medical care, improved socioeconomic conditions, and increased use of technology that helps maintain independence (Murabito, et al., 2008; Schoeni, Freedman, & Martin, 2008).

Because of these trends, a health characteristic that is unique to older adults is a high rate of co-occurrence of multiple chronic conditions, which is termed **comorbidity** (Ferrucci, Giallauria, & Guralnik, 2008). Gerontologists have raised questions about whether the increasing prevalence of chronic conditions among the baby boomer generation will eventually result in poorer health outcomes as this population group ages (Martin et al., 2009). Consequently, gerontological health care providers need to focus on preventing the disabling consequences of chronic illnesses, teaching adults about self-care practices, and supporting optimal functioning and quality of life. Box 1-2 and Figure 1-5 summarize statistics that describe the health characteristics of older adults in the United States.

In recent years, increasing attention has been paid to the negative consequences of health disparities among groups of older blacks and other minorities, as discussed in more detail in Chapter 2. For example, studies found that black older adults have lower levels of health and functioning and are more likely to reside in long-term care facilities with poorer care quality (Cai, Mukamel, & Temkin-Greener, 2010; Spencer et al., 2009). Of particular importance is the wide gap in life expectancy between black males (lowest) and white females (highest). A recent analysis of the longevity gap between black men and white men in the United States indicates that it remained relatively stable at 17% to 18% from beginning to the end of the 20th century (Sloan, Ayyagari, Salm, & Grossman, 2010). See Chapter 4 for more information on life expectancy and race.

Socioeconomic Characteristics

Socioeconomic characteristics that most commonly affect health of older adults include income, education, and occu-

Box 1-2 Stats in Brief: Health Characteristics of People Aged 65+ Years in the United States

Percentage Reporting Good, Very Good, or Excellent Health
- age 65–74   78%
- age 75+   72%

Percentage Needing Help with Personal Care
- age 65–74   3.4%
- age 75–84   6.7%
- age 85+   19.3%

Healthy Body Weight
- age 65–74   30%
- age 75+   42%

Prevalence of Chronic Conditions
- at least one   80%
- two or more   50%

Types of Chronic Conditions
- Diagnosed arthritis (49%)
- Hypertension (41%)
- All types of heart disease (31%)
- Any type of cancer (22%)
- Diabetes (18%)

Source: National Centers for Disease Control and Prevention, Vital and Health Statistics, 2009.

pation, and combinations of these conditions (Matthews, Jagger, Miller, Brayne, & MRC CFAS, 2009).

In particular, poverty and lower educational level can affect healthy aging because these factors are associated with

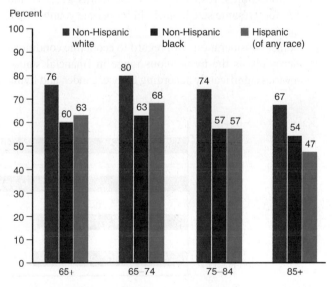

Note: Data are based on a 3-year average from 2004 to 2006. See Appendix B for the definition of race and Hispanic origin in the National Health Interview Study.
Reference population: The data refer to the civilian noninstitutionalized population.

FIGURE 1-5 Percentage of people aged 65+ reporting good to excellent health, by age, race, and Hispanic origin, 2004–2006. (*Source: Centers for Disease Control and Prevention, National Center for Health Statistics, National Health Interview Survey.*)

earlier onset of disease and mortality (Crimmins, Kim, & Seeman, 2009). One analysis of data from 1980 to 2000 found a significant and widening gap in measures of disability, life expectancy, and self-reported health based on educational levels (Meara, Richards, & Cutler, 2008). In this analysis, researchers found that life expectancy in the United States rose by about 3 years for better-educated people, but by only 6 months for less educated during those two decades. Another analysis of data from 1983 to 2003 concluded that educational differences in health varied to some degree by gender and race, with women and blacks experiencing wider disparities (Liu & Hummer, 2008).

Although census data predict gradual and continuing increases in level of education for older adults—with associated better health and higher incomes—many older adults will remain socioeconomically disadvantaged. Limited English proficiency and poor health literacy skills are two variables that are common among older adults and have a negative impact on health and functioning (Bennett, Chen, Soroui, & White, 2009; Lopez-Quintero, Berry, & Neumark, 2009). Figure 1-6 illustrates educational levels of older adults by race and Hispanic origin.

In recent decades, the overall poverty rate for older adults has been declining, but this does not mean that all older people are economically better off today than they were 40 years ago. Gerontologists and sociologists emphasize that statistics about poverty should be interpreted in relation to a broader perspective on the economic conditions of older adults in the United States. One important consideration is that the official "poverty line" varies for the over- and under-65 populations. In 2009, the poverty threshold for people aged 65 years and older was $10,289 and $12,968 for one-person and two-people households, respectively; while it was $11,161 and $14,366 for the same size household for people younger than 65 years.

Another consideration with regard to economic conditions of older adults is the tremendous range in financial status, which varies significantly according to race, gender, and living

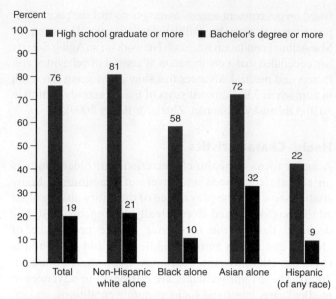

Percent

■ High school graduate or more   ■ Bachelor's degree or more

Note: The term "non-Hispanic white alone" is used to refer to people who reported being white and no other race and who are not Hispanic. The term "black alone" is used to refer to people who reported being black or African American and no other race, and the term "Asian alone" is used to refer to people who reported only Asian as their race. The use of single-race populations in this report does not imply that this is the preferred method of presenting or analyzing data. The U.S. Census Bureau uses a variety of approaches. Reference population: These data refer to the civilian noninstitutionalized population.

FIGURE 1-6 Educational levels of older adults, by race and Hispanic origin, 2007. (*Source: U.S. Census Bureau, Current Population Survey, Annual Social and Economic Supplement.*)

arrangements. Studies found that older women are more likely to be poor than older men and poverty is more common among women aged 75 years and older and those who are widowed or living alone (Gornick, Sierminska, & Smeeding, 2009). Studies also found that length of time in poverty varies by race, with later-life poverty reflecting long-term economic disadvantage for most African American women but for only one-third of white women (Lee & Shaw, 2008). Figure 1-7 illustrates poverty rates for older adults by race and Hispanic origin.

Marital status affects other aspects of older adults' lives in many ways, including economic resources, living arrangements,

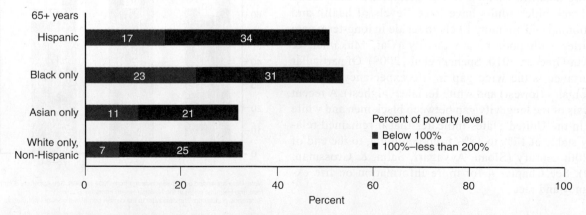

Note: Percent of poverty level is based on family income and family size and composition using U.S. Census Bureau poverty thresholds. Persons of Hispanic origin may be of any race, Black and Asian races include persons of Hispanic and non-Hispanic origin.

FIGURE 1-7 Percent of poverty level for older adults, by race and Hispanic origin: 2007. (*Source: U.S. Census Bureau, Current Population Survey, Annual Social and Economic Supplements.*)

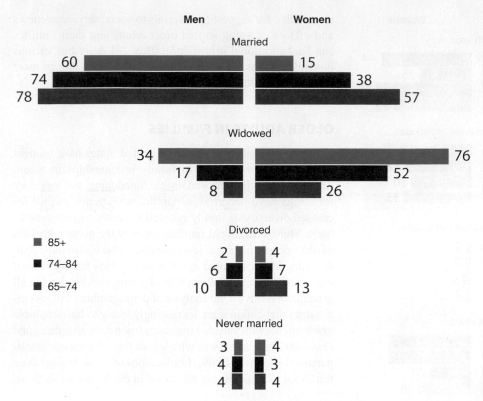

Note: Married includes married, spouse present; married, spouse absent; and separated. Reference population: These data refer to the civilian noninstitionalized population.

FIGURE 1-8 Marital status adults 65+, by sex and age groups, 2007. (*Source: U.S. Census Bureau, Current Population Survey, Annual Social and Economic Supplement.*)

and availability of a caregiver for those who are dependent. Marital status varies significantly by sex and age, as illustrated in Figure 1-8. Box 1-3 summarizes statistics about socioeconomic characteristics of older adults in the United States.

Living Arrangements of Older Adults

Living arrangements for older adults are influenced by such factors as health, marital status, family relationships, and socioeconomic conditions, as indicated in the following statistics from about 2007 (Federal Interagency Forum, 2008):

- Older women were more than twice as likely as men to live alone (39% vs. 19%).
- Older people who live alone are more likely than those who live with a spouse to be in poverty.
- Older black and non-Hispanic white women were more likely than women of other races to live alone.
- Older black men lived alone more than three times as often as older Asian men.
- Older black, Asian, and Hispanic women were more likely than non-Hispanic white women to live with relatives other than a spouse.
- Older Hispanic men were more likely than men of other races to live with relatives other than a spouse.
- The proportion of older adults living in nursing facilities increases with age as follows: 1.3% of those aged 65 to 74 years, 3.8% of those aged 75 to 84 years, and 15.4% of those aged 85 years or older.

Figure 1-9 provides additional details about living arrangements of older adults by sex, race, and Hispanic origin.

The statistic that is most relevant for nurses is that overall, about 90% of the older adult population lives in independent housing settings in the community, with the remaining 10%

Box 1-3 Stats in Brief: Socioeconomic Characteristics of People Aged 65+ Years in the United States

Education	High School	Bachelor's Degree
• 1965	24%	5%
• 2007	76%	20%

Poverty Status in 2008
- Below 100% poverty level   9.0%
- Between 100% and 149%   11.6%
- At or above 150%   78.6%

Marital Status	Men	Women
• Married	72%	42%
• Widowed	14%	42%
• Never married	4%	4%

Language Spoken at Home
- English only   85.9%
- Other   14.1%
- English less than "very well"   8.2%

Source: U.S. Census Bureau, Current Population Survey, 2008.

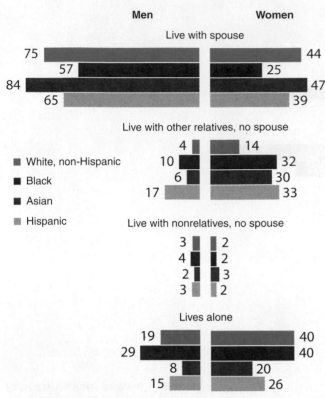

FIGURE 1-9 Living arrangements of noninstitutionalized people aged 65+, by sex and race. (*Source: U.S. Census Bureau, Current Population Survey, Annual Social and Economic Supplement.*)

about equally divided between nursing facilities and settings that provide some assistance with daily needs (e.g., assisted living). Many older adults who live in independent settings receive significant levels of assistance from family members as discussed in the following sections on caregiving. Many also receive significant levels of support from the broad range of community-based services and agencies that increasingly are available (discussed in Chapter 6).

Older adults also have an increasingly wide range of housing options that address the needs of the growing number of older adults who require daily assistance but not full-time care. For example, assisted-living residences are now available in most areas of the country. Although the services provided by these facilities vary widely, basic services generally include a single residential unit, at least one daily meal, and 24-hour availability of assistance. People who live in assisted-living facilities usually need help with three or more daily activities and these services are provided either as part of the care agreement or through other arrangements. In recent years, assisted-living facilities have become a major part of the continuum of health care services for older adults, as discussed in Chapter 6.

Because the range of housing options and community-based services is rapidly increasing, decisions about staying in one's own home or moving to another type of living facility are becoming more complex. Although nurses may not be familiar with all the housing options in their communities, at a minimum, they need to know about the various types of facilities that are commonly available. Moreover, nurses are responsible for suggesting referrals to social service agencies and offices on aging so that older adults and their families can find additional information. Box 1-4 describes various housing options for older adults that are available in most parts of the United States.

OLDER ADULTS IN FAMILIES

Major demographic trends in the United States have brought about important changes in family relationships in recent decades. Trends in improved health, functioning, and longevity for adults have occurred in parallel with trends toward increased diversity of family constellations among all generations. Multigenerational families are now the norm with 10% of older people having at least one child who is also older than 65 years, 25% of people aged 58 to 59 years having at least one living parent, and about half of young children having all grandparents alive. One analysis of demographic changes emphasizes that children are increasingly likely to have multiple grandparents with valuable resources (money, health, time) and fewer siblings and cousins with whom they share these grandparents (Uhlenberg, 2009). Implications of these demographic trends for older adults are discussed in the following sections.

Trends in Caregiving

The increasing numbers of middle-aged adults who simultaneously juggle the demands of caring for older and younger generations are referred to as the **sandwich generation.** Responsibilities of middle-aged adults with parents who depend on them for care (i.e., the sandwich generation) are described demographically by the parent support ratio. According to census data, 10 per 100 people 50 to 64 years of age cared for a family member age 85 years and older. This figure is more than triple the 1960 parent support ratio of 3 per 100, but it is only one-third of the ratio projected for 2030, when the baby boomers begin reaching 85 years of age. Demographics such as these have influenced patterns of family caregiving, particularly for women. The mid-1980s, for example, marked the beginning of an era in which the average woman in the United States spent more time caring for her parents than for her children. Despite the emphasis on women as caregivers for older adults, it is important to recognize that about one quarter of caregivers are men. However, studies show that female caregivers are more likely to provide a higher level of care than male caregivers (defined as helping with at least two activities of daily living and providing more than 40 hours of care per week) (Messecar, 2008).

Since the preindustrial period, nuclear family living arrangements have been predominant in Western Europe and the United States. Typically, younger family members establish separate households after marriage, and older family members attempt to maintain independent households for as long as possible. For much of American history, the "ideal" relationship between older and younger generations in families has been to be far enough away to preserve independent

Box 1-4 Housing Options for Older Adults

Homecare Suite or **In-Law Suite:** A fully functional and accessible modular apartment built as an addition, remodeled in basements, or installed in attached garages.

Shared Housing: A house or apartment shared by two or more unrelated people, with each occupant having a private or semiprivate bedroom. Occupants share expenses and responsibilities, and offices on aging may provide services and coordinate these programs.

Retirement Community: A specially designed residential development occupied by self-sufficient older adults. Recreational programs and support services are usually available.

Cohousing Communities: A residential development of 15 to 25 individually owned houses and commonly owned land and buildings designed to encourage community interaction. These communities typically emphasize individual privacy, resident involvement in planning, and collaborative community management. Intergenerational cohousing communities began in the United States in the 1990s, and in recent years, some communities have been developed for adults older than 50 or 55 years as senior cohousing communities.

The Village: An organized approach, governed by a nonprofit agency, to coordinating and delivering services within a neighborhood to older adults who live in their own homes. These organizations are funded through annual membership fees, and services are provided by volunteers or formal service providers at prenegotiated rates.

Life-Care or **Continuing-Care Retirement Community:** A residential complex designed to provide a wide range of services and accommodations to meet each resident's needs as they change. The development includes independent housing, congregate housing, assisted living, and nursing home care.

Congregate Housing: Individual apartments within a specially designed, multiunit dwelling. Supportive services typically include meals, laundry, housekeeping, limited transportation, and social and recreational activities.

Foster Care or **Board-and-Care Home:** A privately owned group home or small facility, which usually is licensed and regulated by a state agency. Each resident has a private or shared bedroom and use of common space. Services typically include the same ones as in congregate housing, plus assistance with daily care and some type of 24-hour emergency services. Public funding is available for older adults who meet income and health criteria.

Assisted-Living Facility: A residential facility with individual apartments, which typically consists of one to three rooms and a bathroom, and shared space for meals and social activities. Services, licensing, regulation, and funding are similar to those described for foster care homes.

lifestyles but close enough for social support and emotional connectedness. Moreover, this kind of family relationship provides for meeting occasional caregiving needs of family members while allowing for the maintenance of differing lifestyles for both younger and older generations. These family relationships are based on the principle of reciprocity across generations, characterized by mutual assistance and extensive exchanges among kin. The current trend in the United States is that caregiving needs of elders are met primarily by spouses and secondarily by adult children, especially daughters and unmarried children.

In recent years, increased rates of divorce and remarriage among younger generations have resulted in the proliferation of varieties of blended families across several generations. In addition, increased rates of remarriage among older adults who are widowed or divorced have led to increasing numbers of later-life blended families. One consequence of these trends is that family dynamics can become quite complex, particularly when adult stepchildren assume new roles as caregivers or decision makers for dependent older adults. For example, adult children may share caregiving and decision-making responsibilities regarding their impaired parent with a parent's spouse whom they hardly know. Similarly, adult children may assist their parent with caregiving or decision making about a stepparent whom they are just getting to know. Relationships among blended families usually are complicated by concerns regarding financial resources and questions about inheritance.

Expectations and attitudes about caregiving practices also have changed due to societal trends that affect relationships between older adults and their families. In the early 1900s, for example, the tradition of deep involvement in generational assistance, reinforced by strong family and ethnic values, was dominant in American culture. By the mid-1960s, trends were shifting toward a tradition of individualistic values and lifestyles, due in part to the proliferation of public support and services for older Americans. Another major influence has been the increasing numbers of women who have careers independent of their roles in families, which can lead to conflict between the younger generation of adult children and older family members who expect care. Even with complex and evolving social and demographic trends in the United States, studies consistently show that about 80% of care for dependent older adults is provided by family members and other "informal" sources. The term **informal caregiver** refers to the provision of assistance to a family member or friend in a nonprofessional and unpaid role to support the person in a community setting. The current estimate is that between 16% and 30% of Americans are informal caregivers, with the economic value of these services being estimated at $375 billion at any given point in time in 2007 (at an average rate of $10.10/hour) (DeFries, McGuire, Andresen, Brumback, & Anderson, 2009; Houser & Gibson, 2008). Studies indicate that family caregiver support delays or prevents the use of long-term care facilities and also accounts for fewer days in acute care settings (Houser & Gibson, 2008). Spousal and filial responsibilities are traditions that have directed family caregiving in the United States for centuries, and this continues even though the specific dynamics of the care are changing. Cultural Considerations 1-1 summarizes some cultural perspectives related to older adults and family caregiving.

Older Adults as Recipients and Givers of Care

Although much of the literature related to care of older adults focuses on middle-aged women who care for dependent older adults, many older adults themselves are caregivers. A summary of studies indicates that nearly 45% of all primary caregivers are older than 65 years, with 47.4% of spousal primary caregivers being 75 years or older (Messecar, 2008). Many studies focus on **caregiver burden**, which refers to the stresses and negative consequences associated with caregiving. These studies include middle-aged and older adult caregivers, and many of the studies focus on care provided to people with dementia in community settings. Some of the most consistent findings are that people who provide care for adult family members who are chronically ill experience many negative effects including higher levels of stress, anxiety, depression, poor mental and physical health, and lower levels of social interaction and quality of life (Berg & Woods, 2009; Chang, Chiou, & Chen, 2010; Ho, Chan, Woo, Chong, & Sham, 2009). Although fewer studies have focused on positive effects of being a caregiver, most caregivers experience a mixture of negative and positive consequences. Benefits or gains identified in studies center on themes, such as learning new skills; feeling needed, useful, and fulfilled; and adding a sense of purpose or meaning to one's life (Koerner, Kenyon, & Shirai, 2009; Okamoto, Momose, Fujino, & Osawa, 2009). Additional information about caregivers is discussed in Chapter 14 because many of the studies focus on caregiving in relation to people with dementia.

Grandparents Raising Grandchildren

Another phenomenon increasingly addressed by gerontologists; organizations, such as AARP; and the federal government is the dramatic increase in the number of children younger than 18 years living in households maintained by a grandparent with no parent present. These households are referred to as **skipped-generation households**. Households in which children are being raised by both their parents and grandparents are called three-generation, shared-care households. Studies of children's living arrangements and grandparent caregivers provides the following data about grandparents raising grandchildren (Kreider, 2008, Namkung, 2010):

- About 6.5 million children (8.8%) live with at least one grandparent, with 1.6 million living in households headed by grandparents with no parent present.
- 2.2% of children live with grandparents only, compared with 1.8% in 1996.
- 43% of grandparents who live with grandchildren are the primary caregivers for the children.
- African Americans and American Indians/Alaskan Natives were more likely than other groups to be responsible for raising grandchildren.
- Children living in grandparents' households were more likely to be poor, compared with those who lived in households with no grandparents (33.2% vs. 17.3%).
- Children living with a single mother and grandparent were less likely to be poor, compared with those living with a single mother and no grandparents (23% vs. 35%).

Although the overall percentage of older adults and children in these situations is small, the number has been increasing rapidly and significantly in recent decades and there are major implications for children, grandparents, and society. Common reasons for grandparent custody include child abuse; teen pregnancy; parental abuse of drugs or alcohol; and death, disability, mental illness, or incarceration of adult parents. Some studies have found positive effects of becoming a custodial grandparent; however, more studies have documented negative effects (Namkung, 2010). Rewards of grandparent caregiving include role enhancement, sense of purpose in life, motivation to keep physically active, close relationships with younger generations, and satisfaction with maintaining family well-being. Negative consequences include significant stresses, role overload, social isolation, detrimental effects on health, and increased likelihood of being poor. Specifically, studies have found that custodial grandparents were more likely to report more functional limitations, poorer self-rated health, increased prevalence of chronic disease, more depressive symptoms, and lower levels of life satisfaction than noncaregivers (Namkung, 2010).

OLDER ADULTS IN THE WORLD

This chapter has presented characteristics of older adults in the United States that are pertinent to gerontological nursing, but it would be incomplete without a brief perspective on global aspects of aging because the world's population is now aging at an unprecedented rate. Declines in fertility rates and improvements in health and life expectancy that occurred during the 20th century resulted in significant increases in the number and proportion of older adults in most of the world. As these trends continue, as is expected, by 2020 older people will outnumber children for the first time in history (Kinsella & He, 2009).

Much of the information about global aging discusses differences between *developed* countries and *developing* countries because of significantly different conditions that affect population aging in these two types of countries. Organizations, such as census bureaus, the United Nations, and the World Health Organizations, use these terms to differentiate between countries according to level of development. Although there are no universally accepted standards for classifying countries as more or less developed, commonly used criteria include life expectancy, literacy rate, and per capita income. The United Nations classifies Japan, Australia, New Zealand, and all nations in Europe and North America as developed nations, and all other nations of the world as developing nations. World population trends show that the most developed nations have the highest percentages of older adults and the highest median age and some may have more grandparents than young children by 2050. However, many of the developing countries are experiencing more recent and rapid declines in fertility rates, so the proportion of older adults in developing countries is expected to increase significantly during the next decades (Kinsella & He, 2009). Box 1-5 summarizes demographic information about global aging.

Box 1-5 Stats in Brief: Global Aging

Population Changes: People Aged 65+ Worldwide
- 2008   7%
- 2040   14%

World Population Aged 65+ Living in Developing Countries
- 2008   62%
- 2040   76%

Projected Increase in World Population Between 2008 and 2040
- Age 80+   233%
- Age 65+   160%
- All ages   33%

Countries with Highest Proportion of People Aged 65+
- Japan   21.6%
- Italy   20.0%
- Germany   20.0%
- Greece   19.1%

Source: U.S. Census Bureau, An Aging World, 2009.

Chapter Highlights

The Relationship Between Wellness and Aging
- Since the late 1950s, health care professionals have recognized the importance of incorporating wellness goals in their care of older adults; however, there are many conceptual and practical barriers.
- Barriers to promoting wellness in older adults include older adults' negative attitudes about being able to improve, the existence of more serious or pressing health concerns, the focus of health care environments on disease treatment rather than prevention or health promotion, the false attribution of symptoms of pathologic conditions to normal aging processes, and the belief that older adults are not capable of learning and implementing health-promoting behaviors inherent in wellness-oriented care.
- Rather than having a narrow focus on physical health and functioning, wellness-focused nursing considers the older adult's physical, mental, social, and spiritual well-being.
- Definitions of aging can be understood in terms of chronologic age, age identity, or functional age. Addressing functional age is most appropriate in wellness-oriented nursing care.

Attitudes Toward Aging
- Negative images of aging and ageism are pervasive in modern societies (Figure 1-1) and can have a negative impact on care provided to older adults, especially when health care providers—including nurses—base their care on myths and inaccurate information.
- Nurses need to identify myths about older adults (Figure 1-2), examine attitudes toward aging (including their own), and use accurate information as an antidote so they can provide wellness-oriented care for older adults (Table 1-1).

- Cultural perspectives have a significant influence on attitudes about aging, older adults, and family caregiving relationships (Cultural Considerations 1-1).

Debunking Myths: Understanding Realities About Older Adults in the United States
- The older adult population in the United States is increasing, living longer, and reflecting greater diversity (Box 1-1, Figures 1-3 and 1-4).
- Despite a high prevalence of chronic illnesses, most older adults report good to excellent health (Box 1-2, Figure 1-5).
- Socioeconomic characteristics and living arrangements of older adults vary significantly among subgroups (Boxes 1-3 and 1-4, Figures 1-6, 1-7, 1-8, and 1-9).
- The current trend in the United States is that caregiving needs of elders are met primarily by spouses and secondarily by adult children, especially daughters and unmarried children.
- Older adults may be responsible for raising grandchildren in skipped-generation households.
- Declines in fertility rates and improvements in health and life expectancy have led to an aging population worldwide (Box 1-5).

Critical Thinking Exercises

1. Increase your awareness of attitudes toward aging and older adults through the following exercises:
   - During the next 2 weeks, as you go about your usual activities, keep a small notebook handy and jot down examples of images of older adults that you see or hear in the following media: newspapers, magazines, Internet, television, greeting cards, and social conversations. Note whether the images convey a neutral, positive, or negative image.
   - During the next 2 weeks, pay attention to your thoughts and conversations about older adults and identify the perceptions you hold, the terms you use, and the images you convey.
   - Rephrase each of the 20 questions in the Ageism Survey (Figure 1-2) and ask yourself how often you have done any of those activities in the past few months (e.g., "How often did I tell a joke that pokes fun at old people?").
   - Ask an older relative, friend, or acquaintance to fill out the Ageism Survey and discuss his or her experiences.
2. Define old age and aging from each of the following perspectives: chronologic age, age identity, and functional age.
3. Use the Internet to explore one of the sources listed in the "Resources" section and explore additional information about demographic trends and characteristics of older adults in the United States.
4. Use the Internet to explore sources listed in the "Resources" section for information about global aging to find out more information about demographic trends in developed and developing nations.

Resources

For links to these resources and additional helpful Internet resources related to this chapter, visit thePoint. at http://thePoint. lww.com/Miller6e.

Characteristics of Older Adults in the United States

AARP
Federal Interagency Forum on Aging-Related Statistics
National Centers for Health Statistics
National Institute on Aging
Population Reference Bureau
Profile of Older Americans
U.S. Census Bureau

Information about Global Aging

An Aging World, U.S. Census Bureau
Global Action on Aging
United Nations Programme on Ageing
World Health Organization

REFERENCES

Barrett, A. E., & Robbins, C. (2008). The multiple sources of women's aging anxiety and their relationship with psychological distress. *Journal of Aging and Health, 20*(1), 32–65.

Bennett, I. M., Chen, J., Soroui, J. S., & White, S. (2009). The contribution of health literacy to disparities in self-rated health status and preventive health behaviors in older adults. *Annals of Family Medicine, 7,* 204–211.

Berg, J. A., & Woods, N. F. (2009). Global women's health: A spotlight on caregiving. *Nursing Clinics of North America, 44,* 375–384.

Bodner, E. (2009). On the origins of ageism among older and younger adults. *International Psychogeriatrics, 21*(6), 1003–1014.

Bowling, A. (2009). Perceptions of active ageing in Britain: Divergences between minority ethnic and whole population samples. *Age and Ageing, 38,* 703–710.

Boyle, P. A., Barnes, L. L., Buchman, A. S., Bennett, D. A., & Rush Alzheimer's Disease Center & Departments of Behavioral Sciences and Neurological Sciences. (2009). Purpose in life is associated with mortality among community-dwelling older persons. *Psychosomatic Medicine, 71*(5), 574–579.

Butler, R. N. (1969). Ageism: Another form of bigotry. *The Gerontologist, 9,* 243–246.

Butler, R. N. (1975). *Why survive? Being old in America.* New York, NY: Harper & Row.

Butler, R. N., Lewis, M. I., & Sunderland, T. (1991). *Aging and mental health* (4th ed.) New York, NY: Merrill/Macmillan.

Cai, S., Mukamel, D. B., & Temkin-Greener, H. (2010). Pressure ulcer prevalence among black and white nursing home residents in New York state: Evidence of racial disparity? *Medical Care, 48*(3), 233–239.

Chang, H.-Y., Chiou, C.-J., & Chen, N.-S. (2010). Impact of mental health and caregiver burden on family caregivers' physical health. *Archives of Gerontology and Geriatrics, 50,* 267–271.

Chaves, M. L., Camozzato, A. L., Eizirik, C. L., & Kaye, J. (2009). Predictors of normal and successful aging among urban-dwelling elderly Brazilians. *Journal of Gerontology: Psychological Sciences, 64B*(5), 596–602.

Cheng, S. T. (2009). Generativity in later life: Perceived respect from younger generations as a determinant of goal disengagement and psychological well-being. *Journal of Gerontology: Psychological Sciences, 64B*(1), 45–54.

Christensen, K., Doblhammer, G., Rau, R., & Vaupel, J. W. (2009). Ageing populations: The challenges ahead. *Lancet, 374*(9696), 1196–1208.

Christensen, K., Thinggaard, M., McGue, M., Rexbye, H., Hjelmborg, J. V. B., Aviv, A ., . . . Vaupel, J. W. (2009). Christmas 2009: Young

and old; Perceived age as clinically useful biomarker of ageing: Cohort study. *British Medical Journal, 339,* b5262, doi:10.1136/bmj5262.

Collerton, J., Davies, K., Jagger, C., Kingston, A., Bond, J., Eccles, W. P., & Kirkwood, T. B. (2009). Health and disease in 85 year olds: Baseline findings from the Newcastle 85+ cohort study. *British Medical Journal, 399,* b4904, doi:10.1136/bmj.b4904.

Crimmins, E. M., Kim, J. K., & Seeman, T. E. (2009). Poverty and biological risk: The earlier "aging" of the poor. *Journal of Gerontology Series: A Biological Sciences and Medical Sciences, 64*(A), 286–292.

Depp, C. A., & Jeste, D. V. (2006). Definitions and predictors of successful aging: A comprehensive review of larger quantitative studies. *American Journal of Geriatric Psychiatry, 14*(1), 6–20.

DeFries, E. L., McGuire, L. C., Andresen, E. M., Brumback, B. A., & Anderson, L. A. (2009). Caregivers of older adults with cognitive impairment. *Preventing Chronic Disease, Public Health Research, Practice, and Policy, 6*(2), 1–10.

Dillon, D., Ailor, D., & Amato, S. (2009). We're not just playing games: Into aging—an aging simulation game. *Rehabilitation Nursing: The Official Journal of the Association of Rehabilitation Nurses, 34*(6), 248–249.

Dobbs, D., Ecker, J. K., Rubinstein, B., Keimig, L., Clark, L., Frankowski, A. C., & Zimmermen, S. (2008). An ethnographic study of stigma and ageism in residential care or assisted living. *The Gerontologist, 48*(4), 517–526.

Dunn, H. L. (1958). Significance of levels of wellness in aging. *Geriatrics, 13*(1), 51–57.

Dunn, H. L. (1961). *High-level wellness.* Arlington, VA: R.W. Beatty.

Engberg, H., Oksuzyan, A., Jeune, B., Vauper, J. W., & Christensen, K. (2009). Centenarians—A useful model for healthy aging? A 29-year follow-up of hospitalizations among 40,000 Danes born in 1905. *Aging Cell, 8*(3), 270–276.

Federal Interagency Forum on Aging-Related Statistics. (2008). *Older Americans 2008: Key indicators of well-being.* Washington, DC: Government Printing Office.

Ferrucci, L., Giallauria, F., Guralnik, J. M. (2008). Epidemiology of aging. *Radiology Clinics of North America, 46*(4), 643–650.

Gornick, J. C., Sierminska, E., & Smeeding, T. M. (2009). The income and wealth packages of older women in cross-national perspective. *Journal of Gerontology: Social Sciences, 64B*(3), 402–414.

Gruenewald, T. L., Karlamangla, A. S., Greendale, G. A., Singer, B. H., & Seeman, T. E. (2009). Increased mortality risk in older adults with persistently low or declining feelings of usefulness to others. *Journal of Aging and Health, 21*(2), 398–425.

Ho, S. C., Chan, A., Woo, J., Chong, P., & Sham, A. (2009). Impact of caregiving on health and quality of life: A comparative population-based study of caregivers for elderly persons and noncaregivers. *Journal of Gerontology: A Biological Science Medical Sciences, 64A*(8), 873–879.

Houser, A., & Gibson, M. J. (2008). *Valuing the invaluable: The economic value of family caregiving, 2008 Update.* Washington, DC: AARP Public Policy Institute.

Kang, S. K., & Chasteen, A. L. (2009). The moderating role of age-group identification and perceived threat on stereotype threat among older adults. *International Journal of Aging and Human Development, 69*(3), 201–220.

Kinsella, K., & He, W. (2009). *An aging world: 2008* (U.S. Census Bureau, International Population Reports, P95—09-1). Washington, DC: Government Printing Office.

Koerner, S. S., Kenyon, D. Y. B., & Shirai, Y. (2009). Caregiving for elder relatives: Which caregivers experience personal benefits/gains? *Archives of Gerontology and Geriatrics, 48,* 238–245.

Kreider, R. M. (2008). *Living arrangements of children: 2004* (U.S. Census Bureau, Current Population Reports, P70–s114). Washington, DC: Government Printing Office.

Laditka, S. B., Corwin, S. J., Laditka, J. N., Liu, R., Tseng, W., Wu, B., . . . Ivey, S. L. (2009). Attitudes about aging well among a diverse group of older Americans: Implications for promoting cognitive health. *The Gerontologist, 49*(S1), S30–S39.

Lee, S., & Shaw, L. (2008). *From work to retirement: Tracking changes in women's poverty status.* Washington, DC: AARP Public Policy Institute.

Lerolle, N., Trinquart, L., Bornstain, C., Tadie, J. M., Imbert, A., Diehl, J. L., . . . Guérot E.

(2010). Increased intensity of treatment and decreased mortality in elderly patients in an intensive care unit over a decade. *Critical Care Medicine, 38*(1), 59–64.

Levy, B. R., & Leifheit-Limson, E. (2009). The stereotype-matching effect: Greater influence on functioning when age stereotypes correspond to outcomes. *Psychology and Aging, 24*(1), 230–233.

Levy, B. R., Ashman, O., Slade, M. D. (2009). Age attributions and aging health: Contrast between the United States and Japan. *Journal of Gerontology: Psychological Sciences, 64B*(3), 335–338.

Lineweaver, T. T., Berger, A. K., & Hertzog, C. (2009). Expectations about memory change across the life span are impacted by aging stereotypes. *Psychology and Aging, 24*(1), 169–176.

Liu, H., & Hummer, R. A. (2008). Are educational differences in U.S. self-rated health increasing?: An examination by gender and race. *Social Science Medicine, 67*(11), 1898–1906.

Logsdon, R. G., Hochhalter, A. K., & Sharkey, J. R. (2009). From message to motivation: Where the rubber meets the road. *The Gerontologist, 49*(S1), S108–S111.

Lopez-Quintero, C., Berry, E. M., & Neumark, Y. (2009). Limited English proficiency is a barrier to receipt of advice about physical activity and diet among Hispanics with chronic diseases in the United States. *Journal of the American Dietetic Association, 109*(10), 1769–1773.

Manton, K. G. (2008). Recent declines in chronic disability in the elderly U.S. population: Risk factors and future dynamics. *Annual Review of Public Health, 29*, 9–113.

Martin, L. G., Freedman, V. A., Schoeni, R. F., & Andreski, P. M. (2009). Health and functioning among baby boomers approaching 60. *Journal of Gerontology: Social Sciences, 64B*(3), 369–377.

Martin, R., Williams, C., & O'Neill, D. (2009). Retrospective analysis of attitudes to ageing in the economist: Apocalyptic demography for opinion formers? *British Medical Journal,* doi:10.1136/bmj.b4914.

Matthews, F. E., Jagger, C., Miller, L. L., Brayne, C., & MRC CFAS. (2009). Education differences in life expectancy with cognitive impairment. *Journal of Gerontology A Biological Medical Sciences, 64A*(1), 125–131.

McGuire, S. L., Klein, D. A., & Chen, S. L. (2008). Ageism revisited: A study measuring ageism in East Tennessee, USA. *Nursing and Health Sciences, 10*(1), 11–16.

Meara, E., Richards, S., & Cutler, D. (2008). The gap gets bigger: Changes in mortality and life expectancy by education, 1981–2000. *Health Affairs Journal, 27*(2), 350–360.

Messecar, D. C. (2008). Family caregiving. In E. Capezuti, D. Zwicker, M. Mezey, & T. Fulmer (Eds.), *Evidence-based geriatric nursing protocols for best practice* (3rd ed., pp. 127–160). New York, NY: Springer Publishing Co.

Morley, J. E. (2009). Successful aging or aging successfully. *Journal of the American Medical Directors Association, 10*(2), 85–86.

Murabito, J. M., Pencina, M. J., Zhu, L., Kelly Hayes, M., Shrader, P., & D'Agostion, R. B. (2008). Temporal trends in self-reported functional limitations and physical disability among the community-dwelling elderly population: The Framingham heart study. *American Journal of Public Health, 98*(7), 1256–1262.

Musaiger, A. O., & D'Souza, R. (2009). Role of age and gender in the perception of aging: A community-based survey in Kuwait. *Archives of Gerontology and Geriatrics, 48*(2009), 50–57.

Namkung, E. H. (2010). *Grandparents raising grandchildren: Ethnic and household differences in health and service use.* Paper presented at the Society for Social Work and Research 14th Annual Conference.

Neugarten, B. L. (1978). The rise of the young-old. In R. Gross, B. Gross, & S. Seidman (Eds.), *The new old: Struggling for decent aging* (pp. 47–49). Garden City, NY: Anchor Press/Doubleday.

Okamoto, K., Momose, Y., Fujino, A., & Osawa, Y. (2009). Life worth living for caregiving and caregiver burden among Japanese caregivers of the disabled elderly in Japan. *Archives of Gerontology and Geriatrics, 48*, 10–13.

Olshansky, S. J., Goldman, D. P., Zheng, Y., Rowe, J. W. (2009). Aging in America in the twenty-first century: Demographic forecasts from the MacArthur Foundation Research Network on an Aging Society. *The Milbank Quarterly, 87*(4), 842–862.

Palmore, E. (2005). Three decades of research on ageism. *Generations, 29*(3), 87–90.

Plath, D. (2009). International policy perspectives on independence in old age. *Journal of Aging and Social Policy, 21*(2), 209–223.

Prevc, P., & Doupona, T. M. (2009). Age identity, social influence and socialization through physical activity in elderly people living in a nursing home. *Collegium Antropologicum, 33*(4), 1107–1114.

Rees, J., King, L., & Schmitz, K. (2009). Nurses' perceptions of ethical issues in the care of older people. *Nursing Ethics, 16*(4), 436–452.

Rowe, J. W., & Kahn, R. L. (1997). Successful aging. *The Gerontologist, 37*, 433–440.

Schafer, M. H., & Shippee, T. P. (2010). Age identity, gender, and perceptions of decline: Does feeling older lead to pessimistic dispositions about cognitive aging? *Journals of Gerontology Series B, 65B*(1), 91–96.

Schoeni, R. F., Freedman, V. A., & Martin, L. G. (2008). Why is late-life disability declining? *The Milbank Quarterly, 86*(1), 47–89.

Silva, M. G., & Boemer, M. R. (2009). The experience of aging: A phenomenological perspective. *Revista Latino-Americana de Enfermagem, 17*(3), 380–386.

Sloan, F. A., Ayyagari, P., Salm, M., & Grossman, D. (2010). The longevity gap between black and white men in the United States at the beginning and end of the 20th century. *American Journal of Public Health, 100*(2), 357–363.

Spencer, S. M., Schultz, R., Rooks, R. N., Albert, M., Thorpe, R. J., Brenes, G. A., . . . Newman, A. B. (2009). Racial differences in self-rated health at similar levels of physical functioning: An examination of health pessimism in the Health, Aging, and Body Composition Study. *Journal of Gerontology: Social Sciences, 64B*(1), 87–94.

Uhlenberg, P. (2009). Children in an aging society. *Journal of Gerontology: Social Sciences, 64B*(4), 489–486.

Vincent, J. A. (2008). The cultural construction old as a biological phenomenon: Science and anti-aging technologies. *Journal of Aging Studies, 22*(2008), 331–339.

Wilson, D. M., Thurston, A., & Lichlyter, B. (2010). Should the oldest-old be admitted to the intensive care unit and receive advanced life-supporting care? *Critical Care Medicine, 38*(1), 303–304.

Zikic, L., Jankelic, S., Milosevic, D. P., Despotovic, N., Erceg, P., & Davidovic, M. (2009). Self-perception of health (SPH) in the oldest-old subjects. *Archives of Gerontology and Geriatrics, 49*(Suppl. 1), 245–249.

CHAPTER 2

Addressing Diversity of Older Adults

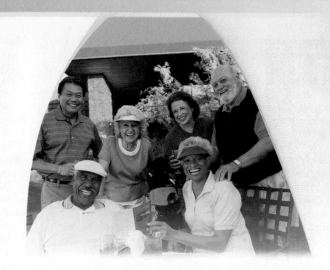

LEARNING OBJECTIVES

After reading this chapter, you will be able to:

1. Discuss the importance of providing linguistically and culturally competent care for older adults.
2. Perform a cultural self-assessment.
3. Describe three major health belief systems that influence cultural perspectives on health and wellness.
4. Describe health disparities that affect older adults of different cultural groups.
5. Identify sources of information that nurses can use to improve their cultural competence.
6. Describe characteristics of the cultural groups of older adults in the United States.

KEY POINTS

cultural competence	health belief system
cultural self-assessment	health disparities
ethnogeriatrics	linguistic competence

The increasing diversity that is characteristic of all age groups in the United States affects almost every facet of health care because cultural background significantly influences values, communication, health beliefs and health-related behaviors, and many other aspects of daily life. Nurses who care for older adults from racially and ethnically diverse backgrounds need to recognize that seven or more decades of cultural influences significantly affect their health beliefs and behaviors as well as their relationships with health care providers and their receptivity to interventions. Although it is beyond the scope of this text to present all the data and address all the implications related to cultural diversity of older adults, the intent of this chapter is to discuss major implications of population trends in relation to nursing care of older adults. This chapter provides overviews of diverse groups of older adults in the United States; however, as with any information related to cultural diversity, it is imperative to recognize that, at best, the overviews provide basic statistics about particular groups. Each group is composed of many individuals and each individual has some characteristics that are common to the group and many that are not. Because overviews do not apply to all individuals within the group, nurses need to avoid stereotypes and generalizations as they care for individual older adults.

CULTURAL DIVERSITY IN THE UNITED STATES

As discussed in Chapter 1, remarkable changes have occurred in the age-related demographics of all countries because of increased life expectancy among most groups and decreased fertility rates among many groups. At the same time that the trend toward population aging has been occurring worldwide, a trend toward increasing diversity by race and ethnicity has been occurring in the United States, notably a gradual shift from African Americans being the largest minority group to Hispanics becoming the largest minority group. This is attributable to major changes in immigration patterns following the 1965 Immigration Act that abolished the national origins quota system. The percent of immigrants coming from Europe decreased from 75% in 1960 to 13% in 2007 and the percent coming from Asia or Latin America increased from 19% to 80% during this same period (Grieco, 2010). In addition to these changes in immigration patterns, high fertility rates among immigrant groups contribute to the increasing cultural diversity in the United States. Projections indicate that by mid-21st century, about one-half of the U.S. population will be non-Hispanic white and one-fourth will be Hispanic, with 15% African American, and 8% Asian, as illustrated in Figure 2-1 (U.S. Census Bureau, 2008). Information about increasing diversity of the older adult population is provided in the sections of this chapter on overviews of cultural groups.

The increasing diversity that is characteristic of the general U.S. population also is reflected in the health care workforce, and is especially noticeable in nursing staff, including nursing assistants, who provide care for older adults in community

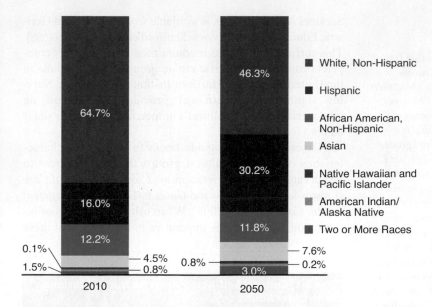

FIGURE 2-1 Actual and projected distribution of U.S. population by race/ethnicity, 2010 and 2050. (*Source: U.S. Census Bureau, 2008, U.S. Interim Projections by Age, Sex, Race, and Hispanic Origin.*)

and long-term care settings. In urban home care settings, care is often provided by caregivers who have recently come to the United States and have not learned to speak English fluently. In these situations, communication barriers between care providers and care recipients are a challenge that needs to be addressed. Thus, it is important to recognize that cultural diversity in health care settings encompasses a wide range of situations, and each situation requires a high degree of **cultural competence** on the part of the health care provider.

CULTURAL COMPETENCE

Since the 1950s, transcultural nursing (i.e., the provision of nursing care across cultural boundaries) has focused on the comparative study of different cultural groups. Although transcultural nursing is an important specialization, the demographic trend toward ever expanding diversity requires that *all* health care professionals are culturally competent. Every nurse–client encounter involves some degree of cultural differences because of the unique values and characteristics of each individual. Consequently, nurses, nursing organizations, and schools of nursing are among the groups that are taking action to ensure the provision of culturally competent care. The Holistic Nursing Scope and Standards of Practice define cultural competence as "the ability to deliver health care with knowledge of and sensitivity to cultural factors that influence the health behavior and the curing, healing, dying, and grieving process of the person" (Mariano, 2009, p. 47). Holistic nursing views cultural competence as essential for improving health and eliminating **health disparities** (Engebretson & Headley, 2009; Maddalena, 2009). Many organizations, such as the Gerontological Society of America and AARP, are emphasizing the need to address cultural diversity in the aging population. In 2003, the American Geriatrics Society published a position statement on **ethnogeriatrics**, which it defined as the component

of geriatrics that integrates the influence of race, ethnicity, and culture on health and well-being of older adults. This position paper, which was updated in 2006, emphasizes that the increasing diversity of older adults in the United States necessitates that health care professionals and systems provide ethnoculturally appropriate care while avoiding over generalizations and stereotyping (American Geriatrics Society, 2006).

Performing a Cultural Self-Assessment

Nursing texts emphasize that cultural competence is an ongoing process, rather than an end point, in which the nurse continuously strives to work effectively within the cultural context of the client (Andrews, 2008a). This process is often described as a progression from judgmental attitudes and practices to positive approaches. For example, Purnell and Paulanka (2008) describe a cultural competence continuum that begins with *unconscious incompetence* as a state of not being aware that one is lacking knowledge about another culture. When the person becomes aware of this knowledge gap, he or she progresses to a state of *conscious incompetence* and takes actions to learn about the cultural group. The person progresses to a stage of *conscious competence* by verifying generalizations and incorporating culture-specific interventions in care. The final stage is *unconscious competence* when knowledge of the cultural group is fully integrated into one's thinking and approach.

Although health care professionals rarely achieve high levels of cultural competency in relation to a broad spectrum of different ethnic/cultural groups, they are expected to achieve cultural competency in relation to the specific cultural groups for whom they provide care. Moreover, they are expected to avoid stereotyping by respectfully probing to determine the extent to which cultural views and practices influence their attitudes and perceptions, as well as the care they provide. An initial step in this process is achieved through a **cultural self-assessment**,

A Student's Perspective

After completing the cultural assessment, I learned that I do not have a thorough grasp on my own culture. We learned in class that nurses must be aware and knowledgeable about their own culture before they can relate to their clients. I have not gotten that one under wraps yet. I do not know, for example, what religious group that I best fit in with. I know that it is necessary to firmly understand your own beliefs and background before you can help a client be comfortable with theirs, yet I obviously do not! Doing the cultural assessment does make me aware of biases. I do feel uncomfortable thinking about immigrants, in that, I do not know who I define as immigrants or where I believe they come from. I also tend to imagine "we are all the same." When in reality all cultures are very different in positive ways, and to generalize is to say that the things that make cultures different are unimportant, when that is not true.

It is definitely the time to answer these questions about culture. Not only is it important for me to identify with my culture, but I also need help in developing an understanding of other people's cultures. Doing this assessment is only the first step; I must continue to question what I believe, where I come from, and who I relate to. Then I can help my clients.

Erin H.

which is an awareness-raising tool for gaining insight into the health-related values, beliefs, attitudes, and practices that one holds (Andrews, 2008a). Box 2-1 describes a cultural self-assessment that is particularly applicable for nurses caring for older adults. It is important to recognize that people can internalize social stigma and prejudices that apply to members of one's own groups. Thus, the self-assessment includes questions to increase one's awareness of internalized stigma.

Obtaining Information About Culturally Diverse Groups

In addition to using a cultural self-assessment, nurses can increase their cultural competency by using pertinent evidence-based sources of information. Types of published works that are particularly useful in this regard are (1) research on incidence of specific conditions in different population groups, (2) studies that examine the effectiveness of a treatment in a specific patient population, (3) studies that compare similar actions or outcomes of two or more culturally diverse groups, and (4) randomized clinical trials to determine the extent to which specific treatments ameliorate health disparities among diverse populations. These kinds of studies are increasingly more available and many are cited throughout this text when they are pertinent to care of older adults.

Nursing texts on transcultural nursing, such as Andrews and Boyle (2008), are good sources of comprehensive information about cultural competence that is both theoretical and clinically relevant. Another excellent resource, *A Core Curriculum in Ethnogeriatrics* (2nd ed.), which was funded by the Bureau of Health Professions Health Resources and

Services Administration, is available from the Stanford Geriatric Education Center (www.Stanford.edu/group/ethnoger/). This curriculum contains modules related to culturally competent care for 12 specific ethnic groups of older adults in the United States. The Hartford Institute for Geriatric Nursing (http://consultgerirn.org) provides information on ethnogeriatrics and cultural competence related to older adults.

Nurses also can use guide books to learn about characteristics of specific cultural groups that are pertinent to health care. Two such references are *Culture & Clinical Care* (Lipson & Dibble, 2005) and *Guide to Culturally Competent Health Care* (Purnell, 2009). When using any sources of information, however, it is imperative to recognize that these

---

Box 2-1 Cultural Self-Assessment for Nurses Working With Older Adults

What Self-Identity Influences My World View?
- With what sociocultural and religious groups do I most closely identify?
- What does it mean to belong to these groups?
- Is there any stigma associated with any of these groups?
- What negative and positive images are associated with these groups?
- What do I like and dislike about these groups and my sociocultural identity?

How Has My Cultural Background Influenced Me?
- How has (does) the society in which I grew up (currently live in) influenced the dominant values that I now hold?
- What is my perception of concepts such as time, work, leisure, health, family, and relationships?
- How do my perceptions differ from those of people who come from different cultural backgrounds?

What Is My Attitude Toward People, Especially Older Adults Who
- are immigrants?
- have difficulty with the English language?
- have difficulty communicating?
- have a cultural background different from my own?
- look or act like the stereotype of people who are gay, lesbian, or transgender?

What Are My Attitudes About and Experiences With Health Practices That Differ From My Own?
- Do (did) members of my family have health care practices that differ(ed) from conventional Western medicine practices (e.g., herbs, poultices, folk remedies)?
- Do (did) they consult with folk, indigenous, religious, or spiritual healers?
- How do I feel about alternative or complementary health care practices for myself and for older adults?

How Well Do I Communicate and Understand?
- What do I do and how do I feel when I have difficulty understanding people whose accents and primary language are different from my own?
- What have I learned about myself because of this self-assessment?

resources can describe general characteristics of a particular group, but they cannot describe the unique way in which each individual is a member of the group. These generalizations, in fact, can be problematic if they lead to "homogenized" rather than "individualized and customized" approaches to the person receiving health care services (Vaughn, 2009). Nurses need to recognize that the culture of each individual person is based on his or her membership in many groups and is internalized in a unique and personal way. Thus, nurses need to be knowledgeable about different cultural groups, but they need to use this information as a backdrop for exploring the ways in which individuals identify with the characteristics of the various cultural groups to which they belong. This is achieved by communicating a nonjudgmental attitude and asking open-ended questions to elicit information about each person's life experiences and cultural influences.

In this text, culturally specific information pertinent to nursing care of older adults is discussed in the following sections of this chapter and highlighted in other chapters in Cultural Considerations boxes and Diversity Notes. Nurses are encouraged to supplement this information by reading journals and other references, and by linking to the Internet resources available at http://thePoint.lww.com/Miller6e. In addition, many of the organizations listed at the end of other chapters provide culturally appropriate educational materials and resources in languages other than English (discussed in more detail in Chapter 5). These materials can be important resources for health promotion interventions and are usually available at little or no cost. In addition, all health care professionals are encouraged to contact local organizations to obtain culturally specific information about groups that reside in their locale.

A Student's Perspective

I came from a highly educated, Christian, Caucasian family and this affects how I see the world both consciously and unconsciously. Education is a very important part of my life. My Christian upbringing makes me value honesty, justice, compassion, and forgiveness. I was raised to have an open mind and not judge people until I got to know them. I think that has been the most important idea that I live my life around.

One thing I learned was how I see everyone who was not born in the United States and those who do not speak English as immigrants. I get very frustrated when I don't understand people because of their heavy accent or inability to speak English. Because one of my grandmothers used plenty of home remedies, I was exposed to alternative medicine from an early age. I think it is important to take into consideration other's beliefs and incorporate them as best as you can into their care. I am sure I will continue to discover my true values and beliefs as I grow in nursing. I think it is a good idea to keep reviewing my own cultural beliefs so that I become aware of them and how they affect my practice.

Sarah L.

Linguistic Competence in Care of Older Adults

Linguistic competence, which refers to health care services that are respectful of and responsive to a person's linguistic needs, is one small part of cultural competence. This concept is important for gerontological nurses because they frequently work with older adults whose primary language differs from their own. Immigrants who come to the United States as adults may be particularly disadvantaged because they may not have the same opportunities to learn English as do school-age children. Even when older adults are able to speak English, the high prevalence of low levels of health literacy can have negative health effects (Cordasco, Asch, Franco, & Mangione, 2009). The challenge of communicating with people who do not speak the same language or dialect is magnified when the person also has dementia or sensory impairments, as is often the case in long-term care settings.

Because the Civil Rights Act of 1964 upholds the rights of individuals with limited English proficiency to have equal access to health and social services programs, health care providers must ensure effective use of interpretation services. In 2001, the U.S. Office of Minority Health published *National Standards for Culturally and Linguistically Appropriate Services*, which are commonly referred to as CLAS and are available at www.omhrc.gov. The CLAS standards include 10 recommendations related to culturally competent care and 4 mandates related to the provision of language access services. One requirement is that health care institutions provide 24-hour no-cost language assistance services for individuals who are not able to speak or understand the English language.

Gerontological nurses have developed an excellent evidence-based protocol, called Interpreter Facilitation for Individuals with Limited English Proficiency, that provides comprehensive guidelines to facilitate the effective use of language interpretation services with older adults who have limited English proficiency (Enslein, Tripp-Reimer, Kelley, Choi, & McCarty, 2002). Nurses need to be aware of interpreter resources that should be available in all health care settings that receive federal funds. For example, the Language Line Services immediate telephone interpretation services for subscribers. In situations where no interpreters are available, nurses can obtain immediate fee-based telephone interpretation services from Language Line Services by calling 1-800-752-6096. Box 2-2 summarizes guidelines for using interpreters in health care settings with older adults.

CULTURAL PERSPECTIVES ON WELLNESS

As discussed in Chapter 1, nurses have numerous opportunities to promote wellness for older adults, even under the most challenging of circumstances, through holistic nursing interventions to improve physical comfort and psychological and spiritual growth. To achieve this, nurses need to have a good understanding of the meaning of health and wellness to each individual older adult. Nurses can explore this with older adults by asking questions such as "What does it mean to you to be healthy?" or "How do you achieve wellness in your life?" If appropriate, nurses can explore this topic from the perspective of cultural diversity with a question such as "I'm interested in knowing more about how Chinese people view wellness. Can you tell me your thoughts about this?"

Because definitions of health and wellness are rooted in the **health belief systems** held by one's cultural group, it is helpful to understand the different types of worldviews held by groups. A worldview is a way of viewing, perceiving, and interpreting one's experiences. One major component of a worldview is the health belief system of a group, which includes their health-related attitudes, beliefs, and practices (Andrews, 2008b). Cultural Considerations 2-1 summarizes key aspects of the three major health belief systems that underpin health beliefs and health-related behaviors of individuals. It is important to recognize that many people integrate beliefs from two or all of these paradigms, but some people are firmly entrenched in one health belief system. Nurses need to be aware of the health beliefs that influence their clients, so they can adapt their interventions accordingly. For example, when caring for people who hold a strong holistic perspective, nurses need to find out if the condition is viewed as "hot" or "cold" and identify the appropriate "hot" or

---

Box 2-2 Guidelines for Using Interpreters

Before the Interaction

- Whenever possible, use the services of a professional interpreter. Avoid using visitors or staff from auxiliary services unless permission to do so has been obtained from both the older adult and the interpreter.
- Given that there are more than 140 languages spoken in North America, be certain that the correct language and dialect have been identified before arranging for an interpreter. For example, does the person speak Cantonese or Mandarin Chinese?
- If an interpreter for the primary language is unavailable, determine whether the older adult speaks other languages. For example, many older adults from Vietnam and some African nations are also fluent in French.
- Be aware of age, gender, and socioeconomic class considerations in selecting an interpreter. In general, it is best to use an interpreter who is the same gender and of the same approximate age and socioeconomic class as the older adult.
- Organize your thoughts and plan ahead to ensure that the most important topics are covered.
- Allow sufficient time for the interaction and expect that it will take longer than an interaction with an older adult for whom English is the primary language.

During the Interaction

- Review the importance of confidentiality.
- Talk to the older adult, not the interpreter.
- Talk about only one topic at a time.
- Use short sentences and simple vocabulary.
- Use the active voice. Avoid vague modifiers.
- Avoid professional jargon, idioms, and slang.
- Be aware that many words do not translate into another language. For instance, the English word *depression* has no equivalent in many Asian and other languages.

CULTURAL CONSIDERATIONS 2-1
Major Health Belief Systems

Magico-Religious Paradigm

- Supernatural forces dominate the fate of the world and all those in it depend on the actions of supernatural forces (e.g., God, gods).
- Origins of illness include sorcery, breach of a taboo, intrusion of a disease object, intrusion of a disease-causing spirit, and loss of soul.
- Illness is initiated by a supernatural agent with or without justification, or by a person who practices sorcery or engages the services of sorcerers.
- *Health is* a gift or reward given as a sign of God's blessing and goodwill.
- Health and illness belong first to the community and then to the individual, so there is a strong sense of community.
- Common among Latino, African, Caribbean, African American, and Middle Eastern groups.

Holistic Paradigm

- Forces of nature must be kept in balance or harmony.
- Human life is only one aspect of nature and a part of the general order of the universe.
- The whole person is viewed in the context of the total environment.
- Disease is caused by an imbalance or disharmony between the human, geophysical, and metaphysical forces of the universe.
- Illness is not an intruding agent but is a natural part of life's rhythmic course; health and illness are both natural parts of a continuum.
- Diseases of civilization (e.g., unemployment, discrimination, ghettos, suicide) are just much illnesses as are biomedical diseases.
- *Health* and *healing reflect* the quality of wholeness associated with healthy functioning and well-being.
- Common among Asian, North American, Indian, (also espoused by Florence Nightingale).

Scientific (Biomedical) Paradigm

- Life is controlled by a series of physical and biochemical processes that can be studied and manipulated by humans.
- Principles of determinism: a cause-and-effect relationship exists for all natural phenomena.
- Principles of mechanism: life processes can be controlled through mechanical, genetic, and other engineered interventions.
- Principles of reductionism: all life can be reduced or divided into smaller parts (e.g., the mind and body are two distinct entities).
- Disease is a breakdown of the human machine as a result of stress, internal damages, or external trauma or invasion.
- *Health is* the absence of disease.
- Common among most Western cultures, including the United States and Canada.

Source: Andrews, M. M. (2008b). The influence of cultural and health belief systems on health care practices. In M. M. Andrews & J. S. Boyle. *Transcultural concepts in nursing care* (pp. 66–81). Philadelphia, PA: Lippincott, Williams & Wilkins.

"cold" remedy to correct the imbalance and restore body functioning.

HEALTH DISPARITIES

In recent years, there has been increasing awareness of major health disparities among racial and ethnic minorities, and this has significant implications for gerontological health care because much of the data points toward lower levels of health and functioning in the population of non-white older adults. Health disparities are defined as significant differences with regard to the rates of disease incidence, prevalence, morbidity, mortality, or life expectancy between one population and another. Figure 2-2 illustrates health disparities for diabetes and heart disease for five groups of Americans. Most of the initial research on health disparities focused on African Americans, but more recent studies have identified major differences in health and functioning for other racial and ethnic groups. The most widely identified health disparities affecting older adults are listed in Cultural Considerations 2-2. Despite the increasing emphasis on eliminating health disparities, studies have found very little progress in many indicators, such as the longevity gap between black and white men (Sloan, Ayyagari, Salm, & Grossman, 2010). A study of progress toward the *Healthy People 2010* goal of eliminating health disparities found that, in fact, the disparities between non-Hispanic blacks and whites widened for most of the health status indicators during a 15-year period (Orsi, Margellos-Anast, & Whitman, 2010).

A common theme related to health disparities is that these are especially pronounced for diseases that can be

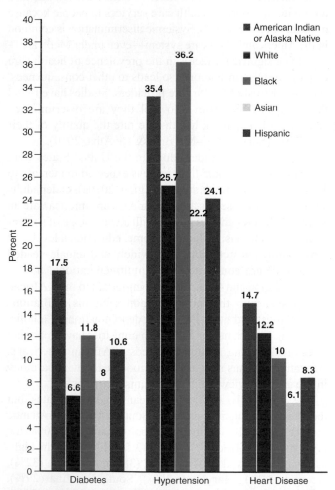

FIGURE 2-2 Percentage of adults aged 18+ years diagnosed with diabetes or heart disease, by race and ethnicity. *(Source: Centers for Disease Control and Prevention, National Health Interview Survey, 2004–2008.)*

CULTURAL CONSIDERATIONS 2-2

Major Health Disparities Affecting Older Adults

African Americans as Compared With White Americans

- Life expectancy: 1.3 (men) and 1.1 (women) years less
- Excess prevalence: stroke, cancer, arthritis, diabetes, glaucoma, hypertension, alcoholism, heart disease, cerebrovascular disease
- Excess mortality rate: stroke (41.2%), heart disease (30.1%) cancer (25.4%)
- Pneumococcal vaccination coverage: 36.1% (vs. 60.6%)
- Influenza vaccination coverage: 52% (vs. 70.2%)
- Needing assistance with personal care: 10.3 (vs. 5.7%)

Hispanics/Latinos as Compared With White Americans

- Pneumococcal vaccination coverage: 23.8% (vs. 60.6%)
- Influenza vaccination coverage: 46.7% (vs. 70.2%)
- Excess prevalence: diabetes, malnutrition, tuberculosis, asthma
- Excess mortality rate: diabetes 1.6 times higher (highest for Puerto Ricans, then Mexican Americans, and Cuban Americans)
- Needing assistance with personal care: 9.2% (vs. 5.7%)

Asian/Pacific Americans as Compared With White Americans

- Tuberculosis: highest case rates of any racial or ethnic population
- Excess prevalence: diabetes, hypertension, tuberculosis, heart disease, hepatitis B, chronic obstructive pulmonary disease, and certain cancers (lung, breast, liver, cervical, colorectal)
- Asian American women are the only group for which cancer outweighs heart disease as the leading cause of death

American Indian and Alaska Native

- Highest prevalence of diabetes than any other group, with excess prevalence of related complications (e.g., blindness, lower extremity amputations, end-stage renal disease)
- Excess prevalence of arthritis, cancer, cataracts, alcoholism, tuberculosis, kidney disease, rheumatoid arthritis, and liver and gallbladder disease
- Excess mortality rates for cancer, diabetes, pneumonia, tuberculosis, chronic liver disease, suicide, and homicide

Source: U.S. Department of Health and Human Services. (2010). *National Healthcare Disparities Report.* Rockville, MD: Agency for Healthcare Research and Quality. AHRQ Publication No. 10–004.

---

prevented through relatively safe, inexpensive, and effective interventions, such as vaccinations (Logan, 2009). Studies have found significant underutilization of pneumonia and influenza immunizations for minority and ethnic older adults as well as worse health outcomes and higher mortality rates in these same groups (Biello, Rawlings, Carroll-Scott, Browne, & Ickovics, 2010; Hutchins, Fiscella, Levine, Ompad, & McDonald, 2009; Li & Mukamel, 2010). One condition that causes health disparities, especially for preventable diseases, is the fact that health promotion materials and programs typically are developed for white people and these approaches may not be effective for people of other cultural backgrounds. Much progress has been made in recent years in identifying evidence-based approaches to disease prevention and health promotion for specific diverse groups. Nurses can find many health education to use for health promotion interventions for specific diverse groups through the links at http://thePoint. lww.com/Miller6e.

OVERVIEW OF CULTURAL GROUPS OF OLDER ADULTS IN THE UNITED STATES

To provide culturally competent care, nurses need to learn about the cultural groups in their patient populations. Although the study of aging in the United States has focused almost exclusively on white Americans, researchers are increasingly addressing interrelationships among race, ethnicity, aging, and health. Studies regarding cultural aspects of aging began with a focus on African Americans during the 1960s and then extended to Hispanic Americans in the 1970s and to other groups in the 1980s. Because little or no census data about various subgroups was available until the early 2000s, researchers are just beginning to address issues related to aging in these population groups. More recently, nonprofit organizations and gerontologists are addressing aging-related concerns of other diverse groups, such as rural, homeless, and incarcerated older adults.

Even today, terminology used in reference to subgroups is inconsistent, and definitions of specific groups vary tremendously. For example, Native Hawaiians are categorized with Pacific Islanders in the U.S. Census, but as Native Americans in the Older Americans Act and in other contexts. Categories defined by the U.S. government for the 2000 census are as follows:

- *American Indian and Alaska Native*: People who descended from any of the original people of North, South, or Central America, and who maintain their tribal affiliation or community attachment
- *Asian American*: People who descended from any of the original people of the Far East, Southeast Asia, or the Indian subcontinent (this includes Asian Indian, Chinese, Filipino, Korean, Japanese, Vietnamese)
- *Black or African American*: People who descended from any of the black racial groups of Africa (this includes Kenyan, Nigerian, Haitian)
- *Hispanic or Latino*: A person of Cuban, Mexican, Puerto Rican, South or Central South American, or other Spanish culture or origin, regardless of race
- *Native Hawaiian and Other Pacific Islander*: People who descended from any of the original peoples of Hawaii, Guam, Samoa, or other Pacific islands
- *Multiracial*: People having origins in two or more of the federally designated racial categories
- *White*: People who descended from any of the original peoples of Europe, the Middle East, or North Africa (e.g., Arab, Irish, German, Lebanese, Near Easterner).

Although much progress has been made in research related to diverse groups of older adults, many subgroups continue to be lumped together. Thus, it is important to realize that conclusions from studies may not apply to all the subgroups that are categorized as one. For example, considerable health disparities exist among the different Hispanic groups, with Puerto Ricans experiencing a higher prevalence of chronic conditions than other groups. However, most epidemiologic research has focused on Mexican Americans because this is the largest U.S. group and conclusions may not apply to Puerto Ricans or other subgroups (Tucker et al., 2010). Information about the four largest minority groups of older adults is presented in the following sections. Nurses can use this information to learn about the cultural traditions of their patient populations but, as stated earlier, must be careful not to generalize or stereotype on the basis of a person's race or ethnicity.

African Americans

African Americans are descendents of Africans who were forcibly brought to the United States and bound into slavery between 1619 and 1860. By the end of the 19th century, more than 10 million Africans had been sold as slaves. Slavery, therefore, became the way of life that formed the roots of African American (black) culture in a European American (white) society. Inherent effects of slavery included racism, poverty, and social and psychological obstacles.

Racism continues in society today and has a particularly negative impact on African Americans. A consequence of racism that has a significant impact on health care is institutional racism, which is the collective failure of organizations to provide appropriate health care services to people because of racial or ethnic factors. Systemic discrimination is common in the American health care system—even under Medicare—and it is a significant factor in the prevalence of health care disparities. Discrimination also leads to other consequences, such as mistrust of health care providers. Studies have found that African Americans who feel they are discriminated against while receiving health care rate the quality of their care lower (Sorkin, Ngo-Metzger, & De Alba, 2010).

In 2008, 8.3% of older adults in the United States were African Americans, and this figure is expected to increase to 11% by 2050 (Administration on Aging, 2010a). Older adults who identify themselves as black or African American are an extremely heterogeneous group, with a wide range of socioeconomic conditions, including income, educational level, and jobs. Family constellations vary widely and female-headed households are common, as are multigenerational households. Religion and spirituality are important to most African Americans, with the most common religious affiliations being Baptist and other Protestant denominations, Catholic, and Islam. Church nurses and parish ministries have important roles in addressing health care needs of African Americans. African Americans may associate good health with harmony in life and may view illness as a punishment for sin.

Geographically, African Americans live in all states, but their largest populations are in the Southeast and mid-Atlantic regions, especially in large metropolitan areas. In 2008, the highest number lived in New York (3.5 million) and the highest proportion lived in Mississippi (38%), Louisiana (32%), Georgia (31%), Maryland (30%), South Carolina (29%), and Alabama (27%) (U.S. Census Bureau, 2009a). African Americans generally speak Standard English, but many also speak Black English (Ebonics) or another dialect. Black English is more common in urban areas, whereas Creole dialect is more common in the rural South.

All age groups of African Americans experience significant health disparities, but those who are older experience serious cumulative effects (refer to Cultural Considerations 2-2). In 2006, African Americans had the highest age-adjusted all-causes death rate of all races/ethnicities (Office of Minority Health & Health Disparities, 2010). Factors contributing to poor health outcomes among African Americans include discrimination, cultural barriers, and lack of access to health care. Major consequences of these health disparities include decreased life expectancy and increased levels of disability and poor health. Older African Americans experience the cumulative effects of these health disparities. In 2004, older blacks accounted for 11% of all nursing home residents and were more likely to be totally dependent in activities of daily living compared with whites (29% and 24%, respectively). Differences in functional status were likely associated to the fact that blacks were more likely to reside in facilities that had serious deficiencies, such as low staffing (Jones, Sonnenfeld, & Harris-Kojetin, 2009).

*M*rs. A. is an 81-year-old African American who lives with her daughter, Mildred, and teenage great-grandson in a two-bedroom apartment in a large metropolitan area of Ohio. Mildred works as a nursing assistant in a nearby nursing home and often works double shifts. Mrs. A. was born in Alabama and lived there until 20 years ago, when her husband died and she moved in with her daughter (who lived alone at the time). Seven years later, Mildred took on responsibility for raising her infant grandson, who is now 13 years old. Mrs. A. has glaucoma, arthritis, and hypertension, and she had a stroke several years ago. She admits to having "a little problem with my memory," but Mildred says "She remembers what she wants to remember." Mrs. A. takes an over-the-counter analgesic as needed for her arthritis and has two prescription medications for hypertension. She also uses prescription eye drops twice daily. Mrs. A. has her blood pressure checked by the parish nurse about once monthly; she sees a doctor and nurse practitioner at a neighborhood clinic for checkups about twice yearly. The parish nurse often tells her that her blood pressure is "a little on the high side" and encourages her to see her doctor, but Mrs. A. has difficulty getting appointments because she depends on Mildred to take her there. Mrs. A. is about 30 pounds overweight and she walks very slowly. When she is out of the house, Mildred provides a supportive hand to assist her with steadiness and mobility. Mildred shops for groceries, but Mrs. A. prepares most meals for the family.

THINKING POINTS

- How might Mrs. A.'s living arrangements influence her health and functioning, both positively and negatively?
- What factors are likely to influence the kind of health care Mrs. A. receives?
- If you were the parish nurse, what actions would you take to decrease health risks and promote quality of life for Mrs. A.?
- What additional resources could be used to improve Mrs. A.'s situation?

Hispanics or Latinos

Because the federal government counts race and Hispanic origin as two separate categories, the census categorizes people by race and by whether or not they are Hispanic or Latino. Thus, the category of Hispanic includes many heterogeneous groups that immigrated from these countries. U.S. distribution of the Hispanic or Latino population in 2007 was 64.2% Mexican, 9.1% Puerto Rican, 3.5% Cuban, 3.2% Salvadoran, 2.7% Dominican, 1.9% Guatemalan, 1.8% Columbian, 1.2% Ecuadorian, 1.2% Honduran, 1% Peruvian, and 10.2% other groups of less than 1% each (Grieco, 2010). Although these groups have some characteristics in common, they actually represent culturally diverse groups that are categorized together for reasons such as census and research. One manifestation of this within-group diversity that is pertinent to population aging is the wide range of median ages for different subgroups. For example, in 2004, the median age for Hispanics as a group is 9 years younger than that of the U.S. population, but the median age for the Cuban Hispanics is 5 years older than the total population (U.S. Census Bureau, 2007b).

According to the Administration on Aging (2010b), 6.8% of the older adult population was Hispanic in July 2008, and by 2019, Hispanics will be the largest racial/ethnic minority group of older adults. By 2050, they will account for 20% of older adults in the United States. In 2008, 70% of Hispanics aged 65 and older lived in four states: California (27%), Texas (19%), Florida (16%), and New York (9%) (Administration on Aging, 2010b).

Hispanics have high regard (*respecto*) for people by virtue of their age, service, or experience, and this carries over to a strong respect for older people. Hispanic groups have a strong sense of family and they tend to place the needs of the group or family over those of the individual. Hispanics, like African Americans, are more likely than whites to be living with family or extended family and less likely to be living in a nursing home. Older Hispanic Americans, especially those who are Puerto Rican, have higher poverty rates than whites. The educational level of older Hispanics is lower than that of whites or African Americans. Most Hispanics in the United States speak both Spanish and English. Differing immigration patterns of these groups has led to different proportions of elderly, with a high proportion among Cubans and a lower proportion among Mexicans and Puerto Ricans.

Mexicans

The initial wave of Mexican immigrants came during the early 1900s to what was then the southwest territory of the Untied States because of political turmoil in Mexico and U.S. economic opportunities building railroads. A second wave of immigrants came during the *bracero* period (1940s to 1960s) as experienced farm laborers to work in cotton, sugar beet, and other agricultural fields. The people who came during the *bracero* period currently comprise the population of older Mexican Americans. Recent Mexican immigrants are younger people, including many who are undocumented immigrants. This group will contribute to the significant increase in older Hispanics that is expected to occur over the next decades.

Puerto Ricans

Puerto Ricans first came in the 1830s and began settling in New York City, but they did not come in great numbers until after World War II. In 1917, Puerto Ricans were granted citizenship if they agreed to mandatory military service. By the 1970s, more than 1 million Puerto Ricans had immigrated to more than 20 cities, motivated primarily by economics, employment, social mobility, and family relationships. Currently, more than 3 million Puerto Ricans live in the United States, with more than half living in the northeastern area. Fluctuating economic conditions in recent years has led to a pattern of Puerto Ricans moving back and forth, which is made easier by the fact that they are U.S. citizens in America and in Puerto Rico.

Cubans

The Republic of Cuba is a multiracial country with people primarily of Spanish and African descent, but also of Chinese, Haitian, and Eastern European origins. Cubans initially immigrated to the United States in the late 1800s to work in the tobacco industry. A second influx occurred between 1940 and 1950 when Cubans came to help with the war industry. The largest number of Cuban emigres came to the United States between 1959 and 1979 when many middle- and upper-class citizens fled Cuba for political reasons. This accounts for the higher number of older Cubans in relation to younger Cubans. They are most highly concentrated in Florida but also have significant numbers in New Jersey, New York, Illinois, and California. Because three or four generations of family often live together, many older adults live with other family members.

*B*oth Mr. and Mrs. H. are 64-year-old Mexican Americans who came to an urban area of Texas to live with their son, Jose, and daughter-in-law, Maria, about 10 years ago. Mr. and Mrs. H. provide child care for their four grandchildren, Jose works as a farm laborer, and Maria does domestic work. Mr. and Mrs. H. prefer to speak and read in Spanish, and all family members speak Spanish in the home, but they can speak English well enough to communicate when necessary. Jose and Mr. H. each smoke a couple of packs of cigarettes a day. None of the family members has health insurance, but this is not of concern to Mr. and Mrs. H. because they have relied on folk healers for many years and this has been effective for them. In their *curandismo* (traditional healing) system, Mrs. H. is the first person consulted and she applies the remedies that have been passed on to her from her mother and grandmother. Her remedies are directed toward restoring balance between hot and cold, and she also encourages prayers and lighting of candles at church. In the rare instances when a family member has not gotten better within a couple of days, Mrs. H. takes him or her to a *yerbero* (herbalist) for herbs and other remedies. Once, when Maria had a more serious "female" problem, Mrs. H. took her to a *curandero* (folk healer), who was able to cure the problem.

You are a community health nurse in the county where Mr. and Mrs. H. reside and you are told to develop a planning committee for a health fair, which is being held at and cosponsored by the Catholic church attended by many of the community's Mexican Americans. The county health department received a grant from the National Institutes of Health to identify people most at risk for cancer, diabetes, and hypertension as part of the *Healthy People 2010* initiative. At least part of the motivation for receiving this grant was to cut the cost of providing care for people who are not diagnosed until these diseases are advanced. Statistics verify that Hispanics in your county have unusually high rates of diabetes, hypertension, and lung and breast cancer. Statistics also confirm that the cost of treating these conditions is disproportionately high because of complications from untreated and undiagnosed cases. The goal of this health fair, which is part of a larger initiative, is to screen for diabetes and to motivate people to return to future fairs for additional preventive measures. Your target population for this health fair is Hispanic people aged 45 years and older.

THINKING POINTS

- Who would you want to be on your committee?
- What factors will significantly influence participation in this health fair, both positively and negatively? What plans would you suggest for overcoming barriers to participation?
- What health topics would you be sure to address for health promotion?

- How might you incorporate a family perspective in the plans for the health fair?
- What could be done to incorporate folk healers in the planning and implementation of the health fair? What are the benefits and risks in doing this?
- What additional information would you want to have so that you could proceed with planning a successful health fair? How would you go about finding this information?

Asians and Pacific Islanders in the United States

The category of "Asians and Pacific Islanders," like the category of "Hispanics," refers to numerous diverse subgroups of people clustered together for purposes of simplifying data. The 2000 census data distinguish between the Asian and the Native Hawaiian and other Pacific Islander population, but previous census data, and much of the available information about U.S. subgroups, lump together at least 30 subgroups in the one category. In 2008, the largest groups of Asians and Pacific Islanders were Chinese (3.62 million), Filipino (3.09 million), Asian Indians (2.73 million), Vietnamese (1.73 million), Koreans (1.61 million), Japanese (1.3 million), and Native Hawaiian and other Pacific Islanders (U.S. Census Bureau, 2010). Subgroups of Native Hawaiian and other Pacific Islander are Polynesian (63.5%), Micronesian (25.1%), Melanesian (5.7%), and smaller groups (5.7%) (U.S. Census Bureau, 2007c). People in these groups speak more than 100 languages and are very diverse. In 2007, 60% of Asians and Pacific Islander and older Americans lived in California (41%), Hawaii (9.85), and New York (9.2%).

Despite the great diversity among Asian and Pacific Islander groups, some general characteristics can be identified. As a group, Asian older adults have higher levels of education than other groups, but they also have higher levels of poverty (12% for Asians vs. 9.4% for all elderly) (Administration on Aging, 2009a). Asian and Pacific Islander cultures are very family oriented and place a strong value on care of older family members. Asian older adults are less likely to live alone than the older population in general in the United States. Most American-born Asians speak English, but some immigrants speak only their native language or are bilingual.

In Asian cultures, health is viewed as a state of spiritual and physical harmony, and illness occurs when the yin and yang are out of balance. "Yin" refers to female energy and is associated with wet, cold, and dark; "yang" refers to male energy and is associated with dry, hot, and light. Asian Americans generally enjoy exceptionally good health and longevity, with women experiencing the longest life expectancy (85.8 years) of any other ethnic group. However, significant health disparities also exist for this group as a whole compared with whites, as outlined in Cultural Considerations 2-2. One study found that unhealthy lifestyle behaviors and subsequent adverse health outcomes account for at least some of the health disparities among Native Hawaiian and Pacific Islander groups (Moy, Sallis, & David, 2010). Although most information about health status and disparities has combined all or many of these groups for pooled data, some recent studies are addressing subgroups. For example, a study of seven major ethnic groups in Hawaii found a 13-year gap between the longest (Chinese) and shortest (Samoans) life expectancy at birth (Park, Braun, Horiuchi, Tottori, & Onaka, 2009). Park and colleagues conclude that these findings confirm the need to conduct ethnic-specific research.

Chinese

The Chinese first migrated as laborers between 1840 and 1882, after which immigration of Chinese people to America was suspended until 1924, when annual quotas were established. Many of these immigrants came for political or socioeconomic reasons and had little or no education. In 1965, the Quota Act was abolished and many professional and highly educated Chinese came to the United States. Many Chinese live in metropolitan areas; the states with the largest Chinese populations are California, New York, Hawaii, and Texas.

Filipinos

Filipinos came in three waves, beginning in the early 1700s when the "pioneer" group came to New Orleans. This first wave continued through the early 1900s and included agricultural workers in Hawaii and the western states. Beginning in 1934, Filipino immigrants were limited to an annual quota of 50. The second wave of Filipino immigrants occurred between 1946 and 1965 when the annual quota was raised to 100. During this period, many became U.S. citizens by joining the armed services or coming as students, professionals, or war brides. The third wave began after quotas were expanded and includes a large proportion of families and young professionals.

Asian Indians

Asian Indians (also called East Indians) began coming to the United States in the late 1900s as laborers in the lumber, farming, shipping, and railroad industries. This first wave of immigrants continued coming until they were barred from these jobs by Asian Immigration Act of 1917. Many left the country at that time and by the time the ban was lifted in 1946, only 1500 Asian Indians remained in the United States (Lipson & Dibble, 2005). After the U.S. immigration laws were changed in the mid-1960s, a second wave of highly educated and technically trained Asian Indians began arriving.

Vietnamese

The Vietnamese began arriving in the mid-1970s seeking political refuge because of the Vietnam War. Second and third waves of Vietnamese, Cambodians, and Laotians have come as refugees, including many older adults and other extended family members. A fourth wave of immigrants began after

American Homecoming Act of 1987, which provided for entry of former South Vietnamese military officers, political detainees, and children of American servicemen and their mothers and close relatives.

Koreans
Koreans began immigrating to the United States in the 1900s, particularly to Hawaii, where they sought plantation work. Between 1950 and 1965, a second major wave of Koreans came, including many war brides of American servicemen. After 1965, many middle-class and college-educated Koreans, including many health care professionals, came.

Japanese
Japanese people began immigrating to America in 1885, and immigration peaked in the early 1900s. In 1924, they were barred from entering the United States, and in 1942, all Japanese people living in the United States were relocated to internment camps. Immigration resumed in the 1950s and increased after 1965 when immigration restrictions were eased. Japanese Americans are the only immigrant group whose members identify themselves according to their generation of birth in the United States. Generation groupings are *issei*, first-generation immigrants; *nisei*, first American-born generation; *sansei*, third generation; and *yonsei, gosei*, and *rokusei* for fourth, fifth, and sixth generations, respectively.

Mrs. C. is a 76-year-old Chinese American widow who lives in an apartment in the Chinatown section of San Francisco. She has lived within the same 1-mile radius since her parents brought her to San Francisco from Mainland China when she was 9 years old. All three of her children are married; two live about an hour away, and the other one lives on the East Coast. Although she can speak and read English, she prefers to use her native Chinese dialect, and all of her reading materials are in Chinese. She completed a high-school education in Chinatown and married a Chinese immigrant when she was 19 years old. She served as her husband's primary caregiver after he developed lung cancer several years ago until his death last year.

Mrs. C. is enrolled in the On Lok Senior Health Program, a health maintenance organization that provides a wide range of health and social services. She attends a daily meal program and sees the nurse at the center for blood pressure checks every month. She has hypertension, arthritis, and coronary artery disease. Mrs. C. sees a local herbalist every few weeks to obtain the herbal medicines that will keep her yin and yang energies in balance, and she chooses foods according to their yin and yang characteristics. She periodically has acupuncture treatments when

her arthritis bothers her. Although Mrs. C. believes she can control her heart problem and high blood pressure with herbs and diet, she takes her two medications as prescribed because the nurse at the On Lok clinic has emphasized that these pills are essential for keeping her energy in balance.

Mrs. C. recently had a stroke and received medical treatment and rehabilitation services. She is being discharged to her apartment with a referral to the On Lok home care services for skilled nursing and speech, physical, and occupational therapies. Discharge orders also include the need to instruct Mrs. C. in a low-sodium diet. In addition to having some aphasia and left-sided paralysis, Mrs. C. has some residual memory impairment from the stroke. Before discharge from the rehabilitation program, she said she would not need any home health aide assistance because she expected that her daughter and daughter-in-law would take turns coming over every day and that they would take care of her. You are the nurse assigned to do the initial assessment and your visit is scheduled for the day after discharge, when the daughter-in-law will be there. Although you have been a visiting nurse for several years, you have recently moved to San Francisco and you began working for On Lok 2 weeks ago.

THINKING POINTS

- What cultural factors might influence Mrs. C.'s acceptance of you, as the skilled care nurse, and of home care services in general?
- What would you do to gain cultural competence to work more effectively with Mrs. C. and other patients in the On Lok health care program?
- What are your specific health care concerns for Mrs. C., and what strategies would you use to develop an effective and acceptable care plan?

American Indians and Alaska Natives
The 2000 U.S. census defined "American Indian and Alaska Native" as people having origins in any of the original populations of North, South, or Central America and who maintain a tribal affiliation or community attachment. They are the only minority group that is indigenous to the United States and they comprise more than 500 federally recognized tribes and an additional 100 to 200 unrecognized tribes. As of July 2008, there were 4.9 million American Indians and Alaska Natives, comprising 1.6% of the total population (U.S. Census Bureau, 2009b). Tribal groups of American Indians and Alaska Natives that comprise 1% or more of this population are Cherokee (15.4%), Navaho (10.7%), Chippewa (4.3%), Pueblo (3.2%), Apache (3.1%), Sioux (3.1%), Lumbee

(2.8%), Choctaw (2.6%), Iroquois (2.4%), Pima (2.3%), Blackfeet (1.8%), Eskimo (1.7%), Creek (1.3%), and Tohono O'Odham (1%) (U.S. Census Bureau, 2007a).

Median age for American Indian and Alaska Native population, which is counted as one group, is 7 years younger than that of the total United States; only 8% are 65 years old and older. In 2007, 51% of American Indian and Native Alaska older adults lived in California (13.8%), Oklahoma (11.2%), Arizona (9.4%), New Mexico (6.5%), Texas (5.7%), and North Carolina (4.3%) (Administration on Aging, 2009b). The typical older American Indian and Alaska Native is poor, has less than a high-school education, lives in a rural area, and may speak little or no English, and is likely to speak one of the more than 150 indigenous languages that continue to be spoken.

American Indians and Alaska Natives experience major health discrepancies, as outlined in Cultural Considerations 2-2. Of particular concern is the high prevalence of diabetes, which increased by 27% between 1995/1996 and 2005/2006 (Jernigan, Duran, Ahn, & Winkleby, 2010). A health discrepancy that is unique to this population group is the excess morbidity and mortality associated with accidents, suicides, and homicides. In 2005, accidents accounted for more than double the percentage of death (11.7%) compared with other groups combined, and age-adjusted suicide rates were 1.73 times as high as corresponding rates for all persons combined (Barnes, Adams, & Powell-Griner, 2010). Factors that contribute to poorer health among American Indians and Alaska Natives include geographic isolation, economic conditions, cultural barriers, and suspicion toward traditional spiritual beliefs. The National Indian Council on Aging has developed health promotion materials that address diabetes, elder abuse, caregiver stress, and other health disparities for use with American Indian and Alaska Native groups. Nurses can find these and other health promotion materials through the organizations listed at the end of this chapter.

*M*rs. I. is a 72-year-old Navajo who lives with her daughter and son-in-law. In accordance with Navajo traditions, Mrs. I. believes that health is closely linked with being in harmony with the environment, family members, and supernatural forces. She regularly attends native healing ceremonies and protects her family and herself from sickness through songs, stories, rituals, prayers, and sand paintings. Mrs. I.'s mother kept a medicine bundle, called a *jish*, containing stones, feathers, arrowheads, and corn pollen and used this for healing and blessings. Mrs. I.'s elder sister now uses the *jish* that was passed on from their mother. Mrs. I. has had diabetes and hypertension for several years, and is about 30 pounds over her ideal weight. She receives medical care at the Indian Health Service, where you are

the nurse. During a recent visit, you found Mrs. I.'s blood pressure was 164/98 mm Hg; her random blood sugar level as measured on the glucometer was 196 mg/dL. You know from previous visits that Mrs. I. does not want to take any prescription medications because she thinks they are not in harmony with spiritual forces. When you explain that both her blood sugar and blood pressure are high, she promises you that she will ask her older sister to use the *jish* for healing. You know from your experience with the Indian Health Service that nurses have been successful in persuading Navajos to perform physical exercise if it is viewed in a larger cultural context. For example, when the nurse consulted a tribal leader in developing an exercise program, the American Indians at a community health center were receptive to incorporating mild aerobic exercise into their daily routines in the form of traditional dance movements.

THINKING POINTS

- What cultural factors are likely to influence Mrs. I.'s understanding of diabetes and hypertension?
- How would you use metaphors and cultural knowledge to help Mrs. I. understand her diabetes and hypertension?
- What questions would you ask Mrs. I. to identify teaching strategies and other interventions that might be successful with regard to her diabetes and hypertension?
- What strategies are likely to be successful in implementing dietary and lifestyle interventions for Mrs. I.?
- What steps would you take to improve your cultural competence in working with Mrs. I.?

OLDER ADULTS IN OTHER DIVERSE GROUPS

It is important to recognize that the concept of cultural competence encompasses all groups of people, including one's own group because people can be influenced by internalized stigma. As already discussed, nurses need to periodically perform a cultural self-assessment and learn about other cultural groups. Some cultural differences are quite obvious (e.g., people of different colored skin or a different spoken language), but many differences are subtle, not noticed, or even purposefully hidden (e.g., sexual orientation, religious affiliations). Thus, nurses need to learn about groups of older adults that may be less visible and smaller in numbers but with unique needs. In recent years, gerontologists are identifying the needs of some of these groups, such as those considered rural or homeless. Other groups, such as those who are discriminated against because of sexual orientation, are advocating on their own behalf to identify and address their unique needs. Information about some of these groups is discussed in this section, and nurses are encouraged to use the resources listed at the end of this chapter to learn more about these and other groups.

Older Adults in Rural Areas

The U.S. Census Bureau classifies "rural" as all those areas outside of an urbanized area or an urban cluster (i.e., areas that have a population density of at least 1000 people per square mile and are surrounded by blocks that have an overall population density of at least 500 people per square mile). Older adults comprise 15% of all rural populations (vs. 12% total), but in one-fourth of these areas, they make up 18% of the population (Jones, Kandel, & Parker, 2007). Population trends that influence the current and evolving composition of rural America are as follows: (1) younger adults have been and are moving out of farming areas to urban areas, (2) long-term residents of rural areas are aging in place, and (3) retirees of the baby boomer generation are relocating to rural areas (NACRHHS, 2008).

Although rural areas in general are not as culturally diverse as urban areas, some are dominated by one or two minority groups as in the following examples (Jones, Kandel, & Parker, 2007):

- Blacks comprise 87% of Jefferson County, Mississippi.
- Almost all of the 50,000 residents of Starr County, Texas, are Hispanic.
- 95% of the 12,500 residents of Shannon County, South Dakota, are Native Americans.
- The majority of residents in Kauai County, Hawaii, are Asian Americans.

Since the 1990s, Hispanics have been the most rapidly growing minority group that is moving into rural areas. This trend is expected to continue (NACRHHS, 2008).

Although significant local differences exist among rural areas, some common characteristics and needs have been identified. Populations in rural regions, including older adults, tend to be poorer and less educated and have worse health outcomes than their urban counterparts. In addition, rural older adults have more limited transportation options and less access to services, including meal and social programs, because of isolation. Health indicators that have been worse among rural (vs. urban) residents for the past two decades include self-reported health, prevalence of chronic conditions, health-related activity limitations, and higher mortality rates (NACRHHS, 2008). One study of older cancer survivors found that overall physical health status was lower for those in rural areas than that of comparable nonrural populations (Beck, Towsley, Caserta, Lindau, & Dudley, 2009). Diet quality of rural older adults also is poor, with one study indicating that fewer than 2% meet the recommended standard for the Healthy Eating Index (Savoca et al., 2009).

Appalachia is a specific, federally defined, rural nonfarming U.S. region established by an act of Congress in 1965. The region spans more than 1500 miles across 13 states: Alabama, Georgia, Kentucky, Maryland, Mississippi, New York, North Carolina, Ohio, Pennsylvania, South Carolina, Tennessee, Virginia, and West Virginia. Much of the designated area lies in mountainous territory, causing geographic isolation and lack of access to health care. Appalachian people have been characterized as white, of British or Scotch-Irish descent, and predominantly fundamentalist Protestant in religion. Appalachia has a higher poverty rate and a lower level of formal education than the general population. Appalachian families maintain strong bonds, and older family members are honored for their role in transmitting their culture to younger generations. Older family members are likely to live with or very close to their children.

Appalachian people may be reluctant to seek medical care, particularly in a hospital, because they view the hospital as a place to go to die. Similarly, they may be reluctant to use rehabilitative services because they tend to view illness as the will of God and disability as an inevitable consequence of aging. These beliefs can present challenges for health care professionals addressing preventive, rehabilitative, or health promotion needs. An important aspect of providing culturally sensitive care is recognizing the ways in which spirituality intertwines with health for people in Appalachia (Diddle & Denham, 2010).

Homeless Older Adults

The category of "older homeless" typically extends downward to the age of 55 years because some researchers have observed that homeless people look and behave as if they were 10 to 20 years older than their actual ages and have significant health problems. Increased homelessness among older adults is associated with increased poverty rates among certain segments and declining availability of affordable housing. Homeless people 65 years old and older are entitled to Medicare and Social Security benefits, but homeless people between the ages of 50 and 64 years usually do not qualify for these benefits unless they have been disabled for 2 years. Characteristics of homeless older adults include significantly higher mortality rates, higher levels of disability, longer length of homelessness, and higher overall rates of chronic illnesses and mental illness than younger homeless adults or older adults who are not homeless (Joyce & Limbos, 2009; Tompsett, Fowler, & Toro, 2009). Since the mid-1980s, social service and health care providers have recognized the need to provide rehabilitative services to address health, social, and behavioral problems of homeless older adults, in addition to addressing their basic needs for food and shelter.

Lesbian, Gay, Bisexual, and Transgender Older Adults

Because 5% to 10% of the adult population identifies as lesbian, gay, bisexual, and transgender (LGBT), all nurses provide care for LGBT elders, even though they may not be aware of this. The acronym LGBT refers to three groups whose sexual orientation is not heterosexual (lesbian, gay, or bisexual) and people who are transgendered. Although sexual orientation and gender identity are distinct entities, they are grouped together under the acronym of LGBT because their common bond is their experience of similar societal stigma, isolation, stereotypes, and prejudices.

Despite the relatively small numbers and invisibility of LGBT older adults, there is growing recognition of the unique barriers, challenges, and inequalities that this group faces. Major progress has been made to address these concerns, as indicated by the following recent events:

- AARP created an Office of Diversity and Inclusion and has a long history of supporting research and programs to identify and address the needs of LGBT adults aged 50 years and older.
- The Administration on Aging awarded a major grant to Services and Advocacy for Gay, Lesbian, Bisexual, and Transgender Elders (SAGE) to develop the nation's first national resource center on LGBT aging.
- The American Society on Aging, LGBT Aging Issues Network, has become a major resource for information, including education and training materials for professionals.
- The Joint Commission added respect for sexual orientation to its patient rights' requirements for assisted living and skilled nursing facilities.
- The National Gay and Lesbian Task Force published a 165-page report, *Outing Age 2010* (Grant, 2010), to promulgate research about critical concerns of LGBT older adults and make recommendations related to key issues, such as health, housing, caregiving, discrimination, and access to services.
- Five major nonprofit organizations published a 90-page report, *Improving the Lives of LGBT Older Adults*, to address the unique circumstances that make successful aging more challenging for this group (LGBT Movement Advancement Project, 2010).

A dominant theme of all these initiatives is on assuring that healthcare providers are culturally competent, which "generally involves not only an acceptance of and respect for difference, but also a degree of understanding of community norms, vulnerabilities and practices" (Grant, 2010, p. 9).

Despite the great diversity among LGBT older adults, one issue they have in common is their experiences of various levels and types of stigma. Even this common experience, however, has been shaped by vastly different sociopolitical forces. For example, cohorts of LGBT older adults older than 70 years entered into young adulthood at a time when nonheterosexual orientation was considered a crime or a mental illness. Detrimental effects of stigmatization—which for some has included the experience of violence—include fear, anxiety, chronic stress, social isolation, and avoidance of needed services and entitlements (LGBT Movement Advancement Project, 2010). Many LGBT people experience their sexual orientation along a continuum and they do not necessarily live as either heterosexual or gay/lesbian during their entire adult lives. Thus, it is important to recognize that older LGBT individuals vary widely in the length of time they have identified themselves as such.

Some LGBT have biologic, adopted, or step children, grandchildren, or great grandchildren and very close relationships with their families. Other LGBT older adults have no biologic family—or have been rejected by their families—but they have strong bonds with their "family of choice." This extended network of family and friends often become the caregivers for older LGBT who need assistance, but all people involved in these situations face social, economic, and legal challenges that do not affect heterosexuals. Older LGBT vary greatly in their intimate relationships and many have had or continue to have monogamous committed partnerships. Relatively few are able to have a legally recognized marriage, and these marriages are not recognized at the federal level. An important aspect of providing culturally competent care for LGBT older adults is using gender-neutral terminology in reference to intimate or partner relationships (as discussed in Chapter 26).

Although some LGBT older adults, especially couples in committed long-term relationships, live very comfortably, LGBT older adults as a group are poorer and less financially secure than other older adults. Many older LGBT have limited income and assets because discrimination limited their job opportunities. Only rarely are LGBT partners able to obtain financial benefits that are similar to those of legally married couples and this has a negative impact on retirement income, assets, and access to health care. One study found that older lesbian couples are twice as likely to be poor compared with heterosexual couples (Goldberg, 2009). The most significant health disparities that affect older LGBT include poorer overall health; lack of access to care; and higher prevalence of cancer, depression, HIV/AIDS, chronic disease and disability, and risky behaviors (e.g., smoking, drug and alcohol abuse) (LGBT Movement Advancement Project, 2010).

Chapter Highlights

Cultural Diversity in the United States
- The population of the United States, including older adults, is increasing in diversity.
- Projections for 2050 estimate that 50% of the U.S. population will be white, 25% Hispanic, 15% black, 8% Asian, and 2% other (Figure 2-1).

Cultural Competence
- All nurses are expected to develop cultural competence by assessing their own attitudes (Box 2-1) and learning about culturally diverse groups.
- All health care providers need to be linguistically competent and to use resources to address needs of patients who are not proficient in English (Box 2-2).

Cultural Perspectives on Wellness

- Nurses need to explore what health and wellness mean to individual older adults.
- Definitions of health and wellness are rooted in the three major health belief systems (Cultural Considerations 2-1).

Health Disparities

- Members of racial or ethnic groups experience many health disparities, and these have significant implications for older adults (Figure 2-2; Cultural Considerations 2-1).

Overview of Cultural Groups of Older Adults in the United States

- Racial and ethnic groups as categorized by the U.S. Census are American Indian and Alaska Native, Asian American, Black or African American, Hispanics or Latinos, Native Hawaiian and Pacific Islanders, and multiracial.
- Nurses can develop cultural competence by educating themselves about the cultural traditions of the older adults in their geographic areas.
- Characteristics of some of these groups are summarized, but it is important to recognize that the larger groups are composed of many subgroups and there is great diversity within these groups.

Older Adults in Other Diverse Groups

- Researchers and nonprofit organizations are identifying and addressing the unique needs of other diverse groups, including rural, homeless, and LGBT older adults.

Critical Thinking Exercises

1. Complete the cultural self-assessment in Box 2-1 and think about whether you have internalized any stigma or prejudices about any of the cultural groups to which you belong.
2. Reflect on your encounters during the past few weeks with people who differ from you culturally. Make a list of the obvious differences and another list of differences that you may not have recognized but most likely existed (e.g., you most likely interacted with someone who was LGBT). Ask yourself how accepting and nonjudgmental you feel about these people.
3. Identify one culturally diverse group that you are likely to work with in your current geographic area. Contact the agencies and organizations that serve these groups and find out what services they offer; ask about unique health care issues affecting these particular groups.
4. Go to the Internet site of a culturally specific organization listed in the Resources and find information that you might use if you were presenting a health education program to a group of older adults who are of a particular cultural background (e.g., Chinese, American Indian, African American). Think about how the health promotion materials for a specific cultural group differ from those that have been developed for whites.
5. Think of the various settings in which you work with older adults and describe what you would do or whom you would call if you needed to communicate with a patient who did not speak English.

Resources

For links to these resources and additional helpful Internet resources related to this chapter, visit thePoint. at http://thePoint.lww.com/Miller6e.

Interpreter Services

National Standards for Culturally and Linguistically Appropriate Services (CLAS)

Cultural Diversity and Health Disparities of Many Groups

AARP, Office of Diversity and Inclusion
American Society on Aging, Network of Multicultural Aging (NOMA), and Serving Elders of Color (SEOC)
Office of Minority Health, U.S. Department of Health and Human Services

Racial and Ethnic Groups

(Chapter 5 lists resources on culturally specific health education materials)
National Asian Pacific Center on Aging
National Caucus and Center on Black Aged
National Hispanic Council on Aging
National Indian Council on Aging

Other Diverse Groups

LGBT Movement Advancement Project
National Gay and Lesbian Task Force
National Rural Health Association
Old Lesbians Organizing for Change (OLOC)
Prime Timers Worldwide
Rural Assistance Center
Services and Advocacy for Gay, Lesbian, Bisexual & Transgender Elders (SAGE)

REFERENCES

Administration on Aging. (2009a). *A statistical profile of Asian older Americans aged 65 and older*. Retrieved from http://aoa.gov/AoARoot/Aging_Statistics/minority_aging/Facts-on-API-Elderly.

Administration on Aging. (2009b). *A statistical profile of American Indian and Native Alaskan elderly*. Retrieved from http://aoa.gov/AoARoot/Aging_Statistics/minority_aging/Facts-on-AINA-Elderly.

Administration on Aging. (2010a). *A statistical profile of Black older Americans aged 65+*. Retrieved from http://aoa.gov/AoARoot/Aging_Statistics/minority_aging/Facts-on-Black-Elderly.

Administration on Aging. (2010b). *A statistical profile of Hispanic older Americans aged 65+*. Retrieved from http://aoa.gov/AoARoot/Aging_Statistics/minority_aging/Facts-on-Hispanic-Elderly.

American Geriatrics Society. (2006). *Position statement on ethnogeriatrics*. Retrieved from http://mericangeriatrics.org/Products/Positionpapers/ethno_committeePF.shtml.

Andrews, M. M. (2008a). Culturally competent nursing care. In M. M. Andrews & J. S. Boyle (Eds.), *Transcultural concepts in nursing care* (5th ed., pp. 15–33). Philadelphia, PA: Lippincott Williams & Wilkins.

Andrews, M. M. (2008b). The influence of cultural and health belief systems on health care practices. In M. M. Andrews & J. S. Boyle (Eds.), *Transcultural concepts in nursing care* (pp. 66–81). Philadelphia, PA: Lippincott Williams & Wilkins.

Andrews, M. M., & Boyle, J. S. (2008). *Transcultural concepts in nursing care* (5th ed.). Philadelphia, PA: Lippincott Williams & Wilkins.

Barnes, P. M., Adams, P. F., & Powell-Griner, E. (2010). *National characteristics of the American Indian or Alaska Native adult population: United States, 2004–2008.* Washington, DC: U.S. Department of Health and Human Services.

Beck, S. L., Towsley, G. L., Caserta, M. S., Lindau, K., & Dudley, W. N. (2009). Symptom experiences and quality of life of rural and urban older adult cancer survivors. *Cancer Nursing, 32*(5), 359–369.

Biello, K. B., Rawlings, J., Carroll-Scott, A., Browne, R., & Ickovics, J. R. (2010). Racial disparities in age at preventable hospitalization among U.S. adults. *American Journal of Preventative Medicine, 38*(1), 54–60.

Cordasco, K. M., Asch, S. M., Franco, I., & Mangione, C. M. (2009). Health literacy and English language comprehension among elderly inpatients at an urban safety-net hospital. *Journal of Health and Human Services Administration, 32*(1), 30–50.

Diddle, G., & Denham, S. A. (2010). Spirituality and its relationships with the health and illness of Appalachian people. *Journal of Transcultural Nursing, 2*(2), 17–12.

Engebretson, J. C., & Headley, J. A. (2009). Cultural diversity and care. In B. M. Dossey, L. Keegan, & C. E. Guzetta (Eds.), *Holistic nursing: A handbook for practice* (5th ed., pp. 573–597). Boston, MA: Jones and Bartlett.

Enslein, J., Tripp-Reimer, T., Kelley, L. S., Choi, E., & McCarty, L. (2002). Interpreter facilitation for individuals with limited English proficiency. *Journal of Gerontological Nursing, 28*(7), 5–11.

Goldberg, N. G. (2009). *The impact of inequality for same-sex partners in employer-sponsored retirement plans.* Los Angeles, CA: University of California School of Law, The Williams Institute.

Grant, J. M. (2010). *Outing age: Public policy issues affecting lesbian, gay, bisexual and transgender elders.* Washington, DC: National Gay and Lesbian Task Force.

Grieco, E. M. (2010). *The American Community Survey Reports: Race and Hispanic Origin of the Foreign-Born Population in the U.S.: 2007.* Washington, DC: U.S. Department of Commerce.

Hutchins, S. S., Fiscella, K., Levine, R. S., Ompad, D. C., & McDonald, M. (2009). Protection of racial/ethnic minority populations during an influenza pandemic. *American Journal of Public Health 100*(Suppl. 2), S261–S270.

Jernigan, V. B., Duran, B., Ahn, D., & Winkleby, M. (2010). Changing patterns in health behaviors and risk factors related to cardiovascular disease among American Indians and Alaska Natives. *American Journal of Public Health, 100,* 677–683.

Jones, A. L., Sonnenfeld, N. L., & Harris-Kojetin, L. D. (2009). *Racial differences in functioning among elderly nursing home residents, 2004.* Washington, DC: U.S. Department of Health and Human Services.

Jones, C. A., Kandel, W., & Parker, T. (2007). Population dynamics are changing the profile of rural areas. *Amber Waves, 5*(2), 31–35.

Joyce, D. P., & Limbos, M. (2009). Identification of cognitive impairment and mental illness in elderly homeless men. *Canadian Family Physician, 55,* 1110–1117.

LGBT Movement Advancement Project. (2010). *Improving the lives of LGBT older adults.* Denver, CO: LGBT Movement Advancement Project.

Li, Y., & Mukamel, D. B. (2010). Racial disparities in receipt of influenza and pneumococcal vaccinations among US nursing-home residents. *American Journal of Public Health, 100*(1), S256–S262.

Lipson, J. G., & Dibble, S. L. (2005). *Culture & clinical care.* San Francisco, CA: University of California Nursing Press.

Logan, J. L. (2009). Disparities in influenza immunization among US adults. *Journal of the National Medical Association, 101*(2), 161–166.

Maddalena, V. (2009). Cultural competence and holistic practice, implications for nursing education practice and research. *Holistic Nursing Practice, 23*(3), 153–157.

Mariano, C. (2009). Holistic nursing: Scope and standards of practice. In B. M. Dossey, L. Keegan, & C. E. Guzetta (Eds.), *Holistic nursing: A handbook for practice* (5th ed., pp. 47–68). Boston, MA: Jones and Bartlett.

Moy, K. L., Sallis, J. F., & David, K. J. (2010). Health indicators of native Hawaiian and Pacific Islanders in the United States. *Journal of Community Health, 35,* 81–92.

NACRHHS (National Advisory Committee on Rural Health and Human Services). (2008, April). *The 2008 Report to the secretary: Rural health and human services issues.* Retrieved from http://ruralcommittee.hrsa.gov.

Office of Minority Health and Disparities. (2010). *Highlights in Minority Health & Health Disparities.* Retrieved from http:www.cdc.gov/omhd/Highlights/Highlight.htm.

Orsi, J. M., Margellos-Anast, H., & Whitman, S. (2010). Black-white health disparities in the United States and Chicago: A 15-year progress analysis. *American Journal of Public Health, 100*(2), 349–356.

Park, C. B., Braun, K. L., Horiuchi, B. Y., Tottori, C., & Onaka, A. T. (2009). Longevity disparities in multiethnic Hawaii: An analysis of 2000 life tables. *Public Health Reports, 124*(4), 579–584.

Purnell, L. D. (2009). *Guide to culturally competent health care* (2nd ed.). Philadelphia, PA: F. A. Davis Co.

Purnell, L. D., & Paulanka, B. J. (2008). *Transcultural health care: A culturally competent approach* (2nd ed.). Philadelphia, PA: F. A. Davis Co.

Savoca, M. R., Arcury, T. A., Leng, X., Bell, R. A., Chen, H., Anderson, A., . . . Quandt, S. A. (2009). The diet quality of rural older adults in the South as measured by Healthy Eating Index-2005 varies by ethnicity. *Journal of the American Dietetic Association, 109*(12), 2063–2067.

Sloan, F. A., Ayyagari, P., Salm, M., & Grossman, D. (2009). The longevity gap between black and white men in the United States at the beginning and end of the 20th century. *American Journal of Public Health, 100*(2), 357–363.

Sorkin, D. H., Ngo-Metzger, Q., & De Alba, I. (2010). Racial/ethnic discrimination in health care: Impact on perceived quality of care. *Journal of General Internal Medicine, 25,* 390–396.

Tompsett, C. J., Fowler, P. J., & Toro, P. A. (2009). Age differences among homeless individuals: adolescence through adulthood. *Journal of Prevention and Intervention in the Community, 37*(2), 86–99.

Tucker, K. L., Mattei, J., Noel, S. E., Collado, B. M., Mendez, J., Nelson, J., . . . Falcon, L. M. (2010). The Boston Puerto Rican Health Study, a longitudinal cohort study on health disparities in Puerto Rican adults: Challenges and opportunities. *BMC Public Health,* doi:10.1186/1471-2458-10-107.

U.S. Census Bureau. (2007a). *The American community—American Indians and Alaska Natives.* Washington, DC: U.S. Department of Commerce.

U.S. Census Bureau. (2007b). *The American community—Hispanics: 2004.* Washington, DC: U.S. Department of Commerce.

U.S. Census Bureau. (2007c). *The American community—Pacific Islanders: 2004.* Washington, DC: U.S. Department of Commerce.

U.S. Census Bureau. (2008). *U.S. Population Projections: National Population Projections.* Retrieved from http://www.census.gov/population/projections/downloadablefiles.html.

U.S. Census Bureau. (2009a). *Facts for features: Black (African-American) history month: February 2010 (CB10 FF.01).* Washington, DC: U.S. Department of Commerce.

U.S. Census Bureau. (2009b). *Facts for features: American Indian and Alaska Native heritage month: November 2009 (CB09-FF.20).* Washington, DC: U.S. Department of Commerce.

U.S. Census Bureau. (2010). *Facts for features: Asian/Pacific American heritage month: May 2010 (CB10-FF.07).* Washington, DC: U.S. Department of Commerce.

U.S. Department of Health and Human Services. (2010). *National healthcare disparities report.* Rockville, MD: Agency for Healthcare Research and Quality. AHRQ Publication No. 10–004.

Vaughn, L. M. (2009). Families and cultural competency, Where are we? *Family and Community Health, 32*(3), 247–256.

CHAPTER 3

Applying a Nursing Model for Promoting Wellness in Older Adults

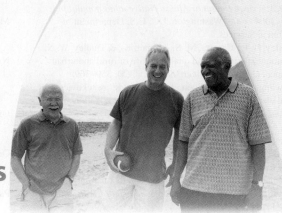

LEARNING OBJECTIVES

After reading this chapter, you will be able to:

1. Discuss the concepts that underpin the Functional Consequences Theory in older adults.

2. Define concepts of age-related changes, risk factors, and functional consequences as they relate to nursing care of older adults.

3. Describe the domains of nursing (i.e., person, nursing, health, environment) in the context of the Functional Consequences Theory.

4. Apply the Functional Consequences Theory to the practice of nursing to promote wellness in older adults.

KEY POINTS

age-related changes

environment

functional consequences

Functional Consequences
   Theory for Promoting
   Wellness in Older Adults

health

nursing

older adult

person

risk factors

wellness outcomes

A s discussed in Chapter 1, myths about aging are insidious and pervasive in society and form the foundation of ageism, which has serious detrimental effects on **older adults.** Nurses are influenced not only by societal myths and ageist attitudes but also by their experiences with older adults in health care settings, which often reinforce the perception that older adults are frail, confused, depressed, and dependent. These attitudes can lead to a sense of pessimism—or even hopelessness—regarding caring for older adults. Fortunately, knowledge can be an effective antidote to ageism, and the theoretical base of information about aging has expanded exponentially during the past half-century (as discussed in

Chapter 4). Research-based information enables health care providers to differentiate between **age-related changes** that are inevitable and **risk factors** that can be addressed or even prevented. Chapters in this text provide research-based information about age-related changes and risk factors affecting a particular aspect of functioning, with emphasis on the changes and factors that nurses can address. Nurses can apply this information to help older adults identify ways of improving functioning and quality of life.

Theories about aging and older adults attempt to answer questions about why and how people age, and they provide a base for identifying the risk factors that health care providers can address. However, they do not address *nursing* care of older adults, as does a nursing theory that explains relationships among the core concepts of **person, nursing, health**, and **environment**. Nurses need discipline-specific nursing theories if they are to enhance health and quality of life when they care for patients (Cody, 2009). The **Functionsal Consequences Theory for Promoting Wellness in Older Adults**, which is delineated in this chapter and used throughout this text, is a theoretical approach that focuses on the role of nurses enhancing health, functioning, and quality of life for older adults.

A NURSING THEORY FOR WELLNESS-FOCUSED CARE OF OLDER ADULTS

During the 1980s, this author proposed a model for gerontological nursing, which was the organizational framework for the first edition of this book (Miller, 1990). Since its inception, this model has emphasized the significant role of nurses in using health education interventions to promote optimal health, functioning, and quality of life for older adults. In the fifth and sixth editions, some terminology has been revised to reflect current emphasis on adding life to years in conjunction with adding years to life. Thus, the model is now called the Functional Consequences Theory for Promoting Wellness in Older Adults. In addition, the revised model reflects and incorporates the increased understanding of wellness that is evolving as an integral aspect of health care. Nurses can apply this model in any situation in which a goal of nursing care is to promote wellness for older adults. The theory was developed to explain questions, such as *"What is unique about promoting wellness for older adults?"* and *"How can nurses address unique wellness needs of older adults?"*

The purpose of nursing theories is to describe, explain, predict, or prescribe nursing care based on scientific evidence. Since the time of Florence Nightingale, nurses have developed theories that address the relationships among the domains of person, nursing, health, and environment. In recent years, nursing theories are increasingly focusing on models that connect the work of theorists, researchers, and practitioners (Marrs & Lowry, 2009). The Functional Consequences Theory is based on a combination of research on aging and health and the author's four decades of providing nursing care for older adults. It also draws on theories that emphasize concepts related to wellness, health promotion, and holistic nursing. When it is applied in this text to specific aspects of functioning, it incorporates the currently available evidence-based practice. Thus, nurses can use this theory as a framework for promoting wellness in older adults because it provides evidence-based information about factors that affect health and quality of life for older adults.

Basic premises of the Functional Consequences Theory are as follows:

- Holistic nursing care addresses the body–mind–spirit interconnectedness of each older adult and recognizes that wellness encompasses more than physiologic functioning.
- Although age-related changes are inevitable, most problems affecting older adults are caused by risk factors.
- Older adults experience positive or negative **functional consequences** because of a combination of age-related changes and additional risk factors.
- Interventions can be directed toward alleviating or modifying the negative functional consequences of risk factors.
- Nurses can promote wellness in older adults through health promotion interventions and other nursing actions that address the negative functional consequences.
- Nursing interventions result in positive functional consequences, also called **wellness outcomes**, which enable older people to function at their highest level despite the presence of age-related changes and risk factors.

This theoretical framework, shown in Figure 3-1, can be illustrated by the following example. Because of age-related visual changes, older adults experience an increased sensitivity to glare and have difficulty seeing clearly when they face bright lights or when lights reflect off shiny surfaces. For instance, it is difficult to see clearly when driving toward the sunlight or reading shopping mall maps that are enclosed in glass cases. In addition to this age-related change, older adults are likely to have disease-related conditions, such as cataracts, that further interfere with their visual abilities. In addition, environmental factors, such as bright lights, highly polished floors, and white or glossy paint, can intensify glare. These age-related changes and risk factors can interfere with

vision to the extent that older adults stop performing activities or perform them unsafely. To counteract these functional consequences, the older person or a nurse can initiate any of the following interventions, which are discussed in Chapter 17:

- Wearing sunglasses and using glare-reducing glasses (self-care)
- Addressing environmental conditions by using adequate nonglare lighting (self-care)
- Obtaining periodic evaluations from an ophthalmologist (self-care)
- Teaching about the use of sunglasses and glare-reducing glasses (nursing action)
- Teaching about environmental modifications (nursing action)
- Taking actions to avoid glare (e.g., not standing in front of a bright window when talking with an older adult) (nursing action)
- Teaching older adults about the importance of having their eyes evaluated at least annually for treatable conditions (nursing action)

Wellness outcomes resulting from these interventions include improved safety, function, and quality of life.

CONCEPTS UNDERLYING THE FUNCTIONAL CONSEQUENCES THEORY

The Functional Consequences Theory draws from theories that are pertinent to aging, older adults, and holistic nursing. The nursing domain concepts of person, environment, health, and nursing are linked together specifically in relation to older adults. Before discussing these domain concepts, however, the concepts of functional consequences, age-related changes, and risk factors are explained. Box 3-1 summarizes the key concepts in the Functional Consequences Theory for Promoting Wellness in Older Adults.

Functional Consequences

Functional consequences are the observable effects of actions, risk factors, and age-related changes that influence the quality of life or day-to-day activities of older adults. Actions include, but are not limited to, purposeful interventions initiated by either older adults or nurses and other caregivers. Risk factors can originate in the environment or arise from physiologic and psychosocial influences. Functional consequences are negative when they interfere with a person's level of function or quality of life or increase a person's dependency. Conversely, they are positive when they facilitate the highest level of performance and the least amount of dependency.

Negative functional consequences typically occur because of a combination of age-related changes and risk factors, as illustrated in the example of impaired visual performance. They also may be caused by interventions, in which case the interventions become risk factors. For example, constipation resulting from the use of an analgesic medication is an

A Nursing Model for Promoting Wellness in Older Adults

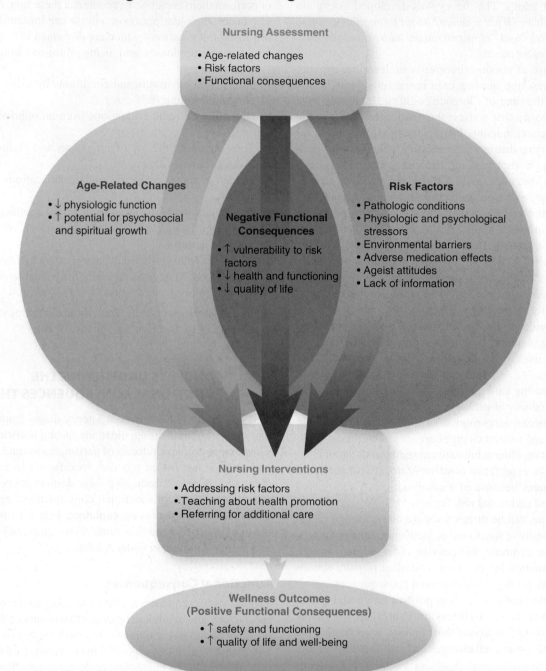

Nursing Assessment

- Age-related changes
- Risk factors
- Functional consequences

Age-Related Changes

- ↓ physiologic function
- ↑ potential for psychosocial and spiritual growth

Negative Functional Consequences

- ↑ vulnerability to risk factors
- ↓ health and functioning
- ↓ quality of life

Risk Factors

- Pathologic conditions
- Physiologic and psychological stressors
- Environmental barriers
- Adverse medication effects
- Ageist attitudes
- Lack of information

Nursing Interventions

- Addressing risk factors
- Teaching about health promotion
- Referring for additional care

Wellness Outcomes (Positive Functional Consequences)

- ↑ safety and functioning
- ↑ quality of life and well-being

FIGURE 3-1 The Functional Consequences Theory for Promoting Wellness in Older Adults. Age-related changes and risk factors combine to cause negative functional consequences. Nurses holistically assess older adults and initiate interventions to counteract or minimize negative functional consequences. Nursing actions result in wellness outcomes.

example of a negative functional consequence caused by an intervention. In this case, the medication is both an intervention for pain and a risk factor for impaired bowel function.

Positive functional consequences can result from automatic actions or purposeful interventions. Often, older adults bring about positive functional consequences when they compensate for age-related changes with or without conscious intent. For example, an older person might increase the amount of light for reading or begin using sunglasses without realizing that these actions are compensating for age-related changes. At other times, older adults initiate interventions in response to a recognized need. In the example cited earlier, improved function would likely result from purposeful interventions, such as cataract surgery or environmental modifications. In a few instances, positive functional consequences are caused directly by age-related changes.

Box 3-1 Concepts in the Functional Consequences Theory for Promoting Wellness in Older Adults

Functional Consequences: Observable effects of actions, risk factors, and age-related changes that influence the quality of life or day-to-day activities of older adults. The effects relate to all levels of functioning, including body, mind, and spirit.
- **Negative Functional Consequences:** Those that interfere with the older adult's functioning or quality of life.
- **Positive Functional Consequences:** Those that facilitate the highest level of functioning, the least dependency, and the best quality of life. When positive functional consequences are the result of nursing interventions, they are called **Wellness Outcomes.**

Age-Related Changes: Inevitable, progressive, and irreversible changes that occur during later adulthood and are independent of extrinsic or pathologic conditions. On the physiologic level, these changes are typically degenerative; however, on psychological and spiritual levels, they include potential for growth.

Risk Factors: Conditions that increase the vulnerability of older adults to negative functional consequences. Common sources of risk factors include diseases, environment, lifestyle, support systems, psychosocial circumstances, adverse medication effects, and attitudes based on lack of knowledge.

Older Adult (Person): A complex and unique individual whose functioning and well-being are influenced by the acquisition of age-related changes and risk factors. When risk factors cause the older adult to be dependent on others for daily needs, their caregivers are considered an integral focus of nursing care.

Nursing: The focus of nursing care is to minimize the negative effects of age-related changes and risk factors and to promote wellness outcomes. Goals are achieved through the nursing process, with particular emphasis on health promotion and other nursing interventions that address the negative functional consequences.

Health: The ability of older adults to function at their highest capacity, despite the presence of age-related changes and risk factors. It is not limited to physiologic function and encompasses psychosocial and spiritual function. Thus, it addresses well-being and quality of life as defined by each older adult.

Environment: External conditions, including caregivers, that influence the body, mind, spirit, and functioning of older adults. Environmental conditions are risk factors when they interfere with function, and they are interventions when they enhance function.

For example, a woman may view the postmenopausal inability to become pregnant as a positive effect of aging. Consequently, sexual relationships may become more satisfying in later adulthood. Similarly, positive functional consequences, such as increased wisdom and maturity, can result from psychological growth in older adulthood. In the context of the nursing process, positive functional consequences are called wellness outcomes because they result from purposeful nursing interventions.

The concept of functional consequences draws on concepts and research regarding functional assessment, which focuses on a person's ability to perform activities of daily living that affect survival and quality of life, as discussed in Chapter 7. From a research perspective, functional assessment provides a framework for research and a method for planning health services for dependent people. From a clinical perspective, health care practitioners view the multidimensional functional assessment as an important component in the care of older people. Evidence-based tools are widely available for assessing specific aspects of functioning and activities of daily living, and there is strong support for using these tools in clinical settings. Nurses can find many standardized, easy-to-use, and up-to-date assessment tools identified as *Best Practices in Care for Older Adults* at the Web site for the Hartford Institute for Geriatric Nursing (http://consultgerirn.org). In addition, many standardized tools are included in the chapters of this book and are cited in the "Resources" sections at the end of chapters available in the Resources provided on thePoint.

Although the Functional Consequences Theory draws on concepts related to functional assessment, its scope is much broader. The Functional Consequences Theory differs from functional assessment in the following ways:

- It distinguishes between age-related changes that increase a person's vulnerability and risk factors that affect function and quality of life.
- It focuses on functional consequences that can be addressed through nursing interventions.
- It focuses on assessment of conditions that affect functioning, rather than simply identifying a person's functional level.
- It leads to interventions that address negative functional consequences.
- It leads to wellness outcomes, such as improved functioning and quality of life.

Age-Related Changes and Risk Factors

A unique challenge of caring for older adults is the need to differentiate between age-related changes and risk factors, because the interventions for age-related changes differ from those for risk factors. Age-related changes cannot be reversed or altered, but it is possible to compensate for their effects so that wellness outcomes are achieved. By contrast, risk factors can be modified or eliminated to improve functioning and quality of life for older adults.

In the Functional Consequences Theory, age-related changes are the inherent physiologic processes that increase the vulnerability of older people to the detrimental effects of risk factors. From a body–mind–spirit perspective, however, age-related changes are not limited to physiologic aspects but include potential for increased cognitive, emotional, and spiritual development. Thus, nurses holistically focus on the whole person by identifying age-related changes that can be strengthened to improve the older adult's ability to adapt to physiologic decline. For example, nurses can work with older adults to strengthen their coping skills, as discussed in

Chapter 12. In addition, nurses have many opportunities to build on the wisdom of older adults, especially their "everyday problem-solving" skills (as discussed in Chapter 11) by teaching about interventions to address risk factors.

The definition of age-related changes in the context of the Functional Consequences Theory draws primarily on research on aging. Biologic theories can help differentiate between age-related and disease-related processes; usually, however, there is some overlap among these processes as discussed in Chapter 4. In addition to biologic theories of aging, other theories about aging and older adulthood can shed light on age-related changes that contribute to the ability of older adults to respond to the challenges of aging. Chapters in Parts 3 and 4 of this book discuss research on age-related changes pertinent to specific aspects of functioning.

Risk factors are the conditions that are likely to occur in older adults and have a significant detrimental effect on their health and functioning. Risk factors commonly arise from environments, acute and chronic conditions, psychosocial conditions, or adverse medication effects. Although many risk factors also occur in younger adults, they are more likely to have serious functional consequences in older adults because of the following characteristics:

- They are cumulative and progressive (e.g., long-term effects of smoking, obesity, inadequate exercise, or poor dietary habits).
- The effects are exacerbated by age-related changes (e.g., effects of arthritis are exacerbated by diminished muscle strength).
- The effects may be mistakenly viewed as age-related changes rather than reversible and treatable conditions (e.g., mental changes from adverse medication effects may be attributed to normal aging or dementia).
- They would not have negative functional consequences in a younger person (e.g., glare or background noise would not affect the vision or hearing of someone who is not experiencing age-related sensory changes).

Researchers and health care providers commonly address risk factors in relation to prevention and treatment of medical conditions. For example, evidence-based practice emphasizes weighing the probable risks versus benefits for pharmacologic or surgical treatments. Similarly, researchers are focusing on identifying factors that increase the chance of developing conditions, such as heart disease, so these risks can be addressed through health promotion interventions.

Nurses incorporate the concept of risk factors in many aspects of the nursing process. For example, many nursing diagnoses, interventions, and outcomes address risk control, risk identification, or risk detection. In particular, nurses identify risk factors that they can address through health promotion interventions. For example, from a holistic perspective, nurses routinely assess for risks associated with stress, smoking, obesity, poor nutrition, and inadequate physical activity. A unique aspect of caring for older adults is the need to assess for risk factors associated with myths or ageist attitudes that can affect interventions. For example, if urinary incontinence is mistakenly attributed to "normal" aging, then the older adult will not receive appropriate evaluation and interventions. Environmental risks are also particularly pertinent to older adults because additional risk factors, such as sensory, mobility, or cognitive impairments, can compromise their safety and functioning. Risk factors are a major focus of the Functional Consequences Theory because nurses have numerous opportunities for promoting wellness by identifying and addressing the many modifiable factors that affect functioning and quality of life for older adults.

Person

In the Functional Consequences Theory, the concept of **person** applies specifically to older adults. Because the holistic approach of the theory views each **older adult** as a complex and unique individual whose functioning and well-being is influenced by many internal and external factors, older adults are not defined simply according to chronologic criteria. From this perspective, an older adult is characterized by the acquisition of physiologic and psychosocial characteristics that are associated with increasing maturity. Physiologic characteristics include slowing down of physiologic processes, compromised ability to respond to physiologic stress, and increased vulnerability to pathologic conditions and other risk factors. Psychosocial characteristics include an increased potential for psychosocial strengths, such as wisdom and creativity, and the potential for advanced levels of personal and spiritual growth.

Because aging is a complex and gradual process involving all aspects of body, mind, and spirit, a person does not suddenly become an older adult at a particular chronologic age. Rather, people who live long enough recognize at some point that they have reached a stage of life that society categorizes as older adulthood. When they reach this point, they may or may not identify with social labels, such as elder, senior, or older adult. Although this concept has the distinct disadvantage of being difficult to measure, it has the advantage of accurately reflecting the realities of older adulthood as a continuum within the life-course continuum. Because people become more heterogeneous rather than homogeneous as they age, any definition of the older adult must, by its nature, be broad. In the context of the Functional Consequences

Theory, an individual is an older adult when he or she manifests several or many functional consequences attributable to age-related changes alone or to age-related changes in combination with risk factors. Stated simply, the accumulation of age-related functional consequences defines someone as an older adult. Moreover, because aging involves many gradual, interacting, and cumulative processes, each older adult experiences his or her own unique continuum. This concept is applied in the progressive case examples in chapters of Parts 3 and 4 of this book, which illustrate the progression of one person from young–old to old–old as he or she is affected by functional consequences pertinent to a particular aspect of functioning.

The older adult is further conceptualized in the context of his or her relationships with others because a person is not an isolated entity but a dynamic being who continually influences and is influenced by the environment and other people. This context is particularly important for older adults, because the more functionally impaired a person is, the more important are support resources and environmental factors. When functional consequences accumulate to the extent that the older adult is very dependent on others for daily needs, nurses shift their primary focus to working with caregivers to identify and implement interventions. Even for older adults who do not rely on others for assistance, this context is important because older people have a long history of interpersonal relationships that influence their health behaviors and well-being. Thus, nurses assess and address the needs of older adults in the context of their relationships.

Although no characteristics apply universally to all older adults, the cumulative effects of aging affect them all and they are all vulnerable to the effects of risk factors. Nurses need to be knowledgeable about the facts and myths about normal aging so that they can implement interventions to address negative functional consequences. Moreover, nurses need to assess each older adult's unique response to the effects of aging and risk factors to implement appropriate interventions to improve function and quality of life. The Functional Consequences Theory emphasizes the importance of identifying and respecting the unique characteristics of each older adult that affect his or her functioning and well-being. This viewpoint is consistent with nursing theories that focus on the need to relate to patients in the context of their unique lived experiences, rather than simply as members of a cultural group (Doane & Varcoe, 2009).

Nursing

The conceptualization of **nursing** in the Functional Consequences Theory draws on many nursing theorists, including the following examples (McEwen & Wills, 2007; Meleis, 2007):

- *Florence Nightingale*: Nurses foster an environment conducive to healing and health promotion.
- *Virginia Henderson*: Nurses provide assistance with daily activities to help gain independence as rapidly as possible.
- *Modeling and Role-Modeling Theory*: Nursing is an interactive, interpersonal process that nurtures strengths to achieve a state of perceived holistic health.
- *Imogene King*: Nurse and client interact to achieve a specific health-related goal.
- *Jean Watson*: Nursing consists of knowledge, thought, values, philosophy, commitment, and action with passion in human care transactions.
- *Martha Rogers*: Nurses promote person–environment interactions for unitary human beings.
- *Margaret Newman*: Nursing is the act of assisting people to use their power to evolve toward higher levels of consciousness.

In addition to drawing on many nursing theories, the concept of nursing in the Functional Consequences Theory is consistent with the American Nurses Association statement on the scope of gerontological nursing, as discussed in Chapter 5.

Health

The Functional Consequences Theory defines **health** as the ability of older adults to function at their highest capacity, despite the presence of age-related changes and risk factors. It encompasses psychosocial as well as physiologic function, including well-being and quality of life as defined by each older adult. In this model, health is individually determined, based on the functional capacities that are perceived as important by that person. For example, one person might define the desired level of function as a capacity for intimate relationships, whereas another might define it as being able to perform aerobic exercise for half an hour daily. Wellness is a closely related concept (defined in Chapter 1) that is used throughout this book in reference to outcomes that address the person's highest potential for well-being.

Some definitions of health that support the conceptualization of health in the Functional Consequences Theory follow (McEwen & Wills, 2007):

- *Florence Nightingale*: to be well, but to be able to use well every power we have
- *Imogene King*: a dynamic life experience involving continuous adjustment to stressors through optimum use of one's resources to achieve maximum potential for daily living
- *Calista Roy*: a state and process of being and becoming integrated and whole
- *Jean Watson*: unity and harmony within the mind, body, and soul; congruence between the self as perceived and the self as experienced
- *Margaret Newman*: expanding consciousness; evolving pattern of the whole of life
- *Rosemarie Parse*: a way of being in the world; the living of day-to-day ways of being
- *Madeleine Leininger*: a state of well-being that is culturally constituted, defined, valued, and practiced by individuals or groups that enables them to function in their daily lives.

Since the 1990s, nurse theorists have been emphasizing the importance of quality of life as a nursing outcome in conjunction with health (DeKeyser & Medoff-Cooper, 2009).

Environment

In the Functional Consequences Theory, environment is a broad concept that includes all aspects of the setting in which the care is provided; for dependent older adults, the environment also includes their caregivers. Some aspects of the conceptualization may seem to be contradictory because the environment can be a source of both negative functional consequences and wellness outcomes. For example, the environment is a risk factor when it interferes with functioning (e.g., glare or poor lighting), but it also can facilitate wellness outcomes when it is used to improve functioning (e.g., grab bars, or bright and nonglare lighting).

The following are some definitions of environment from nursing theories that are pertinent to the Functional Consequences Theory (McEwen & Wills, 2007):

- *Florence Nightingale*: a healthy environment is essential for healing and includes specific aspects such as noise level, cleanliness, and nutritious food.
- *Madeleine Leininger*: the totality of an event, situation, or particular experience that gives meaning to human expressions, interpretations, and social interactions in particular physical, ecologic, sociopolitical, and cultural settings
- *Imogene King*: the background for human interactions, which is both internal and external to the individual
- *Margaret Newman*: all internal and external factors of influences that surround the client or system
- *Calista Roy*: all conditions, circumstances, and influences that surround and affect the development and behavior of humans.

Since the 1970s, gerontologists have studied the influence of the environment on functioning of older adults. For example, the Person-Environment Fit Theory (discussed in Chapter 4) focuses on the interrelationship between the individual person and his or her environment. Gerontologists have used this theory to study the effects of home and neighborhood on many aspects of functioning and quality of life for older adults (Beard et al., 2008; Wahl, Fange, Oswald, Gitlin, & Iwarsson, 2009). Nurses have applied this theory to research related to falls in nursing homes (Hill et al., 2009). Some of the questions that are addressed by gerontologists as well as nurses are as follows:

- How does the environment affect the older adult's level of functioning?
- How does the environment affect the older adult's quality of life?
- Is the environment comfortable for the older adult?
- Is the environment a source of risks that interfere with functioning and well-being of the older adults (e.g., does it increase the risk for falls?)?
- How can the environment be adapted to improve functioning for the older adult?

A Student's Perspective

Today I cared for L.C., who has had two previous cerebrovascular accidents, with the second one leading to left-sided hemiplegia. As I was caring for her, I noticed a few things in her room that may have significance for her. First, I noted that she had poles both by her bed and in the bathroom; both were bolted to the ceiling and the floor. These poles made it easier for L.C. to stand on her own with little assistance from anyone else. I feel that these make her more independent and help her use the strong side of her body. L.C. also had a divided box, with different kinds of tea in each section. I feel that this is significant to her because she is able to have the type of tea she likes whenever she wants it. It allows her to make choices each day and provides one of the comforts of "home." A third item was a triangle pillow that she sleeps on rather than a regular one. This is significant because it allows her to breathe better in the night or whenever she is sleeping. Because L.C. has chronic obstructive pulmonary disease, it is hard for her to breathe.

Kelly Z.

Throughout this text, the Functional Consequences Theory provides a framework for addressing questions such as these as an integral part of the nursing assessment and interventions for specific aspects of functioning.

APPLYING THE THEORY TO PROMOTE WELLNESS IN OLDER ADULTS

In the context of the Functional Consequences Theory, nurses direct their care toward addressing risk factors and promoting wellness outcomes for older adults. The focus and goals of this type of care vary in different settings. For acute care, the focus is on treatment of pathologic conditions that create serious risks; goals include helping vulnerable older adults recover from illness and maintain or improve their level of functioning. For long-term care, the focus is on addressing multiple risk factors that interfere with functional abilities; goals include improved functioning and quality of life. For home and community settings, the focus is on short- and long-term interventions aimed at age-related changes and risk factors; goals include improving or preventing declines in functioning and addressing quality-of-life concerns. In all settings, nurses can incorporate wellness outcomes to address each older adult's personal aspirations toward well-being of body, mind, and spirit.

Nurses apply the nursing process to assess age-related changes and risk factors, identify nursing diagnoses, plan wellness outcomes, implement nursing interventions to achieve wellness outcomes, and evaluate the effectiveness of their interventions. A major focus of nursing care is on educating older adults and the caregivers of dependent older adults about interventions that will eliminate risk factors or minimize their effects. The educational aspects are particularly important when older adults are influenced by myths and misunderstandings about age-related changes. For example, nurses can provide information about the difference between normal aging changes and risk factors to an older person who believes that functional impairments are a necessary consequence of old age and identify ways of minimizing the effects of risk factors and compensating for the effects of age-related changes.

Nurses have developed a middle-range theory for fostering generative quality of life for the elderly that is pertinent to the concepts in the Functional Consequences Theory. According to this model, nurses direct their care toward establishing "patient-centered connections that would result in generative elders who would seek to establish or sustain a variety of connections in response to the forces and processes they encounter on a daily basis" (Register & Herman, 2006, p. 347). Register and Herman suggest the following examples of generative nursing interventions, which are based on this model, to address specific aspects of quality of life for older adults:

- *Metaphysical connectedness*: teaching about guided imagery, journaling activities, and activities that increase self-esteem and a sense of optimism
- *Spiritual connectedness*: arranging transportation to local church services or making referrals to faith-based groups
- *Biologic connectedness*: facilitating participation in congregate meals, doing group exercises to music
- *Connectedness to others*: providing comfort touch, encouraging participation in social and educational activities
- *Environmental connectedness*: encouraging and facilitating activities in nature, referring for transportation resources
- *Connectedness to society*: providing information about support resources, helping older adults develop contingency plans for emergencies.

Providing nursing care for older adults is both challenging and rewarding, despite the common perception that it is futile and discouraging. Although nursing care of older adults is often associated with limited goals, a holistic perspective focuses on the potential of every person to experience wellness by achieving higher levels of psychological or spiritual functioning. Even older adults who have dementia, and other progressive conditions that can profoundly affect psychological function, may have potential for spiritual growth in ways that are not always observable or measurable.

The Functional Consequences Theory helps nurses see older adults as more than an accumulation of age-related physiologic changes and pathologic conditions leading to diminished functioning. Thus, it provides a framework for promoting wellness because it addresses the whole-person needs of the older adult and his or her relationships with self, others, and the environment. It reminds nurses to identify strengths and potentials in relation not only to physical aspects of functioning but also to psychological and spiritual well-being. Moreover, it leads to nursing interventions directed toward achieving wellness outcomes, such as improved quality of life for older adults.

Chapter Highlights

A Nursing Theory for Wellness-Focused Care of Older Adults
- The Functional Consequences Theory explains the unique relationships among the concepts of person, health, nursing, and environment in the context of promoting wellness for older adults.

Concepts Underlying the Functional Consequences Theory
- Combinations of age-related changes and risk factors increase the vulnerability of older people to negative functional consequences, which interfere with the person's level of functioning or quality of life.
- Nurses assess the age-related changes, risk factors, and functional consequences, with particular emphasis on identifying the factors that can be addressed through nursing interventions.
- Wellness outcomes enable older adults to function at their highest level despite the presence of age-related changes and risk factors.

Applying the Theory to Promote Wellness in Older Adults
- Nurses can incorporate wellness outcomes to address each older adult's personal aspirations for well-being of body, mind, and spirit.
- Nurses educate older adults and caregivers about interventions to minimize risk factors or their effects.
- Providing nursing care for older adults is rewarding when approached from a holistic perspective that sees opportunities for wellness in physical, psychological, and spiritual aspects of function.

Critical Thinking Exercises

Bring to your mind a vivid image of an older friend, relative, or patient who is at least 80 years old, and apply the following questions to one obvious functional consequence (e.g., impaired mobility). Develop an opportunity to talk with that person about what you have learned about the Functional Consequences Theory for Promoting Wellness in Older Adults and use Figure 3-1 as a basis for discussion.

1. What age-related changes and risk factors interact to contribute to this functional consequence?
2. What environmental conditions either improve or interfere with the affected aspect of functioning?
3. How can you use your nursing knowledge to improve health and quality of life in relation to that aspect of functioning?

Resources

For links to these resources and additional helpful Internet resources related to this chapter, visit thePoint at http://thePoint. lww.com/Miller6e.

Clinical Tools

American Journal of Nursing and Hartford Institute for Geriatric Nursing
- *How to Try This,* articles and videos

Hartford Institute for Geriatric Nursing
- *Try This: Best Practices in Nursing Care to Older Adults*

Evidence-Based Practice

E. Capezuti, D. Zwicker, M. Mezey, & T. Fulmer (Eds.) (2008). *Evidence-Based Geriatric Nursing Protocols for Best Practice* (3rd ed.). New York: Springer Publishing Co.

Hartford Institute for Geriatric Nursing
National Gerontological Nursing Association (NGNA)
National Guideline Clearinghouse
National Institute of Nursing Research

REFERENCES

Beard, J. R., Blaney, S., Cerda, M., Frye, V., Lovasi, G. S., Ompad, D., . . . Vlahov, D. (2009). Neighborhood characteristics and disability in older adults. *Journal of Gerontology: Social Sciences, 64B,* 252–257.

Cody, W. K. (2009). Nursing theory as a guide to practice. In P. G. Reed & N. B. Crawford Shearer (Eds.), *Perspectives on nursing theory* (5th ed., pp. 160–169). Philadelphia, PA: Wolters Kluwer Health/Lippincott Williams & Wilkins.

DeKeyser, F. G., & Medoff-Cooper, B. (2009). A non-theorist's perspective on nursing theory: Issues of the 1990s. In P. G. Reed & N. B. Crawford Shearer (Eds.), *Perspectives on nursing theory* (5th ed., pp. 59–68). Philadelphia, PA: Wolters Kluwer/Lippincott Williams & Wilkins.

Doane, G. W., & Varcoe, C. (2009). Toward compassionate action: Pragmatism and inseparability of theory/practice. In P. G. Reed & N. B. Crawford Shearer (Eds.), *Perspectives on nursing theory* (5th ed., pp. 111–121). Philadelphia, PA: Wolters Kluwer Health/Lippincott Williams & Wilkins.

Hill, E. E., Nguyen, T. H., Shaha, M., Wenzel, J. A., DeForge, B. R., & Spellbring, A. M. (2009). Person-environment interactions contributing to nursing home resident falls. *Research in Gerontological Nursing, 2,* 287–296.

Marrs, J., & Lowry, L. W. (2009). Nursing theory and practice: Connecting the dots. In P. G. Reed & N. B. Crawford Shearer (Eds.), *Perspectives on nursing theory* (5th ed., pp. 3–12). Philadelphia, PA: Wolters Kluwer Health/Lippincott Williams & Wilkins.

McEwen, M., & Wills, E. M. (2007). *Theoretical basis for nursing* (2nd ed.). Philadelphia, PA: Lippincott Williams & Wilkins.

Meleis, A. I. (2007). *Theoretical nursing: Development and progress* (4th ed.). Philadelphia, PA: Lippincott Williams & Wilkins.

Miller, C. A. (1990). *Nursing care of older adults: Theory and practice.* Glenview, IL: Scott, Forsman/Little, Brown Higher Education.

Register, M. E., & Herman, J. (2006). A middle range theory for generative quality of life for the elderly. *Advances in Nursing Science, 29,* 340–350.

Wahl, H. W., Fange, A., Oswald, F., Gitlin, L. N., & Iwarsson, S. (2009). The home environment and disability-related outcomes in aging individuals: What is the empirical evidence? *The Gerontologist, 49,* 355–367.

4

Theoretical Perspectives on Aging Well

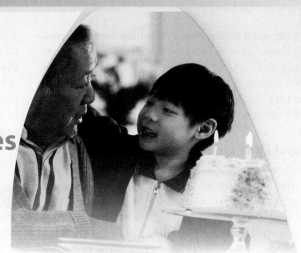

LEARNING OBJECTIVES

After reading this chapter, you will be able to:

1. Describe theoretical perspectives on the relationships among aging, disease, health, and quality of life.

2. Discuss pertinent concepts from biologic theories of aging and their relevance to nursing care of older adults.

3. Discuss pertinent concepts from sociocultural theories of aging and their relevance to nursing care of older adults.

4. Discuss pertinent concepts from psychological theories of aging and their relevance to nursing care of older adults.

K E Y P O I N T S

active life expectancy

activity theory

age stratification theory

apoptosis

biogerontology

biologic aging

caloric restriction theory

compression of morbidity

cross-linkage theory

disengagement theory

free radical theory

gerotranscendence

human needs theory

immunosenescence

life expectancy

life span

person–environment fit theory

program theory of aging

rectangularization of the curve

senescence

subculture theory

wear-and-tear theory

P eople have always looked for answers to universal questions, such as *How long can we live? Why do we age?* and *How can we prevent the unwanted effects of aging?*

Since early times, scientists and philosophers have tried to answer these questions beginning with early theories that addressed **biologic aging**. For example, Aristotle, Hippocrates, Galen, and other early philosopher–scientists associated aging with a decrease in body heat and fluid. As scientists learned more about aging, it became clear that aging is, in fact, an extremely complex and variable process. During the 20th century, theorists explained aging from the following perspectives: (1) biologic age, encompassing measures of functional capacities of vital organ systems; (2) sociologic age, involving the roles and age-graded behaviors of people in response to the society in which they live; and (3) psychological age, referring to the ways in which people adapt to environmental demands.

During the 21st century, the foremost question about aging is *How can we live both long and well?* Gerontologists and health care professionals are focusing their research and practice on the question, *What causes healthy aging?* In addressing this question, researchers and practitioners agree that healthy aging is fundamentally a biopsychosocial process involving multiple contributing factors. Thus, biologic, sociocultural, and psychological perspectives on aging facilitate the understanding of the interplay among these multiple factors (Ryff & Singer, 2009). This chapter focuses on theoretical perspectives that help explain how people can live both long and well, with emphasis on concepts that are most pertinent to the role of nurses in promoting wellness in older adults.

HOW CAN WE LIVE LONG AND WELL?

One way of addressing the question *How long can we live?* is by measuring **life span, life expectancy**, morbidity, and mortality rates. Another way to address this question—and an approach that is particularly relevant to health care practitioners—is through exploring the relationship among aging, health, and disease. Although early theories focused on problems and diseases associated with aging, more recent theories address the relationships among aging, health, and health-related behaviors. Gerontologists and nurse researchers are emphasizing the need to develop a "Healthy Aging Pheno-type" that is based on a holistic and multidisciplinary approach (Franco et al., 2009; Thompson & Voss, 2009). This trend provides a more inclusive explanation of why and how health, mortality, and quality of life change with aging (Bengston, Silverstein, Putney, & Gans, 2009).

Life Span and Life Expectancy

Two measures that gerontologists use to address questions about how long we can live are life span and life expectancy. Life span, defined as the maximum survival potential for a member of a species, is about 116 years for humans. Life expectancy is the predictable length of time that one is expected to live from a specific point in time, such as birth. Life span is relatively fixed, as evident by the barely perceptible extensions that occur over the evolutionary time scale; however, life expectancy has been increasing rapidly to the point that in industrialized countries, it increased as much during the past 100 years as it had increased over the previous 2000 years. For example, in 1900, people surviving to the age of 65 years could expect to live another 12 years, whereas men and women who reached 65 years in 2006 could expect to live an average of 17.4 and 20.3 more years, respectively. For people reaching 85 years in 2006, life expectancy is 6.2 and 7.4 more years for men and women, respectively. People who become centenarians in 2006 have a life expectancy of

2.7 more years. Life expectancy at birth in 1900 was only 47 years and in 2006, it reached a record high of 78.1 years. Figure 4-1 illustrates actual and projected life expectancies at birth and age 65 by race and sex. Although some scientists propose that life expectancy will not exceed 85 years because of an innate program of physiologic decay, other scientists suggest that life expectancy will reach 100 years during the 21st century because of improvements in the environment (Kaplan, Gurven, & Winking, 2009).

DIVERSITY NOTE

Significant sex and race variation exists in life expectancy rates. In 2006, life expectancy for white and African Americans males, respectively, was 76 and 70 years at birth. For white and African American females, respectively, it was 81 and 76.9 years.

Rectangularization of the Curve and Compression of Morbidity

Mortality rates are graphically represented in a survivorship curve, which illustrates the changes occurring in death rates over different periods of time (Figure 4-2). The vertical axis designates the percentage of survivors, whereas the horizontal axis represents the age of survivorship. Since the 1980s, the rate of increase in average longevity has continued to rise, but the pace of increase has slowed down. This change in pace

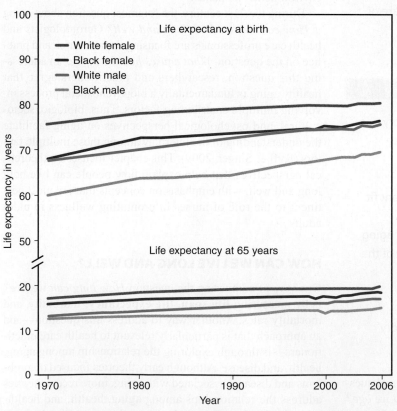

FIGURE 4-1 Life expectancies at birth and age 65, by race and sex: United States, 1970–2006. (*Source: Centers for Disease Control and Prevention, National Center for Health Statistics, National Vital Statistics System. Health, United States, 2009.*)

NOTES: Death rates used to calculate life expectancies for 1997–1999 are based on postsensal 1990-based population estimates; life expectancies for 2000 and beyond are calculated using death rates based on Census 2000.

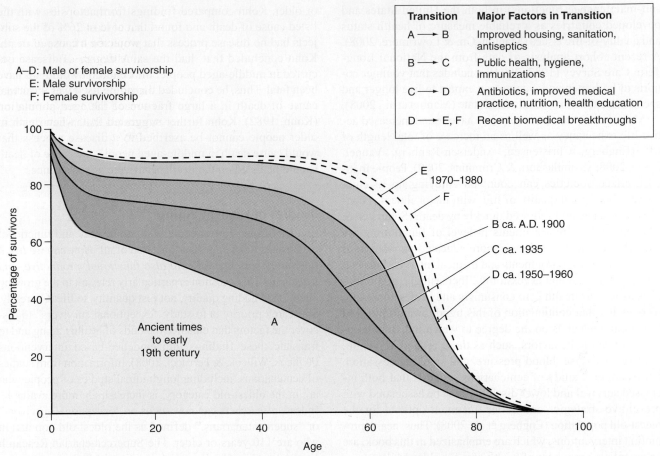

A–D: Male or female survivorship
E: Male survivorship
F: Female survivorship

Transition	Major Factors in Transition
A → B	Improved housing, sanitation, antiseptics
B → C	Public health, hygiene, immunizations
C → D	Antibiotics, improved medical practice, nutrition, health education
D → E, F	Recent biomedical breakthroughs

FIGURE 4-2 Human survivorship curve. (Adapted with permission from Strehler, B. L. (1975). Implications of aging research for society. *Proceedings of the Federation of American Societies for Experimental Biology, 34,* 6.)

has resulted in the squaring of the human survival curve, meaning that life expectancy is not significantly prolonged at the age of 75 or 80 years. This **rectangularization of the curve** is attributed to changes in survival caused by various significant factors occurring at different points in time.

The first major change, during the age of pestilence and famine, resulted from improved housing and sanitation, and the second major change was brought about by the advent of immunization programs and other advances in public health practices during the age of pandemics. The third major change, which occurred between 1960 and 1980, is attributable to biomedical breakthroughs, such as organ transplants, heart–lung machines, and cancer treatments. Recently, gerontologists identified a fourth stage—the age of delayed degenerative diseases—characterized by the later onset of death from diseases that cause disability and chronic illness. Interest in these trends has led to the development of biodemography, which is a subfield of demography that addresses variations in health and mortality that affect populations (Vasunilashorn & Crimmins, 2009). Biodemography is pertinent to health care practitioners because it focuses on the study of quality of life as well as quantity of life.

Although it is clear that increased life expectancy involves a longer time in chronic illness, it is less clear whether this is necessarily associated with a longer time in a state of disability. Thus, the focus of geriatric research and practice shifted from an emphasis on disease processes per se to an emphasis on the functional losses that are of key importance to older people. James Fries, a physician, first brought attention to this concern in an article on the **compression of morbidity**, in which he argued that the onset of significant illness could be postponed, but that one's life expectancy could not be extended to the same extent. Consequently, disease, disability, and functional decline are "compressed" into a period averaging 3 to 5 years before death. Fries and a colleague emphasized that preventive approaches must be directed toward preserving health by postponing the onset of chronic illnesses (Fries & Crapo, 1981).

Active Life Expectancy

Spurred partly by Fries' compression of morbidity hypothesis, gerontologists developed the concept of **active life expectancy**, which is measured on a continuum ranging from inability to perform activities of daily living to full independent functioning, as an indicator of quality of life during later adulthood. Since the 1980s, gerontologists have analyzed data about functional disability (defined as loss of various self-maintenance functions) in both the United States and developed countries as a reliable measure of health status and quality-of-life issues (Manton, Gu, & Lowrimore, 2008). A recent cohort analysis of data from the National Long-Term Care Survey (1982–2004) concludes that younger cohorts of both men and women can expect to live longer and spend more time in a nondisabled state (Manton et al., 2008).

Most, but not all, recent studies have found increased active life expectancy as well as an increase of total length of life (Engberg, Christensen, Andersen-Ranberg, Vaupel, Jeune, 2008; Vasunilashorn & Crimmins, 2009). People in industrialized societies can count on enjoying up to eight decades with good quality of life, with major illnesses confined to old age and followed quickly by death (Settersten & Trauten, 2009). Improvements in level of functioning are attributed to factors such as a more educated population of older adults and environments and medical interventions that improve function and accessibility. Increasingly, gerontologists as well as health care consumers and professionals are recognizing that continuation of this trend toward improved functioning depends on the degree to which individuals engage in healthy behaviors, such as those related to weight, nutrition, exercise, blood pressure, and smoking cessation. For example, a study of centenarians suggests that both increased survival and lower disability may be associated with preventive strategies and better treatment options for the oldest-old population (Engberg et al., 2008). Thus, health promotion interventions, which are emphasized in this book, are an essential component of health care for older adults.

Relationships Among Aging, Disease, and Death

Whether age-associated diseases are inevitable is an important question related to living both long and well. **Biogerontology** is a subspecialty of gerontology that addresses this question. The noted gerontologist Leonard Hayflick described the complex relationship between aging and disease as analogous to the "weak links" in automobiles. According to his analogy, both humans and particular makes and models of cars are characterized by weak links that increase the probability of component failure. For cheap cars, the "mean time to failure" is 4 or 5 years; for Americans born today, it is about 76 years. The weakest links for people in developed countries are the vascular system and the cells in which cancer commonly occurs. As Hayflick (2001–02) stated, "The aging process increases vulnerability to the pathologies that become the leading causes of death" (p. 21).

Attempts to answer questions about the relationships between aging and death have resulted in theories about **senescence**. Senescence refers to the post-reproductive period, which is characterized by a decrease in efficient functioning of an organism with increasing age that leads to an increased probability of death (Ferraro, Shippee, & Schafer, 2009). Kohn (1982) proposed a senescence theory based on postmortem studies of 200 people who died at the age of 85 years

or older. Kohn compared findings from autopsies with the listed cause of death and found that at least 26% of the subjects had no disease process that would be a cause of death. Kohn concluded that, had the same degree of disease occurred in middle-aged people, the condition would not have been fatal. Thus, he concluded that aging itself was the actual cause of death in a large fraction of the aged population (Kohn, 1982). Kohn further suggested that, when death in older people cannot be ascribed to a disease process that would cause death in middle-aged people, the cause of death should be listed on the death certificate as senescence.

Studies of Healthy Aging

Studies of long-lived people who are healthy and functional explore the most important question of all: *How can we live a life that is not only long but also functional, productive, and satisfying?* This question is particularly relevant to the growing attention to adding quality, not just quantity, to life. Currently, a research priority is to study "exceptional survivors" to discover the factors that enhance the odds of healthy aging and to translate these findings into evidence-based interventions (Willcox, Willcox, & Ferrucci, 2008). Information from studies of centenarians, including longitudinal studies of people who are in the oldest-old category, is increasingly more available. Indeed, researchers can now focus on "exceptional survivors" or "supercentenarians," defined as the oldest-old population who are 110 years or older. The Supercentenarian Research Foundation (see the Resources section and   ) maintains a list of age-validated supercentenarians. During 2009 and 2010, between 70 and 90 individuals were listed at any one time, but the foundation noted that the actual estimated number of supercentenarians living worldwide was more likely to be between 300 and 450.

Some studies indicate that even those centenarians who enjoy good health until just before death have underlying multiple pathologies and functional deficits. However, these centenarians have a mechanism of "successful adaptation" that enables them to counteract chronic conditions and postpone the onset of frailty until the very end of maximum life span (Arai et al., 2008). Other studies, however, find an absence of stroke, cancer, and coronary artery disease and little evidence of major organ damage, but the presence of clear signs of "wear-and-tear" conditions, such as compression fractures of the spine (Willcox et al., 2008). Researchers also found that clinically apparent disabilities and major chronic disease (e.g., cancer, diabetes, or cardiovascular disease) were markedly delayed in supercentenarians, often beyond the age of 100 (Willcox et al., 2008).

Gerontologists are attempting to distinguish between those factors that predict survival at different stages of aging. For example, there are fewer factors predictive of mortality among centenarians than for younger groups, but functional capacity and institutionalization are predictors of survival during all decades from the 60s to 100s (Hagberg &

Samuelsson, 2008). A study that followed 100 Swedish centenarians from the age of 100 through 111 found that physiologic reserve and present health and functional status carried more weight as survival predictors than heredity, personality, marital status, or social relationships (Hagberg & Samuelsson, 2008). Current research on centenarians emphasizes that people who survive to 100 years and older are a heterogeneous group with a range of health and functional characteristics (Magnolfi et al., 2009).

HOW DO WE EXPLAIN BIOLOGIC AGING?

Biologic theories of aging address questions about the basic aging processes that affect all living organisms. These theories answer questions, such as *How do cells age?* and *What triggers the process of aging?* Biologic aging is defined as the gradual and progressive decline in functioning that begins in adulthood and ends in death in virtually all animal species (Austad, 2009). All biologic theories attempt to explain the characteristics of age-related changes, and each theory attempts to explain a particular aspect of aging from a particular perspective. Major biologic theories are considered in this chapter, but these are only a sampling of the various perspectives that have been proposed and that continue to evolve.

Wear-and-Tear Theories

The first **wear-and-tear theory** was based on a 19th-century attempt to explain the difference between immortal "germ plasm" cells—those that are capable of reproducing—and mortal "somatic" cells—those that die. In the late 1880s, August Weismann theorized that normal somatic cells were limited in their ability to replicate and function and that death occurred because worn-out tissues could not forever renew themselves. According to this theory, the body can be likened to a machine that is expected to function well during the period of its warranty, but that will wear out at a fairly predictable time. Parts can be fixed or replaced, but eventually, the machine no longer functions because of the extensive accumulation of wear and tear. Like the machine, the longevity of the human body will be affected by the care it receives as well as by its genetic components. Unlike the machine, however, the human body can repair many of its own parts well into old age. Harmful stress factors, such as smoking, poor diet, alcohol abuse, or muscular strain can exacerbate the wearing-out process.

Cross-Linkage Theory

The **cross-linkage theory** proposes that molecular structures that normally are separated may be bound together through chemical reactions. According to this theory, a cross-linking agent attaches itself to a single strand of a DNA molecule and damages that strand. Natural defense mechanisms usually repair the damage, but increasing age weakens these defense mechanisms, allowing the cross-linkage process to continue until irreparable damage occurs. The result is an accumulation of cross-linking compounds that causes mutations in the cell and renders it unable to eliminate wastes and transport ions. This irreversible damage to the cells that form collagen-type substances eventually leads to tissue and organ failure because the protein system becomes inelastic and ineffective.

Free Radical Theory

The **free radical theory**, first proposed in the mid-1950s, has evolved into a major aging theory. Free radicals are highly unstable and reactive molecules that can be produced by normal metabolism, reactions to irradiation, chain reactions with other free radicals, and oxidation of certain environmental pollutants, such as ozone, pesticides, and air pollutants. Free radicals and their conjugated compounds are capable of attacking other molecules because they possess an extra electric charge, or free electron. Because they are so highly reactive, free radicals rapidly interact with and damage cellular components such as lipids, proteins, and nucleic acids. Fortunately, the human body has protective mechanisms that can interfere with oxidation activity and remove and repair damaged cells. Antioxidants, including beta-carotene and vitamins C and E, are one of the major defense mechanisms against oxidative damage from free radicals.

The free radical theory postulates that although most organisms have several mechanisms of antioxidant defense, damage to cells cannot be avoided and increases with age. Defense and repair mechanisms become less effective with age because of increased oxidative burden or inhibited repair/removal systems (Shringarpure & Davies, 2009). Early support for the free radical theory came from the discovery of lipofuscin, a pigmented waste material that is rich in lipids and proteins. Research currently is focusing on interventions to modify or prevent the age-related accumulation of free radicals or to diminish the formation of free radicals.

Neuroendocrine and Immunity Theories

Several biologic theories of aging focus on the primary role of body systems as an underlying cause of aging. For example, neuroendocrine theories are based on the understanding that the neuroendocrine system integrates body functions and facilitates adaptation to changes in both internal and external environments. These theories postulate that numerous alterations of the endocrine system are the underlying cause of age-related changes in organ function. One such theory—the neurotransmitter theory—proposes that an imbalance of nerve impulse–transmitting chemicals in the brain interferes with cell division throughout the body.

Immunity theories, which were first proposed during the 1960s, focus on **immunosenescence**, which is the age-related diminished function of the immune system that increases the susceptibility of older people to diseases. Immunity theories also attempt to explain a relationship between diminished immune functioning and an increase in the body's autoimmune responses. When autoimmunity occurs, the body reacts against itself and produces antibodies in response to its own constituents, which increases the susceptibility of older people to autoimmune diseases such as lupus or rheumatoid arthritis. Many studies that have validated immunity theories also incorporate other biologic theories of aging (Effros, 2009).

Genetic Theories

Genetic theories, which emphasize the role of genes in the development of age-related changes, are one of the most complex types of biologic theories. They are also among the most intensely studied and rapidly evolving types of theories in the 21st century. One of the earliest of the genetic theories is the **program theory of aging**, proposed by Hayflick in the 1960s. This theory states that the life span of animals is predetermined by a genetic program, called a biologic clock, which allows for a maximum of about 110 years in humans (Hayflick, 1965). Hayflick (1974) estimates that normal human cells divide 50 times in this number of years and argues that cells are genetically programmed to stop dividing after achieving 50 cell divisions, at which time they begin to deteriorate. The number of times cell division takes place is different for each species of animal, and the longer a species' life expectancy, the more cell divisions that animal has in its genetic program. Abnormal cells, however, are not subject to this predictable program and can proliferate an indefinite number of times.

The year 2000 saw many advances in genetic research as scientists involved with the Human Genome Project successfully identified the location of each human gene, facilitating the identification of specific genes that influence both biologic aging and age-related diseases. Ongoing developments of the Human Genome Project are likely to contribute significantly to emerging biologic theories of aging, particularly with regard to the complex interactions between aging and disease processes. For example, researchers are identifying genetic variations that alter one's risk of late-life disorders such as prostate cancer, macular degeneration, and type 2 diabetes (Martin, 2009).

Apoptosis Theory

Some biologic theories of aging are based on the relationship between **apoptosis** and aging and were first proposed during the 1970s. According to this theory, apoptosis is a noninflammatory, gene-driven, normal developmental process that occurs continuously throughout life. This process is characterized by cell shrinkage and maintenance of membrane integrity and differs from the inflammatory response to trauma, which is characterized by cell swelling and loss of membrane integrity. When apoptosis is properly regulated, it is beneficial because it helps maintain a balance between cells that should be retained and those that should be eliminated.

Caloric Restriction Theories

Caloric restriction theories are based on numerous animal studies that have found that reducing caloric intake by between 30% and 40% is the one intervention that dramatically increases life span. There is much scientific evidence that severe caloric restriction without malnutrition has many beneficial effects in animals, including enhanced ability to protect cells, increased resistance to stress, and overall longer and healthier life expectancy (Barzilai & Bartke, 2009). However, to date, this research has not been applied to humans.

Conclusions About Biologic Theories and Relevance to Nurses

Some conclusions that can be drawn about the relationships between aging and disease processes include the following:

- Biologic aging affects all living organisms.
- Biologic aging is natural, inevitable, irreversible, and progressive with time.
- The course of aging varies from individual to individual.
- The rate of aging for different organs and tissues varies within individuals.
- Biologic aging is an intrinsic process that is independent of external factors but is strongly influenced by nonbiologic factors.
- Biologic aging processes are different from pathologic processes.
- Biologic aging increases one's vulnerability to disease.

Biologic theories can explain the inevitable consequences of aging as well as the susceptibility of older adults to diseases, such as cancer, osteoarthritis, cardiovascular disease, and neurodegenerative diseases. In addition, these theories attempt to identify the factors that can predict long as well as healthy lives. Although no one theory answers these questions, all biologic theories of aging recognize that aging does not occur as an isolated physiologic process. Rather, it is a multidimensional process that is directly influenced by many interacting factors. Moreover, because of the great variability among people—which increases with aging—no single theory can explain the complex phenomenon of aging that involves many processes and mechanisms.

A primary role of nurses is to help older adults identify and address the modifiable factors that can lead to diseases, disability, and death as well as those health-promoting factors that can contribute to a longer and healthier life. Thus, nurses need to understand not only the relationship between aging and disease but also what "causes" healthy aging and longevity. Biologic theories of aging shed light on the differences between age-related changes and the risk factors that affect the health and functioning of older adults. Nurses then can use this knowledge to implement interventions that promote wellness and a higher level of functioning.

Biologic theories of aging also are applicable to attitudes of health care professionals about aging. If, for example, health care providers hold the perspective of "what do you

A Student's Perspective

One thing I feel I did well during my first week of providing patient care was seeing my patient for the person that she is and not just as a set of problems that needed caring for. I can understand how difficult it may be in today's health care settings to stop for a minute and really "see" the patient. When I cared for Mrs. S., I was able to look past the wrinkles and white hair and see the spunky spirit that she really is. It is easy to just categorize someone in your mind as old, senile, or dependent. One very important lesson that I will take with me for the rest of my career is that you cannot categorize someone because everyone is so different. It's amazing what you can discover if you actually take the time to see people for who they truly are. Taking care of a person holistically means taking care of them physically, psychologically, and spiritually as well.

Sarah L.

*I*magine that you are 72 years old and your mother and father are 96 and 95 years old, respectively, and they live in an assisted-living apartment. You have a brother who died last year at the age of 70 and you have a sister who is 69 years old. You have two children, three grandchildren, and two great-grandchildren. Your mother is moderately obese and has osteoarthritis, hypertension, glaucoma, and type 2 diabetes. Functionally, she uses a walker, needs help with getting in and out of the bathtub, and has some trouble reading but can still see well enough to watch television and get around familiar environments. Your father has hypertension, osteoarthritis, and a recent diagnosis of prostate cancer. Functionally, he is independent in his basic activities of daily living but is quite hearing impaired. Both of your parents have some memory impairment, but the support services at the facility where they live address their needs for meals, medication administration, and reminders about getting to activities.

THINKING POINTS

- Using the concepts of rectangularization of the curve and compression of morbidity, what would you expect the health, functioning, and life expectancy to be for each of the five generations in your family?
- Pick the biologic theory of aging that you think is most applicable for your family and use it to explain to your great-grandchildren why their great-great grandparents are still living.
- Pick a theory about the relationships among age, disease, and death or a theory about active life expectancy and functional health and use it to respond to your mother's statement, "I'm 96 years old—what does it matter if I follow a diabetic diet? If the sugar hasn't killed me so far, then eating two donuts this morning isn't going to kill me. It's old age that will take me, not my diet."
- Pick a theory about the relationships among age, disease, and death or a theory about active life expectancy and functional health and use it to respond to your father's declaration that "Of course, I have prostate cancer! I'm 95 years old!"
- What perspectives on aging would you want your father's primary care provider to use in addressing your father's prostate cancer?

expect, you're old," reversible disease conditions may go untreated. Similarly, if health care providers subscribe to the theory that aging is an ultimately fatal disease, their attitude may reflect a hopelessness that pervades their care for older patients. Biologic theories of aging can be used to point out that such fatalistic perspectives are outdated. Nurses can base their care on a holistic perspective and use studies of healthy and functional oldest-old people to identify health promotion interventions that will improve quality of life for older adults. Nurses often are in positions to serve as teachers and advocates for older adults whose care might be based on outdated or narrow approach that incorrectly equate aging and disease. The Functional Consequences Theory for Promoting Wellness in Older Adults (discussed in Chapter 3) provides a framework for a holistic approach that identifies the risk factors and addresses those that are modifiable in older adults. This book addresses each aspect of functioning from this perspective, with emphasis on those factors that nurses can address through health promotion interventions.

Biologic theories highlight the need for health promotion interventions to prevent disease conditions and minimize the negative effects of aging. However, these theories do not address the significant influence of nursing, medical, and psychosocial interventions that can improve a person's functioning and life expectancy. From a broader perspective, aging is more than an unrelenting progression of cellular deterioration. Survival to old age is an accomplishment that denotes strong will and the ability to adapt. As emphasized throughout this text, older adulthood is a dynamic part of the life span continuum and has the potential to be a most rewarding part of the life cycle, during which one experiences personal growth and self-understanding, fulfillment of potential, and the ability to establish clear priorities. These aspects of aging are addressed in the following sections, which describe sociocultural and psychological theories of aging.

SOCIOCULTURAL PERSPECTIVES ON AGING

Sociocultural theories of aging attempt to explain the interrelationship between older adults and the societies and environments in which they live. Early sociocultural theories viewed older adults in the context of societal problems, but later theories explored the complex interrelationship between older people and their physical, political, and socioeconomic environments. Currently, social gerontologists are developing an integrative approach that examines the broader social context as well as the individual and family perspectives, including cultural, economic, and political influences of all these dimensions (Bass, 2009). The following sections present a sampling of the widely recognized sociocultural theories of aging.

Disengagement Theory

In 1961, Cumming and Henry published the first sociologic theory of aging in their book, *Growing Old: The Process of Disengagement* (Cumming & Henry, 1961). According to **disengagement theory**, a society and older people engage in a mutually beneficial process of reciprocal withdrawal to maintain social equilibrium. This process occurs systematically and inevitably and is governed by society's needs, which override individual needs. Moreover, older people desire this withdrawal and are happy when it occurs. As the number, nature, and diversity of the older person's social contacts diminish, disengagement becomes a circular process that further limits opportunities for interaction. Disengagement theory stimulated many controversies by challenging traditional beliefs about the relationship between a person and society. For instance, there is considerable controversy regarding whether the disengagement process is, in fact, universal, inevitable, and beneficial to the person. Although this theory was initially viewed as an important contribution to social gerontology, it has since been discredited (Johnson, 2009).

Activity Theory

During the early 1970s, social gerontologists built upon the work of Havighurst and Albrecht (1953), which emphasized the relationship between successful aging and keeping active, and proposed the **activity theory**. The activity theory postulates that older people remain socially and psychologically fit if they remain actively engaged in life. For example, one's self-concept is affirmed through activities associated with various roles, and the loss of roles in old age negatively affects life satisfaction. Researchers found that productive activities, such as full-time work and low-level volunteering, had positive effects on the mental health of almost 8000 subjects aged 55 to 66 years (Hao, 2008). Although studies support this theory, its critics claim that it ignores factors such as health and economic disparities that interfere with opportunities for some older adults to engage in activities (Achenbaum, 2009).

> **DIVERSITY NOTE**
>
> A longitudinal study found a positive relationship between activities and decreased mortality in older adults ages 65 to 95 years, with women benefitting most from social and cultural activities (e.g., study circles, organizational activities) and men benefitting most from solitary and cultural activities (e.g., hobbies, gardening) (Agahi & Parker, 2008).

> **A Student's Perspective**
>
> *I think that over the past few weeks, I have really been able to see that it doesn't matter if a person is 90 or 50 or 5, they have a story, a family, a life. They have values and friends and things that are important to them. I think that this is what I will take away from this experience the most. I will try to remember in my nursing career that each patient has a story and that I will be a better nurse if I take the time to find out that story and connect with my patients, no matter what age they are.*
>
> *Erika B.*

Subculture and Age Stratification Theories

The **subculture theory**, first proposed by Rose in the early 1960s, states that old people, as a group, have their own norms, expectations, beliefs, and habits; therefore, they have their own subculture (Rose, 1965). The theory also maintains that older people are less well integrated into the larger society and interact more among themselves, compared with people from other age groups. Moreover, the theory holds that the formation of an aged subculture is primarily a response to the loss of status resulting from old age, which is so negatively defined in the United States that people do not want to be viewed as old. In the aged subculture, individual status is based on health and mobility, rather than on the occupational, educational, or economic achievements that were previously important. Rose (1965) envisioned that one outcome of the aged subculture would be the development of an aging group consciousness that would serve to improve the self-image of older people and change the negative cultural definition of aging.

Because the aged subculture has millions of members in this country, it constitutes a minority group that can organize and make public demands. A group such as the AARP, whose membership exceeds 34 million people, is evidence of the social importance of the aged subgroup. When considered along with the activity theory, the subculture theory supports the perspective that there is a strong relationship between peer group participation and the adjustment process of aging.

The **age stratification theory**, first proposed by Riley, Johnson, and Foner (1972), addresses the interdependencies between age as an element of the social structure and the aging of people and cohorts as a social process. This theory emphasizes the following concepts:

- People pass through society in cohorts that are aging socially, biologically, and psychologically.
- New cohorts are continually being born and each experiences a unique sense of history.
- A society can be divided into various strata according to age and roles.
- Society itself is continually changing, as are the people and their roles in each age stratum.

- A dynamic interplay exists between individual aging and social change.
- Thus, aging people and the larger society are constantly influencing each other and changing both the cohorts and the society.

Emerging Sociocultural Theories

Because gerontologists are recognizing the increasing diversity of older adults not only in the United States but also in many developed countries, more recent theories focus on a broader sociocultural perspective. For example, the purposes of one sociocultural study addressed all the following: (1) cultural values and beliefs that influence how families perceive and give meaning to dementia; (2) influences of culture and other social factors on the level and type of help sought by family caregivers of older people with dementia; and (3) the influence of culture and other social factors on physical functioning, health, and depression of caregivers (Dilworth-Anderson & Cohen, 2009). Topics addressed by cross-cultural sociologic theories include cultural conceptions of time and age, the influence of culture on the aging experience in different societies (Fry, 2009).

Another evolving trend is the theorizing about aging from a feminist perspective. Arguments in support of a feminist perspective emphasize that studies and theories of families focus only on certain kinds of women, specifically those who are derivatives of idealized males. Moreover, these studies and theories also ignore older people because they do not fit within the narrowly defined parameters of the family life cycle (Allen & Walker, 2009). One outcome of this trend is the emergence of feminist gerontology, an inclusive perspective that examines women's experiences from their own standpoints and at the same time allows scholars to derive theories that also incorporate men's experiences. Feminist gerontologists focus their studies on gender, but they also recognize that old men and women exist within the context of their racial-, ethnic-, sexual-, and class-based environments (Calasanti, 2009). Since the 1980s, gerontologists have applied a feminist perspective to legal and ethical aspects of caregiving. For example, one focus of the feminist ethics of care is on the broad and unique needs of the generation of middle-aged women who are responsible for care of their children as well as their parents (Doron, 2009).

Person–Environment Fit Theory

The **person–environment fit theory** considers the interrelationships between personal competence and the environment (Lawton, 1982). According to this theory, personal competence involves the following factors, which collectively contribute to a person's functional ability: ego strength, motor skills, biologic health, cognitive capacity, and sensory–perceptual capacity. The environment is viewed in terms of its potential for eliciting a behavioral response from the person. Lawton asserts that for each person's level of competence, there is a level of environmental demand, or environmental press, that is most advantageous to that person's function. People who function at relatively lower levels of competence can tolerate only low levels of environmental press, whereas people who function at higher levels of competence can tolerate increased environmental demands. An often-quoted correlate is that the more impaired the person, the greater the impact of the environment. This theory is often used in planning appropriate environments for older adults with disabilities.

Relevance of Sociocultural Theories of Aging to Nurses

Sociocultural theories of aging help nurses view older adults in relation to society and environments. Thus, these perspectives contribute to a better understanding of influences, such as culture, family, education, community, ascribed roles, cohort effects, home and living setting, and personal and political economics. These theories remind health care practitioners that there are patterns of similar responses among cohorts, but within those larger patterns, each person is unique. Some older people achieve their identity in a subculture, others may define successful aging in relation to their activities, and still others may find new roles in society.

Sociocultural perspectives encourage nurses to consider not only the cultural needs of individual older adults but also the role of culture in shaping societal attitudes about aging. Feminist-based theories provide a broad and holistic understanding of the needs of older adults as well as their families and caregivers. Information about diverse aspects of aging, such as cultural or gender differences, are discussed throughout this text, and pertinent information gleaned from studies appears in the Diversity Notes. Theories about person–environment interactions are stimulating interest in broadening the environments of institutional settings to include pets and intergenerational activities.

In addition, these theories emphasize the importance of assessing both environmental and psychosocial factors that influence the functioning of an older person. Concepts from the person–environment fit theory help nurses appreciate the importance of environmental adaptations as interventions to improve functional status, especially when working with dependent older adults. Lawton's theory also suggests that when an older person has difficulty, coping interventions can be directed toward improving personal competency or decreasing environmental demands, or both. Some of the risk factors discussed throughout this text identify environmental factors that interfere with the health and functioning of older adults. Similarly, many of the nursing interventions discussed in this text identify ways of modifying the environment to improve the functioning of older adults.

*I*magine that you are 87 years old and have been retired for 10 years. Create an image of yourself at that age, making sure that you incorporate some changes that are likely to occur as you grow older. Describe the people who are an active part of your relationships during a typical month. Describe the activities you would engage in during a typical week for each of the following aspects of your life: leisure activity, physical activity, intellectual stimulation, emotional growth, social interaction, and spiritual nurturing. Are you active in any volunteer organizations? What would your health and functioning be and where would you be living? Based on the image of yourself at 87 years old that you just created, answer the following questions:

THINKING POINTS

- How could you apply either the activity theory or the disengagement theory to your life, as it compares with your life at your present age?
- Would any of the concepts in the subculture or age stratification theories explain your activities and relationships?
- How would the person–environment fit theory explain the relationship between you and your environment?

PSYCHOLOGICAL PERSPECTIVES ON AGING

Psychological theories of aging focus on the psychological factors that affect health, longevity, and quality of life. These theories are especially relevant to psychosocial aspects of aging because they address variables such as learning, memory, feelings, intelligence, and motivation. The following sections review some of the major psychological theories of aging. In addition, relevant psychological theories about wisdom, creativity, cognitive function, spiritual outlook, stress and coping, and depression are discussed in Chapters 11, 12, and 15.

Human Needs Theory

Maslow's hierarchy of needs framework forms the basis of the **human needs theory**, one of the psychological theories that gerontologists use to address the concepts of motivation and human needs. According to Maslow's (1954) theory, the five categories of basic human needs, ordered from lowest to highest, are physiologic needs, safety and security needs, love and belongingness, self-esteem, and self-actualization. The attainment of lower-level needs takes priority over higher-level needs; self-actualization can occur only when lower-level needs are met to some degree. People continually move between the levels but always strive toward higher levels. This theory is particularly applicable to older adults because

Maslow describes self-actualized people as fully mature humans who possess such desirable traits as autonomy, creativity, independence, and positive interpersonal relationships.

Life-Course and Personality Development Theories

Two closely related types of psychological theories or aging are life-course theories, which address old age within the context of the life cycle, and personality development theories, which identify personality types as predictive forces of successful or unsuccessful aging. Both types emphasize that old age is part of a lifelong developmental process, which is embedded in relationships with others (Longino & Powell, 2009).

Carl Jung's (1960) theory categorizes personalities as either extroverted and oriented toward the external world or introverted and oriented toward subjective experiences. A balance between the two orientations, both of which are present to some degree in all people, is essential for mental health. Jung further theorized that people tend to be more extroverted in their younger years because of the nature of the demands and responsibilities associated with family and social roles. As these demands change and diminish, beginning around the age of 40 years, people become more introverted. Jung (1954) describes later adulthood as a period of taking stock, a time during which a person looks backward rather than forward and is responsible for devoting serious attention to self. Successful aging, according to Jung's theory, depends on accepting one's diminishing capacity and increasing number of losses.

Erik Erikson's (1963) original theory about the eight stages of life has been used widely in relation to older adulthood. Erikson defines the stages of life as trust versus mistrust, autonomy versus shame and doubt, initiative versus guilt, industry versus inferiority, identity versus identity diffusion, intimacy versus self-absorption, generativity versus stagnation, and ego integrity versus despair. Each of these stages presents the person with certain conflicting tendencies that must be balanced before he or she can move successfully from that stage. As in other life-course theories, how one stage is mastered lays the groundwork for successful or unsuccessful mastery of the next stage. In works published between 1950 and 1966, Erikson emphasized the life course from childhood to young adulthood; in later publications, however, he reconsidered the meaning of these stages. In 1982, when he was 80 years old, Erikson described the task of old age as balancing the search for integrity and wholeness with a sense of despair. He believed that the successful accomplishment of this task, achieved primarily through life review activities, would result in wisdom.

Peck (1968) expanded Erikson's original theory and divided the eighth stage—ego integrity versus despair—into additional stages occurring during middle age and old age. The stages described by Peck as specific to old age are ego differentiation versus work-role preoccupation, body transcendence versus body preoccupation, and ego transcendence versus ego preoccupation.

Some life-course theories concentrate on middle or later adulthood and address tasks of late life such as the following:

- Adjusting to decreasing physical strength and health
- Coping with physical changes of aging
- Adjusting to retirement and reduced income
- Adjusting to the death of a spouse
- Redirecting energy to new roles and activities, such as retirement, widowhood, and grandparenting
- Establishing an explicit association with one's age group
- Adapting to social roles in a flexible way
- Establishing satisfactory physical living arrangements
- Accepting one's own life
- Developing a point of view about death.

Theory of Gerotranscendence

The theory of **gerotranscendence** was proposed in the early 1990s by Lars Tornstam (1994) and has become widely recognized in Sweden and other Scandinavian countries. This theory proposes that human aging is a process of shifting from a rational and materialistic metaperspective to a more cosmic and transcendent vision. This shift includes the following aspects (Tornstam, 1996):

- Decreased self-centeredness
- Less concern with body and material things
- Decreased fear of death
- Discovery of hidden aspects of self
- Increased altruism
- Increased time spent in meditation and solitude
- Decreased interest in superfluous social interaction
- Urge to abandon roles
- Increased understanding of moral ambiguity
- Increased feelings of cosmic union with the universe
- Increased feelings of affinity with past and coming generations
- A redefinition of one's perception of time, space, and objects.

Theories About Gender and Aging

Over the past decade, some psychological theories of aging have focused on relationships between gender and aging. Some of these studies have addressed diverse populations, such as lesbians, gay men, and transgendered persons. Three purposes of gender-related psychological theories of aging studies have been (1) to compare and contrast male and female performance data, (2) to examine the nature of change in gender roles, and (3) to study the relationship between gender role differences and social roles and social power (Sinnott & Shifren, 2001). Some of the gender-specific aspects of psychology and aging that gerontologists are addressing include intelligence, personality, caregiving, self-efficacy, body attitudes, verbal ability, social ties, self-reported health, sense of control, and medical decision-making processes (Sinnott & Shifren, 2001).

> ### A Student's Perspective
>
> *My comfort level at the nursing home increases each and every week, and I find myself enjoying my time there more and more. Today there was a children's program in the dining room for all the residents. It was very cute. The kids were great, and most of the residents expressed true appreciation and enjoyment while the kids visited. For instance, my patient Mr. B. was chatting with a young boy and his mother. As the boy got more and more involved in the conversation, Mr. B.'s attitude changed completely; he became so happy and engaged with the young boy. I had seen Mr. B. smile a couple of times before, but not to the extent of how he smiled and laughed with the little one. After the boy left, Mr. B. told me that the boy reminded him of his own grandson, whom he doesn't get to see very much. I think it brought Mr. B. joy and a sense of comfort because he felt like he was with his family. Personally, I was quite touched. Sometimes, everyone gets so caught up in current tasks or problems, when really at the end of the day it comes down to making people smile and helping them to enjoy life to the best of one's abilities.*
>
> *Caitlin B.*

One longitudinal study found gender differences in socioeconomic and psychosocial predictors of mortality (Fry & Debats, 2006). For men, the greatest predictors were lower levels of education, perceived control, personal commitment, and physical functioning. For women, the greatest predictors were lower levels of perceived social support and social engagement. The factors that were most influential for men were inconsequential for women, and vice versa. Psychological theories of aging also address gender role development across the life span. They address questions such as *Why is there a gender difference as we age?* (Sinnott & Shifren, 2001). Many researchers believe that gender roles evolve from being narrowly defined in adolescence and younger adulthood to becoming more amorphous in later adulthood. An analysis of research on this subject concluded that gender role development in older adulthood involves transcending roles as they were conceptualized in earlier life and continuing to develop a sense of individual identity, meaning, and community (Sinnott & Shifren, 2001).

Relevance of Psychological Theories of Aging to Nurses

In caring for older adults, nurses can use psychological theories of aging as a framework for addressing certain issues, such as response to losses and continued emotional development. Maslow's hierarchy of needs framework is useful for conceptualizing the nature of interventions in institutional or home settings. For instance, if older adults are unable to purchase food, they are unlikely to feel secure. Likewise, if older adults feel insecure about being able to meet their shelter needs, they are unlikely to have a sense of trust. Older adults who have already met their lower-level needs, however, can be encouraged to focus on higher-level achievements such as self-actualization.

In addition, psychological theories imply that older adults should devote some time and energy to life review and self-understanding. Nurses can facilitate this process by asking sensitive questions and by listening attentively to older adults as they share information about their past. Reminiscence is a positive experience that is essential for continued psychological development, and it can be promoted by nurses either on an individual or group basis.

Life-course models can help nurses identify those areas of personality that are likely to change and those that are more likely to remain stable. Nurses have used life span theories to develop a multidisciplinary theory of thriving (Haight, Barba, Tesh, & Courts, 2002). This model proposes that thriving is achieved when there is concordance between the person and the human and nonhuman environment, that is, when these three elements are mutually engaged, supportive, and harmonious. In contrast, failure to thrive is the result of discordance among these three elements, causing a failure of engagement and mutual support and disharmony (Haight et al., 2002). In addition to these implications, nurses consider implications regarding specific aspects, such as cognitive function and coping responses (see Chapters 11 and 12), in the context of psychological theories of aging.

---

*I*magine, again, that you are 87 years old and add the following information to the description of yourself that you created for the discussion of sociocultural theories. Describe your personality, including, but not limited to, the following characteristics: emotional stability, adjustments to losses, contentedness with life, optimism versus pessimism, engagement in activities versus withdrawal from activities, and feelings of self-efficacy versus feelings of powerlessness. Describe your beliefs about your gender-specific roles (i.e., those aspects of roles that are defined by you being a woman or a man). Based on this image of yourself at 87 years old, answer the following questions:

THINKING POINTS

- Where do you think you would be in Maslow's or Erikson's stages and how would you have moved between the levels in the past decades?
- What aspects of your lifestyle at 87 years old could be explained by the continuity theory?
- How would any concepts in the personality development theories apply to you?
- Based on your own experiences, how has your perception of your role as a woman or man changed over time?

A HOLISTIC PERSPECTIVE ON AGING AND WELLNESS

From a holistic perspective—the one that is most pertinent to promoting wellness—it is necessary to consider the body–mind–spirit interconnectedness of each older adult for whom nurses provide care. Thus, questions about how we can live long and well must be answered in the context of the interplay among the many factors that influence health and aging. This requires an integrated perspective on aging, an avoidance of stereotypes, and a commitment to identifying the factors that most directly affect—both negatively and positively—health and quality of life for each unique older adult. Current theories point to the following determinants of living long and well:

- Inherit good genes.
- Avoid oxidative damage (e.g., from tobacco, environmental conditions).
- Protect from oxidative damage with antioxidants from natural sources (e.g., fruits and vegetables).
- Maintain optimal weight.
- Engage in physical exercise.
- Engage in meaningful social interactions.
- Develop close personal relationships.
- Maintain a sense of spiritual connectedness.
- Reject ageist stereotypes.

The Functional Consequences Theory for Promoting Wellness that was presented in Chapter 3 provides a nursing framework for addressing the factors that affect the health and functioning of older adults. Although it is beyond the scope of any nursing text to address all aspects of body–mind–spirit interconnectedness, nurses can use the functional consequences perspective, in conjunction with information from theories discussed in this chapter, to help older adults answer their own questions about aging. When older adults express resignation in the "What-do-you-expect-you're-old?" outlook, nurses can rephrase that viewpoint and ask "So, what *do* you expect because you are older?" or "What *will* you expect when you are older?" Nurses can challenge ageist stereotypes and approach the question from a holistic perspective that acknowledges the interconnectedness among one's body, one's mind, and one's spirit. From this point of view, nurses can emphasize that even though some degenerative changes affect one's body with increasing age, one's mind and spirit can continue to thrive and even improve.

Because self-responsibility is an essential component of wellness, nurses can ask older adults to identify for themselves those factors that most significantly influence their health and functioning and can focus care on those aspects that are within the scope of nursing. Nurses also need to avoid communicating ageist stereotypes, which requires that we examine our own attitudes about aging and make sure that our nursing care of older adults is based on accurate, theory-based information. Nurses can check their attitudes about their own aging and periodically ask, *What do I expect (or wish) for my own wellness when I am older tomorrow? . . .a week from now? . . .a month from now? . . .a year? . . .10 years? . . .20 years?* Even more important, ask, *What am I doing today that will affect how well I am aging tomorrow? . . .10 years from now?* If we acknowledge that no matter what else is happening, we are aging biologically, we are likely to pay careful attention to health-related behaviors that affect how well we age. Likewise, if we approach our care of older adults holistically, we will be able to identify interventions that promote wellness of body, mind, and spirit.

Chapter Highlights

How Can We Live Long and Well?
- Gerontologists develop theories to answer questions about how and why we age. From a holistic perspective, the most important question is *How can we live a life that is both long and healthy?* Nurses address this question by promoting wellness and facilitating optimal level of functioning for older adults.
- One way of addressing the question *How long can we live?* is by measuring life span, life expectancy, and morbidity and mortality rates.
- Another way to address this question is through exploring the relationship between aging, health, and disease.

How Do We Explain Biologic Aging?
- Biologic theories of aging address questions about basic age-related changes, which are characterized as deleterious, progressive, intrinsic, universal, irreversible, and genetically programmed.
- Biologic theories include genetic, wear-and-tear, immunity, cross-linkage, free radical, neuroendocrine, and apoptosis theories.

Sociocultural Perspectives on Aging
- Sociocultural theories of aging attempt to explain how a society influences its old people and how old people influence their society.
- Sociocultural theories include disengagement, activity, subculture, age stratification, and person–environment fit theories.

Psychological Perspectives on Aging
- Psychological theories of aging provide a framework for addressing certain psychosocial issues that are common among older adults (e.g., responses to losses and continued emotional development).
- Psychological theories include human needs, life-course and personality development, gerotranscendence, and gender theories.

A Holistic Perspective on Aging and Wellness
- Nurses can use theories of aging developed by other disciplines in conjunction with the Functional Consequences Theory (see Chapter 3) to develop and implement a holistic approach to promoting wellness in older adults.

Critical Thinking Exercises

You are assessing an 87-year-old woman who is being admitted to the hospital with congestive heart failure for the third time in the past 2 years. She does not have any cognitive impairment and she lives alone in her own home. When you ask her why she came to the hospital, she states, "I'm 87 years old, you know. Isn't that a good enough reason to be sick? Don't you think you'll be in the hospital when you're my age?"
1. How do you respond to her?
2. What additional assessment information would you want?
3. What health teaching would you think about incorporating into your care plan?

Resources

For links to these resources and additional helpful Internet resources related to this chapter, visit thePoint at http://thePoint.lww.com/Miller6e.

American Federation for Aging Research
Gerontology Research Group
International Longevity Center—USA
National Institute on Aging Information Center
Supercentenarian Research Foundation

REFERENCES

Achenbaum, W. A. (2009). A metahistorical perspective on theories of aging. In V. L. Bengston, M. Silverstein, N. M. Putney, & Gans, D. (Eds.), *Handbook of theories of aging* (2nd ed., pp. 25–38). New York: Springer Publishing Co.

Agahi, N., & Parker, M. G. (2008). Leisure activities and mortality: Does gender matter? *Journal of Aging and Health, 20*(7), 855–871.

Allen, K. R., & Walker, A. J. (2009). Theorizing about families and aging from a feminist perspective. In V. L. Bengston, M. Silverstein, N. M. Putney, & D. Gans (Eds.), *Handbook of theories of aging* (2nd ed., pp. 517–528). New York: Springer Publishing Co.

Arai, Y., Takayama, M., Gondo, Y., Inagaki, H., Yamamura, K., Nakazawa, S., . . . Hirose N. (2008). Adipose endocrine function, insulin-like growth factor-1 axis, and exceptional survival beyond 100 years of age. *Journal of Gerontology: Medical Sciences, 63A*(11), 1209–1218.

Austad, S. N. (2009). Making sense of biological theories of aging. In V. L. Bengston, M. Silverstein, N. M. Putney, & D. Gans (Eds.), *Handbook of theories of aging* (2nd ed., pp. 147–161). New York: Springer Publishing Co.

Barzilai, N., & Bartke, A. (2009). Biological approaches to mechanistically understand the healthy life extension achieved by calorie restriction and modulation of hormones. *Journal of Gerontology: Biological Sciences, 64A,* 187–191.

Bass, S. A. (2009). Toward an integrative theory of social gerontology. In V. L. Bengston, M. Silverstein, N. M. Putney, & D. Gans (Eds.), *Handbook of theories of aging* (2nd ed., pp. 347–374). New York: Springer Publishing Co.

Bengston, V. L., Gans, D., Putney, N. M., & Silverstein, M. (2009). Theories about age and aging. In V. L. Bengston, M. Silverstein, N. M. Putney, & D. Gans (Eds.), *Handbook of theories of aging* (2nd ed., pp. 3–23). New York: Springer Publishing Co.

Calasanti, T. (2009). Theorizing feminist gerontology, sexuality, and beyond: An intersectional approach. In V. L. Bengston, M. Silverstein, N. M. Putney, & D. Gans (Eds.), *Handbook of theories of aging* (2nd ed., pp. 471–485). New York: Springer Publishing Co.

Cumming, E., & Henry, W. (1961). *Growing old: The process of disengagement.* New York: Basic Books.

Dilworth-Anderson, P., & Cohen, M. D. (2009). Theorizing across cultures. In V. L. Bengston, M. Silverstein, N. M. Putney, & D. Gans (Eds.), *Handbook of theories of aging* (2nd ed., pp. 487–498). New York: Springer Publishing Co.

Doron, I. (2009). Jurisprudential gerontology: Theorizing relationships between law and aging. In V. L. Bengston, M. Silverstein, N. M. Putney, & D. Gans (Eds.), *Handbook of theories of aging* (2nd ed., pp. 643–657). New York: Springer Publishing Co.

Effros, R. B. (2009). The immunological theory of aging. In V. L. Bengston, M. Silverstein, N. M. Putney, & D. Gans (Eds.), *Handbook of theories of aging* (2nd ed., pp. 163–177). New York: Springer Publishing Co.

Engberg, H., Christensen, K., Andersen-Ranberg, K., Vaupel, J. W., & Jeune, B. (2008). Improving activities of daily living in Danish centenarians – but only in women: A comparative study of two birth cohorts born in 1895 and 1905. *Journal of Gerontology: Medical Sciences, 63A*(11), 1186–1192.

Erikson, E. H. (1963). *Childhood and society* (2nd ed.). New York: W. W. Norton.

Ferraro, K. F., Shippee, T. P., & Schafer, M. H. (2009). Cumulative inequality theory for research on aging and the life course. In V. L. Bengston, M. Silverstein, N. M. Putney, & D. Gans (Eds.), *Handbook of theories of aging* (2nd ed., pp. 413–433). New York: Springer Publishing Co.

Franco, O. H., Karnik, K., Osborne, G., Ordovas, J. M., Carr, M., & Van Der Ouderaa, F. (2009). Changing course in ageing research: The healthy ageing phenotype. *Maturitas, 63*, 13–19.

Fries, J. F., & Crapo, L. M. (1981). *Vitality and aging: Implications of the rectangularization of the curve.* San Francisco: W. H. Freeman.

Fry, C. L. (2009). Out of the armchair and off the veranda: Anthropological theories and the experience of aging. In V. L. Bengston, M. Silverstein, N. M. Putney, & D. Gans (Eds.), *Handbook of theories of aging* (2nd ed., pp. 499–515). New York: Springer Publishing Co.

Fry, P. S., & Debats, D. L. (2006). Sources of life strengths as predictors of late-life mortality and survivorship. *International Journal of Aging and Human Development, 62*, 303–334.

Hagberg, B., & Samuelsson, G. (2008). Survival after 100 years of age: A multivariate model of exceptional survival in Swedish centenarians. *Journal of Gerontology: Medical Sciences, 63A*(11), 1219–1226.

Haight, B. K., Barba B. E., Tesh, A. S., & Courts, N. F. (2002). Thriving: A life span theory. *Journal of Gerontological Nursing, 28*(3), 14–22.

Hao, Y. (2008). Productive activities and psychological well-being among older adults. *Journal of Gerontology: Social Sciences, 63B*, S64–S72.

Havighurst, R. J., & Albrecht, R. (1953). *Older people.* New York: Longmans, Green.

Hayflick, L. (1965). The limited in vitro lifetime of human diploid cell strains. *Experimental Cell Research, 37*, 614–636.

Hayflick, L. (1974). The longevity of cultured human cells. *Journal of the American Geriatrics Society, 22*, 1–12.

Hayflick, L. (2001–02). Anti-aging medicine hype, hope, and reality. *Generations, 20*, 20–26.

Johnson, M. L. (2009). Spirituality, finitude, and theories of the life span. In V. L. Bengston, M. Silverstein, N. M. Putney, & D. Gans (Eds.), *Handbook of theories of aging* (2nd ed., pp. 659–674). New York: Springer Publishing Co.

Jung, C. G. (1954). Marriage as a psychological relationship. In W. McGuire, H. Reed, M. Fordham, & G. Adler (Eds.) (R. F. C. Hull, trans.), *Collected works: The development of personality* (Vol. 17). New York: Pantheon Books.

Jung, C. G. (1960). The stages of life. In W. McGuire, H. Reed, M. Fordham, & G. Adler (Eds.) (R. F. C. Hull, trans.), *Collected works: The structure and dynamics of the psyche* (Vol. 8, pp. 387–403). New York: Pantheon Books.

Kaplan, H., Gurvan, M., & Winking, J. (2009). An evolutionary theory of human life span: Embodied capital and the human adaptive complex. In V. L. Bengston, M. Silverstein, N. M. Putney, & D. Gans (Eds.), *Handbook of theories of aging* (2nd ed., pp. 39–60). New York: Springer Publishing Co.

Kohn, R. R. (1982). Cause of death in very old people. *Journal of the American Medical Association, 247*, 2793–2797.

Lawton, M. P. (1982). Competence, environmental press, and the adaptation of older people. In M. P. Lawton, P. G. Windley, & T. O. Byerts (Eds.), *Aging and the environment: Theoretical approaches* (pp. 33–59). New York: Springer.

Longino, C. F., & Powell, J. L. (2009). Toward a phenomenology of aging. In V. L. Bengston, M. Silverstein, N. M. Putney, & D. Gans (Eds.), *Handbook of theories of aging* (2nd ed., pp. 375–387). New York: Springer Publishing Co.

Magnolfi, S. U., Noferi, I., Petruzzi, E., Pinzani, P., Malentacchi, F., Pazzagli, M., . . . Marchionni, N. (2009). Centenarians in Tuscany: The role of environmental factors. *Archives of Gerontology and Geriatrics, 48*, 263–266.

Manton, K. G., Gu, X., & Lowrimore, G. R. (2008). Cohort changes in active life expectancy in the U.S., elderly population: Experience from the 1982–2004 National Long-Term Care Survey. *Journal of Gerontology: Social Sciences, 63B*(5), S269–S281.

Martin, G. M. (2009). Modalities of gene action predicted by the classical evolutional theories of aging. In V. L. Bengston, M. Silverstein, N. M. Putney, & D. Gans (Eds.), *Handbook of theories of aging* (2nd ed., pp. 179–191). New York: Springer Publishing Co.

Maslow, A. H. (1954). *Motivation and personality.* New York: Harper & Row.

Peck, R. C. (1968). Psychological developments in the second half of life. In B. L. Neugarten (Ed.), *Middle age and aging* (pp. 88–92). Chicago: University of Chicago Press.

Riley, M. W., Johnson, M., & Foner, A. (1972). *Aging and society. Vol. 3: A sociology of age stratification.* New York: Russell Sage Foundation.

Rose, A. M. (1965). The subculture of the aging: A framework for research in social gerontology. In A. M. Rose & W. Peterson (Eds.), *Older people and their social worlds.* Philadelphia, PA: F. A. Davis.

Ryff, C. D., & Singer, B. (2009). Understanding healthy aging: Key components and their integration. In V. L. Bengston, M. Silverstein, N. M. Putney, & D. Gans (Eds.), *Handbook of theories of aging* (2nd ed., pp.117–144). New York: Springer Publishing Co.

Settersten, R. A., & Trauten, M. E. (2009). The new terrain of old age: Hallmarks, freedoms, and risks. In V. L. Bengston, M. Silverstein, N. M. Putney, & D. Gans (Eds.), *Handbook of theories of aging* (2nd ed., pp. 455–469). New York: Springer Publishing Co.

Shringarpure, R., & Davies, K. J. A. (2009). Free radicals and oxidative stress in aging. In V. L. Bengston, M. Silverstein, N. M. Putney, & D. Gans (Eds.), *Handbook of theories of aging* (2nd ed., pp. 229–243). New York: Springer Publishing Co.

Sinnott, J. D., & Shifren, K. (2001). Gender and aging: Gender differences and gender roles. In J. E. Birren & K. W. Schaie (Eds.), *Handbook of the psychology of aging* (5th ed., pp. 454–476). San Diego: Elsevier Academic Press.

Thompson, H. J., & Voss, J. G. (2009). Health- and disease-related biomarkers in aging research. *Research in Gerontological Nursing, 2*, 137–148.

Tornstam, L. (1994). Gerotranscendence: A theoretical and empirical exploration. In L. E. Thomas & S. A. Eisenhandler (Eds.), *Aging and the religious dimension.* Westport, CT: Greenwood.

Tornstam, L. (1996). Gerotranscendence: A theory about maturing into old age. *Journal of Aging & Identity, 1*, 37–50.

Vasunilashorn, S., & Crimmins, E. M. (2009). Biodemography: Integrating disciplines to explain aging. In V. L. Bengston, M. Silverstein, N. M. Putney, & D. Gans (Eds.), *Handbook of theories of aging* (2nd ed., pp. 63–85). New York, NY: Springer Publishing Co.

Willcox, B. J., Willcox, D. C., & Ferrucci, L. (2008). Secrets of healthy aging and longevity from exceptional survivors around the globe: Lessons from octogenarians to supercentenarians. *Journal of Gerontology: Medical Sciences, 63A*(11), 1181–1185.

Willcox, D. C., Willcox, B. J., Wang, N-C., He, Q., Rosenbaum, M., & Suzuki, M. (2008). Life at the extreme limit: Phenotypic characteristics of supercentenarians in Okinawa. *Journal of Gerontology: Medical Sciences, 63A*(11), 1201–1208.

PART 2

Nursing Considerations for Older Adults

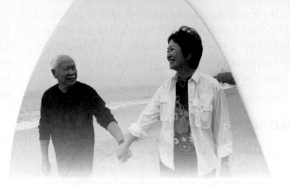

CHAPTER 5

Gerontological Nursing and Health Promotion

LEARNING OBJECTIVES

After reading this chapter, you will be able to:

1. Describe the scope of gerontology and geriatrics.
2. Discuss the practice of gerontological nursing as a specialty.
3. Identify and use resources for improving competence in care of older adults.
4. Describe health promotion programs and interventions that are pertinent to older adults.
5. Identify and use resources for evidence-based health promotion programs for older adults.

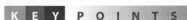

KEY POINTS

geriatrics
gerontology
gerontological nursing
health
health promotion

health-related quality
of life
Transtheoretical Model
wellness

What emerges from the information in Part 1 is an image of older adults as a diverse group of individuals from varied sociocultural backgrounds who are more heterogeneous than homogeneous. What is becoming clear is that, even among the same-age cohorts, as people age, they become less and less like others of the same age. Indeed, the most universal characteristic of increasing age is increasing individuality and diversity. Because the provision of health care and other services to this population is so complicated, several branches of science have evolved to address the

unique issues related to aging and older adults. In recent years, there has been increasing attention to the importance of all nurses becoming competent in addressing the unique health care needs of older adults and applying evidence-based guidelines to nursing practice. There also has been increasing attention to the importance of **health promotion** interventions and the roles of nurses in promoting **wellness**.

GERONTOLOGY AND GERIATRICS

Gerontology is the study of aging and older adults. Gerontology was first recognized as a specialty in the mid-1940s with the establishment of the Gerontological Society of America and the publication of the first issue of the *Journal of Gerontology*. Since its inception, gerontology has addressed problems that "transcend the knowledge and methods of any one discipline or profession" (Frank, 1946, p. 1). Gerontology continues to be multidisciplinary and is a specialized area within various disciplines, such as nursing, psychology, social work, and certain allied health professions. In the early decades of gerontology, researchers and practitioners focused on problems of aging and older adults; but in recent decades, the focus shifted to an emphasis on healthy and successful aging.

In addition to focusing on healthy aging, gerontologists are addressing the increasing diversity among older people, including the increased complexity of caring for older adults in health care settings. Consequently, the health care specialties of geriatric medicine and **gerontological nursing** have emerged. **Geriatrics** is associated with the diseases and disabilities of old people, and geriatric medicine is a subspecialty of internal medicine or family practice that focuses on the medical problems of older people. The American Geriatrics Society was established in 1942 and in its first publication, *Geriatrics*, the editor called for physicians to "alleviate the inevitable deficiencies and limitations inherent in growing old" (Touhy, 1946, p. 17). In 1953, the society changed the name of its journal to the *Journal of the American Geriatrics Society* and broadened its focus to address various issues that affect the **health** and functioning of older adults. These changes reflected the shift in geriatrics from medically oriented care to care that is more preventive—a shift in emphasis from curing to caring. Consistent with this shift in orientation, the current foci of geriatrics include quality-of-life issues, interventions to maintain optimal functioning, and health promotion as a means of delaying the onset of disability.

GERONTOLOGICAL NURSING

Although nurses first recognized the importance of addressing the unique nursing needs of older adults in the early 1900s, geriatric nursing was not considered a subspecialty until the 1960s. By the mid-1970s, the American Nurses Association (ANA) was advocating the use of the term *gerontological nursing*, instead of *geriatric nursing*, to more accurately reflect the broader scope of nursing care rather than a focus on disease conditions. Since the early 2000s, gerontological nursing has been recognized both as a specialty and as an essential and integral component of adult nursing.

Activities of the ANA that supported the growth of gerontological nursing as a specialization include establishing a Council on Gerontological Nursing and developing several documents dealing with standards and scope of practice. Nurses can use the ANA's 2001 *Standards of Professional Gerontological Nursing Performance* as a guide to providing care for older adults (Box 5-1).

Box 5-1 Standards of Professional Gerontological Nursing Performance

I. Quality of Care. The gerontological nurse systematically evaluates the quality of care and effectiveness of nursing practice.

II. Performance Appraisal. The gerontological nurse evaluates his or her own nursing practice in relation to professional practice standards and relevant statutes and regulations.

III. Education. The gerontological nurse acquires and maintains current knowledge applicable to nursing practice.

IV. Collegiality. The gerontological nurse contributes to the professional development of peers, colleagues, and others.

V. Ethics. The gerontological nurse's decisions and actions on behalf of older adults are determined in an ethical manner.

VI. Collaboration. The gerontological nurse collaborates with the older adult, the older adult's caregivers, and all members of the multidisciplinary team to provide comprehensive care.

VII. Research. The gerontological nurse interprets, applies, and evaluates research findings to inform and improve gerontological nursing practice.

VIII. Resource Utilization. The gerontological nurse considers factors related to safety, effectiveness, and cost in planning and delivering patient care.

The American Nurses Credentialing Center (AACN) is another nursing organization that recognizes gerontological nursing as a specialization by offering certification as a gerontological nurse, a clinical specialist in gerontological nursing, or a gerontological nurse practitioner. Even though gerontological nursing certification has been available since 1974, less than 1% of registered nurses are certified in gerontological nursing (National Academy of Sciences, 2008). Three nursing journals are devoted to gerontological nursing, with the first one published in 1979 and the most recent one initiated in 2008, reflecting increasing support for this specialized area of practice.

Gerontological Nursing Education and Practice

Because of the development and growth of gerontological nursing as a specialization, it is now widely recognized that all nurses who work with adults need to be competent in addressing the unique health issues of older adults. For example, during the 1990s, the Association for Gerontology in Higher Education, the National League for Nursing, and the Bureau of Health Professions identified core curriculum and terminal objectives for entry-level professional nurses in the area of gerontological nursing. These competencies, *Older Adults: Recommended Baccalaureate Competencies and Curricular Guidelines for Geriatric Nursing Care*, were first published in 2000 and are updated periodically.

The Comprehensive Geriatric Education Program (CGEP) was authorized through the Nurse Reinvestment Act of 2002 to increase education of health professionals who care for older adults. During the first 5 years of this program, almost 20,000 nurses, nursing students, and other health care professionals received training and education in care of older adults (Douglas-Kersellius, 2009). Despite the increasing efforts to address unique health care needs of older adults, the Institute of Medicine published a report in 2008 emphasizing that much more needs to be done to ensure that all professionals are competent to care for older adults (National Academy of Sciences, 2008).

One way of improving nurse competencies in care of older adults is through continuing education programs. Nursing articles by Barba and Fay (2009); Kowlowitz, Davenport, and Palmer (2009); and McConnell et al. (2009) describe models for continuing education in gerontological nursing. In addition, Palmer et al. (2008) describe clinical simulations that can be used for geriatric nursing continuing education. These peer-reviewed simulations, developed as part of a Health Services and Resources Administration grant, focus on caring for older adults who experience a sudden change in health status, an exacerbation of a chronic condition, or a sentinel event such as a fall. Evaluations found that nurses enjoyed using the simulation, reported increased clinical competency, and significantly increased their knowledge (Kowlowitz et al., 2009). Nurses can use these clinical simulations (available at www.gerosim.org) for continuing education and to improve their geriatric clinical competencies.

Since the early 1990s, the John A. Hartford Foundation has demonstrated a major commitment to improving nursing care of older adults through many initiatives directed toward increased nursing knowledge and evidence-based clinical practice. In 1992, the foundation funded a major initiative called the Nurses Improving Care to the Hospitalized Elderly (NICHE). The NICHE program is ongoing and includes more than 225 hospitals nationwide. It has been shown to improve quality of care for older adults as well as job satisfaction for nurses. Studies of outcomes at NICHE hospitals have demonstrated improvements in clinical care, cost effectiveness, nursing knowledge, and nurse perceptions of the geriatric nursing practice environment and quality of geriatric care (Boltz et al., 2008). In 2007, the Hartford Foundation collaborated with the *American Journal of Nursing* to develop and promulgate a series of 28 cost-free web-based articles and corresponding videos that nurses and nursing students can use to improve their care of older adults. Pertinent videotapes and articles are listed in the Clinical Tool sections of chapters in this book. Figure 5-1 lists milestones in gerontological nursing development and major initiatives directed toward improving nursing knowledge in care of older adults.

Roles for Gerontological Nurses

The concurrent emphasis on the need to improve the quality and cost of health care for the growing numbers of older adults has stimulated the development of new models of care. Most of these models include innovative and expanded roles for nurses. Because these models and the associated roles for gerontological nurses are described in detail in Chapter 6, this section focuses on recent developments related to advanced practice nurses.

A gerontological advanced practice nurse (GAPN) is a registered nurse who holds a degree higher than a baccalaureate and demonstrates clinical expertise in the care of older adults. Categories include gerontological nurse practitioners and gerontological clinical nurse specialists. State boards of nursing define and regulate advanced practice nurses, their roles, certification requirements, and scope of practice. State board requirements differ to some degree, and this causes problems related to consistency and portability (Duffy, 2009). In 2008, the Advanced Practice Registered Nurse (APRN) Work Group and the APRN Joint Dialogue Group published recommendations for nationally recognized standards for education, accreditation, certification, and licensure of APRNs. Criteria that are included in the recommended definition of an APRN include graduate-level education; national certification; advanced clinical knowledge and skills; ability to assume responsibility and accountability for health promotion; and licensure to practice in one of four specific APRN roles, which are certified registered nurse anesthetist, certified nurse-midwife, clinical nurse specialist, or certified nurse practitioner. The regulatory model further specifies that APRNs be qualified to practice with one of six population groups, with one group being adult–gerontology. Each of the six areas of specialization will be certified and regulated by appropriate professional organizations, and the target date for fully implementing this model in all states is 2015 (APRN Consensus Work Group, 2008). It is anticipated that nurses with gerontological specialization will be more in demand than ever because expertise in caring for older adults will be essential to implementing the new model (Duffy, 2009).

Roles of advanced practice nurses include teacher, researcher, consultant, administrator, expert clinician, independent practitioner, care/case manager, individual/group counselor, and multidisciplinary team member/leader. Advanced practice nurses often manage acute and chronic conditions of older adults in their roles as primary care practitioners. GAPNs are knowledgeable about normal aging changes as well as common pathologic conditions of older adults, and their skills include comprehensive assessments of older adults and provision of in-depth prevention and health promotion services. Advanced practice nurses have an important role in long-term care facilities in improving quality of care through direct care and staff education. Their role in providing direct care in long-term care facilities has been expanding since Medicare began covering services of nurse practitioners in 2003.

Evidence-Based Practice for Gerontological Nursing

Standard VII of the ANA *Standards of Professional Gerontological Nursing Performance* mandates that gerontological nurses improve current nursing practice and the future health care for older adults by participating in the generation, testing, utilization, and evaluation of research findings (ANA, 2001). This standard requires nurses at the basic level of practice to ask questions about the care of older adults, participate in studies to address these questions, and apply research findings to improve clinical care of older adults. An important role for gerontological nurses is to examine evidence from systematic literature reviews so that best approaches for care of older adults can be developed (Houde, 2009).

In recent years, resources for evidence-based guidelines have been increasing exponentially and are widely available through reliable Internet sites. Some excellent resources, such as the *Cochrane Review* and the Joanna Briggs Institute, are available only through membership organizations, but many trustworthy guidelines are available through nonprofit agencies, educational institutions, and public agencies (e.g., the National Guideline Clearinghouse). The Hartford Foundation for Geriatric Nursing offers many cost-free resources that specifically address evidence-based nursing care of older adults (available at http://consultgerirn.org/resources). Clinically oriented chapters in this text include evidence-based practice summarizing pertinent evidence-based protocols. In addition, the "Resources" sections at the chapter ends provide information about Internet sites for evidence-based guidelines and clinical practice tools. These sites can be accessed through the**Point**.

Significant events in the growth of gerontological nursing as a specialization

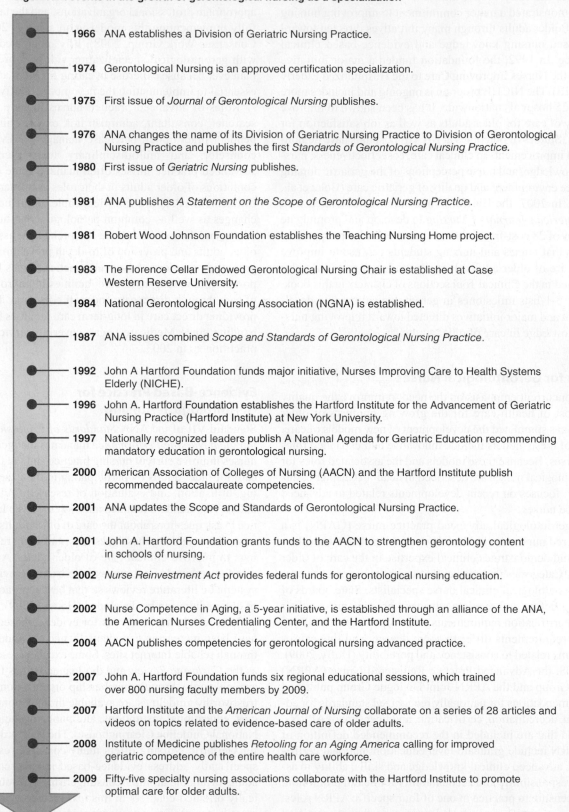

1966   ANA establishes a Division of Geriatric Nursing Practice.

1974   Gerontological Nursing is an approved certification specialization.

1975   First issue of *Journal of Gerontological Nursing* publishes.

1976   ANA changes the name of its Division of Geriatric Nursing Practice to Division of Gerontological Nursing Practice and publishes the first *Standards of Gerontological Nursing Practice.*

1980   First issue of *Geriatric Nursing* publishes.

1981   ANA publishes *A Statement on the Scope of Gerontological Nursing Practice.*

1981   Robert Wood Johnson Foundation establishes the Teaching Nursing Home project.

1983   The Florence Cellar Endowed Gerontological Nursing Chair is established at Case Western Reserve University.

1984   National Gerontological Nursing Association (NGNA) is established.

1987   ANA issues combined *Scope and Standards of Gerontological Nursing Practice.*

1992   John A Hartford Foundation funds major initiative, Nurses Improving Care to Health Systems Elderly (NICHE).

1996   John A. Hartford Foundation establishes the Hartford Institute for the Advancement of Geriatric Nursing Practice (Hartford Institute) at New York University.

1997   Nationally recognized leaders publish A National Agenda for Geriatric Education recommending mandatory education in gerontological nursing.

2000   American Association of Colleges of Nursing (AACN) and the Hartford Institute publish recommended baccalaureate competencies.

2001   ANA updates the Scope and Standards of Gerontological Nursing Practice.

2001   John A. Hartford Foundation grants funds to the AACN to strengthen gerontology content in schools of nursing.

2002   *Nurse Reinvestment Act* provides federal funds for gerontological nursing education.

2002   Nurse Competence in Aging, a 5-year initiative, is established through an alliance of the ANA, the American Nurses Credentialing Center, and the Hartford Institute.

2004   AACN publishes competencies for gerontological nursing advanced practice.

2007   John A. Hartford Foundation funds six regional educational sessions, which trained over 800 nursing faculty members by 2009.

2007   Hartford Institute and the *American Journal of Nursing* collaborate on a series of 28 articles and videos on topics related to evidence-based care of older adults.

2008   Institute of Medicine publishes *Retooling for an Aging America* calling for improved geriatric competence of the entire health care workforce.

2009   Fifty-five specialty nursing associations collaborate with the Hartford Institute to promote optimal care for older adults.

FIGURE 5-1 Significant events in the growth of gerontological nursing as a specialization.

In 1993, the 7-year-old National Center for Nursing Research was elevated to the status of a national institute within the National Institutes of Health (NIH). The National Institute of Nursing Research (NINR) supports multidisciplinary studies on innovative approaches to promoting health and preventing disease, minimizing the effects of acute and chronic illness and disability, and speeding recovery from disease. Since 2000, the NINR has been funding nursing research on topics pertinent to older adults, including care giving issues, independent functioning, quality of life, management of chronic diseases, and care in homes and nursing homes. Nursing Knowledge International, a nonprofit subsidiary of Sigma Theta Tau International (the honor society of nursing), is another nursing organization dedicated to supporting evidence-based knowledge related to nursing care. Nurses are encouraged to visit the Internet sites for these and other organizations listed in the "Resources" section of this chapter for information about nursing research related to older adults.

HEALTH, WELLNESS, AND HEALTH PROMOTION

Nurses often use the terms *health* and *wellness* interchangeably because of the shifting paradigm from the traditional health–illness continuum to a whole-person model. This paradigm shift is evident in holistic nursing definitions of health and wellness. For example, a holistic nursing definition of health is "an individually defined state or process in which the individual (nurse, client, family, group, or community) experiences a sense of well-being, harmony, and unity such that subjective experiences about health, health beliefs, and values are honored; a process of becoming an expanded consciousness" (Mariano, 2009, p. 48). Similarly, a holistic nursing definition of *wellness* is "integrated, congruent functioning aimed toward reaching one's highest potential" (Mariano, 2009). In this text, *health* is defined as the ability of older adults to function at their highest capacity despite the presence of age-related changes and risk factors, whereas *wellness* is an outcome (also called a positive functional consequence) for older adults whose well-being and quality of life is improved through nursing interventions.

The growing emphasis on wellness has resulted not only in increasing recognition of the importance of health promotion but also in a broader focus on self-responsibility. Health promotion refers to programs or interventions that focus on behavior changes directed toward improved health and well-being of individuals, groups, communities, and nations in relation to their environments. Although the concept of health promotion generally includes disease prevention (i.e., risk reduction) and health maintenance (i.e., sustaining a neutral state of health), holistic models also emphasize personal responsibility for health and self-care actions to achieve high-level wellness (Potter & Frisch, 2009). Thus, holistic nursing interventions to promote wellness for older adults inherently involve teaching about actions that are directed toward maintaining and improving all aspects of well-being. Nurses can

use health promotion interventions to enhance wellness by teaching older adults about the following:

- Regularly engaging in several types of physical exercise
- Assuring optimal nutritional intake and avoiding foods associated with risk for disease
- Using stress-reduction methods, such as yoga, meditation, and relaxation
- Fostering healthy relationships with others
- Engaging in self-wellness actions (e.g., getting adequate rest and sleep, taking time for enjoyable activities alone or with others)
- Attending to spiritual growth
- Engaging in holistic wellness practices (e.g., tai chi, imagery, Reiki)

In addition to emphasizing body–mind–spirit interconnectedness, holistic health promotion models also address the relationship between individual behaviors and factors such as motivation, social supports, self-efficacy, quality of life, and cultural and socioeconomic influences. For example, nurses have applied Roy's Adaptation Model to holistic health promotion programs that enhance spirituality and self-efficacy in older adults through physical activity interventions (Rogers & Keller, 2009). In addition, nurses have developed the Health Empowerment Theory and applied it to health promotion interventions that enhance well-being in homebound older adults (Shearer, 2009). Nurses also have applied a lifespan theory, called Selective Optimization With Compensation, to promote self-efficacy, autonomy, and quality of life in health promotion programs for community-living older adults (Grove, Loeb, & Penrod, 2009).

Health Promotion for Older Adults

Health promotion programs are essential not only for preventing chronic conditions but also for reducing mortality. Despite spending more per capita on health care than any other country in the world, the United States has been ranked last among developed nations in preventing avoidable deaths (Zoorob & Morelli, 2008). Studies indicate that 75% of expenditures for health services are associated with preventable chronic conditions, yet only 1% of money spent on health care in the United States is devoted to protecting health and preventing illness and injury (Koffman, Lanza, & Campbell, 2008). Recent reports, such as *Retooling for an Aging America* (National Academy of Sciences, 2008) and *Chronic Care: A Call to Action for Health Reform* (AARP, 2009) strongly advocate for new models of care that focus on health promotion as an integral part of much-needed health care reform.

Many advocacy groups are emphasizing the need to focus more on health promotion and disease prevention in any health system models that are considered part of the health care reform that began in 2008. For example, the official position of the AARP is that we need "to transform our 'sick care' system to a 'health care' system that values and invests in prevention and wellness" (Novelli, 2009). Many organizations are focusing on obesity as a national health issue that needs to be addressed through health promotion. For instance, the American Health Association recently convened a behavioral roundtable to address cardiovascular disease disparities with a focus on the primary prevention of obesity (Wylie-Rosett & Karanja, 2009). The National Center for Chronic Disease Prevention and Health Promotion emphasizes that although much progress has been made in many areas during the past 20 years, health promotion programs that address improved nutrition and increased physical activity are inadequate (Collins, Marks, & Koplan, 2009). An emerging emphasis with regard to health promotion for older adults is on preventing "bounce-back" hospital admissions (i.e., readmission shortly after discharge from a hospital). In one study, the application of a standardized discharge intervention, which included the use of nurse discharge advocates who coordinated plans and prepared patients, lowered readmissions during the first month by about 30% (Jack et al., 2009).

Because of the importance of reducing health care costs, health promotion programs have increasingly focused on evidence-based interventions to prevent, detect, and manage conditions that are leading causes of death and disability (e.g., cardiovascular disease, cancer, stroke). For example, the Centers for Disease Control and Prevention (CDC) is conducting pilot programs to identify people who are at high risk for type 2 diabetes and enroll them in evidence-based diabetes prevention interventions that were identified in a clinical trial (Collins et al., 2009). A Medicare demonstration program that included a strong role for nurses in patient education and individualized health promotion and disease self-management reduced physical functional decline by 54% and could potentially lower total health care expenditures (Meng et al., 2009).

Another focus is on management of chronic conditions that occur more commonly among older adults and affect independent functioning and quality of life. For example, a longitudinal study of well-functioning black and white men and women aged 70 to 79 years found that participation in self-selected exercise activities is independently associated with delaying the onset and progression of frailty (Peterson et al., 2009). Gerontologists also are focusing on health promotion for older caregivers, with emphasis on helping caregivers identify stress-reducing interventions (Lee, 2009).

Even though health promotion interventions are cost-effective ways of preventing disease and disability and improving functioning and quality of life for older adults, older adults as a group receive fewer prevention and screening services than other populations. This is due to inaccurate perceptions that older adults are less responsive to health promotion interventions and that preventive services are less effective after the onset of chronic illness. In reality, health promotion is essential for older adults precisely because they have more chronic conditions, have complex health care needs, and use considerably more health care services than younger adults. Moreover, for the one-fifth of older adults who are in very good health, health promotion programs are essential for supporting continued good health (National Academy of Sciences, 2008).

In addition to having an impact on cost of care, health promotion can have a positive effect on quality of life. A commonly cited goal of gerontological health care is to *add life to years, not just more years to life*, which is synonymous with improved quality of life. The concept of **health-related quality of life** was proposed by the National Center for Chronic Disease and Health Promotion (at the CDC) in 1993 and has been used as a measure of Medicare health outcomes since 2003. Health-related quality of life is measured by a standard set of questions, called "Healthy Days Measures," addressing one's perception of physical and mental health and functioning. Currently, there is increasing attention to improved health-related quality of life as an outcome of health promotion interventions related to specific conditions. For example, a study of visually impaired older adults with comorbidities found that the health promotion intervention of a referral for visual rehabilitation services could have a beneficial effect on the patient's health-related quality of life (van Nispen, de Boer, Hoeijmakers, Ringens, & van Rens, 2009).

Health Promotion Initiatives for Older Adults

During the last four decades, the number of national health promotion initiatives has been increasing and expanding. *Healthy People 2020* (formerly known as *Healthy People 2000* and *Healthy People 2010*) is a well-known program that began in the 1990s and continues today and contains many objectives that are particularly applicable to older adults. The program—designed as a road map for improving the health of all people in the United States—outlines a comprehensive, nationwide agenda for promoting health and preventing illness, disability, and premature death. The two major goals are increasing quality and years of healthy life and eliminating health disparities. For older adults, the first goal is associated with preventing chronic illness as well as exacerbations of existing illnesses. The second goal addresses health disparities that disproportionately affect specific older populations, such as hypertension in African Americans, diabetes in Hispanic and Native American groups, obesity in Hispanic and African American women, and smoking in American Indians and Alaska Natives.

Many governmental and nonprofit organizations, including the CDC, Administration on Aging, American Society on Aging (ASA), and National Council on Aging (NCOA), currently are leading efforts to promote healthy aging, with the recognition that people of all ages can benefit from health-promoting actions. For example, the *Live Well, Live Long: Health Promotion and Disease Prevention for Older Adults* program is a CDC-funded project of the ASA that provides useful information about cultural competence and health literacy as well as specific aspects of health promotion. Nurses can use the web-based modules and resources to teach older adults about diabetes, nutrition, medications, cognitive vitality, physical activity, and safe driving. The *Healthy Aging and Depression* program is another major initiative of the CDC and the National Association of Chronic Disease Directors (NACDD). One goal of this initiative, which began in 2008, is to increase awareness of depression as a major health issue for older adults that can be effectively addressed through community-based programs. The CDC also is sponsoring a major initiative with the Alzheimer's Association, called the *Brain Health Initiative*, to promote cognitive health in diverse populations. This program conducted 75 focus groups and in-depth interviews in English, Spanish, Mandarin, Cantonese, and Vietnamese and with African Americans, American Indians, Asian Americans, Hispanics, non-Hispanic whites, health care practitioners, rural and urban residents, caregivers, and cognitively impaired individuals as an evidence-based framework for designing public health interventions (Laditka et al., 2009). These and other programs that are being implemented through national initiatives are summarized in Box 5-2, along with Web site information about the programs and related resources that nurses can use for health promotion.

Types and Examples of Health Promotion Interventions for Older Adults

Interventions to promote physical and psychosocial well-being include screening programs, risk-reduction interventions, environmental modifications, and health education. This section reviews these types of programs in relation to promoting wellness for older adults. Table 5-1 lists examples of and references for evidence-based programs that have been implemented for older adults. All clinically oriented chapters of this text emphasize health promotion because this is a central focus of the Functional Consequences Model for Promoting Wellness.

Box 5-2 National Health Initiatives and Resources Important to Older Adults

Medicare, www.cms.gov: Covers immunizations and screening services for glaucoma, osteoporosis, and several types of cancer

Brain Health Initiative, www.cdc.gov/aging, www.alz.org: Recommends 44 evidence-based priority action steps to maintain or improve cognitive performance of all adults

Aging States Projects, www.cdc.gov/aging: Provides Opportunity Grants to states to implement evidence-based health promotion and disease prevention programs

Assuring Healthy Caregivers, www.cdc.gov/aging: Provides resources for implementing an evidence-based caregiver intervention program

Healthy Aging Podcast series, www.cdc.gov/aging: Podcast programs about health promotion topics such as smoking, immunizations, and oral health

Healthy Aging and Depression, www.cdc.gov/aging, www.chronicdisease.org: Resources for implementing several evidence-based models for detecting, preventing, and decreasing the severity of depression in older adults

Healthy People 2020, www.HealthyPeople.gov/HP2020: Delineates 10-year national objectives for promoting health and preventing disease

Live Well, Live Long, www.asaging.org/cdc: Provides issue briefs and web-based modules on health promotion for older adults, including information about cultural competency and health literacy

---

Thus, nursing interventions are directed toward improved health, functioning, and quality of life for older adults, with emphasis on teaching older adults and their caregivers about health-promoting activities.

Screening Programs

Screening programs are an essential component of disease prevention because they may detect serious and progressive conditions as early as possible. The National Guideline Clearinghouse publishes numerous evidence-based recommendations for screening related to conditions such as glaucoma, diabetes, hypertension, hyperlipidemia, osteoporosis, hypothyroidism, and many types of cancer. Recommendations focus on conditions that can be accurately detected and effectively treated before they progress to a serious or fatal stage. Cost effectiveness of a screening test is determined according to criteria such as its ability to detect a condition or risk factor at an early stage and without excessive false-positive or false-negative results. Another criteria for recommending a screening test is that early intervention must be superior to waiting until signs or symptoms of disease are present.

A consideration that is particularly pertinent to older adults is the increasing attention to age-based recommendations. For example, screening recommendations for breast, colon, prostate, and cervical cancer are often based on predictions of life expectancy and health status. This is consistent

TABLE 5-1 Examples of Health Promotion Programs for Older Adults

Reference	Example
Abdullah et al., 2008	*Mobile Smoking Cessation Programme:* a pilot program in which trained counselors provide group health education, individual counseling, and a 4-week supply of nicotine replacement therapy for elderly Chinese smokers in Hong Kong
Chiang, Seman, Belza, & Tsai, 2008	*Enhance Fitness:* an evidence-based community exercise program to promote adherence among ethnic older adults
Fleury, Keller, & Perez, 2009	*Mujeres en Accion por Su Salud:* a culturally relevant social support intervention to promote physical activity among Hispanic women
Logsdon, McCurry, Pike, & Teri, 2009	*Resources and Activities for Life Long Independence:* an evidence-based exercise program that uses behavioral principles to improve physical activity in people with mild cognitive impairment
Meng et al., 2009	Medicare demonstration project that used patient education, individualized coaching, and physician care management to reduce decline in physical functioning during the 22-month study period
Neill & Powell, 2009	*Senior Health Mobile Project:* an innovative program to deliver mobile health and wellness services to older adults in rural Idaho
Nguyen et al., 2008	*Silver Sneakers:* Medicare participants were enrolled in a health club as a cost-effective way of improving health; 2 years after the start date, health care costs for participants who used the health club were significantly lower than for those who did not
Novelli, 2009	*Wellness Tour:* A health promotion program of AARP and Walgreens that uses nine buses staffed by trained medical personnel to make 2000 stops in 300 cities to provide 1.3 million free screenings for cholesterol, blood pressure, bone density, glucose levels, waist circumference, and body mass index; educational materials to promote self-responsibility for health
Perez & Fleury, 2009	*Intervencion de Motivacion Para Actividad Fisica:* a culturally relevant motivational intervention to promote physical activity among Hispanic women
Rejeski et al., 2009	*Lifestyle Interventions and Independence for Elders Pilot:* a 10-week group-mediated behavioral program that improved functional status of participants and enhanced long-term rates of adherence
Shenson, Benson, & Harris, 2008	*Sickness Prevention Achieved Through Regional Collaboration (SPARC):* a program that provided immunizations and screening for cancer and cardiovascular disease in collaboration with area agencies on aging
Tan et al., 2009	*Experience Corps:* a program that used a high-intensity senior volunteer program as a health promotion intervention to improve physical activity in high-risk older adults
Wilcox, Dowda, et al., 2009	*Active for Life:* an initiative that evaluated two evidence-based behavioral programs to increase physical activity in almost 2000 older adults from nine community-based organizations

with the current focus on increasing years of healthy living rather than on simply extending the quantity of life. Although the intent of these recommendations is to target those older adults who are most likely to benefit, this does not always happen. One study found that many older women in poor health were screened for cancer, whereas many of those in good health did not receive recommended screenings (Schonberg, Leveille, & Marcantonio, 2008).

Another consideration related to screening programs for older adults is the need to address health beliefs that are likely to influence participation. For example, Korean American women have very low rates of mammography for breast cancer screening. Nursing research indicates that this low rate is attributable to a higher level of perceived barriers and lower levels of perceived seriousness and benefits among older Korean American women (Eun, Lee, Kim, & Fogg, 2009).

Many organizations disseminate guidelines for health promotion interventions, and they are not always in agreement, especially with regard to recommendations for older adults. The American Cancer Society, the United States Preventive Services Task Force, and the Agency for Healthcare Research and Quality are some of the organizations that are prominent in developing and posting guidelines for preventive care. Box 5-3 summarizes some of the more widely agreed-on guidelines for use when educating older adults about health promotion interventions.

Screening for vitamin D deficiency is a major focus of recent research and clinical practice because between 25% and 57% of adults in the United States have low levels of vitamin D (Lee, O'Keefe, Bell, Hensrud, & Holick, 2008). Researchers examining trends in the U.S. population have found that average serum 25(OH)D level dropped from 30 ng/mL between 1988 and 1994 to 24 ng/mL between 2001 and 2004 (Ginde, Liu, & Camargo, 2009). One study of 6000 community-dwelling men between the ages of 65 and 99 years found that one-quarter of the subjects had a vitamin D level lower than 20 ng/mL (Orwoll et al., 2009). Factors that increase the risk for vitamin D deficiency include older age, smoking, obesity, renal or liver disease, and lack of exposure to sunlight. Studies have found that older adults need to maintain a serum 25(OH)D level of at least 30 ng/mL to reduce the risk for falls, cancer, osteoporosis, cognitive impairment, autoimmune deficiencies, cardiovascular disease, and periodontal disease (Buell et al., 2009; Perez-Lopez, 2009; Stechschulte, Kirsner, & Federman, 2009). Studies also indicate that bone health and physical performance of older adults are likely to improve with serum 25(OH)D levels above 50 to 60 ng/mL (Kuchuk, Pluijm, Schoor, Smit, & Lips, 2009). Evidence-based guidelines point to the importance of measuring 25(OH)D levels in all nursing home residents and if the level is below 30 ng/mL, treating aggressively to raise the level (Morley, 2009).

Box 5-3 Guidelines for Prevention and Health Promotion Interventions for Older Adults

Immunizations
For All Older Adults
- **Tetanus-diphtheria** booster shot every 10 years
- **Influenza** annually at beginning of influenza season
- **Pneumovax** once after age 65 years; booster after 5 years if initial vaccination was before age 65 years or if other risk factors are present
- **Herpes zoster** (shingles) once after the age of 60 years, regardless of prior status with exposure or infection

For At-Risk Older Adults
- **Hepatitis A and B**
- **Measles, mumps, rubella** if evidence of lack of immunity and significant risk for exposure
- **Varicella** if evidence of lack of immunity and significant risk for exposure

Screening
For All Older Adults
- **Blood pressure** checks at least annually, more frequently if range is 130–139 mm Hg systolic or 85–90 mm Hg diastolic or if other risk factors are present (e.g., diabetes, African American race)
- **Serum cholesterol** every 5 years, more frequently in people with risk such as personal or family history of cardiovascular disease
- **Fecal occult blood and rectal examination** annually
- **Sigmoidoscopy** every (3 to) 5 years after age 50 years and until age 85 years
- **Visual acuity and glaucoma screening** annually
- **Breast examination:** self-examination monthly, annually by primary care practitioner

For Women
- **Pap smear and pelvic examination:** annually until three consecutive negative exams, then every 2–3 years; discontinue after 65 years of age if three consecutive negative exams
- **Mammogram** annually or biannually between 50 and 69 years, every 1–3 years between 70 and 85 years

For Men
- **Digital rectal examination** annually

For At-Risk Older Adults
- **Blood glucose level**
- **Thyroid function**
- **Heart function (electrocardiography)**
- **Bone density**
- **Mental status assessment**
- **Screening for dementia, depression, substance abuse**
- **Urinary incontinence assessment**
- **Functional assessment**
- **Screening for adverse medication effects and drug interactions**
- **Skin cancer assessment**
- **Fall risk assessment**
- **Pressure ulcer assessment**
- **Elder abuse or neglect assessment**

For Men
- **Prostate-specific antigen (PSA) blood test**

Health Promotion Counseling
For All Older Adults (Unless Contraindicated)
- **Exercise:** at least 30 minutes of moderate-intensity physical activity daily
- **Nutrition:** adequate intake of all vitamins and minerals, especially calcium and antioxidants
- **Dental care and prophylaxis:** every 6 months
- **Protective measures:** seat belts, sunscreens, smoke detectors, fall risk prevention

For Older Adults if Applicable
- **Smoking cessation**
- **Substance abuse cessation**
- **Weight loss**
- **Vitamin supplements or low-dose aspirin**

Risk-Reduction Interventions

Risk-reduction interventions, which are based on an assessment of the risk for developing a particular condition, are directed toward reducing the chance of developing that condition. Some risk-reduction interventions (e.g., vaccinations) are applicable to all older adults, and other interventions vary according to specific risk factors and the health level of an older person. Risk assessment tools have been developed for various conditions pertinent to older adults, including falls, incontinence, heart disease, pressure ulcers, and elder abuse and neglect. These tools often include a rating scale to identify people who are most likely to develop a particular condition so that health care professionals can plan and implement preventive interventions for them. These tools also serve to identify risk factors that can be addressed through preventive interventions.

Even without formal assessment tools, however, health care professionals can usually identify risk factors that can be addressed to prevent disease or disability. Priority usually is given to reducing the risk factors that are most dominant or likely to have the most serious negative consequences. For example, health promotion interventions for a relatively healthy older adult with a history of hypertension, hypercholesterolemia, and family history of heart attacks would address risk factors for heart disease. Health promotion interventions for a frail older adult who is in a skilled care unit and who is recovering from a fractured hip would focus on risk for falls.

For all older adults, risk-reduction interventions include lifestyle factors, such as weight management, optimal nutrition, adequate physical activity, sufficient sleep, avoidance of secondhand smoke, and appropriate stress-relieving techniques. Smoking cessation is a risk-reduction activity for all people who smoke. Health promotion activities to reduce risk may also include the use of over-the-counter medications (e.g., low-dose aspirin), nutritional supplements (e.g., vitamins), and complementary and alternative therapies (e.g., yoga).

Some risk-reduction interventions are recommended for all, or most, older adults. For example, for many years, vaccinations for influenza, pneumonia, and tetanus have been routinely recommended for all older adults. In addition, in 2006, a herpes zoster vaccination for people aged 60 years and older was approved. Results of a large, randomized, placebo-controlled clinical trial found that, compared with placebo, the vaccination reduced the incidence of herpes zoster by 51% and postherpetic neuralgia by 66% (Gelb, 2009).

Environmental Modifications

Environmental modifications are health promotion activities when they reduce risks or improve a person's level of functioning. The Functional Consequences Model for Promoting Wellness addresses environmental modifications as health promotion interventions in relation to many aspects of functioning in clinically oriented chapters of this text. For example, environmental modifications can be effective health promotion interventions when their implementation reduces fall risks (Chapter 22), improves hearing and vision (Chapters 16 and 17), and prevents urinary incontinence (Chapter 19).

Health Education

Health education is an essential component of health promotion because it focuses on teaching people to engage in self-care activities that are preventive and wellness enhancing. For example, a randomized trial found that tailored health education materials were effective in improving self-care behaviors of adults at risk for skin cancer (Glanz, Schoenfeld, & Steffan, 2010). Similarly, an educational intervention to improve recognition of heart attack and stroke symptoms was directed toward improving the ability of older adults to seek immediate medical attention when appropriate (Bell et al., 2009).

Nurses incorporate health education not only in relation to specific conditions but also in relation to lifestyle factors that affect health and functioning. For example, engaging in regular exercise is a major focus of health education because lack of physical activity is well recognized as a risk factor that contributes to numerous unhealthy conditions. Additional topics of health education that are important for all adults are nutrition, dental care, and avoidance of smoking and secondhand smoke (see Chapters 18 and 21). Clinically oriented chapters of this text contain Intervention Boxes with guidelines for teaching older adults and their caregivers about specific aspects of health and functioning (refer to list at the end of the table of contents in the front of this book). Intervention Boxes can also be found on the book's accompanying Web site. Resources for culturally specific health promotion materials that are available from governmental or nonprofit organizations are listed in the "Resources" sections of this and other chapters (e.g., chapters 2 and 20).

Promotion of Physical Activity as a Nursing Intervention for Wellness

Articles about the need for increased physical activity are ubiquitous in lay and professional literature, and physical activity has emerged as the most widely heralded health promotion intervention today. In recent years, there is increasing emphasis on the premise that moderate-intensity physical activity can improve overall health and quality of life and lower the risk for disease (Haskell, Blair, & Hill, 2009; Kruger, Buchner, & Prohaska, 2009; White, Wojcicki, & McCauley, 2009). Studies have found that adequate exercise decreases the risks for stroke, obesity, osteoporosis, sarcopenia, type 2 diabetes, loss of function, and some forms of cancer (Blair & Morris, 2009; Elsawy & Higgins, 2010). Some recent studies about physical activity and older adults are as follows:

- In a sample of 884 adults aged 65 years and older, leisure-time walking was associated with many positive health outcomes, including the prevention of cognitive decline (Prohaska et al., 2009).
- A study of 846 people aged 66 to 98 years at death found that physical activity in middle and later life lowered the risk for dementia, impaired mobility, and the need for inpatient or long-term care (Bonsdorff et al., 2009).
- A longitudinal study of 2205 men indicated that increased physical activity during middle age was associated with reduced mortality to the same level as that associated with smoking cessation (Byberg et al., 2009).
- A meta-analysis found that increased physical activity was associated with modest improvements in quality of life among adults with chronic illnesses (Conn, Hafdahl, & Brown, 2009).
- A pilot study of 102 sedentary adults aged 70 to 89 years at increased risk for cognitive disability showed a positive association between moderate-intensity physical activity and improved cognitive function (Williamson et al., 2009).
- A randomized trial of 544 older adults found statistically significant benefits of participating in a multiple-component physical activity program with regard to self-efficacy, exercise participation, adherence in the face of barriers, and increased upper and lower body strength (Hughes, Seymour, Campbell, Whitelaw, & Bazzarre, 2009).

Despite the wealth of undisputed evidence about the beneficial effects of physical activity for older adults, less than one third of older people in the United States engage in it regularly. Nurses take many roles in promoting physical activity for older adults, in particular, teaching older adults about the health benefits of physical activity. It also is important to teach about public health recommendations for type, frequency, duration, and intensity of physical activity (Wilcox, Sharkey, et al., 2009). Nurses also assess for and address other factors that positively or negatively influence an older adult to participate in regular physical activity. Nurses can use Box 5-4 as a guide to teaching older adults about recommended exercises. The University of Iowa Gerontological Nursing Interventions Research Center has updated its evidence-based protocol related to exercise promotion for older adults (Jitramontree, 2007). See the Evidence-Based Practice Resources section at the end of this chapter.

BOX 5-4 Health Education About Types of Exercise

Type	Definition	Benefits	Intensity	Frequency
Aerobic (e.g., brisk walking, jogging, walking up stairs)	Activity that requires the body to use oxygen to produce the energy necessary for the activity	Lowers blood pressure, strengthens heart muscle, improves lipids and triglycerides, diminishes blood glucose, decreases intra-abdominal fat, decreases risk for cardiovascular disease, improves self-esteem, relieves symptoms of anxiety and depression	Identify your target heart rate by subtracting your age in years from 220 (this is the maximum heart rate) and multiplying by 0.65	2.5 hours weekly of moderate intensity OR 1.25 hours weekly of vigorous intensity (in episodes of at least 10 minutes)
Strength or resistance training (stretch bands, weights, strap-on sandbags, bicep curls, bench presses	Performance of muscle contractions against a resistance that is greater than usual for that muscle; slow and controlled movements of major muscled groups such as arms, back, hips, chest, and shoulders, with exhalation during exertion and inhalation during return to the starting position	Improves balance and diminishes risk for falls, strengthens musculoskeletal system, improves function and independence, decreases risk for osteoporosis, favorably modifies risk factors for cardiovascular disease and type 2 diabetes	You should be able to repeat the movement 8 consecutive times, but not more than 12 times, before experiencing significant muscle fatigue	8–10 different sets of exercises working all major muscle groups, each repeated 8–12 times, several days a week
Stretching (e.g., yoga, range-of-motion exercises)	Activity that improves body flexibility	Increases flexibility, reduces muscle soreness, improves performance of daily activities	Stretch muscle groups, but not to the point of pain, and hold for 10–30 seconds	Repeat each stretch at least 4 times, a minimum of 2–4 times weekly

Notes: Physical activity is any skeletal muscle activity that causes energy expenditure. Exercise refers to structured and repetitive body movements performed with the goal of attaining physical fitness.

THE TRANSTHEORETICAL MODEL OF HEALTH PROMOTION

Health promotion programs that focus on self-care and wellness usually address motivation and personal responsibility as factors that significantly influence health-related behaviors. This is appropriate because disease prevention often requires a change from detrimental health-related behaviors to those that enhance wellness. Once behavior change has been initiated, the new healthier behaviors must be maintained. Initiation and maintenance of these changes involve both motivation and action steps. The more ingrained and rewarding or pleasurable the behaviors that must be changed, the more difficult it is to refrain from these activities. Some unhealthy behaviors, such as cigarette smoking, have a strong addictive component that increases the difficulty of behavior change. Similarly, the more comfortable a person is with the absence of healthy behaviors, such as physical activity, the more difficult it will be to develop healthier behaviors. The role of gerontological health care professionals in health promotion interventions is to lead and support the older person through the stages of change involved in replacing unhealthy behaviors with health-promoting behaviors.

The **Transtheoretical Model** (TTM), developed by Prochaska and DiClemente, has been widely used by health care professionals to explain stages of behavior change. During the last three decades, the TTM has been used successfully in programs for stress management, sun exposure, smoking cessation, medication compliance, alcohol and drug cessa-

tion, diet and weight control, and screening for cancers. Application of this model specifically in gerontological health care settings is described in detail in *Promoting Exercise and Behavior Change in Older Adults* (Burbank & Riebe, 2002).

The TTM is called the "stages-of-change" model because it describes five specific stages through which a person progresses in accomplishing behavior changes. In the first stage, *precontemplation*, the person is unaware of the problem, is in denial of the need for change, or is resistant to change. At this stage, the person has no intention of changing his or her behaviors within the next 6 months. Appropriate health promotion interventions for a person in this stage include providing information about the problem behavior and providing unconditional encouragement for thinking about behavior change. When working with an older adult in this stage, gerontological nurses can offer information, discuss their own beliefs, and help the person identify the personal benefits of the health-promoting behaviors. The nurse also can acknowledge the person's perspective and point out the negative consequences of current behaviors.

The second stage, *contemplation*, is characterized by an intention to change in the foreseeable future, based on some acknowledgment of the negative consequences of current behaviors and positive consequences of different behaviors. The person is likely to ask questions and to seek information about the short- and long-term risks and benefits of various behaviors. He or she is likely to be ambivalent about giving up a rewarding activity or taking on an activity that is viewed as difficult or less enjoyable. During this stage, the gerontological nurse can help the person see that the benefits outweigh the disadvantages, even though the person may not experience the benefits immediately. Appropriate health promotion interventions for this stage include providing additional information about the risks and benefits and exploring with the person how he or she can begin establishing personal goals for a healthier lifestyle. Interventions also include increasing the person's sense of self-efficacy by helping the person to see himself or herself practicing these new behaviors. When working with an older adult in this stage, it is helpful to express confidence in the person's ability to develop health-promoting behaviors.

Stage three, the *preparation* stage, is characterized by some ambivalence about the unhealthy behavior but a stronger inclination to change to healthier behaviors. The person acknowledges the need for change, expresses serious intent to adopt the healthier behaviors within the next month, and begins to identify strategies for implementing them. During this stage, people usually benefit from support from family and friends, and they are likely to state their intentions and seek help from others in accomplishing their goals. Gerontological nurses can support and provide positive reinforcement for the person's intent to change; they also can point out the progress that the person already has made in developing an action plan. An important role for nurses is to assist with developing a plan and identifying the person's goals and small-step strategies to achieve them. Although discussing the barriers to changing behaviors might be necessary, it is important to focus on the benefits of the new behavior. Planning strategies for dealing with anticipated difficulties in implementing the plan is also helpful.

Action, the fourth stage, occurs when the person has already made the behavior change, but the changes have been practiced for less than 6 months. At this stage, people usually do not fully experience the benefits of the new behavior and are vulnerable to resuming prior unhealthy behaviors or giving up the new healthy behaviors. At the same time, they are likely to have high levels of self-efficacy and to feel good about the progress they have made. Health promotion interventions during this stage are directed toward reinforcing the progress that has been made as well as toward identifying any barriers to continuing the healthy behaviors. Gerontological nurses can help the older adult identify motivators, establish a reward system, and plan strategies for overcoming the identified obstacles. They also can ask about support from friends and family and help the person identify ways of extending their support system if necessary.

Stage five, *maintenance*, occurs when the person has continued the healthy behaviors for 6 months or longer. By this time, the person is experiencing positive effects of the healthier behavior and the risk of relapse is less. During this stage, levels of self-efficacy are usually high and the person is motivated to maintain the healthier lifestyle. Because the person has less need for external support, the role of the gerontological nurse diminishes. Health promotion interventions during this stage include reinforcement of progress and positive feedback about the healthier behaviors. In addition, the nurse can ask about any difficulties in maintaining the progress and help the person identify strategies to overcome any difficulties.

*M*rs. H. is 72 years old and visits the local senior center three times weekly for meals and social activities. Once a month she comes to see you to have her blood pressure checked. You have recently studied the TTM and are interested in applying it to your clinical work in the Senior Wellness Program. Mrs. H. takes medication for high blood pressure and has expressed concern about heart disease. When you discuss risk factors for heart disease with Mrs. H., she says that she would like to incorporate more physical activity into her daily life, as long as it doesn't worsen her arthritis. She agrees to begin meeting with you regularly to develop a plan. Table 5-2 shows how you might apply the TTM to your work with Mrs. H.

THINKING POINTS

Precontemplation Stage

- From a health promotion perspective, how would you assess Mrs. H.'s understanding of the role of exercise in prevention of heart disease? What misconceptions would you want to address?
- What are the goals of your teaching interventions at this stage?

Contemplation Stage

- How would you assess Mrs. H.'s perception of the advantages and disadvantages of increased levels of exercise?
- What are the goals of your teaching interventions at this stage?
- What additional teaching points would you incorporate in your health promotion interventions at this time?

Preparation Stage

- What additional assessment questions would you ask Mrs. H.?
- What are the goals of your teaching interventions at this stage?
- What additional teaching points would you incorporate, particularly with regard to Mrs. H.'s concerns about her arthritis?

Action Stage

- What concerns would you have about Mrs. H. during this stage, and what additional questions would you ask?
- What additional teaching points would you make?

Maintenance Stage

- What additional assessment questions would you ask Mrs. H.?
- What additional teaching points would you make?

TABLE 5-2 Applying the Transtheoretical Model to Mrs. H.

Stage	Nurse	Mrs. H.
I: Precontemplation		
Assessment	"I know you're concerned about preventing heart disease because you've talked with me about your high blood pressure and you pay attention to avoiding high-fat foods. How do you think you rate on a scale of 1 to 10, with 1 being the lowest level and 10 being the best, in level of physical activity for preventing heart disease?"	"I would rate myself about 10. I take the dog out for a 5-minute walk every morning. My friend says we don't need more than 10 minutes of walking a day after we're 70 years old."
Intervention	"Did you know that there is extremely good evidence that 30 minutes of physical activity every day—even if it's not done all at once—is a good measure for protecting against heart disease? Would you be willing to read this pamphlet from the American Heart Association and let me know what you think when I see you again next week?"	"I've seen that before, but I'll try to read it this week if I have a chance."
II: Contemplation		
Assessment	"Now that you've had a chance to read that brochure, what's your understanding of the role of physical activity in preventing heart problems?"	"I think the Heart Association is on an exercise kick—they must think we all want to participate in marathons! Maybe they have a point about walking more than 15 minutes a day, but don't they realize that those of us who are in our 70s have a lot of problems walking? Most of us have arthritis. I think that brochure was written for people in their 20s, but on the other hand, maybe they do know what they're talking about."
Intervention	"From what I know, the Heart Association focuses on helping people prevent heart disease through healthy habits. They strongly urge everyone to do physical exercise for 30 minutes every day to keep the heart healthy. Many studies of people of all ages support this recommendation. You already walk 5 minutes with your dog every day, so you've gotten a good start on daily exercise. I bet your dog would love to go just a little farther each day and you would be quite capable of increasing your walk by just a little bit."	"Well, the dog is getting pretty fat, and it would probably do her good to get out for another walk in the evening. But it's hard enough for me to get out once a day with the weather as cold as it is right now. With my arthritis, I think I should wait a couple of months until the weather is warmer."
III: Preparation		
Assessment	"Since we met a couple of months ago, what are your current thoughts about increasing your walking?"	"I've been doing a lot of thinking about what we discussed, and now that spring is finally here, I think it's time to increase my walking time by a little bit each day. I just hope my arthritis doesn't get worse if I walk more."
Intervention	"So, have you thought of a plan that might work for you? Can you identify people who might be helpful in supporting your efforts?"	"Well, to begin with, I thought I could walk for 10 minutes every morning instead of 5—my dog sure would like that. I could increase that by 5 minutes every few weeks until I get up to 30 minutes a day. I've told my daughter that I'm trying to do more walking, and she said she might come over and walk with me and the dog on Saturdays. I do worry about my arthritis, though."
IV: Action		
Assessment	"It's so good to hear that you've been increasing your walking time for 3 months now. Congratulations on getting up to 30 minutes a day. How are you feeling about that?"	"My dog sure likes it, but I'm not sure that it's doing any good for me. I guess it feels good to pay attention to my health, but I haven't noticed that I'm feeling any better physically—at least not yet. My daughter came with me for the first few weeks and that was a good chance to see her, but she hasn't been coming for the last 3 weeks."
Intervention	"You deserve a lot of credit for accomplishing your goal—do you give yourself any rewards? It sounds as though you're disappointed that your daughter stopped walking with you—is there anyone else who might walk with you?"	"I guess I do deserve some credit—I did buy myself a new pair of walking shoes last week. A neighbor lady has talked to me about my walking and she said she'd like to get out there and join me, but I didn't encourage that because I thought my daughter would be coming with me. Maybe I'll invite her along—she could use the exercise, too."
V: Maintenance		
Assessment	"Congratulations on walking for 30 minutes every day for 7 months—that's quite an accomplishment and a nice gift for yourself and your health. You also deserve credit for getting your neighbor to join you at least a couple of days a week. Are you concerned about any temptations to cut down on your walking routine?"	"Thanks for the encouragement—my neighbor says she appreciates me inviting her along, and I enjoy the chance to keep up on neighborhood happenings by chatting with her when we walk. I am a little concerned about keeping up with the walking during the winter. I don't even take the dog out when it snows."
Intervention	"Have you thought about walking in the mall when the weather is bad? I'm not sure if you can take the dog along, but the mall opens every day an hour before the stores open so that walkers can come. I understand there's quite a group that walks there in the mornings."	"That sounds like a good idea—my neighbor mentioned that we might go there in bad weather. I think I'll try that out—maybe if I went to the mall, I could get my daughter to meet me there on Saturdays."

Chapter Highlights

Gerontology and Geriatrics

- Gerontology and geriatrics are areas of professional specialization that have evolved since the mid-1940s to address the unique needs of older adults.
- These specialties initially focused on problems associated with aging, but the current focus is on quality-of-life issues and promoting optimal health and functioning.

Gerontological Nursing

- Gerontological nursing was first recognized as a nursing specialty during the 1960s, and major initiatives continue to encourage the development of this much-needed area of expertise (Box 5-1, Figure 5-1).
- Innovative models of care have paved the way for many roles for gerontological nurses, including opportunities for advanced practice nurses.
- Nurses have many resources for information about evidence-based practice with regard to care of older adults.

Health, Wellness, and Health Promotion

- Nurses have important roles in health promotion interventions, which are essential for preventing chronic conditions, reducing mortality, and improving quality of life for older adults (Box 5-2).
- Many major national initiatives focus on health promotion for older adults and provide valuable resources that nurses can use (Box 5-2).
- Types of health promotion interventions applicable to older adults include screening programs, risk-reduction interventions, environmental modifications, and health education to promote good health practices (Table 5-1, Box 5-3).
- Nurses have important roles in teaching older adults about the benefits of physical activity and promoting exercise (Box 5-4).

The Transtheoretical Model of Health Promotion

- Gerontological nurses can apply the TTM of Health Promotion to address the many disease prevention and health promotion interventions that require a change in health-related behaviors (Table 5-2).
- The TTM describes five specific stages in accomplishing behavior changes: precontemplation, contemplation, preparation, action, and maintenance.

Critical Thinking Exercises

1. Describe the development of gerontological nursing from the 1960s to the present.
2. You are asked to give a presentation to beginning nursing students to recruit them for an elective class called "Nursing for Wellness in Older Adults." What topics would you expect to be covered in this course and what points would you make to encourage them to enlist in this course?
3. You are discussing with your fellow students the choices you will be making about a practice area after graduation. You tell them that you are planning to specialize in gerontological nursing, and they challenge your decision with statements such as "You'll be bored to death taking care of old fogies. Why don't you specialize in something exciting like trauma care? Besides, there's not much to do about the conditions of older folks, and what's the challenge in taking care of people who aren't going to get better?" How do you respond to these statements?
4. Identify one health-related behavior that you would like to change in your life (e.g., smoking cessation, increased level of exercise, decreased dietary fat intake) and develop a care plan for your behavior change using the TTM of Health Promotion (as in the case study).

Resources

For links to these resources and additional helpful Internet resources related to this chapter, visit thePoint at http://thePoint.lww.com/Miller6e.

Clinical Tools

Hartford Institute for Geriatric Nursing
- *Try this: Best Practices in Nursing Care to Older Adults*
  Issue 21 (2007), Immunizations for Older Adults
  Issue 27 (2010), General Screening Recommendations for Chronic Disease and Risk Factors in Older Adults

Evidence-Based Practice

National Guideline Clearinghouse
- Practice guidelines from numerous professional organizations from the United States and many other countries with delineation of level of evidence to support recommendations
- Guideline syntheses for topics such as Alzheimer's disease
- Updated protocol related to exercise promotion (from the University of Iowa Gerontological Nursing Interventions Research Center)

Hartford Institute for Geriatric Nursing
- "*Try This* series of best practice assessment tools (all updated or developed during or after 2007)
- "How to *Try This*" series of 28 cost-free and web-based videos and articles (developed and published between 2007 and 2009) illustrating application of geriatric assessment tools
- Protocols from *Evidence-Based Geriatric Nursing Protocols for Best Practice, 3rd ed.,* by E. Capezuti, D. Zwicker, M. Mezey, & T. Fulmer (Eds.), (2008). New York: Springer Publishing Co.

Health Education

Gerontological Nursing

American Nurses Association (ANA)
Hartford Institute for Geriatric Nursing
National Gerontological Nursing Association (NGNA)

National Institute of Nursing Research
Nurses Improving Care to Health Systems Elders (NICHE)
Sigma Theta Tau International

Health Promotion Materials
African American Health Program: One Healthy Life
Asian American Health Initiative
Lifelong Fitness Alliance (formerly Fifty Plus Fitness Association)
National Alliance for Hispanic Health
National Center for Chronic Disease Prevention and Health Promotion
National Institute on Aging
National Rural Health Association
Native Elder Health Care Resource Center
Office of Disease Prevention and Health Promotion
Office of Minority Health Resource Center
Partnership for Prevention

Note: All these organizations provide culturally specific health education materials, with many in non-English languages.

REFERENCES

AARP. (2009). *Beyond 50.09: Chronic care: A call to action for health reform.* Washington DC: AARP.

Abdullah, A. S. M., Lam, T. H., Chan, S. K., Leung, G. M., Chi, I., Ho, W. W., & Chan, S. S. (2008). Effectiveness of a mobile smoking cessation service in reaching elderly smokers and predictors of quitting. *BMC Geriatrics, 8*(25), 1–9.

American Nurses Association. (2001). *Scope and standards of gerontological nursing practice* (22nd ed.). Washington, DC: Author.

APRN Consensus Work Group & the National Council of State Boards of Nursing APRN Advisory Committee. (July 7, 2008). Consensus Model for APRN Regulation: Licensure, Accreditation, Certification & Education.

Barba, B. E., & Fay, V. (2009). Does continuing education in gerontology lead to changes in nursing practice? *Journal of Gerontological Nursing, 35*(4), 11–17.

Bell, M., Lommel, T., Fischer, J. G., Lee, J. S., Reddy, S., & Johnson, M. A. (2009). Improved recognition of heart attack and stroke symptoms after a community-based intervention for older adults, Georgia, 2006–2007. *Preventing Chronic Disease, 6*(2), 1–11.

Blair, S. N., & Morris, J. N. (2009). Healthy hearts—and the universal benefits of being physically active: Physical activity and health. *Annals of Epidemiology, 19*, 253–256.

Boltz, M., Capezuti, E., Bowar-Ferres, S., Norman, R., Secic, M., Kim, H., . . . Fulmer, T. (2008). Changes in geriatric care environment associated with NICHE (Nurses Improving Care for HealthSystem Elders). *Geriatric Nursing, 29*(3), 176–185.

Bonsdorff, von M. B., Rantanen, T., Leinonen, R., Kujala, U. M., Törmäkangas, T., Manty, M., & Heikkinen, E. (2009). Physical activity history and end-of-life hospital and long-term care. *Journal of Gerontology Medical Sciences, 64A*, 778–784.

Buell, J. S., Scott, T. M., Dawson-Hughes, B., Dallal, G. E., Rosenberg, I. H., Folstein, M. F., & Tucker, K. L. (2009). Vitamin D is associated with cognitive function in elders receiving home health services. *Journal of Gerontology Medical Sciences, 64A*, 888–895.

Burbank, P. M., & Riebe, D. (Eds.), (2002). *Promoting exercise and behavior change in older adults.* New York: Springer.

Byberg, L., Melhus, H., Gedeborg, R., Sundström, J., Ahlbom, A., Zethelius, B., . . . Michaëlsson, K. (2009). Total mortality after changes in leisure time physical activity in 50 year old men: 35 year follow-up of population based cohort. *British Medical Journal, 338*, 1–8.

Chiang, K. C., Seman, L., Belza, B., & Tsai, J. H. C. (2008). "It is Our Exercise Family": Experiences of ethnic older adults in a group-based exercise program. *Preventing Chronic Disease, 5*(1), 1–12.

Collins, J. L., Marks, J. S., & Koplan, J. P. (2009). Chronic disease prevention and control: Coming of age at the centers for disease control and prevention. *Preventing Chronic Disease, 6*(3), 1–9.

Conn, V. S., Hafdahl, A. R., & Brown, L. M. (2009). Meta-analysis of quality-of-life outcomes from physical activity interventions. *Nursing Research, 58*, 175–183.

Douglas-Kersellius, N. V. (2009). The comprehensive geriatric education program. *Journal of Gerontological Nursing, 35*(4), 3–4.

Duffy, E. (2009). The future of the gerontological advanced practice nurse. *Geriatric Nursing, 30*, 71–74.

Elsawy, B., & Higgins, D. O. (2010). Physical activity guidelines for older adults. *American Family Physician, 81*(1), 55–59.

Eun, Y., Lee, E. J., Kim, M. J., & Fogg, L. (2009). Breast cancer screening beliefs among older Korean American women. *Journal of Gerontological Nursing, 35*, 40–50.

Fleury, J., Keller, C., & Perez, A. (2009). Social support theoretical perspective. *Geriatric Nursing, 30*(2S), 211–214.

Frank, L. K. (1946). Gerontology. *Journal of Gerontology, 1*(1), 1–11.

Gelb, L. D. (2009). Reducing the incidence and severity of herpes zoster and PHN with zoster vaccination. *Journal of American Osteopathic Association, 109*(Suppl. 2), S18–S21.

Ginde, A. A., Liu, M. C., & Camargo, C. A. (2009). Demographic differences and trends of vitamin D deficiency in the US population, 1988–2004. *Archives of Internal Medicine, 169*, 626–632.

Glanz, K., Schoenfeld, E. R., & Steffen, A. (2010). A randomized trial of tailored skin cancer prevention messages for adults: Project SCAPE. *American Journal of Public Health, 100*, 735–741.

Grove, L. J., Loeb, S. J., & Penrod, J. (2009). Selective optimization with compensation. *Clinical Nurse Specialist, 23*, 25–32.

Haskell, W. L., Blair, S. N., & Hill, J. O. (2009). Physical activity: Health outcomes and importance for public policy. *Preventive Medicine, 49*(4):280–282.

Houde, S. C. (2009). The systematic review of the literature: A tool for evidence-based policy. *Journal of Gerontological Nursing, 35*, 9–12.

Hughes, S. L., Seymour, R. B., Campbell, R. T., Whitelaw, N., & Bazzarre, T. (2009). Best-practice physical activity programs for older adults: Findings from the National Impact Study. *American Journal of Public Health, 99*, 362–368.

Jack, B. W., Chetty, V. K., Anthony, D., Greenwald, J. L., Sanchez, G. M., Johnson, A. E., . . . Culpepper, L. (2009). A reengineered hospital discharge program to decrease rehospitalization: A randomized trial. *Annals of Internal Medicine, 150*, 178–187.

Jitramontree, E. (2007). *Evidence-based practice guideline: Exercise promotion: Walking in elders.* Iowa City, IA: University of Iowa Gerontological Nursing Interventions Research Center.

Koffman, D. M. M., Lanza, A., & Campbell, K. P. (2008). A purchaser's guide to clinical preventive services: A tool to improve health care coverage for prevention. *Preventing Chronic Disease, 5*(2), 1–6.

Kowlowitz, V., Davenport, C. S., & Palmer, M. H. (2009). Development and dissemination of web-based clinical simulations for continuing geriatric nursing education. *Journal of Gerontological Nursing, 35*(4), 37–43.

Kruger, J., Buchner, D. M., & Prohaska, T. R. (2009). The prescribed amount of physical activity in randomized clinical trials in older adults. *The Gerontologist, 49*, S100–S107.

Kuchuk, N. O., Pluijm, S. M., van Schoor, N. M., Smit, J. H., & Lips, P. (2009). Relationship of serum 25-hydroxyvitamin D to bone mineral density and serum parathyroid hormone and markers of bone turnover in older persons. *Journal of Clinical Endocrinology and Metabolism, 94*, 1244–1250.

Laditka, J. N., Beard, R. L., Bryant, L. L., Fetterman, D., Hunter, R., Ivey, S., . . . Wu, B. (2009). Promoting cognitive health: A formative research collaboration of the Healthy Aging Research Network. *The Gerontologist, 49*, S12–S19.

Lee, C. J. (2009). A comparison of health promotion behaviors in rural and urban community-dwelling spousal caregivers. *Journal of Gerontological Nursing, 35*, 34–40.

Lee, J. H., O'Keefe, J. H., Bell, D., Hensrud, D. D., & Holick, M. F. (2008). Vitamin D deficiency: An important, common, and easily treatable cardiovascular risk factor? *Journal of the American College of Cardiology, 52*, 1949–1956.

Logsdon, R. G., McCurry, S. M., Pike, K. C., & Teri, L. (2009). Making physical activity accessible to older adults with memory loss: A feasibility study. *The Gerontologist, 51*, S94–S99.

Mariano, C. (2009). Holistic nursing: Scope and standards of practice. In B. M. Dossey & L. Keegan (Eds.), *Holistic nursing: A handbook for practice* (5th ed., pp. 47–73). Boston: Jones and Bartlett Publishers.

McConnell, E. S., Lekan, D., Bunn, M., Egerton, E., Corazzini, K. N., Hendrix, C. D., & Bailey, D. E. (2009). Teaching evidence-based nursing practice in geriatric care settings: The geriatric nursing innovations through education institute. *Journal of Gerontological Nursing, 35*, 26–33.

Meng, H., Wamsley, B., Liebel, D., Dixon, D., Eggert, G., & Van Nostrand, J. (2009). Urban-rural differences in the effect of a Medicare health promotion and disease self-management program on physical function and health care expenditures. *The Gerontologist, 49*, 407–417.

Morley, J. E. (2009). Phronesis and the medical director. *American Medical Directors Association, 10*, 149–151.

National Academy of Sciences. (2008). *Retooling for an aging America: Building the health care workforce*. Washington, DC: National Academies Press.

Neill, K. S., & Powell, L. (2009). Mobile interprofessional wellness care of rural older adults: Student outcomes and future perspectives. *Journal of Gerontological Nursing, 35*, 46–52.

Nguyen, H. Q., Ackermann, R. T., Maciejewski, M., Berke, E., Patrick, M., Williams, B., & LoGerfo, J. P. (2008). Managed-Medicare health club benefit and reduced health care costs among older adults. *Preventing Chronic Disease, 5*(1), 1–10.

Novelli, B. (2009). Health care reform hinges on private-sector collaboration. *Preventing Chronic Disease, 6*(2), 1–5.

Orwoll, E., Nielson, C. M., Marshall, L. M., Lambert, L., Holton, K. F., Hoffman, A. R., ... Cauley, J. A. (2009). Vitamin D deficiency in older men. *Journal of Clinical Endocrinology and Metabolism, 94*, 1092–1093.

Palmer, M. H., Kowlowitz, V., Campbell, J., Carr, C., Dillon, R., Durham, C. F., ... Rasin, J. (2008). Using clinical simulations in geriatric nursing continuing education. *Nursing Outlook, 56*, 159–166.

Perez, A., & Fleury, J. (2009). Wellness motivation theory in practice. *Geriatric Nursing, 30*(2S), 15–20.

Perez-Lopez, F. R. (2009). Vitamin D metabolism and cardiovascular risk factors in postmenopausal women. *Maturitas, 62*, 248–262.

Peterson, M. J., Giuliani, C., Morey, M. C., Pieper, C. F., Evenson, K. R., Mercer, V., ... Simonsick, E. M. (2009). Physical activity as a preventive factor for frailty: The health, aging, and body composition study. *Journal of Gerontology Medical Sciences, 64A*, 61–68.

Potter, P. J., & Frisch, N. C. (2009). The holistic caring process. In B. M. Dossey & L. Keegan (Eds.), *Holistic nursing: A handbook for practice* (5th ed., pp. 141–156). Boston: Jones and Bartlett Publishers.

Prohaska, T. R., Eisenstein, A. R., Satariano, W. A., Hunter, R., Bayles, C. M., Kurtovich, E., ... Ivey, S. L. (2009). Walking and the preservation of cognitive function in older populations. *The Gerontologist, 49*, S86–S93.

Rejeski, W. J., Marsh, A. P., Chmelo, E., Prescott, A. J., Dobrosielski, M., Walkup, M. P., ... Kritchevsky, S. (2009). The lifestyle interventions and independence for elderly pilot (LIFE-P): 2-year follow-up. *Journal of Gerontology Medical Sciences, 64A*, 462–467.

Rogers, C., & Keller, C. (2009). Roy's adaptation model to promote physical activity among sedentary older adults. *Geriatric Nursing, 30*, 21–26.

Schonberg, M. A., Leveille, S. G., & Marcantonio, E. R. (2008). Preventive health care among older women: Missed opportunities and poor targeting. *The American Journal of Medicine, 121*, 974–981.

Shearer, N. B. C. (2009). Health empowerment theory as a guide for practice. *Geriatric Nursing, 30*(2S), 4–10.

Shenson, D., Benson, W., & Harris, A. C. (2008). Expanding the delivery of clinical preventive services through community collaboration: The SPARC model. *Preventing Chronic Disease, 5*(1), 1–7.

Stechschulte, S. A., Kirsner, R. S., & Federman, D. G. (2009). Vitamin D: bone and beyond, rationale and recommendations for supplementation. *The American Journal of Medicine, 111*, 793–802.

Tan, E. J., Rebok G. W., Yu, Q., Frangakis, C. E., Carlson, M. C., Wang, T., ... Fried, L. P. (2009). The long-term relationship between high-intensity volunteering and physical activity among older African American women. *Journal of Gerontology Social Sciences, 64B*, 304–311.

Touhy, E. L. (1946). Geriatrics: The general setting. *Geriatrics: Official Journal of the American Geriatrics Society, 1*(1), 17–20.

Van Nispen, R. M., de Boer, M. R., Hoeijmakers, G. J., Ringens, P. J., & van Rens, G. (2009). Co-morbidity and visual acuity are risk factors for health-related quality of life decline: Five-month follow-up EQ-5D data of visually impaired older patients. *Health and Quality of Life Outcomes, 7*(18), 1–9.

White, S. M., Wojcicki, T. R., & McCauley, E. (2009). Physical activity and quality of life in community dwelling older adults. *Health and Quality of Life Outcomes, 7*(10), 1–7.

Wilcox, S., Dowda, M., Dunn, A., Ory, M. G., Rheaume, C., & King, A. C. (2009). Predictors of increased physical activity in active for life program. *Preventing Chronic Disease, 6*(1), 1–6.

Wilcox, S., Sharkey, J. R., Mathews, A. E., Laditka, J. N., Laditka, S. B., Logsdon, R. G., ... Liu, R. (2009). Perceptions and beliefs about the role of physical activity and nutrition on brain health in older adults. *The Gerontologist, 49*, S61–S71.

Williamson, J. D., Espeland, M., Kritchevsky, S. B., Newman, A. B., King, A. C., Pahor, M., ... Miller, M. E. (2009). Changes in cognitive function in a randomized trial of physical activity: Results of the lifestyle interventions and independence for elders pilot study. *Journal of Gerontology Medical Sciences, 64A*, 688–694.

Wylie-Rosett, J., & Karanja, N. (2009). American Heart Association's behavioral roundtable for preventable disparities. *Preventing Chronic Disease, 6*(2), 1–6.

Zoorob, R., & Morelli, V. (2008). Disease prevention and wellness in the twenty-first century. *Primary Care Clinics in Office Practice, 35*, 663–667.

CHAPTER 6

Diverse Health Care Settings for Older Adults

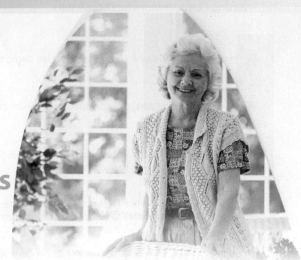

LEARNING OBJECTIVES

After reading this chapter, you will be able to:

1. Describe the services that are included in a continuum of care for older adults.

2. Describe characteristics of several models of acute care programs for older adults.

3. Describe types of nursing home settings, including newer models of care.

4. Describe the types of home care services and explain how people obtain these services.

5. Describe each of the following types of community-based services: adult day centers, respite services, parish nursing, health promotion programs, and management programs.

6. Discuss ways in which each of the following programs facilitate coordination of care: comprehensive models, chronic care models, and care and case management services.

7. Discuss the roles of nurses caring for older adults in acute care, long-term care, and home and community settings.

8. Describe sources of payment for health care services for older adults.

KEY POINTS

acute care for elders (ACE)
adult day centers
aging in place
assisted-living facilities
case management services
continuum of care
culture change
geriatric care manager
hospital-at-home model

intermediate nursing
 home care
long-term care
long-term care insurance
Medicaid
Medicare
medigap
nursing home
Older Americans Act (OAA)

parish nursing
resident-centered care
respite care
restorative care
skilled home care
skilled nursing home care

small-house nursing home
special care units (SCUs)
subacute care units
telehealth
transitional care

Although nurses have always cared for older adults, only since the late 1960s have health care organizations developed programs to address the unique health care needs of older adults. Because of these programs, a **continuum of care** for older adults has gradually evolved, and health care services are increasingly addressing specific needs of older adults during different phases of health and illness. Another outcome of these programs is the emergence of new roles for nurses, particularly for those who specialize in care of older adults. This chapter presents an overview of the continuum of health care services for older adults that began developing in the late 1960s and continues to evolve today; it also discusses roles of nurses working with older adults in these programs.

DEVELOPMENT OF A CONTINUUM OF CARE FOR OLDER ADULTS

The establishment of **Medicare** in 1965 (discussed later in this chapter) stimulated major changes in the delivery of health care services to older adults, and nurses have taken prominent roles in developing health care programs. Although some of these programs arose from an increased concern about health expenditures, many resulted from an increased awareness of the importance of meeting complex care needs of older adults in a way that addresses both financial concerns and quality-of-life issues. Figure 6-1 delineates major trends that stimulated the development of new models of care for older adults since the late 1960s.

A confusing array of terms related to health care services and settings for older adults evolved over the last several

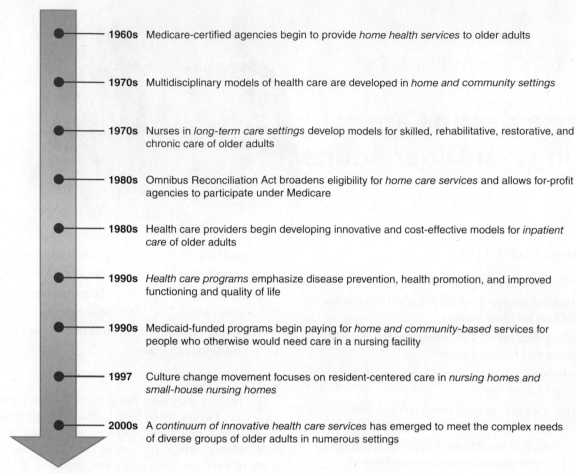

FIGURE 6-1 Significant events that have spurred the development of diverse models of care for older adults.

1960s Medicare-certified agencies begin to provide *home health services* to older adults

1970s Multidisciplinary models of health care are developed in *home and community settings*

1970s Nurses in *long-term care settings* develop models for skilled, rehabilitative, restorative, and chronic care of older adults

1980s Omnibus Reconciliation Act broadens eligibility for *home care services* and allows for-profit agencies to participate under Medicare

1980s Health care providers begin developing innovative and cost-effective models for *inpatient care* of older adults

1990s *Health care programs* emphasize disease prevention, health promotion, and improved functioning and quality of life

1990s Medicaid-funded programs begin paying for *home and community-based* services for people who otherwise would need care in a nursing facility

1997 Culture change movement focuses on resident-centered care in *nursing homes and small-house nursing homes*

2000s A *continuum of innovative health care services* has emerged to meet the complex needs of diverse groups of older adults in numerous settings

decades because of the trends delineated in Figure 6-1. Phrases such as **long-term care**, continuum of care, and **aging in place** refer to various models without standards to define the types of care. Moreover, recent developments with regard to chronic care models and care facilities have added to the confusion. For example, some aging-in-place or continuing care programs require that residents move to a new location within a larger facility or group of facilities when their needs change. Gerontologists and health care practitioners have raised concerns about the application of this concept in these settings, because Shippee (2009) found that within-facility transitions were disruptive to the residents' social interaction, sense of home, and sense of autonomy. Box 6-1 describes pertinent terms and the following sections describe the variety of settings and models that address unique and complex needs of older adults. In addition to describing settings where older adults receive their care, the sections focus on pertinent issues that are currently being addressed to improve quality of health care for older adults. Unique roles for gerontological nurses in various settings are also described.

Box 6-1 Terms Describing Models of Care for Older Adults

Long-term care: In the 1960s, this term referred to nursing homes, which were the only place of care for people with long-term disabilities who could not stay in their own homes. Although the term is still strongly associated with care provided in institutional settings, long-term care services are provided in community settings, such as homes and apartments.

Aging in place: A range of services provided in one setting to address different levels of care as the needs of the older adult change. This concept initially referred to supporting people in their own homes, but it has expanded to include institutional settings that provide a wide range of services.

Continuum of care: Programs that provide comprehensive, coordinated, and multidisciplinary services (e.g., primary and preventive care, acute care, transitional care, rehabilitation services, extended care, respite care, social services, home health care, adult day centers, and care management services). Examples include Life care or continuing care retirement communities (described in Chapter 1) and On Lok Program and the Program of All-inclusive Care for the Elderly (PACE) (described later in this chapter).

ACUTE CARE SETTINGS

Acute care settings are an important part of the continuum of care because of the complexity of care associated with illnesses in older adults (as discussed in detail in Chapter 27). In response to the increasing recognition of the need for specialized geriatric services, many acute care settings have implemented innovative models of care, as discussed in the following sections.

Specialized Geriatric Acute Care Units

Since the early 1980s, hospitals in the United States have been establishing comprehensive geriatric assessment units to provide multidisciplinary assessment and care planning for frail older adults. These programs became more widespread during the early 2000s and were designated as **acute care for elders (ACE)** units.

The underlying premise for these units was that older adults have complex and unique needs that can be addressed by a specially trained multidisciplinary team to prevent functional decline during hospitalization. A meta-analysis of 11 studies of ACE units showed that compared with patients who receive usual hospital care, those who receive care in ACE units had an 18% reduction in functional decline and a better chance of living at home after discharge (Baztan, Suarez-Garcia, Lopez-Arrieta, Rodrigues-Manas, & Rodrigues-Artalejo, 2009). In addition to these benefits, studies found that ACE units could reduce the length of hospital stay (Zelada, Salinas, & Baztan, 2009).

Key elements of ACE units are interdisciplinary team management, patient-centered nursing care, early discharge planning, a specially adapted physical environment, and assessment and interventions for common geriatric syndromes (e.g., mobility, fall risk, self-care, skin integrity, continence, confusion, depression, anxiety). In addition to gerontological nurses, the health care teams in ACE units typically include a geriatrician, pharmacist, social worker, various rehabilitation therapists (e.g., speech, physical, or occupational therapists), and mental health professionals (e.g., psychologists or psychiatrists). Some teams also include a **geriatric care manager** and music, activity, or horticultural therapists.

Although less than 10% of hospitals had implemented strategies to address quality of care issues for older patients before 2008, support for specialized programs is increasing through programs such as the Nurses Improving Care for Healthsystem Elders (NICHE), as described in Chapter 5 (Capezuti, 2008). Since October 2008, the Centers for Medicare & **Medicaid** Services (CMS) has provided financial incentives to improve quality of care in hospitals because they deny payment for certain hospital-acquired conditions that are deemed to be preventable. Three conditions that are included in this category are fall-related injuries, pressure ulcer stages III and IV, and catheter-associated urinary tract infections. These conditions disproportionately affect older adults. Nurses in any acute care setting can identify risk factors for functional decline by using the Hospital Admission Risk Profile (HARP) clinical tool, listed as a clinical tool at the end of this chapter. In addition to ACE units and the NICHE initiative, Capezuti and Brush (2009) identified the following innovative models proven to improve care of hospitalized older adults:

- Hospital Elder Life Program (HELP): focuses on identification and management of delirium in hospitalized older adults
- Dual-function units that provide palliative care within an ACE unit
- Geriatric and orthopedic co-management of patients with fractured hips
- Programs that minimize older patients' time in surgery through a standard protocol
- Specialized trauma teams composed of geriatricians and gerontological advanced practice nurses
- Geriatric-oncology consultation teams or units

Subacute Care Units

Subacute care units are another recent development within acute care settings that address medically complex needs of hospitalized older adults. These programs provide skilled nursing and other skilled care services for patients who need comprehensive rehabilitation after major health altering episodes, such as a stroke or orthopedic surgery. Services in subacute care programs include chemotherapy; intravenous therapy; complex wound care; enteral and parenteral nutrition; speech, physical, and occupational therapies; and management of complex respiratory care (e.g., ventilator, tracheostomy).

Hospital-at-Home Model

The **hospital-at-home model** was introduced in Europe during the 1990s as a cost-cutting measure in response to the increasing demand for hospital admissions. These multidisciplinary programs provide a specific service that requires active participation by health care professionals for a limited time. Types of hospital-at-home models include those that facilitate early discharge from the acute care setting and those that substitute entirely for an inpatient admission. Conditions that are addressed through these models include cellulitis, pneumonia, infusion therapy, postsurgical care, chronic heart failure, and chronic obstructive pulmonary disease. An analysis of 10 randomized trials found that at 3 months there was no significant difference in mortality for patients who received care at home but at 6 months the mortality rate was significantly lower for those patients (Shepperd et al., 2009). Additional findings of Shepperd and colleagues were that these programs were less expensive than admission and patients reported more satisfaction. Another study of four hospital-at-home programs found that participants experienced modest improvements in activities of daily living (ADL), whereas patients who received hospital care for the same problems experienced a decline in ADL (Leff, 2009). Although studies have identified clear advantages to this model, it has received little support from health insurance programs in the United States and has been adopted only by the Veterans Affairs health system and a few managed care systems (Cheng, Mantalto, & Leff, 2009).

Transitional Care Models

The concept of **transitional care** was introduced during the 1990s in reference to specialized units in hospitals that now are called subacute care units. The term is now applied to a broad range of services and settings designed to promote the safe and timely movement of patients through various care settings (Naylor & Keating, 2008). A main goal of transitional care is to provide coordination and continuity of health care across different settings (Graham, Ivey, & Neuhauser, 2009).

Transitional care from acute care settings has gained much attention in recent years because of increasing concerns about frequent hospital readmissions soon after discharge among Medicare recipients. A survey of health care systems in the United States and seven other developed countries found that hospital readmission rates within a short time after discharge were problematic in all countries and this was interpreted as a health risk related to inadequate care during hospital stays and transitions to home (Schoen, Osborn, How, Doty, & Peugh, 2009). Studies have confirmed that many of these rehospitalizations could be prevented if systems were in place to address the underlying issues that contribute to readmissions (Greenwald & Jack, 2009). Studies have also found that the two problems that most often occur during transitions are medication discrepancies and lack of continuity of care (Boling, 2009).

The Re-engineered Hospital Discharge (RED) program is an evidence-based model that hospitals have used successfully to address issues related to transitional care. Patients enrolled in the RED intervention group were 30% less likely to be readmitted or use the emergency room within 30 days of discharge, and the cost of their care was 34% lower than for those patients who received usual care (Jack et al., 2009). The three major components of this model are as follows: (1) a nurse discharge advocate whose primary responsibility is to coordinate discharge plans and communicate with patient/family and all care providers; (2) an after-hospital care plan document that is patient-centered, low-literacy level, and highly pictorial that includes all pertinent information; and (3) telephone follow-up by a clinical pharmacist 3 days post-discharge for teaching and follow-up.

Nurses have developed an easy-to-use and evidence-based screening tool called the Transitional Care Model (TCM): Hospital Discharge Screening Criteria for High Risk Older Adults to identify older adults who are at risk for poorly managed transitions. Studies demonstrate that the use of this tool by nurses resulted in improved patient outcomes and substantial decreases in health care costs (Bixby & Naylor, 2009). The tool is available as part of the *Try This* series of the Hartford Institute for Geriatric Nursing and is listed as a clinical tool at the end of this chapter. Nurses are encouraged to use this tool to identify older adults who need special attention for transitional care interventions. Nurses can make sure that patients/families have information about all the following: presenting problem and final diagnoses; discharge medica-

tions, including schedule, purpose and cautions for each, and changes from preadmission; follow-up appointments; anticipated problems and suggested interventions; 24/7 call-back number; and all care providers (Podrazik & Whelan, 2008).

Roles for Gerontological Nurses in Acute Care Settings

As acute care settings have developed programs to address the unique needs of hospitalized older patients, new roles have emerged for gerontological nurses. Gerontological nurses are likely to serve as consultants and role models for staff nurses and often assist in developing and implementing specialized care programs and protocols for hospitalized older adults. The Hartford Institute for Geriatric Nursing has supported and promoted the Geriatric Resource Nurse (GRN) model as a foundation for improving geriatric care in hospitals. This unit-based model prepares staff nurses as gerontological clinical resources for other nurses so they can identify and address specific geriatric syndromes, such as falls and confusion, and implement interventions that discourage using restrictive devices and promote patient mobility (Capezuti, 2008). Refer to www.nicheprogram.org for information on the GRN model.

NURSING HOME SETTINGS

The term **nursing home**, or *nursing facility,* refers to a residential institutional setting for people who need assistance with several ADL. Nursing homes are licensed by a state or federal agency and must be certified as a Medicare or Medicaid facility if they receive funds from these programs. Nursing homes are required to have continuous on-site supervision by a registered nurse or a licensed practical nurse. In addition to medical care and nursing services, nursing homes must provide dental, podiatry, medical specialty consultation services, and rehabilitation therapies (e.g., physical and occupational therapies). Nursing homes provide many of the same health care services that are provided in acute-care settings; however, the care recipients are called *residents* rather than *patients* because these are residential facilities.

Levels of Nursing Home Care

Nursing home care is generally categorized as skilled (usually short-term) or intermediate care (usually long-term). To qualify for **skilled nursing home care** (sometimes called skilled rehabilitation care), people must meet the following Medicare criteria:

- Have an inpatient hospitalization of at least 3 consecutive days within the previous 30 days for a medical condition that is associated with the need for skilled care
- Have a physician referral for services that must be provided by licensed professionals, such as nurses or therapists
- Require daily skilled care that can be provided appropriately in a Medicare-certified skilled nursing facility

For people who meet the criteria for care in a skilled nursing facility, Medicare will cover all or part of the care for up to 100 days of care, but only if the person continues to require the skilled level of services. Although many older adults require skilled care when they are discharged from acute care settings, they receive only an average of about 23 days of Medicare-covered services because they do not meet the criteria for the full 100 days that might be covered. Typical diagnoses associated with skilled nursing home care are stroke, fractured hip, congestive heart failure, and rehabilitation after acute illnesses (e.g., pneumonia, myocardial infarction). The expectation is that the person will be able to progress to a higher level of functioning and show some recovery from the acute episode.

Intermediate nursing home care refers to nursing services provided for chronically ill people who need assistance with daily activities. In recent years, there is an increasing focus on rehabilitation, or **restorative care**, for chronically ill people who receive long-term nursing home care. For example, nurses have developed the comprehensive nursing rehabilitation program as a model for promoting physical functioning of moderately frail nursing home residents posthospitalization (Grando et al., 2009). Since the late 1980s, the federal government has mandated that nursing facilities provide restorative care, which is an approach that helps residents compensate for functional impairments so their abilities do not decline.

Admission to Long-Term Care

Gerontologists have identified the reasons older people are admitted to nursing homes for long-term care. In contrast to admissions for skilled nursing care that are associated with a hospitalization, these admissions commonly occur after a period of gradual decline in functioning because of a chronic condition, such as dementia. Studies indicate that more severe functional limitations, cognitive impairment, and problematic behaviors in people with dementia are predictors of admission to nursing facilities for long-term care (Cho, Zarit, & Chiriboga, 2009). Additional factors that increase the likelihood of being admitted to a nursing home include white race, female sex, living alone, advanced age, and low socioeconomic status (Martikainen et al., 2009). Since the 1970s, gerontologists have recognized that admission to a nursing home for long-term care is determined not only by the person's level of functioning but also by the availability of capable and willing caregivers. Thus, many older people move to a nursing home not because their condition has changed significantly, but because there has been a change in the availability or abilities of the caregiver. Figure 6-2 illustrates the differences in levels of functioning for older adults residing in nursing facilities, community housing with assistance, and independent housing.

Trends in Nursing Home Care

In recent decades, changes in health care services for older adults have significantly influenced both long-term and short-

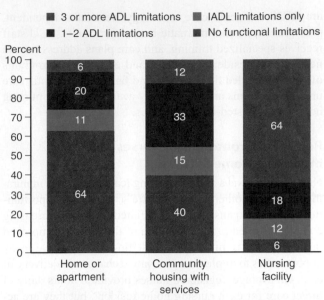

FIGURE 6-2 Percentage of Medicare enrollees age 65+ with functional limitations by residential setting, 2005. (*Source: Centers for Medicare & Medicaid Services, Medicare Current Beneficiary Survey.*)

term nursing home care. On any given day, about 5% of older adults are residing in a nursing facility; however, almost half of people older than 65 years are likely to spend some time in a nursing home. These statistics reflect the following major trends in health care for older adults in the United States:

- Shorter lengths of hospital stays and subsequent increased use of skilled nursing and rehabilitation care in nursing homes
- Higher percentages of nursing home residents returning to community settings
- Increased use of **skilled home care** services
- Increased availability of **assisted-living facilities** and community-based long-term care services that substitute for nursing home care

Because of these trends, most nursing homes provide a combination of skilled care services for short-term residents and intermediate care services for long-term residents. Because the skilled care provided in nursing homes today is similar to the care that used to be provided to patients in hospitals, residents often are able to stay in the nursing facility during acute illnesses rather than being admitted to a hospital. Another result of these trends is that the percentage of long-term residents who are more dependent on assistance with ADL has gradually increased in recent years, because people who are less dependent now receive care in other settings, such as assisted-living facilities.

A recent development in long-term care settings is the establishment of **special care units (SCUs)**, which are separate units designed to address the needs of specific groups of residents who meet explicit admission criteria. More than 3000 nursing homes have SCUs, which account for about 7% of all beds (Burger et al., 2009). Dementia care units, or Alzheimer's units, are a common type of SCU; other types are AIDS, subacute care, oncology, ventilator-dependent, pressure ulcers, and traumatic brain injury units. SCU staff receives specialized training, and care plans address unique needs of the residents. Support and educational programs often are provided for residents and families. Dementia care units or programs are increasingly available in both nursing homes and assisted-living facilities.

Roles for Gerontological Nurses in Nursing Home Settings

Nurses have always assumed strong leadership roles in nursing homes and other long-term care settings, and opportunities for role expansion are associated with the increasing complexity of care. Also, because of the focus on improved quality of care in nursing home settings, nurses have many opportunities to implement innovative changes in delivery of care. On average, registered nurses provide 6 hours daily of direct care for each nursing home resident, but they are accountable for all nursing components of care (Burger et al., 2009). Some of the most common roles for registered nurses in long-term care settings include team leader, nursing supervisor, wellness nurse, director of nursing, and assistant director of nursing. Nurses also have very strong roles in teaching nursing assistants about the best care for nursing home residents. Nurses have developed a model for teaching nursing assistants how to implement a restorative approach to change the way in which care is provided in nursing homes (Resnick et al., 2009). A nurse-led statewide initiative to improve care in nursing facilities resulted in improvements in all of the following quality indicators: falls, weight loss, pressure ulcers, and bedfast status (Rantz et al., 2009).

In the late 1990s, numerous opportunities opened up for advanced practice gerontological nurses when Medicare and Medicaid began to reimburse for nurse practitioner services. In addition to direct care of residents, advanced practice nurses may provide staff education, assist with program development, act as consultants in planning and implementing care, establish support groups for clients and families, and act as advocates for clients and their families. Additional details about roles for advance practice nurses are discussed in Chapter 5.

NEWER MODELS OF NURSING HOME CARE

During the past two decades, health care consumers, providers, and organizations have increasingly focused on concerns about quality of care and quality of life for people who need long-term care. This focus stems in part from consumer pressure that began during the 1970s through the National Citizens Coalition for Nursing Home Reform and, in part, from the Nursing Home Reform Act of 1987 (discussed in Chapter 9). At the same time, there has been increasing concern about cost of care in traditional nursing home settings and an associated interest in developing lower cost—and better quality—alternatives. Because of these concerns,

A Student's Perspective

This week in the nursing home, I found it was important to listen to Mrs. R. while allowing her to make her limitations known to me. I asked if she needed help, and didn't just provide it. I paid close attention to her body language and nonverbal communication. After finding her fast asleep sitting up during breakfast, I woke her and allowed her to tell me what was next. She determined that going to the bathroom and then getting washed would be best. After she was ready, I helped her down to the beauty salon to get her hair done, which is something she does every Friday afternoon. It can be easy to fall into the patient care aspect of a nursing home where you expect them to be on a schedule; however, you have to treat it as their home and allow them to pick and choose their activities and rest periods.

Jillian B.

a new era in nursing home care has evolved. It is referred to as the **culture change** movement.

The Culture Change Movement

The term culture change, which was coined in 1997, in now widely used to describe a major movement toward a slow and comprehensive set of fundamental reforms in the way that nursing homes provide care (Rahman & Schnelle, 2008). A major goal of culture change is to transform the philosophy and practice in nursing homes from an overemphasis on safety, uniformity, and medical care to a consumer-directed focus on health promotion, quality of life, and individualized care (Robinson & Reinhard, 2009; White-Chou, Graves, Godfrey, Bonner, & Sloane, 2009). The term **resident-centered care** is often used with this approach to emphasize personal choice, individualized care, and quality of life for residents of long-term care facilities.

The culture change movement has been gaining momentum, not only in the private sector but also in the public sector. For example, the CMS publishes a self-study tool, called the Artifacts of Culture Change Tool, to help nursing homes assess their progress toward improved quality of care. In addition, the CMS helped launch a voluntary public–private coalition in 2006, called Advancing Excellence in America's Nursing Homes, to address quality of care concerns. This coalition has reported major progress in reducing the use of restraints, decreasing the risk of pressure ulcers, and improving pain management for residents of nursing homes (see www.nhqualitycampaign.org for more information).

In 2009, the CMS issued guidelines for nursing home surveyors that sharpened the focus on residents' rights in key areas including ensuring dignity, offering choices in care and services, accommodating the environment to individual needs and preferences, and creating a homelike environment for residents and visitors. For reports and resources from Advancing Excellence in America's Nursing Home, see the Health Education Resources section at the end of this chapter.

Evidence for Positive Outcomes With Culture Change

Because the culture change movement is a relatively recent development, researchers have not yet established a strong evidence base related to cost and quality of care. One research review identified 16 descriptive studies that evaluated culture change models and noted that the 3 studies with larger samples and quasi-experimental designs found positive improvements in resident, staff, and organizational outcomes (Burger et al., 2009). With the growing interest in culture change, there is a concomitant increase in identifying outcomes of specific interventions. Gerontologists have suggested that researchers begin by studying the effects of interventions that increase resident choice over daily activities because this is a core value of culture change (Rahman & Schnelle, 2008).

In 2007, the Commonwealth Fund, a major supporter of the culture change movement, surveyed directors of nursing in 1435 nursing homes to identify the level of implementation about three aspects of culture change: resident care, physical environment, and staff culture and working environment. Highlights of the survey as reported by Doty, Koren, and Sturla (2008) are as follows:

- There was a positive correlation between implementation of culture change initiatives and greater benefits in terms of staff retention, higher occupancy rates, better competitive position, and improved operational costs.
- Between 30% and 40% of all nursing homes report they are implementing some principle of culture change that fosters resident-directed care.
- Of nursing homes that adopt culture change, 58% allow residents to determine their own daily schedules versus 22% of traditional nursing home.
- Among culture change adopters, 64% implement resident-centered bathing techniques, in contrast to only 37% of traditional nursing homes.
- Some 70% of culture change adopters report that residents are actively involved in decisions about their facility, but only 27% of traditional nursing home do so.
- About 86% of culture change adopters consistently assign the same aides to residents, versus 74% of traditional nursing homes.

The next section describes models of nursing home care that are part of the culture change movement and provide information about evidence-based outcomes of these models.

Pioneer Network

The Pioneer Network in Long-Term Care—which is considered the umbrella organization of the culture change movement—has evolved since 1997 from a landmark meeting of pioneers across the United States with the goal of changing the philosophy of care in nursing homes (White-Chou et al., 2009). The Pioneer Network identifies 13 core values that focus on individualized and holistic care; optimal use of all aspects of the physical, organizational, and psycho/social/spiritual environment; and on-going growth and continuous quality improvement. Two of the most widely implemented models of care that are part of the Pioneer Network are the Eden Alternative and the Green House Project.

The Eden Alternative is a model developed in the mid-1990s by William Thomas, MD, with the intent of creating small group neighborhoods of residents to combat boredom, loneliness, helplessness, and lack of meaning that are common in traditional nursing homes. The Eden Alternative is a comprehensive program of transforming the organizational culture as well as the physical, spiritual, psychosocial, and interpersonal environments of a facility. An essential component is the systematic introduction of pets, plants, and children to create a homelike setting and improve the quality of life of residents. In addition, the Eden Alternative incorporates strategies to engage and empower staff in bringing about the environmental change. Nursing homes that adopt this comprehensive model and pledge to abide by Eden Principles are listed in the Eden Registry. Outcomes of this model that have been identified in studies include enhanced staff retention, increased satisfaction of staff and residents, and reduction in the number of medications and infections (Bowers, Nolet, Roberts, & Edmond, 2009). Nurses can find additional information about this model at www.edenalt.org.

The Green House Project, described as a **small-house nursing home**, has also been promoted by William Thomas, MD, who is the founder of the Eden Alternative and a major leader in the Pioneer Network. The first project opened in 2003 and consisted of four self-contained Green Houses that operated under the license of a sponsoring nursing home in Tupelo, Missouri. Green Houses typically house 7 to12 residents in a home that blends in with neighboring houses. These small-house nursing homes provide a full range of licensed and certified nursing home services to older people with high levels of disability, including those associated with dementia, in a normal household setting. The Green House approach emphasizes relationships and meaning-making in interventions for dementia-related behavioral disturbances. A study of the first 2 years of this model found that residents experienced better outcomes on many dimensions of quality of life and had no declines in health outcomes (Kane & Cutler, 2008). Researchers also have found that families were more satisfied with the care and their own experiences, appreciated increased autonomy and enhanced privacy for the residents, and had no greater family burden (Lum, Kane, Cutler, & Yu, 2008–2009). Overall, early studies of the small-house model identified many benefits for cognitively impaired older adults as well as improved job satisfaction for nurses who work in an environment that promotes holistic and person-centered care (Rabig, 2009).

Assisted-Living Facilities

In addition to the models described in this chapter, many older adults receive a wide range of health care services in assisted-living facilities and continuing-care retirement communities. Because these models are independent community-based housing options, details are discussed in Chapter 1 in the context of living arrangements for older adults. Although assisted-living facilities developed during the 1980s as settings for independent living, some of these facilities have evolved to provide levels of care similar to that provided in nursing homes. Recent studies confirm that the typical assisted living resident is older and more functionally impaired and requires more care than residents who were described in the early studies (Cartwright, Miller, & Volpin, 2009). Because of this trend, some assisted-living facilities are integrally associated with and physically connected to nursing homes and provide a high level of care for residents who no longer meet qualifications for Medicare-covered services.

Another recent development is that some assisted living facilities provide specialized dementia care, and in some of these dementia-care facilities, the level of care has evolved to be similar to that provided in nursing homes. Recent data indicate that more than half of assisted-living residents have dementia and a greater number require daily memory aid. In addition, assisted-living residents often exhibit symptoms of anxiety, depression, and agitation, and two-thirds of residents with cognitive impairment exhibit behavioral problems (Kang, Smith, Buckwalter, Ellingrod, & Schultz, 2010; Teri et al., 2009). End-of-life care is another issue being addressed in assisted living facilities because residents express the desire to die at home. Because of this, many assisted living facilities are now working closely with hospice organizations to provide end-of-life care.

Roles for Nurses in Newer Models of Care

Newer models of care present many challenges, as well as opportunities, for nurses because culture change involves philosophical and organizational changes that affect all staff. For example, the Green House model conceptualizes nurses and other professionals as members of a visiting clinical support team that order and supervise care within their area of professional practice. Nurses do not supervise the direct care staff, but they often assume administrative and consultant roles. In 2009, the Hartford Institute for Geriatric Nursing and the Pioneer Network published an issue paper on *Nurses Involvement in Nursing Home Culture Change: Overcoming Barriers, Advancing Opportunities* (Burger et al., 2009). Highlights of this paper that are pertinent to roles for nurses are as follows:

- Goals and philosophy of culture change are highly compatible with those of nursing because both support and incorporate resident-directed care.
- Intense nursing participation is essential for providing coordinated, evidence-based clinical nursing care in the context of a resident-centered philosophy of care.
- Nurses need to be care-team leaders and role models so they can foster and promote a team approach in which direct-care staff are involved in decision making.
- Exclusion of nurses from decision making about culture change has been the greatest barrier to implementing culture change.

- Nurse managers need to have both clinical and management skills in the decentralized models and they may be unprepared for this role.

Because the culture change movement poses many dilemmas and challenges for nurses, efforts are underway to implement recommendations that address the major issues. Nurses can keep up-to-date with regard to their roles in relation to culture change by exploring information at the Internet sites listed in thePoint and Resources at the end of this chapter.

HOME CARE SERVICES

Trends in Home Care Services

Older people and other dependent populations have always received much of their health care at home, and visiting nurse services have existed in the United States since the 1800s. However, the delivery of home care services dramatically changed after 1965 when Medicare funds became available for these services. In 1975, the **Older Americans Act (OAA)** and Title XX Social Services Act allocated federal funds for home-based services, and the federal Health Services Program funded grants for the establishment, operation, or expansion of programs providing home health services. By the late 1970s, thousands of home care agencies had been established, and their number escalated exponentially during the next two decades.

Although Medicare home health care services were established as a short-term supplement to acute care services for people who needed skilled care, consumers came to view these services as an extension of long-term care for people with chronic illnesses. Two major factors that affected trends in home care services during the 1980s were the removal of many restrictions on Medicare-covered home care services and the implementation of the hospital prospective payment system that resulted in earlier discharges. By the 1990s, home care had become the fastest-growing component of the Medicare program, and costs had increased so drastically that Congress included cost-containment measures in the Balanced Budget Act of 1997. Because of this legislation and other federal mandates, it became increasingly more difficult for people to receive skilled home care services. Studies of the effect of these changes found that fewer Medicare beneficiaries received care, beneficiaries received fewer visits and a shorter care duration, and home care agencies received lower payments for services. These decreases had a more negative impact on beneficiaries who had the following characteristics: poor; female; sicker; nonwhite; served by for-profit agencies; discharged from a skilled nursing or rehabilitation facility; and those with diagnoses of diabetes, skin ulcers, heart failure, or cerebrovascular disease (Murkofsky & Alston, 2009).

At the same time that the federal government was cutting funds for home care, state governments were addressing the high cost of care in nursing homes—which placed a heavy financial burden on state Medicaid programs—by providing more funds for home- and community-based services. Thus, motivated both by cost containment and by consumer preference, state long-term care policy shifted from a focus on institutional care to a focus on noninstitutional services. Although many state-funded programs are limited to people who would be eligible for Medicaid if they were in a nursing home, many affordable services have become widely available through public, private, and nonprofit agencies.

Because of the trends in home care during the past four decades, two types of home care services—skilled home care and long-term home care—have evolved to address different goals. Skilled home care services address the goal of providing treatment for an illness or injury and to help patients regain their independence and become as self-sufficient as possible. For people with long-term chronic health problems, the goal is to maintain the highest level of function and health and to cope with illness or disability (Murkofsky & Alston, 2009). Positive outcomes for older adults who use home care services include the prevention of acute illnesses and better management of acute and chronic conditions.

Skilled Home Care

Home care services provided under Medicare and some other health insurance programs have always been limited to skilled home care and restricted to people who meet all of the following criteria:

- The person must be homebound (i.e., leaving the home requires considerable and taxing effort).
- The services must be ordered by a primary care provider.
- There must be a need for skilled nursing or rehabilitative services.
- The person must require intermittent, but not full-time, care.

For people who meet these criteria, Medicare covers the following types of home care services: skilled nursing, physical therapy, occupational therapy, nutrition counseling, speech–language therapy, medical social work, home health aide, and medical supplies and equipment. In addition to nursing assessment and interventions, skilled nursing services can include case management, medication management, infusion therapy, intravenous antibiotics, and psychiatric nursing care. Examples of home health aide services that can be provided under the directions of a licensed nurse or therapist include assistance with bathing, linen changes, range-of-motion exercises, and assistance with transfers and ambulation. People often qualify for skilled home care after a hospitalization or a stay in a skilled nursing or rehabilitation setting for an acute episode, or they may qualify when they experience a change in their condition but have not needed care in a hospital or nursing home.

Because skilled home care services are meant to be short-term, a major focus is on teaching the older person and caregivers about self-care activities. Typical skilled care recipients are (1) people who are homebound but able to manage most of their daily care at some level of independence and (2) people who, although homebound and dependent in many functional areas, receive help from families, friends, or paid caregivers to supplement the skilled care services. If people reach a level of independence such that they are no longer homebound, they cannot continue receiving skilled care services under Medicare. Likewise, people no longer qualify for skilled care after they achieve self-care goals. Many people receiving skilled care, however, still need some level of home care services after they no longer qualify for Medicare-funded skilled care and services are discontinued.

Long-Term Home Care

A wide spectrum of long-term home care services are available for the large majority of older adults who need home care but do not meet the criteria for Medicare-covered skilled care. At one end of the spectrum is nonskilled care provided by companions, homemakers, and home health aides. The most common services are meal preparation, light housekeeping, assistance with personal care, accompaniment to medical appointments, and grocery shopping and other errands. These services are often supplemented by community-based services such as transportation and home-delivered meals. Frequency of service ranges from periodic to 24 hours daily. A licensed nurse may assess the client and supervise the services, and a registered nurse usually assists with medication management, if needed. At the other end of the spectrum is skilled care for people who need this type of care but do not meet Medicare criteria. Virtually any skilled service available under Medicare is available as a self-pay service, but these services are usually quite expensive.

Sources of Home Care Services

Home care services are available through formal sources (e.g., agencies) or informal sources (e.g., independent caregivers). People who self-pay for home care can obtain services from agencies or from informal sources, but when home care services are covered by insurance or public funds, they traditionally have been provided by agencies under contractual arrangements. This is changing, however, and some states now allow care recipients to choose and direct independent providers (including family members) who are paid under Medicaid.

Agencies usually provide initial assessments, arrange for services, assign workers, provide ongoing supervision, and collect payment for services. They are responsible for hiring, training, directing, scheduling, and firing workers. Some agencies provide a wide range of services, including care management. Other agencies provide only a limited type of service, such as the provision of home health aides. Some so-called agencies, however, are little more than a registry or referral service. When services are obtained from informal sources rather than from agencies, the care recipient or a surrogate decision maker is responsible for performing the organizational tasks that agencies normally perform (e.g., hiring, firing, and supervising the caregiver). In this case, sometimes the aid of a geriatric care management service (discussed later in this chapter) is enlisted to arrange for services and oversee the care. A common way of finding independent caregivers and other home care resources is through a word-of-mouth network, in which names are obtained from friends, families, churches, or local offices on aging.

COMMUNITY-BASED SERVICES FOR OLDER ADULTS

Public and private agencies have provided many types of community support resources for older adults for decades, and the range of these services is continually broadening. For example, home-delivered meals programs have been available in most metropolitan areas for decades, and in recent years various home-delivered groceries and prepared meals have become available for delivery within 24 hours through Internet sites or toll-free phone numbers. Although community-based services are widely available, less than a quarter of older adults take advantage of these programs. Older adults and their caregivers often are not aware of the great variety of services available to meet the health needs of older adults in their own homes. Even when they are aware of the availability of such services, they may not know the eligibility criteria for publicly funded services to which they are entitled. Also, if community-based services are not culturally relevant, older adults or their families may not use them, even when they are aware of their existence. For example, a study found that Mexican Americans were reluctant to use home care services because of the belief that family caregivers can give better and safer care (Crist, Kim, Pasvogel, & Velazquez, 2009). Because the use of these resources may improve the health, functioning, and quality of life of the older adult, nurses need to address any lack of information about these services. Also, nurses need to assess barriers to the use of community services, as discussed in Chapter 13. Nurses in all settings have many opportunities to suggest the use of the community-based services that are described in Box 6-2. Figure 6-3 illustrates the percentage of older adults living in different residential settings according to age groups.

Adult Day Centers

Adult day centers, first developed in the 1970s, have become a major community-based resource for the care of dependent older adults. These centers provide structured social and recreational activities for functionally impaired older people in a group setting. In addition to group social activities, adult day centers provide meals and any of the following services: transportation, medication management, assistance with personal care, and other health-related services and therapies. Adult day centers generally provide supervised care on weekdays for 8 hours a day, with approximately 5 hours of formal programming during that time and 3 hours of social interaction and other unstructured activities. Less commonly, services are available for longer hours and on weekends and holidays.

Box 6-2 Community Resources for Older Adults

National Eldercare Locator (www.eldercare.gov, 800–677-1116). This service provides free information about state or local resources in any part of the United States according to the zip code where services are desired.

Senior Information and Referral Service. This service, which is sometimes referred to as an "Infoline," provides information about agencies to address specific needs.

Area Agency on Aging. Funded through state, county, and local resources, these agencies provide a range of services, including referrals, case management, and non–medical home care workers.

Senior Centers. These community centers provide meals and social and educational programs for older adults.

Home-Delivered Meals. This program provides home delivery of hot meals to homebound people.

Companions and Friendly Visitors. Nonmedical caregivers visit homebound older adults; they also may perform errands or provide escort service to appointments.

Telephone Reassurance. Service providers make scheduled telephone calls to older people to provide support and reminders.

Personal Emergency Response Systems. This emergency response system allows someone to use a remote-control device to initiate a phone call to designated people when assistance is needed (e.g., if the person falls).

Energy Assistance Programs. State and local programs offer financial assistance for utility bills for low-income people.

Home Weatherization and Home Repair Service. Contractors paid by government agencies provide home repairs and maintenance (e.g., insulation, window caulking, and installation) for low-income people.

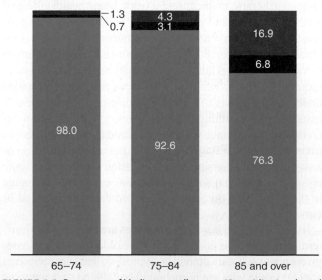

■ Nursing facility
■ Community housing with services
■ Home or apartment

FIGURE 6-3 Percentage of Medicare enrollees age 65+ residing in selected residential settings, by age group, 2005. *(Source: Centers for Medicare & Medicaid Services, Medicare Current Beneficiary Survey.)*

Participants in adult day centers usually are impaired to the point that they need supervision or assistance in several functional areas. Most participants are cognitively impaired, but depression and physical disabilities also are common conditions among adult day center participants. Participants typically live with a family member, but some live independently or in group settings. The goals of these programs are to maintain or improve the functional abilities of impaired older people; to delay or prevent the need for institutional care; to provide relief for caregivers of dependent older adults; and to improve the quality of life for impaired older adults and their caregivers. Researchers have found that adult day centers improve the quality of life for participants and are an important source of support for caregivers (Molzahn, Gallagher, & MvNulty, 2009).

Costs of adult day center programs vary widely, as does the source of payment. Although families have been the primary source of payment for most costs of adult day center care, public funds are increasingly becoming available because of the growing recognition of the benefits and cost-effectiveness of this kind of community-based service. Some programs are subsidized by nonprofit organizations and some have a sliding fee scale. Only a few health insurance policies cover adult day center programs. The Program of All-inclusive Care for the Elderly (PACE) model (discussed later in this chapter) is a very successful, but atypical, model that uses adult day centers as a core component of long-term care services.

Respite Services

Respite care refers to any service whose primary goal is to relieve caregivers periodically from the stress of their usual caregiving responsibilities. Gerontologists first used this term in the late 1970s because of the recognition that caregivers had substantial risk of developing social isolation, clinical depression, psychological distress, and other problems directly related to the burden of caregiving. As such, respite services are provided for people who are living in a home setting and are being cared for by family members or other unpaid help. Goals of respite services include improved well-being for caregivers and delayed institutionalization of dependent older people. Types of respite services include adult day centers, overnight and short-term nursing home care, and provision of in-home companions or home health aides.

Parish Nursing Programs

Parish nursing was established in the early 1970s and has been recognized by the American Nurses Association (ANA) as a specialty practice since 1998. In 2005, the ANA and the Health Ministries Association jointly published *Faith Community Nursing: Scope and Standards of Practice* in recognition of this area of nursing specialization. Parish nursing is a holistic approach to addressing the physical, emotional, and spiritual health care needs of members of church-based congregations, with a focus on health promotion activities such as screenings, education, and increased access to health care.

Health promotion activities commonly provided by parish nurses are blood pressure screening; health education about exercise, weight control, and stress reduction; and some spiritual counseling (King & Tessaro, 2009). Although parish nurse programs serve people of all ages, a high percentage of care recipients are older adults or people with chronic illnesses. Parish nurses have estimated that they spend between half and 100% of their time serving older adults (McCabe & Somers, 2009).

Health Promotion Programs

Because of the growing emphasis on health promotion, many community-based programs address the needs of older adults who are relatively healthy and functional, as discussed in Chapter 5. Senior centers and other places where older adults gather often offer periodic health screenings and other health promotion activities. Among the health promotion activities offered by these programs are blood pressure checks; safe driving courses; smoking cessation classes; health screening (e.g., cancer, vision, hearing); flu shots and other immunizations; medication assessment, management, and education; and various types of exercise, such as walking, aerobics, aquatics, or tai chi. Health education topics include nutrition, stress management, general health care, and seasonal health issues such as hypothermia, heat-related illness, and colds and flu.

Organized group activities, such as senior wellness programs, frequently take place in or are sponsored by community-based senior centers that exist in almost every community. Hospitals and other health care institutions are becoming more involved in providing this kind of program and are employing nurses to address the needs of older adults in the community. Senior centers and health care agencies often cosponsor programs to address specific health issues, such as diabetes, glaucoma, cholesterol, or blood pressure. For example, senior health fairs provide the opportunity for follow-up and referral of identified medical issues. Thus, these programs can provide a valuable health promotion service for older adults and at the same time increase the potential patient base for health care providers.

Roles for Gerontological Nurses in Home and Community Settings

Home care and other community-based services for older adults provide many opportunities for innovative roles for gerontological nurses in various settings. In addition to the usual responsibilities related to assessment and interventions, nurses often have primary responsibility for coordination of care, referrals for additional services, and organization and management of programs. Nurses also have many opportunities for expanding their roles to assess and address the needs of caregivers. In most home and community settings, nurses direct their interventions as much toward the caregivers of dependent older people as toward the older people themselves.

A characteristic of nursing roles in community settings is that nurses typically work in collegial relationships with other members of a multidisciplinary team, including primary care providers, psychiatrists, social workers, physical therapists, and other health care providers to address the needs of older adults as well as their caregivers. Nurses also have many opportunities to work closely with community-based services providers, many of whom have little or no formal training in professional disciplines. For example, senior centers may be the primary resource for meals and transportation, and nurses need to maintain good communication and relationships with people who work in these settings. In many community settings, nurses assume responsibility for training volunteers and teaching services providers about many health-related needs of older adults.

One challenge for nurses in home and community settings is to keep up-to-date with technological advances that increasingly are an integral part of health care services. In addition to increasing use of electronic medical records, technologic advances have significantly influenced the availability of new communication systems that are commonly used in home care. **Telehealth** (also called telemedicine) is the use of audio, video, and Internet-based devices to collect and transmit information for patient assessment through physiologic monitors connected to a computer in the home. Assessment data are then sent through a telephone connection to a nurse or other health care professional who verbally communicates with the patient to obtain additional information. Some systems use videophones to allow for visual as well as audio communication. One current focus of telehealth is management of arrhythmias through the use of telemonitors that can send electrocardiogram information to a call center where a health care professional is alerted to potential problems (Bayne & Boling, 2009). In addition to collecting assessment information, telehealth technology is used to share information, review care plans, and introduce patient teaching materials. Studies indicate that 72% of home care agencies use telehealth to provide cost-effective care for patients with conditions such as diabetes, heart failure, and chronic obstructive pulmonary disease (Vasquez, 2008).

MODELS ADDRESSING COORDINATION OF CARE

Consumer demand for community-based programs and persistent increases in the cost of care have stimulated the development of new models of comprehensive care. These programs receive some federal funds and are organized by nonprofit or health care organizations. In addition, care and **case management services** have evolved to coordinate the wide range of services for older adults.

Comprehensive Models

Since 1979, the federal government has funded innovative models of long-term care for people with chronic conditions that are both comprehensive and cost-effective. These Medicare and Medicaid waiver programs—sometimes called Social Health Maintenance Organizations—provide a wide range of social and medical services on a capitated managed care basis. The prototype of this model is the On Lok Senior Services program, which began in 1971 as one of the first senior day health centers in the Chinatown area of San Francisco. On Lok—Cantonese for "peaceful happy abode"—continues in a greatly expanded form as a successful model of community-based, comprehensive, and cost-effective care for older adults. Since 2005, the On Lok Lifeways program has provided a team of on-site mental and behavioral health professionals. Two of the positive outcomes of this program are fewer admissions for inpatient psychiatric care and improved access to mental health services (Ginsburg & Eng, 2009).

The success of On Lok prompted the development of a similar program, called PACE, in the late 1980s. This program has gradually expanded, and in 1997, the federal government designated PACE models as permanent Medicare and Medicaid providers. In 2000, two private foundations—the Robert Wood Johnson Foundation and the John A. Hartford Foundation—supported the expansion of these models of care. In 2008, 61 PACE programs were operational in 29 states (Mosocco, 2009). The target group for PACE is people who are eligible for both Medicare and Medicaid services, live in the community, and qualify for nursing home care. A typical PACE participant is a female who is 80 years old, has 7.9 medical conditions, and is limited in three or more ADLs (Mosocco, 2009).

Distinguishing features of the model are (1) the provision of comprehensive and community-based long-term care services to nursing-home-eligible clients, (2) an emphasis on preventive services, (3) integrated service delivery through adult day health centers, (4) case management through multidisciplinary teams, and (5) full funding on a capitation basis (similar to health maintenance organizations). Core components of PACE programs are nutrition, transportation, home care, acute care, respite care, primary care, social services, restorative therapies, prescription drugs, long-term care, adult day care, medical specialty care, durable medical equipment, and multidisciplinary case management. This model has demonstrated that the concurrent goals of improved health outcomes and reduced health care expenses can be achieved for frail older adults with complex needs (Hirth, Baskins, & Dever-Bumba, 2009).

Another federal initiative for integrating acute and long-term care is the Evercare model, which two nurse practitioners began as a Medicare pilot program in 1987. In 2004, the federal government gave permanent status to the Evercare projects and by 2008, it was available in 34 states in the continental United States. The Evercare model was initially limited to nursing homes, but it has been expanded to home and community settings. In this model, medical services are covered in all settings, so there is no financial incentive to provide services in a hospital if they can be provided elsewhere.

The Evercare model is made up of nurse practitioners and care managers who guide patients through the health care system. Core care principles of the Evercare model are as follows:

- Nurse practitioners plan and provide care, with attention to the patient's physical, social, and psychological needs.
- Transfers between different health care settings are minimized.
- Health care providers focus on prevention and ensure regular assessments and early detection of illness.
- Care teams advocate for patients and help them get the most from their health insurance benefits.
- Families are encouraged to be actively involved with the care.

Some outcomes of implementing the Evercare model in nursing homes are 45% reduced hospitalizations with no change in mortality, reduced acute episodes in nursing homes, 50% reduction in emergency room admissions, and decreased length of hospital stay by 1 day (Kappas-Larson, 2008).

Chronic Care Models

Although health insurance rarely covers comprehensive continuing care services, there is widespread awareness that medical care for people with advanced chronic conditions drives most health care costs for Medicare beneficiaries. Moreover, many older adults with functional limitations and high chronic illness burden have preventable hospitalizations and receive fragmented care that is not patient-centered (Boling, 2009). Thus, the federal government and health care planners and providers have shown some interest in developing innovative and cost-effective models of care that address the needs of people with chronic medical conditions. For example, the Independence at Home model is a patient-centered approach in which a mobile team of physician, nurse, and social worker provides comprehensive care in the older person's home (DeJonge, Taler, & Boling, 2009).

The Guided Care model has been implemented as a nurse/physician partnership for promoting evidence-based care and self-management for patients with chronic conditions. Initial studies indicate that this model improves quality and efficiency of care and is feasible and acceptable to physicians, patients, and family caregivers (Boult, Giddens, & Frey, 2009). Guided Care nurses use electronic health records and work closely with the patient, family, and primary care physician to implement the following clinical processes: assessments, monitoring, and coaching; provision of evidence-based comprehensive interventions; promotion of self-management; coordination of all care, including transitions; education and support of caregivers; and facilitation of access to community resources (Aliotta et al., 2008). A more recently developed component of the program, called the Guided Care Program for Families and Friends, is currently being implemented and evaluated as a unique approach to support caregivers of older adults with complex health-related needs (Wolff et al., 2009). Nurses can find additional information about the Guided Care model at thePoint, and in the Resources section at the end of this chapter.

Care and Case Management Services

As the range of services for older adults has expanded and health care needs have become more complex, identification of appropriate services and coordination of care has become more necessary and more challenging. Although family members sometimes take on these tasks, they may not be prepared to assume this challenge or they may not have the time or availability to do so. Two societal trends that have affected the ability and availability of families to manage eldercare services are the entry of more women into the paid workforce and the cross-country, or even international, mobility of adult children families away from their hometowns. These factors, along with the significant increase in the number of people aged 85 years and older, have led to the need for independent community-based professional geriatric care management services.

A geriatric care manager serves as the primary care coordinator who is responsible for implementing immediate and long-term plans as the needs of the older adult change. Care management services involve comprehensive assessment, care planning, implementation, monitoring, and reassessment. Care managers typically work not only with older adults but also with other professionals, family members, caregivers, and support resources. When family member are providing care or coordination of services, care managers often provide counseling and education to address the needs of caregivers, who may or may not be older adults themselves. Nurses are in an ideal position to assume the role as a geriatric care manager because they can comprehensively assess the needs for immediate and long-term care services and then plan, coordinate, and oversee the services. Geriatric care managers work either as independent contractors or through nonprofit and for-profit groups and organizations. Internet sites that provide information about geriatric care managers are listed on thePoint.

Case management services are similar to geriatric care management services, but these are provided within an organizational context as part of a broader institution-based program. Hospitals and health insurance companies use case managers to make sure that patients receive the most appropriate and cost-effective services. Case management services also are usually provided as an integral part of comprehensive models, such as the Evercare model, to facilitate continuity and coordination of care. One study found that case management services in comprehensive models were highly valued by patients and their caregivers for improving access to health care, increasing psychosocial support, and improving communication with health care professionals (Sheaff et al., 2009). A review of studies on case management services found that there should be more priority given to implementing case management programs that focus on patient advocacy and that nurses have important roles in developing these programs (Oeseburg, Wynia, Middel, & Reijneveld, 2009).

PAYING FOR HEALTH CARE SERVICES FOR OLDER ADULTS

Sources of payment for health care services are self-pay and government programs or health insurance, such as Medicare, Medicaid, the Veterans Administration, supplemental insurance policies, and comprehensive models (e.g., PACE). Because of the current focus on reforming health care programs to address financial as well as quality issues, new models of care are emerging and it is increasingly more difficult to be knowledgeable about all sources of payment for care. For example, a program called Home Based Primary Care provides comprehensive primary care and interdisciplinary home care services for veterans with complex chronic conditions. Eligibility for this program depends in part on proximity to a Veterans Administration hospital and many areas of the country are not included in the target area (Beales & Edes, 2009).

Despite the complexity and limitations of programs, however, nurses need to know enough about the most common sources of payment for health services so they can understand and address some of the barriers to and challenges of implementing nursing care plans and discharge plans. For example, knowing the Medicare criteria for skilled home care services enables the nurse to make referrals for this type of nursing care when appropriate. The next sections provide an overview of the most common sources of payment for health services for older adults. Nurses are encouraged to keep up-to-date about major sources of health care coverage for older adults. For internet resources, go to thePoint.

Out-of-Pocket Expenses

Despite the major contribution of health insurance programs in paying for health care services, out-of-pocket health care expenses have been increasing steadily in recent decades and that burden falls disproportionately on poor people. Between 1997 and 2005, the median out-of-pocket health care spending as a percentage of income among Medicare beneficiaries increased from 11.9% to 16.1% (Neuman, Cubanski, & Damico, 2009). Older adults with lower incomes and those aged 85 and older experienced disproportionately higher increases in out-of-pocket expenses, as illustrated in Figure 6-4.

Except for the limited coverage for skilled nursing home care, Medicare does not cover costs of care in nursing homes or in assisted-living facilities. Because assisted-living facilities are residential places, however, Medicare will pay for skilled home care services and hospice care for people who meet the criteria for these services. A national survey found that the median rate for a private room was $3185 per month in assisted-living facilities and $6266 per month in nursing homes in 2009 (Genworth Financial, 2010).

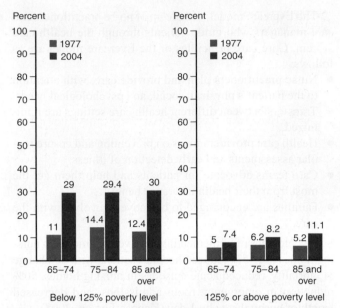

FIGURE 6-4 Out-of-pocket health care expenditures as a percentage of household income for peoples age 65+ by age and income category, 1977 and 2004. (*Source: Agency for Healthcare Research and Quality, Medical Expenditure Panel Survey and predecessor surveys.*)

Medicare

As a federal health insurance program for people who are eligible for Social Security benefits, Medicare covers primarily hospital and physician services, with very limited coverage for some skilled care services in homes and nursing homes (as reviewed previously in this chapter). The original Medicare plan is divided into Part A, funded through payroll taxes, and Part B, financed through monthly premiums paid by beneficiaries and by general revenues. Medicare, therefore, is part of the national budget and is subject to the same political processes that affect other budget items. Thus, the program has changed many times in response to concerns about cost and quality of care and pressure from consumers and health care providers.

A major limitation of the original Medicare program was that it did not cover preventive services. However, in recent years it has been expanded to cover the following preventive services: diabetes education; glaucoma screening; bone density measurements; colorectal cancer screening; mammograms and breast examinations; Papanicolaou test and pelvic examinations; influenza, pneumonia, and hepatitis B vaccinations; and prostate-specific antigen (PSA) tests and digital rectal examinations. Another limitation that is addressed by some Medicare Advantage plans is coverage for vision, hearing, and dental care. Box 6-3 summarizes information about the various Medicare programs that are now available to older adults in the United States.

Medigap Insurance

Because of the many limitations of Medicare as a health insurance program, many older adults purchase **medigap** policies, which are supplemental policies that attempt to fill the

Box 6-3 Medicare Insurance Plans

Original Medicare Part A, Also Called Hospital Insurance

- Available since 1965 without charge; provides hospital care coverage to people who are eligible for Social Security and Railroad Retirement benefits
- Helps pay for inpatient care in a hospital; care in a skilled nursing facility after a hospital stay; skilled home care services; hospice care
- Requires beneficiaries to be responsible for a co-pay amount for most services
- Reimburses hospital and skilled nursing facility fees based on benefit periods, which begin on the first day of hospital admission and end 60 days after the person no longer qualifies for care in a hospital or skilled nursing facility
- Administered by the federal government, Centers for Medicare & Medicaid Services (CMS), so that features are uniform throughout the United States.

Original Medicare Part B, Also Called Supplemental Insurance

- Available since 1965; supplements Medicare Part A for beneficiaries who pay a monthly premium
- Helps pay for outpatient medical care, including doctor visits, diagnostic imaging, and laboratory services; certain ambulance services; some durable medical equipment; some preventive services; and the services of certain specially qualified, nonphysician, health care practitioners (e.g., nurse practitioners)
- Requires beneficiaries to be responsible for monthly premiums and for co-pay amounts
- Managed by the federal government, CMS, so benefits are uniform throughout the United States.

Medicare Advantage Plans (Also Called Medicare Part C)

- Allows beneficiaries to enroll in one of the following types of private insurance plans: health maintenance organization (HMO), preferred provider organization (PPO), or private fee-for-service (PFFS)
- Provides an option for all beneficiaries who are entitled to Part A and enrolled in Part B, beneficiaries can elect to change plans on an annual basis between November 15 and March 31 of the following year
- Covers all benefits covered under Medicare Parts A and B, plus some additional services, such as preventive care and prescription medications
- Regulated and funded by the federal government, but are managed by private insurance companies; more than 3000 plans are available nationwide, with each one serving a specific geographic location.

Medicare Part D

- Available since 2006, provides limited coverage for prescription medications for Medicare beneficiaries
- Requires a monthly premium and cost-sharing amounts
- Applies limits to the annual amount covered and excludes some drugs (e.g., drugs for anorexia, weight control, or relief of symptoms of coughs or colds)
- Offers Medicare beneficiaries a choice of approved drug plans, and each plan varies in coverage for specific drugs. Beneficiaries are expected to compare available plans to determine which one best meets their needs.

gap between the services covered by original Medicare and those that are paid for out-of-pocket. All supplemental policies, which are regulated by federal and state laws, cover the premiums and copayments for services covered by Medicare Parts A and B, but additional benefits vary according to each policy. The National Association of Insurance Commissioners has developed 10 standard plans that insurance companies must follow in the provision of medigap policies. Plan A contains basic benefits, such as coverage for coinsurance payments and additional payments for hospital days. Other plans (B through J) cover Part A deductible and additional services, such as prescription medications, preventive medical care, skilled nursing coinsurance, and medical care in foreign countries.

A relatively new type of supplemental policy is the Medicare Select policy, which provides the same coverage as medigap policies, but only when services are provided by a designated, preferred provider. It is important to know that medigap policies were designed as supplements to original Medicare Parts A and B, and they are appropriate for people who enroll in the more recently developed Medicare Advantage plans. Because health insurance choices have become increasingly complex, nurses can encourage older adults and their caregivers to seek information from nonprofit organizations, such as the ones listed in the Resources at the end of this chapter.

Medicaid

Medicaid legislation was enacted at the same time as Medicare to provide health insurance for poor people. Medicaid is a federal/state partnership that has evolved to become the nation's largest health insurer. In recent years, studies indicate that it pays for care for all the following: two-thirds of nursing home residents, 20% of people younger than 65 with chronic disabilities, more than 25% of children, and more than one-third of all births (Mollica, 2009).

To qualify for Medicaid, people must meet medical and financial criteria, which are established by both state and federal regulations. States limit liquid assets to no more than about $2000, and the value of the home is generally exempt up to a maximum amount. Medicaid rules include strict policies to prevent the transfer of assets from one family member to another for 5 years before applying for Medicaid; however, the income and assets of a spouse are usually exempt from these restrictions. Because the cost of nursing home care is usually around $200/day, many older adults with modest incomes meet the eligibility criteria because they have limited assets and high medical expenses.

Although states have some discretion about what services are covered by Medicaid, the federal government mandates that certain medical services, including skilled home care and all levels of nursing home care, are covered for all eligible adults. Initially, Medicaid paid primarily for care in institutional rather than community-based settings; however, in the early 1990s, the focus shifted toward paying for community-based services for people who otherwise would need nursing home care. In the early 2000s, many states started reducing financial support for home- and community-based programs because of state budget crises. This is unfortunate because studies confirm that cutting funds to these programs results in higher use of more costly services, such as nursing facilities (D'Souza, James, Szafara, & Fries, 2009). Studies have also found that the provision of community-based services is cost effective because older adults use these services intermittently rather than requiring public support for nursing home care for the rest of their lives (Chapin, Baca, Macmillan, Rachlin, & Zimmerman, 2009). Medicaid funds often are available for home care services for people who otherwise would need nursing home care, but the cost of home care must be lower than the cost of care in an institutional setting.

Older Americans Act

The Older Americans Act (OAA) was enacted in 1965 to support programs to help older adults remain independent in their own homes and communities. Most of the OAA funds are allocated to nutrition services, which provide congregate and home-delivered meals, with lesser amounts allocated for a range of other services including homemaker, personal care, case management, transportation, chore, and adult day care. In recent years, OAA funds have been allocated for the National Family Caregiver Support Program, which provides services for caregivers, including training, counseling, and respite care. In 2006, the OAA Reauthorization Act included major provisions for improving coordination and delivery of long-term services and supports. This reauthorization act also funded an initiative called the Administration on Aging's Choice for Independence to provide information and support for consumers with regard to long-term care services. Another component of the OAA, the Nursing Home Diversion program, provided grants to states in 2007 and 2008 to provide services for people who are at high risk for nursing home placement but are not eligible for Medicaid (Accius, 2008). OAA-funded programs vary significantly among the states and localities, but they are administered through local senior centers. Nurses can generally find information about these programs by contacting social workers in health care organizations. Nurses also can suggest that older adults and their families explore these resources by contacting social workers in health care institutions or community-based organizations, such as senior centers.

Long-Term Care Insurance

Long-term care insurance policies are designed to cover some long-term care expenses that are not covered by health insurance programs. When long-term care insurance policies were first promoted in the late 1980s, they were unregulated and many of the policies contained large loopholes and significant barriers to receiving benefits. In recent years, many states enacted laws mandating standards suggested by the National Association of Insurance Commissioners. Suggested requirements for long-term care insurance policies include inflation protection and caps on rates. A good long-term care policy will provide payment for a range of options, including home care services, assisted-living facilities, and nursing home care. In addition, policies should be open enough that they include services that may be developed in the future but are not available at the time the policy is initiated. For example, the first long-term care policies that were developed were limited to nursing home care because few other options were available at that time. A major drawback of this type of insurance for older people is that the premiums are based on the age of the person when he or she initially signs up for the policy. For most older adults, therefore, the cost of the policy will outweigh the benefits.

Chapter Highlights

Development of a Continuum of Care for Older Adults
- After the establishment of Medicare and Medicaid in 1965, many new models of care emerged to address diverse health care needs of older adults (Figure 6-1).
- Terms such as aging in place, continuum of care, and long-term care are used to describe the focus of various settings of care for older adults (Box 6-1).

Acute Care Settings
- Acute care for elders (ACE) units address the complex needs of hospitalized older adults though multidisciplinary assessments and interventions.
- Subacute care units address the medically complex needs of hospitalized older adults.
- The hospital-at-home model provides cost-effective care for older adults with complex medical needs that can be addressed in a home setting.
- Transitional care is a term that is used in relation to models that provide coordination and continuity when patients move from one setting to another.
- The Geriatric Resource Nurse model prepares staff nurses as clinical resources for other nurses so they can address common geriatric syndromes, such as falls and confusion.

Nursing Home Settings
- Nursing homes are licensed residential institutional settings that provide a combination of skilled nursing for short-term post-hospital residents and intermediate care services for long-term residents.
- The reasons older adults need long-term nursing home care usually involve a combination of a gradual decline in functioning due to chronic conditions and the lack of caregivers who can provide the care at home.
- For people who meet the criteria, Medicare covers all or part of skilled nursing home care for a limited time.
- In recent decades, the level of dependency of nursing home residents has increased and special care units have been established to meet the needs of specific groups.

- Nurses in nursing home settings often assume teaching and leadership roles.

Newer Models of Nursing Home Care
- The culture change movement was initiated in 1997 with the goal of transforming the philosophy and practice in nursing homes to emphasize resident-centered care.
- Early studies of outcomes of culture change indicate that this approach results in positive improvements for residents, staff, and the nursing facility.
- The Pioneer Network in Long-Term Care promotes the development of culture change models, such as The Eden Alternative and the Green House Project.
- Assisted-living facilities were developed in the 1980s as settings for independent living, but in recent years some have evolved to provide a high level of care or specialized care.
- Newer models of care associated with culture change present many challenges as well as opportunities for nurses.

Home Care Services
- Because of many changes in health care trends during the past four decades, two types of home care services have emerged to address different needs: skilled home care and long-term home care.
- Skilled home care services provide short-term skilled nursing or rehabilitative services for homebound people who meet specific criteria.
- Long-term home care includes a wide spectrum of services ranging from nonskilled care such as meal preparation and grocery shopping to full-time hands-on nursing care.
- People obtain home care services through formal sources, such as agencies, or informal sources, including independent caregivers and family and friends.

Community-Based Services for Older Adults
- A wide variety of community-based services are available through public and private agencies (Box 6-2).
- Adult day centers provide structured activities for functionally impaired older people in a group setting.
- The primary goal of respite services is to relieve caregivers periodically from the stress of their usual caregiving responsibilities.
- Parish nursing is a holistic approach to addressing the physical, emotional, and spiritual health care needs of members of church-based congregations.
- Health promotion programs provide organized screening and health education services in community settings, such as senior centers.
- Nurses have many opportunities for innovative roles in establishing and implementing programs to address health-related needs of older adults in community settings.
- Nurses in home and community settings are likely to use telehealth technology for assessment or management of chronic conditions.

Models Addressing Coordination of Care
- Since the 1980s, the federal government has funded new models of comprehensive care, such as the Program of All-Inclusive Care for the Elderly (PACE) and the Evercare model.
- Chronic care models are currently being developed and promoted as cost-effective models of care that address the needs of people with chronic medical conditions.
- Geriatric care management services involve comprehensive assessment, care planning, implementation, monitoring, and reassessment to address immediate and long-term needs of older adults.
- Case management services are provided within the context of institution-based programs to ensure that patients receive the most appropriate and cost-effective services.

Paying for Health Care Services for Older Adults
- Sources of payment for health care services are self-pay, public funds for people who qualify, and insurance policies for people who have them.
- Medicare is the health insurance program that covers hospital and medical care and some skilled care services for people who are eligible for Social Security (Box 6-3).
- Medigap insurance is available from many sources to supplement Medicare coverage.
- Medicaid is a federal/state partnership that was established to provide medical care for poor people, but it has become the primary source of payment for nonskilled long-term care for older adults.
- The Older Americans Act funds services to help older adults remain independent in their own homes; in recent years, it has expanded to include programs that support caregivers and provide services for people who are at high risk for nursing home placement but are not eligible for Medicaid.
- Long-term care insurance policies are available to cover the cost of some long-term care services, but the costs outweigh the potential benefits for most older adults.

Critical Thinking Exercises

1. Mrs. S. is 84 years old and was recently diagnosed with dementia. She is able to care for herself as long as someone reminds her to eat her meals and take her medications. Two months ago, she began living with her daughter who works full time and is involved with several church-related activities. Three days a week, Mrs. S's daughter takes her to an adult day center at 8:30 and picks her up at 4:30. Twice weekly, Mrs. S. receives home-delivered meals. Find local resources for the types of services delineated in Box 6-2 and obtain information about four or five additional services that Mrs. S.'s daughter may need to use.
2. Mrs. F. is a resident in the skilled care section of the nursing home where you work. She had been living alone in her own home before being admitted to the hospital with a fractured hip 4 weeks ago. She has regained much of her independence

and walks with a walker and one-person assist. She expects to ambulate independently using a walker within 2 weeks, at which time she expects to return to her own home. She asks you what kind of services would be available in her home. What additional information would you want to know before you answered her questions? What information would you give to her? What suggestions would you make?

3. Your grandmother, who is 64 years old, asks your advice about health insurance choices that she needs to make before her next birthday. How would you explain her choices and what suggestions would you make to her? Use Box 6-3 and find additional information from organizations listed in the Resources section.

4. Explore information about culture change at www. pioneernetwork.net and print a copy of the Artifacts of Culture Change document in Appendix A. Apply as much information from this document as you can to evaluate a nursing facility where you have visited or done clinical work.

Resources

For links to these resources and additional helpful Internet resources related to this chapter, visit the Point. at http://thePoint. lww.com/Miller6e.

Clinical Tools

American Journal of Nursing and Hartford Institute for Geriatric Nursing
- *How to Try This,* article and video: The Hospital Admission Risk Profile (HARP), by C. Graf, *American Journal of Nursing, 108(8)*, 62–68.

Hartford Institute for Geriatric Nursing
- *Try This: Best Practices in Nursing Care to Older Adults* Issue 26 (2009). The Transitional Care Model (TCM): Hospital Discharge Screening Criteria for High Risk Older Adults

Nurses Improving Care for Healthsystem Elders (NICHE)
- Information about the Geriatric Registered Nurse model (from the Hartford Institute)

Health Education

Administration on Aging, Eldercare Locator
AARP
Advancing Excellence in America's Nursing Homes coalition
Advancing Excellence Campaign
American Association of Homes and Services for the Aging
American Health Care Association
Center for Excellence in Assisted Living
Centers for Medicare & Medicaid Services
Guided Care
National Association of Professional Geriatric Care Managers
National Citizens Coalition for Nursing Home Reform
National Institute on Aging
National PACE Association
Pioneer Network

REFERENCES

Accius, J. (2008). *The role of the Older Americans Act in providing long-term care.* Washington, DC: AARP Public Policy Institute.

Aliotta, S. L., Grieve, K., Giddens, J. F., Dunbar, L., Groves, C., Frey, K., & Boult, C. (2008). Guided care: A new frontier for adults with chronic conditions. *Professional Case Management, 13*, 151–158.

Bayne, C. G., & Boling, P. A. (2009). New diagnostic and information technology for mobile medical care. *Clinics in Geriatric Medicine, 25*, 93–107.

Baztan, J. J., Suarez-Garcia, F. M., Lopez-Arrieta, J., Rodrigues-Manas, L., & Rodrigues-Artalejo, F. (2009). Effectiveness of acute geriatric units on functional decline, living at home, and case fatality among older patients admitted to hospital for acute medical disorders: Meta-analysis. *British Medical Journal, 338*, doi:10.1136/bmj.b50.

Beales, J. L., & Edes, T. (2009). Veteran's Affairs home based primary care. *Clinics in Geriatric Medicine, 25*, 149–154.

Bixby, M. B., & Naylor, M. D. (2009). The Transitional Care Model (TCM): Hospital discharge screening criteria for high risk older adults. *Try This: Best Practices in Nursing Care to Older Adults.* Hartford Institute for Geriatric Nursing. Retrieved from http://consultgerirn/resources.

Boling, P. A. (2009). Care transitions and home health care. *Clinics in Geriatric Medicine, 25*, 135–148.

Boult, C., Giddens, J., & Frey, K. (2009). *Guided care: A new nurse-physician partnership in chronic care.* Baltimore: Johns Hopkins University.

Bowers, B., Nolet, K., Roberts, T., & Edmond, S. (2009). *Implementing change in long-term care: A practical guide to transformation.* The Commonwealth Fund. Retrieved from http://www.commonwealthfund.org/Content/Innovations/Tools/2009/Apr/Implementing-change.

Burger, S. G., Kantor, B., Mezey, M., Mitty, E., Kluger, M., Algase, D., . . . Rader, J. (2009). *Nurses involvement in nursing home culture change: Overcoming barriers, advancing opportunities.* The Hartford Institute for Geriatric Nursing Coalition for Geriatric Nursing Organizations & The Pioneer Network. Retrieved from http://hartfordign.org.

Capezuti, E. (2008). Optimizing care for hospitalized adults. *Geriatric Nursing, 29*, 27–29.

Capezuti, E., & Brush, B. L. (2009). Implementing geriatric care models: What are we waiting for? *Geriatric Nursing, 30*, 204–206.

Cartwright, J. C., Miller, L., & Volpin, M. (2009). Hospice in assisted living: Promoting good quality of care at end of life. *The Gerontologist, 49*, 508–5516.

Chapin, R., Baca, B., Macmillan, K., Rachlin, R., & Zimmerman, M. (2009). Residential outcomes for nursing facility applicants who have been diverted: Where are they 5 years later? *The Gerontologist, 49*, 46–56.

Cheng, J., Mantalto, M., & Leff, B. (2009). Hospitals at home. *Clinics in Geriatric Medicine, 25*, 79–91.

Cho, S., Zarit, S. H., & Chiriboga, D. A. (2009). Wives and daughters: The differential role of day care use in the nursing home placement of cognitively impaired family members. *The Gerontologist, 49*, 57–67.

Crist, J. D., Kim, S. S., Pasvogel, A., & Velazquez, J. H. (2009). Mexican American elders' use of home care services. *Applied Nursing Research, 22*, 26–34.

DeJonge, K. E., Taler, G., & Boling, P. A. (2009). Independence at home: Community-based care for older adults with severe chronic illness. *Clinics in Geriatric Medicine, 25*, 155–169.

Doty, M. M., Koren, M. J., & Sturla, E. (2008). *Culture change in nursing homes: How far have we come?* The Commonwealth Fund. Retrieved from http://www.commonwealthfund.org/publications_show.htm?doc_id=684709.

D'Souza, J. C., James, M. L., Szafara, K. L., & Fries, B. E. (2009). Hard times: The effects of financial strain on home care services use and participant outcomes in Michigan. *The Gerontologist, 49*, 154–165.

Genworth Financial. (2010). *Genworth 2010: Cost of care survey.* Retrieved from http://www.genworthfinancial.com.

Ginsburg, I. F., & Eng, C. (2009). On-site mental health services for PACE (Program of All-inclusive Care for the Elderly) centers. *Journal of the American Medical Directors Association, 10*, 277–280.

Graham, C. L., Ivey, S. L., & Neuhauser, L. (2009). From hospital to home: Assessing the transitional care needs of vulnerable seniors. *The Gerontologist, 49*, 23–33.

Grando, B. T., Buckwalter, K. C., Maas, M. L., Brown, M., Rantz, M. J., & Conn, V. S. (2009). A trial of a comprehensive nursing rehabilitation program for nursing home residents post-hospitalization. *Research in Gerontological Nursing, 2*, 12–19.

Greenwald, J. L., & Jack, B. W. (2009). Preventing the preventable: Reducing rehospitalizations through coordinated, patient-centered discharge processes. *Professional Case Management, 14*, 135–140.

Hirth, V., Baskins, J., & Dever-Bumba, M. (2009). Program of all-include care (PACE): Past, present, future. *Journal of the American Medical Directors Association, 10*, 155–160.

Jack, B. W., Chetty, V. K., Anthony, D., Greenwald, J. L., Sanchez, G. M., Johnson, A. E., . . . Culpepper, L. (2009). A reengineered hospital discharge program to decrease rehospitalizations. *Annals of Internal Medicine, 150*, 178–187.

Kane, R. A., & Cutler, L. J. (2008). *Sustainability and expansion of small-house nursing homes: Lessons from the Green Houses in Tupelo, MS. Division of Health Policy and Management, School of Public Health, University of Minnesota.* Retrieved from http://www.sph.umn.edu

Kang, H., Smith, M., Buckwalter, K. C., Ellingrod, V., & Schultz, S. K. (2010). Anxiety, depression, and cognitive impairment in dementia-specific and traditional assisted living. *Journal of Gerontological Nursing, 36*(1), 18–30.

Kappas-Larson, P. (2008). The Evercare story: Reshaping the health care model, revolutionizing long-term care. *Journal for Nurse Practitioners, 4*(2), 132–136.

King, M. A., & Tessaro, I. (2009). Parish nursing: Promoting healthy lifestyles in the church. *Journal of Community Nursing, 26*, 22–24.

Leff, B. (2009). Comparison of functional outcomes associated with hospital at home care and traditional acute hospital care. *Journal of the American Geriatrics Society, 57*, 273–278.

Lum, T. Y., Kane, R. A., Cutler, L. J., & Yu, T. C. (2008–2009). Effects of Green House nursing homes on residents' families. *Health Care Financing Review, 20*, 35–51.

Martikainen, P., Moustgaard, H., Murphy, M., Einiö, E. K., Koskinen, S., Martelin, T., & Noro, A. (2009). Gender, living arrangements, and social circumstances as determinants of entry into and exit from long-term institutional care at older ages: A 6-year follow-up study of older Finns. *The Gerontologist, 49*, 34–45.

McCabe, J., & Somers, S. (2009). Faith community nursing: Meeting the needs of seniors. *Journal of Community Nursing, 26*, 104–109.

Mollica, R. L. (2009). *Taking the long view: Investing in Medicaid home and community-based services is cost-effective.* Washington, DC: AARP Public Policy Institute.

Molzahn, A. E., Gallagher, E., & McNulty, V. (2009). Quality of life associated with adult day centers. *Journal of Gerontological Nursing, 35*(8), 37–46.

Mosocco, D. (2009). Introducing the PACE concept: Managed care for the frail older adult. *Home Healthcare Nurse, 27*, 423–428.

Murkofsky, R. L., & Alston, K. (2009). The past, present, and future of skilled home health agency care. *Clinics in Geriatric Medicine, 25*, 1–17.

Naylor, M., & Keating, S. A. (2008). Transitional care: Moving patients from one care setting to another. *American Journal of Nursing, 108*, 58S–63S.

Neuman, T., Cubanski, J., & Damico, A. (2009) *Revisiting 'Skin in the Game' among Medicare beneficiaries*. The Kaiser Family Foundation. Retrieved from http://www.kff.org.

Oeseburg, B., Wynia, K., Middel, B., & Reijneveld, S. A. (2009). Effects of case management for frail older people or those with chronic illness. *Nursing Research, 58*, 201–210.

Podrazik, P. M., & Whelan, C. T. (2008). Acute hospital care for the elderly patient: Its impact on clinical and hospital systems of care. *Medical Clinics of North America, 92*, 387–406.

Rabig, J. (2009). Home again: Small houses for individuals with cognitive impairment. *Journal of Gerontological Nursing, 35*(8), 10–15.

Rahman, A. N., & Schnelle, J. F. (2008). The nursing home culture-change movement: Recent past, present, and future directions for research. *The Gerontologist, 48*, 142–148.

Rantz, M. J., Cheshire, D., Flesner, M., Petroski, G. F., Hicks, L., Alexander, G., . . . Thomas, S. (2009). Helping nursing homes "at risk" for quality problems: a statewide evaluation. *Geriatric Nursing, 30*, 238–249.

Resnick, B., Gruber-Baldini, A. L., Galik, E., Pretzer-Aboff, I., Russ, K., Hebel, J. R., & Zimmerman, S. (2009). Changing philosophy in long-term care: Testing of the restorative care intervention. *The Gerontologist, 49*, 175–184.

Robinson, K. M., & Reinhard, S. C. (2009). Looking ahead in long-term care: The next 50 years. *Nursing Clinics of North America, 44*, 253–262.

Schoen, C., Osborn, R., How, S. K., Doty, M. M., & Peugh, J. (2009). Experiences of patients with complex health care needs in eight countries. *Health Affairs (Millwood), 28*(1), w1–w16.

Sheaff, R., Boaden, R., Sargent, P., Pickard, S., Gravelle, H., & Roland, M. (2009). Impacts of case management for frail elderly people: A qualitative study. *Journal of Health Services Research Policy, 14*, 88–95.

Shepperd, S., Doll, H., Angus, R. M., Clarke, M. J., Iliffe, S., Kalra, L., . . . Wilson, A. D. (2009). Avoiding hospital admission through provision of hospital care at home: A systematic review and meta-analysis of individual patient data. *Canadian Medical Association Journal, 180*, 175–182.

Shippee, T. P. (2009). "But I am not moving": Residents' perspectives on transitions within a continuing care retirement community. *The Gerontologist, 49*, 418–427.

Teri, L., McKenzie, G. L., LaFazia, D., Farran, C. J., Beck, C., Huda, P., . . . Pike, K. C. (2009). Improving dementia care in assisted living residences: Addressing staff reactions to training. *Geriatric Nursing, 30*, 153–163.

Vasquez, M. S. (2008). Down to the fundamentals of telehealth and home healthcare nursing. *Home Healthcare Nurse, 26*, 280–287.

White-Chou, E. G., Graves, W. J., Godfrey, S. M., Bonner, A., & Sloane, P. (2009). Beyond the medical model: The culture change revolution in long-term care. *Journal of the American Medical Directors Association, 10*, 370–378.

Wolff, J. L., Rand-Giobannetti, E., Wegener, S., Palmer, S., Reider, L., Frey, K., . . . Boult, C. (2009). Caregiving and chronic care: The Guided Care Program for Families and Friends. *Journal of Gerontology: Medical Sciences, 64A*, 785–791.

Zelada, M. A., Salinas, R., & Baztan, J. J. (2009). Reduction of functional deterioration during hospitalization in an acute geriatric unit. *Archives of Gerontology and Geriatrics, 48*, 35–39.

CHAPTER 7

Assessment of Health and Functioning

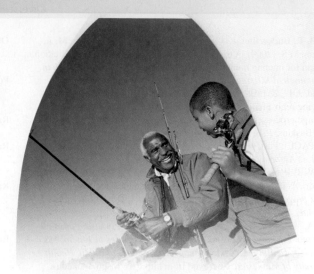

LEARNING OBJECTIVES

After reading this chapter, you will be able to:

1. Discuss factors that contribute to the complexity of assessing older adults.
2. Identify resources for nursing assessment tools.
3. Perform a functional assessment of an older adult.
4. Describe how the older adult's environment, use of adaptive and assistive devices, and cognitive abilities can affect functioning.
5. Explain how nurses can assess and address concerns about safe driving in older adults.

K E Y P O I N T S

activities of daily living (ADLs)
comprehensive geriatric assessment
everyday competence
functional assessment

instrumental activities of daily living (IADLs)
Minimum Data Set (MDS) for Resident Assessment and Care Screening

Assessment of health and functioning of older adults is an essential and complex component of nursing care. This chapter discusses the general approach to assessing the older adult's health and functioning and provides tools for **functional assessment**. In addition, because health and functioning significantly affect the ability to drive a motor vehicle—which is a major safety concern with implications for society and individual older adults—this chapter discusses how nurses can assess and address risk factors that interfere with safe driving in older adults.

ASSESSING HEALTH OF OLDER ADULTS

A major challenge of caring for older adults is the complexity of assessing their health, especially from a comprehensive and holistic nursing perspective. Several factors contribute to the complexity of assessing health and functioning of older adults:

- Older adults commonly have one or more chronic conditions in addition to any acute health conditions for which they are being assessed. These conditions often interact, causing older adults' health to fluctuate unpredictably.
- Manifestations of illness, even acute illness, tend to be obscure and less predictable in older adults than in younger adults. For example, in older adults, one of the most common manifestations of illness or an adverse medication effects is a change in behavior or mental status.
- For any one manifestation of illness in an older adult, there are usually several possible explanations. For example, changes in function can be caused by a combination of several of the following conditions: acute illness, psychosocial factors, environmental conditions, age-related changes, a new chronic illness, an existing chronic illness, or an adverse effect of medication(s) or other treatments.
- Treatments are often directed toward the symptoms while the source of a problem is obscure and unresolved. This approach can mask the underlying problem even further and cause additional complications (e.g., when adverse medication effects are not recognized as such and are treated with additional medications).
- Cognitive impairments can make it difficult for older adults to accurately report or describe a physiologic problem and there may be few or no reliable sources of information.
- In many cases, by the time illness in an older adult is detected and addressed, the underlying physiologic disturbance is in an advanced stage, and additional complications have developed.
- Myths and misunderstandings can lead health care providers, family members, or older adults to falsely attribute treatable conditions to aging.

Because of all of these factors, nurses must take a detective-like approach to assessing older adults. This approach requires nurses to assess all aspects of the person's body, mind, and spirit to look for clues—which are usually many and complicated and range from subtle to obvious—to underlying causes of changes in health or functioning. The Functional Consequences Model for Promoting Wellness in Older Adults is described in Chapter 3 and applied to specific aspects of functioning throughout this text. Nurses can use these detailed guides to assess older adults holistically and to plan and implement nursing interventions directed toward improved functioning and quality of life (refer to list in Table of Contents). Nurses also can refer to information in Chapter 27 about unique and atypical manifestations of illness in older adults.

Clinically oriented chapters of this text also include information about normal age-related variations that nurses need to consider when assessing specific aspects of health and functioning. In addition, nurses can use Table 7-1 as a guide to age-related variations in laboratory values that are pertinent to overall nursing assessment of older adults.

NURSING ASSESSMENT TOOLS

Since the late 1980s, the Hartford Institute for Geriatric Nursing has been in the forefront of developing, promulgating, and updating evidence-based and easy-to-use nursing assessment tools for use in various settings. These assessment guides, which are called *Try this: Best Practices in Nursing Care to Older Adults,* and a series of 28 cost-free web-based articles and corresponding videos demonstrating the application of these tools is available online at http://consultgerirn.org/resources. These tools do not replace a comprehensive assessment but are useful for identifying specific areas to address in the care plan. Assessment tools from the Hartford Foundation and other reliable sources are listed in the Clinical Tools sections at the ends of chapters in this book.

Nurses in home care settings have addressed the need for a simple-to-use functional assessment tool that can be used to measure quality of care and changes in level of functioning in older adults. For example, the "SHOW ME" functional assessment tool can be used to assess functioning in the following areas: **S**hirt & **S**hoes, **H**ike to bathroom, **O**rganization and use of grooming utensils, **W**alk through home in all areas needed for ADLs/IADLs, **M**edications, and **E**ating and making meals (Narayan, Salgado, & VanVoorhis, 2009).

✚ Wellness Opportunity

When assessing older adults, nurses try to identify the conditions that affect not only health status and level of functioning but also quality of life.

ASSESSING FUNCTION OF OLDER ADULTS

A functional assessment is an integral component of a holistic assessment because an essential part of promoting wellness for older adults is identifying areas where function can be

A Student's Perspective

During my first week with Mr. M., I was able to sit with him while he was having breakfast, and I used this time to consider his strengths and weaknesses. While studying his interactions with others, I observed that he had difficulty being understood. He struggled to articulate his various wants and needs. This seemed to lead Mr. M. being more isolated than would otherwise be the case. One of his strengths was his ability to feed himself. Initially, I had hoped to read his chart more before meeting him. However, this interaction allowed me a more accurate assessment of his abilities than what would have been recorded in his chart.

After breakfast, we returned to his room to do oral care and to shave. After this, I helped transfer Mr. M. to his bed and he asked for a drink, which I gave him and he started choking. I was terrified, but fortunately my senior student was with me and together we managed the situation and he was okay. I learned from this experience to assess the person's entire environment before addressing patient needs and desires. Mr. M. choked because I gave him a cup of water that was not thickened.

Kimberly S.

improved. Functional assessment refers to the measurement of a person's ability to fulfill responsibilities and perform self-care tasks. It is associated with a rehabilitation approach, rather than a medical diagnosis approach, because it emphasizes improved functioning in daily life. For example, a functional assessment for a person with hemiparesis resulting from a stroke focuses on the limitations and abilities of the person in carrying out his or her usual activities so that a care plan can be developed to meet goals for improved functioning.

Using Functional Assessment Tools

Functional assessment tools have their roots in 1920s when workers' compensation programs needed to determine a cash value to impairments that affected loss of function in jobs. Initially, there were no standards for this and the determination was based solely on a physician's opinion. When rehabilitation services were developed two decades later, tools were needed to measure changes in functional abilities. In recent years, health care practitioners have increasingly recognized the value of functional assessment, particularly with regard to rehabilitation services, chronic conditions, and geriatric care. Because functional ability is one of the most sensitive indicators of health in older adults, standards for evidence-based practice mandate that nurses incorporate functional assessments into all patient-care assessments (Kresevic, 2008). Figure 7-1 lists major trends that have lead to the use of functional assessment tools in gerontological health care settings today.

Functional assessment scales measure the following six **activities of daily living (ADLs)**, which are the tasks involved with meeting one's basic needs independently: toileting, feeding, dressing, grooming, bathing, and ambulation. In addition, they measure more complex tasks that are essential in

TABLE 7-1 Age-Related Variations in Laboratory Values

Test Values, Ages 20–40 Years	Age-Related Changes	Considerations
Serum		
Albumin, 3.5–5 g/dL	Younger than age 65: higher in men Older than age 65: equal levels that then decrease at same rate	Increased dietary protein intake needed in older patients if liver function is normal; edema: a sign of low albumin level
Alkaline phosphatase, 13–39 IU/L	Increases 8–10 IU/L	May reflect liver function decline or vitamin D malabsorption and bone demineralization
Beta globulin, 2.3–3.5 g/dL	Increases slightly	Increases in response to decrease in albumin if liver function is normal; increased dietary protein intake needed
Blood urea nitrogen Men: 10–25 mg/dL Women: 8–20 mg/dL	Increases, possibly to 69 mg/dL	Slight increase acceptable in absence of stressors, such as infection or surgery
Cholesterol, 120–220 mg/dL	Men: increases to age 50, then decreases Women: lower than men until age 50, increases to age 70, then decreases	Rise in cholesterol level (and increased cardiovascular risk) in women as a result of postmenopausal estrogen decline; dietary changes, weight loss, and exercise needed
Creatine kinase, 17–148 U/L	Increases slightly	May reflect decreasing muscle mass and liver function
Creatinine, 0.6–1.5 mg/dL	Increases, possibly to 1.9 mg/dL in men	Important factor to prevent toxicity when giving drugs excreted in urine
Creatinine clearance, 104–125 mL/min	Men: decreases; formula: (140 − age) × kg body weight/72 × serum creatinine Women: 85% of men's rate	Reflects reduced glomerular filtration rate; important factor to prevent toxicity when giving drugs excreted in urine
Glucose tolerance (fasting plasma glucose) 1 hour: 160–170 mg/dL 2 hr: 115–125 mg/dL 3 hr: 70–110 mg/dL	Rises faster in first 2 hours, then drops to baseline more slowly	Reflects declining pancreatic insulin supply and release and diminishing body mass for glucose uptake (Rapid rise can quickly trigger hyperosmolar hyperglycemic nonketotic syndrome. Rapid decline can result from certain drugs, such as alcohol, beta-adrenergic blockers, and monoamine oxidase inhibitors.)
Hematocrit Men: 45%–52% Women: 37%–48%	May decrease slightly (unproven)	Reflects decreased bone marrow and hematopoiesis, increased risk of infection (because of fewer and weaker lymphocytes and immune system changes that diminish antigen—antibody response)
Hemoglobin Men: 13–18 g/dL Women: 12–16 g/dL	Men: decreases by 1–2 g/dL Women: unknown	Reflects decreased bone marrow, hematopoiesis, and (for men) androgen levels
High-density lipoprotein, 80–310 mg/dL	Levels higher in women than in men but equalize with age	Compliance with dietary restrictions required for accurate interpretation of test results
Lactate dehydrogenase, 45–90 U/L	Increases slightly	May reflect declining muscle mass and liver function
Leukocyte count, 4300–10,800/mcL	Decreases to 3100–9000/mcL	Decrease proportionate to lymphocyte count
Lymphocyte count T cells: 500–2400/mcL B cells: 50–200/mcL	Decreases	Decrease proportionate to leukocyte count
Platelet count, 150,000–350,000/mm³	Change in characteristics: decreased granular constituents, increased platelet-release factors	May reflect diminished bone marrow and increased fibrinogen levels
Potassium, 3.5–5.5 mEq/L	Increases slightly	Requires avoidance of salt substitutes composed of potassium, vigilance in reading food labels, and knowledge of hyperkalemia's signs and symptoms
Thyroid-stimulating hormone, 0.3–5 mcIU/mL	Increases slightly	Suggests primary hypothyroidism or endemic goiter at much higher levels
Thyroxine, 4.5–13.5 mcg/dL	Decreases 25%	Reflects declining thyroid function
Triglycerides, 40–150 mg/dL	Range widens: 20–200 mg/dL	Suggests abnormalities at any other levels, requiring additional tests such as serum cholesterol
Triiodothyronine, 90–220 ng/dL	Decreases 25%	Reflects declining thyroid function
Urine		
Glucose, 0–15 mg/dL	Decreases slightly	May reflect renal disease or urinary tract infection (UTI); unreliable check for older diabetic people because glucosuria may not occur until plasma glucose level exceeds 300 mg/dL
Protein, 0–5 mg/dL	Increases slightly	May reflect renal disease or UTI
Specific gravity, 1.032	Decreases to 1.024 by age 80	Reflects 30%–50% decrease in number of nephrons available to concentrate urine

Laboratory values that are not affected by increased age:

- Prothrombin time
- Partial thromboplastin time
- Serum chloride
- Serum carbon dioxide
- Serum acid phosphatase
- Aspartate aminotransferase
- Total serum protein

From *Handbook of geriatric nursing care* (2nd ed., Appendix B, pp. 627–629) (2003). Philadelphia, PA: Lippincott Williams & Wilkins.

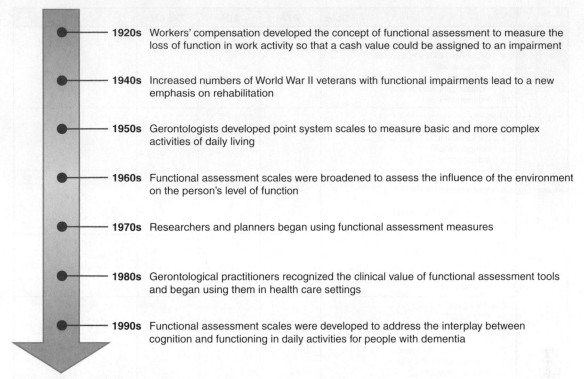

FIGURE 7-1 Significant trends that led to the development and use of functional assessment tools in gerontological health care settings.

community-living situations. These complex tasks, designated as **instrumental activities of daily living (IADLs)**, include shopping, laundry, transportation, housekeeping, meal preparation, money management, medication management, and use of telephone. Assessment of ADL performance is important in determining the level of assistance needed on a daily basis and is particularly helpful in addressing long-term care needs. Likewise, an evaluation of IADLs is important in determining the level of assistance needed by people in independent or semi-independent settings.

Some functional assessment tools document changes that occur over time and identify factors that influence functional abilities. For example, the functional assessment tool illustrated in Figure 7-2 was developed by nurses in a geriatric rehabilitation setting and can be used to measure a person's functional status at different times.

An initial functional assessment, which is performed at the time of admission (ADM), provides information on which goals for care are based. The form also includes a column for information about the person's reported level of function before admission, which is helpful in determining the person's potential level of function. At the time of discharge, the reassessment information enables the staff to determine whether the goals were met. In settings in which post-discharge follow-up is possible, or in settings in which the person is readmitted at different times, the same assessment form is used to measure changes over time. Each category of activity is assigned a numeric value based on the criteria listed in Boxes 7-1 and 7-2. The numeric values are then used

as a guide to measure progress toward goals as the person's level of function changes.

The functional assessment form in Figure 7-2 differs from many others in several ways. First, it allows for measurement of changes over time. The three time designations indicated on the form signify the period prior to admission (PTA), the ADM, and the day of discharge (DISCH). The unmarked columns may be used at any time after discharge, or upon readmission. In a rehabilitative or long-term care setting, these measurements over time are particularly helpful in evaluating progress and reevaluating goals. Second, it includes a scale for documenting mental status because it is essential to ascertain the effects of cognition on functioning. Third, for each category, the number 1 rating is used to indicate that the person does not depend on others but depends on some adaptive device or equipment for independent function in that area. The adaptive device might be as small as a shoehorn or as complex as an electric wheelchair. The importance of this designation is that the staff is then aware that the person has compensated for a deficit, but that the compensatory mechanism must be available for the person's use.

Nurses obtain information for the functional assessment from several sources. When older adults are able to provide reliable information about their level of function before admission, the nurse obtains data for the column marked "PTA" by interviewing the patient/resident within 24 hours of the admission to the care facility. When, as is often the case, older adults are not able to provide this information, the nurse interviews a family member or other person who is knowledgeable about

		Date	PTA	ADM	DISCH		
Personal Care	Bathing 5 completely dependent 4 dependent with some assist 3 heavy partial 2 light partial 1 independent with devices 0 independent						
	Dressing 5 complete assist 3 partial assist 1 compensated 0 independent						
	Mouth care 5 totally unable to do 3 some assist 1 independent with device 0 independent						
	Hair care 5 completely unable 3 some assist 1 independent with device 0 independent						
	Dietary intake 5 total assist 4 assist with feeding 3 supplements 2 set up/encouragement 1 independent with device 0 independent						
Mobility	Transfer 5 completely unable 4 3-person/portalift 3 2-person 2 1-person 1 independent with devices 0 independent						
	Ambulation 5 completely unable 4 3-person assist 3 2-person assist 2 1-person assist 1 independent with devices 0 independent						
	Bed 5 unable to move in bed 3 needs assist 1 independent with device 0 independent						
Mental Status	Mental 5 totally impaired 4 assist with simple tasks 3 assist with complex tasks 2 inconsistent 1 compensated 0 no impairment						

FIGURE 7-2 Functional assessment of older adults. This form allows for recording changes over time. The three time designations indicated on the form signify the period prior to admission (PTA), the time of admission (ADM), and the day of discharge (DISCH). The unmarked columns may be used at any time after discharge, or upon readmission. (Used with permission from Fairview General Hospital, Cleveland, OH.) (*continued*)

the person's level of function before admission. Nurses directly observe the person's current level of function in performing ADLs to complete the columns marked "ADM" and "DISCH." In institutional settings, nurses must obtain much of the information on IADLs by questioning the older adult or his or her caregivers because many of these activities pertain only to

community-based settings. The source of information is noted on the chart, and any discrepancies between objective and subjective information also are noted.

In interviewing the older adult or caregiver, it is important to ask for specific details about how tasks are accomplished, rather than ask open-ended questions such as "Do you have

		Date	PTA	ADM	DISCH		
Elimination	*Bladder* 5 completely incontinent 3 occasionally incontinent 1 continent with assist/device 0 continent/independent						
	Bowel 5 completely incontinent 3 occasionally incontinent 1 continent with assist/device 0 continent/independent						
	Assist/device codes A bedside commode E ostomy I catheter, intermittent B bathroom F incontinence pads J verbal cuing/supervision C urinal G catheter, external K other_____ D bedpan H catheter, indwelling						
Instrumental Activities of Daily Living	*Meal preparation* 5 unable to do 3 assist/supervise 1 independent with resources 0 independent						
	Shopping 5 unable to do 3 assist/supervise 1 compensated 0 independent						
	Telephone 5 unable to do/doesn't have 3 assist 1 independent with device 0 independent						
	Transportation 5 completely homebound 3 assist 1 arranges own 0 independent						
	Medications 5 unable to take 3 assist 1 independent 0 doesn't use						
	Housekeeping 5 unable to do 3 assist 1 independent with resources 0 independent						
	Laundry 5 unable to do 3 assist 1 independent with resources 0 independent						
	Money management 5 unable to handle 3 assist 1 independent with resources 0 independent						
	Total Points						

FIGURE 7-2 (continued)

any difficulty with . . .?" Also, it is important to find out whether the task is meaningful to the person, rather than assuming that the person wants or needs to do the task. For example, in the IADL categories, a person who lives with other people might never have to participate in grocery shopping or money management. Therefore, assessment information, particularly regarding IADLs, must be considered in relation to the person's support system and living arrangements.

Wellness Opportunity

Nurses identify factors that affect the older adult's quality of life by asking a question such as "Are there enjoyable activities that you used to do but are no longer able to do because of health problems?"

Assessing Activities of Daily Living

The following areas of function are those generally considered in an assessment of ADLs: grooming, bathing, dressing,

Box 7-1   Criteria for Assessing Activities of Daily Living (ADLs)

Bathing
5 Unable to assist in any way
4 Able to cooperate but cannot assist
3 Able to wash hands, face, and chest with supervision; needs help with completing the bath
2 Able to wash face, chest, arms, and upper legs; needs help with completing the bath
1 Bathes self but requires devices (e.g., long-handled sponge)
0 Bathes self-independently

Dressing
5 Needs total assistance
4 Needs total supervision but is able to dress self if clothing articles are given one at a time or set out in the order they are needed
3 Needs reminding and encouragement and some assistance with clothing selection, but can dress with little supervision
2 Dresses self, but needs help with activities requiring fine motor skills (e.g., zippers, shoelaces)
1 Dresses self, using assistive devices (e.g., zipper pullers, long-handled shoehorn)
0 Dresses independently

Mouth Care
5 Cannot perform oral hygiene but requires that it be done by others
4 Needs total supervision; needs toothpaste put on brush
3 Needs reminding and some supervision
2 Needs reminding but is otherwise independent
1 Performs oral hygiene using devices (e.g., toothbrush with built-up handle)
0 Performs oral hygiene independently

Hair Care
5 Cannot perform hair care but requires that it be done by others
4 Needs total supervision
3 Needs some assistance with daily care
2 Performs daily care independently but needs assistance with washing hair
1 Performs hair care using devices (e.g., hairbrush with built-up handle)
0 Performs all hair care (including washing) independently

Dietary Intake
5 Cannot prepare or obtain food; cannot feed self; nutritional requirements would not be met without total assistance
4 Needs assistance in obtaining and preparing food; needs total supervision with eating, but can feed self; nutritional requirements would not be met adequately without assistance
3 Needs assistance in tasks that involve complex skills (e.g., cutting meat, opening packages, preparing and obtaining food), but feeds self; nutritional needs would be met partially without assistance
2 Requires some assistance with obtaining and preparing food, but eats independently; would maintain adequate nutrition with encouragement or a little assistance
1 Needs assistive devices for food preparation and consumption (e.g., plate rings, rocker knife); adequately maintains nutritional requirements
0 Requires no assistance

Transfer Mobility
5 Cannot transfer, except with extreme difficulty
4 Needs assistance of three people for transfers, or needs two people and a lifting device
3 Needs the assistance of two people
2 Needs the assistance of one person
1 Transfers independently with a device (e.g., sliding board)
0 Transfers independently

Ambulation
5 Completely unable to walk
4 Walks with the assistance of three people
3 Walks with the assistance of two people
2 Walks with the assistance of one person
1 Walks independently with device (e.g., walker, quad cane)
0 Walks independently

Bed Mobility
5 Unable to move in bed
4 Needs the assistance of two people
3 Needs the assistance of one person
2 Needs to be encouraged and supervised
1 Moves independently with device (e.g., uses side rails or trapeze)
0 Moves independently in bed

Mental Status
5 Has extremely poor memory function; cannot follow directions; has minimal ability to identify and express needs; requires a totally structured environment
4 Has obvious memory impairment that interferes with daily life; has poor judgment and may undertake inappropriate actions; may be aware of the deficit and, consequently, may be anxious or depressed; can participate in daily routine but needs supervision; requires a strong orientation and reminder program
3 Fluctuates between levels two and four; unpredictable on a routine basis; requires monitoring and some supervision; may engage in risky behaviors at times
2 Minimal short-term memory loss; able to perform most daily tasks with only minimal reminding or supervision; has good-to-fair judgment and occasionally needs assistance, but does not engage in any risky behaviors
1 Is dependent on self-initiated reminders and cues for daily activities
0 No observable impairment in memory; no cognitive or psychosocial impairment that interferes with daily activities

Bladder and Bowel Elimination
5 Consistently soils self
4 Needs supervision and assistance on a regular basis
3 Needs reminding on a regular basis
2 Generally controls elimination; has accidents no more than once a week
1 Maintains control of elimination with devices (listed in Figure 11-1)
0 Fully continent without any assistance

---

eating, elimination, and mobility. The assessment format illustrated in Figure 7-2 further specifies these activities as follows: bathing, dressing, mouth care, hair care, dietary intake, transfer mobility, ambulation, bed mobility, and bladder and bowel elimination. In addition, a brief mental status assess-

ment is included on the ADL form. Including mental status in the functional assessment rather than using a separate mental status assessment tool reinforces the fact that cognitive function is an integral component of ADLs. In addition, it helps to determine whether ADL impairments are attributable, at least

Box 7-2 Criteria for Assessing Instrumental Activities of Daily Living (IADLs)

Meal Preparation

5 Unable to prepare even simple meals
4 Can assist with meal preparation
3 Prepares meals but cannot obtain groceries
2 Prepares meals with reminding or supervision
1 Prepares meals and obtains food using resources (e.g., specialized equipment, Meals on Wheels program, transportation to the grocery store)
0 Independent in obtaining and preparing food

Grocery Shopping

5 Cannot participate in shopping
4 Can accompany someone else and assist with food selection
3 Can shop and select appropriate food with some supervision
2 Can shop but has difficulty obtaining transportation
1 Is able to arrange for necessary help with shopping
0 Shops independently

Telephone Use

5 Cannot dial or answer the phone, or carry on a routine phone conversation
4 Can talk on the phone but cannot dial or answer it
3 Can use the phone with assistance (e.g., help in dialing)
2 Can use the phone with supervision
1 Depends on adaptive devices for telephone activities (e.g., automatic dialing system, speaker phone)
0 Independent in phone-related activities

Transportation

5 Does not leave home, even for medical care
4 Leaves home only for medical care or in rare circumstances
3 Needs assistance in arranging for transportation and needs special accommodations (e.g., wheelchair lift)
2 Needs assistance in arranging for transportation but can get in and out of cars with little or no help
1 Arranges for own transportation but depends on others for any transportation other than walking
0 Independent in traveling from one place to another (e.g., drives a car)

Medications

5 Unable to obtain or take medications without assistance or complete supervision
4 Cannot obtain medications but can take them with assistance or supervision
3 Can obtain and take medications with reminders from others or with a system set up by others
2 Can obtain and take medications with a self-initiated reminder or setup system
1 Safely takes and prepares all medications
0 Does not use medications

Housekeeping

5 Cannot perform any routine household tasks
4 Can assist with household tasks (e.g., bed making, dusting, vacuuming)
3 Can perform household tasks if supervised during the activity
2 Can perform household tasks if encouraged to do so
1 Arranges for housekeeping assistance
0 Is independent in all routine tasks

Laundry

5 Cannot perform any laundry tasks
4 Can assist with folding clothes; cannot wash or iron clothes
3 With assistance, can perform laundry tasks adequately
2 Can perform laundry tasks with supervision and reminding
1 Arranges for laundry to be done
0 Completes all laundry tasks independently

Money Management

5 Unable to manage any aspect of finances
4 Can handle simple cash transactions but no other financial transactions (e.g., writing checks)
3 Can write checks with supervision or assistance; cannot handle any higher-level transactions (e.g., bank withdrawals)
2 Maintains checkbook, pays bills appropriately, and understands currency exchanges, but needs some assistance or supervision with these tasks
1 Arranges for someone else to handle financial matters
0 Handles all finances independently

---

in part, to cognitive impairments, rather than primarily to physical limitations. See Box 7-1 for the functional assessment criteria for each of the ADLs, as well as for mental status.

Assessing Instrumental Activities of Daily Living

IADLs are less important in institutional settings than they are in community settings. In institutional settings, however, an assessment of IADLs is an important consideration in discharge planning. When older adults cannot perform IADLs independently, caregivers often provide the assistance that enables the person to remain in a community setting. Often when older adults cannot perform IADLs and have no caregiver to help with the task, community resources are available to meet these needs. Home-delivered meals programs, for example, might be appropriate for older adults who have difficulty with shopping or meal preparation. Community resources usually can be arranged with one or two phone calls, and they can be effective and efficient ways of improving an older adult's ability

to perform IADLs. See Box 7-2 for assessment criteria for the IADLs that are included in Figure 7-2.

Assessing Function in Cognitively Impaired Older Adults

Because cognitive status and psychosocial functioning can significantly affect one's level of functioning, it is particularly challenging to assess function in older adults who have any cognitive or psychosocial limitations (e.g., dementia, delirium, depression). Some functional assessment scales have been developed specifically for people with dementia in a variety of settings and at all levels of cognitive impairment. These tools address the interplay between cognition and abilities to perform ADLs. For example, the Cleveland Scale for Activities of Daily Living (CSADL) divides each ADL into smaller components to identify specific effects of the underlying cognitive deficit. Studies have found that this instrument, illustrated in Figure 7-3, is reliable and valid as a

CLEVELAND SCALE FOR ACTIVITIES OF DAILY LIVING (CSADL)

Name or ID of Subject _____   Date _ _ / _ _ / _ _   Rater _____
                                                                       m m d d y y

Name of Informant _____

Relation of Informant to Subject (Circle one.)   Contact with Subject   Interview Type

1 Spouse   4 Friend or other family   1 2 days/week   1 Visit
2 Child   5 Professional: _____   2 3–4 days/week   2 Telephone
3 Sibling   6 Other: _____   3 5 or more days/week

To administer this scale, the rater must be thoroughly familiar with the Manual, which includes the full instructions. Place rating in blank after each item number. Several items have specific rating instructions. In particular, some require special questioning if the subject is rated as dependent (rating of 1, 2, or 3).

Rating	Meaning of Rating
0	**Never Dependent.** [S] does this effectively, quite independently, without any direction or help.
1	**Sometimes Dependent.** [S] usually does this independently, but sometimes or in some situations [S] needs direction or help.
2	**Usually Dependent.** [S] usually requires some direction or help, but sometimes or in some situations [S] does it independently.
3	**Always Dependent.** [S] always requires direction or help. [S] never does it independently.
9	Cannot rate because of insufficient information

Bathing

1. ____   Initiates bath or shower with appropriate frequency and at appropriate times

2. ____   Prepares bath/shower (draws water of proper temperature, ensures soap and towel are present, etc.)

3. ____   Gets in and out of tub or shower

4. ____   Cleans self

Toileting

5. ____   Able to physically control timing of urination

6. ____   Able to physically control timing of bowel movements

7. ____   Recognizes need to eliminate

8. ____   After toileting, cleans and re-clothes self appropriately

Personal Hygiene and Appearance

9. ____   Initiates personal grooming with appropriate frequency and at appropriate times

10. ____   Washes hands and face

11. ____   Brushes teeth

12. ____   Combs hair, shaves (as appropriate)

FIGURE 7-3 The Cleveland Scale for Activities of Daily Living (CSADL). This functional assessment form was specifically designed for use with people with Alzheimer's disease. (Used with permission from the University Memory and Aging Center, Case Western Reserve University, Cleveland, OH. © 1994.)

Dressing

13. _____   Initiates dressing at appropriate time

14. _____   Selects clothes

15. _____   Puts on garments, footwear, etc.

16. _____   Fastens clothing (buttons, shoelaces, zippers, etc.)

Eating

17. _____   Initiates eating at appropriate times of day and with appropriate frequency

18. _____   Carries out physical acts of eating (including using utensils)

19. _____   Eats with acceptable manners, e.g. with appropriate speed, does not speak with food in mouth, etc.

20. _____   Prepares own meals (includes cooking on stove). *This item requires special questioning.*

Mobility

21. _____   Initiates actively moving about the environment, as opposed to sitting, not attempting to get about, etc.

22. _____   Actively moves about environment (with or without assisting device)

22a.   Does subject have physical limitations of mobility? *(Circle one of following codes.)*

    0   No physical limitations of mobility

    1   Yes, there are physical limitations of mobility. *(Circle all that apply.)*

Needs assistance of other persons to walk	Trouble getting in or out of bed	Other Mobility Problems
Needs cane	Trouble getting in or out of chair	*(describe):*
Needs walker	Trouble getting on or off toilet	
Needs wheelchair	Trouble climbing or descending stairs	

Medications

23. _____   Takes medications as scheduled and in correct dosages. *If subject has taken no medications during prior year, rate item as 9. This item requires questioning.*

Shopping

24. _____   Does necessary grocery shopping, buying appropriate items and quantities. *This item requires special questioning.*

25. _____   Does necessary clothes shopping, buying appropriate items and quantities. *This item requires special questioning.*

Travel

26. _____   Finds way about in familiar surroundings

27. _____   Orients to unfamiliar surroundings without undue difficulty

28. _____   Travels beyond walking distance (i.e., driving own vehicle or using public transportation)

29. _____   Drives motor vehicle. *This item requires special questioning.*

FIGURE 7-3 (continued)

Hobbies, personal interests, employment

30. _____   Initiates activities of personal interest (e.g. card playing, woodworking, others). *This item requires special questioning.*

31. _____   Carries out such activities. *This item requires special questioning.*

32. _____   Does subject work for pay? *If subject does not work because of having reached an age appropriate to retirement from his or her occupation, rate 9. This item requires special questioning.*

Housework/home maintenance (as appropriate to individual situation)

33. _____   Initiates work around house as needed. *This item requires special questioning.*

34. _____   Carries out work effectively, e.g. cleanly, neatly, accurately, efficiently*This item requires special questioning.*

Types of work done *(Don't score, just circle)*

Dish washing	Vacuuming	Mowing lawn
Sweeping	Scrubbing floors	Gardening
Personal laundry	Small home repairs	Minor car care
Other types of work *(Describe):*		

Telephone

35. _____   Looks up numbers

36. _____   Dials numbers

37. _____   Answers phone

38. _____   Takes messages

Money Management

39. _____   Pays for purchases (selecting appropriate amount and determining correct change). *This item requires special questioning.*

40. _____   Manages financial responsibilities beyond paying for immediate purchases (e.g., paying monthly bills, managing checking or savings account, etc.). *This item requires special questioning.*

Communication Skills

41. _____   Spontaneously expresses thoughts and needs to others

42. _____   Responds accurately to spoken instructions and conversation

43. _____   Reads and understands single words and short phrases (signs, lists, etc.)

44. _____   Reads and understands complex material (books, newspapers, etc.)

45. _____   Writes short phrases (lists, brief messages)

46. _____   Writes complex material (letters, diary, etc.)

FIGURE 7-3 (continued)

Social Behavior

47. _____ Behaves in a socially appropriate manner. Socially inappropriate behaviors encompass a **wide** range of behavior, including but not limited to such things as making rude remarks, belching, touching private parts, showing little regard for personal privacy, etc. For this item, dependency refers to the extent to which other people must direct or manage the subject to ensure that he or she behaves in a socially appropriate fashion.

Other Problems — Are there any situations in which patient does not behave in an independent and responsible fashion that have not been covered by these questions? *(Circle one of following codes.)*

48.   0   No other dependent behaviors

       1   Yes, there are other dependent behaviors. *(Please provide details below.)*

QUALITY OF INTERVIEW (Rater's Judgment)

Interview appeared valid   0

Some questions about interview, but it is probably acceptable   1

Information from interview is of doubtful validity   2

Rater should record the basis for judging the interview of questionable or doubtful validity.

Comments:

FIGURE 7-3 (continued)

measurement of functional deficits in people with Alzheimer's disease (Mack & Patterson, 2006).

Wellness Opportunity

When assessing the impact of cognitive abilities on functioning, nurses can try to identify simple interventions, such as putting labels on drawers, that can improve the person's self-esteem by promoting independence.

Assessing the Use or Potential Use of Adaptive and Assistive Devices

The actual or potential use of items such as mobility aids (e.g., canes, walkers, wheelchairs) and adaptive equipment (e.g., grab bars) should be assessed as factors that can significantly affect safety, functioning, and quality of life for older adults. Physical, occupational, and rehabilitation therapists are skilled in assessing for the use of these aids, but nurses need to be familiar with the array of adaptive and assistive devices so that they can make recommendations or facilitate referrals for further evaluation. Many innovative and inexpensive devices are available through catalogues or Internet sites and can be used to improve functioning and independence in daily activities. Additional assistive devices are illustrated and discussed in many chapters of this book (e.g., see Chapters 16, 17, 22).

Nurses also can identify problems related to the use of assistive devices and request further evaluation by a qualified

TABLE 7-2 Negative Effects of Improper Wheelchair Fit

Seating Problem	Result on Body	Potential Effect
Wheelchair too high	Feet do not touch the floor Unable to self-propel Pelvis moves forward	Edema and decreased circulation in legs Decreased activity Poor sitting posture
Poor back support	Compression of trunk, chest, abdomen Sliding out of chair Increased pelvic tilt	Skin breakdown on back and sacrum Impaired gastrointestinal and respiratory function
Wheelchair too heavy	Difficulty moving chair	Decreased activity
Wheelchair too wide	Pelvic shifting laterally Forward leaning Difficulty using hand rims	Shear stress on skin Poor posture, circulation Decreased mobility
Seat not firm enough ("sling" effect)	Scoliosis Sliding out of chair	Poor posture, circulation Shear stress on skin
Footrest too high	Poor femoral support Unequal pressure distribution Increased ischial tuberosity	Poor posture Skin breakdown

From Rader, J., Jones, D., & Miller, L. (2000). The importance of individualized wheelchair seating for frail older adults. *Journal of Gerontological Nursing, 26*(11), 24–31.

therapist. For example, nurses can assess comfort and function of wheelchairs because improper fit leads to specific problems such as those summarized in Table 7-2. In addition, improper wheelchair fit is likely to cause pain, fatigue, discomfort, agitation, and decreased tolerance for using a wheelchair (Rader, Jones, & Miller, 2000).

COMPREHENSIVE GERIATRIC ASSESSMENTS

As gerontologists and health care providers began addressing the complexity of care for older adults, they recognized the need for assessment models that were more comprehensive than those that focused specifically on particular aspects of health or functioning (refer to Chapter 6 for a description of these programs). Thus, in the early 1980s, standardized tools for **comprehensive geriatric assessments** were developed, but they were not widely implemented at that time. In 1987, the Omnibus Budget Reconciliation Act (OBRA) mandated that all Medicaid- and Medicare-funded nursing homes begin using a standardized assessment form as part of the effort to improve quality of care through regulation and inspections. This form, known as the **Minimum Data Set (MDS) for Resident Assessment and Care Screening**, includes several hundred items that document 18 areas of functioning, such as medical, mental, and social characteristics of nursing home residents. Since 1990, all nursing homes that receive Medicare or Medicaid funds have been using the MDS, which has been updated twice, with the most recent version implemented in October 2009. A major advantage of the MDS is that it requires nursing home staff to assess the health and functional status of each resident on admission to identify problems and strengths and to reassess every 3 months and document any changes (Shin & Sherer, 2009).

Because the use of the MDS as an assessment instrument has been successful in improving care in nursing homes, the federal government and accrediting organizations (e.g., the Joint Commission) have promoted the use of standardized assessment tools in all gerontological health care settings. Since the 1990s, all federally funded home care agencies have been mandated to use a home version of the MDS (MDS-HC). In Italy, the MDS-HC is used as an integral part of community-based team assessment and care management services, and this has led to a reduced rate of admissions to hospitals and nursing facilities (Wieland & Ferrucci, 2008).

The value of the MDS has been internationally recognized and both the nursing home and home care versions have been translated, validated, and implemented in many countries, including Canada, Australia, and Asian and European countries. Gerontologists have cited the MDS as a prototype assessment instrument that established a new philosophy and approach to care of older adults and laid the groundwork for evidence-based geriatric assessment and management (Bernabei, Landi, Graziano, Liperoti, & Gambassi, 2008).

Wellness Opportunity

Keep in mind that formal assessment tools fulfill requirements for documentation, but their primary purpose is to improve care and quality of life for older adults.

ASSESSING OLDER ADULTS IN RELATION TO THEIR ENVIRONMENTS

In addition to assessing the older adult's health and functioning, nurses need to be aware of environmental factors that influence the person's safety, functioning, and quality of life. Researchers and practitioners increasingly are addressing the interrelationship between people and their environments, and this is particularly pertinent to care of older adults. In the late 1990s, the term **everyday competence** was used to describe the effects of cultural, physical, cognitive, emotional, social, and contextual factors on a person's daily functioning. This is particularly important to consider when assessing older adults because these factors can appreciably hinder or improve functional abilities. For example, environmental factors that significantly affect hearing, vision, and mobility are discussed in Chapters 16, 17, and 22, respectively.

Home assessments provide an excellent base for assessing the relationship between older adults and their environments. These assessments are essential not only for identifying fall risks (as discussed in Chapter 22) but also for identifying environmental conditions that positively or negatively affect safety, functioning, and quality of life. For example, proper lighting is essential for performing enjoyable activities such as reading, playing cards, and engaging in hobbies. Similarly, the ability to regulate the temperature is important not only as a safety consideration for preventing hypothermia and hyperthermia but also for comfort. During home visits, it is especially important for nurses to respect autonomy and privacy and be nonjudgmental, and at the same time be able to identify all factors that affect the person's functioning and quality of life. Nurses can use Box 7-3 as a guide to assessing home environments for safety and optimal functioning.

Box 7-3 Guidelines for Assessing the Safety of the Environment

Illumination and Color Contrast
- Is the lighting adequate but not glare producing?
- Are the light switches easy to reach and manipulate?
- Can lights be turned on before entering rooms?
- Are night lights used in appropriate places?
- Is color contrast adequate between objects, such as a chair and the floor?

Hazards
- Are there highly polished floors, throw rugs, or other hazardous floor coverings?
- If area rugs are used, do they have a nonslip backing, and are the edges tacked to the floor?
- Are there cords, clutter, or other obstacles in pathways?
- Is there a pet that is likely to be running underfoot?

Furniture
- Are chairs the right height and depth for the person?
- Do the chairs have armrests? Are tables stable and of the appropriate height?
- Is small furniture placed well away from pathways?

Stairways
- Is lighting adequate?
- Are there light switches at the top and bottom of the stairs?
- Are there securely fastened handrails on both sides of the stairway?
- Are all the steps even?
- Are the treads nonskid?
- Should colored tape be used to mark the edges of the steps, particularly the top and bottom steps?

Bathroom
- Are grab bars placed appropriately for the tub and toilet?
- Does the tub have skid-proof strips or a rubber mat in the bottom?
- Has the person considered using a tub seat?
- Is the height of the toilet seat appropriate?
- Has the person considered using an elevated toilet seat?
- Does the color of the toilet seat contrast with surrounding colors?
- Is toilet paper within easy reach?

Bedroom
- Is the height of the bed appropriate?
- Is the mattress firm at the edges to provide enough support for sitting?
- If the bed has wheels, are they locked securely?
- Would full or partial side rails be a help or a hazard?
- When side rails are in the down position, are they completely out of the way?

- Is the pathway between the bedroom and bathroom clear of objects and adequately illuminated, particularly at night?
- Would a bedside commode be useful, especially at night?
- Is a light near the bed, and does the person have sufficient physical and cognitive ability to turn it on before getting out of bed?
- Is furniture positioned to allow safe use of assistive devices for ambulation?
- Is a telephone situated near the bed?

Kitchen
- Are storage areas used to the best advantage (e.g., are objects that are frequently used in the most accessible places)?
- Are appliance cords kept out of the way?
- Are nonslip mats used in front of the sink?
- Are the markings on stoves and other appliances clearly visible?
- Does the person know how to use the microwave safely?

Assistive Devices
- Is a call light available, and does the person know how to use it?
- What assistive devices are used?
- Would the person benefit from any assistive devices that are not being used?
- Are assistive devices being used safely and properly, or do they present additional hazards?

Temperature
- Is the temperature of the room(s) comfortable?
- Can the person read the markings on the thermostat and adjust it appropriately?
- During cold months, is the room temperature high enough to prevent hypothermia?
- During hot weather, is the room temperature cool enough to prevent hyperthermia?

Overall Safety
- How does the person obtain objects from hard-to-reach places?
- How does the person change overhead light bulbs?
- Are doorways wide enough to accommodate assistive devices?
- Do door thresholds create hazardous conditions?
- Are telephones accessible, especially for emergency calls? Would it be helpful to use a cordless portable phone?
- Would it be helpful to have some emergency call system available?
- Does the person wear sturdy shoes with nonskid soles?
- Does the person keep a list of emergency numbers by the phone?
- Does the person have an emergency exit plan in the event of fire?
- Are smoke alarms present and operational?
- Is there a carbon monoxide detector in an appropriate place (if the house has gas appliances, wood burning stoves, or another object that produces carbon monoxide)?

ASSESSING AND ADDRESSING DRIVING SAFETY

The ability to drive a vehicle safely is an aspect of daily living that merits special consideration when assessing older adults. Driving at an advanced age is a major focus of attention, not only for health care providers but also for all members of society. For example, studies have identified driving as one of the top 10 tough ethical issues associated with dementia (Dobbs, Harper, & Wood, 2009). Commentaries and news articles frequently address issues about people who continue to drive when they are in their 80s and 90s. Regardless of age, most driving-related problems arise from chronic conditions that affect cognitive abilities or neurologic or musculoskeletal function. However, even healthy older adults need to compensate for age-related changes in vision and other areas of function that affect driving, as discussed in Chapter 17.

Older drivers who recognize changes in their abilities usually self-regulate their driving behavior through actions such as minimizing their exposure to hazardous situations by restricting when, where, and under what conditions they drive (Ross et al., 2009). Studies have identified the following self-regulation techniques used by older drivers: trip planning, reducing mileage, and avoidance of difficult driving situations, such as high traffic or freeway driving (Morgan, Winter, Classen, McCarthy, & Awadzi, 2009).

Decisions about driving are very complex because they are associated with many psychosocial implications, as discussed in Chapter 12. Many studies have found that "driving retirement" is associated with many negative consequences and diminished quality of life. Specific negative consequences associated with driving cessation include decreased social contacts; decreased self-esteem; increased depressive symptoms; and loss of control, freedom, dignity, and independence (Kerschner, 2009; Croston, Meuser, Berg-Weger, Grant, & Carr, 2009). Despite the many negative consequences associated with cessation of driving, however, a few positive consequences have been identified. Positive themes identified in one study included, increased time with family or significant other, increased community participation, strengthened social ties, a heightened sense of personal safety, and feelings of relief (Pellerito, 2009).

Increasingly, nurses are among the health care professionals responsible for addressing concerns about driving, not only as a personal safety issue for older adults but also as a moral obligation to protect society. As with other aspects of functioning, nurses are responsible for identifying potential risk factors for unsafe driving. Moreover, nurses need to be knowledgeable about resources for assessing and addressing this risk. Because decisions about driving are multidimensional, nurses work closely with other care providers, such as physicians and social workers, to address this important issue from a broad perspective. Thus, health care providers facilitate referrals not only for assessments of driving but also for interventions that help people retain safe driving skills as long as possible.

Identifying Risks and Consequences

When motor vehicle accident rates are adjusted for miles driven, drivers older than 80 years represent a crash risk that is higher than that of teenage drivers (O'Connor, Kapust, & Hollis, 2008). Health care providers are responsible for identifying conditions that can affect driving skills, such as medical conditions, functional limitations, medication use, alcohol consumption, and changes in habits or personality. In addition, they are responsible for identifying risk factors for unsafe driving when they perform physical, functional, or mental status assessments. Functional abilities that are strongly associated with safe driving in older adults include vision deficits, head and neck flexibility, speed of information processing, emotional functioning, and mental status including attention and visuospatial memory (Baldock, Berndt, & Mathias, 2008). Even healthy older adults are likely to experience the following conditions that can affect driving safety (Edwards et al., 2009; Horswill et al., 2008; O'Connor et al., 2008):

- Diminished field of vision
- Decreased visual acuity
- Increased sensitivity to glare
- Diminished musculoskeletal abilities
- Difficulty switching attention between tasks
- Slower motor response
- Delayed reaction time
- Diminished ability to perceive hazards

To identify risks for unsafe driving, nurses can inquire about recent vehicular accidents, dents and scratches in the car, and any legal actions related to unsafe driving or driving under the influence. Nurses also can inquire about behavioral indicators for unsafe driving, such as getting lost, reacting too slowly, showing poor judgment, driving at inappropriate speeds, miscalculating speed or distance, going through stop signs or lights, etc. During the assessment, nurses need to identify the older adult's perception of his or her driving abilities. Studies have found that drivers who overestimate their driving abilities and have high levels of confidence are likely to create significant safety risks for themselves and others

(MacDonald, Myers, & Blanchard, 2008). When appropriate, nurses can also obtain information from family members who are likely to have observations and concerns. Nurses can encourage older adults to use self-assessment tools, such as the *Roadwise Review*, which is listed in the Health Education About Driving section, to assess their driving strengths and weaknesses (Myers, Blanchard, MacDonald, & Porter, 2008).

Health care professionals also assess nonmedical reasons that older adults limit or stop driving, such as concerns about crime, accidents, or road conditions and feeling more vulnerable to experiencing difficulties in traffic (Friedland & Rudman, 2009). In addition, based on a holistic approach, nurses assess psychosocial implications of driving cessation, as well as practical implications, such as need for alternative means of transportation.

> **Wellness Opportunity**
>
> Nurses can promote personal responsibility by assessing the older adult's awareness of driving issues and their willingness to consider addressing these concerns.

Addressing Risk Factors

Addressing risk factors that interfere with safe driving is an important health promotion activity that should be integrated into health care programs, preferably before significant safety concerns arise (Friedland & Rudman, 2009). When risks are identified, nurses also try to identify contributing factors that can be addressed through appropriate interventions. For example, when vision impairments affect driving, older adults may benefit from a referral to an ophthalmologist, as discussed in Chapter 17. Similarly, because hearing impairments can affect safety while driving, nurses can discuss the importance of interventions to improve hearing, as discussed in Chapter 16. In addition to addressing specific risk factors, health promotion programs should help older adults make informed choices about mobility transitions so that they can retain dignity and independence (DiStefano, Lovell, Stone, Oh, & Cockfield, 2009).

Another approach to improving driving safety for some older adults is to address medication-related issues when these are likely to have a negative impact on driving. When adverse effects of medications affect safe driving, nurses can encourage older adults to discuss this with the prescribing practitioner to explore options. For example, it may be possible to adjust dosing of medications to minimize their effects on driving. Some over-the-counter medications, such as diphenhydramine (Benadryl), can interfere with safe driving even during the day after an evening dose.

When pathologic conditions affect neuromuscular functioning, nurses may suggest a referral for physical or occupational therapy to improve particular aspects of functioning that affect driving. For example, an older person with arthritis or Parkinson's disease may benefit from working with a therapist who has additional training for driving rehabilitation. Even if the therapist does not have special training, the older adult can focus on the goal of improved safety and functioning for driving skills as part of the therapy program. Older adults may be more motivated to participate in exercises prescribed by physical or occupational therapists if they see a connection between the therapies and maintaining safe and independent functioning.

> **Wellness Opportunity**
>
> Nurses can promote quality of life for older adults by creatively identifying appropriate and acceptable ways of improving an older adult's ability to continue driving safety.

When nurses identify safety risks, they must assess the older adult's awareness and degree of cooperation for further assessment. If older adults self-restrict their driving to eliminate safety risks, health care professionals need to reassess the situation periodically. However, when any significant risks are identified, a referral to occupational therapy may be necessary for further evaluation and possible interventions. When medically warranted, these referrals are covered by Medicare and other health insurance plans.

When suggesting this kind of referral, nurses can emphasize that the purpose is not to take away the person's driving privileges but rather to identify interventions to improve safety for the person and others. Recommendations fall within a wide range and may include having no or few driving restrictions, adding adaptive devices to the vehicle, participating in driving rehabilitation therapy, or refraining from driving. Examples of recommended driving restrictions that are based on specific performance errors include no highways, familiar areas only; daytime or fair weather driving only, limited to short times (e.g., 20 minutes); drive only with navigator; and no passengers or distractions (e.g., radio) (Freund & Petrakos, 2008). Researchers have found that because driving restrictions can prolong the safe-driving period for older adults, this can be an effective intervention for supporting independence and delaying the need for a move to an institutional setting (Nasvadi & Wister, 2009).

Referring to Community Resources

Nurses need to be familiar with the range of programs for driving safety, education, and rehabilitation to facilitate referrals. Driving evaluation programs, which usually are administered by occupational therapy departments, provide appropriate follow-up when the person can benefit from education and rehabilitation. A recent review of 20 years of research related to driving and older adults suggests that efforts should be directed toward teaching older adults to drive safely rather than quitting driving (Eberhard & Mitchell, 2009). The American Occupational Therapy Association developed an older driver initiative to support research, education, and practice to address the needs of older drivers (Stav, 2008). Driving rehabilitation programs typically provide evaluation, recommendations, and follow-up for people with conditions that affect their driving. Adaptive driving equipment that is

...ludes pedal extenders, distance sensors, left ...s, steering wheel adaptations, touch pads to ...y controls, and spot mirrors to compensate ...ual and range-of-motion deficit.

Driving education programs are available through organizations such as AARP (Mature Driving Program) and the American Automobile Association (Safe Driving for Mature Operators). Numerous Internet resources provide excellent information about driving assessments and interventions to improve driving safety for older adults. Some of the resources that are most relevant to nurses are listed in the Health Education About Driving section of this chapter.

In addition to suggesting programs that directly address safe driving, nurses can suggest programs that provide transportation for older adults. Public transportation is generally available only in urban and suburban areas, and older adults rely on it for less than 5% of their transportation needs (McCarthy, 2009). However, senior centers, which are available in every area of the country under the Area Agency on Aging, generally provide transportation services and information about local resources.

Nurses also can address psychosocial implications by suggesting referrals to programs that help older adults cope with the loss or decrease of driving privileges. For example, one study found that a support group for people with dementia was effective in ameliorating many of the negative consequences associated with loss of driving privileges (Dobbs et al., 2009).

Working With Caregivers

Families are likely to seek guidance from nurses and other health care professionals to address their safety concerns about driving abilities of an older adult. A study of caregivers of cognitively impaired older adults emphasized the importance of health care professionals providing information to family caregivers about resources for addressing the issue of driving (D'Ambrosio et al., 2009). Another study of family caregivers identified the following most frequently cited concerns: driving alone, driving at night, not paying attention, driving long distances, driving too fast or too slow, and being too old to drive (Kostyniuk, Molnar, & Eby, 2009). One way of addressing caregivers' concerns about driving safety is to provide information about resources that families can use to approach this issue. For example, some of the organizations listed in the Health Education About Driving section provide guides for helping families talk with older members about driving as a health issue. Nurses also can refer family of people with dementia to caregiver support groups, which can be effective in helping them address driving-related issues (Stern et al., 2008).

Chapter Highlights

Assessing Health of Older Adults
• Assessment of older adults is a multidimensional process addressing the complex interactions among

older adults, their health, and all contextual factors (e.g., culture, environments, medical conditions, adverse medication effects).
• Factors that contribute to the complexity of assessing older adults include multiple interacting conditions, unique manifestations of illness, treatments that mask the underlying problem, inaccurate or inadequate sources of information, and myths and misunderstandings about aging.
• Nurses need to be aware of age-related variations in laboratory values for older adults (Table 7-1).

Nursing Assessment Tools
• Evidence-based nursing assessment tools and web-based articles demonstrating the use of many of these tools are widely available (See Clinical Tools at end of chapter).

Functional Assessment
• A functional assessment is a formal process of measuring a person's ability to fulfill responsibilities and perform self-care tasks (Figure 7-1).
• Functional assessment tools focus on the person's ability to perform ADLs and IADLs, as illustrated in Figure 7-2 and Boxes 7-1 and 7-2.
• Assessment of the home environment is important for identifying factors that affect safety, comfort, functioning, and quality of life (Box 7-3).
• Assessing the use of adaptive equipment and assistive devices is important for identifying factors that affect safety, comfort, and functioning (Table 7-1).
• Some assessment tools address the effect of cognitive impairment on ability to perform activities of daily living (Figure 7-3).
• Nurses can suggest the use of innovative and inexpensive devices to improve functioning and promote independence.

Comprehensive Geriatric Assessments
• The MDS is used in nursing facilities and home care agencies to document 18 areas of functioning.

Assessing Older Adults in Relation to Their Environments
• Everyday competence is a term that describes the effects of cultural, physical, cognitive, emotional, social, and contextual factors on a person's daily functioning.
• Home assessments are essential for identifying risks for safety and interventions to improve functioning (Box 7-3).

Assessing and Addressing Driving Safety
• Nurses have an important role in identifying risk factors that compromise safe driving in older adults.
• Common risk factors include conditions that affect vision, cognition, motor responses, and reaction time.
• Nurses address risk factors by facilitating referrals for further evaluation or for programs related to driving safety, education, and rehabilitation.

Critical Thinking Exercises

1. Identify an older adult who has some functional impairment but no cognitive impairment and perform a functional assessment on him or her, using Figure 7-2.
2. Identify another older adult (in a clinical setting or someone you know personally) who has some functional impairment as well as some cognitive impairment and perform a functional assessment on him or her, using Figure 7-3.
3. Identify an older adult (in a clinical setting or someone you know personally) who has risk factors that affect his or her driving safety; then explore one or more of the health education to find information applicable to addressing concerns about safe driving for this person.
4. View the video on monitoring functional status in hospitalized older adults, which can be found at www.nursingcenter.com, and identify ways in which you can apply the information in clinical settings.

Resources

For links to these resources and additional helpful Internet resources related to this chapter, visit thePoint, at http://thePoint.lww.com/Miller6e.

Clinical Tools

American Journal of Nursing and Hartford Institute for Geriatric Nursing
- *How to Try This,* article and video: Fulmer SPICES, by T. Fulmer, *American Journal of Nursing, 107*(10), 40–48.
- *How to Try This,* article and video: Monitoring functional status in hospitalized older adults, by M. Wallace & M. Shelkey, *American Journal of Nursing, 108*(4), 64–70.
- *How to Try This,* article and video: The Lawton instrumental activities of daily living scale, by C. Graf, *American Journal of Nursing, 108*(4), 52–60.

Cleveland Scale for Activities of Daily Living
Hartford Institute for Geriatric Nursing
- *Try This: Best Practices in Nursing Care to Older Adults* Issue 1 (2007), SPICES: An Overall Assessment Tool for Older Adults
  Issue 2 (2007), Katz Index of Independence in Activities of Daily Living (ADL)
  Issue 23 (2007), The Lawton Instrumental Activities of Daily Living (IADL) Scale

Evidence-Based Practice

Kresevic, D. M. (2008). Assessment of function. In E. Capezuti, D. Zwicker, M. Mezey, & T. Fulmer (Eds.), *Evidence-based geriatric nursing protocols for best practice* (3rd ed., pp. 23–40). New York: Springer Publishing Co.

Health Education About Driving

American Automobile Association (AAA): *AAA Roadwise Review*
AARP: "55 Alive" (classes for older adults about driving)
American Medical Association (resources on safe driving and helping older drivers)
American Occupational Therapy Association (information about driving evaluation and rehabilitation)
Association for Driver Rehabilitation Specialists (directory of certified driver rehabilitation specialists in the United States and Canada)
Beverly Foundation Senior Transportation Library (information about transportation options, rural transportation, and transportation for people with dementia)
CarFit (educational program to improve older adult driving safety, with emphasis on evaluating the "fit" of vehicles for individuals)
DriveWell Toolkit
Driving Safely While Aging Gracefully, National Highway Traffic Safety Administration
Grand Driver (advice about safe driving practices for older adults)
Hartford: Family Conversations With Older Drivers (to help families talk with older adults about driving safety)
Safe and Reliable Mobility Equipment, National Mobility Equipment Dealers Association
Senior Drivers (numerous reports and resources for consumers, providers, and researchers on aging and driving)

REFERENCES

Baldock, M. R. J., Berndt, A., & Mahias, J. L. (2008). The functional correlates of older drivers' on-road driving test errors. *Topics in Geriatric Rehabilitation, 24,* 204–223.

Bernabei, R., Landi, F., Graziano, O., Liperoti, R., & Gambassi, G. (2008). Second and third generation assessment instruments: The birth of standardization in geriatric care. *Journal of Gerontology: Medical Sciences, 63A,* 308–313.

Croston, J., Meuser, T. M., Berg-Weger, M., Grant, E. A., & Carr, D. B. (2009). Driving retirement in older adults with dementia. *Topics in Geriatric Rehabilitation, 25,* 154–162.

D'Ambrosio, L. A., Coughlin, J. F., Mohyde, M., Carruth, A., Hunter, J. C., & Stern, R. A. (2009). Caregiver communications and the transition from driver to passenger among people with dementia. *Topics in Geriatric Rehabilitation, 25,* 33–42.

DiStefano, M., Lovell, R., Stone, K., Oh, S., & Cockfield, S. (2009). Supporting individuals to make informed personal mobility choices. *Topics in Geriatric Rehabilitation, 25,* 55–72.

Dobbs, B. M., Harper, L. A., & Wood, A. (2009). Transitioning from driving to driving cessation: The role of specialized driving cessation support groups for individuals with dementia. *Topics in Geriatric Rehabilitation, 25,* 73–86.

Eberhard, J. W., & Mitchell, C. G. B. (2009). Recent changes in driver licensing rates, fatality rates, and mobility options for older men and women in the United States and Great Britain. *Topics in Geriatric Rehabilitation, 25,* 88–98.

Edwards, J. D., Myers, C., Ross, L. A., Roenker, D. L., Cissell, G. M., McLaughlin, A. M., & Ball, K. K. (2009). The longitudinal impact of cognitive speed of processing training on driving mobility. *The Gerontologist, 49,* 485–494.

Freund, B., & Patrakos, D. (2008). Continued driving and time to transition to nondriver status through error-specific driving restrictions. *Gerontology & Geriatrics Education, 29,* 326–335.

Friedland, J., & Rudman, D. L. (2009). From confrontation to collaboration: Making a place for dialogue on seniors' driving. *Topics in Geriatric Rehabilitation, 25,* 12–23.

Horswill, M. S., Marrington, S. A., McCullough, C. M., Wood, J., Pachana, N. A., McWilliam, J., & Raikos, M. K. (2008). The hazard perception ability of older drivers. *Journal of Gerontology: Psychological Sciences, 63B,* P212–P218.

Kerschner, H. K. (2009). Transportation transitions and older adults. *Topics in Geriatric Rehabilitation, 25,* 173–178.

Kostyniuk, L. P., Molnar, L. J., & Eby, D. W. (2009). Safe mobility of older drivers: Concerns expressed by adult children. *Topics in Geriatric Rehabilitation, 25,* 24–32.

Kresevic, D. M. (2008). Assessment of function. In E. Capezuti, D. Zwicker, M. Mezey, & T. Fulmer (Eds.), *Evidence-based geriatric nursing protocols for best practice* (3rd ed., pp. 23–40). New York: Springer Publishing Co.

MacDonald, L., Myers, A. M., & Blanchard, R. A. (2008). Correspondence among older drivers' perceptions, abilities, and behaviors. *Topics in Geriatric Rehabilitation, 24,* 239–252.

Mack, J. L., & Patterson, M. B. (2006). An empirical basis for domains in the analysis of dependency in the activities of daily living (ADL): Results of a confirmatory factor analysis of the Cleveland Scale for Activities of Daily Living (CSADL). *Clinical Neuropsychologist, 20,* 662–667.

McCann, J. A. S. (2003). *Handbook of geriatric nursing care* (2nd ed.). Philadelphia, PA: Lippincott Williams & Wilkins.

McCarthy, D. P. (2009). Transitioning from driver to passenger. *Topics in Geriatric Rehabilitation, 25,* 1–2.

Morgan, C. M., Winter, S. M., Classen, S., McCarthy, D. P., & Awadzi, K. D. (2009). Literature review on older adult gender differences for driving self-regulation and cessation. *Topics in Geriatric Rehabilitation, 25,* 99–117.

Myers, A. M., Blanchard, R. A., MacDonald, L., & Porter, M. M. (2008). Process evaluation of the American Automobile Association *Roadwise Review* CD-ROM. *Topics in Geriatric Rehabilitation, 24,* 224–238.

Narayan, M. C., Salgado, J., & VanVoorhis, A. (2009). SHOW Me: Enhancing OASIS functional assessment. *Home Healthcare Nurse, 27*(1), 19–23.

Nasvadi, G. C., & Wister, A. (2009). Do restricted driver's licenses lower crash risk among older drivers: A survival analysis of insurance data from British Columbia. *The Gerontologist, 49,* 474–484.

O'Connor, M. G., Kapust, L. R., & Hollis, A. M. (2008). DriveWise: An interdisciplinary hospital-based driving assessment program. *Gerontolgy & Geriatrics Education, 29,* 351–362.

Oxley, J., & Charlton, J. (2009). Attitudes to and mobility impacts of driving cessation: differences between current and former drivers. *Topics in Geriatric Rehabilitation, 25,* 43–54.

Pellerito, J. M. (2009). The effects of driving retirement on elderly men and women living in metropolitan Detroit. *Topics in Geriatric Rehabilitation, 25,* 135–153.

Rader, J., Jones, D., & Miller, L. (2000). The importance of individualized wheelchair seating for frail older adults. *Journal of Gerontological Nursing, 26*(11), 24–31.

Ross, L. A., Clay, O. J., Edwards, J. D., Ball, K. K., Wadley, V. G., Vance, D. E., . . . Joyce, J. J. (2009). Do older drivers at-risk for crashes modify their driving over time? *Journal of Gerontology: Psychological Sciences, 64B*(2), 163–170.

Shin, J. H., & Scherer, Y. (2009). Advantages and disadvantages of using MDS data in nursing research. *Journal of Gerontological Nursing, 35,* 7–16.

Stav, W. B. (2008). Occupational therapy and older drivers: Research, education, and practice. *Gerontology & Geriatrics Education, 29,* 336–350.

Stern, R. A., D'Ambrosio, L. A., Mohyde, M., Carruth, A., Tracton-Bishop, B., Hunter, J. C., ... Coughlin, J. F. (2008). At the crossroads: Development and evaluation of a dementia caregiver group intervention to assist in driving cessation. *Gerontology & Geriatrics Education, 29,* 363–382.

Wieland, D., & Ferrucci, L. (2008). Multidimensional geriatric assessment: Back to the future. *Journal of Gerontology: Medical Sciences, 63A,* 272–274.

CHAPTER **8**

Medications and Other Bioactive Substances

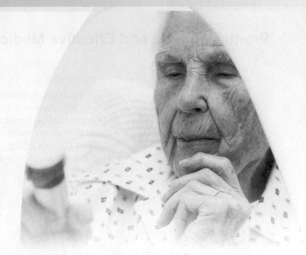

LEARNING OBJECTIVES

After reading this chapter, you will be able to:

1. Examine age-related changes and risk factors that affect the action of medications in the body and the skills involved with taking them.

2. Discuss considerations about safety and efficacy of herbs and other bioactive substances that are pertinent to care of older adults.

3. Describe interactions that can occur between medications and other bioactive substances.

4. Identify the adverse medication effects that are likely to occur in older adults.

5. Describe the purposes of a medication assessment and explain how to perform a comprehensive medication assessment.

6. Identify nursing interventions directed toward enhancing the therapeutic effectiveness of medications, reducing the risks for adverse effects, and minimizing the negative functional consequences of these effects.

KEY POINTS

adverse medication effects
anticholinergic adverse
  effects
Beers criteria
clearance rate
cytochrome P-450 enzyme
  system
"donut hole"
drug-induced
  parkinsonism
elimination half-time

herbs
generic medications
inappropriate
  medications
Medicare Part D
medication
  nonadherence
medication reconciliation
pharmacodynamics
pharmacokinetics
polypharmacy

potentially inappropriate
  medications
prescribing cascade

prescription assistance
  programs
tardive dyskinesia

Although the topic of bioactive substances and the older adult is not a distinct category of function in the same sense as physiologic and psychosocial aspects of function (e.g., vision and cognition), it can be addressed from a similar perspective. Thus, this chapter presents information about age-related changes, risk factors, and functional consequences related to bioactive substances and the behaviors associated with taking them relative to older adults. Like other chapters, it addresses the role of nurses in assessing and managing bioactive substances in the context of the functional consequences theory for promoting wellness.

INTRODUCTION TO BIOACTIVE SUBSTANCES

The bioactive substances that are most relevant to care of older adults are prescription and over-the-counter medications, vitamins and minerals, and **herbs** and homeopathic remedies. Nurses need to be aware of the special considerations related to commonly used types of bioactive substances so that they can promote safe and effective use for older adults.

Considerations Regarding Medications

Effects of medications in the body are usually considered in relation to **pharmacokinetics** (i.e., how the drug is absorbed, distributed, metabolized, and excreted) and **pharmacodynamics** (i.e., how the body is affected by the drug at the cellular level and in relation to the target organ). Absorption refers to the passage of a medication from its site of introduction, usually the gastrointestinal tract, into the general circulation. Absorption of oral medications can be affected by diminished gastric acid, increased gastric pH, delayed gastric emptying, and the presence of other substances (e.g., food, nutrients, inert ingredients of medications). Because most oral medications are absorbed by passive diffusion across the

Promoting Safe and Effective Medication Use in Older Adults

Nursing Assessment

- Medication-taking patterns
- Use of all bioactive substances (herbs, vitamins, minerals)
- Barriers to adherence
- Cultural considerations
- Therapeutic and adverse medication effects

Age-Related Changes

- ↓ body water
- ↓ lean tissue
- ↑ body fat
- ↓ serum albumin
- ↓ liver and renal function
- Altered receptor sensitivity

Negative Functional Consequences

- Less predictable therapeutic effects
- ↑ risk for adverse effects
- ↑ risk for interactions

Risk Factors

- Pathologic processes
- Functional impairments
- Polypharmacy
- Inadequate monitoring
- Financial barriers
- Insufficient recognition of adverse effects

Nursing Interventions

- Teaching about safe and effective medications
- Teaching about herbs and other bioactive substances
- Decreasing the number of medications

Wellness Outcomes

- Improved safety and effectiveness of medications
- Prevention or alleviation of interactions and adverse effects
- Improved quality of life

small intestine—a process that is not pH dependent—they are not usually affected by any alterations in gastric acidity. The unique chemical properties of each medication determine the degree to which it is susceptible to any gastrointestinal changes, regardless of age. For example, pH-sensitive medications, such as penicillin and ferrous sulfate, are more likely to be affected by altered gastric acid levels or by prolonged exposure to these acids because of delayed emptying.

Two measures of the efficiency of metabolism and elimination of a drug are **elimination half-time** and **clearance rate**. Elimination half-time (also called serum half-life) is the time required to decrease the drug concentration by one half of its original value. It takes five half-times to reach steady-state concentrations after a drug is initiated or to completely eliminate a drug from the body after a drug is discontinued. The clearance rate measures the volume of blood from which the drug is eliminated per unit of time. An increase in serum half-time or a decrease in clearance rate may result in accumulation of the drug. The result is that the therapeutic effect is likely to be altered, and the risk of adverse effects is likely to be increased.

Considerations Regarding Herbs and Homeopathy

The use of complementary and alternative medicine (CAM) is increasing dramatically in the United States, especially among women, older adults, and people with chronic conditions. Most studies have confirmed the increasing use of CAM during the last two decades to the point that more than 90% of the elderly have now used CAM (Cherniack et al., 2008). All health care practitioners need to know what products their patients are using so that they can address concerns about safety, effectiveness, and potential interactions. This is particularly important with regard to bioactive substances, such as herbs and other dietary supplements, in relation to interactions with medications. In addition, health care practitioners need to be prepared to address questions that their patients may ask about alternative practices, as discussed in the Nursing Interventions section of this chapter.

Although herbs, homeopathy, and folk remedies are viewed as "nontraditional" or "alternative" approaches to preventing and treating illness, these remedies have been used for centuries in many non-Western cultures. Both herbal and homeopathic products have physiologic actions; however, herbal products are of particular concern because their actions can be similar to those of prescription and over-the-counter medications. Thus, they can produce beneficial effects, adverse effects, and interactions. This section presents an overview of herbs and homeopathic remedies; additional aspects of herbs are discussed throughout this chapter with regard to physiologic considerations, adverse effects, and herb–medication interactions. Pertinent aspects also are addressed in the sections on Nursing Assessment and Nursing Interventions.

DIVERSITY NOTE

Among African Americans, CAM use is a combination of European, Native American, and African customs; African Americans and Native Americans view spirituality as integral to the prevention of illness and maintenance of health (Moquin, Blackman, Mitty, & Flores, 2009).

Herbs

Herbs were perhaps the original over-the-counter products, used by people who found these medicinal remedies in their natural environments. Herbs (also called botanicals or phytotherapies) are plant-based products that have medicinal properties. Herbs and many other pharmaceutical preparations have common origins in nature. Examples of plant-derived medications that are commonly used today include

antibiotics, anticholinergics, anticoagulants, antihypertensives, antineoplastic agents, aspirin, and digoxin (Plotnikoff, 2010).

Information about the pharmacokinetics and pharmacodynamics that applies to medications (discussed later in the section on Changes That Affect the Action of Bioactive Substances in the Body) also applies to the action of herbs in the body. This is particularly pertinent with regard to herbs that are metabolized by the liver, because metabolism of substances in the liver is affected by many factors, including diet and genetic variations. Thus, it is important to keep in mind that even when taken alone, herbs can be affected by the same age-related changes and risk factors that affect medications in older adults.

Most people who use herbs believe that they are safe because they are commonly available natural products that can be purchased without a prescription (Snyder, Dundas, Kirkpatrick, & Neill, 2009). Despite this common perception, however, herbs and other biologically active agents can cause problems, particularly for people who also take medications. As with all bioactive substances, nothing is taken without risk and the risk increases in proportion to the number of substances consumed. Because herbs as well as many medications have common origins in plants, some herbs are similar in bioactivity to over-the-counter or prescription medications and can increase the risk for adverse effects and drug interactions. Table 8-1 lists some herbs and medications that have similar bioactivity, and medication–herb interactions are addressed in the section on Medication Interactions.

TABLE 8-1 Drugs and Herbs With Similar Bioactivity

Drug	Herb
Aspirin	Birch bark Willow bark Wintergreen Meadowsweet
Anticoagulants	Dong quai Feverfew Garlic Ginkgo biloba Wintergreen
Caffeine	Guarana Kola nut
Ephedrine	Ephedra
Estrogen	Black cohosh Fennel Red clover Stinging nettle
Lithium	Thyme Purslane
Monoamine oxidase inhibitors	Ginseng St. John's wort Yohimbe
Nicotine	Lobelia
Calcium channel blockers	Angelica

A factor that complicates safety issues is the limited amount of testing performed that meets the standards established by the U.S. Food and Drug Administration (FDA) for medications. Because herbs are categorized as dietary supplements, there is no requirement that they be tested for safety or efficacy, and the labels do not necessarily include reliable information about additional ingredients, potential harmful effects, quantity of active ingredients, or suitability of form for human use. Manufacturers are required to ensure the accuracy of the ingredient list; however, there have been many cases of adulteration and contamination of supplements. In response to these concerns, the United States Pharmacopoeia (USP) has established a quality verification program to assure consumers that they are buying a quality product that has been held to rigorous standards. This voluntary program ensures that all ingredients of a dietary supplement (1) maintain consistent quality in every batch; (2) meet manufacturers' claims for identification, strength, purity, and quality; (3) are manufactured in accordance with appropriate good manufacturing practices; and (4) meet requirements for acceptable limits of contamination.

The verification process involves extensive evaluation and review of products and on-going audits of the manufacturing process. Products that meet these rigorous standards display a USP Verified Mark (illustrated in Figure 8-1) on the label. Nurses can educate themselves and their patients to buy only those products with this mark to ensure they are buying a product that is of high quality and true to its label. The USP Web site (see Resource list at the end of this chapter) lists up-to-date information about which products have been verified by USP, including information about where to purchase these products.

Dietary supplements are generally safe if they are obtained from reliable sources, but some bioactive substances are

TABLE 8-2 Potential Adverse Effects of Some Herbs	
Black cohosh	Bradycardia, hypotension, joint pains
Bloodroot	Bradycardia, arrhythmia, dizziness, impaired vision, intense thirst
Boneset	Liver toxicity, mental changes, respiratory problems
Coltsfoot	Fever, liver toxicity
Dandelion	Interactions with diuretics, increased concentration of lithium or potassium
Ephedra	Anxiety, dizziness, insomnia, tachycardia, hypertension
Feverfew	Interference with blood clotting mechanisms
Garlic	Hypotension, inhibition of blood clotting, potentiation of antidiabetic drugs
Ginseng	Anxiety, insomnia, hypertension, tachycardia, asthma attacks, postmenopausal bleeding
Ginkgo biloba	Increased anticoagulation
Goldenseal	Vasoconstriction
Guar gum	Hypoglycemia
Hawthorn	Hypotension
Hops, skullcap, valerian	Drowsiness, potentiation of antianxiety or sedative medications
Kava	Damage to the eyes, skin, liver, and spinal cord from long-term use
Licorice	Hypokalemia, hypernatremia
Lobelia	Hearing and vision problems
Motherwort	Increased anticoagulation
Nettle	Hypokalemia
Senna	Potentiation of digoxin
Yohimbe	Anxiety, tachycardia, hypertension, mental changes

likely to have adverse effects and the risk for adverse effects is increased for people with certain conditions, such as a history of stroke, glaucoma, diabetes, hypertension, heart disease, thyroid disorder, and any disorder requiring anticoagulation therapy. Another concern is that herbs and other dietary supplements have the potential for interactions with other drugs. Types of medications that are most likely to interact with herbal products include antidepressants, sedative–hypnotics, and drugs with a narrow therapeutic range (e.g., digoxin and theophylline). There also is increasing concern about the effects of herbs during periods of physiologic stress. For example, because surgical care can be complicated by effects of herbs that interfere with coagulation, or prolong the effects of anesthetics, or cause electrolyte disturbances, surgeons generally recommend that all herbs and supplements be discontinued at least 2 weeks prior to surgery when possible (Barnett, 2009). Some of the more serious effects of herbs (listed in Table 8-2) include altered liver function, electrolyte imbalance, elevated blood pressure, diminished blood clotting mechanisms, and alterations of the heart rate and rhythm. Less serious adverse effects include nausea, vomiting, and other gastrointestinal symptoms from oral preparations, especially if they are taken with medications that have similar adverse effects. Table 8-3 lists some of the herbs more commonly used by older adults.

Homeopathic Remedies

Three concepts are crucial to understanding homeopathy, as a German physician, Samuel Hahnemann, initially

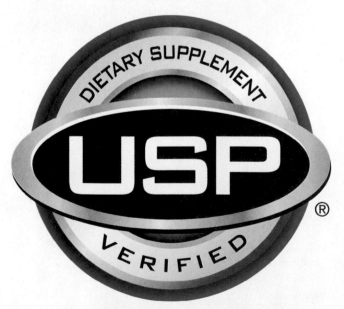

FIGURE 8-1 The United States Pharmacopoeia (USP) mark affixed to approved dietary supplements is an assurance of quality.

TABLE 8-3 Selected Herbs: Indications, Actions, and Cautions

Herb	Uses	Actions and Precautions
Bilberry	The German E Commission approves bilberry for acute non-specific diarrhea and topical treatment of mild inflammation of the mouth, throat, and oral mucosa. Concentrated extracts are used for retinopathy (diabetic and hypertensive), venous insufficiency, and varicose veins.	High doses may inhibit platelet aggregation; monitor anticoagulants if patient is taking larger dosages. Avoid in patients with hemorrhagic disorders.
Black cohosh	The German E Commission approves preparations of fresh or dried rhizome for menopausal symptoms (hot flashes, night sweats, sleep disturbances, irritability).	Monitor liver function every 6 months because of possible hepatotoxicity. Several NIH clinical trials are in progress that may answer the question of whether long-term use of black cohosh causes endometrial hyperplasia.
Cat's claw	Osteoarthritis of the knee and rheumatoid arthritis.	Avoid in patients with organ transplants, lymphocytosis, or autoimmune disease. Use with caution with antiplatelet therapy, hypertensive medication, and medications that suppress immune response. Inhibits chromosome P-450 CYP3A4 enzyme in vitro. May dilate peripheral blood vessels and increase heart rate.
Chamomile	The German E Commission approves chamomile for inflammation of GI tract and GI spasms. Topical preparation use includes inflammation of skin and mucous membranes and bacterial skin diseases.	Contraindicated with allergy to chamomile. No herb–drug interactions reported in the literature.
Echinacea	The German E Commission approves for supportive therapy for colds and infections of the respiratory and urinary tract.	Caution when coadministering with drugs dependent on CYP3A or CYP1A2 for elimination. Contraindicated in progressive systemic diseases (e.g., HIV, AIDS, tuberculosis, multiple sclerosis, leukocytosis). Avoid in patients taking immunosuppressant drugs (e.g., transplant patients).
Evening primrose	Atopic dermatitis and eczema. May improve blood flow and nerve conduction deficits in diabetes.	Possible interaction with antipsychotic medications and inhibition of anticonvulsants.
Garlic	The German E Commission approves garlic use to lower cholesterol levels, prevent hardening of arteries, and treat minor respiratory infections.	Inhibits platelet aggregation; may increase risk of bleeding when taken with warfarin, aspirin, or NSAIDs. Discontinue garlic supplementation 7–14 days prior to surgery, except for garlic used in cooking.
Ginger	The German E Commission approves for prevention of motion sickness. Anti-inflammatory.	Contraindicated in active gallbladder disease. Discontinue supplementation 7–14 days before surgery, except for ginger used in cooking.
Ginkgo biloba	Standardized ginkgo extract has a positive German E Commission monograph for degenerative and vascular dementia, peripheral artery occlusive disease, vertigo, and tinnitus. Ginkgo leaf has a null German E Commission monograph.	American Herbal Products Association contraindicates use with monoamine oxidase (MAO) inhibitors. Potential for interaction with anticoagulant and antiplatelet medications (e.g., warfarin, aspirin). Rare case reports of spontaneous bleeding. Potential to increase blood glucose levels in type 2 diabetes. Discontinue 7–14 days before surgery.
Ginseng	The German E Commission and World Health Organization (WHO) recognize ginseng as a tonic, prophylaxis, or restorative agent for invigoration during times of fatigue, exhaustion, stress, and convalescence.	May cause hypoglycemia or increase blood pressure. Avoid with MAO inhibitors. Contraindicated in acute asthma or acute infection.
Hawthorn	The German E Commission approves hawthorn leaf with flower for the treatment of congestive heart failure.	May potentiate action of digitalis and beta-blockers.
Horse chestnut	The German E Commission approves horse chestnut for treatment of chronic venous insufficiency, night cramps, and itching.	Monitor bleeding times in patients taking anticoagulants.
Kava	Used for treatment of anxiety.	May cause hepatotoxicity (leading to transplants and deaths). Has high potential for drug interactions, including decreased effectiveness of warfarin and potentiation of barbiturates.
Licorice	The German E Commission approves the use of licorice root for inflammation of the upper respiratory tract and gastric/duodenal ulcers.	Contraindicated in liver disorders, congestive heart failure, or edema. Avoid prolonged use of higher dosages. Licorice can increase blood pressure. Potential interactions with diuretics, corticosteroids, and antihypertensives.

(continued)

TABLE 8-3 Selected Herbs: Indications, Actions, and Cautions (*continued*)

Herb	Uses	Actions and Precautions
Saw palmetto	The German E Commission and USP (U.S. Pharmacopoeia) recognize saw palmetto as treatment for benign prostatic hypertrophy.	No reported drug interactions. Does not appear to affect prostate-specific antigen (PSA) levels.
St. John's wort	The German E Commission recognizes use in mild-to-moderate depressive moods, anxiety, and nervousness.	Not indicated for use in severe depression. Phototoxicity is extremely rare but can occur in light-skinned people. Potential for decreased cyclosporine levels; decreased effectiveness of warfarin; possible decreased digoxin levels; reduced levels of protease inhibitors (e.g., indinavir); decreased levels of simvastatin. Avoid in patients taking multiple medications.
Valerian	Used as a mild sleep-promoting agent in nervous, restlessness, and anxiety-related sleep disturbances.	In theory, there is potential additive effect when taken with central nervous system depressants.

proposed it two centuries ago. First, there is the law of similars, or "like cures like." According to this concept, homeopathy treats an illness by stimulating the body's self-healing abilities through the use of a small amount of a substance similar to that which caused the illness. For example, quinine can produce symptoms of malaria in a healthy person, and it can cure malaria when administered in minute doses. The second key concept is that the more a substance is diluted, the more potent it becomes. Based on this concept, homeopathic remedies are diluted repeatedly, and each dilution is vigorously shaken to increase its potency. The third concept is that illnesses are highly individualized, and, therefore, the treatment must be individualized. Based on this principle, homeopathic practitioners focus on treating the person, not the disease, and they spend a lot of time interviewing and assessing patients before prescribing a homeopathic remedy. Homeopathy is widely used in India, Russia, Mexico, and European countries, and it is gaining acceptance in the United States as a safe alternative to conventional medicine.

Although most homeopathic remedies are now available for self-treatment, a few are available only through health care practitioners. Unlike herbs, homeopathic remedies are regulated by the FDA as over-the-counter products. Remedies come in a variety of single-substance or combination forms, including powders, wafers, small tablets, and alcohol-based liquids. Over-the-counter homeopathic products are too weak to cause adverse effects, and there are very few precautions, interactions, or contraindications that apply to these products. People who are taking homeopathic remedies are advised to limit the amount taken and the length of time they are consumed. Other precautions include avoiding food, caffeine, beverages, toothpaste, and mouthwashes for 15 to 60 minutes before and after taking the substance. Also, oils of camphor, eucalyptus, and peppermint should be avoided during homeopathic treatments. Information about homeopathic remedies and homeopathic practitioners can be obtained from the National Center for Complementary and Alternative Medicine (see Health Education in Resources section).

 ## AGE-RELATED CHANGES THAT AFFECT BIOACTIVE SUBSTANCES IN OLDER ADULTS

Age-related changes that affect bioactive substances in older adults are discussed in relation to those that affect the actions of the agents in the body, and those that affect the skills involved with taking them. The factors that have the most significant impact on the effectiveness of bioactive substances in older adults are not age-related changes, but risk factors, and are considered in the section on Risk Factors.

Changes That Affect the Action of Bioactive Substances in the Body

An age-related decline in glomerular filtration rate, which begins in early adulthood and progresses at an annual rate of 1% to 2%, may affect the concentrations of bioactive substances in the body, particularly those that are cleared through the kidneys. For example, diminished renal function can decrease the clearance of water-soluble medications that depend on glomerular filtration (e.g., gentamicin) or tubular secretion (e.g., penicillin) for their removal. Likewise, the consequences of diminished renal function will be greater on substances that readily reach toxic levels because they have a narrow therapeutic index (e.g., digoxin). Box 8-1 lists some medications that are likely to be affected by age-related renal changes.

An age-related decline in hepatic blood flow that begins around the age of 40 years can affect serum concentration and volume of distribution of substances that are metabolized more extensively by the liver, even in healthy older adults. This change slows down the delivery of medications that normally are rapidly metabolized. In addition to age-related changes, many other factors affect the liver metabolism of substances in people of all ages. The specific effect of age-related liver changes on the metabolism of bioactive agents is unclear because factors such as diet, caffeine, smoking, alcohol, genetic variations, and pathologic conditions are likely to simultaneously affect the metabolism of substances and exert a stronger influence than any age-related factors. Box 8-1 also lists some

Box 8-1 Effects of Age-Related Changes on Medication Effectiveness

Decreased Clearance Caused by Renal Changes
Amantadine
Amoxicillin
Ampicillin
Atenolol
Ceftriaxone
Cephalexin
Chlorpropamide
Cimetidine
Ciprofloxacin
Colchicine
Digoxin
Enalapril
Furosemide
Glyburide
Hydrochlorothiazide
Levofloxacin
Lisinopril
Metformin
Ranitidine

Decreased Clearance Caused by Hepatic Changes
Acetaminophen
Amitriptyline
Barbiturates
Benzodiazepines
Codeine
Labetalol
Lidocaine
Meperidine
Morphine
Phenytoin
Propranolol
Quinidine
Salicylates
Theophylline
Warfarin

Increased Concentrations Caused by Changes in Body Composition
Cimetidine
Digoxin

Ethanol (alcohol)
Gentamicin
Morphine
Propranolol
Quinine
Warfarin

Decreased Concentrations Caused by Changes in Body Composition
Phenobarbital
Prazosin
Thiopental
Tolbutamide

Increased Receptor Sensitivity (Increased Potency)
Angiotensin-converting enzyme (ACE) inhibitors
Diazepam
Digoxin
Diltiazem
Enalapril
Felodipine
Levodopa
Lithium
Midazolam
Morphine
Temazepam
Verapamil
Warfarin

Decreased Receptor Sensitivity (May Have Delayed Signs of Toxicity)
Beta-blockers
Bumetanide
Dopamine
Furosemide
Isoproterenol
Propranolol
Tolbutamide

medications whose clearance is likely to be delayed because of age-related liver changes.

In recent years, there has been increasing attention paid to the role of the **cytochrome P-450 enzyme system**, which is composed of many specific enzymes responsible for the metabolism of medications and other bioactive substances, including herbs, nutrients, and nicotine. The cytochrome P-450 system is particularly important with regard to interactions between herbs, medications, and other substances because competition at the enzyme sites can affect clearance. Pathways most commonly involved with pharmaceutical agents are 1A2, 2C9, 2C19, 2D69, and 3A4. Clearance of substances that depend on the cytochrome P-450 system is likely to be delayed to a small degree because of age-related changes and to a greater degree when two or more bioactive agents compete at these enzyme sites. Table 8-4 lists examples of some commonly used drugs and herbs according to their metabolic pathway.

An age-related decrease in total body water and an increase in the proportion of body fat to lean body mass can alter the action of bioactive substances in older adults. Between the ages of about 20 and 80 years, the following changes in body composition occur: body fat gradually increases by 15% to 20%, lean tissue decreases by about 20%, and total body water is reduced by 10% to 15%. Because these age-related changes in body composition will affect substances according to their degree of fat or water solubility, agents that are distributed primarily in body water or lean body mass may reach higher serum concentrations in older adults and their effects may be more intense. Similarly, the serum concentration of highly fat-soluble substances, which are distributed and stored in fat tissue, may be lowered, and these agents have an increased tendency to accumulate in adipose tissue. Consequently, fat-soluble substances may have a prolonged duration of action, be more erratic in their effects, and have less intense immediate effects. Box 8-1 also lists some medications whose concentrations are likely to be increased or decreased because of age-related changes in body composition.

As bioactive substances are distributed and metabolized in the body, some molecules are bound to serum albumin and other proteins, so the bound portion becomes inactive while the unbound molecules remain active. Because the unbound portion is the amount available for metabolism, tissue perfusion, and renal excretion, the protein-binding capacity of an agent is an important determinant of its potential for both therapeutic and adverse effects. The degree of protein binding of each substance varies, with some medications, such as warfarin, having a protein-binding capacity of 99%. The binding capacity of substances that are highly protein bound can be influenced by diminished serum albumin levels in older adults. Additional factors that affect the degree of protein binding for any agent include the strength of the binding and the number of chemicals competing for the binding sites.

Although gerontologists disagree about the extent and cause of decreased serum albumin levels in older adults, it is generally agreed that the level diminishes by as much as 20% in the later decades of life. Diminished serum albumin levels are associated with a combination of factors, including malnutrition, pathologic processes, decreased mobility, and age-related liver changes. Regardless of the cause, a decrease in the serum albumin level will lead to an increased amount of the active portion of protein-bound substances. Medications that are highly protein bound, which are commonly taken by older adults, are most strongly affected. This effect is intensified when more than one protein-bound substance is consumed because the agents compete for the same sites. Medications

TABLE 8-4 Metabolic Pathways of Some Commonly Used Bioactive Substances

CYP1A2	CYP2C9	2C19	2D6	3A4	2C8
amitriptyline*	carbamazepine	ginkgo	bupropion	alprazolam	gemfibrozil
caffeine	cranberry	carbamazepine	celecoxib	clarithromycin	phenobarbital
charbroiled food	diazepam	fluoxetine	codeine	erythromycin	rifampin
clomipramine	ginkgo	omeprazole	oxycodone	estrogens (oral)	quercetin
echinacea	isoniazid	phenytoin	cimetidine	felodipine	
estradiol	phenobarbital		sertraline	fentanyl	
imipramine	phenytoin		sildenafil	St. John's wort	
nicotine	St. John's wort		simvastatin	caffeine	
St. John's wort	warfarin		tamoxifen	progesterone/	
theophylline			garlic	progestins	
				grapefruit	
				pomegranate	

*Words in italics indicate that the drug or herb has been involved in a drug interaction of clinical relevance or associated with a strong drug interaction warning.

that are most likely to have adverse effects when they are taken together or when serum albumin levels are low include aspirin, digoxin, furosemide, nonsteroidal anti-inflammatory drugs (NSAIDs), hypoglycemics, phenytoin, sertraline, and sulfonamides.

Independent of any changes that affect pharmacokinetics, age-related changes in receptor sensitivity can influence pharmacodynamics and cause older adults to be more or less sensitive to particular substances. For example, an increased sensitivity of the older brain to centrally acting psychotropic medications may potentiate both the therapeutic and adverse effects of these drugs. This is particularly true for benzodiazepines, which have stronger sedative effects in older adults. Box 8-1 lists examples of drugs that have increased or decreased sensitivity in older adults. Age-related change in homeostatic mechanisms, such as thermoregulation, fluid regulation, and baroreceptor control over blood pressure, also can affect pharmacodynamics. For example, inefficient fluid regulation may alter the action of medications, such as lithium, that are particularly sensitive to fluid and electrolyte balance.

Body size is an additional factor that can add to the effects of age-related changes and influence the action of bioactive substances in the body. Because body size can affect both the therapeutic and adverse effects of substances, doses need to be adjusted for older adults who are small or have lost or are losing weight. This consideration is particularly important for older adults who are losing muscle mass or have decreased renal function.

Changes That Affect Behaviors Related to Taking Bioactive Substances

For any adult, all the following factors affect the appropriate use of bioactive substances:

- Motivation
- Knowledge about the purpose of the substance
- Cultural and psychosocial influences
- Ability to obtain correct amounts (influenced by factors such as cost, accessibility)
- Ability to distinguish the correct container
- Ability to read and comprehend directions
- Ability to hear and remember verbal instructions
- Knowledge about correct timing for consumption
- Ability to follow the correct dosage regimen
- Physical ability to remove the substance from the container and administer it
- Ability to swallow oral preparations
- Additional skills related to coordination, manual dexterity, and visual acuity for substances that are administered nasally, transdermally, subcutaneously, or by other methods.

Even for healthy older adults, age-related changes and functional impairments often interfere with these skills. For example, hearing or vision changes can interfere with the ability to understand instructions and read directions, especially labels on bottles. Any limitations in fine motor movement of the hands may interfere with the ability to remove lids from containers, especially when the lids are tamper resistant. Although the skills related to taking bioactive substances are sometimes influenced by age-related changes, more often they are influenced by risk factors that commonly occur in older adults.

 ### RISK FACTORS THAT AFFECT BIOACTIVE SUBSTANCES

By approximately age 75, even the healthiest of older adults have age-related changes that affect pharmacokinetic and pharmacodynamic processes in their bodies. Even more significant, however, are the numerous risk factors that have even greater effects on behaviors of older adults relative to taking bioactive substances. Risk factors can be the result of the patient's own attitudes, level of knowledge, and socioeconomic circumstances, or they can be attributed to outside sources (e.g., health care providers).

The consumption of more than one bioactive substance greatly increases the potential for adverse and altered therapeutic effects. Because older adults take a disproportionately greater number of medications than do younger people, they are more susceptible to adverse or altered effects. Additional risks arise from myths and misunderstandings that affect the medication consumption patterns of older adults. Finally, certain factors unrelated to age, such as weight, sex, and smoking habits, combine with age-related changes and risk factors to increase further the risk of adverse and altered effects.

◆ Wellness Opportunity

Nurses provide holistic care when they explore the wide range of factors that affect bioactive substances and substance-taking behaviors.

Pathologic Processes and Functional Impairments

Because the purpose of any medication is to relieve or control symptoms of pathologic conditions, it can be assumed that people who take medications have at least one disease-related process. The increased prevalence of chronic conditions in older adults adds to their vulnerability to medication–disease interactions and to the complexity of prescribing the safest and most appropriate medications. For example, pain management for the many older adults who have both osteoporosis and hypertension is complicated by the fact that studies indicate that NSAIDs can induce significant increases in systolic blood pressure (White, 2009). It is important to recognize that medication–disease interactions that affect pharmacokinetics and pharmacodynamics can be asymptomatic but clinically important. For example, chronic renal disease may be identified only by laboratory values but can significantly affect the concentration and clearance of some medications. In general, people with chronic renal disease need to take most of their medications at lower doses and longer intervals to obtain a constant blood level (Olyaei & Bennett, 2009).

Medication–disease interactions manifest themselves in any of the following ways:

- Pathologic processes can exacerbate age-related changes that would otherwise have little or no impact on the medication. For example, malnutrition further decreases serum albumin, thereby increasing both the therapeutic and adverse effects of highly protein-bound medications.
- Pathologic processes can alter therapeutic and adverse effects of substances. For instance, congestive heart failure decreases both the metabolism and the excretion of most medications.
- Bioactive substances can cause serious adverse effects for people with pathologic conditions. For example, anticholinergics may cause urinary retention in men with prostatic hyperplasia.

Pathologic conditions not only influence the action of substances in the body but also contribute to nonadherence, especially in combination with functional limitations. For example, dementia can significantly affect the older adult's ability to understand directions, remember instructions, and self-manage medication regimens. Dysphagia is an example of a physical limitation that can interfere with the ability to take substances orally.

Behaviors Based on Myths and Misunderstandings

Myths and misunderstandings influence attitudes held by older adults, as well as their caregivers, about the consumption of bioactive substances. An attitude that can be potentially harmful for older adults is that medications, particularly over-the-counter products, provide a "quick fix" for any uncomfortable symptom. For example, messages promoting constipation remedies can reinforce false beliefs about bowel function and lead to laxative abuse. Although adults of any age can be influenced by these attitudes, older adults are more likely than their younger counterparts to experience negative consequences because they are more vulnerable to adverse effects and drug interactions.

Another potentially harmful belief is that over-the-counter remedies are always safe, even in extra-strength doses. Although over-the-counter preparations may be relatively safe for healthy younger adults, they often create problems for older adults, particularly with pathologic conditions and combined with other substances. For example, over-the-counter preparations for colds and insomnia typically contain anticholinergic ingredients that are strongly associated with delirium and other serious adverse effects in older adults. In these situations, the addition of a seemingly harmless over-the-counter product to an already complex regimen of prescription medications can be the factor that tips the scale of safety and causes a serious adverse effect, such as delirium. NSAIDs are another category of over-the-counter drugs that commonly have serious adverse effects in older adults, either alone or with other substances (e.g., anticoagulants, prednisone). This can be especially problematic for people with hypertension because NSAIDs can increase blood pressure by causing sodium and fluid retention (Cooney & Pascuzzi, 2009). Acetaminophen is another commonly used over-the-counter product that can have serious adverse effects, including liver failure and death, when used in high doses.

Attitudes and expectations about medications as quick-fix remedies also can influence the prescribing patterns of primary care practitioners. For example, when over-the-counter remedies are ineffective, people expect their health care practitioners to provide an otherwise unobtainable remedy—a prescription—for their discomfort. Sometimes, a nonpharmacologic remedy is safer than, and just as effective as, a prescription medication, but these remedies usually demand more of the practitioner's time and some degree of patient motivation. For example, it is easier to prescribe an antihypertensive than to advise about diet and exercise interventions. Another factor contributing to the reluctance of practitioners to suggest nonpharmacologic remedies is that there are more controlled clinical trials supporting the use of medications. Sleep and anxiety complaints are examples of conditions that respond to nonpharmacologic treatments, but these are often addressed by prescription medications because of the attitudes of the patient or primary care practitioner.

◆ Wellness Opportunity

By taking time to identify an older adult's beliefs about illness and treatments (including pharmacologic and nonpharmacologic approaches), nurses pave the way for teaching about the safest and most effective interventions.

Communication Barriers

Another factor that may contribute to an increased use of prescriptions by older adults is their own reluctance to challenge or question the primary care practitioner because they perceive him or her as "all-knowing." Although the image of the infallible physician is subsiding, older adults are still inclined to accept advice from prescribing practitioners without question.

Communication barriers and lack of confidence in one's communication skills may further inhibit someone from discussing treatment options with a health care practitioner. Because medical knowledge has been expanding at a tremendous pace in recent years, treatment decisions have become increasingly more complex. Consequently, older adults may hesitate to ask questions about medical decisions out of fear of appearing ignorant. Hearing and vision impairments also may interfere with patient-directed discussions of a treatment plan. Other communication barriers, such as an attitude of impatience on the part of the health care practitioner, also may thwart discussion. In addition, poor command of the English language, on the part of either the older adult or the health care practitioner, can interfere with a discussion of health issues and lead to misunderstandings. Language barriers and a low education level can present major impediments to many treatment decisions, including medication adherence.

Lack of Information

Despite the fact that older adults are the primary consumers of prescription and over-the-counter medications, our knowledge about medication effects in older adults is insufficient and still in an early phase. Before the 1980s, research on the influence of age on the action of specific medications was virtually nonexistent and pharmaceutical companies determined normal adult doses based on clinical trials of healthy younger men. In addition, the few studies of age-related influences on medications were cross-sectional rather than longitudinal and identified age differences rather than age-related changes. Although many clinical drug trials now include older subjects, they do not include medically frail or very old adults.

Information about adverse effects and medication–medication interactions also is lacking, especially for newly approved drugs. Because the FDA requires only limited testing of medication–medication interactions, these interactions are often identified only after the medication has been on the

market for several years. Similarly, most adverse drug effects are not identified until a drug has been available for several months to years because clinical trials are not high powered enough to detect low incidences of safety risks (Zarowitz, 2008). Thus, any recently approved medication should be used cautiously in older adults because of the increased risk of adverse effects and unpredictable interactions. Examples of medications that are likely to cause serious adverse effects when consumed with another medication include alcohol, analgesics, anticoagulants, anticholinergics, digoxin, phenytoin, theophylline, and warfarin.

In 1982, the USP, which sets the official standards for medications in the United States, established a geriatrics advisory panel to examine age-related influences on medication action. Since the late 1980s, three trends have emerged in the pharmaceutical industry that are beneficial for older adults: (1) pharmaceutical companies began testing medications on older adults; (2) they began focusing on **adverse medication effects**, including medication interactions; and (3) because of the emphasis on adverse reactions, new medications are now developed and promoted not only for their therapeutic effectiveness but for their lack of unwanted effects. Also, since 1997, pharmaceutical companies have been required to include a separate geriatric-use section in drug labeling.

Inappropriate Prescribing Practices

During the late 1980s, geriatricians began to address medication-related problems in older adults because of widespread concerns about the large numbers as well as the types of drugs prescribed for this population. The phrase **potentially inappropriate medications** (PIMs) refers to medications that pose more risks than benefits for older adults, particularly when safer alternatives exist. In 1991, an international panel of experts used consensus criteria to identify drugs that should not be used by frail older adults (Beers et al., 1991). According to these explicit criteria, called the **Beers criteria**, medications are deemed inappropriate if they are ineffective or have poor safety profiles, or if better drugs are available (Beers et al., 1991).

The updated 2002 Beers criteria lists medications that should not be prescribed for older adults because they are less effective or pose a higher risk than other available medications. A second part lists medications that should not be prescribed to older adults with specific medical conditions. These criteria have been widely used in the United States and worldwide to guide research and clinical practice, and they are recommended as a best practice tool by the Hartford Institute for Geriatric Nursing (Molony, 2009). In addition, the Centers for Medicare and Medicaid and other organizations commonly use the Beers criteria as a quality indicator when evaluating geriatric services.

Some common themes in the Beers criteria include the following:

● Anticholinergic drugs and drugs with anticholinergic properties are inappropriate because of toxicity and

TABLE 8-5 Research Evidence: Prevalence of Potentially Inappropriate Medications

Reference	Country	Research Findings
Agashivala & Wu, 2009	USA	Based on data analysis of 11,940 nursing home residents, those receiving psychoactive potentially inappropriate medications (PIMs) had an increased risk of falls compared with those taking no or other psychoactive drugs
Barton, Sklenicka, Sayegh, & Yaffe, 2008	USA	22% of 100 older adults evaluated at a memory disorders clinic were taking at least one medication that could interfere with cognitive function (most common: benzodiazepines, oxybutynin, amitriptyline, fluoxetine, diphenhydramine)
Berdot et al., 2009	France	32% of 6343 community-dwelling older adults used at least one PIM at baseline; over a 3-year period, PIM was associated with an increased risk of falls (most commonly implicated medications: benzodiazepines, other psychotropics, anticholinergics
Brekke et al., 2009	Norway	18.4% of 85,836 older adults in outpatient settings were taking one or more PIM (most common: NSAID combined with another drug, long-acting benzodiazepine)
Buck et al., 2009	USA	23% of 61,251 older adults in two outpatient settings were receiving a PIM (most common: propoxyphene and fluoxetine)
Carey et al., 2008	UK	Data from records of about 230,000 older adults in 201 general practices in 2005 found that 28.3% were taking at least one PIM
Chen et al., 2009	Taiwan	19.3% of 1,429,463 older adults who visited emergency departments received at least one PIM annually (most common: short-acting nifedipine, muscle relaxants and antispasmodics, antihistamines, and ketorolac)
Fick, Mion, Beers, & Waller, 2009	USA	40% of almost 18,000 community-dwelling older adults filled prescriptions for one PIM and an additional 13% had prescriptions for two or more PIMs
Hosia-Randell, Muurinen, & Pitkala, 2008	Finland	34.9% of almost 2000 nursing home residents regularly used at least one PIM (most common: benzodiazepines, hydroxyzine, nitrofurantoin)
Prudent et al., 2008	France	28% of 1176 patients aged 75 years and older took at least one PIM during the 2 weeks prior to hospitalization
Radosevic, Gantumur, & Viahovic-Palcevski, 2008	Croatia	25% of 225 hospitalized older adults received at least one PIM (most common: amiodarone, diazepam)
Rothberg et al., 2008	USA	49% of almost 500,000 older adults in 384 hospitals received at least one PIM and 6% received three or more PIMs (most common: promethazine, diphenhydramine, propoxyphene)
Rupawala, Kshirsager, & Gogtay, 2009	India	8% of adverse drugs events in patients aged 65 years and older were attributable to a PIM
Schuler et al., 2008	Austria	Record review of 543 hospitalized patients aged 75 years and older found the following related to preadmission medications: 65.8% possible drug–drug interactions, 58.4% taking more than six drugs, 36.3% unnecessary drugs, 30.1% PIMs, 23.4% wrong dose, and 17.8% adverse reactions

serious side effects (e.g., seizures, delirium, agitation, hallucinations, cardiac arrhythmias, cognitive impairment, and urinary retention).

- Tricyclic antidepressants are inappropriate not only because of anticholinergic effects but also because of their increased volume of distribution and slowed metabolism, which are particular concerns for older adults with cardiac conditions.
- Antipsychotic medications can produce extrapyramidal and anticholinergic effects, as well as **tardive dyskinesia**, even with low doses and short-term use.
- Barbiturates are inappropriate, except as anticonvulsants, because their high protein-binding capacity can lead to accumulation and toxicity.
- Benzodiazepines, especially those that have been on the market the longest (e.g., diazepam, chlordiazepoxide, flurazepam) have a high risk for accumulation and toxicity because of their prolonged half-life in older adults.

In recent years, numerous studies have used the Beers criteria to analyze prescribing patterns and health outcomes of PIMs. For example, one recent study found that medical and total health care costs were significantly higher for those older adults taking PIMs than for those in control group (Stockl, Le, Zhang, & Harada, 2010). Table 8-5 summarizes some recent studies of the prevalence of PIM across various settings and in many countries.

Despite the increasing recognition of the value of the Beers criteria during the past two decades, inappropriate prescribing continues to be prevalent and problematic, particularly for psychotropic drugs. The use of psychotropic drugs in long-term care facilities has been a particular focus of concern since 1987, when the Nursing Home Reform Act mandated that the Health Care Financing Administration addresses this issue. Despite efforts to improve prescribing practices, however, studies indicate that little progress has been made. One study found that almost one-third of 6103 elderly nursing home residents with dementia received an antipsychotic medication, mainly atypical agents (Kamble, Chen, Sherer, & Aparasu, 2009). Studies also have found that psychotropic medication use is disproportionately more prevalent among community-living older adults than in younger age groups and that a very high percentage of assisted living residents receive at least one psychotropic medication (Lindsey, 2009).

Polypharmacy and Inadequate Monitoring of Medications

Polypharmacy refers to the inappropriate and often unnecessary prescribing of multiple medications that results in negative outcomes (Planton & Edlund, 2010). Studies have consistently found that older adults in the United States account for one-third or more of prescription medications and a larger percentage of over-the-counter medications. One recent review of studies found that 29.4% of community-dwelling older adults are prescribed six or more medications, 15.7% are prescribed **inappropriate medications**, and 9.3% took six or more medications and that also included at least one inappropriately prescribed drug (Bushardt, Massey, Simpson, Arial, & Simpson, 2008). There is even greater concern about polypharmacy among older adults in institutional settings. The high level of medication use is primarily associated with the increased prevalence of chronic illness among older adults, and although it is usually appropriate and therapeutic, it can lead to drug interactions and adverse medication effects. Thus, geriatricians emphasize the importance of prescribing medication regimens according to evidence-based criteria about therapeutic effectiveness and adverse effects of the medications as well as on the research on effectiveness of safe nonpharmacologic treatments. For example, Morley (2009) suggests that one simple way to reduce drug use in nursing homes would be to install bright lights (i.e., 1060 to 2000 lux) and introduce regular exercise programs.

As the number and sources of medications increase, the need for monitoring becomes more important, from the time of the initial prescription until the termination of treatment. The following risk factors could potentially interfere with medication monitoring in older adults:

- Patient consultations with multiple health care providers, who usually do not communicate with each other about the patient's care
- Health care practitioners' lack of information about medications obtained from a variety of sources (i.e., prescription medications offered by friends and relatives, or nonprescription products, such as herbs, nutritional supplements, and over-the-counter products)
- Health care practitioners' lack of information about a patient's nonadherence to a treatment regimen
- A patient's fear of disclosing information about folk remedies or medications obtained from sources other than the prescribing health care practitioner
- A patient's reluctance to disclose information about self-directed changes in the medication regimen
- An assumption by the patient or health care practitioner that once most medications are started, they should be continued indefinitely
- An assumption by the patient or health care practitioner that once an appropriate medication dosage is established, it will not need to be changed
- An assumption by the patient or health care practitioner that a lack of adverse effects early in the course of treatment indicates that adverse effects will never occur
- Changes in the patient's weight, especially weight loss, which may affect pharmacokinetic processes
- Changes in the patient's daily habits (e.g., smoking, activity level, or nutrient and fluid intake), which may affect pharmacokinetic processes
- Changes in the patient's mental–emotional status, which may affect medication consumption patterns
- Changes in the patient's health status, which may affect medication actions, increasing the potential for adverse effects.

Medication Nonadherence

Medication nonadherence (also called noncompliance) refers to medication-taking patterns that differ from the prescribed pattern, including missed doses, failure to fill prescriptions, or medications taken too frequently or at inappropriate times. Although nonadherence is often viewed as a problem specific to older adults, studies indicate that 50% of adults of any age do not take drugs as prescribed (Williams, Manias, & Walker, 2008). A study of 2640 men with benign prostatic hyperplasia found that only 40% adhered to prescribed medications and that younger men were more likely to discontinue their medication regimens in contrast to older men (Nichol, Knight, Wu, Barron, & Penson, 2009).

Factors that can contribute to nonadherence include depression, cognitive impairment, isolated living situation, financial considerations, disease category, adverse medication effects, complex medication regimen, inadequate understanding of the medication regimen, and the use of two or more prescribing practitioners or pharmacies. A study of attitudes of older adults about medications found that adherence with taking multiple medications was significantly influenced by not experiencing adverse effects and by perceptions about the "goodness" of the medication regimen (Moen et al., 2009). Consequences of nonadherence include hospitalization, exacerbation of disease conditions, and increased risk for mortality for these patients (Conn et al., 2009; Ho et al., 2008).

DIVERSITY NOTE

Studies have found lower adherence to antihypertensive medications among younger people, men, and blacks (Krousel-Wood, Muntner, Islam, Morisky, & Webber, 2009).

Financial Concerns Related to Prescription Drugs

In recent years, increasing attention has been paid to the disproportionate and rapid increase in the cost of prescription drugs, which has been far exceeding the rate of inflation of other health services. For example, in 2006, the annual rate of increase for prescription spending was 9%, whereas the increases for hospital care and physician services were 7% and 6%, respectively (Centers for Medicare & Medicaid Services, 2008). In 2007, the average retail cost of a prescription drug was $69.91, representing an annual increase of 6.9% during the previous decade. During this same period, the percent of older adults taking prescription medications increased from 86% to 91% (Kaiser Family Foundation, 2008).

Major concerns about prescription drug costs led to the legislation creating the **Medicare Part D** prescription drug program, which became effective in January 2006. Now, everyone enrolled in Medicare has a choice of at least one type of prescription drug insurance coverage and as of January 2008, about 90% of Medicare recipients had drug coverage. Low-income Medicare beneficiaries may qualify for full prescription drug coverage under Medicaid, or for substantial subsidies with no monthly premiums. However, there are fewer choices about these plans and the enrollment process is more cumbersome, so many of the people who are eligible for these subsidies are not enrolled.

Unlike the basic publicly funded and government administered Medicare program, Medicare Part D plans are offered by private insurance companies. Between 40 and 50 Medicare stand-alone prescription drug plans are available in each state, with an average premium of $39 per month in 2010 (Kaiser Family Foundation, 2009). Plans vary according to the specific drugs they cover (especially generic vs. trade names), and the process for determining the most cost-effective plan for each person is especially complicated for those who take several or more medications. Although there are many Internet-based resources for helping consumers select the most cost-effective plan, people who cannot readily navigate the Internet are at a major disadvantage. Thus, older adults often rely on families, caregivers, or community-based resources to help them select a prescription drug plan.

In addition to paying a monthly premium, which increases every year, many plans require co-pays and deductibles and at least 80% of plans include a period during which the plan provides little or no coverage. Under the standard benefit plan, this "**donut hole**" period begins after an enrollee has paid $2830 (2010 criterion) for prescriptions, and insurance coverage resumes after the enrollee has spent an additional $4550 in drug costs (including deductibles and co-pays). Based on these figures, an older adult with prescription drug coverage could still incur about $7000 in out-of-pocket costs for prescriptions in 2010. The conditions or drug classes associated with highest out-of-pocket drug costs include dementia, diabetes, osteoporosis, antidepressants, angiotensin-converting enzyme (ACE) inhibitors, angiotensin-receptor blockers, and proton pump inhibitors. Analysis of the first years of Medicare Part D indicated that this benefit has the positive effects of decreased out-of-pocket expenditures and modest increases in drug utilization (Yin et al., 2008).

Insufficient Recognition of Adverse Medication Effects

Another problem specific to older adults is that adverse effects are likely to be misinterpreted or not recognized as such because of their similarity to age-related changes or commonly occurring pathologic conditions. When an older adult experiences an adverse medication reaction, two or three potential causes other than the medication usually can be identified. The term **prescribing cascade** has been applied to the following commonly occurring scenario: an adverse drug reaction is misinterpreted as a new medical condition, a drug is prescribed for this condition, another adverse drug effect occurs, the patient is again treated for the perceived additional medical condition, and the sequence perpetuates new adverse events. A common and serious example of the prescribing cascade is the use of medications to treat **drug-induced parkinsonism**, which is a potentially reversible condition that commonly occurs in older adults who are taking haloperidol, phenothiazines, and other antipsychotics (Alvarez & Evidente, 2008; Thanyi & Treadwell, 2009). Although adverse effects are not unique to older adults, they occur more commonly with increasing age and are more likely to be attributed erroneously to pathologic conditions or age-related changes and circumstances. Table 8-6 summarizes adverse medication effects that are likely to remain unrecognized in older adults because of their similarity to age-related changes.

> **✦ Wellness Opportunity**
>
> Nurses promote wellness when they challenge ageist attitudes and identify adverse effects falsely attributed to aging or pathologic conditions.

MEDICATION INTERACTIONS

Medications can interact with any other biologically active substance, including other medications, herbs, nutrients, alcohol, caffeine, and nicotine. These interactions occur not only with prescription medications but also with commonly used over-the-counter products, including antacids, analgesics, and remedies for coughs, colds, and sleep problems. Outcomes of medication interactions with other substances include altered or erratic therapeutic effect, increased potential for adverse effects, and, in rare cases, a decreased potential for adverse effects.

Medication–Medication Interactions

The risk of adverse effects from interactions between two or more medications increases exponentially according to the number of medications being consumed. Because older adults are more likely than younger people to take two or more medications concurrently, they are at increased risk for medication–medication interactions. Medication–medication interactions are typically caused by competitive action at binding sites, but they can be caused by any mechanism that influences the

TABLE 8-6 Some Adverse Medication Effects That May Remain Unrecognized in Older Adults

Manifestation	Medication Type	Specific Examples
Cognitive impairment	Antidepressants; antipsychotics; antianxiety agents; anticholinergics; hypoglycemics; over-the-counter (OTC) cold, cough, and sleeping preparations	Perphenazine, amitriptyline, chlorpromazine, diazepam, chlordiazepoxide, benztropine, trihexyphenidyl, cimetidine, digoxin, barbiturates, tolazamide, tolbutamide, chlorpheniramine, diphenhydramine
Depression	Antihypertensives, antiarthritics, antianxiety agents, antipsychotics	Reserpine, clonidine, propranolol, indomethacin, haloperidol, barbiturates
Urinary incontinence	Diuretics, anticholinergics	Furosemide, doxepin, thioridazine, lorazepam
Constipation	Narcotics, antacids, antipsychotics, antidepressants	Codeine, chlorpromazine, calcium carbonate, aluminum hydroxide, amoxapine
Vision impairment	Digitalis, antiarthritics, phenothiazines	Digoxin, indomethacin, ibuprofen, chlorpromazine
Hearing impairment	Mycin antibiotics, salicylates, loop diuretics	Gentamicin, aspirin, furosemide, bumetanide
Postural hypotension	Antihypertensives, diuretics, antipsychotics, antidepressants	Guanethidine, furosemide, propranolol, chlorpromazine, imipramine, clonidine
Hypothermia	Antipsychotics, alcohol, salicylates	Haloperidol, aspirin, alcohol, fluphenazine
Sexual dysfunction	Antihypertensives, antipsychotics, antidepressants, alcohol, antihypertensives	Timolol, clonidine, thiazides, haloperidol, amitriptyline, alcohol, cimetidine, propranolol, methyldopa
Mobility problems	Sedatives, antianxiety agents, antipsychotics, ototoxic medications	Chloral hydrate, diazepam, furosemide, gentamicin
Dry mouth	Anticholinergics, corticosteroids, bronchodilators, antihypertensives	Chlorpromazine, haloperidol, prednisone, furosemide, sertraline, theophylline
Anorexia	Digitalis, bronchodilators, antihistamines	Digoxin, theophylline, diphenhydramine
Drowsiness	Antidepressants, antipsychotics, OTC cold preparations, alcohol, barbiturates	Amitriptyline, haloperidol, chlorpheniramine, secobarbital
Edema	Antiarthritics, corticosteroids, antihypertensives	Ibuprofen, indomethacin, prednisone, reserpine, methyldopa
Tremors	Antipsychotics	Haloperidol, chlorpromazine, thioridazine

absorption, distribution, metabolism, or elimination of any of the medications. It is important to recognize that medications in a particular class of drugs can have the same therapeutic outcomes but differ significantly in potential for interactions because they have different bioactive pathways. For example, cimetidine (Tagamet) was the first drug in the class of histamine-2 receptor antagonists and had been widely used before drug interactions were widely recognized. Now, cimetidine is not recommended in the elderly because it is associated with clinically important interactions due to inhibition of CYP-450 enzymes (Zarowitz, 2009).

Effects of medication–medication interactions include increased or decreased serum levels of either one or both of the medications, with subsequent altered therapeutic effects and increased risk of adverse or toxic effects. Geriatricians and researchers are particularly concerned about interactions with warfarin (Coumadin) because of the increasing use of this drug on a long-term basis for prevention of thrombosis by people who also take other medications, including over-the-counter analgesics. A review of almost 200 studies of warfarin found strong evidence of potentially serious interactions with the following medications, which are commonly used by older adults: omeprazole, amiodarone, lipid-lowering agents, selective serotonin reuptake inhibitors, antibiotics (including azoles, macrolides, and quinolones), and NSAIDs (including selective ones) (Holbrook et al., 2005). Another focus of recent studies is on medication–medication interactions that decrease the effectiveness of clopidogrel (Plavix). Studies have found adverse clinical outcomes and decreased platelet inhibition when clopidogrel was administered with

calcium-channel blockers or with most proton pump inhibitors (Juurlink, Gomes, Ko, Szmitko, & Mamdani, 2009; Siller-Matula, Lana, Christ, & Jilma, 2008). Table 8-7 summarizes specific mechanisms of medication–medication interactions and examples of each type that are most likely to occur in older adults.

Medications and Herbs

Many medication–herb interactions have been identified in recent years because of the increased use of herbs and increased attention to interactions. Studies have found that the aspirin and warfarin are the two medications that most commonly interact with herbs (Holcomb, 2009). Although the more widely recognized medication–herb interactions are sometimes listed in pharmacology references, the FDA does not require identifying or publishing information about these interactions because these products are classified as dietary supplements. In general, herbs should be used very cautiously with anticoagulants and medications for diabetes and in people with compromised renal or hepatic function. Another concern, for example, is the stimulation of the cytochrome P-450 system by St. John's wort, which can significantly affect the metabolism of statin (cholesterol lowering) medications (Gordon, Beeker, & Rader, 2009). One survey of almost 1800 patients found that garlic, valerian, kava, ginkgo, and St. John's wort accounted for more than two-thirds of the potential clinically significant interactions between dietary supplements and prescription medications (Sood et al., 2008). This same study found that the four types of medications that accounted

TABLE 8-7 Types and Examples of Medication–Medication Interactions

Type of Interaction	Interaction Example	Effect
Binding effect (e.g., an oral drug diminishes the absorption of another drug in the stomach)	Magnesium- or aluminum-containing antacids may bind with tetracycline in the stomach	Decreased effects of tetracycline
Metabolism interference effect (e.g., one drug interferes with liver metabolism of another drug)	Ciprofloxacin and anticonvulsants inhibit metabolism of warfarin	Increased effects of warfarin
Metabolism enhancing effect (e.g., one drug activates the drug-metabolizing enzymes in the liver)	Phenobarbital increases metabolism of warfarin	Decreased effects of warfarin
Elimination interference effect (e.g., one drug interferes with the renal elimination of another drug)	Furosemide can interfere with elimination of salicylates	Increased effects of salicylates
Elimination enhancement effect (e.g., renal reabsorption is blocked because of altered urinary pH)	Sodium bicarbonate can enhance excretion of lithium, tetracyclines, and salicylates	Decreased effects of lithium, tetracycline, or salicylate
Competitive or displacement effect (e.g., two drugs compete at receptor sites)	Diphenhydramine may interfere with effect of cholinergic agents (e.g., tacrine, donepezil)	Decreased effects of tacrine or donepezil
Potentiating effect (e.g., two drugs produce greater effects when taken together even though they have different actions)	Acetaminophen taken with codeine has a greater analgesic effect than either medication taken alone	Increased analgesic effect
Additive effect (e.g., two drugs produce greater effect because they have similar action)	Verapamil or diltiazem may have additive effect when taken with a beta-blocker	Increased effect on blood pressure

for 94% of potentially clinical significant interactions were antithrombotic, sedative, antidepressant, and antidiabetic agents. Other studies found that St. John's wort is the dietary supplement that most commonly is associated with interactions, with the most serious interactions occurring with anticoagulants, cardiovascular medications, oral hypoglycemics, and antiretrovirals (Gardiner, Phillips, & Shaughnessy, 2008). Refer to Table 8-3 for common interactions and precautions regarding herbs.

Medications and Nutrients

Interactions between medications and nutrients can affect either the nutrient or the medication. Because the influence of medications on nutrients is addressed in Chapter 18, this chapter focuses on the effects of nutrients on medications. In the context of medication–nutrient interactions, the term nutrient includes foods, beverages, enteral formulas, and dietary supplements. Commonly consumed foods and beverages that can affect medications include cocoa, coffee, fiber, alcohol, protein, cabbage, grapefruit juice, caffeinated tea, and Brussels sprouts. In addition, food preparation methods, such as charcoal broiling, can affect certain medications. Medication–nutrient interactions affect people of all ages; however, they are likely to have more serious consequences in older adults because they occur in combination with age-related changes and other risk factors.

Absorption of medications in the stomach can be altered by any of the following mechanisms: decreased stomach secretions, delayed transit time, slowed gastric emptying, or competitive binding of molecules. In many situations, the effect of the nutrient is to diminish the absorption of the medication, causing the serum levels to be lower than expected. In other situations; however, the effect on the medication is delayed absorption, which increases the time required to

reach peak serum levels, but does not necessarily affect the total amount absorbed. In some situations, delayed gastric emptying increases the amount of medication that is absorbed before it passes into the small intestine. Examples of some common medication–nutrient interactions, including those involving absorption, are listed in Table 8-8.

Another medication–nutrient interaction that is the focus of much attention is the effect of certain beverages on medications that are metabolized through the P-450 enzyme system.

TABLE 8-8 Medication–Nutrient Interactions

Effect on Medication	Example of Interaction Effect
Delayed absorption rate, no effect on amount absorbed	Ingestion of food may delay absorption of cimetidine, digoxin, and ibuprofen.
Reduced rate and amount of absorption	Calcium decreases absorption of tetracycline. A high-protein or high-fiber meal decreases absorption of levodopa. Grapefruit juice can decrease absorption of antifungals and antihistamines.
Reduced absorption because of nonnutrient components	Caffeinated tea and fiber intake interfere with iron absorption.
Increased absorption	High-fat foods increase serum levels of griseofulvin.
Decreased therapeutic effect	Vitamin K decreases the effectiveness of warfarin. Charcoal broiling of foods diminishes the effectiveness of aminophylline or theophylline.
Increased rate of metabolism	A high-protein diet increases the metabolism of theophylline.
Increased concentrations and bioavailability	Potential effect of grapefruit juice and amiodarone, atorvastatin, buspirone, calcium channel blockers, carbamazepine, diazepam, lovastatin, simvastatin, and triazolam.

Grapefruit juice in particular has been the focus of many clinical studies in recent years because it contains compounds that affect one of the P-450 isoforms. A review of studies related to the interaction between medications and grapefruit juice concluded that the interaction has not been clearly established and is not clinically significant in people who have normal liver function and for medications that have a wide therapeutic range (McCloskey, Zaiaken, & Couris, 2008). Some examples of interactions that have been observed in studies are listed in Table 8-8.

Medications and Alcohol

Alcohol interacts with medications in the same way as other central nervous system depressants, but health care practitioners do not always inquire about a patient's use of alcohol, and even when people are asked, they might not accurately acknowledge the amount of alcohol used. Alcohol is consumed not only in beverages but also in over-the-counter preparations, some of which contain up to 40% alcohol. Categories of over-the-counter preparations that are most likely to contain alcohol include mouthwashes, vitamin and mineral tonics, and liquid cough and cold preparations. When taken with medications, alcohol can alter the therapeutic action of medications and increase the potential for adverse effects. The combination of alcohol and medications also can cause vitamin deficiencies (e.g., retinol) (Ferreira & Weems, 2008). Older adults may be more susceptible to medication–alcohol interactions because age-related changes in receptor sensitivity and body composition lead to higher serum levels of alcohol than those in a younger person who consumes an equivalent amount of alcohol. In addition, any condition that decreases the secretion of the stomach enzymes that metabolize alcohol can increase the concentration of alcohol in the blood. Table 8-9 lists some of the medication–alcohol interactions that can occur in older adults.

DIVERSITY NOTE

Increased age and female gender are factors that increase the bioavailability of alcohol after it is consumed (Ferriera & Weems, 2008).

Medications and Caffeine

Medication–caffeine and medication–nicotine interactions have received little attention, despite the widespread use of caffeine and nicotine and the fact that interactions between these substances and medications can be as harmful as medication–medication interactions. Caffeine is found not only in food and beverages but also in many over-the-counter analgesics and cold preparations. Most medication–caffeine interactions affect the action of the medication rather than that of the caffeine; however, a few medications alter caffeine metabolism and increase its serum half-time. Table 8-10 lists examples of medication–caffeine interactions.

Medications and Nicotine

Medication–nicotine interactions can be associated with tobacco smoking, smokeless tobacco, and the many nicotine-based products that are increasingly being used as substitutes for smoking. Nicotine can affect medications through any of the following actions: vasoconstriction, stimulation of the central nervous system, activation of neuroendocrine pathways, increased gastric acid secretions, and altered metabolism of liver enzymes. Most often, the medication–nicotine interaction interferes with the therapeutic action of the medication, and smokers may require higher doses of a medication than nonsmokers to achieve the same therapeutic effects. Prescribing practitioners may need to adjust medication doses not only for smokers but also when the use of nicotine products is discontinued. Even a change from smoking tobacco to a nicotine product can affect some medications because

TABLE 8-9 Medication–Alcohol Interactions

Type of Interaction	Example of Interaction Effect
Altered metabolism of benzodiazepines when combined with alcohol	Increased psychomotor impairment and adverse effects
Altered metabolism of barbiturates and meprobamate when combined with alcohol	Central nervous system depression
Competition between alcohol and chloral hydrate at metabolic sites	Increased serum levels of alcohol and chloral hydrate
Altered metabolism of alcohol when combined with chlorpromazine	Increased serum levels of alcohol and acetaldehyde; increased psychomotor impairment
Enhanced vasodilation as a result of a combination of alcohol and nitrates	Severe hypotension and headache, enhanced absorption of nitroglycerin
Altered hepatic gluconeogenesis, which influences the action of oral hypoglycemics, as a result of alcohol	Potentiation of oral hypoglycemics by alcohol

TABLE 8-10 Medication–Caffeine Interactions

Type of Interaction	Example of Interaction Effect
Caffeine-induced increase in gastric acid secretion	Decreased absorption of iron
Caffeine-induced gastrointestinal irritation	Decreased effectiveness of cimetidine; increased gastrointestinal irritation from corticosteroids, alcohol, and analgesics
Altered caffeine metabolism	Prolonged effect of caffeine when combined with ciprofloxacin, estrogen, or cimetidine
Caffeine-induced cardiac arrhythmic effect	Decreased effectiveness of antiarrhythmic medications
Caffeine-induced hypokalemia	Exacerbated hypokalemic effect of diuretics
Caffeine-induced stimulation of the central nervous system	Increased stimulation effects from amantadine, decongestants, fluoxetine, and theophylline
Caffeine-induced increase in excretion of lithium	Decreased effectiveness of lithium

Effect of Nicotine	**Example of Interaction Effect**
Altered metabolism	Decreased efficacy of analgesics, lorazepam, theophylline, aminophylline, beta-blockers, and calcium channel blockers
Vasoconstriction	Increased peripheral ischemic effect of beta-blockers
Central nervous system stimulation	Decreased drowsiness from benzodiazepines and phenothiazines
Stimulation of antidiuretic hormone secretion	Fluid retention, decreased effectiveness of diuretics
Activation of neuroendocrine pathways	Interacts with insulin, aggravates insulin resistance, interferes with alpha-blockers
Increase in platelet activity	Decreased anticoagulant effectiveness (heparin, warfarin); increased risk of thrombosis with estrogen use
Increased gastric acid secretion	Decreased or negated effects of H_2 antagonists (cimetidine, famotidine, nizatidine, ranitidine)
Effect of hydrocarbons in tobacco smoke on CYP-450 enzyme system	Cessation of tobacco smoking can increase concentrations of clozapine, olanzapine, theophylline, warfarin, even when a nicotine product is initiated

TABLE 8-11 Medication–Nicotine Interactions

hydrocarbons in tobacco smoke can affect drugs that are metabolized by the CYP-450 enzyme system. A review of studies found that dosage adjustments are clearly indicated for warfarin, olanzapine, clozapine, and theophylline when a patient changes smoking habits (Schaffer, Yoon, & Zadezensky, 2009). This is important not only for patients who voluntarily quit smoking but also for those who temporarily change smoking habits because of hospitalization or other short-term circumstances. Table 8-11 lists some common medication–nicotine interactions.

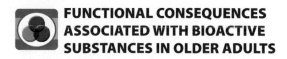

FUNCTIONAL CONSEQUENCES ASSOCIATED WITH BIOACTIVE SUBSTANCES IN OLDER ADULTS

The major functional consequence affecting bioactive agents in healthy older adults who take only one substance is an increased potential for both altered therapeutic action and adverse effects. Older adults who take more than one substance or have other risk factors are likely to have additional functional consequences, such as interactions with other substances and a higher risk for altered therapeutic action and adverse effects. Age-related changes and risk factors also affect consumption patterns, increasing the possibility of nonadherence and its associated consequences.

Altered Therapeutic Effects

Age-related changes alone can alter the therapeutic action of some substances; however, most of the altered therapeutic effects that occur in older adults are caused by risk factors, such as polypharmacy. Consequently, the therapeutic effectiveness

of substances is less predictable, even in healthy older adults. The main implication is that bioactive agents need to be monitored more closely in older adults, especially initially and when there is any change in the person's medical status or treatment regimen. Thus, the commonly accepted principle for geriatric drug prescribing is "start low and go slow."

Increased Potential for Adverse Effects

Adverse medication effects (also called adverse drug events) are the unintended and undesired outcomes of a medication that occur in doses normally used in humans. Consequences of adverse medication effects include a decline in function, an increased risk for falls and fractures, an increased number of visits for health care services, admission to a hospital or prolongation of a hospital stay, and death. There is much agreement that adverse medication effects occur commonly, have serious consequences, and frequently are avoidable. In recent years, there has been increasing attention on adverse medication effects as a preventable cause of hospitalizations particularly for older adults. One study, in which 8.37% of the hospital admissions were attributed to adverse medication effects, identified the following important risk factors: polypharmacy, self-medication, and use of antithrombotics and antibiotics (Olivier et al., 2009).

A multicenter study of almost 13,000 unplanned hospital admissions in the Netherlands found that 5.6% were medication related and concluded that 46.5% were potentially preventable (Leendertse, Egberts, Stoker, & Van Den Bemt, 2008). This study identified the following determinants of preventable medication-related hospitalizations: cognitive impairment, four or more comorbidities, dependent living situation, impaired renal function, nonadherence, and polypharmacy. Types of medications most frequently cited as causes of admission are anticoagulant/antiplatelet drugs, antidiabetic drugs, NSAIDs, and central nervous system agents. Box 8-2 lists some factors that could increase risk for altered medication effects.

Several aspects of adverse medication effects are particularly important for the care of older adults. As discussed in

 Box 8-2 Factors That Increase the Risk for Adverse Medication Effects

- Increased numbers of medications
- Frailty
- Malnourishment or dehydration
- Multiple illnesses
- An illness that interferes with cardiac, renal, or hepatic function
- Cognitive impairment
- History of medication allergies or adverse effects
- Fever, which can alter the action of certain medications
- Recent change in health or functional status
- Medications in any of the following categories: anticoagulant/antiplatelet, antidiabetics, NSAIDs, central nervous system drugs

the section on Risk Factors (and listed in Table 8-6), adverse effects may not be recognized as such because they are similar to the manifestations of pathologic conditions or they are mistakenly attributed to aging. Three concerns of particular importance are anticholinergic toxicity, changes in mental status, and tardive dyskinesia.

Anticholinergic Adverse Effects

In recent years, geriatricians have increasingly recognized that older adults are particularly susceptible to the **anticholinergic adverse effects** from medications, including some medications that are not widely recognized as having anticholinergic effects in the body. Research reviews have consistently identified anticholinergic agents as a causative factor for delirium and other types of cognitive impairment in older adults (Campbell et al., 2009; Wright et al., 2009). Many over-the-counter agents commonly used for coughs, colds, and sleep problems contain anticholinergic ingredients. In fact, even nonprescription antihistamines are likely to have potent anticholinergic actions that can be stronger than those of some prescription drugs. Anticholinergic toxicity also can occur from systemic absorption of commonly used topical medications or ophthalmic agents (e.g., mydriatics and cycloplegics). Common types of medications with anticholinergic properties include antidepressants, antihistamines, antiparkinson agents, antipsychotics, cardiovascular agents, gastrointestinal agents, and urinary antispasmodics (see Box 8-3 for examples). Researchers emphasize the importance of reducing anticholinergic medications as a modifiable risk factor that can reduce negative functional consequences (Rudolph, Salow, Angelini, & McGlinchey, 2008).

Even drugs with weak anticholinergic activity can cause the usual adverse effects (i.e., falls, dizziness, constipation, dry eyes, dry mouth, mental changes, and urinary retention). In recent years, there has been increasing attention to the role of anticholinergic medications as a major contributing factor for both the occurrence and severity of delirium (Maldonado, 2008). There also is increasing attention to the potential role of anticholinergics as a risk factor for dementia. A longitudinal study of almost 7000 community-dwelling older adults in France found that anticholinergic drugs were associated with an increased risk for cognitive decline and dementia (Carriere et al., 2009). In this same study, discontinuation of anticholinergic drugs was associated with a decreased risk.

Another concern related to anticholinergics is that their pharmacologic action counteracts the effects of cholinesterase inhibitors, which are prescribed as a primary treatment for dementia. Despite the evidence that this combination should be avoided, studies indicate that these types of medications are often prescribed concomitantly. A study of more than 3000 nursing home residents who were taking cholinesterase inhibitors found that 46.7% of these residents were also taking anticholinergic drugs, most of which had a very high level of anticholinergic action (Modi et al., 2009). Another study found that 9% of 731,105 community-dwelling Swedes aged

Box 8-3 Examples of Medications With Anticholinergic Effects	
Antidepressants Amitriptyline Desipramine Imipramine Mirtazapine Nortriptyline Paroxetine Trazodone ***Antihistamines*** Chlorpheniramine Diphenhydramine Hydroxyzine Loratadine Meclizine Promethazine ***Antiparkinson Agents*** Benztropine Trihexyphenidyl ***Antipsychotics*** Chlorpromazine Clozapine Fluphenazine Haloperidol Prochlorperazine Promethazine Quetiapine Risperidone	***Cardiovascular Agents*** Captopril Digoxin Dipyridamole Isosorbide dinitrate Nifedipine ***Gastrointestinal Agents*** Belladonna Cimetidine Dicyclomine Hyoscyamine Loperamide Ranitidine ***Urinary Antispasmodics*** Oxybutynin Tolterodine ***Miscellaneous Agents*** Amantadine Atropine Meclizine Theophylline Warfarin

75 years or older taking cholinesterase inhibitors were also taking anticholinergics, but only 5% of the subjects who were not taking cholinesterase inhibitors were taking anticholinergics (Johnell & Fastbom, 2008).

Altered Mental Status

Although medications can cause mental changes in anyone, older adults are at increased risk for medication-induced altered mental status because of age-related changes and risk factors. In addition, when older adults experience changes in their mental status, these changes are likely to be attributed to dementia or another pathologic condition, rather than being recognized as adverse medication effects. Nurses need to be alert to the possibility that even a simple over-the-counter product, such as diphenhydramine, is a common cause of mental changes in older adults.

Delirium is an acute confusional state that can be precipitated by any medication or by medication interactions (refer to Chapter 14 for further discussion of delirium). Older adults are particularly susceptible to medication-induced delirium because of altered neurochemical activity in the brain. Moreover, some pathologic conditions (e.g., dementia, dehydration, malnutrition, head injury, or central nervous system infection) can increase the risk for medication-induced

TABLE 8-12 Mechanisms of Action for Mental Changes Caused by Adverse Medication Effects

Mechanism of Action	Examples
Anticholinergic effects	Atropine, scopolamine, antihistamines, antipsychotics, antidepressants, antispasmodics, antiparkinsonian agents
Decreased cerebral blood flow	Antihypertensives, antipsychotics
Depression of respiratory center	Central nervous system depressants
Fluid and electrolyte alterations	Diuretics, alcohol, laxatives
Altered thermoregulation	Alcohol, psychotropics, narcotics
Acidosis	Diuretics, alcohol, nicotinic acid
Hypoglycemia	Hypoglycemics, alcohol, propranolol
Hormonal disturbances	Thyroid extract, corticosteroids
Depression-inducing action	Reserpine, methyldopa, indomethacin, barbiturates, fluphenazine, haloperidol, corticosteroids

delirium. Even at nontoxic serum levels, or at doses considered normal, medications can cause mental changes in older adults. It is important to keep in mind that medication-induced mental changes do not always subside immediately after the offending medication is discontinued. In some cases, it may take several weeks or even months after the medication is decreased or discontinued for mental function to return to the premedication level. Some medications that are likely to cause mental changes in older adults, as well as the mechanisms underlying these adverse actions, are listed in Table 8-12.

Tardive Dyskinesia and Drug-Induced Parkinsonism

Tardive dyskinesia refers to a constellation of rhythmic and involuntary movements of any of the following: the trunk and extremities and the jaw, lips, mouth, and tongue (referred to as oro-buccal-lingual). The earliest signs are usually fine, wormlike movements of the tongue. Other early signs include chewing, grimacing, lip smacking, jaw clenching, eye blinking, and side-to-side jaw movements. Studies have concluded that tardive dyskinesia is caused by medications that block dopamine receptors in the brain, such as antipsychotics (Chou & Friedman, 2006).

Manifestations can begin as early as 3 to 6 months after initiation of antipsychotic medications, and they persist even after the causative agent is discontinued. Tardive dyskinesia deserves special attention with regard to older adults for the following reasons:

- For people taking antipsychotic medications, prevalence ranges from approximately 35% of community-residing older adults to more than 80% of institutionalized older adults (Chou & Friedman, 2006).
- Advanced age correlates with both an earlier onset and increased severity of tardive dyskinesia.
- The chance of reversing tardive dyskinesia decreases with increasing age.

- When combined with age-related changes and risk factors, tardive dyskinesia can seriously impair the older adult's ability to perform activities of daily living (ADLs).
- The risk of tardive dyskinesia can be eliminated by avoiding the use of antipsychotics when nonpharmaceutical therapies could be effective, as with behavioral and psychological symptoms of dementia.

Drug-induced parkinsonism is the occurrence of Parkinson-like manifestations as an adverse medication effect. Manifestations can be reversed if the offending drug is stopped, but many times the condition is misdiagnosed as Parkinson disease and treated inappropriately with an antiparkinson medication. Risk factors for development of drug-induced parkinsonism include older age, female gender, cognitive impairment, family history of Parkinson disease, coexistence of tardive dyskinesia, and taking certain medications (e.g., haloperidol, metoclopramide, risperidone, phenothiazines) (Alvarez & Evidente, 2008; Thanyi & Treadwell, 2009).

Antipsychotics in People With Dementia

The strong association between serious adverse effects and the so-called first-generation antipsychotics (e.g., haloperidol and thioridazine) has spurred the development of the so-called atypical antipsychotics, which include clozapine, risperidone, olanzapine, quetiapine, amisulpride, and ziprasidone. Although some studies suggest that the newer antipsychotics reduce the risk of tardive dyskinesia or drug-induced parkinsonism, other studies found that older adults with dementia are likely to have serious adverse effects even from the newer atypical antipsychotics. Reviews of studies have concluded that relative to atypical antipsychotics, patients treated with first-generation antipsychotics have an increased incidence of cardiac arrhythmias and extrapyramidal symptoms. However, the use of atypical antipsychotics is associated with an increased risk of hyperglycemia, venous thromboembolism, and aspiration pneumonia, and any type of antipsychotic is associated with increased risk of all-cause mortality and cerebrovascular events (Trifir, Spina, & Gambassi, 2009). People with dementia and Parkinson disease or dementia with Lewy bodies are especially prone to developing serious adverse effects from any antipsychotic medication (Schwab, Messinger-Rapport, & Franco, 2009). Refer to Chapter 14 for further discussion of this topic.

DIVERSITY NOTE

Female sex and African American race are possible risk factors for tardive dyskinesia (Chou & Friedman, 2006).

NURSING ASSESSMENT OF MEDICATION USE AND EFFECTS

Nurses assess medication regimens and medication-taking behaviors of older adults to accomplish the following:

- Determine the effectiveness of the medication regimen
- Identify any factors that interfere with the correct regimen

- Ascertain risks for adverse effects or altered therapeutic actions (with particular attention to older adults at increased risk)
- Detect adverse medication effects
- Identify teaching needs with regard to medications.

During a medication assessment, nurses should clarify the prescribed medication regimen and identify actual medication-taking behaviors so that they can assess for adherence to the treatment regimen.

Communication Techniques for Obtaining Accurate Information

Some of the many barriers to obtaining accurate information about medications and medication-taking behaviors include time limitations, complex medication regimens, and lack of a trusting relationship. Because medication assessments can be very time-consuming, and because the older adult may not think of all the information during the first interview or may initially be reluctant to reveal accurate information, it may be necessary to conduct the medication assessment over the course of two or more visits. In addition, older adults may be reluctant to answer questions about their medications because they perceive this information, including information about the use of alcohol, as being very private. Many older adults have learned not to ask questions about their health care because they are unsure of what to ask or they falsely believe that they are not entitled to medical information. Although most older adults appreciate the opportunity to discuss medications with a nurse, they initially may hesitate to ask questions or share information. Some of this reluctance may be caused by fear of being judged, especially if the prescribed regimen is not being followed exactly, or if the person uses folk remedies, alternative therapies, or over-the-counter medications. When people do not follow the medication regimen exactly as prescribed, they are likely to recite the orders rather than describe their actual medication-taking behaviors. Another factor that contributes to this reluctance is anxiety about discussing the underlying reason for not following the regimen. For example, older adults who cannot afford medications may be embarrassed to discuss their limited finances.

Nurses can address the barriers by asking open-ended questions in a matter-of-fact way and conveying a nonjudgmental attitude during the medication interview. They should also keep in mind that they need to elicit information about the use of herbs, folk remedies, over-the-counter preparations, and complementary and alternative care practices. For example, "What do you do to help you sleep?" is more open-ended than "Do you take any medications for sleep?" because the latter may be interpreted only in relation to prescription medications.

Another interview technique is to use leading questions related to potential risk factors that interfere with the older person's ability to take medications accurately. For example, because the high cost of medications is a commonly acknowledged problem, nurses can ask a question such as "I know that some of these medications that are prescribed for you can be quite expensive; do you have any problems with getting them?" Similarly, asking a question such as "I know you don't drive—are you able to have your medications delivered, or do you have someone who helps you get them from the pharmacy?" may elicit information about transportation barriers.

Nurses should ask additional questions about the person's ability to take his or her medications as prescribed based on specific observations. For example, if a nurse observes that a pill is very large, a question such as "Do you have any trouble swallowing these capsules?" might be appropriate. Similarly, if the nurse knows that the older adult has limited hand strength, an appropriate assessment question would be "Do you have any difficulty getting the caps off your medication bottles?" Another technique for eliciting information is to ask about the person's method of organizing medications. For example, people taking medications often have a method of organizing their regimen by using divided medication boxes or written charts or schedules. They usually are willing to show this organizational system to the nurse and, in fact, may be proud to discuss their method with the nurse during the medication assessment.

> **Wellness Opportunity**
>
> Nurses can build on their trusting relationship with older adults to encourage open discussion of factors that interfere with adherence to medication regimens.

Scope of a Medication Assessment

Medication assessments include information about all of the following:

- Prescription and over-the-counter medications, used orally and by all other routes (e.g., nasal, aural, topical, optical, injectable, dermal methods)
- Medications that are used only sporadically, or as needed
- Vitamins, minerals, and dietary supplements (including doses and frequency)
- Alcohol, caffeine
- Tobacco smoking, use of nicotine products (including information about recent changes)
- Folk remedies and CAMs, including all herbal products and homeopathic remedies.

Information about doses of vitamins and minerals is important because megavitamins can be harmful, and even low doses can cause interactions or have adverse effects (e.g., iron or calcium carbonate can be constipating). Information about the brand names of over-the-counter medications can help identify additives that may be causing problems or increasing the risk of altered medication action (e.g., analgesics with caffeine, antacids with lactose, or bronchodilators with sulfites). Information about folk remedies and complementary and alternative health care practices can help identify health beliefs that affect adherence and other aspects of medication-taking behaviors.

Nurses also need to assess the person's understanding of the purpose of medications; doing so provides information about his or her understanding of health status and medical conditions. As with other parts of the medication assessment, it is essential to phrase questions in as open-ended and non-judgmental a manner as possible. Asking "What do you take this pill for?" with a tone of curiosity will likely elicit more information than asking questions such as, "What do you take for your heart?" or "Why do you take furosemide?"

Obtaining information about allergies and adverse reactions is essential because anyone with a history of medication-related problems will need to be closely monitored, especially if the medications being administered are similar to those that caused the reaction. Sometimes people state that they are allergic to a medication, but when they are asked about the symptoms, they describe an adverse effect, rather than an allergic reaction. Therefore, rather than simply documenting that the person is allergic to a certain medication, nurses should document the specific reaction that occurred. Nurses can use Box 8-4 as a guide to assessing medications regimens and medication-taking behaviors.

Nurses should also obtain and document information about the person's perception of and preferences for various forms of medications because this information can influence prescribing decisions, especially when there are several options that may be equally effective. Similarly, nurses should identify any cultural factors that might influence medication-taking behaviors. For example, according to some Asian traditions, illness is perceived as an imbalance of hot and cold forces. If the illness makes the body hot, then the remedy should make it cooler. Cultural Considerations 8-1 lists some cultural factors that are pertinent to a medication assessment.

Another component of a comprehensive medication assessment is obtaining information about various sources of health care. This information is particularly important when someone receives care from more than one health care practitioner, as is often the case. Nurses can ask nonjudgmentally about whether the person receives care from non-Western health care practitioners, such as herbalists, spiritual healers, naturopathic practitioners, or Ayurvedic doctors. Cultural Considerations 8-2 summarizes some culturally specific sources of health care and treatment modalities that older adults might use.

Wellness Opportunity

Nurses promote personal responsibility for health by encouraging discussion of various sources of care.

Box 8-4 Guidelines for Medication Assessment

Information About the Therapeutic Agents
- Prescription pills, liquids, injections, eye drops, ear drops, nasal sprays, transdermal methods, and topical preparations
- Over-the-counter preparations that are used regularly or occasionally
- Vitamins, minerals, and nutritional supplements
- Pattern of alcohol, caffeine, or tobacco use
- Herbs and herbal preparations
- Homeopathic remedies
- Home folk remedies
- Sources of health care, including complementary and alternative practitioners.

Interview Questions to Assess Medication-Taking Behaviors
- How would you describe your usual daily routine for taking medications and remedies, beginning when you get up in the morning?
- Is there anything else you do or use to treat illness or to maintain your health, such as using herbs, ointments, home remedies, or nutritional supplements?
- Are you taking anyone else's medications?
- What do you do when you miss a dose of medication?
- What do you take for constipation? What do you do to help you sleep (or to alleviate any other identified problem)?
- How do you get your prescriptions filled? (Where do you get your remedies?)
- Do you have any difficulty taking your pills?
- What method do you use to keep track of your medications and remedies?
- Is there anything you do to help you remember to take your medicines or remedies at the appropriate time?

Interview Questions to Assess the Person's Understanding of the Purpose of Medications and Other Remedies
- What is this medication (or herb, etc.) for?
- For medications (or remedies) that are used as needed (PRN): How do you decide when to take this pill (or remedy)?
- What did your health care practitioner tell you about this medication (or herb, etc.)?
- What problems were you having when the health care practitioner prescribed this medication (or suggested that you use this remedy)?

Interview Questions to Elicit Additional Information
- Are there any medications or remedies you were taking at one time but are no longer taking?
- Have you ever had an allergic reaction, or any other bad reaction, to a medication or remedy? (If yes, describe what happened.)
- Where do you store your medications and remedies?

Questions and Observations Based on Reading of Prescription Labels
- Who is the prescribing health care practitioner?
- If there is more than one health care practitioner, does each practitioner know all the medications that are being used?
- Are any medications the same or similar and prescribed by different health care practitioners?
- If the dates on various prescriptions are different, were the later medications supposed to be added to the medication regimen, or were they intended to replace previously prescribed medications?
- Are the date of the last refill and the number of pills in the bottle consistent with the prescribed regimen?

CULTURAL CONSIDERATIONS 8 - 1

Cultural Considerations With Regard to Medication Assessment and Interventions

- Teaching about medications should be done in the context of culturally based beliefs about health, illness, and remedies.
- Medications that are not readily available or that are available by prescription only in the United States may be available over the counter in other countries, such as Mexico, Canada, and Latin America.
- Older Hispanic people may view wine and other forms of alcohol as a food staple, not a social drug, because they may be used as a healthy alternative to potentially contaminated water in their home country.
- People of Vietnamese and other cultural groups may view injections as being more effective than pills, and pills as being more effective than drops.
- People of Asian, Latino, and Middle Eastern heritage believe it is important to take medicine with certain foods or beverages (e.g., tea or warm water rather than cold water) to provide the necessary balance.
- Some Chinese and other Asian people may have the following preferences:
  Balms and ointments rather than pills for local pain.
  Teas and soups rather than antacids for indigestion.
  Herbs rather than prescription drugs.

- The following differences in response to medications may occur:
  Arab Americans may require a lower dose of antiarrhythmics, antihypertensives, neuroleptics, and psychotropics and a higher dose of opioids.
  Asian/Pacific Islanders may require a lower dose of neuroleptics, antidepressants, lithium, fat-soluble medications.
  Blacks with hypertension respond better to diuretics, calcium antagonists, and alpha-blockers and are less responsive to beta-blockers and ACE inhibitors.
  Blacks are more susceptible to extrapyramidal side effects of psychotropic drugs such as haloperidol.
  Hispanics may require lower dosage and experience higher incidence of adverse effects of tricyclic antidepressants.

Source: Andrews, M. M. (2008). Cultural competence in health history and physical examination. In M. M. Andrews & J. S. Boyle. *Transcultural concepts in nursing care.* Philadelphia, PA: Lippincott Williams & Wilkins.

Observing Patterns of Medication Use

In addition to using good communication techniques, nurses obtain essential assessment information by reviewing the person's array of medications. When nurses conduct the medication assessment in the home setting, they can ask to see all the medications that the older person uses. In settings other than the home, the nurse can ask the older adult ahead of time to bring in all of his or her medications. In community settings, nurses might sponsor a "brown bag" medication review session. Program participants are asked to bring all their med-

ications to an educational session, during which the nurse provides group education and individual assessment and counseling regarding the medications. Because older people often are very comfortable discussing medications with their peers, this method is both nonthreatening and quite effective.

Direct observation of medication containers provides useful information about adherence, dates of original prescription and refills, duplication of similar medications, and pharmaceutical treatments for pathologic conditions. For example, if three types of antihypertensive medications have

---

CULTURAL CONSIDERATIONS 8 - 2

Culturally Specific Health Care Sources and Practices

Cultural Group	Sources of Care*	Health Practices*
African Americans	Home remedies, faith and root healers (herbalists)	Folk remedies (e.g., teas, herbs); magic or voodoo (especially in rural areas)
Amish	Folk healers (braucher orbrauch-doktor)	Physical manipulation, massage, herbs, teas, reflexology
Native Americans/ Alaskan Natives	Native practitioners, shaman	Roots, herbs, physical modalities (e.g., purification rituals), sacred objects
Chinese	Herbalists, acupuncturists	Herbs, food, beverages, and other remedies to balance yin and yang
Christian scientists	Christian science practitioners and nurses	Medications are not used, focus is on hygiene measures
Filipino	Folk healers (hilot)	Prayer, exorcism, hot/cold balance
Hindu	Traditional healers (nattuvaidhyars)	Ayurvedic medicine (herbs and roots)
Japanese	Herbalists	Herbs, prayer at temple, church, or small shrines at home
Mexicans	Folk healer (curandero) or spiritualist (espirituista)	Herbs, teas, soups, rituals, physical modalities (massage, manipulation), prayer, candles
Puerto Ricans	Healers (espiritistas and santeros)	Tea, herbs, folk remedies, liquid astringent
Russians	Folk remedies	Herbal teas, sweet liquor, physical modalities (oils, ointments, enemas, mud baths)
Vietnamese	Asian physicians, folk healers, spiritual healers, magicians (sorcerers)	Herbs, acupuncture, cup suctioning, skin pinching

*In the United States, Western practitioners and medicine often are used with these sources of care and health practices.
Sources: Andrews, M. M., & Boyle, J. S. (2008). *Transcultural concepts in nursing care.* Philadelphia, PA: Lippincott Williams & Wilkins.
Purnell, L. D. (2009). *Guide to culturally competent health care.* Philadelphia, PA: F. A. Davis Company.

been prescribed at different times, the nurse can inquire whether the second or third medication was supposed to replace or supplement the original medication. Nurses can also assess whether the bottles contain the original medications, and ask additional questions when the contents are not consistent with expectations. For example, if the label indicates that the original prescription was for 30 pills, but it has not been refilled for 1 year, the nurse might inquire about the reason. Patients may explain that they cannot afford the prescription or they cannot manipulate the childproof lid. Another purpose for examining medication containers is to discover information about sources of care and duplication of medications. It is not unusual to find that patients are getting prescriptions from more than one health care practitioner. Sometimes, patients have the same or similar medications from different sources or under more than one name (e.g., generic and brand names).

Linking the Medication Assessment to the Overall Assessment

The nurse uses information from the medication interview with the overall health assessment in several ways. First, information about past and present medication patterns can provide clues to identified problems or complaints. For example, if the person complains of morning lethargy or experiences mental changes, the nurse can inquire about the use of medications with anticholinergic properties, including over-the-counter products (e.g., diphenhydramine). Information about changes in health-related behaviors can also shed light on current problems, such as the recurrence of symptoms that once were controlled by medications. For example, if an insulin-dependent diabetic stopped smoking, it is important to consider whether the dose of insulin needs to be decreased. Recent medication-taking behaviors also may account for health problems that are residual or latent adverse medication effects. A common example of a residual adverse effect is the onset of diarrhea after a course of antibiotics.

Second, nurses use the overall health assessment as a base of information to determine the expected and actual outcomes of medications. These outcomes are evaluated through subjective and objective assessment information. For example, analgesic effectiveness is measured according to reported level of pain relief, and the effectiveness of antihypertensive medications is judged according to lowered blood pressure readings.

Third, the overall assessment, including functional aspects, helps answer the question "Can the person or caregivers safely and effectively administer medications?" This complex question involves an assessment of all aspects of medication-taking behaviors, as described in the sections on age-related changes and risk factors. The environment also should be assessed in relation to certain conditions, such as the accessibility of water and the availability of a refrigerator (if necessary for medication storage) that can affect medication-taking behaviors. The overall assessment also might provide information about financial limitations, mobility, or transportation problems that interfere with obtaining medications.

Fourth, if the home environment can be observed as part of the overall assessment, important clues to health problems and medication-taking behaviors may be disclosed. For example, observing that nitroglycerin is stored on a sunny window sill may explain why the medication is not effective in relieving angina. An assessment of the home environment may lead to additional pertinent information. For example, when the nurse observes over-the-counter preparations and folk remedies in the home, she or he has the opportunity to ask about the use of these items.

Finally, the overall health assessment serves as the basis for identifying many factors that can increase the risk for non-adherence, altered therapeutic effects, and adverse medication effects. For example, the nursing assessment of the older adult's cognitive abilities and abilities to perform daily activities provides valuable information about factors that can significantly influence medication-taking behaviors. Similarly, the nursing assessment of depression and other psychosocial aspects of functioning can provide important information about motivational and behavioral factors that can influence medication-taking behaviors.

Identifying Adverse Medication Effects

The first, and sometimes most difficult, step in alleviating adverse medication effects is to recognize their existence. Because many adverse effects are subtle and superimposed on one or more symptoms of illness, they may be attributed to pathologic conditions rather than to the treatment of the condition. Nurses often are the first to recognize adverse medication effects because they generally spend more time with patients than do primary care practitioners. Nurses also are more attentive to long-term monitoring of changes in day-to-day function, in contrast to the medical practitioner's focus on acute illness. Especially in long-term care and home settings, the nurse is the health professional most likely to notice subtle changes in function that may be attributable to adverse medication effects.

Health care practitioners may hesitate to discuss adverse medication effects with patients for any of the following reasons: (1) they may be uncertain about the potential adverse effects of a prescribed drug, especially when newer medications are prescribed; (2) they may assume that the power of suggesting possible adverse effects will become a self-fulfilling prophecy; or (3) they may fear that the patient will choose not to take the medication. The nurse can serve as an "interpreter" between the prescribing practitioner and the patient by emphasizing the medication's benefits as well as pointing out the problems that are most likely to arise. The nurse also can provide health education about ways to avoid adverse effects. For example, if a medication is likely to cause stomach irritation, taking the medication after meals or with milk may prevent this effect. Nurses do not automatically initiate a discussion of all the potential adverse effects of a medication, but when a change in health status is potentially related to adverse medication effects, nurses can raise that possibility.

Changes in mental status are a potentially devastating adverse medication effect that is often overlooked as such, especially when superimposed on existing dementia. Medication-induced mental status changes (e.g., confusion, lethargy, depression, or agitation) can be sudden and obvious, or subtle and gradual. For example, delirium or hallucinations usually are very obvious, but they may be attributed mistakenly to pathologic processes rather than to medication effects. Thus, whenever an older person experiences an alteration in mental status, medication intake must be assessed carefully. Besides considering all prescription drugs, alcohol and over-the-counter medications (especially those with anticholinergic agents) must be considered as potential contributing factors. When medications are a potential cause of altered mental status, consideration must be given to discontinuing or lowering the dose of the medication. Assessment also addresses the possibility that the altered mental state interferes with proper dosing (e.g., when memory impairment contributes to over-dosing or underdosing). Another aspect of assessing the relationship between mental changes and medications is to recognize that it may take days or even months after discontinuation of the medication before mental status returns to baseline. The resolution time depends on the particular medication involved, the length of time it was consumed, and the person's general health status.

NURSING DIAGNOSIS

When the nursing assessment identifies factors that interfere with safe and accurate medication self-administration (e.g., cognitive or functional impairments affecting medication-taking ability), an applicable nursing diagnosis is Ineffective Self Health Management. This diagnosis is defined as a "pattern of regulating and integrating into daily living a therapeutic regime for treatment of illness and its sequelae that is unsatisfactory for meeting specific health goals" (NANDA International, 2009, p. 58). Related factors that might be identified include complex medication regimens, inadequate social supports, adverse effects of medication(s), lack of money or transportation, and lack of understanding of instructions. The nursing diagnosis of Noncompliance may be appropriate in some situations, but nurses need to be sure it is not associated with a judgmental attitude on the part of the health care provider.

If the nursing assessment identifies adverse effects of medications, particularly those that affect one's safety or quality of life, the nurse might address these through a nursing diagnosis that is specific to the adverse effect. Examples of these diagnoses include Confusion, Constipation, Urinary Incontinence, Imbalanced Nutrition, Impaired Memory, Ineffective Thermoregulation, Sleep Pattern Disturbance, and Risk for Falls because of medication-related falls and postural hypotension. These nursing diagnoses are discussed in other chapters of this text.

PLANNING FOR WELLNESS OUTCOMES

Wellness outcomes pertinent to medications and older adults include Adherence to Therapeutic Regimens and Identification and Prevention of Adverse Effects. Nurses can use any of the following Nursing Outcomes Classification (NOC) terminology in their care plans: Compliance Behavior, Health Promoting Behaviors, Knowledge: Medication, Medication Response, Risk Detection, and Self-Care: Nonparenteral Medication.

 ## NURSING INTERVENTIONS TO PROMOTE HEALTHY MEDICATION-TAKING PATTERNS

Nursing interventions for older adults who are taking medications focus on teaching about both the therapeutic and adverse effects and on addressing any factors that interfere with adherence to the therapeutic regimen. In addition, when appropriate, nurses teach older adults about effectively communicating with their prescribing practitioners, and they provide information about the use of other bioactive substances, such as herbs and homeopathic remedies. Nurses can consider using any of the following Nursing Interventions Classification (NIC) terminology in care plans: Health Education, Medication Management, Risk Identification, Self-Care Assistance: IADL, and Teaching: Prescribed Medication.

Implementing Evidence-Based Interventions

Nurses and other health care professionals have routinely incorporated strategies for the safe and effective administration of medications, including prescription and over-the-counter products, in many settings. In recent years, however, more attention has been paid to evaluating the effectiveness of various strategies with emphasis on preventing adverse drug events and improving adherence. An extensive literature review of interventions used to assess and improve medication adherence in older adults emphasized that interventions need to be multifaceted and address the patient's beliefs and preferences as well as practical factors, such as motivation and cognitive abilities (Banning, 2009). Research reviews of interventions to improve medication management in home settings identified the following evidence-based strategies (Center for Home Care Policy & Research, 2009; Shearer, 2009):

- Reminder strategies: alarm clock, location of medications, written reminders, phone calls
- Packaging, memory, organizing aids: pill boxes, blister packs
- Fewer number of medications: use long-acting/sustained release doses, decrease the number of medications for a single health condition, discontinue cautionary medications
- Medication simplification: remove unused medications, use one pharmacy for all medications, use nondrug alternatives to reduce medications, coordinate doses with usual activities
- Patient teaching: repeated and multifaceted to include ways to simplify regimens and increase convenience.

Evidence-Based Practice 8-1 summarizes an evidence-based protocol for reducing adverse drug events and provides information about resources for additional evidence-based protocols (Zwicker & Fulmer, 2008). The following sections describe practical interventions that nurses can use to promote adherence, prevent adverse effects, and encourage safe and effective medication-taking behaviors in older adults.

Medication reconciliation is an evidence-based intervention that has been widely implemented in health care settings and has been mandatory in hospital settings since January 2006. Medication reconciliation is the process of identifying a patient's medication errors, such as omissions, duplications, dosing errors, or drug interactions during transitions in care. The three steps involved in the process are as follows: (1) verification by collecting an accurate list; (2) clarification of questions about drugs, doses, frequency, and other pertinent information; and (3) reconciliation of any discrepancies or concerns by communicating with prescribing practitioners. This process is warranted because studies show that half of hospitalized patients have at least one medication discrepancy on admission and that almost one-quarter of patients experience an adverse drug event after discharge, most of which could be prevented through better communication (Cua & Kripalani, 2008). Although the initial focus of medication reconciliation was on hospital admissions and discharges, it is imperative that this process be done during any transition, even within the same facility. A study of the clinical outcomes of a home-based reconciliation program for people discharged from a skilled care facility found that a formal medication reconciliation progress can decrease mortality (Delate, Chester, Stubbings, & Barnes, 2008). Nurses can find clinical tools and additional information about medication reconciliation protocols in the Resources section at the end of this chapter and in the Internet Resources available on thePoint.

Teaching About Medications

Medications are safest and most therapeutic when they are taken as prescribed and when the regimen is periodically reevaluated for maximum effectiveness and minimal risk of adverse reactions. An effective way to initiate health education

---

Evidence-Based Practice   8-1
Reducing Adverse Drug Events

Statement of the Problem

- Older adults are increasingly more susceptible to adverse drug events, which result in four times as many hospitalizations than in younger persons
- Reasons for medication-related problems: age-related physiologic changes that alter pharmacokinetics and pharmacodynamics, polypharmacy, incorrect doses of medications, inappropriate use of medications to treat symptoms that are not disease specific, adverse drug reactions and interactions, nonadherence, medication errors

Recommendations for Nursing Assessment

- Tools to evaluate ability to self-administer medications (Drug Regimen Unassisted Grading Scale) and to identify potential problems associated with inappropriate medications (Beers criteria), adverse effects and interactions with other drugs and herbs (computer/PDA programs), renal function (Cockroft Gault Formula)
- Assessment of pharmacokinetics and pharmacodynamics: absorption, distribution, metabolism, clearance
- Assessment strategies: brown bag method, medication reconciliation process, Beers criteria
- Assessment of certain high-risk medications in the following categories: warfarin, antihypertensives, psychoactive drugs, anticholinergics, cardiotonics, and over-the-counter products
- Comprehensive medication assessment includes nicotine, alcohol, all nonprescription products, folk remedies

Recommendations for Nursing Interventions

Address Adherence Issues
- Attempt a trial of nonpharmacologic interventions when addressing new symptoms
- Work with pharmacists and prescribing practitioners to reduce the complexity of medication regimens
- Address issues related to access, cost, support resources, and other factors that interfere with taking medications as prescribed
- Identify and address health-related barriers, including cognitive, affective, and functional abilities
- Identify beliefs, concerns, and problems related to medication regimen.

Address Adverse Drug Events
- Consider possibility that new symptoms could be adverse drug reactions
- Collaborate with interdisciplinary team to reduce adverse effects and interactions, many of which are preventable
- Monitor for toxicity
- Review drug regimen whenever falls occur

SOURCE: Zwicker, D. E., & Fulmer T. (2008). Reducing adverse drug events (2008). In E. Capezuti, D. Zwicker, M. Mezey, & T. Fulmer (Eds.), *Evidence-based geriatric nursing protocols for best practice* (3rd ed., pp. 257–308). New York: Springer Publishing Co.

about medications is to have the person write a list of all medications and over-the-counter agents taken and to include a history of medication allergies and adverse effects. Nurses can emphasize that this information should be available to health care practitioners during all interactions because it is essential that all practitioners keep track of the person's medications. This list is especially important when more than one health care practitioner is involved. Nurses should explain that a medication list facilitates communication and reminds the health care practitioner periodically to reevaluate the medication regimen. Nurses can discuss each medication on the list and provide appropriate information based on assessment of the person's knowledge and understanding.

Because older adults may be reluctant to question their health care practitioners, nurses can suggest pertinent questions for discussion with prescribing practitioners. In addition, nurses can teach older adults and their caregivers about obtaining medication-related information from knowledgeable sources, such as pharmacists. People need to understand that prescribing practitioners are skilled in diagnosing illnesses and deciding the most appropriate interventions, and that pharmacists are the health care practitioners who are most knowledgeable about the specific actions and interactions of medications. Nurses can use Box 8-5 to teach older adults about which medication questions are best answered by prescribing practitioners and which are best addressed by pharmacists.

Because good communication skills are essential to obtaining answers to the questions listed in Box 8-5, nurses can suggest ways of communicating effectively with pharmacists and other health care practitioners. For example, nurses can

help older adults develop a list of questions about specific medications that they can discuss with pharmacists or health care practitioners. In home settings, nurses can serve as role models of appropriate communication by calling the pharmacist or prescribing practitioner to discuss medications in the presence of the older adult or caregiver.

 Wellness Opportunity

Nurses find opportunities to empower older adults by teaching them effective ways of communicating with health care providers so that they can knowledgeably observe for therapeutic and adverse medication effects.

Teaching About Herbs and Other Bioactive Substances

As discussed in the Nursing Assessment section, nurses need to ask about the use of herbs and other bioactive substances so that they can observe for and teach about interactions and adverse effects, when appropriate. Although information about the use of complementary and alternative therapies needs to be an integral part of the assessment, nurses cannot know all the details about these products. At a minimum, however, they need to know how to teach about these remedies, just as they teach about pharmacologic and medical interventions. Nurses can use Box 8-6 as a tool to teach their patients about general precautions for the use of herbs and homeopathic remedies, such as being aware of potential interactions and adverse effects and making sure that all health

 Box 8-5 Tips on Safe and Effective Medication Use

Carry an up-to-date list of all your medications, including herbs and over-the-counter preparations, and show the list to your health care practitioner(s).

When your health care practitioner suggests a medication, ask if there is any way to take care of the problem without medication.

Ask your health care practitioner the following questions about each new, regularly scheduled medication:
- What is the reason for taking the medication?
- How will I know if it's doing what it's meant to do?
- How soon can I expect to feel the beneficial effects?
- What will happen if I don't take it?
- How often am I supposed to take it?
- How long should I continue taking it?
- What should I do if I miss a dose?
- When will you want to see me again, and what will you want me to tell you so that you can determine whether the medication is effective?

Ask your health care practitioner the following questions at follow-up visits:
- Do I still need to take this medication?
- Can the dosage be reduced?

Ask your health care practitioner the following questions about each medication that is prescribed on an "as-needed" (PRN) basis:
- What is the reason for taking the medication, and how should I determine whether I need the medication?
- How often can I take it? Is there a range of frequency?
- What is the maximum dose I can take within 24 hours?
- What should I do if the medication does not relieve the symptoms (e.g., if chest pain continues after taking several nitroglycerin tablets)?

Ask your pharmacist the following questions:
- What are the generic and brand names for this medication?
- Is it likely to interact with the other medications I'm taking?
- Is it likely to interact with herbs, cigarettes, alcohol, or any nutrient?
- What is the best time of day to take it?
- Does it matter if I take it before or after meals?
- Are there any side effects I should watch for?
- Is there anything I can do to minimize the risk of side effects (e.g., taking the medication with milk or meals to reduce stomach irritation)?
- Is there anything I should avoid while I'm taking this medication (e.g., milk, certain foods, driving)?
- Are there any special instructions for storing this medication?

Box 8-6 Tips on the Use of Herbs and Homeopathic Remedies

- Before treating any symptom with a nonprescription product, make sure you are not overlooking a condition that requires medical attention.
- Discuss the use of any nonprescription product with your primary health care provider(s).
- Be cautious about substituting herbs or any over-the-counter product for prescribed medications.
- Seek information from objective sources and check any warnings on the label or package.
- Keep in mind that dietary supplements are not fully regulated by the FDA.
- Purchase only those dietary supplements (e.g., vitamins, minerals, herbs) that have a recognized mark of quality verification on the label.
- Observe for beneficial and harmful effects.
- Report any possible side effects to your primary health care provider for evaluation.
- Introduce only one new substance at a time.
- Start with a low dose and increase the dose gradually.
- Doses may need to be lowered when combining two or more herbs or an herb and a medication.
- Some herbs are for short-term use only.
- Some herbs need to be taken for 1–3 months before effects are noticed (e.g., ginkgo biloba, St. John's wort).

- Herbs can interact with all of the following: other herbs, food, beverages, caffeine, nutrients, prescription medications, and over-the-counter medications.
- Some herbs are contraindicated in people with the following conditions: stroke, glaucoma, diabetes, hypertension, heart disease, thyroid disorder, and any bleeding disorder or condition requiring anticoagulation.
- Some herbs are most effective when taken on an empty stomach.
- Many herbs can cause gastrointestinal effects (e.g., anorexia, nausea, diarrhea).
- Some herbs, especially those that are applied externally, can cause skin rashes.
- Herbs can cause allergic reactions.
- Some herbs are extremely toxic, or fatal, if ingested.
- A few herbs, or ingredients in herbs, can be toxic when taken in large doses or for a long time (e.g., Oregon grape, used for prostatitis, may cause heart failure).
- A few herbs are thought to be carcinogenic.
- Herbs that are used for anxiety or insomnia should not be taken before driving a car.
- Be skeptical about exaggerated claims; if it sounds too good to be true, it probably is!

Source: U.S. Food and Drug Administration.

care practitioners are aware of all over-the-counter products that are used.

Another important nursing role—and a way of promoting personal responsibility—is teaching patients about reliable sources of information on which they can base decisions about self-care practices. The National Institutes of Health (NIH) established an Office of Alternative Medicine to fund research and provide evidence-based information about complementary and alternative practices. Nurses can keep up to date on developments and find reliable information that is pertinent to the care of older adults by periodically checking the NIH Web site (www.nccam.gov). In addition, the FDA Web site (www.fda.gov) provides a wealth of evidence-based information about prescription and over-the-counter products and also publishes a consumer-oriented guide to evaluating Internet-based health information.

Addressing Factors That Affect Adherence

When older adults have trouble adhering to their medication regimen, nurses can work with them and their caregivers to identify ways to improve adherence. For example, unit-dose medication systems, which have been widely used in institutional settings, are becoming more available for use in home settings, and may be helpful in improving medication adherence, especially when medication regimens are complex. A variety of simple "pill organizers" (i.e., containers with separate compartments designated for each day of the week and with one or more compartments for each day) are widely available in stores. In addition, more sophisticated devices to

enhance independence and improve adherence are available and may be particularly helpful for people with cognitive or functional impairments. For example, human voice recordings, telephone–computer services, and beeping watches or key chains can be used to remind the person to take medications at designated times. Medication-dispensing systems, which can be filled monthly and programmed to dispense medications at specific times, also are available. Internet sites that provide information about these more technologically advanced systems are listed in the Resources section available on thePoint. Nurses can encourage older adults and their caregivers to investigate different types of devices and systems (such as those depicted in Figure 8-2) that can be used to improve medication adherence.

Wellness Opportunity

Nurses promote self-responsibility by addressing factors that interfere with adherence and, at the same time, supporting independence.

Even with the increased availability of prescription drug benefits through Medicare, older adults and people with chronic conditions are burdened by the high and increasing cost of prescription medications. Thus, nurses often need to address financial barriers that affect adherence to medication regimens because even a person who has an adequate income may decide that a medication is not worth the high cost, especially on an ongoing basis. Many of the newer medications are developed because they are safer or more effective than

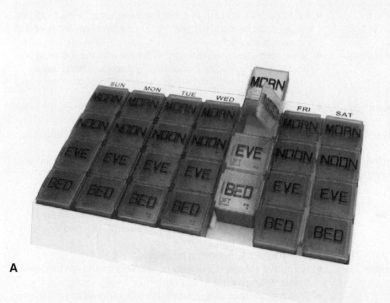

A

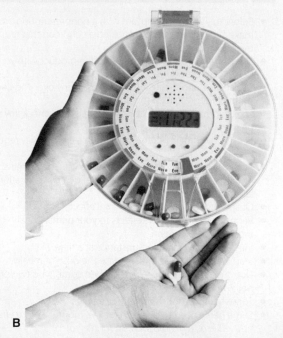

B

JOE SAMPLE   1/1
Take April 16, 2009   @09:00 AM

Colace   100MG   Qty 1
red oval capsule n 512

Glucophage   500MG   Qty 1
white round tablet BMS 6060

Motrin   600MG   Qty 1
white oblong tablet 600

Norvasc   5MG   Qty 1
white octagonal tab NOR

Prilosec   20MG   Qty 1
purple oblong capsule 742

C1

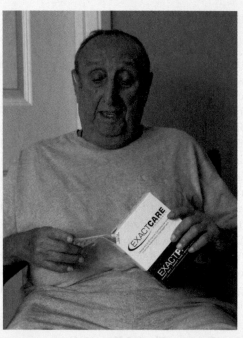

C2

FIGURE 8-2 Examples of devices and systems designed to improve medication adherence and independence. (**A**) One of the many types of simple pill organizers available in stores. (**B**) An automatic pill dispenser with a tamper-proof locking system and an audible alarm, with 28 compartments that can be programmed for taking medications up to four times a day. (**C**) An individualized dosing system for prescription and nonprescription medications, for use in homes and institutions, with each tear-apart compartment printed with patient name, date and time of administration, medication name and dose, and pill description. *(Figures A & B courtesy of ActiveForever.com. Figure C, courtesy of ExactCarepharmacy.com.)*

older medications; however, they usually are more expensive. Nurses can encourage older adults to be candid with their health care practitioners and ask about the availability of less costly but equally safe and effective medications.

One way of addressing high costs is to use **generic medications**, which are regulated by the FDA and required to be

bioequivalent (i.e., identical) to their brand-name counterparts in dosage form, safety, purity, strength, quality, intended use, performance characteristics, and route of administration. Generic drugs can be manufactured when the patent on a brand-name drug expires; they become more widely available as patents expire. About three-fourths of drugs are currently available in generic form in the United States today. In addition to the major cost savings of generic drugs, another important advantage is that they have a long track record of being used, so there is much information about therapeutic and adverse effects and interactions with other bioactive substances. In recent years, questions have been raised about the clinical equivalence of generic versus brand-name drugs, particularly with regard to those with narrow therapeutic ranges. A systematic review of 47 studies—including 38 randomized, controlled trials—confirmed that generic drugs are as safe and effective as brand-name drugs (Kesselheim et al., 2008). Studies also have confirmed that FDA-approved bioequivalence standards assure that generic drugs are therapeutically equivalent to the brand-name counterparts (Davit et al., 2009). Nurses can use this evidence-based information to encourage older adults to ask their prescribing practitioners about generic drugs that are appropriate for treating their conditions. The FDA provides complete and up-to-date information about the equivalency of all generic drugs at www.fda.gov/cder.

Additional ways of decreasing the cost of medications include obtaining free samples of medications from prescribing practitioners and enrolling in **prescription assistance programs**, which provide medications at little or no cost to consumers. Until recently, it was difficult to obtain information about these programs; however, in April 2005, the Partnership for Prescription Assistance was established to increase awareness and improve access. This partnership provides a single point of access to about 500 organizations, including pharmaceutical companies that provide free or low-cost medications to people who earn less than 200% of the federal poverty level. Nurses can teach about the increasing availability of prescription assistance programs and encourage older adults and their caregivers to explore this valuable resource at www.pparx.org.

Decreasing the Number of Medications

Because the chance of adverse medication effects increases in proportion to the number of medications consumed, a key intervention is to decrease the number of medications to as few as possible. This intervention is important not only for preventing adverse effects but also for improving adherence (Banning, 2009). Nurses accomplish this by coordinating the efforts of the prescriber(s) to discontinue duplicate medications or medications that are no longer appropriate and by educating the older person about the judicious use of medications that are not medically necessary. In community-based settings, nurses can teach older adults to review their medications with their health care practitioners at every visit. In home settings and long-term care facilities, nurses can assure that medication regimens are reviewed at least every 3 months and whenever there is a change in the patient's condition. In any setting, nurses have many opportunities to raise questions about medication regimens and to communicate with prescribing practitioners about medications.

When older adults are admitted to the hospital, they often are under the care of primary care practitioners who were not the ones who prescribed the medications taken before the admission. Nurses usually obtain the medication history, and the prescribing practitioner may automatically order the medications that are listed on the admission assessment. Because the hospital admission is an ideal time to reevaluate the safety, efficacy, and necessity of medications, nurses should ask older adults or their caregivers about the purpose and potential adverse effects of each medication. This assessment, which should be done with the medication reconciliation process, may provide important clues to medications or interactions that contributed to or directly caused the problem for which the patient is hospitalized.

When medications are prescribed for behavioral reasons rather than for a medical condition, nurses can teach older adults and their caregivers about these medications and about nonpharmacologic alternatives. For example, caregivers of people with dementia may use medications to address behaviors that might respond equally well to nonpharmacologic interventions that do not have any risk of adverse effects. Once these medications are prescribed, they are likely to be used over long periods without reevaluation. Nurses need to recognize that the efficacy may diminish (e.g., with hypnotics), the underlying reason may resolve or change (e.g., with situational anxiety), and adverse effects may develop gradually and not be recognized (e.g., with anticholinergic agents). Thus, it is imperative to review periodically all medications and to consider whether nonpharmacologic approaches could be used to address the symptoms or behaviors. Behavioral problems are one example of the types of symptoms that can be managed medically but might be managed just as well, and with fewer risks, through nonpharmacologic interventions. Other types of problems that can often be managed without pharmacologic agents are those related to sleep, comfort, anxiety, and chronic illnesses.

In community settings, it is important to make sure that older adults and caregivers understand the appropriate use of medications that are prescribed as needed (i.e., as needed). For example, a caregiver of someone with dementia may be instructed to give a behavior-modifying medication when the person becomes agitated. Although the episodes of agitation may be precipitated by environmental factors (e.g., noise or overstimulation), the caregiver might not realize that nonpharmacologic interventions could be equally effective and carry no risk of adverse effects. In contrast to this situation, a caregiver may withhold medications that could improve the quality of life for the older person and for himself or herself because of misunderstandings or lack of information about the appropriate use of medications. Nurses can teach caregivers about nonpharmacologic interventions, as well as the appropriate use of medications for behavior management, particularly for people with dementia (discussed in Chapter 14).

In institutional settings, nurses must establish clear criteria for administering medications for behavior management. These criteria must be based primarily on the patient's needs, rather than those of the staff. In home settings, different criteria for behavioral medication might be justified, and the needs of the caregivers may take precedence over the needs of the dependent older adult. For example, if nighttime waking of a dependent older person interferes with the caregiver's sleep, medication intervention might be warranted. In an institutional setting, however, the nursing staff that is paid to provide around-the-clock care might try nonpharmacologic interventions, or allow the person to be awake at night, rather than immediately turning to the use of medications.

◆ Wellness Opportunity

Nurses promote wellness by talking with older adults and their caregivers when appropriate about choosing interventions, such as relaxation techniques, that can improve health and quality of life, rather than using medications.

EVALUATING EFFECTIVENESS OF NURSING INTERVENTIONS

Nurses evaluate interventions related to medication management according to the degree to which the older adult follows a safe and effective medication regimen. This process involves an evaluation of medication-taking behaviors as well as an evaluation of the therapeutic effects of the medication. Another evaluation criterion is the extent to which negative functional consequences, such as interactions and adverse effects, are prevented, alleviated, or controlled. In home settings, nurses can evaluate the effectiveness of their interventions by observing the medication-taking patterns of the older adult. In any setting, nurses can evaluate the knowledge of safe and effective use of prescription and over-the-counter medications. Another measure of effectiveness is the degree to which barriers to adherence are eliminated or addressed.

Mrs. M., who is 76 years old, is being discharged to her home after a stay in a nursing home for rehabilitation after a stroke. Residual problems from the stroke include left-sided weakness and visual–perceptual difficulties. In addition to the stroke, Mrs. M.'s diagnoses include glaucoma, depression, and congestive heart failure. Her medications include the following: multivitamin, one tablet daily; furosemide, 20 mg, two tablets daily; Ecotrin, 81 mg daily; Plavix, 75 mg daily; Cardizem, 60 mg, three times daily; Lopressor, 50 mg twice daily; Zocor, 40 mg at bedtime; Zoloft, 50 mg at bedtime; and Timoptic, 0.25% twice daily. The nursing home regimen for administering the medications is as follows:

7:30 AM:	Cardizem 60 mg
	Furosemide 20 mg, 2 tablets
	Ecotrin 81 mg
	Timoptic, 0.25% in each eye
9:00 AM:	Lopressor 50 mg
1:00 PM:	Multivitamin, 1 tablet
	Cardizem 60 mg
3:30 PM:	Furosemide 20 mg, 2 tablets
7:30 PM:	Timoptic, 0.25% in each eye
	Cardizem 60 mg
	Plavix 75 mg
9:00 PM:	Lopressor 50 mg
	Zoloft 50 mg
	Zocor 40 mg daily

NURSING ASSESSMENT

Your assessment reveals that, before her hospitalization and nursing home stay, Mrs. M. administered her medications independently, but the only medications she took were the eye drops, furosemide (20 mg once daily), and digoxin, which she is no longer taking. The functional assessment indicates that Mrs. M. has weakness and limited use of her left arm and hand, causing difficulty performing tasks that require fine motor movements. She has full use of her right upper extremity, and she is right-hand dominant. She ambulates independently, but slowly, with a walker. A mental status assessment reveals that Mrs. M. is alert, oriented, and has no memory deficits; however, her abstract thinking and time perception have been impaired by the stroke. She has some expressive aphasia, but she seems to understand instructions, especially if ideas are reinforced by using concrete examples and demonstrations.

Mrs. M. expresses motivation to take her medications, but she admits to being overwhelmed by the complexity of the regimen, stating that at the nursing home, they administered her medications at six different times. She is also concerned about self-administering her eye drops because she used to use her left hand to hold her eyelids open. With regard to furosemide, she says she does not like taking it twice a day because it makes her go to the bathroom too much. While at the nursing home, she has not had any trouble with incontinence, but she worries about what she'll do at home because there is no bathroom on the first floor. She asks whether she can take the entire dose of furosemide at night so that she will only have to get up during the night to go to the bathroom, which is located near the bedroom.

In response to your questions about medication management routines before her stroke, Mrs. M. reports using a compartmentalized medication container and taking her two medications and the eye drops after breakfast, around 9:30 AM. She would administer the second dose of eye drops around 9:30 PM, before getting ready for bed. She had no difficulty remembering the medications because she kept the pill container and one bottle of eye drops near the toaster, and she kept a second bottle of eye drops on her nightstand. Now, however, she expresses concern about the number of times she must take medications if the regimen remains the same as in the nursing home, and she thinks she will need six pill containers but is not sure where she should put all of them. Mrs. M. also tells you that she is worried about paying for so many medications because when she signed up for Medicare Part D, she was taking only two generic medications and eye drops. Now that she is on so many new pills—and she knows that some are very expensive—she needs to have her prescription drug plan reviewed and perhaps changed.

Mrs. M. lives with her husband, who is physically healthy but has early-stage Alzheimer's disease. Their daughter lives nearby and visits two or three times weekly to assist with grocery shopping, laundry, and household chores. She also provides transportation to stores and appointments.

NURSING DIAGNOSIS

You decide on a nursing diagnosis of Noncompliance because Mrs. M. expresses a desire to take her medications, but several factors deter adherence to the current regimen. Related factors include functional impairments, complex medication regimens, negative side effects of furosemide, and concern about the cost of medications.

NURSING CARE PLAN FOR MRS. M.

Expected Outcome	Nursing Interventions	Nursing Evaluation
Mrs. M.'s medication routine will be simplified.	• Work with the pharmacist and the prescribing practitioner to simplify the medication regimen. • Discuss with Mrs. M.'s prescribing practitioner the problem of the complexity of the regimen and the cost of medications. Ask Mrs. M.'s prescribing practitioner if she can take Cardizem CD, 180 mg daily, rather than Cardizem, 60 mg three times a day. (This will be less expensive and will eliminate two doses of medication daily.) • Ask the pharmacist about combining medications to allow twice-daily administration. • Assist Mrs. M. in establishing a routine for self-administering medications that will fit in with her usual activities. • At least 3 days before discharge from the nursing home, arrange for Mrs. M. to assume responsibility for her own medication management, using pill containers that she herself fills.	• Mrs. M. will be able to follow a twice-daily medication dosing schedule.
Mrs. M.'s concerns about furosemide will be addressed.	• Explain the importance of taking furosemide, as ordered, to control congestive heart failure effectively. • Suggest that Mrs. M. obtain a portable commode for use downstairs during the day.	• Mrs. M. will take furosemide as directed and will not experience difficulty with urinary incontinence.

(case study continues on page 144)

NURSING CARE PLAN FOR MRS. M. *(continued)*

Expected Outcome	Nursing Interventions	Nursing Evaluation
Mrs. M.'s concerns about the cost of medications will be addressed.	• Encourage Mrs. M. to talk with her primary care practitioner about her concerns over the cost of the prescribed medications. • Suggest that Mrs. M. talk with her usual pharmacist about her current prescription drug plan and ask if there might be a better plan for her.	• Mrs. M. will be able to afford her prescribed medications.
A system for self-administering eye drops will be identified.	• Ask an occupational therapist to evaluate Mrs. M.'s ability to self-administer her eye drops and to identify any assistive devices that may increase her independence and reliability in performing this task. • Have Mrs. M. practice self-administering her eye drops before she is discharged from the nursing home, with staff providing whatever assistance is necessary. • Talk with Mrs. M. about the possibility of her husband assisting with the eye drop procedure if she is unable to do this independently. • Ask Mrs. M.'s ophthalmologist whether the eye drop regimen can be simplified to once-daily dosing by prescribing an extended-action eye drop formula.	• Mrs. M. will self-administer her eye drops or will receive the assistance she needs for eye drop administration from her husband.

THINKING POINTS

- What are the factors that influence Mrs. M.'s ability to manage her medications independently?
- What additional assessment information would be helpful in establishing a plan for Mrs. M. to manage her medications independently?
- What health education would you provide to address Mrs. M.'s concerns about the cost of her medications?
- What steps would you take to ensure that expected outcomes are achieved after Mrs. M. is back in her own home?

Chapter Highlights

Introduction to Bioactive Substances

- Effects of bioactive substances in the body in relation to pharmacokinetics and pharmacodynamics
- Herbs and medications with similar bioactivity (Table 8-1)
- Potential adverse effects of herbs (Table 8-2)
- Herbs commonly used by older adults: uses, actions, and precautions (Table 8-3)
- Homeopathic remedies

Age-Related Changes That Affect Bioactive Substances in Older Adults

- Decreased clearance due to changes in the kidneys and liver (Box 8-1)
- Metabolism by the cytochrome P-450 system (Table 8-4)
- Effects of changes in body composition (Box 8-1)
- Medications affected by serum albumin levels
- Effects of changes in receptor sensitivity (Box 8-1)
- Changes that affect medication-taking behaviors

Risks Factors That Affect Bioactive Substances

- Pathologic processes and functional impairments (medication–disease interactions, effects on the ability to take substances)
- Behaviors based on myths and misunderstandings (attitudes about and expectations for bioactive substances)
- Communication barriers between older adults and prescribing practitioners
- Lack of information
- Inappropriate prescribing practices (Beers criteria)
- Polypharmacy and inadequate monitoring
- Medication nonadherence
- Financial concerns related to prescription drugs (Medicare Part D)
- Insufficient recognition of adverse effects (Table 8-6)

Medication Interactions

- Medication–medication interactions (Table 8-7)
- Medication–herb interactions (Table 8-3)
- Medications and nutrients (Table 8-8)
- Medications and alcohol (Table 8-9)
- Medications and caffeine (Table 8-10)
- Medications and nicotine (Table 8-11)

Functional Consequences Associated With Bioactive Substances in Older Adults

- Altered therapeutic effects
- Increased potential for adverse effects (Box 8-2)
- Adverse effects of anticholinergic medications (Box 8-3)
- Increased potential for altered mental status (Table 8-12)
- Increased potential for tardive dyskinesia

Nursing Assessment of Medication Use and Effects

- Communication techniques for obtaining accurate information (open-ended, nonjudgmental)
- Scope of a medication assessment (all bioactive substances, older adult's understanding of regimen, preferences) (Box 8-4)
- Cultural considerations (factors that influence medication-taking behaviors, culturally specific health care sources and practices) (Cultural Considerations 8-1 and 8-2)
- Patterns of medication use
- Medication assessment as it relates to the overall assessment
- Factors in identifying adverse medication effects

Nursing Diagnoses

- Ineffective Self Health Management
- Instrumental Self-Care Deficit
- Noncompliance
- Readiness for Enhanced Self Health Management

Planning for Wellness Outcomes

- Knowledge: Medication
- Self-care: Non-Parenteral Medication
- Compliance Behavior

Nursing Interventions to Promote Healthy Medication-Taking Patterns

- Implementing evidence-based interventions (Evidence-Based Practice 8-1)
- Teaching about medications (Box 8-5, patient teaching tool)
- Teaching about herbs and other bioactive substances (Box 8-6, patient teaching tool)
- Addressing factors that affect adherence (Figure 8-2)
- Decreasing the number of medications

Evaluating Effectiveness of Nursing Interventions

- Medication-taking behaviors that are safe and effective
- Prevention, alleviation, or control of negative functional consequences (e.g., interactions, adverse effects).

Critical Thinking Exercises

1. You are asked to give a half-hour presentation on "Medications and Aging" to a local senior citizens group. Describe the following:
   - What points would you cover about age-related changes?
   - How would you address the risk factors that affect medication action and medication-taking behaviors?
   - What tips would you give about taking medications?
   - What educational materials would you use?
   - How would you involve the group participants in the discussion?
2. Carefully read the interview questions in Box 8-4 and decide which questions you would use and how you would phrase the questions in your own words for each of the following situations:
   - You are doing an admission interview for a 78-year-old man who lives alone and has been admitted to the hospital for the third time in 18 months for congestive heart failure.
   - You are working in a Senior Wellness program in an urban setting with a large number of older adults who were born in Mexico. You are preparing for 15-minute interviews with older adults who have agreed to participate in an educational session to which they must bring all their pills in a bag and ask the nurse about them.
3. Carefully read the information in Boxes 8-5 and 8-6 and describe what information you would be likely to use in each of the following situations.
   - Discharge planning for the 78-year-old man described in Exercise 2, bullet 1.
   - Health education for people described in the Senior Wellness program in Exercise 2, bullet 2.

Resources

For links to these and additional helpful Internet resources related to this chapter, visit thePoint. at http://thePoint.lww.com/Miller6e.

Clinical Tools

American Journal of Nursing and Hartford Institute for Geriatric Nursing
- *How to Try This,* article and video: Molony, S. L. (2009). Monitoring medication use in older adults. *American Journal of Nursing, 109,* 68–78.

Hartford Institute for Geriatric Nursing
- *Try This: Best Practices in Nursing Care to Older Adults* Issue 16.1 (2008 Revised), Beers Criteria for potentially inappropriate medication use in older adults. Part I: 2002 criteria independent of diagnoses or conditions. Issue 16.2 (2008 Revised) Beers Criteria for potentially inappropriate medication use in older adults. Part II: 2002 criteria considering diagnoses or conditions.

Medications Management in Home Health Care Toolkit
- Evidence-based protocols for addressing common medications problems

Evidence-Based Practice

Zwicker, D., & Fulmer, T. (2008). Reducing adverse drug events. In E. Capezuti, D. Zwicker, M. Mezey, & T. Fulmer (Eds.), *Evidence-Based Geriatric Nursing Protocols for Best Practice,* (3rd ed., pp. 257–308). New York: Springer Publishing Co.

National Guideline Clearinghouse
- Medication management guideline
- Improving medication management for older adult clients
- Substance misuse and alcohol use disorders

Health Education

AARP
American Botanical Council
Centers for Medicare and Medicaid Services
Food and Drug Administration (FDA)
Herb Research Foundation
National Center for Complementary and Alternative Medicine
National Council on Aging Center for Healthy Aging
National Council on Patient Information and Education
Partnership for Prescription Assistance
Therapeutic Products Directorate (Canada)
United States Pharmacopoeia (USP)

REFERENCES

Agashivla, N., & Wk, U. (2009). Effects of potentially inappropriate psychoactive medications on falls in US nursing home residents: Analysis of the 2004 National Nursing Home Survey database. *Drugs and Aging, 26*(10), 853–860.

Alvarez, M. V. G., & Evidente, V. G. H. (2008). Understanding drug-induced parkinsonism, separating pearls from oysters. *Neurology, 70,* e32–e34.

Andrews, M. M. (2008). Cultural competence in health history and physical examination. In M. M. Andrews & J. S. Boyle (Eds.), *Transcultural concepts in nursing care,* (5th ed., pp. 34–65). Philadelphia, PA: Lippincott Williams & Wilkins.

Banning, M. (2009). A review of interventions used to improve adherence to medication in older people. *International Journal of Nursing Studies, 46*(11), 1505–1515.

Barnett, S. R. (2009). Polypharmacy and perioperative medications in the elderly. *Anesthesiology Clinics, 27,* 377–389.

Barton, C., Sklenicka, J., Sayegh, P., & Yaffe, K. (2008). Contraindicated medication use among patients in a memory disorders clinic. American *Journal of Geriatric Pharmacotherapy, 6*(3), 147–152.

Beers, M. H., Oslander, J. G., Rollingher, J., Brooks, J., Reuben, D., & Beck, J. C. (1991). Explicit criteria for determining potentially inappropriate medication use by the elderly. *Archives of Internal Medicine, 151,* 1825–1832.

Berdot, S., Bertrand, M., Dartigues, J. F., Fourrier, A., Tavernier, B., Richie, K., & Alpérovitch, A. (2009). Inappropriate medication use and risk of falls—A prospective study in a large community-dwelling elderly cohort. *BMC Geriatrics, 9,* 30. doi:10.1186/1471-2318-9-30.

Brekke, M., Rognstad, S., Staraad, J., Furu, K., Gjelstad, S., Bjorner, T., & Dalen, I. (2008). Pharmacologically inappropriate prescriptions for elderly patients in general practice: How common? Baseline data from The Prescription Peer Academic Detailing (Rx-PAD) study. *Scandinavian Journal of Primary Health Care, 26*(2), 80–85.

Buck, M. D., Atreia, A., Brunker, C. P., Jain, A., Suh, T. T., Palmer, R. M., . . . Wilcox, A. B. (2009). Potentially inappropriate medication prescribing in outpatient practices: Prevalence and patient characteristics based on electronic health records. *American Journal of Geriatric Pharmacotherapy, 7*(2), 84–92.

Bushardt, R. L., Massey, E. B., Simpson, T. W., Arial, J. C., Simpson, K. N. (2008). Polypharmacy: Misleading, but manageable. *Clinical Interventions in Aging, 3*(2), 383–389.

Campbell, N., Boustani, M., Limbil, T., Ott, C., Fox, C., Maidment, I., . . . Gulati, R. (2009). The cognitive impact of anticholinergics: A clinical review. *Clinical Interventions in Aging, 4,* 225–233.

Carey, I. M., DeWilde, S., Harris, T., Victor, C., Richards, N., Hilton, S. R., & Cook, D. G. (2008). What factors predict potentially inappropriate primary care prescribing in older people? Analysis of UK primary care patient record database. *Drugs and Aging, 25*(8), 693–706.

Carriere, I., Fourrier-Reglat, A., Dartiques, J. F., Rouaud, O., Pasquier, F., Ritchies, K., & Ancelin, M. L. (2009). Drugs with anticholinergic properties, cognitive decline, and dementia in an elderly general population: The 3-city study. *Archives of Internal Medicine, 169*(14), 1317–1324.

Center for Home Care Policy & Research (2009). Medication management: Evidence brief. *Home Healthcare Nurse, 27*(6), 379–386.

Centers for Medicare & Medicaid Services. (2008). National Health Expenditure Accounts, Historical. www.cms.hhs.gov/NationalHealthExpendData.

Chen, Y. C., Hwang, S. J., Lai, H. Y., Chen, T. J., Lin, M. H., Chen, L. K., & Lee, C. H. (2009). Potentially inappropriate medication for emergency department visits by elderly patients in Taiwan. *Pharmacoepidemiology and Drug Safety, 18*(1), 53–56.

Cherniack, E. P., Ceron-Fuentes, J., Florez, H., Sandals, L, Rodriguzx, O., & Palacios, J. C. (2008). Influence of race and ethnicity on alternative medicine as a self-treatment preference for common medical conditions in a population of multi-ethnic urban elderly. *Complementary Therapies in Clinical Practice, 14,* 116–123.

Chou, K. L., & Friedman, J. H. (2006). Tardive syndrome in the elderly. *Clinics in Geriatric Medicine, 22,* 915–933.

Conn, V. S., Hafdahl, A. R., Cooper, P. S., Ruppar, T. M., Mehr, D. R., Russell, C. L. (2009). Interventions to improve medication adherence among older adults: Meta-analysis of adherence outcomes among randomized controlled trials. *The Gerontologist, 49*(4), 447–462.

Cooney, D., & Pascuzzi, K. (2009). Polypharmacy in the elderly: Focus on drug interactions and adherence in hypertension. *Clinical Geriatric Medicine, 25,* 221–233.

Cua, Y. M., & Kripalani, S. (2008). Medication use in the transition from hospital to home. *Annals of the Academy of Medicine, 37*(2), 136–141.

Davit, B. M., Nwakama, P. E., Buelher, G. J., Conner, D. P., Haidar, S. H., Patel, D. T., . . . Woodcock, J. (2009). Comparing generic and innovator drugs: A review of 12 years of bioequivalence data from the United State Food and Drug Administration. *Annuals of Pharmacotherapy, 43,* 1583–1597.

Delate, T., Chester, E. A., Stubbings, T. W., & Barnes, C. A. (2008). Clinical outcomes of a home-based medication reconciliation program after discharge from a skilled nursing facility. *Pharmacotherapy, 28*(4), 444–452.

Ferreira, M. P., & Weems, M. K. S. (2008). Alcohol consumption by aging adults in the United States: Health benefits and detriments. *Journal of the American Dietetic Association, 108,* 1668–1678.

Fick, D. M., Mion, L. C., Beers, M. H., & Waller, J. (2009). Health outcomes associated with potentially inappropriate medication use in older adults. *Research in Nursing & Health, 31*(1), 42–51.

Gardiner, P., Phillips, R., & Shaughnessy, A. F. (2008). Herbal and dietary supplement–drug interactions in patients with chronic illnesses. *American Family Physician, 77*(1), 73–78.

Gordon, R. Y., Beeker, D. J., & Rader, D. J. (2009). Reduced efficacy of Rosuvastatin by St. John's Wort. *The American Journal of Medicine, 122*(2), e1–e2.

Ho, P. M., Magid, D. J., Shetterly, S. M., Olson, K. L., Maddox, T. M., Peterson, P. N., . . . Rumsfeld, J. S. (2008). Medication nonadherence is associated with a broad range of adverse outcomes in patients with coronary artery disease. *American Heart Journal, 155,* 772–779.

Holbrook, A. M., Pereira, J. A., Labiris, R., McDonald, H., Douketis, J., Crowther, M., & Wells, P. S. (2005). Systematic overview of warfarin and its drug and food interactions. *Archives of Internal Medicine, 165,* 1095–1105.

Holcomb, S. S. (2009). Common herb-drug interactions: What you should know. *The Nurse Practitioner, 34*(5), 21–29.

Hosia-Randell, H. M., Muurinen, S. M., Pitkala, K. H. (2008). Exposure to potentially inappropriate drugs and drug-drug interactions in elderly nursing home residents in Helsinki, Finland: A cross-sectional study. *Drugs and Aging, 25*(8), 683–692.

Johnell, K., & Fastbom, J. (2008). Concurrent use of anticholinergic drugs and cholinesterase inhibitors: Register-based study of over 700,000 elderly patients. *Drugs and Aging, 25*(10), 871–877.

Juurlink, D. N., Gomes, T., Ko, D. T., Szmitko, P. E., Mamdani, M. M. (2009). A population-based study of the drug interaction between proton pump inhibitors and clopidogrel. *Canadian Medical Association, 180*(7), 713–718.

Kaiser Family Foundation. (2008). Prescription drug trends. www.kkf.org

Kaiser Family Foundation. (2009). Medicare Part D data spotlight: The coverage gap. www.kkf.org.

Kamble, P., Chen, H., Sherer, J. T., Aparasu, R. R. (2009). Use of antipsychotics among elderly nursing home residents with dementia in the US: An analysis of National Survey Data. *Drugs and Aging, 26*(6), 483–492.

Kesselheim, A. S., Misono, A. S., Lee, J. L., Stedman, M. R., Brookhart, M. A., Choudhry, N. K., & Shrank, W. H. (2008). Clinical equivalence of generic and brand-name drugs used in cardiovascular disease: A systematic review and meta-analysis. *Journal of the American Medical Association, 300*(21), 2514–2526.

Krousel-Wood, M. A., Muntner, P., Islam, T., Morisky, D. E., & Webber, L. S. (2009). Barriers to and determinants of medication adherence in hypertension management: Perspective of the Cohort Study of Medication Adherence Among Older Adults. *Medical Clinics of North America, 93*, 753–769.

Leendertse, A. J., Egberts, A. C. G., Stoker, L. J., & Van Den Bemt, P. M. (2008). Frequency of and risk factors for preventable medication-related hospital admissions in the Netherlands. *Archives of Internal Medicine, 168*(17), 1890–1896.

Lindsey, P. (2009). Psychotropic medication use among older adults, what all nurses need to know *Journal of Gerontological Nursing, 35*(9), 28–38.

Maldonado, J. R. (2008). Delirium in the acute care setting: Characteristics, diagnosis and treatment. *Critical Care Clinics, 24*, 657–772.

McCloskey, W. W., Zaiken, K., & Couris, R. R. (2008). Clinically significant grapefruit juice-drug interactions. *Nutrition Today, 43*(1), 19–26.

Modi, A., Weiner, M., Craign, B. A., Sands, L. P., Rosenman, M. B., Thomas, J. (2009). Concomitant use of anticholinergics with acetylcholinesterase inhibitors in Medicaid recipients with dementia and residing nursing homes. *Journal of the American Geriatric Society, 57*(7), 1238–1244.

Moen, J., Bohm, A., Tillenius, T., Antonov, K., Nilsson, J. L., Ring, L. (2009). "I don't know how many of these (medications) are necessary"—A focus group study among elderly users of multiple medicines. *Patient Education and Counseling, 74*(2), 135–141.

Molony, S. L. (2009). How to try this: Monitoring medication use in older adults. *American Journal of Nursing, 109*(1), 68–78.

Moquin, B., Blackman, M. R., Mitty. E., & Flores, S. (2009). Complementary and alternative medicine (CAM). *Geriatric Nursing, 30*(3), 196–203.

Morley, J. E. (2009). Polypharmacy in the nursing home. *Journal of American Medical Directors Association, 10*, 289–291.

NANDA International. (2009). *Nursing diagnoses: Definitions and classification 2009–2011.* Oxford, UK: Wiley-Blackwell.

Nichol, M. B., Knight, T. K., Wu, J., Barron, R., & Penson, D. F. (2009). Evaluating use patterns of and adherence to medications for benign prostatic hyperplasia. *Journal of Urology, 181*(5), 2214–2221.

Olivier, P., Bertrand, L., Tubery, M., Lauque, D., Montastruc, J. L., & Lanevre-Mestre, M. (2009). Hospitalizations because of adverse drug reactions in elderly patients admitted through the emergency department: A prospective survey. *Drugs and Aging, 26*(6), 475–482.

Olyaei, A. J., & Bennett, W. M. (2009). Drug dosing in the elderly patients with chronic kidney disease. *Clinics in Geriatric Medicine, 25*, 459–527.

Planton, J., & Edlund, B. J. (2010). Strategies for reducing polypharmacy in older adults. *Journal of Gerontological Nursing, 36*(1), 8–12.

Plotnikoff, G. A. (2010). Herbal medicines. In M. Snyder & R. Lindquist (Eds.), *Complementary & alternative therapies in nursing* (6th ed., pp. 4221–438). New York: Springer Publishing Company.

Prudent, M., Drame, M., Jolly, D., Trenque, T., Parioie, R., Mahmoudi, R., . . . Novella, J. L. (2008). Potentially inappropriate use of psychotropic medications in hospitalized elderly patients in France: Cross-sectional analysis of the prospective, multicentre SAFEs cohort. *Drugs and Aging, 25*(11), 933–946.

Purnell, L. D. (2009). *Guide to culturally competent care* (2nd ed.). Philadelphia, PA: F. A. Davis Co.

Radosevic, N., Gantumur, M., & Viahovic-Palcevski, V. (2008). Potentially inappropriate prescribing to hospitalized patients. *Pharmacoepidemiology and Drug Safety, 17*(7), 733–737.

Rothberg, M. B., Pekow, P. S., Liu, F., Kore-Gorodzicki, B., Brennan, M. J., Bellantonio, S., . . . Lindenauer, P. K. (2008). Potentially inappropriate medication use in hospitalized elders. *Journal of Hospital Medicine, 3*(2), 91–102.

Rudolph, J. L., Salow, M. J., Angelini, M. C., & McGlinchey, R. E. (2008). The anticholinergic risk scale and anticholinergic adverse effects in older persons. *Archives of Internal Medicine, 168*(5), 508–513.

Rupawala, A. H., Kshirsager, N. A., & Gogtay, N. J. (2009). A retrospective analysis of adverse events in the elderly in a tertiary referral center in Mumbai (Bombay), India. *Indian Journal of Medical Sciences, 63*(5), 167–173.

Schaffer, S. D., Yoon, S., & Zadezensky, I. (2009). A review of smoking cessation: Potentially risky effect on prescribed medications. *Journal of Clinical Nursing, 18*(11), 1533–1540.

Schuler, J., Duckelmann, C., Beindl, W., Prinz, E., Michalski, T., Pichler, M. (2008). Polypharmacy and inappropriate prescribing in elderly internal-medicine patients in Austria. *Wien Kin Wochenschr, 120*(23–24), 733–741.

Schwab, W., Messinger-Rapport, B., & Franco, K. (2009). Psychiatric symptoms of dementia: Treatable, but no silver bullet. *Cleveland Clinic Journal of Medicine, 26*(3), 167–174.

Shearer, J. (2009). Improving oral medication management in home health agencies. *Home Health Care Nurse, 27*(3), 184–191.

Siller-Matula, J. M., Lana, I., Christ, G., & Jilma, B. (2008). Calcium-channel blockers reduce the antiplatelet effect of clopidogrel. *Journal of the American College of Cardiology, 52*(19), 1557–1563.

Snyder, F. J., Dundas, M. L., Kirkpatrick, C., & Neill, K. S. (2009). Use and safety perceptions regarding herbal supplements: A study of older persons in southeast Idaho. *Journal of Nutrition for the Elderly, 28*(1), 81–95.

Sood, A., Sood, R., Brinker, F. J., Mann, R., Loehrer, L. L., & Wahner-Roedler, D. L. (2008). Potential for interactions between dietary supplements and prescription medications. *American Journal of Medicine, 121*(3), 207–211.

Stockl, K. M., Le, L., Zhang, S., & Harada, A. S. (2010). Clinical and economic outcomes associated with potentially inappropriate prescribing in the elderly. *American Journal of Managed Care, 16(1)*, e1–e10.

Thanvi, B., & Treadwell, S. (2009). Drug induced parkinsonism: A common cause of parkinsonism in older people. *Postgraduate Medical Journal, 85*(1004), 322–326.

Trifir, A. G., Spina, E., & Gambassi, G. (2009). Use of antipsychotics in elderly patients with dementia: Do atypical and conventional agents have a similar safety profile? *Pharmacological Research: The Official Journal of the Italian Pharmacological Society, 59*(1), 1–12.

White, W. B. (2009). Defining the problem of treating the patient with hypertension and arthritis pain. *American Journal of Medicine, 122*(Suppl 5.), S3–S9.

Williams, A. F., Manias, E., & Walker, R. (2008). Adherence to multiple, prescribed medications in diabetic kidney disease: A qualitative study of consumers' and health professionals/perspectives. *International Journal of Nursing Studies, 45*(12), 1742–1756.

Wright, R. M., Roumani, Y. F., Boudreau, R., Newman, A. B., Ruby, C. M., Studenski, S. A., . . . Hanlon, J. T. (2009). Impact of central nervous system (CNS) medication use on cognition decline in community dwelling older adults: Findings from the health, aging and body composition study. *Journal of the American Geriatric Society, 57*(2), 243–250.

Yin, W., Basu, A., Zhang, J. X., Rabbani, A., Meltzer, D. O., & Alexander, G. C. (2008). The effect of the Medicare Part D prescription benefit on drug utilization and expenditures. *Annals of Internal Medicine, 148*, 169–177.

Zarowitz, B. J. (2008). Black Box warnings—Implications in practice. *Geriatric Nursing, 29*(6), 402–409.

Zarowitz, B. J. (2009). Pharmacologic consideration of commonly used gastrointestinal drugs in the elderly. *Gastroenterology Clinics of North America, 38*(2009), 547–562.

Zwicker, D., & Fulmer, T. (2008). Reducing adverse drug events. In E. Capezuti, D. Zwicker, M. Mezey, & T. Fulmer (Eds.), *Evidence-based geriatric nursing protocols for best practice* (3rd ed., pp. 257–308). New York: Springer Publishing Co.

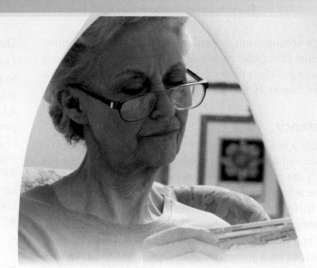

CHAPTER 9

Legal and Ethical Concerns

LEARNING OBJECTIVES

After reading this chapter, you will be able to:

1. Define the following terms: autonomy, competency, and decision-making capacity.

2. Describe the following advance directives: living wills, medical directives, and durable power of attorney for health care.

3. Discuss ethical issues that nurses commonly address when caring for older adults.

4. Describe cultural considerations that affect autonomy, decision making, and advance directives.

5. Describe nursing responsibilities regarding advance directives and decisions about care.

KEY POINTS

advance directives

artificial nutrition and
    hydration

autonomy

competency

decision-making capacity

do not resuscitate (DNR)
    order

durable power of attorney
    for health care

executive control functions

guardianship

health care proxy

incompetent

living wills

Minimum Data Set (MDS)

Nursing Home Residents'
    Bill of Rights

Omnibus Budget
    Reconciliation Act
    (OBRA) of 1987

Patient Self-Determination
    Act

values clarification

In the past several decades, various legislative efforts have addressed the rights of older adults and their quality of life. During the early 1980s, state and federal governments began addressing issues related to vulnerable elders. Later in that decade, legislative efforts focused on issues related to end-of-life decisions, the rights of patients and nursing home residents, and the quality of care provided under Medicaid and Medicare programs. Many of these legislative and policy initiatives have created ethical issues for gerontological health care practitioners. For example, nurses commonly address questions about the extent to which an older person is able to make decisions about his or her health care. Although legislation can provide legal guidelines for these questions, laws do not resolve ethical dilemmas that arise when no advance directive is provided or when conflicts exist about how an advance directive should be interpreted or implemented. The next sections review some of the pertinent legal and ethical issues that are relevant to nursing care of older adults. Additional legal and ethical considerations regarding vulnerable or abused elders are addressed in Chapter 10.

AUTONOMY AND RIGHTS

Autonomy is the personal freedom to direct one's own life as long as it does not infringe on the rights of others. An autonomous person is capable of rational thought and is able to recognize the need for problem solving. The person can identify the problem, search for alternatives, and select a solution that allows his or her continued personal freedom, as long as it does not cause any harm to another's rights or property. Loss of autonomy and, therefore, loss of independence, is a very real fear among the elderly. Moreover, for older adults with dementia and other conditions that affect decision-making abilities, loss of autonomy is an inevitable reality that is addressed by families and health care professionals.

Because autonomy is highly valued in many European and North American cultures and there is no easy way to evaluate decision-making abilities—which can fluctuate from day to day—questions often arise about medical interventions and health care decisions. Thus, nurses need to be familiar with legal and ethical guidelines related to **competency** and **decision-making capacity**. Nurses have a responsibility to assist older adults and their families, often as impartial mediators, when issues concerning personal autonomy arise. However, if the safety of the older person is threatened because of risky behaviors arising from impaired decision-making abilities, nurses must refer older people to the appropriate community agencies (e.g., Adult Protective Services) for further evaluation (see Chapter 10).

Competency

Competency is a legal term that refers to the ability to fulfill one's role and handle one's affairs in a responsible manner. All adults are presumed to be competent, and state laws designate the age of competency—usually 18 years—for participating in legally binding decisions. Because competent people are guaranteed all the rights granted by the U.S. constitution and state laws, all adults who have not been declared **incompetent** by a judge have the legal right to make their own decisions about medical treatment and health care. However, families or health care providers often raise questions about an older person's ability to make reasonable decisions, particularly when the person is cognitively impaired.

When questions are raised about a person's ability to participate in health care decisions, a legally appointed, surrogate decision maker, if one has been designated, assumes decision-making responsibility (see the discussion of "**health care proxy**" in the section on Advance Directives). In the absence of a surrogate decision maker or when conflicts exist among the people involved with making and implementing decisions, a petition can be filed with probate court to determine whether the person is competent. Often, these petitions are filed because a health care provider (usually a physician) is concerned that appropriate decisions be made for a person who does not seem able to make reasonable medical decisions independently. Usually a family member files the petition, but if no qualified family member is available, or if family members are in conflict about the petition, an attorney or other person may file. If the court determines that the person is incompetent (i.e., incapable of making decisions on his or her own behalf), the judge assigns either a partial or a full **guardianship** (also called a *conservatorship*).

With a partial guardianship, the incompetent person is permitted to make limited decisions; with a full guardianship, the person loses all of his or her rights to make such decisions. Although court action can revoke or reverse a guardianship, the guardianship typically remains in place until the incompetent person dies. Usually, guardianship is initiated only as a last resort when no other legal intervention is appropriate because it is a drastic measure that takes away rights and entails court proceedings and ongoing court monitoring. Most often the need for guardianship can be avoided if a person makes his or her wishes known in a comprehensive and legally binding manner, including the appointment of a surrogate decision maker, before any questions arise about his or her mental capacities. In the absence of these documents, however, or when conflict arises about the ability of designated people to honor the person's wishes, legal and ethical issues are generally addressed through probate court proceedings, such as guardianship.

Decision-Making Capacity

Decision-making capacity is a measure of a person's ability to make an informed and logical decision about a particular aspect of his or her health care. In contrast to competency—which is determined by a court of law—decision-making capacity is determined by health care practitioners and it relates to a single decision rather than a global determination of one's ability to manage one's own affairs (Carroll, 2010). The following abilities are widely recognized by legal and health care practitioners as essential components of decision-making capacity (Beattie, 2009):

- Understanding: ability to comprehend information that is relevant to the decision and ability to demonstrate that comprehension
- Appreciation: ability to apply the understanding to one's own situation
- Reasoning: ability to use the information to consider alternatives and the associated consequences
- Expressing a choice: ability to communicate the decision to others.

Additional characteristics that should be considered are stability over time and consistency with the person's usual beliefs and values.

Determination of decision-making capacity should not be based on a particular diagnosis or the person's chronologic age. This is especially important with regard to older adults who have dementia because studies have found that there is a significant lack of knowledge about the relationship between this diagnosis and one's decision-making capacity (Beattie, 2009). Rather than drawing conclusions about decision-making capacity based on age or diagnosis, determination of this multifaceted ability should be based on a careful evaluation of the person's ability to understand the issues involved in a specific situation, to weigh the pros and cons of choices, and to communicate about them. For example, a person with dementia may be able to decide about the appointment of a surrogate decision maker but may not be able to participate in a complex decision about medical treatment options for cancer. In this situation, it might be reasonable for the person to designate a family member to make the treatment decision. Nurses have dual roles in helping surrogate decision makers involve the older adult as much as possible, and at the same time supporting the decision maker in assuming responsibility for decisions.

Determination of decision-making capacity also recognizes that cognitive abilities can fluctuate from day to day and hour to hour and may be significantly influenced by factors that can be addressed. Thus, health care professionals need to search for treatable conditions that interfere with capacity, including delirium, dementia, depression, and polypharmacy (Walaszek, 2009). Thus, an important role of nurses is to promote optimal decision-making capacity by identifying and addressing the factors that influence cognitive functioning and is within the realm of nursing responsibilities (e.g., sensory impairments, medication effects). For example, even such a relatively simple measure as ensuring that a hearing-impaired person uses his or her hearing aid may improve communication and thereby have a positive effect on decision-making abilities. Similarly, if a person with dementia has better cognitive abilities in the morning or when he or she is rested, then efforts can be made to discuss health care decisions during this time, rather than when the person is more confused.

The phrases *decisional autonomy* and *executional autonomy* are sometimes used in relation to the concept of decision-making capacity. Decisional autonomy is the ability and freedom to make decisions without external influence, and executional autonomy (also called executive autonomy) is the ability to implement the decisions (Collopy, 1988). These concepts call attention to the complexity of assessing decision-making capacity and the importance of evaluating a person's ability not only to make reasonable decisions but also to carry out all of the actions necessary for implementing them. This point is particularly important in relation to people with impaired **executive control functions**, which are the cognitive skills involved in successfully planning and carrying out goal-oriented behavior, such as self-care tasks. Conditions that are likely to cause impaired executive control functions include dementia, major depression, Parkinson's disease, and traumatic brain injury. These situations are particularly difficult to evaluate because the person may retain the capacity to understand and make decisions (decisional autonomy) but may not have the capacity to carry them out (executive autonomy). Chapter 13 discusses guidelines for nursing assessment of executive control functions.

ADVANCE DIRECTIVES

Advance directives (also called *advance medical directives*) are legally binding documents that allow competent people to document what medical care they would or would not want to receive if they were not capable of making decisions and communicating their wishes. Advance directives also enable people to appoint a health care proxy (also called a *proxy decision maker*), who is a person responsible for communicating his or her wishes if he or she becomes incompetent or unable to communicate them. Studies have found that older adults are generally ready and eager to discuss advance care planning and that the best time for doing this is during periods of relative wellness (Malcomson & Bisbee, 2009).

Advance directives are implemented on the basis of the **Patient Self-Determination Act (PSDA)**, which was enacted by Congress in 1990 and became effective on December 1, 1991. The primary intent of this congressional legislation is to protect health care consumers by requiring that providers do all of the following:

- Inform patients of their right to refuse treatments and make health care decisions
- Provide written information about their state's provisions for implementing advance directives

- Ask each person whether an advance directive has been completed
- Include documentation of patients' advance directives in their medical records
- Provide education for the staff and the community on advance directives

The PSDA applies to all hospices, hospitals, home health agencies, extended care facilities, and health maintenance organizations that receive federal funds. Because of this legislation, nurses in all settings routinely inquire about advance directives and facilitate communication about patients' wishes.

Many advocacy groups encourage all adults to establish advance directives and to make their wishes known to their families and health care providers regarding health care decisions, particularly end-of-life care issues. For example, the organization Aging With Dignity promotes the use of the *Five Wishes* document for use as an advance directive document (see the Resources section). The *Five Wishes* document addresses the following:

- Who you want to make care decisions for you when you cannot make them?
- What kind of medical treatment you want or not want?
- What is the level of comfort you want?
- How you want people to treat you?
- What you want your loved ones to know?

This document was introduced in 1997 with support from the Robert Wood Johnson Foundation and is now widely accepted in the United States as an advance directive. Even if the document does not meet state requirements for an advance directive, people can use it in conjunction with state-issued forms (Aging with Dignity, 2009).

Advance directive documents must be drawn up when the person is capable of understanding their intent, and they become effective only when the person lacks the capacity to make a particular health-related decision. Thus, it is imperative to address advance directives before the onset of any condition, such as dementia, that can affect functioning and cognitive abilities. Studies have found that the cognitive abilities required for competent medical decision-making capacity begin to decline even during early stages of dementia (Okonkwo et al., 2008). When the diagnosis of dementia has already been made, it is imperative that decision-making capacity be evaluated and documented specifically in relation to the task of executing advance directive documents (Mayo & Wallhagen, 2009).

All states and the District of Columbia have laws requiring all adults to have advance directive documents, but this issue is often overlooked. Although many studies cite a very low prevalence rate for advance planning documents, one study found that there has been a progressively upward trend, especially in long-term care facilities (Daaleman et al., 2009). Most states require a periodic update of the advance directives (e.g., every 5 to 7 years). State laws vary regarding the scope and other details (e.g., type of document included, conditions under which it applies) of advance directives, and not all states honor out-of-state advance directives. This policy is particularly problematic for older adults who travel between or reside in more than one state. Nurses need to have up-to-date information about their own state's legal requirements for advance directives, which is widely available in health care institutions. Common types of advance directives are discussed in the following sections.

Living Wills and Do Not Resuscitate (DNR) Orders

Living wills are legal documents whose purpose is to allow people to specify the type of medical treatment they would want or not want if they become incapacitated as a result of terminal illness. Living wills evolved as a component of the first right-to-die statute, which was enacted in 1976 in California. People must be competent to initiate a living will, and they can revoke or change it at any time. A major goal of living wills is to affirm the right of a person to refuse treatment, but they do not always specify the particular type of treatment that can be refused. In addition to expressing wishes about refusal of treatment, living wills may express the person's preferences about pain management, organ donation, place of death, and specific treatments he or she would want to receive.

A limitation of living will directives is that they apply only to situations in which the person is considered terminally ill, whereas advance directives apply to a broader range of circumstances (e.g., irreversible brain damage or temporary incapacity) that do not meet criteria for being a terminal illness, as previously discussed. Definitions of terminal illness are not always clear, and there may be disagreement about whether the person is terminally ill. In general, someone is considered to be terminally ill when a physician determines that his or her predictable life expectancy is 6 months or less. Some laws or policies require that two physicians document that the person is terminally ill.

Most states and the District of Columbia recognize the validity of living wills, but the scope and details of living wills differ from state to state. For example, some states require that living wills specifically address certain procedures, such as the withholding or withdrawal of artificial sustenance. Advocacy groups and health care professionals are encouraging all adults to draw up living wills and to take steps to ensure that all their health care providers have copies of these documents. For a membership fee, the United States Living Will Registry (listed in the Resources section) electronically stores living wills and health care proxy documents and provides immediate access to living will documents.

A **do not resuscitate (DNR) order** is a very specific type of medical directive that compels health care providers to refrain from cardiopulmonary resuscitation if the person is no longer breathing and has no heartbeat. Sometimes, families, as well as health care professionals, mistakenly associate DNR orders with directives to withhold other medical treatments. For example, they may raise questions about sending the person to a hospital or not requesting certain diagnostic or treatment procedures simply because a DNR order is in place. Thus, nurses have important roles in clarifying this document with the patient and the health care proxy so that additional and appropriate advance medical directives are in place to cover the circumstances that are most likely to arise.

Some states have enacted laws that allow variations of the DNR order, with the most common one being Comfort Care DNR (also called, DNR-Comfort Care, CC/DNR, or Comfort Care Only DNR). These legal interventions direct health care professionals (including emergency care workers and first responders) to provide designated comfort care measures but not resuscitative therapies (e.g., cardioversion, chest compression, artificial airway, resuscitative drugs, drugs to correct heart rhythm) if the person is in full respiratory or cardiac arrest or if the person is near this condition. Examples of comfort care measures that are defined in these documents are oxygen therapy, positioning, airway suctioning, pain medication, control of bleeding, and emotional support of patient and family. State procedures for implementing these documents usually require that they be signed by a primary care practitioner and encourage people to make sure these directives are readily available whenever they may be needed. Some states have also implemented identification procedures with the use of officially recognized bracelets, wallet cards, or other items.

In addition to focusing on the right to refuse treatments, medical directives address the person's desire for medical treatment that should be provided in certain circumstances. These directives can provide instructions about specific interventions, such as antibiotics, food and nutrition, and admission to the hospital. These documents afford reassurance to people who fear that treatments or pain control and comfort measures will not be provided when they are sick and cannot express their own wishes. Medical directives cannot guarantee that a medical intervention will be provided regardless of the circumstances; however, they provide legal assurance that the person's preferences will be considered. Because of the inability to predict medical treatments that might become available, and because of the changing health condition of the person executing the document, medical directives should be reviewed and updated periodically.

Durable Power of Attorney for Health Care

A **durable power of attorney for health care** is an advance directive that takes effect whenever someone cannot, for any reason, provide informed consent for health care treatment decisions. Because it enables a surrogate health care decision maker, also called a health care proxy (as previously discussed), to represent the person during any time of incapacity, it is often considered the most important advance directive. Like other powers of attorney, the durable power of attorney for health care must be initiated when the person is competent, and it takes effect only when the person is incapacitated. The document is used with other advance directives to provide the proxy with written guidelines stating the person's wishes on issues such as the termination of life support. It is imperative that the health care proxy has a copy of all advance directives and periodically discusses the person's wishes about medical treatments and end-of-life issues. Because language in advance directive documents can sometimes be vague, nurses should encourage older adults to discuss their wishes with their primary care provider, other health care workers, and their designated surrogate before a crisis develops.

LEGAL ISSUES SPECIFIC TO LONG-TERM CARE SETTINGS

As the regulator of Medicare and Medicaid programs, Congress is responsible for ensuring that dollars expended for health care are well spent. In response to public concern about the quality of care in nursing homes during the 1960s, Congress mandated an Institute of Medicine study entitled *Improving the Quality of Care in Nursing Homes,* which was published in 1986. Recommendations of the study included the increased use of registered nurses, the use of standardized resident assessments, and the implementation of training and certification for nurse's aides. Subsequently, the Nursing Home Reform Act was included as part of the **Omnibus Budget Reconciliation Act (OBRA) of 1987**. This legislation has had far-reaching consequences, including increased emphasis on residents' rights and quality of life and major initiatives to improve quality of care (as discussed in Chapter 6). The provisions of OBRA that apply to nursing homes were developed through joint efforts of the Health Care Financing Administration, the National Citizens Coalition for Nursing Home Reform, the American Association for Retired Persons, representatives from the long-term care industry, and health care professionals.

OBRA states that each resident in a long-term care facility is to be at his or her highest practicable level of physical, mental, and psychosocial well-being, and that the long-term care facility is to accomplish this goal in an atmosphere that emphasizes residents' rights. To assist facilities in accomplishing this task, OBRA mandates that all Medicaid- and Medicare-funded facilities use a standardized form, known as the **Minimum Data Set (MDS)** for Resident Assessment and Care Planning. This form includes a Resident Assessment Instrument (RAI), which is a structured, multidimensional resident assessment and problem identification system. OBRA requires that within 14 days of admission, and at least annually thereafter, nursing facility staff performs a comprehensive, interdisciplinary assessment of every resident. Also, a care plan must be developed from that assessment, with the goal of continually evaluating the resident's highest functional level and preventing any deterioration unless it is assessed and clearly documented as unavoidable. A primary responsibility of nurses is to ensure that the comprehensive assessment is performed at the appropriate times. Also, the nurse must ensure that the assessment tool is used as a basis for planning care that addresses

the changing needs of the resident. By October 1991, the RAI was being used in all Medicaid- and Medicare-funded nursing homes; in 1995, a second version of the MDS was developed to replace the first version.

In addition to addressing the development and documentation of care plans in nursing homes, OBRA strengthened the government oversight of nursing homes and addressed the many issues related to quality of care, which had been a focus of consumer advocacy groups since the 1970s. Improvements in nursing home care that have been attributed to the enactment of OBRA include decreased use of indwelling catheters, decreased prevalence of dehydration and pressure ulcers, increased presence of geriatricians and nurse practitioners, and reduced use of physical restraints and psychotropic drugs.

The **Nursing Home Residents' Bill of Rights** is one of the components of OBRA that has had the most far-reaching consequences for nursing home staff and residents. Under this provision, federal law requires that all residents of long-term care facilities are informed of their rights and that all long-term care facilities must have a mechanism in place for addressing complaints if residents think that their rights have been compromised. Moreover, facilities must post the Residents' Bill of Rights and the resources for investigating complaints in a prominent place. According to this law, "the resident has a right to a dignified existence, self-determination, and communication with and access to persons and services inside and outside the facility" (Code of Federal Regulations, Title 42, Section 483.10). Box 9-1 lists some of the rights explicitly defined by this bill. The National Long-Term Care Ombudsman program advocates for rights of residents of nursing homes, assisted-living facilities, and board and care homes and investigates complaints. This program is established under the Older American Act and is available in every part of the United States (see the Resources section for additional information).

ETHICAL ISSUES COMMONLY ADDRESSED IN GERONTOLOGICAL NURSING

Ethical Issues in Everyday Care of Older Adults

Although ethical issues are often associated with life-or-death situations, nurses are increasingly recognizing that many daily care issues related to patients' values, preferences, and quality of life involve ethical dilemmas. Nurses also deal with ethical decisions related to organizational issues, such as time constraints and limitations that interfere with the provision of best quality of care. Some questions posed by Burkhardt and Keegan (2009) in their discussion of holistic nursing ethics are as follows:

- Am I wise and courageous enough to perceive and respect others' differences and honor them as I honor my own beliefs?
- What does the patient want?
- Does the patient understand his or her choices?
- Is the patient being coerced?

Box 9-1 Some Rights of Nursing Home Residents

The Right to Be Fully Informed
- The right to daily communication in their language
- The right to assistance if they have a sensory impairment
- The right to be notified in advance of any plans to change their room or roommate
- The right to be fully informed of all services available and the charge for each service

The Right to Participate in Their Own Care
- The right to receive adequate and appropriate care
- The right to participate in planning their treatment, care, and discharge
- The right to refuse medications, treatments, and physical and chemical restraints
- The right to review their own record

The Right to Make Independent Choices
- The right to make personal choices, such as what to wear and how to spend their time
- The right to reasonable accommodation of their needs and preferences
- The right to participate in activities, both inside and outside the nursing home
- The right to organize and participate in a resident council

The Right to Privacy and Confidentiality
- The right to private and unrestricted communication with any person
- The right to privacy in treatment and in personal care activities
- The right to confidentiality regarding their medical, personal, or financial affairs

The Right to Dignity, Respect, and Freedom
- The right to be treated with the fullest measure of consideration, respect, and dignity
- The right to be free from mental and physical abuse
- The right to self-determination

The Right to Security of Possessions
- The right to manage their own financial affairs
- The right to be free from charge for services covered by Medicaid or Medicare

Rights During Transfers and Discharges
- The right to remain in the facility unless a transfer or discharge is necessary, appropriate, or required
- The right to receive a 30-day notice of transfer or discharge

The Right to Complain
- The right to present grievances without fear of reprisal
- The right to prompt efforts by the nursing home to resolve grievances

The Right to Visits
- The right to immediate access by their relatives
- The right to reasonable visits by organizations or individuals providing health, social, legal, or other services

Adapted from the U.S. Code of Federal Regulations, Title 42, Section 483.10.

- What does quality of life mean for this patient?
- How are others responding to the patient's perceptions of quality of life?
- Does having the technology always mean it should be used?

A process of **values clarification** is a tool that nurses can use to guide ethical decision making in everyday nursing practice. Values clarification is an ongoing process in which an individual increases his or her awareness of what is important and just—and why (Burkhardt & Keegan, 2009). Nurses apply this process to themselves in their professional roles and they also use it as a nursing intervention in their practice. Nurses can use values clarification to develop a "caring consciousness" that fosters a humanistic caring approach that is especially important for working with older adults (Gallagher-Lepak & Kubsch, 2009).

Ethical Issues Specific to Long-Term Care Settings

The increasing attention to quality of care in long-term care settings in recent years has led to more emphasis on autonomy, individual rights, and quality of life for residents (as discussed in Chapter 6). Ethical issues are often associated with these approaches because it is not always easy to balance needs of individual residents with those of others and the institution itself. Ethical issues also are associated with questions about safety versus freedom. For example, conflicts arise when a resident with a history of falls desires to walk freely around the facility, but staff members want to limit that person's activity to reduce the risk of falls. Additional examples of ethical decisions that nurses in long-term care settings commonly address include

- Using restrictive measures to address concerns about safety
- Restricting cigarette smoking
- Allowing residents to refuse treatments, social activities, and food or fluid
- Providing more care assistance than necessary because it is more time-efficient for the staff
- Scheduling resident care practices for the convenience of the staff rather than according to individual preferences
- Accommodating residents who wish to express sexual interests and activities.

Long-term care settings address these ethical issues by establishing policies and procedures that are based on best practices. An important nursing responsibility is to involve residents and their surrogate decision makers in developing a plan that is safe, individualized, and appropriate for addressing everyday ethical issues.

Ethical Issues Related to Artificial Nutrition and Hydration

Nurses who care for older adults whose health is at risk due to their limited ability to chew and swallow frequently address ethical issues about **artificial nutrition and hydration**, and these issues have become more controversial in recent years. Artificial nutrition and hydration refers to methods of bypassing the upper gastrointestinal to deliver nutritional substances. A percutaneous endoscopic gastrostomy (PEG) tube (sometimes referred to as a "feeding tube") is a surgically inserted tube that is used to deliver nutrients directly to the stomach. This procedure was initially developed in the 1980s for short-term use in pediatric patients, but it is now used for patients of all ages and conditions and is considered the most appropriate and common method for providing long-term enteral nutrition (Kuo, Rhodes, Mitchell, Mor, & Teno, 2009). In recent years, enteral nutrition has become widely recognized as a life-sustaining treatment that should be considered for patients who cannot meet their nutritional needs by mouth. PEG tubes are now commonly considered for people with dementia when their ability to safely chew and swallow becomes compromised. Studies have found that the prevalence rate for PEG tubes in nursing home residents with advanced cognitive impairment is between 18% and 34% nationally, with substantial state variation from 7.5% to 40% (Kuo et al., 2009). Two-thirds of nursing home residents who have PEG tubes have them inserted during a hospitalization for an acute illness for conditions such as pneumonia, dehydration, and dysphagia (Kuo et al., 2009).

Because enteral feeding has become such a commonly used life-sustaining treatment for people with advanced dementia, many studies have addressed safety, efficacy, and outcome issues associated with this intervention. A recent Cochrane review concluded that despite the large number of patients receiving this intervention, there is insufficient evidence of the benefits of enteral tube feeding for people with advanced dementia and data are lacking with regard to adverse effects (Sampson, Candy, & Jones, 2009). Many other studies and literature reviews conclude that the use of feeding tubes in patients with advanced dementia does not result in improved outcomes, such as the prevention of aspiration pneumonia and pressure sores (Delegge, 2009). Also, the position statement of the Board of the American Geriatrics Society states that feeding tubes are unlikely to provide medical benefits or improved comfort in patients with advanced dementia. Another consideration is that people who are still able to enjoy the sensation of food are deprived of that simple pleasure when feeding tubes are used.

Sometimes, the discussion about tube feeding is initiated because caregivers must provide considerable and time-consuming assistance with oral hydration and nutrition. Another reason for initiating discussion about tube feeding is concern about hunger and discomfort, which is typically associated with the poor intake that commonly occurs during advanced dementia. However, when patients with chronically declining conditions are impaired to the extent that their nutritional status is significantly affected, they are usually in the terminal stage. There is much research to support the view that withholding artificial hydration and nutrition at this stage is not associated with suffering as long as good oral care and desired sips of water are provided. One literature review concluded that artificial nutrition and hydration did not improve comfort or meet the objectives of reducing hunger or thirst (Suter, Rogers, & Strack, 2008).

Despite evidence to the contrary, families who make the decisions for cognitively impaired patients may have unrealistically optimistic expectations about benefits of a feeding tube. Thus, when families face complex decisions about feeding tubes, nurses are responsible for providing up-to-date information and answering questions about the advantages and disadvantages of artificial fluid and nutrition. They can teach families that assisting with feeding and providing the benefits of social interaction and enjoyment of food may be a more compassionate approach than using feeding tubes, even if caloric intake is reduced. In many situations, the appropriate intervention is "comfort feeding only," which ensures the person's comfort through an individualized feeding care plan (Palecek et al., 2010). Nurses also can facilitate referrals for evaluation and treatment by a speech therapist who can advise about swallowing and the safest and most effective ways of providing nutrients by mouth. Registered dieticians are another resource because they make recommendations on providing, withdrawing, or withholding nutrition for individual situations and they also serve as active members of institutional ethics committees (American Dietetic Association, 2008).

The American Nurses Association Code for Nurses emphasizes respect for all persons, which includes honoring their wishes regarding treatment decisions (American Nurses Association, 2001). In 2008, the Hospice and Palliative Nurses Association specifically addressed the issue of withholding and/or withdrawing life-sustaining therapies, including parenteral and enteral nutrition and hydration, in a position statement (Hospice and Palliative Care Nurses Association, 2009). Nurses can use this statement, which is summarized in Box 9-2, to guide them in their care of older adults and discussions with caregivers.

CULTURAL ASPECTS OF LEGAL AND ETHICAL ISSUES

In the United States, one major area of concern relative to the cultural aspects of legal and ethical issues is the need to accommodate people who do not speak English. Language barriers can significantly increase the difficulty of understanding advance directives and participating in complex decisions about treatment and other aspects of care. Even when advance directives are available in the person's primary language, it is difficult to communicate the intent of these documents when there are conflicting cultural views on decisions about health care choices. Interventions to address language barriers are discussed in Chapter 2. Nurses also can use the *Five Wishes* document, which is available in more than 20 languages, as a base for discussing advance directives (see Resources section).

Another major issue with regard to advance directives and decision making is that the PSDA and other legal requirements

---

Box 9-2 Position Statement of Hospice and Palliative Nurses Association: Withholding and/or Withdrawing Life-Sustaining Therapies

Every person with decision-making capacity has the right to initiate any medical therapy that offers reasonable probability of benefit and to withhold and/or withdraw any medical therapy.

Patients have the right to appoint a surrogate decision maker.

It is the duty of the health care team to honor any previously communicated advance directive, including those that appoint a surrogate decision maker if the patient loses decision-making capacity.

Patients who lack decisional capacity and who do not have a previously designated surrogate decision maker should have one named in accordance with state, local, and institutional regulations.

Parents/guardians have legal authority to make decisions regarding treatment for their children if they are younger than 18 years, and the parents/guardians are considered to have their child's best interest at heart.

All life-sustaining therapies may be withheld or withdrawn.

Palliative care nurses shall assist as needed to facilitate decision making and advocate care that is consistent with the stated wishes of the patient and his/her surrogates.

Source: Hospice and Palliative Nurses Association. (2009). Withholding and/or withdrawing life-sustaining therapies. *Journal of Hospice and Palliative Nursing, 11,* 131.

---

are strongly biased toward Anglo-centric cultures, and it is important to recognize that there are significant cultural differences with regard to patterns of decision making about medical interventions and health care services. A review of literature found that cultural groups with family-centered decision making or with less trust in health care professionals were less likely to have advance directives than groups that valued individual autonomy (Thomas et al., 2008). For example, some families may believe that it is a sign of respect to protect an elder from the burdens of receiving information about his or her health status, or from making decisions about medical interventions and long-term care plans. This attitude may be in conflict with that of health care professionals who believe that all competent adults are entitled to information about their own health. Thus, nurses need to identify and accept individual and family decision-making preferences when they discuss advance directives and other aspects of health care decisions.

It is crucial to be sensitive to cultural differences when discussing not only advance directives but also all end-of-life issues. Many studies have found that African Americans are more reluctant than other groups to accept hospice services or complete advance directives, and some studies have attempted to identify reasons for this. Johnson, Kuchibhatia, and Tulsky (2008) explored this issue and found that these differences were associated with a combination of beliefs and values, including greater preferences for life-sustaining therapies, less comfort discussing death, greater distrust of the health care system, and spiritual beliefs that conflicted with goals of hospice care. Another study concluded that African American nursing home residents would benefit from discussions within their families and cultural communities about

A Student's Perspective

In working with "G.," an 82-year-old Chinese woman, I have learned a lot about her background. She and her three brothers, two sisters, and parents were all born in China. Her parents moved the children to Jakarta, a city in Indonesia, which was a Dutch colony at the time, to get a better education. Chinese culture emphasizes respect for elders, especially the father, who is head of the family. G. giggles and comments, "When father said 'eat that,' we ate it, whether we liked it or not." As an adult, she worked for a time in the front lobby of the U.S. embassy as a translator. Her position led her on many journeys throughout the world, working in Russia, Germany, France, and eventually to the United States. G. didn't marry until she was 70, when she married an American. She now lives in a quiet neighborhood with her husband.

A difficulty in learning more about G. and her culture regarding health care has been her acceptance of her disease process. Her cultural background taught her to view authority figures, such as physicians, with incredible esteem. Until I learned more about her culture, I wasn't always certain she understood what was being said because she would sit with her head down and only nod, or simply say, "yes." I now realize those behaviors are her way of showing respect to an authority figure. She seldom looks you in the eye, another form of showing respect. She is also hesitant to ask questions so as not to appear disrespectful. G. looks to her husband many times to make decisions for her.

Deborah L.

goals of end-of-life care (Ott, 2008). Other studies also have concluded that improved communication by culturally competent health care providers about end-of-life care is an intervention for addressing racial and ethnic disparities in the completion of advance directives (Ko & Lee, 2009; Reynolds, Hanson, Henderson, & Steinhauser, 2008; Rich, Gruber-Baldini, Quinn, & Zimmerman, 2009).

Cultural Considerations 9-1 summarizes some cultural considerations related to legal and ethical aspects of gerontological nursing care.

ROLE OF NURSES REGARDING LEGAL AND ETHICAL ISSUES

Nurses have important roles with regard to implementing advance directives and facilitating decisions about care. Although these issues are often addressed within the context of a multidisciplinary team and always with the primary care practitioner, nurses have unique and important responsibilities, which are reviewed in the following sections.

Implementing Advance Directives

Evidence-based guidelines emphasize the importance of communication and education by nurses to facilitate completion of advance directives and to dispel myths and misperceptions about these documents (Mitty & Ramsey, 2008). Studies have

CULTURAL CONSIDERATIONS 9-1

Cultural Considerations Related to Legal and Ethical Aspects of Care

Cultural Factors That Influence Ethical Decision Making

- The intent of advance directives is based on Western values of individual autonomy, but many cultures believe that the fate of human beings is beyond their control.
- Values of filial piety and respect for authority of one's elders—rather than the model of individual autonomy—guide decisions about care in traditional Asian cultures.
- In collectivist cultures (e.g., the Xhosa tribe in South Africa), tribal elders make decisions about care of their members, based on distribution of human and material resources.
- Traditional Chinese and many other cultures rely on family members and their physicians to make decisions, rather than expecting to receive information and being involved in decision making.
- Ethnoreligious groups, including Jews, Muslims, and Hindus, are likely to base end-of-life decisions on their beliefs on the sanctity of life.
- Religious beliefs may take precedence over scientific reasoning (e.g., opposition of blood transfusions as a life-saving measure by members of Jehovah's Witnesses).
- Some groups may prefer their own religious and spiritually based healing practices to those of scientific medicine (e.g., Christian scientists) (Pacquiao, 2008).

Cultural Considerations Related to Ethical and Legal Issues in Specific Groups

- *African Americans:* It is important to include women and extended family members in decision making and dissemination health information.
- *Amish:* Grandparents and other extended family are involved with health care decisions, which are based on consideration of the type of health problem, accessibility of health care services, and perceived cost of the care.
- *Appalachian:* Individuals may abdicate self-responsibility for decision making and prefer that physicians take charge of their care completely.
- *Arab:* Older males assume decision-making roles; most patients expect physicians to select treatments.
- *Bosnian:* Health care providers need to give detailed explanations of tests and procedures; trust is a major issue.
- *Chinese:* Each family has a recognized male head who has great authority and assumes all major responsibilities.
- *Cuban:* Traditional patriarchal family structure is the most important social unit and the primary spokesperson needs to be involved in decision making.
- *European American:* There is great variation among families, but high value is generally placed on egalitarian relationships and decision making;

advance directives allow patients to specify their wishes and designate a decision maker.
- *Filipino:* Because planning for one's death is taboo, many are adverse to discussing advance directives or living wills.
- *German:* Extended family should be included in decision making.
- *Greek:* Older people hold positions of respect; extended nuclear family members should be included in decision making.
- *Haitian:* The family council, composed of influential family members, is an important unit for decision making.
- *Hindu:* The patriarchal joint family, based on the principle of superiority of men over women, is the primary authority for decisions.
- *Hmong:* Traditional decision making requires that the male head of the family or clan make decisions for family members; individuals do not have the right to make their own decisions about health care.
- *Iranian:* The father and/or older male siblings have authority to make decisions for family.
- *Irish:* Families make end-of-life decisions and these are usually influenced by all the following: their definition of extraordinary means, financial considerations, quality of life, and effects on the family.
- *Italian:* Traditional families recognize the father's absolute authority and they accept his decisions as law.
- *Japanese:* Discussion of serious illness and death is taboo, so it is difficult to obtain information.
- *Jewish:* Rabbis may be included in making decisions about health care (e.g., organ donation or transplant).
- *Korean:* Older adults are frequently consulted on important family matters as a sign of respect for their experience.
- *Mexican:* Families are not necessarily patriarchal, but men are expected to be the spokesperson for the family, so it is important to ask who makes which decisions.
- *Navajo Indian:* Tribes are matrilineal, with the grandmothers and mothers at the center of decision making.
- *Puerto Rican:* Adults, especially women, may prefer to consult with close family members before making health care decisions.
- *Russian:* It is important to ask clients whom they want to include in medical decisions because extended family is very important.
- *Somali:* Discussing advance directives and end-of-life care is taboo because faithful Muslims believe that Allah will determine how long a person will live; thus, these issues should be addressed indirectly.
- *Turkish:* Traditional families are patriarchal but less traditional ones are more egalitarian, so it is important to identify the family spokesperson and accept decision-making patterns without judgment.
- *Vietnamese:* Women often make family health care decisions.

(*Source:* Purnell, L. D. [2009]. *Guide to culturally competent health care* [2nd ed.]. Philadelphia, PA: F. A. Davis Co.)

found that older adults are very comfortable with their health care providers initiating a discussion of advance directives and, in fact, view this discussion as a way of being in charge of end-of-life care (Jackson, Roinick, Asche, & Heinrich, 2009). Health care professionals need to understand that communication about advance directives is a long-term process that begins with listening, occurs periodically, and incorporates discussions about personal values and goals of care (Messinger-Rapport, Baum, & Smith, 2009). In addition to working directly with older adults and their caregivers, nurses have a key role in ensuring that documents are readily accessible to health care providers (Alfonso, 2009). All health care providers should know what advance directives cover. When

they care for people over long periods, they should periodically review and discuss the documents with the older adult or his or her proxy. In addition, nurses should encourage people to provide copies of advance directives to their family members, designated surrogate, and anyone likely to be involved with decisions about their medical care. When written advance directives do not exist, nurses can initiate a discussion of relevant medical care and end-of-life treatment preferences and document any statements made that express a patient's wishes.

Another role for nurses is addressing barriers to effective implementation of advance directives. Studies have found that the perception of advance directives as irrelevant and the need for information from health care professionals are two major barriers to implementation of advance directives (Hirschman, Kapi, & Karlawish, 2008; Schickedanz et al., 2009). A meta-analysis of studies that looked at interventions for addressing barriers found that the provision of verbal information over multiple sessions was the most successful intervention (Bravo, Dubois, & Wagneur, 2008). Nurses are in key positions to address these barriers by initiating discussions with and providing educational materials to older adults and their caregivers. Evidence-based guidelines emphasize that "nurses in virtually every kind of health care delivery setting can take the initiative to review the document with patients annually and in the event of a significant change of condition" (Mitty & Ramsey, 2008, p. 551). By integrating this teaching into their usual care, nurses can communicate that advance directives are an important tool for maintaining autonomy and ensuring that one's wishes are honored.

Facilitating Decisions About Care

Nurses play key roles not only in implementing advance directives but also in working with family members and other caregivers who are involved with making decisions related to care and treatment issues. Advance directives designate surrogate decision makers, but the surrogates do not always have a good understanding of the person's wishes and this can be a barrier to appropriate implementation. Studies have found that family surrogates feel burdened when they need to make end-of-life decisions, and this perception of burden is compounded when they are uncertain about the patient preferences (Braun, Beyth, Ford, & McCullough, 2008). Nurses and other health care professionals need to facilitate discussions about advance directives between older adults and their surrogate decision makers because this can improve the chance that their preferences will be understood and honored (Glass & Nahapetyan, 2008; Moorman & Carr, 2008). Nurses facilitate these discussions by providing accurate information on rights and statutes, addressing questions about care options, listening to the needs and concerns of all involved, attending to concerns about end-of-life care, and acting as liaisons with primary care providers when necessary.

As discussed previously, decisions about care are particularly complicated when working with older adults who have cognitive impairments. Evidence-based guidelines for nurses

---

Box 9-3   Model for Facilitating Decisions About the Care of People With Dementia

Step I: Assess the Decision-Making Situation
- What is the decision-making ability of the person with dementia?
- What are the typical decision-making patterns in the family?
- Who influences the decision making, either directly or indirectly?
- How do family relationships help or hinder the decision-making process?
- Are there patterns of passive nondecisions as well as active decisions?
- What is each person's perception of the situation?
- How objective are the perceptions of the various decision makers?
- What does each person in the decision-making process have to gain or lose based on various decisions?

Step II: Obtain Consensus About Problems and Needs
- Have each person involved with the care describe the problems and needs from their perspective.
- Provide additional assessment information about the needs of the person with dementia.
- Address the needs of the caregivers as well as the needs of the person with dementia.
- Summarize the identified needs of the older adult and the caregivers.

Step III: Discuss Potential Resources
- Ask caregivers to suggest potential solutions and resources.
- Identify resources for the caregivers' needs as well as for those of the person with dementia.
- Supplement the family's knowledge about resources and potential solutions.
- Discuss the positive and negative consequences of each option for the person with dementia and for the caregivers.
- As the family members discuss solutions, assess their attitudes about using various services and spending family resources to purchase services.

- Provide information about the long-range benefits that the caregivers might not perceive.
- Summarize important points on paper or a blackboard for all participants to review.

Step IV: Agree on a Plan of Action
- Obtain agreement about the most appropriate actions to take.
- Emphasize the fact that any plan of action will be given a trial period and should not be viewed as a permanent decision.
- Suggest a time frame and criteria for evaluating the plan of action.
- Identify one or two people who will evaluate the plan and make appropriate changes.

Step V: Involve the Person With Dementia
- Discuss the ability of the person with dementia to understand the decision.
- Identify the most realistic level of involvement for the person with dementia.
- Identify the best approach to take in involving the person with dementia.
- Identify the roles of caregivers and professionals in assisting the person with dementia to understand the decision.

Step VI: Summarize the Plan and Clarify Roles
- Review and summarize the plan of action.
- Have the caregivers state their roles in very specific terms.
- Clarify the role of the nurse and other professionals.
- Assure caregivers that you will be available for further discussion and problem solving, or provide the name of someone who can assume this role.

summarize the following nursing care strategies for health care decision making (Mitty & Post, 2008):

1. Communicate with patient, family, and surrogate decision makers to improve their understanding of treatment options.
2. Be sensitive to racial, ethnic, religious, and cultural influences with regard to care decisions, disclosure of information, and end-of-life planning.
3. Be aware of available resources for conflict resolution.
4. Assess and document the patient's ability to state preferences, follow directions, make simple choices, and communicate consistent care wishes.
5. Assess and document fluctuations in patient's mental status and factors that affect it.
6. Assess the patient's understanding specifically in relation to a particular decision (e.g., ask what the patient understands about the risks and benefits of the intervention).
7. Use appropriate decision aids.
8. Help the patient express what he or she understands about the clinical situation and the potential outcomes.
9. Help the patient identify who should participate in discussions and decisions.

Another important role of nurses is to involve other professionals and support resources when complex decisions must be made or when the decision makers seek additional help. In some settings, an interdisciplinary team—composed of a social worker, a religious leader, therapists, nurses, and a primary care provider—may provide information and support to proxy decision makers. Decision-making assistance from professionals may relieve families and proxy decision makers of some of the guilt they could experience when making and implementing decisions, particularly difficult end-of-life decisions. Hospitals and long-term care facilities that are accredited by the Joint Commission (formerly the Joint Commission on Accreditation of Healthcare Organizations [JCAHO]) are required to have ethics committees that provide a formal mechanism for addressing medical ethical dilemmas within their institutions. Nurses also take a strong role in supporting and facilitating decisions about care during chronic conditions and end-of-life care. In particular, nurses provide information about the best types of services (e.g., hospice programs, palliative care) or place of care (e.g., hospital admission for nursing home residents when medical problems arise). Box 9-3 summarizes a nursing model for facilitating decisions about long-term care for people with dementia. Some of the many excellent health education that are available for nurses and consumers about advance directives and ethical decisions are listed on thePoint (see Resources section for more information).

Chapter Highlights

Autonomy and Rights
- Autonomy is the personal freedom to direct one's own life as long as it does not infringe on the rights of others.
- Adults have the right to make health-related decisions unless they have been declared incompetent by a judge.
- If an adult's decision-making capacity is questionable, his or her rights can be protected through legal documents, such as advance directives.

Advance Directives
- Legal documents (e.g., living wills, DNR orders) make a person's wishes relative to medical treatments known to care providers and surrogate decision makers.
- Nurses play an important role in making sure these documents are available and their instructions are followed.

Legal Issues Specific to Long-Term Care Settings
- Since the federal government enacted OBRA legislation in the 1980s, nursing homes are required to meet certain standards of care and to document assessments and care plans.
- Positive consequences of OBRA in nursing homes include decreased use of indwelling catheters, reduced use of physical and chemical restraints, and fewer cases of dehydration and pressure ulcers.
- The Nursing Home Bill of Rights states that residents are entitled to dignity, self-determination, and the opportunity to communicate.
- Autonomy issues are frequently addressed by nurses in long-term care settings; balancing the rights of residents with institutional needs often poses a challenge.

Ethical Issues Commonly Addressed in Gerontological Nursing
- Values clarification is a tool that nurses can use as they address ethical issues in everyday care of older adults.
- Nurses are often involved in decisions about artificial hydration and nutrition.
- Assisting with care decisions during chronic illness is one of the most challenging aspects of nursing.

Cultural Aspects of Legal and Ethical Issues
- Language barriers are important to consider when discussing advance directives.
- Nurses should identify culturally influenced patterns of decision making when discussing advance directives and end-of-life care with patients and their families.

Role of Nurses Regarding Legal and Ethical Issues
- Nurses communicate with older adults about advance directives, inform other members of the health care team about advance directives, and address barriers to implementing advance directives.
- Nurses facilitate decision making about advance directives by providing information about advance directives and care options to older adults and to proxy decision makers.

Critical Thinking Exercises

1. You have been assigned to work with Mrs. M., an 85-year-old, white, widowed woman who is in the hospital with congestive heart failure. Her son and daughter tell you that

they would like to arrange for her to be discharged to a nursing home because they don't think she takes her medications correctly, and they are tired of her being admitted to the hospital every couple of months "to get her straightened out." The son and daughter live in another state and visit only when their mother is in the hospital. Mrs. M. has told you that she thinks her son and daughter would like to have her "put away in one of those homes" but she is adamantly opposed to leaving her home. She also has told you that they think she is "senile" and that she should stop driving her car, but she thinks she is quite capable of living alone, driving her car, and taking care of herself. Your observations are that she needs a lot of direction to take medications and participate in self-care activities, and she seems to be somewhat confused later in the day. What steps would you take to address her competency and decision-making abilities?

2. A Mexican American woman, 78 years old, is being admitted to the hospital with hemiplegia after a stroke. There are no advance directives on her chart. What information would you want to know before you approached her about a living will and durable power of attorney for health care? How would you explain these documents to her?

3. Mr. S. is 78 years old and has been admitted for hip surgery after a fall-related fracture. He has had dementia for 5 years and his family provides care for him in his home. His son is his durable power of attorney for health care, but he will not make any decisions unless his three sisters agree to them. Mr. S. does not have any other advance directives and the family says he never talked much about what medical care services he would want. He always told his family that they could make whatever decisions are best for him. The physician has asked the family to consider placement of a PEG tube because Mr. S.'s food and fluid intake are inadequate to meet his needs and one pressure area is beginning to develop on his buttocks. Mr. S.'s son and one daughter think that their father would have wanted to have every intervention possible in such a situation, and they think the PEG tube will improve his comfort and prevent the pressure ulcer. The other two daughters adamantly state that their father would never agree to such an invasive procedure and they are not sure it will make him any more comfortable. They also worry about complications from having the tube. You are a member of the multidisciplinary team that is meeting with the family to help them come to a decision about a PEG tube. What points would you want to make during this family conference?

Resources

For links to these resources and additional helpful Internet resources related to this chapter, visit thePoint at http://thePoint. lww.com/Miller6e.

Clinical Tools

Consumer's Tool Kit for Health Care Advance Planning
American Bar Association Commission on Law and Aging

Evidence-Based Practice

Mitty, E. L., & Post, L. F. (2008). Health care decision making. In E. Capezuti, D. Zwicker, M. Mezey, & T. Fulmer (Eds.), *Evidence-Based Geriatric Nursing Protocols for Best Practice* (3rd ed., pp. 521–538). New York: Springer Publishing Co.
Mitty, E. L., & Ramsey, G. C. (2008). Advance Directives. In E. Capezuti, D. Zwicker, M. Mezey, & T. Fulmer (Eds.), *Evidence-Based Geriatric Nursing Protocols for Best Practice* (3rd ed., pp. 539–563). New York: Springer Publishing Co.

Health Education

AARP
Aging With Dignity
American Association of Colleges of Nursing, End-of-Life Nursing Education
Consortium Project (ELNEC)
American Bar Association Commission on Law and Aging
American Bar Association, Senior Lawyers Division
American Nurses Association, Center for Ethics & Human Rights
National Long-Term Care Ombudsman Program
National Senior Citizens Law Center
United States Living Will Registry

REFERENCES

Alfonso, H. (2009). The importance of living wills and advance directives. *Journal of Gerontological Nursing, 35*(10), 42–45.
American Dietetic Association. (2008). Position of the American Dietetic Association: Ethical and legal issues in nutrition, hydration, and feeding. *Journal of the American Dietetic Association, 108*(5), 873–882.
American Nurses Association. (2001). *Code for Nurses with Interpretive Statements.* Kansas City, MO: American Nurses Association.
Beattie, E. (2009). Research participation of individuals with dementia. *Research in Gerontological Nursing, 2*(2), 94–102.
Braun, U. K., Beyth, R. J., Ford, M. E., & McCullough, L. B. (2008). Voices of African American, Caucasian, and Hispanic surrogates on the burdens of end-of-life decision making. *Journal of General Internal Medicine, 23*(3), 267–274.
Bravo, G., Dubois, M. F., & Wagneur, B. (2008). Assessing the effectiveness of interventions to promote advance directives among older adults: A systematic review and multi-level analysis. *Social Science and Medicine, 67*(7), 1122–1132.
Burkhardt, M. A., & Keegan, L. (2009). Holistic ethics. In B. M. Dossey & L. Keegan (Eds.), *Holistic nursing: A handbook for practice* (5th ed., pp. 125–137). Boston, MA: Jones and Bartlett Publishers.
Carroll, D. W. (2010). Assessment of capacity for medical decision making. *Journal of Gerontological Nursing, 36*(5), 47–52.
Collopy, B. J. (1988). Autonomy in long term care: Some crucial distinctions. *The Gerontologist, 28*(Suppl.), 10–17.
Daaleman, T. P., Williams, C. S., Preisser, J. S., Sloane, P. D., Biola, H., & Zimmerman, S. (2009). Advance care planning in nursing homes and assisted living communities. *American Medical Directors Association, 10*, 243–251.
Delegge, M. H. (2009). Tube feeding in patients with dementia: Where are we? *Nutrition in Clinical Practice: Official Publication of the American Society for Parenteral and Enteral Nutrition, 24*(2), 214–216.
Gallagher-Lepak, S., & Kubsch, S. (2009). Transpersonal caring, a nursing practice guideline. *Holistic Nursing Practice, 23*(3), 171–182.
Glass, A. P., & Nahapetyan, L. (2008). Discussions by elders and adult children about end-of-live preparation and preferences. *Preventing Chronic Disease Public Health Research, Practice, and Policy, 5*(1), 1–8.
Hirschman, K. B., Kapi, J. M., & Karlawish, J. H. T. (2008). Identifying the factors that facilitate or hinder advance planning by persons with dementia. *Alzheimer Disease and Associated Disorders, 22*(3), 293–298.

Hospice and Palliative Nurses Association. (2009). HPNA Position Paper: Withholding and/or withdrawing life-sustaining therapies. *Journal of Hospice and Palliative Nursing, 11*, 131–132.

Jackson, J. M., Roinick, S. J., Asche, S. E., & Heinrich, R. L. (2009). Knowledge, attitudes, and preferences regarding advance directives among patients of a managed care organization. *The American Journal of Managed Care, 15*(3), 177–186.

Johnson, K. S., Kuchibhatia, M., & Tulsky, J. A. (2008). What explains racial differences in the use of advance directives and attitudes toward hospice care? *Journal of the American Geriatrics Society, 56*(10), 1953–1958.

Ko, E., & Lee, J. (2009). End-of-life communication: Ethnic differences between Korean American and non-Hispanic white older adults. *Aging and Health, 21*(7), 967–984.

Kuo, S., Rhodes, R. L., Mitchell, S. L., Mor, V., & Teno, J. M. (2009). Natural History of feeding-tube use in nursing home residents with advanced dementia. *Journal of American Medical Directors Association, 10*, 264–270.

Malcomson, H., & Bisbee, S. (2009). Perspectives of healthy elders on advance care planning. *Journal of the American Academy of Nurse Practitioners, 21*(1), 18–23.

Mayo, A. M., & Wallhagen, M. I. (2009). Considerations of informed consent and decision-making competence in older adults with cognitive impairment. *Research in Gerontological Nursing, 2*(2), 103–110.

Messinger-Rapport, B. J., Baum, E. E., & Smith, M. L. (2009). Advance care planning: Beyond the living will. *Cleveland Clinic Journal of Medicine, 76*(5), 276–285.

Mitty, E. L., & Post, L. F. (2008). Health care decision making. In E. Capezuti, D. Zwicker, M. Mezey, & T. Fulmer (Eds.), *Evidence-based geriatric nursing protocols for best practice* (3rd ed., pp. 521–538). New York: Springer Publishing Co.

Mitty, E. L., & Ramsey, G. C. (2008). Advance directives. In E. Capezuti, D. Zwicker, M. Mezey, & T. Fulmer (Eds.), *Evidence-based geriatric nursing protocols for best practice* (3rd ed., pp. 539–563). New York: Springer Publishing Co.

Moorman, S. M., & Carr, D. (2008). Spouses' effectiveness as end-of-life health care surrogates: Accuracy, uncertainty, and errors of overtreatment or undertreatment. *The Gerontologist, 48*(6), 811–819.

Okonkwo, O. C., Griffith, H. R., Copeland, J. N., Belue, K., Lanza, S., Zamrini, E. Y., . . . Marson D. C. (2008). Medical decision-making

capacity in mild cognitive impairment, a 3-year longitudinal study. *Neurology, 71*, 1474–1480.

Ott, B. B. (2008). Views of African American nursing home residents about living wills. *Geriatric Nursing, 29*(2), 117–124.

Pacquiao, D. F. (2008). Cultural competence in ethical decision-making. In M. M. Andrews & J. S. Boyle (Eds.), *Transcultural concepts in nursing care* (5th ed., pp. 408–423). Philadelphia, PA: Lippincott Williams & Wilkins.

Palecek, E. J., Teno, J. M., Casarett, D. J., Hanson, L. C. Rhodes, R. L., & Mitchell, S. L. (2010). Comfort feeding only: A proposal to bring clarity to decision-making regarding difficulty with eating for persons with advanced dementia. *Journal of the American Geriatrics Society, 58*, 580–584.

Reynolds, K. S., Hanson, L. C., Henderson, M., & Steinhauser, K. E. (2008). End-of-life care in nursing home settings: Do race or age matter? *Palliative and Support Care, 6*(1), 21–27.

Rich, S. E., Gruber-Baldini, A. L., Quinn, C. C., & Zimmerman, S. I. (2009). Discussion as a factor in racial disparity in advance directive completion at nursing home admission. *Journal of American Geriatric Society, 57*(1), 146–152.

Sampson, E. L., Candy, B., & Jones, L. (2009). Enteral tube feeding for older people with advanced dementia. *Cochrane Database of Systematic Reviews (online), (2)*, CD007209.

Schickedanz, A. D., Schillinger, D., Landefeld, C. S., Knight, S. J., Williams, B. A., & Sudore, R. L. (2009). A clinical framework for improving the advance care planning process: start with patients' self-identified barriers. *Journal of American Geriatric Society, 57*(1), 31–39.

Suter, P. M., Rogers, J., & Strack, C. (2008). Artificial Nutrition and Hydration for the terminally ill, a reasoned approach. *Home Health Care Nurse, 26*(1), 23–29.

Tallahassee, F. L. (2009). Aging with dignity. *Five wishes*. Retrieved from www.agingwithdignity.org/five-wishes.php

Thomas, R., Wilson, D. M., Justice, C., Birch, S., & Sheps, S. (2008). A literature review of preferences for end-of-life care in developed countries by individuals with different cultural affiliations and ethnicity. *Journal of Hospice and Palliative Nursing, 10*(3), 142–160.

Walaszek, A. (2009). Clinical ethics issues in geriatric psychiatry. *Psychiatric Clinics of North America, 32*(209), 343–359.

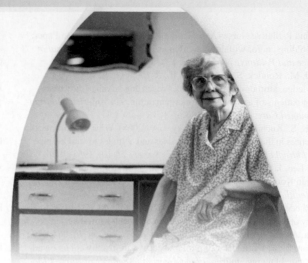

CHAPTER **10**

Elder Abuse and Neglect

LEARNING OBJECTIVES

After reading this chapter, you will be able to:

1. Define the various types of elder abuse.
2. Identify risk factors that contribute to elder abuse and neglect.
3. Describe nursing assessment aimed toward identifying elder abuse and neglect as well as risks for abuse and neglect.
4. Describe the nurse's opportunities for interventions for elder abuse in different practice settings.
5. Discuss the range of nursing and legal interventions directed toward preventing and alleviating elder abuse.

KEY POINTS

abandonment

adult protective services
  law

domestic violence

emotional (psychological)
  abuse

neglect

physical abuse

self-abuse

self-neglect

sexual abuse

Certain members of any population are vulnerable to abuse and **neglect** by virtue of being physically or psychosocially impaired or subjugated. In industrialized societies today, vulnerable groups are protected and cared for through legislative mandates and social programs. In the United States and many other countries, for example, children and people with developmental disabilities have been protected for many decades.

OVERVIEW OF ELDER ABUSE AND NEGLECT

In recent decades, additional groups have been recognized as needing protection: victims of **domestic violence** and abused or neglected older people. Although the problem of abused or neglected older adults is not new, elder abuse has received increased attention as a social problem.

Characteristics of Elder Abuse

Definitions of elder abuse have changed over time in response to shifts in political climate, public sentiment, available funding, and increasing knowledge and professional interest. This section discusses widely recognized characteristics of elder abuse and the following section discusses the historical recognition of elder abuse.

The National Research Council (2003, p. 1) defines elder mistreatment as "(a) Intentional actions that cause harm or create a serious risk of harm, whether or not intended, to a vulnerable elder by a caregiver or other person who stands in a trust relationship to the elder, or (b) failure by a care-giver to satisfy the elder's basic needs or to protect the elder from harm." This definition was developed to address the historic ambiguities over what constitutes elder abuse and to foster empirical investigation of the subject using comparable research design. Although an admirable goal, the definition does not address issues identified by clinicians and evident in state statutes (Pillemer et al., in press).

The National Center on Elder Abuse (2009b) recognizes three basic categories of elder abuse (i.e., domestic elder abuse, institutional elder abuse, and **self-neglect** or **self-abuse**) and seven major types or forms (i.e., **physical abuse, sexual abuse**, emotional or psychological abuse, neglect, **abandonment**, financial or material exploitation, and self-neglect). Self-neglect in this classification includes behaviors of older adults that threaten their health or safety (National Center on Elder Abuse, 2009a).

Internationally, the concept of elder abuse has almost unlimited boundaries, as evidenced by the United Nations Second World Assembly on Aging (United Nations Economic and Social Council, 2002). This World Assembly viewed elder abuse as encompassing virtually anything that causes harm or distress to an older person and that occurs in a relationship with a trust expectation. This includes acts as wide ranging as direct forms of aggression to denial of dignity to older people (United Nations Economic and Social Affairs,

2008). Other examples of ever-expanding views of elder abuse include newspaper articles depicting older disaster victims as suffering from elder abuse and legal services advertisements labeling compromised quality of care in long-term care facilities as elder abuse.

Efforts are currently underway to provide greater clarity to the meaning and dimensions of elder abuse. Conrad (2009), for example, has applied sophisticated research methods, such as concept mapping, to financial exploitation. After national and local groups of elder abuse experts identified relevant statements for the construct, the statements were sorted, rated, and depicted as conceptual maps. Then focus groups of practitioners and older adult service consumers reviewed these items, and elder abuse victims refined them before the items were subjected to tests of validity and reliability. The resulting older adult financial exploitation measure is intended to aid in the assessment of the problem by both clinicians and researchers.

Historical Recognition of a Social Problem

Awareness of elder abuse as a social problem began in the 1950s and 1960s as the writings of Geneva Mathiasen and Gertrude Hall introduced the concept of protecting vulnerable adults. Centers such as the Benjamin Rose Institute in Cleveland, Ohio, developed the concept in the early 1970s through initial demonstration projects, usually specifically related to self-neglect. Awareness of physical abuse, however, did not surface until the late 1970s, and awareness of other types of elder abuse followed. The late 1980s witnessed the growing criminalization of elder abuse, a movement that continues through today. With it, consumer fraud aimed at older adults, including scams and con games, was subsumed under elder abuse. Concurrently, recognition of domestic violence in later life as an elder abuse form served to shift the practice paradigm to empowering victims and holding perpetrators accountable.

The 1990s brought the medicalization of elder abuse, with physicians increasingly dominating problem intervention, sometimes with a criminal justice twist, as in the establishment of forensic centers and markers related to elder abuse. In this context, too, elder abuse has come to be seen as a public health matter, with interventions assuming a prevention lens. Finally, elder abuse has become a global concern. First recognized in the United States, Great Britain, and Canada, elder abuse became an international problem by the late 1990s, as evidenced by the establishment of the International Network for the Prevention of Elder Abuse in 1997 and its World Elder Abuse Awareness Day in 2006, an event commemorated in countries worldwide every year since.

Reports of elder abuse are increasing, and it is now recognized as a major social and health problem and a significant aspect of family violence. This increasing attention can be attributed to reasons such as the following:
- The older adult population has been increasing rapidly, with the most vulnerable groups of older people (i.e., those who are 85 years of age and older) increasing at the fastest rate.
- Adult children increasingly are called upon to care for their elderly parents; however, some lack the capacity, skills, resources, availability, or physical proximity to undertake this responsibility successfully.
- Researchers and clinicians are directing more attention to the problems that affect the most vulnerable older adults, leading to more information and publications.
- Educational efforts have made professionals and the public more aware of reporting laws and adult protective services.
- Congressional hearings and educational programs have stimulated public and professional interest in the issue.
- Organizations, such as the National Committee for the Prevention of Elder Abuse and the National Adult Protective Services Association, have promoted professional networking and advocated for public policy addressing elder abuse.

Gerontological nurses have been in the forefront of research, publications, and practice innovations in elder abuse. Nursing journals have featured articles on elder abuse since the 1970s and, clinically oriented nursing texts on elder abuse have been coauthored by nurses since the 1980s. Since the mid-1980s, nursing has been represented in the field of elder abuse through the research of such scholars as Terry Fulmer, Linda Phillips, and Elizabeth Podnieks. Nurses also have developed important clinical tools and protocols, particularly in the areas of screening and assessment.

Prevalence and Causes

Elder abuse is neither a rare nor an isolated phenomenon in the United States or elsewhere. Rather, all indicators suggest that maltreatment of vulnerable older adults is widespread and occurs among all subgroups. Although estimates of elder abuse range generally from 2% to 10% for the United States (National Research Council, 2003) and 3% to 28% worldwide (Cooper, Selwood, & Livingston, 2008), it is difficult to be confident about the accuracy of these estimates because of significant underreporting and differing definitions of elder abuse and neglect. Studies suggest that most maltreatment is repeated, is seldom reported to authorities, and represents more than one form of abuse.

Two recent nationally representative elder abuse prevalence studies suggest high rates overall and for particular forms. Laumann, Leitsch, and Waite (2008) asked a sample of 3005 community-dwelling adults aged 57 to 85 years about any recent experience of verbal, financial, or physical mistreatment. Nine percent of respondents reported verbal, 3.5% financial, and 0.2% physical mistreatment by a family member in the past year. Acierno (2009) surveyed an even larger sample (5777 adults aged 60 years and older) about recent mistreatment across five forms: neglect as well as emotional, physical, sexual, and financial abuse. The results suggested that about 1 in 10 community-dwelling, cognitively intact older adults experienced neglect or emotional, physical, or sexual abuse during the past year. The rate increased to 1 in 7 when financial exploitation was included. Among the various abuse forms, financial exploitation and emotional abuse were the most common and sexual abuse the least.

Although the problem can affect any older person, the typical reported elder abuse victim is a socially isolated and physically or cognitively impaired woman of advanced age who lives alone or with the abuser and depends on the abuser for care. Other studies have identified profiles of abused elders by type of abuse. For example, victims of self-neglect are likely to have the following characteristics: older age; living alone; socially isolated; inadequate economic resources; and having dementia, mental illness, substance abuse, or hoarding behaviors (Choi, Kim, & Asseff, 2009; Dyer, Goodwin, Pickens-Pace, Burnett, & Kelly, 2007; Ernst & Smith, in press; Nathanson, 2009). Finally, there may be some association between type of abuse and the sex of the perpetrator, with men being more likely to exploit or physically abuse elders and women being more likely to physically neglect or psychologically abuse elders.

Studies of specific types of maltreatment indicate that elder abuse results from multiple, interrelated variables. Brandl et al. (2007) summarized the characteristics associated with victims and perpetrators (Box 10-1), emphasizing that perpetrator characteristics were more powerful predictors of abuse occurrence than victim characteristics. Research on the causes of elder abuse points in the following directions:

- Causation varies by form of abuse.
- The etiology of any form of abuse is a composite of several interrelated variables.
- The origins of elder abuse are found in both the victim and the perpetrator as well as in the relationship between the two.
- The etiology of elder abuse differs from that suggested for other abused populations in important ways (e.g., elder abuse is uniquely associated with ageism).

Cultural Considerations

As a worldwide issue, elder abuse is being addressed in the context of the basic human right to be free from violence in

---

Box 10-1   Elder Abuse Profiles

Characteristics of the Perpetrator
- Alcohol abuse
- Mental illness
- History of violence or hostility
- Financial or housing dependence on the victim
- Lack of social supports

Characteristics of the Victim
- Social isolation
- Chronic illness or functional limitation
- Cognitive impairment
- Shared living arrangement with the perpetrator
- Problem behaviors

CULTURAL CONSIDERATIONS 10-1

Studies of Cultural Variation and Commonality With Regard to Elder Abuse

- Korean Americans were more likely to blame the victims for their abuse and more resistant to seeking outside help than whites or African Americans (Moon & Benton, 2000).
- The only study of Native American elders in an urban setting found that 10% definitely or probably and an additional 7% possibly had been abused, with women nine times more likely to be physically abused than men, and elder abuse victims four times more likely to be dependent on others for food than nonvictims (Buchwald et al., 2000).
- Older African Americans were likely to emphasize physical abuse when giving examples of extremely abusive behavior (Tauriac & Scruggs, 2006).
- A study of four ethnic groups in two urban areas found comparability among European Americans, African Americans, Puerto Ricans, and Japanese Americans in the importance placed on psychological abuse and neglect as forms of mistreatment (Anetzberger, Korbin, & Tomito, 1996).
- African American and working class Caucasian older women are more likely than Latina and upper income Caucasian women to identify financial abuse as an aspect of elder mistreatment (Daykin & Pearlmutter, 2009).
- Asian Indians were found to consider ignoring and not visiting the worst things that family members can do to elderly people (Nagpaul, 1997).
- An investigation of two geographically distinct Plains Indian reservations revealed that elder abuse was more common in the reservation that had the higher unemployment and substance abuse rates and little potential income from the land (Krassen Maxwell & Maxwell, 1992).
- African Americans often perceive placing older relatives in nursing homes as an act of abuse (Patterson & Malley-Morrison, 2006).
- In studies examining within-group differences among two Native American groups and five white American groups in North Carolina, differences were noted with regard to perceptions of the boundaries of elder abuse (Hudson, Armachain, Beasley, & Carlson, 1998; Hudson et al., 2000).

---

the home. Much of the focus is on cultural variations in definitions of elder abuse, and many studies in the United States center on attitudes toward elder abuse across different ethnic communities (Malley-Morrison, Nollido, & Chawla, 2006) (Cultural Considerations 10-1). For various reasons, most studies on elder abuse across ethnic and other cultural groups were conducted in the 1990s.

Cultural variation extends beyond race and ethnicity, of course. Although research in this area is minimal, some studies suggest that some groups may be more vulnerable to elder abuse, especially self-neglect, because of social isolation. For example, a homophobic social environment may cause older gays and lesbians to live in hiding, place a high value on independence, and avoid contact with senior service providers. Recent research by Walsh, Olson, Ploeg, Lohfeld, and MacMillan (in press) in Canada using focus group interviews with older lesbians revealed concern about losing their sexual orientation identity in moving to a nursing home. Respondents also voiced fear of discrimination and potential extreme isolation in institutional settings.

Although understanding cultural variations in the incidence and interpretations of elder abuse is important, nurses also should remember that individuals vary. Not all members of a cultural, religious, or minority group behave according to reported trends.

 ## RISK FACTORS FOR ELDER ABUSE AND NEGLECT

Because risk for elder abuse and neglect is associated with a combination of characteristics and circumstances in the victim and perpetrator, identification of all risk factors is very complex. Most often, several risk factors must be present and these generally develop over a long period. Characteristics that tend to be common to most elder abuse situations are invisibility of the problem, vulnerability of the older person, and psychosocial and caregiver risk factors.

Invisibility and Vulnerability

In contrast to most problems affecting older adults, one of the major risk factors for elder abuse is its invisibility. Despite the increasing attention given to elder abuse, the vast majority of cases are unreported, even in states with good reporting and intervention models. Factors that contribute to this invisibility and underreporting include the following:

- Older people generally have less contact with the community than do other segments of the population.
- Older people are reluctant to admit to being abused or neglected, because they fear reprisal or believe that alternative situations may be worse than the abusive one.
- Many myths and negative stereotypes associated with old age foster a strong denial of aging and an even stronger denial of the social problems associated with vulnerable older people.

Vulnerability is associated with a combination of social, personal, situational, and environmental factors. For example, elders may have significant psychosocial limitations resulting from conditions such as dementia, depressions, and mental illness. These conditions can increase their vulnerability to self-neglect or abuse or exploitation by others; they also can affect the ability to seek help from others. Another factor that leads to vulnerability is the absence of close relatives or other support people who are able and willing to provide adequate and appropriate assistance.

✚ Wellness Opportunity

By sensitively communicating care and concern, nurses encourage vulnerable older adults to talk about conditions that can be addressed to prevent abuse or neglect.

Psychosocial Factors

Impaired cognitive function is one of the most common characteristics of abused older adults. Considerable attention has been focused on dementia as a risk factor for self-neglect as well as psychological and physical abuse (Cooper et al., 2009). Impaired judgment, lack of insight, inability to make safe decisions, and loss of contact with reality are specific impairments that can lead to abuse and neglect. One study found that mistreatment was detected in 47.3% of a sample of 129 persons with dementia and their caregivers (Wiglesworth et al., 2010). Wiglesworth and colleagues found the following variables associated with increased occurrence of abuse: aggressive behaviors of the person with dementia and caregiver's anxiety, depression, lower education, and higher perceived burden. In addition to dementia, depression and delirium are other conditions that can increase the risk for elder abuse and neglect. Characteristics of depression that contribute to its role in self-neglect include social isolation, a negative outlook, and lack of interest in self-care.

When the older adult denies the cognitive impairment or refuses help or evaluation, the risk for elder abuse increases. Older people who live alone and are aware of their impairments may be afraid of acknowledging them, because they fear that they have an untreatable problem that will require a move to a long-term care facility. This fear may lead to social isolation, the overlooking of treatable or reversible causes of impairment, or a progressive but unnecessary decline in function.

Long-term mental illness also may predispose an older adult to abuse or neglect, especially in combination with other factors, such as dementia or the loss of a significant social support. Additional risk factors arise from social and environmental sources. The absence of a support system is one of the most common contributing factors to self-neglect, especially in people in their 80s, 90s, or older who may have outlived most of the people who once provided support and tangible services. This is especially problematic for people who have been lifelong recluses or who have no children or extended family.

Caregiver Factors

Caregiving itself does not cause elder abuse; however, it can lead to abuse when those assuming the caregiving role are incapable of doing so because of life stresses, pathologic characteristics, personality characteristics, insufficient resources, or lack of understanding of the older adult's condition. Caregivers who perpetrate abuse often exhibit some of the same risk factors associated with abused elders, particularly if the caregivers themselves are older adults. Caregiver factors associated with elder abuse include poor health, cognitive impairment, social isolation, dependence and coresidence, and poor interpersonal relations with the dependent elder. It is not unusual to have a mutually neglectful or abusive situation when an older married couple has several of the psychosocial risk factors just identified and is, in addition, socially isolated. For example, a couple who both have dementia may unintentionally abuse each other and neglect themselves.

*M*rs. B. is an 82-year-old divorced and widowed mother of four. She lives in a senior citizens' apartment located in the downtown area of a large city. The building is regularly serviced by subsidized transportation to grocery stores and shopping malls and has a nutrition center on the ground floor. Mrs. B.'s eldest son died in an accident 12 years ago. Her daughter lives 65 miles away but visits once a week to do the grocery shopping and other errands. Two sons live within 4 miles of their mother's apartment. Mrs. B. lived in the home of one son and his wife until they argued 1 year ago. The other son lives alone in a small apartment and visits his mother two or three times weekly and frequently takes her to lunch or dinner. Mrs. B. has been hospitalized for major depression eight times since her eldest son's death. She also has been diagnosed as having hypertension, rheumatoid arthritis, and type 2 diabetes.

Mrs. B. was referred to a home health agency for follow-up after her last hospital stay because her medication regimen, which she had followed for 6 years, had been changed while she was in the hospital. At the time of discharge, Mrs. B. was given a 30-day supply of medications set out in daily-dose medication containers for her. She was to take glyburide, 2.5 mg once a day; propranolol, 40 mg twice a day; paroxetine, 25 mg once a day; folic acid, 1 mg once a day; and methotrexate, 2.5 mg four tablets each Wednesday. Scheduled medication times were 8 AM and 8 PM. The home health nurse was to instruct Mrs. B. in her medication regimen, including what medications she was to take, how she was to take them, what each medication was expected to do, and possible side effects. The nurse was also to assess Mrs. B.'s ability to follow instructions and her adherence to the medication regimen.

Because Mrs. B.'s vision was impaired from diabetes, she had difficulty managing her complex medication regimen. The visiting nurse arranged for unit-dose packaging for Mrs. B.'s prescriptions and visited twice a day for 2 days to observe Mrs. B.'s ability to take her medications accurately. On the third morning, the nurse telephoned Mrs. B. at 8:15 AM and asked Mrs. B. if she had any problems taking her pills. Mrs. B. happily reported that she had taken all the pills, including the four methotrexate tablets, without any difficulty. The nurse then scheduled Mrs. B. to be seen three times a week for ongoing assessment for several weeks.

THINKING POINTS

- What are the factors that contribute to the risk of Mrs. B. becoming abused or neglected?

- What are the factors that protect Mrs. B. from becoming abused or neglected?
- As the visiting nurse, what concerns would you have about Mrs. B. when you discharge her from home care, and how would you address these concerns?

ELDER ABUSE AND NEGLECT IN NURSING HOMES

Awareness of elder abuse in nursing homes erupted during the early 1970s when many exposes on the subject were published. Two widely read exposes were Ralph Nader's study group report on nursing homes *Old Age: The Last Segregation* (Townsend, 1970) and *Tender Loving Greed* (Mendelson, 1974). However, perhaps no depiction was so vivid and disheartening as novelist's May Sarton's (1973) *As We Are Now*, written in the aftermath of visiting a friend in a New Hampshire facility. During this period, too, Congress held hearings on fire and other safety issues for nursing home residents, culminating in a series of reports printed 1974–1976 and titled *Nursing Home Care in the United States: Failure in Public Policy*. By the end of the decade, Bruce Vladeck (1980, pg 3,4) summarized the results of these efforts: "The typical nursing home is a much better place than it was a few years ago. . . . But the indifference, neglect, and physical abuse of patients continues. . . ."

Although evidence-based data are sparse, available studies indicate that elder abuse in nursing homes and other institutional settings is a widespread and hidden problem (Gittler, 2008). Although state reporting laws vary, the local adult protective services agency and the nursing home ombudsman program investigate the report. When an abuse report is substantiated, further investigation is carried out by the state agency responsible for licensure and certification and also by the state professional licensing authority when the abuse is committed by a professional (Gittler, 2008). A recent random sample survey of family members with an elderly relative in a nursing home found that 21% of these residents were neglected on at least one occasion in the last year (Zhang et al., 2010). In addition, a Michigan study comparing elder abuse rates across care settings (nursing home, assisted living, and paid home care) discovered that moving from paid home care to nursing home care more than tripled the odds of neglect, even when adjusting for health condition. Indeed, nursing homes were found to have the highest rates for all forms of elder abuse (Page, Conner, Prokhorov, Post, & Fang, in press). Families of nursing home residents have identified neglect and caretaking mistreatment as the two most frequent types of abuse reported (Griffore, Barboza, Oehmke, & Post, 2009).

Elder abuse in nursing homes is rarely reported to authorities, despite the many state and federal laws aimed at protecting residents from mistreatment (Gittler, 2008). Categorically, these include federal Medicare/Medicaid certification laws, state licensing laws, federal and state elder abuse laws, such as **adult protective services laws** and criminal laws, federal and state health care fraud and abuse laws, and long-term care ombudsman laws (both the Federal Older Americans Act and state-enabling laws). Studies of nursing home employees revealed that when elder abuse was not reported, it was typically for one of the following reasons: staff stress and burnout; inadequate staff education or training on elder abuse; difficulty in making a determination about whether or not a situation should be reported; barriers to making a report; or a belief that some elder abuse situations happen because staff are overworked, inexperienced, or frustrated in handling difficult residents (McCool, Jogerst, Daly, & Xu, 2009; Shinan-Altman & Cohen, 2009).

Although research is just beginning to unravel elder abuse risk factors in nursing homes, the National Center of Elder Abuse (2005) developed a list of facility factors based on available studies. It includes no abuse prevention policy, insufficient staff screening, inadequate staff education and training, staff shortages and turnover, and few visitors. Moreover, DeHart, Webb, and Cornman (2009) identified necessary staff competencies to prevent elder abuse based upon interviews with direct care workers. They include understanding elder abuse risk factors along with acquiring communication, relationship building, and coping skills.

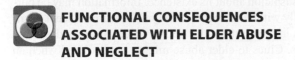

FUNCTIONAL CONSEQUENCES ASSOCIATED WITH ELDER ABUSE AND NEGLECT

Older people who have several risk factors are likely to become victims of elder abuse, as illustrated by the following case examples:

1. A middle-aged alcoholic man hit his aged father during an argument. In turn, both were beaten by their sons/grandsons, who wanted money for drugs.
2. An elderly woman never left home because she feared her memory lapses would prevent her from finding the way back. When she did venture out, she fell on the porch, and the local office on aging was called. Outreach workers found she had no food in the house and was malnourished.
3. An unemployed couple kept their impaired grandparents confined to the house, refusing them visitors, abandoning them for days without adequate food, and denying them help for fear of losing access to their Social Security checks.
4. A son visited his mother in the nursing home and sexually assaulted her when staff members were not present.
5. A depressed elderly woman refused to take a needed medication with the result that her legs became so swollen that she could not leave her chair.
6. A woman in her 80s—who was weak, incontinent, and had hypertension—was abandoned in an emergency department with a note reading "Totally dependent! Handle with care."

These situations illustrate various forms of abuse, which are defined below (National Center on Elder Abuse, 2009b):

- **Physical abuse:** use of physical force that may result in bodily injury, physical pain, or impairment
- **Sexual abuse:** nonconsensual sexual contact of any kind with an elderly person
- **Emotional (psychological) abuse:** infliction of anguish, pain, or distress through verbal or nonverbal acts
- **Neglect:** refusal or failure to fulfill any part of a person's obligations or duties to an elderly person
- **Abandonment:** desertion of an elderly person by an individual who has assumed responsibility for providing care for the elder, or by a person with physical custody of the elder
- **Self-neglect:** behavior of an elderly person that threatens his/her own health or safety

Specific actions that are defined in state elder abuse laws include undue influence, unreasonable confinement, violation of rights, and denying privacy or visitors.

Self-neglect and self-abuse are forms of elder abuse that differ from other types in that they have no perpetrator other than the older person himself or herself. In cases of self-neglect, the older person fails to meet essential needs, usually because of such factors as serious functional impairments or the desire to die. One study found that self-neglect was strongly associated with poor coping abilities of people with chronic conditions (Gibbons, 2009). In cases of self-abuse, the older person causes injury or pain to herself or himself, including body mutilations.

Although until recently the elder abuse literature usually did not address situations that were mutually abusive or neglectful, nurses working in home settings have long encountered situations in which two people, often a married couple, abuse each other or are both neglected. These situations may be rooted in a long-term, mutually abusive relationship but usually evolve because of gradual declines in the functional abilities of both people. They also may be associated with the poor coping skills of a spouse or caregiver who is faced with increasing demands and little or no outside help. Many of these situations are now being recognized as aspects of domestic violence.

Since the late 1980s, domestic violence in later life has been recognized as another aspect of elder abuse. Some of this attention arose from the battered women's movement of the 1970s and some is related to attention on the issue by national organizations such as AARP. Research indicates that domestic violence against older women may be more common than suspected. For example, a cross-sectional study of 842 community-dwelling elderly women found that nearly half had experienced physical, psychological, or sexual abuse since turning 55 years of age, many repeatedly (Fisher & Regan, 2006). Another random sample study of 370 women ages 65 and older from a health care system found that 26.5% had experienced partner violence at some time and 2.2% within the past year (Bonomi et al., 2007).

Programs that address domestic violence as an aspect of elder abuse are few and rare, especially in rural areas. Barriers to the use of available services include inaccessibility of some shelters and reluctance of older victims to leave abusive relationships because of long-term attachment to the perpetrators. A recent study exploring help seeking in a domestic violence situation among women aged 50 years and older revealed several themes for service agencies to consider when intervening with this population. They include the importance of family and friends, trust placed in physicians, discomfort with labeling behavior as domestic violence, and value of outreach in appropriate places, such as the offices of primary care physicians, home care agencies, and within the faith community (Leisey, Kupstas, & Cooper, 2009).

DIVERSITY NOTE

Rural culture can affect help-seeking behavior in domestic violence situations. For instance, victims may stay in abusive relationships because they live in small, insulated communities with nearby family and strong social networks, especially if violence is an accepted part of life.

Although rape and other sexual violence perpetrated against older people received some attention during the late 1970s, the focus at that time was on sexual assault by strangers. During the 1990s, sexual assault by family members and paid caregivers became a widely recognized aspect of elder abuse. Reports of sexual assault against older people are not common, but the resulting physical and emotional consequences can be severe and long lasting (Poulos & Sheridan, 2008). Research on reported sexual abuse found the typical victim to be an older woman residing in a nursing facility (Teaster & Roberts, 2004). The first national study of sexual abuse in care facilities discovered that the typical perpetrator was a man (78.4%) aged 56 (range 19 to 96) and almost as likely to be another resident (41%) as facility staff (43%). His victim suffered from various illnesses (most commonly Alzheimer's disease 64%, heart disease 45%, and/or diabetes 16%) and had disabling conditions (usually cognitive 48%, psychiatric 40%, and/or physical 38%). Nearly half of the victims required assistance in all activities of daily living (ADLs), and two-thirds could not ambulate independently. Sexual abuse most often was represented by molestation, which was four times more frequent than vaginal rapes, the second usual form (Ramsey-Klawsnik, Teaster, Mendiondo, Marcum, & Abner, 2008). Most cases are never prosecuted because of insufficient evidence or because victims are unable to participate in the prosecution (Burgess, Ramsey-Klawsnik, & Gregorian, 2008).

*W*hen Mr. P.'s wife died, this frail man sought care in the home of a neighbor who offered both board and care in exchange for his monthly Social Security check. In reality, the neighbor provided neither, but locked Mr. P. in the basement and gave him little food. If he complained about the treatment or refused to sign over the income or property, the caregiver hit or kicked him. After 4 years, the situation was discovered and reported to the county protective services agency. Mr. P. later sat in the social worker's office and sadly commented, "So this is what it's like to be a protective case."

THINKING POINTS

- What type(s) of abuse does this case represent?
- What are some of the psychosocial consequences that Mr. P. is likely to have experienced in the past 4 years?
- What are some factors that contribute to this situation going on for 4 years?

NURSING ASSESSMENT OF ABUSED OR NEGLECTED OLDER ADULTS

Elder abuse is not so much assessed as it is detected, so nurses often must assume the role of detective. Because elder abuse by its very nature is a hidden problem, assessment begins with a suspicion about its existence. Information may be purposefully withheld, and it is rarely volunteered, except in situations in which the older person or caregiver is desperate for help. Clues to elder abuse might first be noted when an older person is seen in an emergency department or admitted to a hospital. Most often, a home visit is an essential component of the assessment process, and gaining admission to the home usually is the first assessment challenge. Many times, the situation deteriorates so gradually that it is hard to determine the onset of abuse. In questionable situations, people who suspect that elder abuse is occurring may ignore the clues in hopes that the situation will resolve by itself.

Wellness Opportunity

Nurses pay particular attention to the older adult's relationships with others so that they can detect clues to elder abuse.

Unique Aspects of Elder Abuse Assessment

Assessment of elder abuse differs from usual nursing assessment in several respects. First, a major goal is to determine whether legal interventions are appropriate or necessary, in contrast to situations in which the primary focus is on specific health needs. In situations in which abuse is suspected, the immediate assessment focus is on the safety of the older person. This approach is similar to critical care nursing, in which basic life-sustaining needs are addressed immediately and other needs are considered later.

Second, realistic goals for elder abuse situations often are quite limited. Health care professionals sometimes have to accept basic safety as the only goal, especially when the elder and caregiver insist on choices that are not consistent with those recommended by health care workers. An assessment of risks to safety is essential, therefore, because choice of legal interventions is based partially on the degree of risk. Because the determination of safety often is based on medical and nursing information, the role of the nurse is especially important. In home settings in particular, the nurse may be the only health care professional who directly assesses the situation, and the nursing assessment may be the major determinant of recommendations for legal intervention.

Third, cases of elder abuse generally involve some element of resistance from the older person or caregiver(s). Only in rare situations do abused elders or their caregivers seek assistance from health care professionals. Although it might be impossible to establish a trusting relationship, the nurse must try, at the very least, to establish an accepting relationship. The initial assessment, therefore, is aimed at identifying ways of gaining access and at least passive acceptance.

Fourth, in contrast to most health care situations, the nurse may be viewed as a threat rather than a help. Thus, it may be difficult to gain access or to obtain adequate assessment information. When nurses are viewed as the "bad guy," they need to minimize the perceived threat even before the initial contact. Nurses can accomplish this by identifying someone who acknowledges that a problem exists and is willing to facilitate the assessment process. Any of the following people can be helpful in gaining access and acceptance:

- Neighbors or friends
- Relatives (especially family members who do not live in the problematic home setting)
- Staff from senior centers, offices on aging, or health care or community agencies
- Physicians or any other health professionals
- Church-based people (e.g., clergy, parish nurses).

Fifth, when legal interventions are being considered, the legal rights of the person and the caregivers must be addressed. Nurses and other workers involved in elder abuse cases usually are uncomfortable making decisions that involve the rights of other adults. In institutional settings, legal and ethical decisions are guided by medical information and institutional policies, and the role of the physician usually is the most important. In home settings, however, there are few clear guidelines and little or no physician input.

Finally, the personal safety of the nurse is an assessment consideration in many elder abuse situations, especially when the nurse visits homes where the caregiver is a known or suspected perpetrator. In any situation that places a nurse at risk, an essential component of the assessment is ensuring that protections are in place for the nurse. For example, nurses can arrange their visits in conjunction with protective service workers visits or, if warranted, law enforcement officers. Some communities have law enforcement officers who are specially trained to deal with elder abuse situations. When-

ever nurses visit patients in places where the nurses' safety may be threatened, they need to be vigilant about potential risks and always be attentive to an escape route.

> **Wellness Opportunity**
>
> When making home visits, nurses pay particular attention to self-wellness by protecting themselves from risks.

Physical Health

The nursing assessment of physical abuse and neglect focuses on the following: nutrition, hydration, bruises and injuries, degree of frailty, and presence of pathologic conditions. The following sections discuss each of these aspects in relation to elder abuse and neglect.

Nutrition and Hydration

Nutrition and hydration are important in determining not only the existence of physical neglect but also the seriousness and urgency of the situation. In community settings, nutrition and hydration status are crucial in determining if time allows for working with the elder in the home setting. The guidelines discussed in Chapter 18, particularly in Table 18-2 (Causes and Consequences of Nutrient Deficiencies), can be applied to the detection of malnutrition and dehydration.

Skin turgor over the extremities is not necessarily a reliable indicator of hydration, especially for very old people or for people who have lost weight. Examination of the mucous membranes and an assessment of skin turgor over the sternum or abdomen provide more accurate clues to dehydration. The absence of thirst sensation is not necessarily an indicator of adequate hydration because older people may have a diminished thirst response. On the other hand, the presence of thirst sensation is a positive indicator of dehydration, a physiologic disturbance, or an adverse medication effect. If a urine sample can be obtained, a measurement of specific gravity will provide information about hydration. When a urinometer is not available, a visual examination of urine concentration provides some clues about hydration.

When indicators of malnutrition or dehydration are identified, the next step is to determine whether the hydration or nutritional status can be improved adequately without removing the person from the setting. The role of the nurse can be especially important in assessing not only the nutrition and hydration status but also the measures required to alleviate these risks immediately. Sometimes, the provision of water and food is the most important intervention in neglect situations. In addition, this intervention is inexpensive and readily available and can be quite effective in establishing a relationship with a hungry or thirsty person.

Injuries, Bruises, and Other Physical Harm

Assessment of indicators of physical harm is an important aspect of the detection of neglect or physical abuse. Any of the following conditions can be indicators of abuse or self-neglect:

leg ulcers; pressure ulcers; dependent edema; poor wound healing; burns from stoves, cigarettes, or hot water; and bruises, swelling, or injuries from falls, especially repeated falls. More than one of these indicators at the same time, or over a short period of time, should raise high levels of suspicion about neglect. The possibility of drug or alcohol abuse also should be considered when any of these indicators is identified, especially if the person is also depressed or socially isolated. To detect physical abuse, the nurse should look for any indication of injury caused by people who live with or visit a vulnerable older adult. Examples are marks from cuts, bites, burns, or punctures; bruises or injuries, especially of the face, head, or trunk; bruises on both upper arms, as would result from being grabbed or shaken harshly; or bruises that reflect the shape of objects, like belts or hairbrushes. If evidence of injuries from falls is present, the nurse must consider the possibility that the person was shoved or otherwise caused to fall by someone else.

Nurses routinely assess the presence and characteristics of bruises, with particular attention to the onset of new bruises and the progression of bruises. Changes in color have traditionally been considered indicators of the age of bruises, with the expectation that they progress from blue/black to green, then yellow, with red appearing at any time. A few studies have addressed progression of accidental bruises in relation to child abuse, but there is little research on bruises in older adults. In 2002, Mosqueda and colleagues conducted a landmark study on the life cycle of bruises in older adults (Mosqueda, Burnright, & Liao, 2005). Trained research assistants performed daily head-to-toe examinations of 101 older adults during the initial 14-day inspection period to identify the onset of new bruises. Seventy-three subjects had 108 bruises, which were documented and examined daily for up to 6 weeks. Researchers screened subjects to exclude any possibility of abuse and they considered variables such as medications, fall history, and medical conditions. The following findings from this study are pertinent to nursing assessment of bruises in older adults (Mosqueda et al., 2005):

- Accidental bruises occur in a predictable pattern in older adults, with nearly 90% appearing on extremities.
- No accidental bruises were observed on the neck, ears, genitalia, buttocks, or soles of the feet.
- Bruise duration varied from 4 to 41 days, with 81% resolving by day 11.
- Red, yellow, and purple are the most common discolorations during the early phase, but they can last throughout the life of the bruise.
- Yellow discoloration can begin within the first 24-hours after onset, tends to increase over time, and was the most common color in bruises after 3 weeks.
- Subjects were more likely to know the cause when the bruises occurred on their trunks than when it was on their extremities.
- The most commonly reported cause was bumping into something.

- Subjects with compromised function and those on medications known to affect coagulation were more likely to have multiple bruises, with no differences in size, color, or location.

A study of 67 older adults who were determined to have been physically abused found that 72% of the subjects had bruises (Wiglesworth et al., 2009). When findings were compared with the earlier study by Mosqueda et al., (2005), researchers found that the victims were more likely to know the cause of the bruising and that the bruises were larger than 5 cm and more likely to occur on the face, lateral right arm, and the posterior torso (Wiglesworth et al., 2009). Nurses can use the illustration of most common sites of accidental bruising (Figure 10-1) to help identify bruises that are more likely to be associated with abusive situations. In addition, nurses can review the photographs of elder abuse victims that the National Center on Elder Abuse posts on its Web site (www.ncea.aoa.gov) for educational purposes.

Nurses also assess for indicators of abuse caused indirectly, as by a caregiver who gives the person excessive amounts of alcohol or drugs, especially psychoactive medications. Sometimes caregivers who abuse drugs or alcohol will give these substances to the people for whom they care, especially if the dependent person is not able or willing to refuse. Another sign of abuse is excessive use of psychoactive medications solely for the caregiver's benefit so that the elder

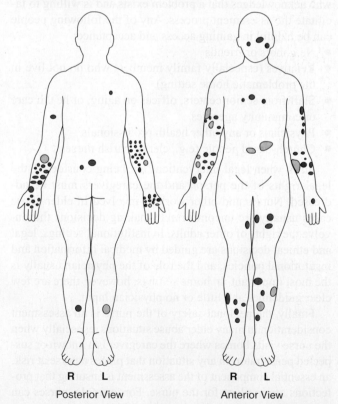

R   L   R   L
Posterior View   Anterior View

FIGURE 10-1 Most common sites of accidental bruises in older adults. (From Mosqueda, L., Burnright, K., & Liao, S. (2005). The life cycle of bruises in older adults. *Journal of the American Geriatrics Society, 53,* 1339–1343. Used with permission from Wiley-Blackwell.)

is more easily managed. Nurses are likely to observe any of the following indicators of overmedication in an elder: ataxia, somnolence, clouded mentation, slurred speech, staggering gait, or extrapyramidal manifestations.

Aspects of physical neglect may include withholding therapeutic medications or interfering with medical care. For example, caregivers may decide not to purchase prescriptions or provide nursing care, medical equipment, or comfort items because they do not want to spend the money, even though this care is necessary. If the older adult has not freely chosen to forego treatments, medications, or assistance, then this may constitute physical neglect. If the caregiver is likely to inherit the money that is being saved, this may represent financial exploitation as well.

Degree of Frailty

The degree of frailty of the older adult is another consideration in assessing actual or potential abuse or neglect. For example, an older adult who is slightly obese and fully ambulatory would not have the same degree of risk for fall-related injuries as one who weighs only 78 pounds and ambulates unsteadily with a walker. Similarly, if the 75-year-old wife of an alcoholic man can easily escape to safety when he becomes violent, and she chooses to remain in the situation, she would not necessarily be considered a protective case. In contrast, if the woman is cognitively impaired, physically frail, or unable to move quickly, and is the target of violence when her husband is inebriated, the situation could be defined as elder abuse.

Pathologic Conditions

In certain medical conditions, it is essential to assess the ability to follow medical regimens and the consequences of noncompliance. For example, consequences can be quite serious if an elder has diabetes or congestive heart failure and cannot take medications correctly. Nurses also assess whether the medical regimen can be modified to improve compliance and support the elder's ability to remain in an independent setting. For example, in an acute care setting, a therapeutic regimen might require the administration of some medications before meals and others after meals, and others three or four times a day at different times. Although this might be ideal for optimal effectiveness, elders or caregivers in a home setting may not be able to comply. A thorough nursing assessment can lead to interventions, such as patient education or simplification of the regimen, to achieve adequate compliance.

Activities of Daily Living

A major focus of assessment in elder abuse situations is to determine the necessity for legal interventions. Therefore, a nursing assessment of the person's potential for safe performance of activities of daily living (ADLs) is extremely important. This is particularly important when assessing self-neglect because impairments in instrumental ADLs are strongly associated with this type of abuse (Naik, Burnett, Pickens-Pace, & Dyer, 2008).

For community-living older adults, it is essential to assess the home environment and the elder's level of functioning in that environment. In addition, nurses often need to obtain information from caregivers. Home care workers provide valuable information, and they usually are more objective than family members. In some circumstances, it may be appropriate to involve occupational or physical therapists in the home assessment. When a difference of opinion exists, or when it is difficult to determine the safety of the situation, it may be helpful to have a team conference that includes all of the people who function in assessment or caregiving capacities and who have some degree of objectivity. In cases of suspected elder abuse, the assessment team may include many informal sources of help, such as family and neighbors, as well as formal sources of help, such as nurses and social workers.

Personal dress, hygiene, and grooming are among the most visible and commonly appraised aspects of daily function. People often are viewed as neglected when they do not comply with socially defined standards of cleanliness, particularly when an unpleasant odor is noted. In elder abuse situations, nurses need to consider that poor hygiene and grooming are important reflections of many underlying problems, but they are not necessarily indicators of safety concerns. When families and health care or social service workers initially work with a neglected older person who is in need of much personal care, they often are tempted to begin by assisting the person with bathing and grooming. Although the workers may view this as a socially acceptable way to begin, the elder may perceive this as a threat to their pride and independence. Thus, nurses assess not only the impact of poor hygiene on the elder's health but also the consequences of imposing assistance when the elder is unwilling to accept help or acknowledge a hygiene problem. The nurse may determine that efforts to deal with personal hygiene would interfere with the short-term goal of establishing a relationship and the long-term goal of assisting with other aspects of daily function. Thus, nurses may need to begin by addressing nutrition, hydration, and safety, while deferring attention to personal care issues associated with the most resistance.

Adequate nutrition, hydration, and an ability to obtain help in an emergency are the basic human needs that are most often called into question in cases of elder abuse. Other basic needs may also be compromised, usually in relation to specific functional impairments and environmental circumstances. For instance, it is imperative to address bowel and bladder elimination for people who are confined to bed or a chair. For people with mobility limitations or serious vision impairments, safe ambulation and the ability to avoid falls are important considerations. Table 10-1 summarizes some of the specific functional and environmental conditions that present risks to basic needs.

Psychosocial Function

Information in Chapters 13 (Psychosocial Assessment), 14 (Delirium and Dementia), and 15 (Depression) is pertinent

TABLE 10-1   Risks to Safety Associated With Functional Limitations

Functional Limitation	Risks to Safety
Any mental or physical impairment, especially combined with social isolation and lack of a support system	Nutrition and hydration
Mobility limitations or seriously impaired vision, especially combined with poor judgment	Falls
Cognitive impairments in ambulatory people	Wandering, getting lost
Compromised mobility	Pressure sores
Cognitive impairment, especially poor judgment	Inability to get help
Poor judgment, especially when living in an unsafe neighborhood	Basic safety and security

to assessing psychosocial function in relation to elder abuse. In addition, an important aspect of psychosocial function for abuse situations is assessment of the elder's capacity for reasonable judgments about self-care. This is difficult because the determination of someone's ability to make appropriate judgments is based, at least in part, on subjective criteria and opinions. People whose judgment is impaired to the point that they are at serious risk, especially if they do not acknowledge the risk, are usually considered incompetent or incapacitated. Thus, the crucial element of psychosocial assessment for elder abuse cases is a determination of risk (i.e., danger to the person) rather than a determination of whether other people would judge the decision as *good* or *appropriate*. When the competence of an older adult to make safe decisions regarding self-care is in doubt, nurses may be legally bound to make reports or consider other legal interventions. There are no federal guidelines for determining the mental capacity of abused or neglected older adults, and the legal criteria differ from state to state. The ethical and legal considerations related to elder abuse are discussed later in this chapter and more extensively in Chapter 9.

Wellness Opportunity

Nurses promote self-determination for older adults by respecting their rights to make decisions about their care, as long as their actions do not jeopardize safety for themselves or others.

Support Resources

Support resources include those people, such as caregivers and friends, who influence a person's physical and psychosocial function. Some or all of the support people may directly cause the abusive situation or may actively or passively contribute to it. Therefore, nurses assess the support resources in terms of both helpful and detrimental effects. In addition, support resources not currently being used are identified as potential sources of help.

When the caregivers who perpetrate the abuse are also the support resources, nurses assess the potential for working with them to alleviate the negative consequences. Although it is not always easy to work with abusive caregivers, it may be even more difficult to eliminate their influence over an older adult. During the assessment, therefore, nurses identify any strengths of the caregiver and any willingness to change the situation voluntarily. If the caregiver is extremely stressed, then respite, along with individual or group support and counseling, may be effective interventions. In mutually abusive situations in which the designated caregiver also is abused or neglected, the nurse tries to identify any outside sources of support that have not been tapped. For example, in a mutually abusive situation involving a socially isolated married couple, the nurse might identify a relative or friend who is willing to assist with caregiving or decision-making responsibilities.

Because a caregiver's lack of knowledge can be an underlying factor in elder abuse, nurses assess the caregiver's understanding of the elder's needs. For example, caregivers may have good intentions when they use adult briefs for the control of incontinence and do not change them frequently, but they may not understand the potential for skin breakdown. Caregivers may administer excessive amounts of psychoactive medications because they do not understand the correct dosing schedule or the potential adverse effects. This is especially common when medications are ordered on an as-needed basis and the caregiver has not been given clear guidelines for determining when the medication is needed, or what the most effective dosage is. In these situations, nursing assessment of the caregiver's knowledge is especially important because educational interventions, role modeling, or the provision of additional services may alleviate the abuse.

In situations of neglect, there usually are very few support services to assess, and the task of the nurse is to identify potential sources of help and the barriers that interfere with the use of these resources. The assessment of barriers to the use of resources is discussed in Chapter 13 and is summarized in Box 13-8. It is especially important to identify these barriers because simple interventions, such as provision of information or assistance with transportation, may be effective in eliminating them. Cultural influences also must be assessed in relation to the use of support resources, as discussed in Chapter 2.

Environmental Influences

As with other aspects of elder abuse, the primary purposes of assessing the environment are to identify the factors that create risks and to determine which of these factors can be alleviated through interventions. With regard to the immediate living conditions, the nurse assesses whether minimal standards of safety and cleanliness are being maintained. When nurses assess home environments that are terribly cluttered, they must make some determination of both the meaning and the consequences of the clutter. A massive collection of clutter from hoarding reflects an underlying disorder and may or may not be a risk factor that needs to be addressed. Consequences of hoarding range from socially unacceptable appearances to serious risks to health and safety. Therefore, the nurse must assess the person's ability to maneuver in the environment during daily activities, as well as the person's safety in emergency situations, such as a fire. When nurses and other workers are initially exposed to massive amounts of clutter, their first inclination may be to think of a way to eliminate some of it. If this reaction is communicated to the resident of the cluttered home, however, it may become impossible to establish an accepting relationship, and the older adult may reject any further interventions. In assessing the home environment, therefore, nurses must be nonjudgmental, except in circumstances in which the risks are so great that immediate action must be taken.

Nurses also assess the neighborhood environment for its impact on the safety of the person. This is especially important when the older person lives in an area of high crime or extreme isolation and is vulnerable by virtue of impaired judgment, physical frailty, or a combination of physical and psychosocial impairments. People who are only moderately forgetful may be safe in an apartment or a suburban neighborhood where neighbors watch out for them. In a high-crime neighborhood, however, forgetting to lock the doors or to take other precautions may place the person at increased risk for physical harm, financial exploitation, or other serious abuses. Likewise, in a rural environment, social isolation may increase the risks for vulnerable elderly people.

Finally, seasonal conditions can influence the degree of risk for self-neglect in people who have dementia and live in climates characterized by extreme heat or cold. For example, a person who does not pay utility bills may not be in any danger as long as the weather is mild, but when the temperature turns cold, that person would be at risk for hypothermia. The same is true for people who occasionally wander outside without dressing appropriately. As long as the neighborhood is safe and the weather is mild, they may be relatively safe; however, they may be at increased risk during the cold months or very hot months, especially if they do not wear proper clothing. Nurses also assess any of the risk factors for hypothermia or heat-related illness.

Threats to Life

The most immediate consideration in determining whether legal interventions are necessary is the assessment of threats to life. Situations often are viewed as being of crisis proportions when they are first discovered, and the immediate reaction of the person who discovers the situation may be to remove a person from the environment. Many times, however, the person may not want to leave, or there may be no better setting in which the person can receive care immediately. In these situations, the nurse may be asked to assess the urgency and seriousness of the situation and to provide an opinion about whether legal interventions are justified. The nurse often is the person who can either convince the elder to accept help or convince the caregivers and social workers that the present situation is tolerable. For instance, when nurses determine that the situation is not life-threatening, they can reassure the person that they are trying to improve the situation and support the person remaining as safe and independent as possible. Examples of threats that nurses commonly assess in elder abuse situations include the following:

- History of physical violence on the part of the caregiver, especially when the elder is unable to escape or otherwise be protected
- Untreated wounds or infections
- Inability to administer insulin correctly
- Progressive gangrene or ulcerated conditions
- Inability to adhere to therapeutic regimens
- Consistent wandering in unsafe neighborhoods or in very cold weather
- Misuse (usually unintentional) of certain medications, such as digitalis or insulin
- Excessive use of drugs or alcohol, either self- or caregiver-induced.

In situations in which the caregiver is the abuser, the nurse and other team members must assess whether the caregiver presents a threat to the life of the dependent older person.

When nurses do not have firsthand knowledge of the abused or neglected older person before being notified of a crisis situation, the first consideration is whether this is objectively a crisis or merely a crisis in the eyes of the person who just discovered the situation. Situations that appear the most appalling may actually represent a gradual deterioration over several months or years. Therefore, the initial assessment is aimed at determining any immediate threats to the life of the abused elder, such as malnutrition, dehydration, or an untreated medical condition. Finally, suicide potential must be assessed, especially in self-neglected elders who also are depressed and expressing feelings of hopelessness. Nurses can apply all of the principles of suicide assessment, discussed in Chapter 15, to abused and neglected elders.

Cultural Aspects

Definitions and perceptions of elder abuse and neglect are influenced to a great extent by cultural norms. For example, Asian Indians may consider not visiting an older family member to be a form of psychological neglect, but Anglo Americans may consider it a way of respecting privacy and autonomy. Cultural factors also have a strong influence on caregiver roles and responsibilities. Most families have culturally influenced expectations about which family members should provide care to dependent older adults and about whether it is acceptable to enlist the aid of paid caregivers. In some families, there may be conflicts about these expectations, particularly between older and younger generations. Sometimes, these conflicts may need to be identified and addressed before elder abuse or neglect can be resolved.

Nurses must identify cultural factors that influence the care that is provided—or not provided—to older adults. Cultural Considerations 10-2 lists some of the assessment questions that should be considered in identifying cultural influences. When assessing family caregiver relationships,

CULTURAL CONSIDERATIONS 10 - 2

Cultural Considerations in Assessing Elder Abuse and Neglect

- What are the family and cultural expectations concerning family care-givers? (e.g., Is it acceptable to employ paid caregivers, or are family members expected to provide all the care?)
- Do family members differ in their perceptions about caregiving responsibilities?
- What are the family and cultural perspectives on autonomy and independence?
- Do family members differ in their perspectives on autonomy and independence?
- How are decisions made about care of the older adult? (e.g., Is it a patriarchal or matriarchal family?)
- Who are the acceptable sources of social support and personal assistance?
- Who are the acceptable sources of health care (e.g., herbalists, spiritual healers, Native American practitioners)?
- What are the acceptable health care practices (e.g., herbs, homeopathy, acupuncture, faith healing, folk remedies)?
- Are there language barriers that influence the care that is provided or that limit the number of care providers?
- How does skin color affect assessment of bruises, pressure sores, and other skin changes?

nurses should be sensitive to cultural variations in perspectives on family caregiving and respect differences, but they also must address abusive situations. In addition, cultural assessment information on the following topics should be considered: communication and psychosocial assessment (see Chapter 13), nutrition (see Chapter 18), dementia (see Chapter 14), and depression (see Chapter 15).

*M*rs. K. is 80 years old and had resided in a nursing facility for 1 year until she recently was discharged at her request but "against medical advice" with no prescriptions for her medications or medical referral for home care. She has complex health conditions, including osteoarthritis, coronary artery disease, congestive heart failure, chronic obstructive pulmonary disease (COPD), depression, and insulin-dependent diabetes. Although alert and oriented, Mrs. K. has major deficits in her ability to perform daily living tasks. She also depends on a walker for ambulation and has a history of falling, including a fall that resulted in a hip fracture and her admission to a nursing facility.

Mrs. K.'s support system is limited. Her son lives in another state but functions as power of attorney and provides some telephone reassurance. Her daughter is estranged from Mrs. K., and at their last meeting was verbally abusive to her. Mrs. K.'s older brother visits a few times weekly to help with meal preparation, grocery shopping,

transportation, and medication pickups; however, his own health problems prevent him from providing more help.

Shortly after returning home, Mrs. K.'s precarious health status rapidly deteriorated. She became severely short of breath, requiring continuous oxygen. She began to hallucinate in the evening, believing that she alone had the responsibility of feeding all of the children in the neighborhood. As her fears increased, so too did the calls to her brother. Eventually, she made several calls every night, overwhelming and exhausting him.

THINKING POINTS

- What form(s) of elder abuse is (are) represented?
- What are signs or indicators of abuse that you as a nurse would be able to identify?
- What factors contribute to Mrs. K.'s current risks?
- How will you proceed in conducting a nursing assessment of Mrs. K.?
- What barriers might you encounter in conducting the assessment? How will you overcome them?

NURSING DIAGNOSIS

Because elder abuse and neglect is so broad and complex, various nursing diagnoses are applicable, depending on the situation. A nursing diagnosis that would apply to many elder abuse situations where family members are caregivers is Disabled Family Coping. This is defined as "behavior of significant person (family member or other primary person) that disables his or her capacities and the client's capacities to effectively address tasks essential to either person's adaptation to the health challenge" (NANDA International, 2009, p. 253). Related factors include changes in family roles, unrealistic expectations about caregiving, and changes in the health status of the older adult. If the nursing assessment identifies stressors related to family caregiving, the nursing diagnosis of Caregiver Role Strain might be applicable. Related caregiver factors include ineffective coping patterns, functional or cognitive impairments, and insufficient resources (e.g., respite, financial assets, assistance with care). Related factors involving the dependent older adult include increased dependence and the presence of difficult or unsafe behaviors (e.g., paranoia, wandering, incontinence).

The nursing diagnosis of Risk for Injury might be used for older adults who are in self-neglecting situations, especially if the person lives alone and is physically and psychosocially impaired. The nursing diagnosis of Decisional Conflict might apply to abused or neglected older adults who live in an environment that places them at risk for harm because they are unable to make decisions about alternative environments. Related factors include fear, lack of information about alternatives, and impaired decision-making ability.

PLANNING FOR WELLNESS OUTCOMES

Nurses direct care for abused or neglected older adults toward addressing the complex needs of the elder as well as those of the family caregivers. Some Nursing Outcomes Classification (NOC) terminology that is likely to pertain to the abused older adult includes Abuse Cessation, Abuse Protection, Abuse Recovery Status, Neglect Cessation, Risk Control, Self-Care Status, and Social Support. Outcomes related to abusive caregivers or family members include Abusive Behavior Self-Restraint, Caregiver Emotional Health, Caregiver-Patient Relationship, Caregiver Stressors, Caregiver Endurance Potential, Family Coping, Family Social Climate, Knowledge: Health Resources, Role Performance, and Stress Level.

NURSING INTERVENTIONS TO ADDRESS ELDER ABUSE AND NEGLECT

From a health care perspective, abused elders can be described as the intensive care patients of the community because they require the highest level of skill from a variety of professionals. Unlike intensive care patients in hospitals, however, the team members are not specialized health care professionals but rather are community-based workers and people who provide informal support. Nurses often assume the role of coordinator or team leader in implementing interventions that address the older adults, the caregivers, and the environment for these inherently complex and challenging situations.

Because of the extensive scope of elder abuse, there are numerous Nursing Interventions Classification (NIC) terms that could be applicable to both the abused or neglected elder and the caregiver. Some that would be appropriate in most situations are Abuse Protection Support: Elder, Crisis Intervention, Referral, and Risk Identification for the elder; and Caregiver Support, Coping Enhancement, Referral, Role Enhancement, and Teaching for caregivers.

Interventions in elder abuse situations may involve legal actions when decision-making abilities of the older adult are impaired. Many situations involve caregivers who are not competent decision makers or are not acting in the best interest of the elder. Thus, many cases of elder abuse involve legal and ethical questions about the competency of the elder and the caregivers. Nurses often have a key role in advocating for the older adult and may feel unprepared or uncomfortable either making or participating in decisions that affect the rights of others. Similarly, nurses may feel torn between the right of the person to refuse treatment and the obligation to report abuse and neglect situations, as discussed later in this chapter.

Interventions for elder abuse are implemented in community settings, over a long period of time, by a team of formal and informal care providers. Nurses working in home and community settings have the most direct opportunities for both the prevention of and interventions for elder abuse. Home-delivered meals and nursing and medical strategies are interventions that are usually readily accepted and effective for addressing abused older adults in community settings. Nurses in institutional settings are likely to use interventions such as education and support of caregivers and facilitation of referrals to appropriate community agencies. Because the opportunities for intervention in institutional settings are quite different from those in community settings, each of these areas is discussed separately in the following sections.

Interventions in Institutional Settings

Nurses in acute and long-term care settings can intervene in cases of elder abuse when they interact with caregivers, who often seek advice from nurses about ways of providing care. For example, nurses can encourage caregivers to use a period of institutionalization to reevaluate the demands of the situation and to consider resources for support and assistance. Family may express ambivalence about managing the older adult's care at home, or they may be unsure or unrealistic about their own ability to provide appropriate care or to cope with the stress of the situation. In some cases, caregivers may be seeking approval for not providing care at home. In these situations, nurses can facilitate communication among all the decision makers, including the primary care provider, the older adult (if appropriate), and the various family members who are responsible for care. Sometimes, it is appropriate to suggest individual counseling or support groups or make referrals for social services, particularly when caregivers are very stressed about care-related decisions.

When elder abuse is rooted in the caregiver's lack of information, nurses can be a role model and teach about appropriate caregiving measures. When caregivers need additional health education or support services, nurses can initiate a referral to a home care agency for follow-up. Nurses also try to identify needs for skilled nursing care because health insurance usually covers these services. When nurses have serious questions about the adequacy of a discharge plan, they can refer to a protective service agency for further assessment and ongoing services.

Interventions in Community Settings

Families caring for people with dementia in home settings have identified professional advice about understanding and handling memory problems as an important interventions for preventing elder abuse (Selwood, Cooper, Owens, Blanchard, & Livingston, 2009). Nurses in community settings have many opportunities for teaching caregivers about adequate care through role modeling and verbal and written instruction. For example, if caregivers have trouble managing complex medication regimens, nurses can use charts and organizers to facilitate compliance. Nurses also can educate caregivers about basic care needs, such as nutrition, exercise, and elimination. For example, nurses may suggest innovative ways of meeting the nutritional requirements of an elderly person who does not eat adequately. Home care nurses have the advantage of observing many creative and effective techniques used by caregivers that have never been described in any nursing texts. Thus, experienced home care nurses are continually expanding their repertoire of techniques for physical care and behavioral management, and these techniques can then be passed on to other family caregivers.

When elder abuse is rooted in caregiver stress, nurses can suggest services and help find ways of providing care so that the caregiver can use these resources for self-care. The following are examples of services aimed at reducing caregiver stress or dealing with caregiver problems:

- Alcoholics anonymous for caregivers with alcoholism
- Individual counseling to learn coping skills
- Alzheimer's Association for support and education groups
- In-home or day care for respite.

Home health aides are the service providers who are most likely to care for abused elders in home settings, but they often are ill prepared to detect or address elder abuse. Nurses who provide home-based services, therefore, have a tremendous responsibility to help home care workers recognize and intervene in elder abuse situations. For example, nurses can teach about detecting clues to elder abuse, and they can address concerns about questionable conditions. If nurses cannot openly discuss the situation during home visits, they may have to arrange for a phone conversation with the home care worker. In situations in which the older adult requires a significant degree of physical care or supervision, the services of a home health aide may be the most effective means of preventing elder abuse. Often, however, the retention of a home health aide in challenging situations depends largely on the degree of support and guidance provided by a professional nurse.

Nurses in other community settings, such as clinics or senior centers, have opportunities to intervene in elder abuse. For example, parish nurses may be the only contact for older adults who neglect themselves or care for a dependent spouse and are not aware of the many resources to address their needs. Nurses can prevent or alleviate elder abuse by facilitating referrals for appropriate community-based resources, such as adult day care or group or home-delivered meals. Even if nurses are not familiar with specific community services,

they can discuss the advantages of various types of services and encourage older adults to call their local office on aging. At a minimum, however, nurses need to be familiar with the phone number for the area agency on aging that serves as an information center about local resources in every geographic area of the United States. Information about local agencies on aging also is available by calling the Eldercare Locator at (800) 677-1116.

Wellness Opportunity

Nurses help caregivers maintain self-wellness by identifying ways of alleviating stress associated with the demands of caregiving.

Interventions in Multidisciplinary Teams

In many community settings, nurses are part of multidisciplinary teams that implement interventions to address complex elder abuse situations. For example, many hospitals have elder abuse teams, and community agencies offer protective or case management services to older people and their families. Multidisciplinary teams for elder abuse generally include professionals who offer the perspectives of law, nursing, medicine, psychiatry, social work, and rehabilitation therapy. Additional disciplines are included if the situation requires. When legal interventions are being considered, the multidisciplinary team must conduct a complete assessment, including assessment of the person's ability to function safely in the home environment, the involvement of the family and significant others in meeting basic needs, and the ability of the older person to participate in developing a safe and realistic plan of action.

If nurses are not part of a multidisciplinary team, they sometimes need to be creative in finding other professionals with whom they can work. For example, when nurses work with people who are homebound, they may need to identify resources for an initial medical evaluation or for ongoing monitoring. In many areas of the country, primary care providers are resuming the practice of making home visits. In addition, with the growing demand for home health services, an increased number of diagnostic tests are performed in the home (e.g., radiography, blood tests, and electrocardiography). In many situations, these diagnostic tests are essential for determining whether involuntary care measures are justified. For instance, if the older adult refuses to go out of the home, blood tests or radiography done in the home may provide the evidence needed to determine whether a hospitalization is warranted.

Multidisciplinary teams provide a holistic perspective, which is essential for thoroughly assessing the problem and determining appropriate solutions. They facilitate collaboration in handling complex and difficult cases. Finally, they help develop professional relationships, enabling the establishment of more effective approaches to elder abuse prevention and treatment within an organization or community (Anetzberger, Dayton, Miller, McGreevey, & Schimer, 2005). In recent years, specialized teams have evolved to address particular elder abuse forms or situations. Among them are financial abuse specialist teams (FASTs), rapid response FASTs, older adult hoarding teams, fatality or death review teams, and medically focused teams (Nerenberg, 2008; Koenig, Leiste, Spano, & Chapin, in press).

Referrals

Nurses often facilitate referrals for services that improve functioning for the older adult and decrease the burden of caregiving responsibilities. For instance, speech, physical, and occupational therapies may be useful in improving the older person's ability to communicate, ambulate, and perform ADLs. Referrals for skilled home care services usually are made at the time of discharge from an institution; however, the older adult or family may have refused the services at that time. Older adults who are not admitted to health care facilities may not know they qualify for skilled home care services, and a nurse making a home visit may be the first health professional to suggest these resources. Although older adults or their families may not know about or may have refused such services, nurses need to assess their willingness to accept help as conditions change.

Nurses also assess whether recent changes in the elder qualify the person for skilled home care services. For example, a change in medications might qualify a person for skilled nursing care, and a fall might qualify a person for skilled physical therapy. Staff in home care agencies usually are happy to discuss skilled care services with anyone who calls for information. Nurses also can advise about the possibility of having services covered by health insurance, and they can obtain orders from the primary care provider for those services that are covered under Medicare or other health insurance programs.

Another important role for nurses is suggesting types of medical equipment, disposable supplies, and assistive devices to improve function and safety for the elder and ease caregiver burden. For example, caregivers may respond positively to suggestions from the nurse about obtaining and using grab bars for preventing falls in the bathroom. Some durable medical equipment is covered by health insurance, and medical supply companies usually are quite helpful in advising people about specific equipment.

Prevention and Treatment Interventions

Abused elders and their caregivers or abusers typically need a wide range of interventions, which can be categorized according to basic function:

- Core, or essential, integrative services
- Emergency services, during crises or just before or after abuse or neglect occurs
- Support services for managing the problem and improving the situation
- Rehabilitative services to address problems of either the victim or the perpetrator
- Preventive services, including programs directed toward changing society in ways that diminish the likelihood of maltreatment or self-neglect.

Figure 10-2 identifies some of the specific types of services, arranged by function, that may be needed in elder abuse situations. Nurses are the health care professionals who are most accepted and qualified for implementing or arranging for many of the services for both the caregivers and abused or neglected older person(s).

Financial exploitation is an aspect of elder abuse that can be prevented through relatively simple and widely available measures to protect assets. For example, nurses can suggest that a trusted family member establishes a joint account with the older adult and keep track of all transactions. Out-of-town families can oversee financial transactions through online banking. Nurses can find information about programs directed toward prevention of financial abuse and exploitation at the Internet sites listed in the Resources section at the end of this chapter. For example, the National Center on Elder Abuse maintains an up-to-date list "Promising Practices to Prevent Financial Abuse" describing programs that are available in many states.

*M*r. and Mrs. G. have been married for over 50 years and have six children, four of who live in their area. Because of Mrs. G.'s memory loss in recent years, Mr. G. has allowed home care workers into the house to help her with eating and to perform personal care. The workers report that Mr. G. yells at his wife when she forgets things. On more than one occasion, they witnessed him attempting to force feed her when she failed to eat an entire meal. After the couple has gone to their bedroom in the evening, the night workers have reported hearing screams, crying, and slapping sounds coming from behind the closed bedroom door. In the morning, Mrs. G. had bruises on her body and bumps on her head. When asked, Mr. G. denied hitting his wife. Mrs. G. cried when questioned, never providing an explanation for her injuries.

Mr. G. is reluctant to consider additional services, such as adult day care, fearing that the couple's savings will evaporate. He had Mrs. G. change doctors several times in recent years because "they don't do anything to really help her." The children who live nearby have said that they do not want to get involved in their parents' situation. They describe years of their father physically and verbally abusing their mother and fear what might happen if any action is taken now.

THINKING POINTS

- What interventions might be helpful in addressing the elder abuse evident in this situation?
- What is the role of the home care nurse in introducing and implementing these interventions?
- What barriers might be encountered in acceptance of the interventions?
- As the home care nurse in this situation, how will you help to overcome these barriers?

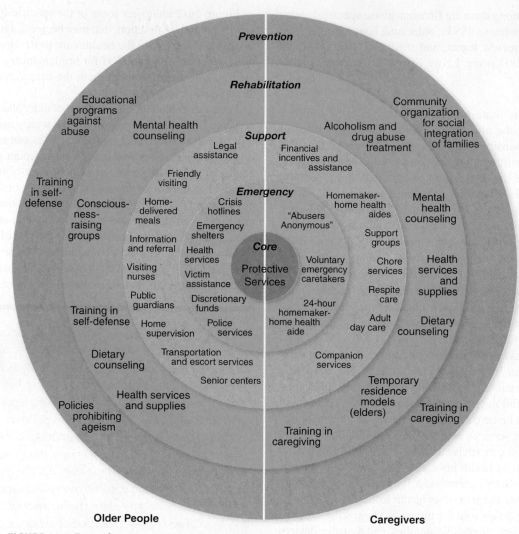

FIGURE 10-2 Types of services needed by abused older adults and their caregivers. (Used with permission from Anetzberger, G. J. (2010). *Report of the Elder Abuse Project: Recommendations for addressing the problem of elder abuse in Cuyahoga County*. Cleveland, OH: Federation for Community Planning. Originally published in 1982.)

LEGAL INTERVENTIONS

Most elder abuse situations require consideration of voluntary or involuntary legal interventions. Whenever feasible, problems should be remedied without the use of involuntary legal intervention. Because voluntary legal interventions require the consent of the older person, they cannot be initiated if the person is not mentally competent. Competent adults can revoke voluntary legal interventions at any time. Money management, power of attorney, and various types of bank accounts, such as joint or direct deposit, are all interventions of this nature. Other legal interventions that are useful for mentally competent older adults are discussed in Chapter 9.

Some legal interventions, such as guardianship or civil commitment, are either voluntary or involuntary but are most commonly used on an involuntary basis when the older person's safety or property is in jeopardy. Because these legal interventions involve a much more extensive loss of personal freedom than voluntary ones, they should be used with

extreme caution. A key consideration in the choice of legal interventions is determining the competency of the person to make decisions, as discussed in Chapters 9 and 13. Some measures, such as guardianship, may be easier to initiate than to discontinue. Others, such as civil commitment, may be accompanied by long-term stigma, even when the intervention is terminated.

Involuntary legal interventions are used when mental impairments—such as limited insight, judgment, memory, or cognition—affect the ability of older people to function safely and meet their basic human needs. In general, involuntary legal intervention is indicated when assessment reveals all of the following conditions:

- Decisions must be made about the older person's health, living arrangements, money, or property.
- The older person is not capable of making reasonable decisions.
- There is a risk to the older person's health, safety, money, or property.

- The risk would be reduced or eliminated if someone else were empowered to make and implement decisions.

Legal interventions that address the abuser include domestic violence law and the criminal code. Adult protective services law is particularly limited when considerable property needs protection, the maltreatment is significant and repeated, the older person's mental impairment is substantial and permanent, or the goal is to prevent maltreatment rather than to treat it. Under these conditions, other legal interventions should be considered with, or as alternatives to, adult protective services.

◆ Wellness Opportunity

Nurses support autonomy for older adults by identifying the least invasive legal interventions, while also ensuring the least amount of endangerment.

Adult Protective Services

Philosophically, adult protective services law provides protection for the person who is abused, for the person offering assistance, and for society from possible dangers posed by the person. Because there are no federal guidelines or specific funding, provisions of elder abuse reporting and adult protective services laws differ among the 50 states. Although states vary in dealing with the complex problem of elder abuse, purposes of state laws for protecting vulnerable older people include the following:

- Facilitating the identification and referral of abuse or neglect
- Conveying public and centralized authority for addressing protective matters
- Establishing a system of protective services to prevent, correct, or discontinue abuse or neglect
- Permitting, under certain circumstances, involuntary access to the suspected victim of abuse for the purpose of investigation and service delivery.

Usually, local departments of social services receive reports of abuse, but in some states, departments of aging or prosecutors' offices receive them.

The scope of reports includes neglect; exploitation; and physical, sexual, and psychological abuse; in several states, laws include abandonment and cruel punishment. In most states, reporting suspected abuse is mandatory for health, social service, and safety professionals and paraprofessionals. Most state laws protect the confidentiality of reports and the identity of all people involved in making them. The typical penalty for failure to report is a charge of a misdemeanor, with or without financial penalty. In some states, however, failure to report can result in imprisonment, civil liability for damages, or notification of the state licensing board.

The public authority responsible for implementation must investigate promptly; sometimes, the law mandates a response within 24 to 72 hours. Investigation generally includes a home visit with the alleged victim and consultation with people knowledgeable about the situation. Interventions for at-risk older people can include health care, support services, protective placement, emergency care, or financial management. Most laws emphasize due process, self-determination, least restrictive interventions, and voluntary acceptance of services by mentally competent adults. Although protective service workers have the primary responsibility for implementing elder abuse laws, nurses have essential roles in reporting and collaborating, assessing, consulting, testifying in court, and providing care. Nursing responsibilities associated with each of these roles are discussed in the next sections.

Reporting and Collaborating

Nurses are the health care workers most commonly identified as mandatory reporters in adult abuse and protective services laws. This is appropriate because the usual duties assumed by nurses place them in a key position for witnessing the consequences of abuse and neglect. In addition, a primary role of nurses is to foster collaboration between health care professionals as abuse reporters and adult protective service or law enforcement officials as abuse investigators or service providers.

Mandatory reporting laws do not require reporters to *know* whether abuse or neglect has occurred, but merely to report it if they *suspect* its occurrence. The responsibility for problem verification rests with the public agency charged with law implementation, not with the reporter or referral source. Suspecting elder abuse means detecting signs of violence, such as bruises, welts, or fractures. It also means recognizing conditions associated with neglect or deprivation, such as frostbite, malnutrition, dehydration, oversedation, mental changes, or uncontrolled medical conditions.

Because most reporting laws provide immunity for mandatory reporters, nurses who act in good faith and without malicious intent can report suspected cases without fear of liability. Some laws offer immunity in the workplace; in these cases, nurses cannot be fired, transferred, or demoted for making a report. In all states, responsibility for making the report rests with the individual nurse, so nurses cannot delegate reporting to anyone else. The nurse alone has the responsibility for reporting, and for the consequences—both legal and moral—of failing to do so. Even though individual nurses are responsible for reporting, most agencies and hospitals have established protocols to clarify roles and enhance the credibility of the report. Excellent examples of elder abuse detection protocols are available, and they should be considered for use by nurses in all health care settings involving multiple professions and levels of authority. Box 10-2 illustrates a typical protocol for hospital- or agency-based nurses.

Assessing

Protective service workers often call upon nurses to assess their clients, especially when there is concern about endangerment or questions about the effects of neglect or abuse.

Box 10-2 Sample Protocol for Nurses With Regard to Elder Abuse

Assessment

- Use usual assessment forms and observe for clues to elder abuse.
- If there is reason for suspicion, use a formal elder abuse assessment tool.
- Observe and interview caregivers and caregiver–client interactions.
- Analyze data that raise a suspicion of abuse, neglect, or exploitation.
- Consider whether objective findings fit the explanation.

If Abuse and/or Neglect Are Suspected, Consult the Abuse Detection Team

- Report pertinent findings to the team leader and the primary care provider as soon as possible.
- Summarize findings from the assessment guide on progress notes.
- Determine the need to report abuse or neglect to authorities.
- Document additional facts, and whether a report was made, in the progress notes.
- Document discussions with the client and caregivers.

Follow-up Actions

- Summarize action steps taken and recommended by team.
- Implement any security measures to protect the client.
- Implement appropriate interventions.

Nurses commonly are involved with assessments of clients who are newly referred or experiencing a change in health status. Nurses are the preferred health care worker for such assessments because of their holistic approach, their availability through nursing agencies, their willingness to make home visits, and the relative ease with which older people usually accept nurses.

Because assessment was discussed earlier in this chapter, only one aspect requires further examination here. Formal elder abuse assessment instruments are used to collect and organize all pertinent information; summarize observations; and provide a base for planning referrals, services, or legal actions. These tools assess and document all of the following:

- Background data (e.g., client's name and address)
- Signs of maltreatment or self-neglect according to type (e.g., bruises or welts in cases of suspected physical abuse)
- Severity of signs (e.g., an immediate life threat)
- Indicators of maltreatment intentionality (e.g., a caregiver who will not allow the nurse to be alone with the client)
- Symptoms of acute or chronic illness or impairment (e.g., incontinence)
- Functional incapacity (e.g., an inability to dress or toilet without assistance)
- Aggravating social conditions (e.g., a client who lives alone and is socially isolated)
- Source of information (e.g., agency referral)
- Recommended action (e.g., referral of the case to home health care service providers)

Fulmer (2008) and colleagues developed an elder assessment instrument that currently is recommended as a *Try This: Best Practices in Nursing Care to Older Adults* tool by the Hartford Institute for Geriatric Nursing. Additional information and a cost-free video demonstrating the application of this tool in a clinical setting is available through collaboration of the Hartford Institute and the *American Journal of Nursing* at http://consultgerirn.org/resources or at www.nursingcenter.com.

Consulting

In addition to providing direct assessment, nurses often provide consultation when questions arise regarding the health status of clients. Typical questions relate to medications, continence, nutrition and hydration, and disease signs. Often, consultation services are part of networks among service providers in a given community; sometimes, they are formally organized through clinical consultation teams that are integral parts of protective services coalitions. Another role for nurses is in staff education for protective services workers on topics such as health assessment, recognition of endangerment, and disease prevention and detection.

Testifying in Court

Although very few cases of elder abuse involve court actions, adult protective service workers may need legal assistance to gain access, deliver services, or obtain a comprehensive assessment. In these situations, the older person usually is mentally impaired and unable to make decisions that would alleviate or eliminate the neglect or abuse. Legal intervention may also be appropriate when older adults in life-endangering circumstances refuse help. Before legal interventions are permitted, the protective service worker must present evidence to a judge or referee about all of the following:

- Abuse or neglect
- Need for protective services
- Inability to gain voluntary cooperation
- No other way to alleviate the problems.

Most of the evidence is provided by physicians, mental health providers, and protective service workers; however, nurses are sometimes asked to testify or submit reports about their assessments or services.

Testimony involves two types of evidence: direct observation and expert opinion. Nurses are likely to be called upon to provide in-person testimony about their direct observations because they can provide a professional assessment of the health status or function of the older person. In addition, nursing documentation about assessments and care plans may be used as evidence in court proceedings. Thus, nurses need to carefully, accurately, and objectively document all pertinent information with the understanding that their documentation may be used in legal proceedings.

Providing Care

As discussed in the nursing interventions section of this chapter, nurses provide essential care and treatment for abused

Elder Abuse and Neglect | CHAPTER 10 | 181

and neglected older people. They help correct conditions caused by maltreatment and self-neglect, and they prevent their recurrence through such activities as treating injuries, monitoring medication, educating caregivers, obtaining assistive devices, and facilitating service referrals. In this role, as in others, nurses work cooperatively with other professionals and with paraprofessionals and use their knowledge and expertise to help the victims of elder abuse.

Ethical Issues

Ethical issues related to abused and neglected elders are similar to ethical issues in medicine and other fields. Rather than having clear answers and absolute rights and wrongs, there are usually differing perspectives and different implications, depending on what course of action is taken. Law, community pressures, and personal concepts of professionalism lead to the erroneous assumption that a problem, such as maltreatment or self-neglect, can be easily or simply resolved. Protective situations involving older people are rarely easily resolved.

Surrounding ethical issues in adult protective services is the fact that all adults in American society have rights—including freedom from intrusion, the right to fair treatment, freedom from unnecessary restraint, and the right to self-determination—but these rights can be taken away through the use of legal measures. Professionals often face a dilemma when they need to initiate legal measures that take away the rights of other adults. For example, unless an older adult has been judged to be incompetent by a court of law, he or she has the right to be protected from intrusion, even by well-intentioned professionals. In adult-protective service situations, this right is threatened and services can be imposed on an older person who does not willingly agree to assistance.

Another dilemma involves the characteristics of protective situations that sometimes make respecting personal rights so difficult. The following are examples of situations that present ethical dilemmas in relation to respecting personal rights:

- In situations that are urgent or dangerous, it is hard to walk away, even when the older person asks to be left alone.
- Public pressure to do something, no matter what, places pressure on care providers who are trying to resolve the situation while respecting the rights of the older person.
- Contradictory societal values may pit individual rights against other values, such as paternalism and protectionism.
- Because nursing is directed toward helping others, it is difficult to deal with vulnerable elders who do not accept help, especially when the lack of help has detrimental consequences.
- It may be necessary to make serious decision based on little information because the older adult may be cognitively impaired, the situation may require immediate actions, or pertinent information may be withheld by the older person or the caregivers.
- The questionable mental status of many abused or neglected elders places decision-making responsibility in the hands of other people. Involuntary legal interventions may unnecessarily deprive the person of certain rights, but inaction can mean that basic human needs are not being met adequately, or at all.
- The intrusive nature of legal interventions, including mandatory reporting, can deprive people of their fundamental rights.

Nurses can apply the hierarchy of principles summarized in Box 10-3 to address ethical dilemmas about particular situations. These principles of adult protective services are arranged from the most to the least important considerations with regard to interventions for abused or neglected elders.

Adult protective services are fraught with ethical dilemmas. Some of these dilemmas are related to the five basic roles—reporter, investigator, service provider, administrator, and planner—assumed by professionals. Each role has a particular sphere of responsibility in addressing elder abuse and neglect. The reporter detects the situation and describes it to someone authorized by law to deal with it. The investigator is the legal agent who assesses the situation and determines the need for protective services. The service provider offers interventions for correcting or discontinuing maltreatment or self-neglect. The administrator manages a protective services

---

Box 10-3 Principles of Adult Protective Services

I. **Freedom Over Safety.** The client has a right to choose to live at risk of harm, providing she or he is capable of making that choice, harms no one, and commits no crime.

II. **Self-Determination.** The client has a right to personal choices and decisions until such time that she or he delegates, or the court grants, the responsibility to someone else.

III. **Participation in Decision Making.** The client has a right to receive information to make informed decisions and to participate in all decision making affecting her or his circumstances to the extent that she or he is able.

IV. **Least Restrictive Alternative.** The client has a right to service alternatives that maximize choice and minimize lifestyle disruption.

V. **Primacy of the Adult.** The worker has a responsibility to serve the client, not the community people concerned about appearances, the landlord concerned about crime, or the family concerned about finances.

VI. **Confidentiality.** The client has a right to privacy and secrecy.

VII. **Benefit of Doubt.** If there is evidence that the client is making a reasoned choice, the worker has a responsibility to see that the benefit of doubt is in her or his favor.

VIII. **Do No Harm.** The worker has a responsibility to take no action that places the client at greater risk of harm.

IX. **Avoidance of Blame.** The worker has a responsibility to understand the origins of any maltreatment and to commit no action that would antagonize the perpetrator and so reduce the chances of terminating the maltreatment.

X. **Maintenance of the Family.** The worker has a responsibility to deal with the maltreatment as a family problem, if the perpetrator is a family member, and to try to find the necessary family services to resolve the problem.

Anetzberger, G. J. (1999). Ethical issues in personal safety. In T. F. Johnson (Ed.), *Handbook on ethical issues in aging* (pp. 187–219). Westport, CT: Greenwood Press.

TABLE 10-2 Ethical Questions and Suggested Solutions Regarding Abused Elders

Ethical Question/Implications	Suggested Solution
When do I report elder abuse? (If I report too soon, I may needlessly invade someone's privacy. If I wait, the situation may worsen.)	Report elder abuse when you believe that, without intervention, the situation will deteriorate or endanger the elder.
What if my report places the elder in more danger, or labels someone inaccurately? What if it causes the elder to shy away from me and my agency?	Report elder abuse if you believe that the protective services system can reduce the risk better than the current interventions.
How do I decide if the elder or the caregiver receives priority? (If my priority is the elder, I may alienate his or her family members, who serve as the primary sources of care. If my priority is the family, then the care plan may be contrary to the elder's wishes and may not adequately respect his or her rights.)	With certain exceptions, the elder should receive priority. These exceptions are limited to circumstances in which the elder has been judged to be incompetent by a court of law or is endangering others by his or her behavior.
Is it more important to maintain standards of confidentiality than to comply with a reporting law?	State law takes precedence over professional standards.
Does the right of an elder to refuse services extend to total self-neglect and intentional suicide? How can I know that endangered elders clearly understand the consequences of their self-neglect? How can I accept abandoning the situation?	Ethical dilemmas such as these often can be resolved through the use of a hierarchy of values or principles, such as those summarized in Box 10-3.
Can emergency services be thrust upon an elder who would have refused them under ordinary circumstances? If the elder's life is endangered, then is it not my primary responsibility to use my nursing skills in life-saving ways, no matter what the elder chooses? Even if the elder might have refused services in the past, does that mean he or she absolutely would refuse them now?	If the elder is incapable of deciding whether to accept or reject emergency services, then these services should be provided, subject to the constraints of the protective services law. This offers the elder essential protection, but recognizes his or her right to refuse ongoing services when the emergency has subsided and he or she is capable of making decisions on his or her own behalf.

program. Finally, the planner develops policies and programs, as well as community education initiatives, aimed at preventing or treating the problem.

Professional workers in each of these roles face different ethical issues. Issues of the reporter role include questions about making a report and the consequences of doing so. The role of the investigator involves confronting questions about privacy, openness, and confidentiality. The service provider deals with issues about the rights of the elder, the rights of the caregivers, and the degree of risk for the elder. Program planners and administrators face dilemmas about service priorities and funding, staff, and other critical resources. Nurses most often deal with ethical issues in their roles as reporters, investigators, and service providers. Table 10-2 identifies some of the ethical problems, as well as related solutions, that nurses may encounter in their roles in adult protective services.

EVALUATING EFFECTIVENESS OF NURSING INTERVENTIONS

Nursing care of abused or neglected older adults is evaluated by the extent to which nursing goals are achieved. If a nursing goal is to alleviate the contributing factor of unnecessary dependence, the care is evaluated by whether the older adult is functioning at a higher level of independence. If a nursing goal is to address caregiver stress, the nursing care might be evaluated by the caregiver accepting help with the care, attending caregiver support groups, and expressing less stress about his or her caregiving responsibilities. When the nursing goal is to protect an incompetent older adult from harm, nursing care might be evaluated by the extent to which the least restrictive legal interventions are implemented. In such cases,

nursing care is evaluated in terms of protecting the older adult from harm while also protecting his or her rights.

*R*ecall that Mrs. B. is 82 years old and lives in a senior citizens apartment. After 2 months of receiving skilled nursing visits, Mrs. B. was discharged from the home care agency because she was successfully managing her medications and other aspects of functioning adequately. Several months after she was discharged, the nurse in the wellness clinic at the senior citizens apartment noted a change in her mannerisms, accompanied by slurred speech and an unbalanced gait. Mrs. B. had bruises on her arms, knees, and forehead, but insisted that she had not fallen. After further investigation, the nurse found that her blood pressure was 210/104 mm Hg and that her blood glucose level was 410 mg/dL on the glucometer that the nurse kept in the clinic. A pill count revealed that Mrs. B. had not taken her medications for 2½ days. After a consultation with her primary care provider, Mrs. B. was admitted to the hospital. Tests revealed that she had suffered a stroke, resulting in left-sided weakness and short-term memory loss.

Mrs. B. left the hospital against medical advice and returned to her apartment, initially refusing visits from the home health nurse. She insisted that her children come and administer her medications and prepare her meals because she was unable to do this for herself. Mrs. B. reasoned that she had cared for her children when they were young, so they should come when she needed them. The children tried to assist Mrs. B. for 4 days but were unable to meet both her demands and those of their jobs and families. Mrs. B. reluctantly agreed to a visit from the home health nurse who had visited her before. She expected that she would see the nurse once and that the nurse would "make my children do right."

Mrs. B.'s children were present for the initial assessment. Mrs. B. was unable to stand or transfer to the commode without help. She could not use her chart and color-coded boxes to take her pills. Mrs. B. flatly refused to consider admission to a nursing facility to receive therapy to regain her strength, and she would not consider living with her daughter or either son. The family told the nurse that they were exhausted and on the "verge of a breakdown" and could not continue to provide the care that Mrs. B. needed. The nurse explained to Mrs. B. that it was not safe for her to remain in her apartment without assistance. She suggested that she hire an aide until other arrangements could be made, because her children were not obligated to lose their jobs or jeopardize their family relationships to care for her. Mrs. B. accused her children of being greedy and caring only about themselves. She said that children have a duty to care for their parents and that she wasn't going to "have strangers doing the things that decent children should be doing." She directed her concluding remarks at the nurse, stating, "What's more, I don't need you to come back either, because all you want to do is side with my children."

THINKING POINTS

- What strategies would you use to establish a relationship with Mrs. B.?
- What additional assessment information would you want to obtain, and how would you obtain it?
- What would your next steps be in working with Mrs. B.?
- How would you work with the family?
- What other resources would you involve in planning and providing care for Mrs. B.?
- What criteria would you use for making a referral for adult protective services?

Chapter Highlights

Overview of Elder Abuse and Neglect
- Seven major forms of elder abuse defined by the National Center on Elder Abuse are physical abuse, sexual abuse, emotional or psychological abuse, neglect, abandonment, financial or material exploitation, and self-neglect.

- Awareness of elder abuse as a social problem began in the 1950s and 1960s and is now recognized as a major social and public health problem and a significant aspect of domestic violence.
- Studies of causes of elder abuse indicate that it differs from other forms of abuse and is complex (Box 10-1).
- Cultural differences in family and caregiver roles affect definitions of elder abuse (Cultural Considerations 10-1).

Risk Factors for Elder Abuse and Neglect
- Elder abuse is usually related to multiple risk factors that develop over a long period
- Invisibility and vulnerability are two risk factors that occur in most situations of abuse or neglect
- Common psychosocial risk factors: impaired cognition, long-term mental illness
- Caregiver factors: psychosocial impairments.

Elder Abuse and Neglect in Nursing Homes
- Elder abuse has been recognized as a problem in nursing homes since the 1970s, and studies indicate that it is widespread and underreported.

Functional Consequences Associated With Elder Abuse and Neglect
- Definitions: neglect, physical abuse, sexual abuse, emotional or psychological abuse, abandonment, self-neglect
- Domestic violence, rape, and sexual violence are unique aspects of elder abuse

Nursing Assessment of Abused or Neglected Older Adults
- Unique aspects of elder abuse assessment: safety, limited goals, resistance, nurse viewed as threat, legal and ethical considerations, safety of nurse
- Physical health: nutrition, hydration, indicators of physical harm (Figure 10-1), degree of frailty, pathologic conditions
- Activities of daily living: assess in relation to safety, basic needs, vulnerability (Table 10-1)
- Psychosocial function: impaired cognition, judgments about self-care
- Support resources: caregivers who also are perpetrators, lack of resources, barriers to using services
- Environmental influences: home, neighborhood, seasonal factors
- Threats to life: degree of endangerment and ability to alleviate risks
- Cultural aspects: family and cultural expectations, perspectives on caregiving, barriers to assessment (Cultural Considerations 10-2)

Nursing Diagnosis
- Disabled Family Coping
- Caregiver Role Strain
- Risk for Injury
- Decisional Conflict

Planning for Wellness Outcomes
- Quality of Life
- Abuse Cessation, Protection, Recovery Status
- Neglect Cessation
- Risk Control
- Caregiver Stressors, Emotional Health, Endurance Potential
- Family Coping
- Social Support

Nursing Interventions to Address Elder Abuse and Neglect
- Role of the nurse in institutional settings (teaching care-givers, discharge planning, addressing caregiver stress)
- Role of the nurse in community settings (teaching, super-vising, providing direct care, working with home health aides, facilitating referrals)
- Role of the nurse in multidisciplinary teams
- Facilitating referrals (services for older adults and care-givers, medical equipment)
- Prevention and treatment interventions (types of core services, programs for preventing financial abuse; Figure 10-2)

Legal Interventions
- Voluntary and involuntary
- Adult protective services (Box 10-2): reporting and collaborating, assessing, consulting, testifying in court, providing care
- Ethical issues: principles of adult protective services (Box 10-3)
- Ethical questions and suggested solutions (Table 10-2)

Evaluating Effectiveness of Nursing Interventions
- Higher level of functioning of older adult
- Alleviation of caregiver stress
- Use of least restrictive legal interventions
- Protection of the older adult

Critical Thinking Exercises

1. Identify factors in each of the following categories that currently contribute to elder abuse and neglect in the United States:
   - Demographic statistics
   - Changes in families
   - Health care systems
   - Health status and other characteristics of older adults
   - Social awareness
2. What is different about the nursing assessment of abused or neglected elders compared with the nursing assessment of other older adults?
3. What do you believe about family caregiving responsibil-ities? How would you deal with a family whose values about caregiving differ significantly from yours?
4. What are your beliefs about the degree of risk a frail elder should be allowed to take?
5. Under what circumstances should an elder be denied the right to remain in his or her own home?

Resources

For links to these resources and other helpful Internet resources related to this chapter, visit thePoint. at http://thePoint.lww.com/Miller6e.

Clinical Tools

American Journal of Nursing and Hartford Institute for Geriatric Nursing,
- *How to Try This,* article and video: Screening for mistreat-ment of older adults. *American Journal of Nursing, 108*(12), 52–59.

Hartford Institute for Geriatric Nursing
- *Try This: Best Practices in Nursing Care to Older Adults* Issue Number 15 (2008), Elder Mistreatment Assessment

Evidence-Based Practice

National Guideline Clearinghouse
- Elder abuse prevention

Center of Excellence on Elder Abuse and Neglect

Health Education

National Center on Elder Abuse—Administration on Aging
National Committee for the Prevention of Elder Abuse
American Bar Association—Commission on Law and Aging
Center of Excellence on Elder Abuse and Neglect
USC Ageworks CME on Elder Abuse and Neglect
National Adult Protective Services Association
National Clearinghouse on Abuse in Later Life
National Long-Term-Care Ombudsman Resource Center
ElderCare Locator

REFERENCES

Acierno, R. (2009, June 15). *Prevalence findings: The National Institute of Justice national elder mistreatment study.* Paper presented at the An-nual National Institute of Justice Conference, Arlington, VA.

Anetzberger, G. J. (1999). Ethical issues in personal safety. In T. F. John-son (Ed.), *Handbook on ethical issues in aging* (pp. 187–219). West-port, CT: Greenwood Press.

Anetzberger, G. J., Dayton, C., Miller, C. A., McGreevey, J. F., Jr., & Schimer, M. (2005). Multidisciplinary teams in the clinical manage-ment of elder abuse. *Clinical Gerontologist, 28*(1/2), 157–171.

Anetzberger, G. J., Korbin, J. E., & Tomito, S. K. (1996). Defining elder mistreatment in four ethnic groups across two generations. *Journal of Cross-Cultural Gerontology, 11*, 187–211.

Bonomi, A. E., Anderson, M. L., Reid, R. J., Carrell, D., Fishman, P. A., Rivara, F. P., & Thompson, R. S. (2007). Intimate partner violence in older women. *The Gerontologist, 47*(1), 34–41.

Brandl, B., Dyer, C. B., Heisler, C. J., Otto, J. M., Steigel, L. A., & Thomas, R. W. (2007). *Elder abuse detection and intervention: A col-laborative approach.* New York: Springer Publishing Co.

Buchwald, D., Tomita, S., Hartman, S., Furman, R., Dudden, M., & Manson, S. M. (2000). Physical abuse of urban Native Americans. *Journal of General Internal Medicine, 15*, 562–564.

Burgess, A. W., Ramsey-Klawsnik, H., & Gregorian, S. B. (2008). Com-paring routes of reporting in elder sexual abuse cases. *Journal of Elder Abuse & Neglect, 20*, 336–352.

Choi, N. G., Kim, J., & Asseff, J. (2009). Self-neglect and neglect of vul-nerable older adults: Reexamination of etiology. *Journal of Geronto-logical Social Work, 52*(2), 171–187.

Conrad, K. (2009, June 15). *Client self-report measure of financial ex-ploitation.* Paper presented at the Annual National Institute of Justice Conference, Arlington, VA.

Cooper, C., Selwood, A., & Livingston, G. (2008). The prevalence of elder abuse and neglect: A systematic review. *Age & Ageing, 37*(2), 151–160.

Cooper, C., Selwood, A., Blanchard, M., Walker, Z., Blizzard, R., & Livingston, G. (2009). Abuse of people with dementia by family carers: Representative cross sectional survey. *British Medical Journal, 338,* b155, doi: 10.1136/bmj.b155.

Daykin, E., & Pearlmutter, S. (2009). Older women's perceptions of elder mistreatment and ethical dilemmas in adult protective services: A cross-cultural, exploratory study. *Journal of Elder Abuse & Neglect, 21,* 15–57.

DeHart, D., Webb, J., & Cornman, C. (2009). Prevention of elder mistreatment in nursing homes: Competencies for direct-care staff. *Journal of Elder Abuse & Neglect, 21*(4), 360–378.

Dyer, C. B., Goodwin, J. S., Pickens-Pace, S., Burnett, J., & Kelly, P. A. (2007). Self-neglect among the elderly: A model based on more than 500 patients seen by a geriatric medicine team. *American Journal of Public Health, 97*(9), 1671–1676.

Ernst, J. S., & Smith, C. A. (in press). Adult protective services clients confirmed for self-neglect: Characteristics and service use. *Journal of Elder Abuse & Neglect, 23*(1).

Fisher, B. S., & Regan, S. L. (2006). The extent and frequency of abuse in the lives of older women and their relationship with health outcomes. *The Gerontologist, 46,* 200–209.

Fulmer, T. (2008). Screening for mistreatment of older adults. *American Journal of Nursing, 108*(12), 52–59.

Gibbons, S. W. (2009). Theory synthesis for self-neglect. *Nursing Research, 58,* 194–200.

Gittler, J. (2008). Governmental efforts to improve quality of care for nursing home residents and to protect them from mistreatment: A survey of federal and state laws. *Research in Gerontological Nursing, 1*(4), 264–284.

Griffore, R. J., Barboza, G. E., Oehmke, L. B., & Post, L. A. (2009). Family members' reports of abuse in Michigan nursing homes. *Journal of Elder Abuse and Neglect, 21,* 105–114.

Hudson, M. F., Armachain, W. D., Beasley, C. M., & Carlson, J. R. (1998). Elder abuse: Two Native American views. *The Gerontologist, 38,* 538–548.

Hudson, M. F., Beasley, C., Benedict, R. H., Carlson, J. R., Craig, B. F., Herman, C., & Mason, S. C. (2000). Elder abuse: Some Caucasian-American views. *Journal of Elder Abuse & Neglect, 12*(1), 89–114.

Koenig, T. L., Leiste, M. R., Spano, R., & Chapin, R. K. (in press). Multidisciplinary team perspectives on older adult hoarding and mental illness. *Journal of Elder Abuse and Neglect, 24*(4).

Krassen Maxwell, E., & Maxwell, R. J. (1992). Insults to the body civil: Mistreatment of the elderly in two Plains Indian tribes. *Journal of Cross-Cultural Gerontology, 7,* 3–23.

Laumann, E. O., Leitsch, S. A., & Waite, L. J. (2008). Elder mistreatment in the United States: Prevalence estimates from a nationally representative study. *Journal of Gerontology: Social Sciences, 63B*(4), S248–S254.

Leisey, M., Kupstas, P. K., & Cooper, A. (2009). Domestic violence in the second half of life. *Journal of Elder Abuse & Neglect, 21,* 141–155.

Malley-Morrison, K., Nolido, N. E.-V., & Chawla, S. (2006). International perspectives on elder abuse: Five case studies. *Educational Gerontology, 32,* 1–11.

McCool, J. J., Jogerst, G. J., Daly, J. M., & Xu, Y. (2009). Multidisciplinary reports of nursing home mistreatment. *American Medical Directors Association, 10*(3), 174–180.

Mendelson, M. A. (1974). *Tender loving greed: How the incredibly lucrative nursing home "industry" is exploiting America's old people and defrauding us all.* New York: Alfred A. Knopf.

Moon, A., & Benton, D. (2000). Tolerance of elder abuse and attitudes toward third-party intervention among African American, Korean American, and white elderly. *Journal of Multicultural Social Work, 8,* 283–303.

Mosqueda, L., Burnright, K., & Liao, S. (2005). The life cycle of bruises in older adults. *Journal of the American Geriatrics Society, 53,* 1339–1343.

Nagpaul, K. (1997). Elder abuse among Asian Indians: Traditional versus modern perspectives. *Journal of Elder Abuse & Neglect, 9*(2), 77–92.

Naik, A. D., Burnett, J., Pickens-Pace, S., & Dyer, C. B. (2008). Impairment in instrumental activities of daily living and the geriatric syndrome of self-neglect. *The Gerontologist, 48,* 388–393.

NANDA International. (2009). *Nursing diagnoses: Definitions and classification 2009–2011.* Oxford, UK: Wiley-Blackwell.

Nathanson, J. N. (2009). Animal hoarding: Slipping into the darkness of co-morbid animal and self-neglect. *Journal of Elder Abuse & Neglect, 21*(4).

National Center on Elder Abuse. (2005). *Nursing home abuse risk prevention profile and checklist.* Washington, DC: National Association of State Units on Aging.

National Center on Elder Abuse. (2009a). Elder abuse/mistreatment defined. Retrieved June 28, 2009, from www.ncea.aoa.gov/NCEAroot/Main_Site/FAQ/Basics/Definition.aspx.

National Center on Elder Abuse. (2009b). Major types of elder abuse. Retrieved June 28, 2009, from www.ncea.aoa.gov/NCEAroot/Main_Site/FAQ/Basics/Types_of_Abuse.aspx.

National Research Council. (2003). *Elder mistreatment: Abuse, neglect, and exploitation in an aging America.* Washington, DC: The National Academies Press.

Nerenberg, L. (2008). *Elder abuse prevention: Emergency trends and promising practices.* New York: Springer Publishing Co.

Page, C., Conner, T., Prokhorov, A., Post, L., & Fang, Y. (in press). The effect of care setting on elder abuse: Results from a Michigan survey. *Journal of Elder Abuse & Neglect, 23*(3).

Patterson, M., & Malley-Morrison, K. (2006). A cognitive-ecological approach to elder abuse in five cultures: Human rights and education. *Educational Gerontology, 32,* 73–82.

Pillemer, K., Breckman, R., Sweeney, C. D., Brownell, P., Fulmer, T., Berman, J., . . . Lachs, M. S. (in press). Practitioners' views on elder mistreatment research priorities: Recommendations from a research-to-practice consensus conference. *Journal of Elder Abuse & Neglect, 23*(2).

Poulos, C. A., & Sheridan, D. J. (2008). Genital injuries in postmenopausal women after sexual assault. *Journal of Elder Abuse & Neglect. 20,* 323–335.

Ramsey-Klawsnik, H., Teaster, P. B., Mendiondo, M. S., Marcum, J. L., & Abner, E. L. (2008). Sexual predators who target elders: Findings from the first national study of sexual abuse in care facilities. *Journal of Elder Abuse & Neglect, 20,* 353–376.

Sarton, M. (1973). *As we are now.* New York: W. W. Norton.

Selwood, A., Cooper, C., Owens, C., Blanchard, M., & Livingston, G. (2009). What would help me stop abusing? The family carer's perspective. *International Journal of Psychogeriatrics, 21,* 309–313.

Shinan-Altman, S., & Cohen, M. (2009). Nursing aides' attitudes to elder abuse in nursing homes: The effect of work stressors and burnout. *The Gerontologist, 49,* 674–684.

Tauriac, J. J., & Scruggs, N. (2006). Elder abuse among African Americans. *Educational Gerontology, 32,* 37–48.

Teaster, P. B., & Roberts, K. A. (2004). Sexual abuse of older adults: APS cases and outcomes. *The Gerontologist, 44,* 788–796.

Townsend, C. (1970). *Old age: The last segregation.* New York: Grossman.

United Nations Economic and Social Affairs. (2008). *Guide to the national implementation of the Madrid International Plan of Action on Aging.* New York: United Nations Headquarters.

United Nations Economic and Social Council. (2002, February 25–March 1). *Abuse of older persons: Recognizing and responding to abuse of older persons in a global context.* Document of the Commission for Social Development presented at the Second World Assembly on Aging, New York.

Vladeck, B. C. (1980). *Unloving care: The nursing home tragedy*. New York: Basic Books.

Walsh, C. A., Olson, J., Ploeg, J., Lohfeld, L., & MacMillan, H. L. (in press). Elder abuse and oppression: Voices of marginalized elders. *Journal of Elder Abuse & Neglect, 23*(1).

Wiglesworth, A., Austin, R., Corona, M., Schneider, D., Liao, S., Gibbs, L., & Mosqueda, L. (2009). Bruising as a marker of physical elder abuse. *Journal of the American Geriatrics Society, 57*, 1191–1196.

Wiglesworth, A., Mosqueda, L., Mulnard, R., Liao, S., Gibbs, L., & Fitzgerald, W. (2010). Screening for abuse and neglect of people with dementia. *Journal of the American Geriatrics Society, 58*, 493–500.

Zhang, Z., Schiamberg, L. B., Oehmke, J., Barboza, G. E., Griffore, R. J., Post, L. A., . . . Mastin, T. (2010). Neglect of older adults in Michigan nursing homes. *Journal of Elder Abuse & Neglect, 22*(3).

Promoting Wellness in Psychosocial Function

PART 3

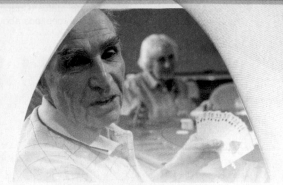

CHAPTER 11

Cognitive Function

LEARNING OBJECTIVES

After reading this chapter, you will be able to:

1. Describe age-related changes that affect cognitive abilities.
2. List risk factors that influence cognitive function in older adults.
3. Discuss the functional consequences associated with cognition in older adults.
4. Identify nursing interventions to help older adults maintain or improve cognitive abilities.

KEY POINTS

age-associated memory
  impairment
automatic and effortful
  processing theory
cognitive reserve
contextual theories
continuum of processing
crystallized intelligence
developmental
  intelligence
empowering model
everyday problem solving

executive functions
fluid intelligence
memory
metamemory
neuroplasticity
paradox of well-being
scaffolding theory of aging
  and cognition
socioemotional selectivity
stage theories
wisdom

Cognition involves the processes of thinking, learning, and remembering. Myths about cognitive aging are pervasive and long-standing in the society and can be detrimental to older adults. Indeed, the adage that "you can't teach

an old dog new tricks" underlies some of the most widely held—and inaccurate—perspectives on older adults' cognition. Research in recent decades supports a more optimistic view of cognitive aging and identifies interventions that improve cognition. One of the most significant ways in which nurses can promote wellness for older adults is by correcting myth-based views and encouraging older adults to engage in activities that foster cognitive fitness.

 ## AGE-RELATED CHANGES THAT AFFECT COGNITION

Current theories about aging and cognition differ significantly from those that were first proposed during the 1960s. Initial cross-sectional studies, which were based on tests designed to predict school performance in children, led to the conclusion that a decline in cognitive abilities was a normal part of the aging process. By the mid-1980s, results of longitudinal studies began showing that intellectual function remained the same or improved up to the age of 50 or 60 years, after which it gradually declined. In recent decades, researchers have focused on the interplay between cognitive abilities and factors such as emotions, environment, life experiences, and socioeconomic conditions. Gerontologists are particularly interested in identifying interventions that improve cognitive abilities in older adults because studies indicate that the brain has the ability to change.

As with many other aspects of function in older adults, gerontologists are trying to distinguish between the cognitive changes that occur in healthy older adults and those that are associated with pathologic processes such as dementia (discussed in Chapter 14). Age-related changes affecting cognition can be understood in terms of physical changes in the central nervous system and in theories about intelligence, **memory**, and psychological development that attempt to explain the relationship between aging and cognition.

Promoting Cognitive Wellness in Older Adults

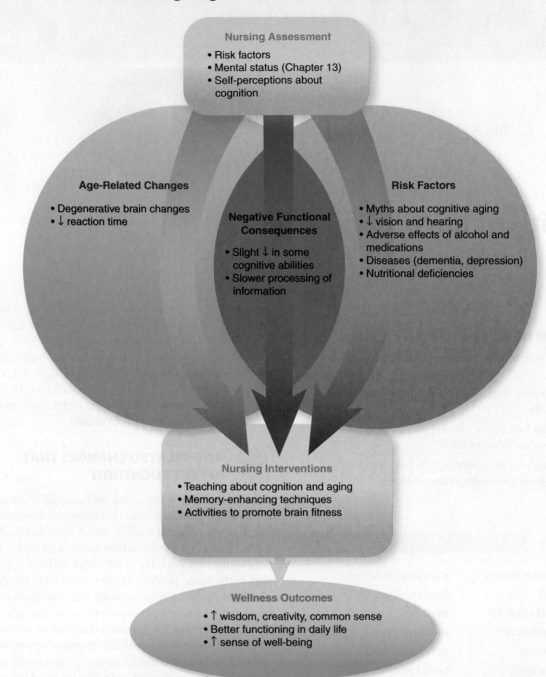

Nursing Assessment

- Risk factors
- Mental status (Chapter 13)
- Self-perceptions about cognition

Age-Related Changes

- Degenerative brain changes
- ↓ reaction time

Negative Functional Consequences

- Slight ↓ in some cognitive abilities
- Slower processing of information

Risk Factors

- Myths about cognitive aging
- ↓ vision and hearing
- Adverse effects of alcohol and medications
- Diseases (dementia, depression)
- Nutritional deficiencies

Nursing Interventions

- Teaching about cognition and aging
- Memory-enhancing techniques
- Activities to promote brain fitness

Wellness Outcomes

- ↑ wisdom, creativity, common sense
- Better functioning in daily life
- ↑ sense of well-being

Central Nervous System

Knowledge about brain aging is gleaned from many types of studies, including clinical, neuropsychological, neuropathologic, and neurochemical investigations. Initial studies of brain aging relied on autopsy findings, but recent major advances in noninvasive neuroimaging techniques (e.g., functional magnetic resonance imaging) have significantly broadened the knowledge base. Recent studies continue to identify age-related changes in the brain, but they are incon-

clusive with regard to the impact of these changes on cognition. Current research findings are discussed here.

Loss of white matter is frequently noted on brain imaging tests, and these changes affect global functioning in older adults; however, studies indicate that these changes are due to small vessel disease associated with vascular risk factors rather than age-related changes alone (Inzitari et al., 2009). Studies have also found decreased cerebral blood flow and cortical volume loss, particularly in the frontal lobes, but

A Student's Perspective

The residents at Heritage continue to amaze me with their stories. There is so much one can learn just by listening, and the residents just want to share their stories and have our company more than anything—at least that is the impression I continually receive from them. They are all friendly, open people who are no different than the rest of us, but they have gained a large amount of knowledge over the years that many of us who are students probably have not acquired yet.

Megan S.

some studies suggest that the brains of older adults may be able to compensate for these changes (Sorond, Schnyer, Serrador, Milberg, & Lipstiz, 2008). Additional age-related changes in the brain and central nervous system that potentially affect cognitive abilities are reduced brain weight, diminished cerebral blood flow, enlarged ventricles and wider sulci, loss and shrinkage of neurons, reduced neurotransmitters or their binding sites, and accumulation of lipofuscin in nerve cell bodies. In addition to directly affecting cognitive skills, these age-related changes cause a slower reaction time and affect the speed of processing information.

Gerontologists are emphasizing that age-related degenerative changes in the neural structures do not totally determine cognitive abilities because cognitive potential can remain even when neural structures are compromised (Willis, Schaie, & Martin, 2009). Researchers have proposed the **scaffolding theory of aging and cognition** as a way of explaining the adaptive response of the brain to the declining neural structures and function. According to this theory, scaffolding is a normal process that involves the development and use of complementary and alternative neural circuits to achieve a cognitive goal (Goh & Park, 2009). This process protects cognitive abilities despite the presence of age-related changes (Park & Reuter-Lorenz, 2009).

The term **neuroplasticity** (also called *neural plasticity*) refers to the physiologic ability of the brain and neural circuits to change and develop in response to environmental stimuli. The closely related concept of **cognitive reserve** refers to the capacity to continue to function at an adequate cognitive level despite the presence of age-related or pathologic processes that affect the neural structures (Vance & Wright, 2009; Willis et al., 2009). Neuroplasticity is defined as positive when it promotes neuronal connections and increases cognitive reserve and as negative when it inhibits neuronal connections and decreases cognitive reserve (Vance & Wright, 2009). Gerontologists increasingly are emphasizing that cognitive development can occur at every stage of human development; however, older adults have more constraints and limits that need to be addressed (Willis et al., 2009). Studies based on the cognitive reserve model indicated that participation in creative activities (e.g., art, storytelling, dance classes) and leisure time cognitive activities (e.g., reading, writing, group discussions, playing music) is associated with delayed onset of memory decline and improved cognition in older adults (Hall et al., 2009; McFadden & Basting, 2010).

Although research on brain aging provides the biologic base of information, psychological theories explain differences in cognitive abilities, as discussed in the following sections.

Fluid and Crystallized Intelligence

Cattell and Horn theory of fluid and crystallized intelligence, first proposed in the late 1960s, is one of the first theories that attempted to explain age-related changes in some cognitive abilities. **Fluid intelligence** depends primarily on central nervous system functioning and a person's inherent abilities, such as memory and pattern recognition. Fluid intelligence is associated with the cognitive skills of integration, inductive reasoning, abstract thinking, and flexible and adaptive thinking. This cognitive characteristic enables people to identify and draw conclusions about complex relationships. **Crystallized intelligence** refers to cognitive skills, such as vocabulary, information, and verbal comprehension, that people acquire through culture, education, informal learning, and other life experiences. This cognitive characteristic is strongly associated with **wisdom**, judgment, and life experiences.

According to this theory, fluid and crystallized intelligence develop concurrently during infancy and childhood and are indistinguishable as the central nervous system is maturing. Age-related changes in neural structures cause a decline in fluid intelligence. Crystallized intelligence, however, continues to develop during adulthood because of accumulated experiences and learning. Crystallized intelligence, except for those processes that depend on the speed of response, does not decline with age, and it may even increase because of experiences that improve wisdom. Although fluid intelligence is thought to decline with increased age, a recent longitudinal study of 626 adults found that a strong sense of self-direction in work situations prevented declines in verbal memory and inductive reasoning, which are two aspects of fluid intelligence (Yu, Ryan, Schaie, Willis, & Kolanowski, 2009).

Memory

Memory is often conceptualized as a computer-like information-processing system in which information is first perceived, then stored, and finally retrieved when needed or wanted. *Primary memory* has a short duration and a very small capacity, and it serves as a holding tank for events of the immediate past few seconds rather than as a true memory storage system. Information in the primary memory can be either recalled for a brief time or transmitted to long-term storage. *Secondary memory* has longer duration and, therefore, is more important in terms of retrieval, as well as storage, of information. Retrieval of information from storage is referred to as remote, tertiary, or very–long-term memory processing, and skills involved are classified as *recall memory* and *recognition memory*. Some theories associated with these concepts suggest that older people remember events of long ago better than recent events; however, studies indicate that both types of memory decline equally but older adults have a larger store of information about events of long ago (Botwinick, 1984). Studies have also found that older adults can remember the events that occurred but have more difficulty remembering the context in which they took place (Cansino, 2009).

More recently, gerontologists have viewed the information-processing model as too simplistic because it ignores the milieu in which the memory operates. Thus, newer **contextual theories** address variables that can affect memory. For example, slower speed of processing is an age-related change that can significantly affect memory and other cognitive skills. Other variables that can affect memory include motivation, expectations, experiences, education, personality, task demands, learning habits, intellectual skills, sociocultural background, physical and mental health, and style of processing information. Recent studies found that memory and other cognitive skills of older adults are equal to or better than those of younger adults under some conditions (Labouvie-Vief, 2009). For example, older adults have better memory recall and recognition than do younger adults when the information or emotional stimuli are positive in comparison to stimuli that are negative (Blanchard-Fields & Kalinauskas, 2009). Similarly, older adults are capable of using complex cognitive skills when the situation is highly interesting or has personal relevance (Hess, Leclerc, Swaim, & Weatherbee, 2009).

Another theoretical approach emphasizes encoding and analyzing rather than storage and retrieval aspects of memory. According to this perspective, memory is a **continuum of processing**, ranging from shallow to deep levels; the deeper the level at which information is stored, the longer the memory will last. Any of the following variables can affect the depth of storage (Botwinick, 1984):

- Processing techniques, ranging from the shallowest levels used for sensory information to the deepest levels used for highly abstract information
- Elaboration, or quality, of processing conducted at any depth level
- Distinctiveness of the information, which depends partially on how well it is learned
- Depth and elaboration of retrieval processes.

Several studies based on this framework concluded that older adults have decreased memory function because of faulty processing mechanisms (Botwinick, 1984). A recent study suggested that the age-related reduction in memory accuracy is associated, at least in part, from poorer encoding (Pansky, Goldsmith, Koriat, & Pearlman-Avnion, 2009).

Another theoretical perspective that views memory as a continuum is the **automatic and effortful processing theory**, which was proposed by Hasher & Zacks (1979). At one end of the continuum is automatic processing, or those tasks that do not require attention or awareness and do not improve with practice. At the other end is effortful processing, or those tasks that demand high levels of attention and cognitive energy. With practice, effortful tasks require less attention and

become more automatic. According to this theory, aging does not affect automatic memory because these tasks require little or no cognitive energy. Effortful memory, however, declines with age because the limited cognitive resources that are available for memory functions begin to decline in early adulthood. Studies have confirmed declines in effortful processes (e.g., selective attention, mental imagery, verbal fluency, language production, and verbal and visuospatial working memory) and no declines in automatic cognitive functions (e.g., picture recognition and implicit and procedural memory) (Carstensen, Mickles, & Mathers, 2006).

Metamemory refers to self-knowledge and perceptions about memory, cognitive function, and development of memory. Metamemory is important in everyday activities because if people know what they can remember and how much effort they will need to remember certain things, they can plan efficient and effective strategies for remembering. Because older adults tend to perceive themselves as less competent than younger adults or less competent than they actually are in many cognitive tasks, gerontologists emphasize the importance of addressing ageist attitudes that contribute to negative self-stereotypes about cognitive abilities (Levy & Leifheit-Limson, 2009).

◆ Wellness Opportunity

Nurses can influence attitudes by conveying positive beliefs about the ability of older adults to improve memory skills.

Adult Psychological Development

Theories about psychological development postulate that the thinking of older adults becomes increasingly complex and shows progressive reorganization of intellectual skills (Labouvie-Vief & Blanchard-Fields, 1982). For example, a recent focus of these theories is on cognitive abilities associated with decision making and **everyday problem solving**. Conclusions from studies of decision-making skills are as follows (Mariske & Margrett, 2006):

- Affect and motivation are strong predictors of decision making in older adults.
- Older adults are more selective in the information they use for decision making (i.e., they base decisions on less information).
- Older adults require more time to make decisions that are equal in quality to those of younger adults, but they may choose to spend the same or less time.
- Increased task complexity is associated with more error and more inconsistencies for both older and younger adults.
- Task expertise and prior experience contribute to better decisions for both older and younger adults.

Nurses can apply conclusions from these studies when they involve older adults in decisions about self-care.

Stage theories of adult cognitive development were first developed during the 1970s as an extension of Piaget theory of intellectual development in children and adolescents. One such theory postulated that children and adolescents focus on acquiring knowledge, and adults focus on applying knowledge in the following stages (Schaie, 1977–1978):

- *Achieving stage* (early adulthood): adults apply acquired knowledge to demands and commitments, such as career and family; they use their intellectual abilities to establish their independence and develop goal-oriented behaviors.
- *Responsible stage* (late 30s to early 60s): adults integrate long-range goals and attend to the needs of their family and society.
- *Executive stage* (a subset of the responsible stage): applies to people who have high levels of social responsibilities.
- *Reintegration stage* (later adulthood): intellectual tasks are to simplify life and select only those responsibilities that have meaning and purpose; older adults ask "Why should I know?" rather than "What should I know?"

More recently, Cohen (2005) developed an **empowering model** based on studies of more than 3000 older adults. This model describes the following four phases of mature aging:

- *Midlife reevaluation* (early 40s to late 50s): people confront their sense of mortality; plans and actions are shaped by a quest or crisis; brain changes spur developmental intelligence.
- *Liberation* (late 50s to early 70s): people feel a new sense of inner liberation; development in information-processing part of the brain increases desire for novelty; plans and actions are shaped by personal freedom; retirement allows time for new experiences.
- *Summing up* (late 60s through 80s): people are motivated to share wisdom; plans and actions are shaped by a desire to find meaning; brain development improves capacity for autobiographical expression; people may feel compelled to attend to unfinished business and unresolved conflicts.
- *Encore* (late 70s to the end of life): plans and actions are shaped by the desire to restate and reaffirm major themes and to explore novel variations on those themes; brain changes promote positive emotions and morale; the desire to live well to the very end has a positive impact on others.

Gerontologists have also focused on the **paradox of well-being**, which describes the phenomenon of older adults suffering significant losses of health, cognition, and social functioning but reporting high levels of well-being and positive emotions (Labouvie-Vief, 2009). The **socioemotional selectivity** theory addresses this question in the context of motivation. According to this theory, older adults recognize that time is limited, so they are motivated to pursue emotional satisfaction. Thus, they shift their focus from the pursuit of knowledge and information gathering and concentrate on relationships that are closer and more intimate (Labouvie-Vief, 2009).

Another current focus is on wisdom as an aspect of cognitive function, which is viewed as "a special type of expertise about the meaning of life and the pragmatics of how things work in a particular situation" (Zarit, 2009). A working definition of wisdom as an integral aspect of adult development includes the following (Knight & Laidlaw, 2009, p. 684):

- An accumulation of "knowing how" expertise over "knowing what"

- A greater ability to integrate and balance emotion and reason
- An awareness of the many contexts of life and how they change over the years
- An acceptance of uncertainty in life and an understanding of how to handle this
- An understanding of the relativism of individual values and an increased tolerance for individual differences.

A similar concept is **developmental intelligence**, defined as "the maturing of cognition, emotional intelligence, judgment, social skills, life experience, and consciousness and their integration and synergy" (Cohen, 2005, p. 35). Cohen's view of cognitive aging, which is both optimistic and research based, emphasizes that many older adults display the age-dependent quality of wisdom because they integrate all the components of developmental intelligence.

> **Wellness Opportunity**
>
> Nurses acknowledge the wisdom of older adults by asking questions such as "Do you have some words of wisdom to share about that valuable experience?"

 ## RISK FACTORS THAT AFFECT COGNITIVE WELLNESS

A multitude of internal and external conditions can affect cognitive function in people of all ages, but older adults are particularly vulnerable to these risk factors. Nurses need to pay particular attention to identifying the risk factors that are reversible and the ones that can be addressed through health promotion interventions.

Personal, Social, and Attitudinal Influences

Numerous personal characteristics affect cognitive abilities in people of any age, and researchers have tried to identify those that most significantly affect older adults. Years of formal education is the factor most consistently associated with cognitive performance in older adults, and this association is independent of race and sex and cultural, geographic, or other variables (Kaufman, Kaufman, Lui, & Johnson, 2009; Wilson et al., 2009). Other factors that affect cognitive function include occupation, education, social relations, race and ethnicity, hearing and vision problems, leisure and intellectual activities, and lifestyle factors (e.g., nutrition, physical activity) (Friedman et al., 2009; Hakansson et al., 2009; Nikolova, Demers, & Beland, 2009).

Ageism and diminished expectations of older adults in modern societies can negatively affect cognitive function. Studies indicate that older adults internalize stereotypes about memory decline as an inevitable outcome of aging and that these perceptions have adverse effects on their cognitive abilities (Hess, Hinson, & Hodges, 2009; Levy & Leifheit-Limson, 2009). In addition, these studies found that the negative effects of stereotypes were the strongest for the older adults with higher levels of education (Hess, Emery, & Queen, 2009).

Physical and Mental Health Factors

Many chronic conditions and other aspects of physical health affect cognitive abilities in older adults. Examples of chronic conditions associated with impaired cognitive function include thyroid disorders, diabetes, dementia, and cardiovascular disorders. The effect of pathologic conditions on cognitive function is reviewed further in Chapter 14.

Nutritional status is widely recognized as a health factor that can affect cognitive function regardless of a person's age. For example, low levels of beta-carotene, and vitamins B, C, and D are associated with poor cognitive function. Researchers have focused much attention on nutritional factors that affect cognition because these can often be addressed through relatively simple interventions. The following conclusions are based on recent studies:

- A longitudinal study of 436 women aged 70 to 80 years at baseline found that anemia was associated with poorer baseline performance and more precipitous declines in cognitive abilities (Deal, Carison, Xue, Fried, & Chaves, 2009).
- Data from almost 3000 community-living men and women older than 60 years found that poorer nutritional status was associated with increased risk of cognitive impairment (Lee et al., 2009).
- A study of 980 community-living men and women aged 65 to 99 years found that low serum vitamin D levels were associated with poorer performance on tests of executive function and attention/speed of processing but not with memory tests (Buell et al., 2009).
- A study of more than 3000 men between the ages of 40 and 79 years found that serum vitamin D levels lower than 35 nmol/L were associated with poorer performance on a test of cognitive function (Lee et al., 2009).
- Studies indicate that cognitive abilities of older adults may be adversely affected by serum vitamin B levels above the traditional cutoff for deficiency (Smith & Refsum, 2009).
- A study of 1358 Puerto Ricans aged 45 to 75 years in Massachusetts found that food insecurity was associated with lower cognitive performance (Gao, Scott, Falcon, Wilde, & Tucker, 2009).
- A longitudinal study of almost 1500 women aged 70 years and older with type 2 diabetes found that higher intakes of saturated and trans fat since midlife and lower polyunsaturated to saturated fat ratio was associated with worse cognitive decline (Devore et al., 2009).

Sensory impairment is another aspect of health that affects cognitive processes because hearing or vision deficits limit the quantity and quality of information received from the environment. Because sensory input significantly influences learning and other cognitive processes, nurses need to ensure optimal visual and hearing conditions when communicating with older adults (as discussed in Chapters 16 and 17).

Researchers are also focusing on mental health factors that can affect cognitive function. Psychological stress, especially if prolonged, is a health factor that can suppress the development of new neurons (Cohen, 2005). Studies have found that anxiety impairs cognitive abilities by causing excessive worry and self-doubts and by interfering with attention and the speed of processing (Beaudreau & O'Hara, 2009). Depression and even subclinical variations in depressive symptoms are strongly associated with impaired cognitive function (especially memory), as discussed in Chapter 15. Depression contributes to negative self-expectations and interferes with attention and concentration, which are two cognitive skills that significantly affect memory.

Some studies focus on a combination of health-related factors, with emphasis on health behaviors that promote good cognitive function. Data from a 17-year study of more than 5,000 men and women with initial mean age of 44 years found an association between the number and duration of unhealthy behaviors and lower scores on measures of cognitive function in later life (Sabia et al., 2009). Other studies have found that healthy lifestyle behaviors (e.g., nonsmoking, physical activity, vegetable consumption, and social engagement) are associated with maintaining good cognitive function (Lee, Kim, & Back, 2009; Williamson et al., 2009; Yaffe et al., 2009). A recent review of studies concluded that epidemiologic studies, short-term randomized controlled trials, and biologic research suggest that physical activity improves cognitive functioning in older adults (Rolland, vanKan, & Vellas, 2010).

Medication Effects

Prescription and over-the-counter medications can interfere with memory and other cognitive functions in a variety of ways. For example, anticholinergic ingredients, contained in numerous prescription and over-the-counter medications, significantly affect memory and other cognitive functions and are a common cause of changes in mental status in older adults (Carriere et al., 2009). Because many medications have anticholinergic effects, researchers and clinicians have paid particular attention in recent years to the cumulative effects of these medications on acetylcholine, which is a neurotransmitter that directly affects cognitive function. Chapter 8 provides detailed information about anticholinergics and other types of medications that can interfere with cognitive function. Refer to Table 8-12 for information about specific medications and the modes of action that affect cognitive function.

Smoking and Environmental Factors

Researchers are also examining risk factors such as smoking and exposure to environmental toxins. Studies have found that chronic smoking and exposure to secondhand smoke are associated with increased risk of cognitive decline (Azizian, Monterosso, O'Neill, & London, 2009; Llewellyn, Lang, Langa, Naughton, & Matthews, 2009). A longitudinal study found that at baseline, smokers scored lower than nonsmokers on tests of cognitive function. At 5-year follow-up, the decline among smokers was significantly greater (Noovens, Van Gelder, & Verschuren, 2008). Studies also found an association between occupational exposure to lead and progressive declines in cognitive function, even after an average 16 years after the exposure ended (Stewart et al., 2006). Studies are also addressing questions about whether exposure to environmental toxins, such as solvents, mercury, pesticides, and cigarette smoke, causes progressive and long-term damage that mimics the aging process (Rowland & McKinstry, 2006).

Wellness Opportunity

From a holistic perspective, nurses help older adults identify risk factors, such as nutrition and over-the-counter medications, that can be addressed through self-care actions.

FUNCTIONAL CONSEQUENCES AFFECTING COGNITIVE FUNCTION

Healthy older adults will not experience any significant cognitive impairment that interferes with daily life, but they will notice minor deficits in some aspects of cognitive function and improvements in other aspects. Longitudinal studies have identified patterns of cognitive change that are likely to occur even in the absence of any pathologic processes. These changes can be summarized as follows (Carlson, Xue, Zhou, & Fried, 2009; Caserta et al., 2009):

- Aspects of cognition that are involved with perceptual speed and numerical ability begin to decline during the third decade and continue to decline at a modest linear rate.
- Episodic memory (i.e., memory of personally experienced events) may begin to decline as early as the third or fourth decade.
- Decline of verbal ability and tasks of inductive reasoning during the fifth or sixth decade.
- Changes that begin during earlier and middle adulthood are gradual and do not reach a level of significance until the seventh or eighth decade, at which point they may continue to decline.
- **Executive functions** (e.g., problem-solving skills, inhibition, and flexibility) show considerable age-related declines.
- Word lexicon and general knowledge improve well into the sixth decade and remain stable during later adulthood.

It is important to keep in mind that these conclusions about patterns of change are based on well-designed studies, but gerontologists emphasize that there is a great deal of individual variation in cognitive changes, with some older adults showing no decline and a small percentage even showing improvement in cognitive abilities. Gerontologists also emphasize that studies focusing only on age-related cognitive changes do not address the strong interplay between cognition and other factors. For example, researchers have found that social expertise and emotional processing and regulation remain stable and may even improve with increased age (Blanchard-Fields & Kalinauskas, 2009). Thus, cognitive function in older adults must be considered in relation to social, emotional, and other factors.

CULTURAL CONSIDERATIONS 11-1

Cultural Factors and Cognitive Function

- It is important to recognize that the standards of intellectual performance used in the United States have been developed for English-speaking white Americans.
- It is important to recognize that cognitive abilities are highly influenced by health, education, and socioeconomic status and that these factors and cultural factors are interrelated.
- Cultural and language factors may influence an older adult's perception and description of memory problems.

This perspective is supported by recent studies that indicate that "healthy older brains are often as good as or better than younger brains in a wide variety of tasks" (Cohen, 2005, p. 4). Cohen cites the following evidence-based findings that support an optimistic view of cognitive aging:

- New brain cells form throughout life.
- Experience and learning enable the brain to "resculpt" itself.
- Emotional circuitry of the brain matures and becomes more balanced during older adulthood.
- Functions of the left and right hemispheres of the brain become more integrated in older adults.

Another important consideration is that conclusions about cognitive aging do not necessarily address cultural factors and, therefore, are limited by the factors cited in Cultural Considerations 11-1.

An important implication of the findings discussed in this section and the section on risk factors is that numerous conditions affect cognitive function in older adults, and nurses can address many of these variables through educational interventions. In addition, nurses need to adapt their teaching methods to compensate for age-related changes in cognition that can affect learning. Box 11-1 summarizes some of research-based conclusions about cognitive aging that are most relevant for identifying and implementing health education interventions for older adults.

Wellness Opportunity

Nurses promote wellness by encouraging older adults to identify ways in which their cognitive abilities have improved (e.g., wisdom based on experiences).

NURSING ASSESSMENT OF COGNITIVE FUNCTION

Formal assessment of intellectual performance involves administering psychometric tests, but nurses can informally assess memory and cognitive skills. In addition to assessing the intellectual performance of older adults, nurses can assess for risk factors that are likely to interfere with cognitive function. Because nursing assessment of cognition is an integral part of the psychosocial assessment, it is addressed comprehensively in Chapter 13 rather than in this chapter. Nursing

Box 11-1 Functional Consequences Affecting Cognition in Older Adults

Cognitive Abilities in Healthy Older Adults

- Skills that stay the same or improve: wisdom, creativity, common sense, coordination of facts and ideas, and breadth of knowledge and experience
- Skills that decline slightly and gradually: abstraction, calculation, word fluency, verbal comprehension, spatial orientation, inductive reasoning, and episodic memory
- Word finding may be more difficult (i.e., "tip-of-the-tongue" experiences), but total vocabulary increases
- Remote memory remains intact and holds a large store of information about the past
- Factors that interfere with cognitive function: anxiety, depression, diminished sensory input, poor health, negative beliefs, ageist attitudes, pathologic processes (e.g., dementia)
- Factors that improve cognitive function: good nutrition, physical exercise, mental stimulation, challenging leisure activities, strong social networks, and activities that provide a sense of control and mastery.

Learning Abilities

- Older adults are as capable of learning new things as younger people, but the speed with which they process information is slower.
- Older adults are more cautious in their responses and make more errors of omission.
- Potential barriers to learning in older adults include distractions, sensory deficits, lack of relevance, teacher–learner age differences, and values that are incongruent with new knowledge.

assessment of impaired cognitive function is addressed in Chapter 14 (Delirium and Dementia).

NURSING DIAGNOSIS

Healthy older adults are able to maintain good cognitive function; however, many older adults experience memory deficits that affect their overall functioning. In these situations, nurses can use the nursing diagnosis of Impaired Memory, which is defined as the "inability to remember or recall bits of information or behavioral skills" (NANDA International, 2009, p. 173). Nursing diagnoses related to cognitive impairment associated with dementia, confusional states, and other serious cognitive impairments are discussed in Chapter 14.

Wellness Opportunity

Nurses can use the wellness nursing diagnosis of Readiness for Enhanced Knowledge for older adults who are motivated to improve their cognitive skills.

PLANNING FOR WELLNESS OUTCOMES

A wellness-oriented outcome criterion related to cognitive function is that older adults take responsibility for addressing risk factors and compensating for age-related cognitive changes. Examples of outcomes related to risk factors would be that older adults compensate for sensory deficits (e.g., using

A Student's Perspective

At the beginning of the 5 weeks at Friendship Village, I didn't know what to expect. I assumed we would just be taking vital signs and making small talk with a few of the clients. I didn't realize I would learn so much by just listening to the life story of someone who is 96 years old. I realized that many of these individuals have had quite the amazing life and have a lot of wisdom and knowledge to pass down.

Needless to say, my expectations changed dramatically! They went from just getting the 5 weeks over with, to me not wanting to leave after the 5 weeks. Many of the residents were still "with it" and could remember a lot about their childhood and past experiences. This is the information that I did my best to take in. How did they get to live to be 96 years old and be able to look back on their life and be proud of their accomplishments. That's the life I want to live!!

Kim V.

a hearing aid) and engage in physically and mentally stimulating activities. Older adults can compensate for age-related cognitive changes by using memory-enhancing techniques. Nurses can use the following Nursing Outcomes Classification (NOC) terminology for outcomes related to cognitive wellness: Cognition, Concentration, Information Processing, Knowledge: Health Promotion, Leisure Participation, Hearing Compensation Behavior, and Vision Compensation Behavior.

Wellness Opportunity

Personal well-being is a wellness outcome that nurses can promote by supporting personal responsibility for actions that improve cognitive abilities.

NURSING INTERVENTIONS TO PROMOTE COGNITIVE WELLNESS

Nurses have key roles in teaching older adults about the following evidence-based strategies for cognitive health and vitality (Akbaraly et al., 2009; Kamijo et al., 2009; Yevchak, Loeb, & Fick, 2008):

- Proper nutrition: Include foods high in antioxidants (e.g., fruits and vegetable) and omega-3 fatty acids (e.g., fatty fish); restrict salt, cholesterol, and saturated fat; limit caloric intake to maintain a healthy weight.
- Mental exercise: Engage in new learning experiences that are appealing and challenging.
- Physical exercise: Include moderate aerobic activity, strengthening exercises, and flexibility and balance exercises.
- Take part in challenging leisure activities (listed in order of most to least effective): dancing, playing board games, playing a musical instrument, doing crossword puzzles, reading.
- Choose activities in which there is a sense of control and mastery: learning computer skills, a new language, or how to play a musical instrument.

- Develop strong social networks: Maintaining social relationships with family and friends.

Many of the health promotion interventions discussed throughout this text provide specific examples of these types of activities. For example, interventions for cardiovascular wellness (see Chapter 20) are particularly relevant to promoting optimal cognitive function. Also, because vision and hearing impairments can interfere with cognitive abilities, any interventions directed toward improving sensory function (discussed in Chapters 16 and 17) may also be effective in improving cognitive function.

Nurses can apply the following Nursing Interventions Classification (NIC) terminology for interventions related to cognitive wellness: Activity Therapy, Communication Enhancement: Hearing Deficit, Communication Enhancement: Visual Deficit, Exercise Promotion, Health Education, Learning Facilitation, Learning Readiness Enhancement, Meditation Facilitation, Progressive Muscle Relaxation, Role Enhancement, Self-Awareness Enhancement, Self-Responsibility Enhancement, and Teaching: Individual.

> ◆ **Wellness Opportunity**
>
> Nurses promote personal responsibility for wellness by helping older adults identify ways of incorporating "brain fitness" activities into their daily lives.

Teaching About Memory and Cognition

Teaching older adults about techniques to maintain or improve cognitive skills is within the realm of nursing responsibilities, in the same way as is teaching about maintaining and improving physical function. In recent years, governmental and non-profit organizations have developed several major initiatives to promote cognitive health in older adults. For example, The Healthy Brain Initiative: A National Public Health Road Map to Maintaining Cognitive Health is an ongoing program of the National Institutes of Health that addresses cognitive health as a public health issue for older adults. This program emphasizes the importance of teaching older adults about healthy lifestyle practices, including good nutrition and adequate physical activity, that are effective in preventing cognitive decline (Anderson, Logsdon, Hochhalter, & Sharkey, 2009). Nurses can access educational materials from this and other initiatives listed in the Resources section at the end of this chapter to use when they teach older adults about healthy brain aging.

The concept of metacognition suggests that an understanding of one's own cognitive processes can influence performance. For example, someone who wants to remember a list of names needs both the intent to remember and knowledge about techniques for remembering. Studies find that memory training can be effective in improving metamemory, memory knowledge, and objective memory performance in older adults (Bottiroli, Cavallini, & Vecchi, 2008; Langbaum, Rebok, Bandeen-Roche, & Carlson, 2009; Smith, 2009). Speed-of-processing training is another intervention that is effective in improving cognitive abilities that affect everyday functioning, including driving (Vance, 2009).

In addition to addressing memory training techniques, health education also needs to address beliefs about cognition and aging because these can significantly influence one's ability to learn. Thus, health education needs to include all the following aspects:
- Correcting myths and misinformation
- Providing accurate information about age-related changes
- Communicating positive expectations
- Identifying goals for self-learning
- Providing information about techniques to enhance cognitive abilities
- Identifying the techniques that are most effective for the individual.

In community and long-term care settings, group sessions can effectively and efficiently address many psychosocial aspects of aging, including cognitive function. Nurses can use the model developed by Turner Geriatric Services at the University of Michigan for either single- or multiple-session programs for older adults. A training manual provides information about developing memory training programs, and it includes lesson plans and handouts for group leaders (Fogler & Stern, 2005). Box 11-2, which outlines a sample presentation for older adults based on the material from the Turner Geriatric Clinic, can be used to educate older adults about techniques for memory enhancement.

> ◆ **Wellness Opportunity**
>
> Nurses holistically address learning needs of older adults by encouraging participation in group programs, which have the additional benefit of offering social support.

Improving Concentration and Attention

When one's ability to attend to the environment and concentrate on visual and auditory cues is limited, the ability to learn and remember is also impaired. Thus, techniques such as relaxation, imagery, and meditation, which enhance attention and concentration, may also improve memory and learning. Likewise, any method that reduces environmental distractions may also improve one's cognitive abilities. Mindfulness (also called *mindfulness meditation*), which is the practice of focused awareness of the environment and one's reactions to it, is a self-care practice that can improve cognitive function and overall well-being. Many self-help books describe techniques for meditation, mindfulness, and relaxation as ways of opening the mind to new learning. Nurses can teach the relaxation technique outlined in Chapter 24 to older adults for a variety of uses, including the enhancement of mental skills. Nurses also promote personal responsibility for cognitive wellness by encouraging older adults to identify self-care practices that improve attention.

Encouraging Participation in Mentally Stimulating Activities

Because there is much evidence that participation in mentally stimulating activities is effective for promoting cognitive

Box 11-2 Memory Training for Older Adults

Introduction
- Forgetting is a normal part of life for all people, but memory skills can be learned. The purposes of this program are to look at some reasons people forget things and to discuss ways of improving memory skills.
- When older adults are forgetful, they may blame it on old age, rather than seeing it as something that happens to everyone, regardless of age.
- Memory problems can be viewed as a challenge. Anyone can improve his or her memory, but as with any other skill, an effort must be made.

Stages of Memory
- *Sensory memory* lasts only a few seconds. It involves the awareness of information obtained through vision, hearing, smell, taste, and touch.
- *Short-term memory* is your working memory, or what is in your conscious thoughts. This, too, is very brief and contains small amounts of information. For example, this type of memory allows you to recall a telephone number as you dial it.
- *Long-term memory* is the memory bank, or what you depend on whenever you need to retrieve information. This memory bank is almost limitless and contains information you just learned, as well as information from long ago.

Memory Changes and Aging
- Aging is blamed for a lot of memory problems, but very few changes occur solely because of aging.
- In older adulthood, the processes of learning new information and recalling old information slow down a little. The overall ability to learn and remember, however, is not significantly affected in healthy older people.

Factors That Interfere With Memory
As people grow older, an increasing number of factors may interfere with their ability to remember, including the following:
- Not being attentive to the situation. This might be attributable, for example, to the fact that the situation is not relevant to you
- Being distracted by a lot of things that interfere with your ability to concentrate. For example, this might be the result of worry or anxiety
- Feeling stressed
- Having a physical illness or being tired
- Having vision, hearing, or other functional impairments that interfere with the ability to obtain information
- Feeling sad or depressed, or coping with loss or grief
- Not being intellectually stimulated (principle of "use it or lose it!")
- Not having cues to help you remember
- Not organizing information for easy retention; not being organized in daily life
- Taking medications or alcohol that interfere with mental abilities
- Not being physically fit (e.g., as a result of poor nutrition or lack of exercise)

Ways of Improving Memory Skills
- Write things down (e.g., use lists, calendars, and notebooks).
- Use auditory cues (e.g., timers, alarm clocks) combined with written cues.
- Use environmental cues. For instance, you might remove something from its usual place, then return it to its normal location after it has served its purpose as a reminder.

- Assign specific places for specific items and keep the items in their proper place (e.g., keep keys on a hook near the door).
- Put reminders in appropriate places (e.g., place shoes that need to be repaired near the door).
- Use visual images. ("A picture is worth a thousand words.") Create a picture in your mind when you want to remember something; the more unusual the picture, the more likely it is that you will remember.
- Use active observation: pay attention to details of what is going on around you and be alert to the environment.
- Make associations, or mental connections. (For example, the phrase "spring ahead, fall back" can be recalled to ensure accuracy in changing clocks for seasonal time changes [from daylight savings time to standard time and vice versa].)
- Make associations between names and mental images (e.g., Carol and Christmas carol).
- Rehearse items you want to remember by repeating them aloud or writing the information on paper.
- Use self-instruction; say things aloud (e.g., "I'm putting my keys on the counter so I remember to turn off the stove before I leave.").
- Divide information into small parts that can be remembered easily. (For instance, to remember an address or a zip code, divide it into groups [seven hundred sixty, fifty-five].)
- Organize information into logical categories (e.g., shampoo and hair spray, toothpaste and mouthwash, soap and deodorant).
- Use rhyming cues (e.g., "In 1492, Columbus sailed the ocean blue.").
- Use first-letter cues and make associations. (For example, to remember to buy carrots, apples, radishes, pickles, eggs, and tea bags, remember the word CARPET.)
- Make word associations. (For instance, to remember the letters of your license plate, make a word, such as camel, out of the letters CML.)
- Search the alphabet while focusing on what you are trying to remember. (For example, to remember that someone's name is Martin, start with names that begin with A and continue naming names through the alphabet until your memory is jogged for the correct one.)
- Make up a story to connect things you want to remember. (For instance, if you have to go to the cleaners and the post office, create a story about mailing a pair of pants.)

Conclusion
- Do not try to remember all of these techniques—you will need another method just to remember them all!
- Select a few techniques that you like, and use these whenever appropriate or needed.
- Minimize any distractions; pay attention to one thing at a time.
- Give yourself time to remember; forgetfulness is most likely to occur when you are in a hurry. Try to prepare in advance, when you have time to concentrate.
- Maintain some sense of organization in your daily life, and devise systems to organize routine tasks, such as taking medications.
- Carry a notepad or a calendar, and use written records so you do not have to rely entirely on mental cues.
- Relax and maintain a sense of humor. If you become anxious about your memory and are convinced you cannot remember, then you will create a self-fulfilling prophecy.

(Adapted with permission from Fogler, J., & Stern, L. [2005]. Improving your memory: How to remember what you're starting to forget. Baltimore: Johns Hopkins University Press.)

wellness, nurses can encourage older adults to participate in adult learning activities. In some settings, nurses can address health-related concerns of older adults through group health education programs, which have the additional benefit of providing social support. A process for implementing a nurse-led health education group is delineated in Chapter 12.

Nurses can also promote the use of computers by older adults for mental stimulation and practical benefits, such as increased communication with others and the acquisition of information that is relevant to their health and daily functioning. A health communication project called "Partnering with Seniors for Better Health" found that older adults in a low socioeconomic community were capable of learning to use the Internet for health information. Moreover, 95% of the participants reported that they felt more confident exploring and evaluating health information on the Internet, that they planned on using Internet-based health information to manage their chronic illnesses, and that they had learned more about prescription drugs and Medicare benefits and would share this information with others (Chu, Huber, & Mastel-Smith, 2009).

Nurses can encourage older adults to participate in educational opportunities in their local communities. Some universities and colleges (particularly community colleges) offer reduced-rate or no-fee courses for students 60 years and older. Some programs also offer associate degrees, certification programs, or a general equivalency diploma (GED). The Institutes for Learning in Retirement (ILR) is a community-based organization for retirement-age learners that develops and implements educational programs in affiliation with a college or university. These sessions typically involve homework and usually are held for a few hours weekly for several months. Less formal education programs often are available through local senior centers and adult education programs affiliated with local school districts. Older adults can contact local colleges and information to find courses that are offered under this program.

Exploritas is a nonprofit organization that was founded in 1975 (called Elderhostel until 2009) to provide opportunities for lifelong learning by combining travel and education at a reasonable cost. In 2009, this program offered an extraordinary range of topics and formats in a wide range of affordable accommodations throughout the United States and in more than 90 other countries. Nurses can encourage older adults to obtain additional information about this and other programs that are listed in the Resources section at the end of this chapter.

Wellness Opportunity

Nurses promote personal responsibility by helping older adults identify activities that address their unique learning needs based on their life experiences and current interests.

Box 11-3 Guidelines for Health Education for Older Adults

Conditions That Promote Learning

- Supportive and rewarding contexts (e.g., praise and positive feedback) in contrast to those that are neutral, challenging, or critical
- Environment that is pleasant, familiar, brightly lit, with little or no background noise and as few distractions as possible
- Personally relevant information that builds on prior experiences
- Information that is concrete rather than abstract
- Shorter, more frequent sessions

Presentation Methods Most Conducive to Learning

- Self-paced rate that allows time for assimilation
- Presentation of one idea at a time
- Emphasis on integration and application of knowledge and experience, rather than on acquisition of irrelevant information
- Visual aids for material that lends itself to thoughtful analysis
- Auditory aids, alone or with visual aids, for information that is factual
- Advance organizers, such as outlines, overviews, and written cues
- Reinforcement of the value of using organizing aids

Adapting Health Education Materials

Much of the research on cognitive aging has centered on factors that affect learning in older adulthood. Because many nursing interventions include patient teaching or health education, information about cognitive aging can be used to adapt educational methods and materials to older adults. For example, nurses facilitate learning through the following adaptations: (1) allowing older adults enough time to process information, (2) providing small amounts of information over several sessions, (3) making referrals for home care nurses to follow up on teaching, (4) eliminating distractions in the learning environment, and (5) relating the information to past experiences and acquired wisdom (Cutilli, 2008). The suggestions presented in this text for communicating with older adults and compensating for hearing and vision deficit (see Chapters 13, 16, and 17) can be applied to health education. Nurses can apply the guidelines in Box 11-3 to educational interventions for older adults.

Adaptations of health education materials may also be necessary to ensure they are culturally appropriate. Many teaching materials are available in languages other than English. For instance, many of the federal government sites listed in the Resources section of Chapter 5 and other chapters provide health education materials in Spanish. Because there is growing emphasis on addressing needs of culturally diverse populations, nurses need to check the resources periodically and inquire about the availability of teaching materials for specific groups. Nurses can contact organizations, local hospitals, home care agencies, and long-term care facilities or check Internet sources to inquire about health education materials available to address learning needs of culturally diverse populations in their service area. For example, organizations and state governments have developed advance directive forms and teaching tools that address learning needs of specific cultural groups, as discussed in Chapter 9. Chapter 2 of this text further addresses the topic of culturally sensitive health education.

EVALUATING EFFECTIVENESS OF NURSING INTERVENTIONS

Effectiveness of nursing interventions is evaluated by the degree to which older adults are able to use their cognitive abilities to meet their daily needs. For example, older adults who forget to keep appointments might learn to use a calendar or other organizational aids to remember the appointments. In these situations, the effectiveness of interventions is measured by how well these persons remember to keep appointments. Effectiveness of nursing interventions also can be measured subjectively, based on the degree to which older adults express positive perceptions of their cognitive abilities and satisfaction with interventions, including self-care actions.

M rs. C. is 71 years old and lives alone in her own home. She attends a local senior wellness clinic for blood pressure checks, health screenings (e.g., cholesterol levels), and her annual flu shot. During her monthly visit for a blood pressure check, she confides that she is embarrassed about missing a doctor's appointment last week. She says she has been noticing increased difficulties with memory, and one of her friends has told her that she probably has Alzheimer disease. She asks if there is a place where she can get a test for Alzheimer disease.

N U R S I N G   A S S E S S M E N T

Your nursing assessment indicates that Mrs. C. has missed a couple of health care appointments during the past year. She said she missed a dental appointment 6 months ago when she was very worried about her daughter, who was undergoing diagnostic tests for a lump in her breast. Last week, when she missed her doctor's appointment, she had been busy shopping for presents for her grandson's wedding. When you ask about additional problems with memory, Mrs. C. admits that she has more difficulty re-

membering people's names than she used to have. You do not identify any risk factors that might affect Mrs. C.'s cognitive abilities (e.g., depression, medication effects, poor nutrition). Mrs. C. has never used calendars, and she says she remembers her doctor's appointments by keeping the appointment cards in her desk drawer along with her bills and her checkbook. She says that she checks her appointment cards every month, but she had not noticed the cards for the two appointments she missed.

N U R S I N G   D I A G N O S I S

You use the nursing diagnosis of Health-Seeking Behaviors because Mrs. C. is interested in learning about memory training skills to assist her in remembering appointments. Mrs. C.

has a poor understanding of age-related cognitive changes, and she indicates that she is interested in learning about ways to improve her memory.

N U R S I N G   C A R E   P L A N   F O R   M R S .   C .

Expected Outcome	Nursing Interventions	Nursing Evaluation
Mrs. C. will express an interest in improving her memory skills.	• Use information in Box 11-1 to teach Mrs. C. about age-related changes that affect cognitive abilities. • Discuss the difference between dementia and **age-associated memory impairment**. • Emphasize that memory skills can be developed through memory training techniques.	• Mrs. C. will agree to participate in a discussion of memory training skills.

Expected Outcome	Nursing Interventions	Nursing Evaluation
Mrs. C. will use memory training techniques to improve her functional level.	• Give Mrs. C. a copy of Box 11-2 and review the information. • Assist Mrs. C. in identifying one or two strategies for remembering appointments (e.g., begin using a calendar). • Assist Mrs. C. in identifying one or two strategies for remembering the names of people she meets (e.g., using visual images).	• Mrs. C. will report success in using a method for remembering appointments. • Mrs. C. will report success in using a method for remembering names of people.

THINKING POINTS

- What factors are likely to be contributing to Mrs. C.'s forgetting about her appointments?
- What is the most effective way of using information in Boxes 11-1 and 11-2 to facilitate learning for Mrs. C?
- What additional interventions would you suggest for Mrs. C?

Chapter Highlights

Age-Related Changes That Affect Cognition

- Central nervous system: degenerative changes in brain, slower reaction time
- Fluid intelligence (inductive reasoning, abstract thinking) declines, but crystallized intelligence (wisdom and judgment) improves
- Some, but not all, memory functions decline in healthy older adults
- Models of adult psychological development describe phases of mature aging

Risk Factors That Affect Cognitive Wellness

- Personal and social influences: education, socioeconomic factors, ageism
- Physical and mental health factors: chronic conditions, nutritional status
- Adverse medication effects, especially from anticholinergics

Functional Consequences Affecting Cognitive Function (Box 11-1)

- Cognitive skills that decline with age: perceptual speed, numerical ability, episodic memory, verbal ability, inductive reasoning, executive functions
- Cognitive skills that improve with age: word lexicon, general knowledge
- Rapid or significant declines are due to pathologic processes (e.g., strokes, dementia)
- Cultural factors and cognitive function (Cultural Considerations 11-1)

Nursing Assessment of Cognitive Function

- Refer to Chapter 13

Nursing Diagnosis

- Readiness for Enhanced Knowledge
- Health-Seeking Behaviors

Planning for Wellness Outcomes

- Cognition
- Concentration
- Health Beliefs
- Health-Seeking Behavior
- Information Processing
- Knowledge: Health Promotion
- Leisure Participation

Nursing Interventions to Promote Cognitive Wellness

- Evidence-based strategies for cognitive health: nutrition, mental exercise, physical exercise, challenging leisure activities, strong social networks, activities that foster a sense of control and mastery
- Teaching about memory and cognition for individuals and groups (Box 11-2)
- Improving concentration and attention (mindfulness, imagery, relaxation)
- Encouraging participation in mentally stimulating activities (computers, classes)
- Adapting health education materials (Box 11-3)

Evaluating Effectiveness of Nursing Interventions

- Expresses satisfaction with improved cognitive abilities
- Able to use cognitive skills in daily activities

Critical Thinking Exercises

1. Identify the factors in your own life that interfere with cognitive function.
2. What memory aids do you use in your life? Are they effective? Would you like to develop additional memory aids?
3. You are working in a senior center and have suggested that the center sponsor a series of classes on the memory problems of older adults. This suggestion is based on your observation that many of the older adults have asked you questions about memory problems, and some are

concerned about Alzheimer disease. Address each of the following issues:

- The center director is a firm believer in the adage, "You can't teach an old dog new tricks." How would you convince the director that the classes you wish to offer are worthwhile?
- How would you structure the sessions (number and length of sessions, number of participants, and so forth)?
- Describe the content you would cover and the approach you would use for each topic. Include information about normal cognitive aging, risk factors for impaired cognitive function, and techniques for improving memory and other aspects of cognition.
- What audiovisual aids, including written materials, would you use?
- How would you adapt your teaching method and materials for the group?
- How would you evaluate the sessions?

Resources

For links to these resources and other helpful internet resources related to this chapter, visit thePoint* at http://thePoint.lww.com/Miller6e.

Clinical Tools (See Chapter 13)

Health Education

AARP, Brain Games
American Society on Aging, MindAlert Program
Exploritas (formerly called Elderhostel)
Healthy Brain Initiative, Centers for Disease Control and Prevention
Turner Geriatric Clinic

- Publications include *Improving Your Memory: How to Remember What You're Starting to Forget* and *Teaching Memory Improvement to Adults*

REFERENCES

Akbaraly, T. N., Portet, F., Fustinoni, S., Dartigues, J-F., Artero, S., Rouaud, O., . . . Berr C. (2009). Leisure activities and the risk of dementia in the elderly, results from the three-city study. *Neurology, 73*, 854–861.

Anderson, L., Logsdon, R. G., Hochhalter, A. K., & Sharkey, J. R. (2009). Introduction to the special issue on promoting cognitive health in diverse populations of older adults. *The Gerontologist, 49*(S1), S1–S2.

Azizian, A., Monterosso, J., O'Neill, J., & London, E. D. (2009). Magnetic resonance imaging studies of cigarette smoking. *Handbook of Experimental Pharmacology, 192*, 113–143.

Beaudreau, S. A., & O'Hara, R. (2009). The association of anxiety and depressive symptoms with cognitive performance in community-dwelling older adults. *Psychological Aging, 24*(2), 507–512.

Blanchard-Fields, F., & Kalinauskas, A. (2009). Theoretical perspectives on social context, cognition, and aging. In V. L. Bengston, M. Silverstein, N. M. Putney, & D. Gans (Eds.), *Handbook of theories of aging* (2nd ed., pp. 261–276). New York: Springer.

Bottiroli, S., Cavallini, E., & Vecchi, T. (2008). Long-term effects of memory training in the elderly: A longitudinal study. *Archives of Gerontology and Geriatrics, 47*, 277–289.

Botwinick, J. (1984). *Aging and behavior* (3rd ed.). New York: Springer.

Buell, J. S., Scott, T. M., Dawson-Hughes, B., Dallai, G. E., Rosenberg, T. H., Folstein, M. F., & Tucker, K. L. (2009). Vitamin D is associated with cognitive function in elders, receiving home health services. *The Journals of Gerontology A: Biological Sciences, Medical Sciences, 64*(8), 888–895.

Cansino, S. (2009). Episodic memory decay along the adult lifespan: A review of behavioral and neurophysiological evidence. *International Journal of Psychophysiology, 71*, 64–69.

Carlson, M. C., Xue, Q-L., Zhou, J., & Fried, L. P. (2009). Executive decline and dysfunction precedes declines in memory: The Women's Health and Aging Study II. *The Journals of Gerontology A: Biological Sciences, Medical Sciences, 64*(1), 110–117.

Carriere, I., Fourrier-Reglat, A., Dartigues, J. F., Rouaud, O., Pasguier, F., Ritchie, K., & Ancelin M-L. (2009). Drugs with anticholinergic properties, cognitive decline, and dementia in an elderly general population: The 3-city study. *Archives of Internal Medicine, 169*(14), 1317–1324.

Carstensen, L. L., Mikels, J. A., & Mather, M. (2006). Aging and the intersection of cognition, motivation, and emotion. In J. E. Birren & K. W. Schaie (Eds.), *Handbook of the psychology of aging* (6th ed., pp. 343–362). San Diego, CA: Academic Press.

Caserta, M. T., Bannon, Y., Fernandex, F., Giunta, B., Schoenbery, M. R., & Tan, J. (2009). Normal brain aging: Clinical immunological, neuropsychological, and neuroimaging features. *International Review of Neurobiology, 84*, 1–19. doi: 10.1016/S0074-7742(09)00401-2.

Chu, A., Huber, J., & Mastel-Smith, B. (2009). "Partnering with Seniors for Better Health": Computer use and internet health information retrieval among older adults in a low socioeconomic community. *Journal of the Medical Library Association, 97*(1), 12–19.

Cohen, G. D. (2005). *The mature mind: The positive power of the aging brain*. New York: Basic Books.

Cutilli, C. C. (2008). Teaching the geriatric patient, making the most of "cognitive resources" and "gains." *Orthopaedic Nursing, 27*(3), 195–198.

Deal, J. A., Carison, M. C., Xue, O. L., Fried, L. P., & Chaves, P. H. (2009). Anemia and 9-year domain-specific cognitive decline in community-dwelling older women: The Women's Health and Aging Study II [published online ahead of print August 13, 2009]. *American Geriatric Society, 57*(9), 1604–1611.

Devore, E. E., Stampfer, M. J., Breteler, M. M., Rosner, B., Hee Kang, J., Okereke, O., . . . Grodstein, F. (2009). Dietary fat intake and cognitive decline in women with type 2 diabetes. *Diabetes Care, 32*(4), 635–640.

Friedman, D. B., Laditka, J. N., Hunter, R., Ivey, S. L., Wu, B., Laditka, S. B., . . . Mathews, A. E. (2009). Getting the message out about cognitive health: A cross-cultural comparison of older adults' media awareness and communication needs on how to maintain a healthy brain. *The Gerontologist, 49*(S1), S50–S60.

Fogler, J., & Stern, L. (2005). *Improving your memory: How to remember what you're starting to forget* (3rd ed.). Baltimore: Johns Hopkins University Press.

Gao, X., Scott, T., Falcon, L. M., Wilde, P. E., & Tucker, K. L. (2009). Food insecurity and cognitive function in Puerto Rican adults. *American Journal of Clinical Nutrition, 89*(4), 1197–1203.

Goh, J. O., & Park, D. C. (2009). Neuroplasticity and cognitive aging: The scaffolding theory of aging and cognition. *Restorative Neurology and Neuroscience, 27*(5), 391–403.

Hakansson, K., Rovio, S., Helkala, E-L., Vilska, A-R., Winblad, B., Soininen, H., . . . Kavipelto, M. (2009). Association between mid-life marital status and cognitive function in later life: Population based cohort study. *British Medical Journal, 339*, b2462. doi:10.1136/bmj.b2462.

Hall, C. B., Lipton, R. B., Sliwinski, M., Katz, M. J., Derby, C. A., & Verghese, J. (2009). Cognitive activities delay onset of memory decline in persons who develop dementia neurology. *American Academy of Neurology, 73*(5), 356–361.

Hasher, L., & Zacks, R. T. (1979). Autonomic and effortful processes in memory. *Journal of Experimental Psychology: General, 108*, 356–388.

Hess, T. M., Hinson, J. T., & Hodges, E. A. (2009). Moderators of and mechanisms underlying stereotype threat effects on older adults' memory performance. *Experimental Aging Research, 35*(2), 153–177.

Hess, T. M., Emery, L., & Queen, L. (2009). Task demands moderate stereotype threat effects on memory performance. *Journal of Gerontology: Psychological Sciences, 64B*(4), 482–486.

Hess, T. M., Leclerc, C. M., Swaim, E., & Weatherbee, S. R. (2009). Aging and everyday judgments: The impact of motivational and processing resource factors. *Psychological Aging, 24*(3), 735–740.

Inzitari, D., Pracucci, G., Poggesi, A., Carlucci, G., Barkhof, F., & Chabriat, H. (2009). Changes in white matter as determinant of global functional decline in older independent outpatients: Three-year follow-up of LADIS (leukoaraiosis and disability) study cohort. *British Medical Journal, 339,* b2477. doi:10.1136/bmj.b2477.

Kamijo, K., Hayashi, Y., Sakai, T., Yahiro, T., Tanaka, K., & Nishihira, Y. (2009). Acute effects of aerobic exercise on cognitive function in older adults. *Journal of Gerontology: Psychological Sciences, 64B*(3), 356–363.

Kaufman, A. S., Kaufman, J. C., Lui, X., & Johnson, C. K. (2009). How do educational attainment and gender relate to fluid intelligence, crystallized intelligence, and academic skills at ages 22–90 years? *Archives of Clinical Neuropsychology, 24*(2), 153–163.

Knight, B. G., & Laidlaw, K. (2009). Translations theory: A wisdom-based model for psychological interventions to enhance well-being in later life. In V. L. Bengston, M. Silverstein, N. M. Putney, & D. Gans (Eds.), *Handbook of theories of aging* (2nd ed., pp. 693–705). New York: Springer.

Labouvie-Vief, G. (2009). Dynamic integration theory: Emotion, cognition, and equilibrium in later life. In V. L. Bengston, M. Silverstein, N. M. Putney, & D. Gans (Eds.), *Handbook of theories of aging* (2nd ed., pp. 277–293). New York: Springer.

Labouvie-Vief, G., & Blanchard-Fields, F. (1982). Cognitive aging and psychological growth. *Ageing and Society, 2,* 183–209.

Langbaum, J. B. S., Rebok, G. W., Bandeen-Roche, K., & Carlson, M. C. (2009). Predicting memory training response patterns: Results from ACTIVE. *Journal of Gerontology: Psychological Sciences, 64B*(1), 14–23.

Lee, D. M., Tajar, A., Ulubaev, A., Pendleton, N., O'Neill, T. W., O'Connor, D. B., . . . Wu, F. C. (2009). Association between 25-hydroxyvitamin D levels and cognitive performance in middle-aged and older European men. *Journal of Neurology, Neurosurgery and Psychiatry, 80*(7), 772–779.

Lee, K. S., Cheong, H-K., Kim, E. A., Kim, K. R., Oh, B. H., & Hong, C. H. (2009). Nutritional risk and cognitive impairment in the elderly. *Archives of Gerontology and Geriatrics, 48*(1), 95–99.

Lee, Y., Kim, J., & Back, J. H. (2009). The influence of multiple lifestyle behaviors on cognitive function in older persons living in the community. *Preventive Medicine, 48*(1), 86–96.

Levy, B. R., & Leifheit-Limson, E. (2009). The stereotype-matching effect: Greater influence on functioning when age stereotypes correspond to outcomes. *Psychology and Aging, 24*(1), 230–233.

Llewellyn, D. J., Lang, L. A., Langa, K. M., Naughton, F., & Matthews, F. E. (2009). Exposure to secondhand smoke and cognitive impairment in non-smokers: National cross sectional study with cotinine measurement. *British Medical Journal, 338,* b462. doi:10.1136/bmj.b462.

Mariske, M., & Margrett, J. A. (2006). Everyday problem solving and decision making. In J. E. Birren & K. W. Schaie (Eds.), *Handbook of the psychology of aging* (6th ed., pp. 315–342). San Diego, CA: Academic Press.

McFadden, S. H., & Basting, A. D. (2010). Healthy aging persons and their brains: Promoting resilience through creative engagement. *Clinics in Geriatric Medicine, 26,* 149–161.

NANDA International. (2009). *Nursing diagnoses: 2009–2010.* Hoboken, NJ: John Wiley & Sons.

Nikolova, R., Demers, L., & Beland, F. (2009). Trajectories of cognitive decline and functional status in the frail older adults. *Archives of Gerontology and Geriatrics, 48,* 28–34.

Noovens, A. C., Van Gelder, B. M., & Verschuren, W. M. (2008). Smoking and cognitive decline among middle-aged men and women: The Doetinchem Cohort Study. *American Journal of Public Health, 98*(12), 2244–2250.

Pansky, A., Goldsmith, M., Koriat, A., & Pearlman-Avnion, S. (2009). Memory accuracy in old age: Cognitive, metacognitive, and neurocognitive determinants. *European Journal of Cognitive Psychology, 21*(2/3), 303–329.

Park, D. C., & Reuter-Lorenz, P. (2009). The adaptive brain: Aging and neurocognitive scaffolding. *Annual Review of Psychology, 60,* 173–196.

Rolland, Y., vanKan, G. A., & Vellas, B. (2010). Healthy brain aging: Role of exercise and physical activity. *Clinics in Geriatric Medicine, 26,* 75–87.

Rowland, A. S., & McKinstry, R. C. (2006). Lead toxicity, white matter lesions, and aging. *Neurology, 66,* 1464–1466.

Sabia, S., Nabi, H., Kivimaki, M., Shipley, M. J., Marmot, M. G., & Singh-Manoux, A. (2009). Health behaviors from early to late midlife as predictors of cognitive function: The Whitehall II study. *American Journal of Epidemiology, 170*(4), 428–437.

Schaie, K. W. (1977–1978). Toward a stage theory of adult cognitive development. *Journal of Aging and Human Development, 8,* 129–138.

Smith, A. C., & Refsum, H. (2009). Vitamin B-12 and cognition in the elderly. *American Journal of Clinical Nutrition, 89*(2), 707S–711S.

Smith, G. E. (2009). A cognitive training program based on principles of brain plasticity: Results from the Improvement in Memory with Plasticity-based Adaptive Cognitive Train (IMPACT) study. *Journal of American Geriatrics Society, 57*(4), 594–603.

Sorond, F. A., Schnyer, D. M., Serrador, J. M., Milberg, W. P., & Lipstiz, L. A. (2008). Cerebral blood flow regulation during cognitive tasks: Effects of healthy aging. *Cortex, 44,* 179–184.

Stewart, W. F., Schwartz, B. S., Davatzikos, C., Shen, D., Liu, D., Wu, X., . . . Youssem, D. (2006). Past adult lead exposure is linked to neurodegeneration measured by brain MRI. *Neurology, 66,* 1476–1484.

Vance, D. E. (2009). Speed of processing in older adults: A cognitive overview for nursing. *Journal of Neuroscience Nursing, 41,* 290–296.

Vance, D. E., & Wright, M. A. (2009). Positive and negative neuroplasticity, implications for age-related cognitive declines. *Journal of Gerontological Nursing, 35*(6), 11–18.

Williamson, J. D., Espeland, M., Kritchevsky, S. B., Newman, A. B., King, A. C., Pahor, M., . . . Miller, M. E. (2009). Changes in cognitive function in a randomized trial of physical activity: Results of the Lifestyle Interventions and Independence for Elders Pilot Study. *Journals of Gerontology A: Biological Sciences Medical Sciences, 64A*(6), 688–694.

Willis, S. L., Schaie, K. W., & Martin, M. (2009). Cognitive plasticity. In V. L. Bengston, M. Silverstein, N. M. Putney, & D. Gans (Eds.), *Handbook of theories of aging* (2nd ed., pp. 295–322). New York: Springer.

Wilson, R. S., Hebert, L. E., Scherr, P. A., Barnes, L. L., Mendes de leon, C. F., & Evans, D. A. (2009). Educational attainment and cognitive decline in old age. *Neurology, 72,* 460–465.

Yaffe, K., Fiocco, A. J., Lindquist, K., Vittinghoff, E., Simonsick, E. M., Newman, A. B., . . . Harris, T. B. (2009). Predictors of maintaining cognitive function in older adults: The Health ABC study. *Neurology, 72*(23), 2029–2035.

Yevchak, A. M., Loeb, S. J., & Fick, D. M. (2008). Promoting cognitive health and vitality: A review of clinical implications. *Geriatric Nursing, 29*(5), 302–310.

Yu, F., Ryan, L. H., Schaie, K. W., Willis, S. L., & Kolanowski, A. (2009). Factors associated with cognition in adults: The Seattle Longitudinal Study. *Research in Nursing and Health, 32*(5), 540–550.

Zarit, S. H. (2009). A good old age: Theories of mental health and aging. In V. L. Bengston, M. Silverstein, N. M. Putney, & D. Gans (Eds.), *Handbook of theories of aging* (2nd ed., pp. 675–691). New York: Springer.

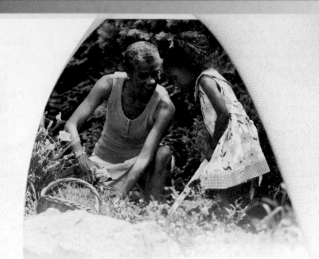

CHAPTER 12

Psychosocial Function

LEARNING OBJECTIVES

After reading this chapter, you will be able to:

1. Identify the life events that commonly occur in older adulthood.

2. Discuss theories related to stress and coping as they apply to older adults.

3. Identify the risk factors and cultural factors that influence psychosocial function in older adults.

4. Describe the functional consequences associated with psychosocial function in older adults.

5. Identify nursing interventions that promote psychosocial wellness in older adults.

6. Describe how to teach a "healthy aging class" for a small group of older adults.

KEY POINTS

culture-bound syndrome
elderspeak
infantilization
learned helplessness
life events
life review
loneliness
reminiscence

selective optimization with
    compensation
self-esteem
socioemotional selectivity
    theory
spirituality
stress
stressors

Although the physiologic changes and chronic illnesses associated with older adulthood may affect a person's functional abilities, the psychosocial changes are often the most challenging and demanding in terms of coping energy. Of course, many psychosocial challenges are strongly associated with compromised health and physical functioning, but some are attributable to changes in roles, relationships, and living environments. Because many of the psychosocial changes are inevitable and somewhat predictable, older adults can prepare for and respond to psychosocial changes by developing and using effective coping strategies. Nurses can promote psychosocial wellness by supporting effective coping mechanisms and assisting in the development of new coping strategies.

 ## LIFE EVENTS: AGE-RELATED CHANGES AFFECTING PSYCHOSOCIAL FUNCTION

Life events are the major changes that occur at various times during the life cycle and significantly affect daily life. Certain events are commonly associated with different periods in one's life. For example, younger adults are likely to experience the following life events: establishing a career, moving away from the nuclear family, committing to a partner, creating a home, and beginning a family. The major life events of younger adulthood are familiar to us through either personal experiences or the shared experiences of friends. People usually view these events as positive gains and choose them purposefully. By contrast, life events of older adulthood might be unknown, unexpected, inevitable, and, in fact, unwanted or even feared. Thus, older adults may experience a greater fear of losing control over their lives. In addition, life events during older adulthood are likely to involve losses of significant others and objects that have been part of life for many decades. Moreover, they tend to occur close together, with less time available to adjust to each event. Some life events evolve into chronic stresses. Dealing with ageist attitudes and behaviors of others is a life event that is specific to older adults.

Life events that are most likely to occur during older adulthood include retirement, relocation, chronic illness and functional impairments, decisions about driving a vehicle, widowhood, death of friends and family, and confronting ageist attitudes. Figure 12-1 illustrates some of the major life events that are likely to occur in older adulthood, as well as the related consequences. Although most of the consequences are negative, some consequences can be positive. For example, because of these life events, older adults may focus on achieving integrity and meaning in life, and they may develop a greater acceptance of things that cannot be controlled. The illustration attempts to show the interrelatedness among the life events of older adulthood.

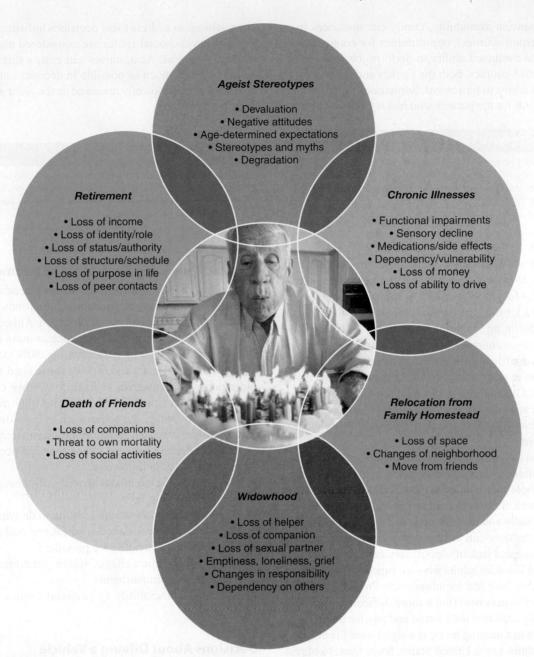

Ageist Stereotypes

- Devaluation
- Negative attitudes
- Age-determined expectations
- Stereotypes and myths
- Degradation

Retirement

- Loss of income
- Loss of identity/role
- Loss of status/authority
- Loss of structure/schedule
- Loss of purpose in life
- Loss of peer contacts

Chronic Illnesses

- Functional impairments
- Sensory decline
- Medications/side effects
- Dependency/vulnerability
- Loss of money
- Loss of ability to drive

Death of Friends

- Loss of companions
- Threat to own mortality
- Loss of social activities

Relocation from Family Homestead

- Loss of space
- Changes of neighborhood
- Move from friends

Widowhood

- Loss of helper
- Loss of companion
- Loss of sexual partner
- Emptiness, loneliness, grief
- Changes in responsibility
- Dependency on others

FIGURE 12-1 Psychosocial challenges of older adulthood.

Wellness Opportunity

Nurses promote wellness by asking older adults to talk about the meaning of life events that they have experienced.

Retirement

Retirement from employment is often viewed as a milestone that marks the passage into older adulthood. The age of 65 years is the traditional retirement age; however, there is a growing trend toward "bridge employment" involving a transition from full-time to part-time employment before retirement. Studies have found that bridge employment facilitates adjustment to retirement by helping older adults structure their time, offering opportunities for supplemental income, and developing new routines and interests before full retirement (Mehrotra & Wagner, 2009).

Societal attitudes can influence one's adjustment to retirement, particularly in societies with a strong work ethic. In these societies, working people have a higher status than unemployed people and, among working people, status is based on the kind of job one holds and the salary one earns. Therefore, when people retire, they inevitably cope with a change in social status, and the psychosocial challenge may be the greatest for people whose **self-esteem** (the extent to which one perceives oneself to be worthy or significant) and self-concept are based on job status. The following factors commonly influence the decision to retire: health, financial assets, job conditions, pension availability, family circumstances (e.g., caregiving responsibilities), opportunities for continued employment, and continued ability to perform job responsibilities. For married couples, both the worker and the spouse, or partner, must adjust to retirement. Sometimes the adjustment is more difficult for the partner who has not been employed.

DIVERSITY NOTE

Women, minority workers, and people who live in rural areas are likely to have a sporadic work history and lower-paying jobs throughout their adult lives. They also may have lower retirement assets (Mehrotra & Wagner, 2009).

Relocation

Another common psychosocial adjustment for older adults is the decision to move from the family home because of factors, such as loss of spouse, lack of available assistive services, lack of a kinship network or caregiver, chronic conditions and declining functional abilities, and cognitive impairment or psychiatric illness. Increased dependence on others because of health problems is a common reason for older adults to move to a facility where they can receive support services. Older adults whose adult children have moved to another location may relocate to be closer to them. Or older adults may choose to move to a desirable geographic location after they retire.

In addition to family and personal factors, many environmental conditions influence the decision to move. For example, older people in urban areas may find they are unsafe or socially isolated because the neighborhood around them has changed gradually and they are no longer surrounded by people with whom they can easily relate. In rural areas, geographic distance and lack of support services can have serious consequences for older adults who are functionally impaired, especially if they have few social supports. Problems also arise for older homeowners who find it more difficult to physically and financially maintain their home and pay for utilities.

Relocation to a nursing home is a significant life event for some older adults. In the United States, fewer than 5% of people aged 65 years or older reside in nursing facilities at any one time, but they have a 39% to 49% chance of being admitted to a nursing facility at some time (Stone, 2006). Nurses caring for older adults in hospitals and nursing homes have important roles in assisting older adults and their families with relocation decisions and adjustments.

When discussing issues related to living arrangements for older adults, nurses need to recognize that in the U.S. health care system, decisions about long-term care are often based on a narrow medical perspective rather than a broader psychosocial one. This is especially pertinent when decisions need to be made soon after the older adult experiences an abrupt change in health status and does not have strong caregiver resources. In these situations, relocation to a nursing facility may be recommended, but these decisions should be viewed as short-term rather than permanent. Nurses are in

key positions to address these decisions holistically by ensuring that psychosocial issues are considered along with the medical concerns. Also, nurses can ensure that older adults are involved as much as possible in decisions and that these decisions are periodically reviewed as the older adult's needs change.

Wellness Opportunity

Nurses promote psychosocial wellness by encouraging older adults to express their feelings about decisions related to long-term care plans and by helping them identify effective ways of coping, even when they are not happy about the decision.

Chronic Illness and Functional Impairments

Another major life adjustment for many older adults is coping with chronic illnesses and functional limitations, particularly limitations that curtail their independence. Although the large majority of older adults experience one or more chronic conditions that affect their daily functioning, 80% to 90% of people aged 65 to 75 years and 60% of those aged 85 years and older perceive themselves as healthy (Østbye et al., 2006). Most functional limitations necessitate only minor adjustments in daily living, but some, such as considerable cognitive, mobility, or visual impairments, significantly increase one's dependence on others. Other consequences of chronic illnesses include the following:

- Threats to self-esteem and altered self-concept
- Changes in lifestyle
- Unpredictability about one's ability to do what one wants
- Expenditures for assistance, medications, and medical care
- Frequent trips to health care providers
- Adverse medication effects, which sometimes cause further functional impairments
- Increased vulnerability to personal crimes and fear of crime.

Decisions About Driving a Vehicle

Decisions about driving a vehicle represent one of the most emotionally charged issues relating to functional impairment that older adults, their families, and health care professionals face. In the United States, access to an automobile and the possession of a valid driver's license not only provide transportation but also serve as significant indicators of autonomy. In fact, for many older adults, the ability to drive is synonymous with independence, and the possession of a driver's license, even one that goes unused, is a symbol of one's ability to shield oneself from dependence on others. Studies confirm that driving cessation is a stressful experience for many older adults, leading to depression, isolation, loss of identity, loss of self-esteem, feelings of diminished self-worth, and diminished life satisfaction and quality of life (Kostyniuk, Molnar, & Eby, 2009; Oxley & Charlton, 2009). Studies also indicate that driving status is a strong predictor of nursing home placement and of 3-year mortality risk (Edwards, Perkins, Ross, & Reynolds, 2009).

The loss of an independent means of transportation affects every aspect of an older person's life, from the acquisition of food and medicine to opportunities for social interaction. Because of this far-reaching impact, families and older persons may avoid dealing with driving-related issues. Family members may be reluctant to suggest that an older relative give up driving for a number of reasons. For example, family members may not want to assume an authority role, or they may lack acceptable alternatives for transportation. It is not surprising, then, that older adults and their families may avoid or resist the decision to stop driving. Neither is it surprising that when older adults give up or significantly curtail their driving, they face a difficult psychosocial challenge that may be viewed as a major life event.

Widowhood

The example of widowhood as a life event of older adulthood illustrates all of the characteristics discussed earlier. For most older couples, widowhood is inevitable, and the chances are greater that women become widowed more than men. When widowhood occurs, additional consequences follow. Common additional consequences include the following:

- Loss of companionship and intimacy
- Loss of one's sexual partner
- Feelings of grief, loneliness, and emptiness
- Increased responsibilities
- Increased dependence on others
- Loss of income and less efficient financial management
- Changes in relationships with children, married friends, and other family members.

When a marriage or partnership has lasted for many decades, as is common in people who are in their 70s and 80s, the impact of the loss can be tremendous, and the feelings of grief, **loneliness**, and emptiness may be overwhelming. Despite the major impact of widowhood, however, some studies have found that spousal bereavement is associated with higher risk of mortality among middle-aged, but not older, adults (Aldwin, Hofer, & McCammon, 2006). Another study found that older women experienced a negative impact on health and well-being soon after the loss of their spouse but that this was followed by a shift into a new and positive life phase of learning to live alone (Young & Cochrane, 2004).

Another characteristic of widowhood in older adulthood is that the chance of remarriage diminishes with advancing age. This is especially true for women because there are disproportionately fewer older men than older women due to greater longevity of women. In addition to the "shortage" of eligible men, other reasons that widows do not remarry are loyalty to their deceased husbands, family issues, and a preference for their newly independent lives (Cattell, 2009). Even when widows or widowers do remarry, they need to adjust to entirely different roles with a new partner. If the married couple had clearly divided roles, as is common in the cohort of

people who are old today, loss of the partner means an adjustment in important day-to-day tasks. For example, older couples often divide tasks so that only one of the two manages money, drives the vehicle, cleans the house, shops for groceries, and does household repairs and maintenance. When the person responsible for a task no longer performs the role, the other person may be unable, unwilling, or unprepared to assume this role.

Wellness Opportunity

When applicable, nurses encourage older adults to talk about their experience of widowhood by opening the conversation with a question such as, "How is your life different since your partner passed away?"

Death of Friends and Family

Like other life events of older adulthood, the loss of friends and family becomes inevitable with each year. Many people who are in their 90s have outlived most, if not all, of their friends and many of their relatives. Indeed, people who are in their 90s may not even know anyone who is older than they are. Moreover, as people are confronted with the death of others who are younger than or similar to them in age, they become increasingly aware of their own mortality. Older people may read obituaries and death notices in the newspaper as a daily activity. Although families may view this activity as a morbid preoccupation, it may, in fact, be an effective way for older people to learn what is happening to their friends. Because meaningful social relationships are an important predictor of well-being for older adults, loss of family and friends is likely to have a negative impact on psychosocial wellness. However, older adults who are able to adjust their expectations and do not feel a sense of social isolation may fare better than those who perceive themselves as socially isolated and disconnected (Cornwell & Waite, 2009).

Ageist Attitudes

A life adjustment that, by its nature, is unique to older adulthood is the acceptance of being old. Because of the ageist attitudes common in modern industrialized societies, many older adults deny that they are old. Ageism can lead to prejudices, fear of aging, and feelings of devaluation and degradation (as discussed in Chapter 1). Studies indicate that positive or negative aging stereotypes affect older adults' decisions and behaviors in beneficial or detrimental ways, respectively (Levy & Leifheit-Limson, 2009). Consequences of negative age-based stereotypes include impaired memory and decreased cognitive performance, declining will to live and diminished positive affect, negative effects on physical health (e.g., increased cardiovascular stress), and behavioral changes such as decreased walking speed and shaky handwriting (Kang & Chasteen, 2009). When negative ageist stereotypes are pervasive in a society, people with a good self-acceptance of being old may feel that it is socially unacceptable to admit that it is okay to be old.

Because of these societal attitudes, older adults may be confronted with age-determined expectations that dictate appropriate social behaviors. For example, public displays of affection are viewed as socially appropriate for teenagers and younger adults. However, when older adults hold hands or kiss in public, observers are likely to make comments like, "Isn't that cute, look at that old couple holding hands." Having sexual relationships outside of a marriage is another action that is generally overlooked when done by young adults, but that is likely to be criticized when done by older adults.

As an example of age-determined expectations, consider the following scene: a gray-haired man, who was clearly an older adult, was wearing headphones and listening to music on a portable radio. He was briskly moving along in a combination dance–walk tempo on a public sidewalk in an urban area. Observers remarked that the old man looked like he needed psychiatric care, whereas they ignored several teens nearby who were dancing and listening to music blaring from loudspeakers. The only apparent difference between the older adult and the teens was that the younger people were listening to louder music and demonstrating less control in their movements. The primary difference, however, was in the age-determined expectations in the eyes of the beholders!

Wellness Opportunity

Nurses can promote positive attitudes about aging by talking about people who are examples of successful aging.

THEORIES ABOUT PSYCHOSOCIAL FUNCTION IN OLDER ADULTS

Theories about aging and psychosocial function address questions such as, How do emotions develop over the life course? What influences the way older adults respond to life events? Are certain life events more stressful for older adults? How do coping patterns change in older adulthood? The following sections focus on several of the widely accepted theories about emotional development, stress, coping, and the response of older adults to stressful events. In keeping with the perspective of this text, these theories are used to explain the age-related changes that can cause positive or negative functional consequences with regard to psychosocial function. Additional psychological theories pertinent to older adults are discussed in Chapter 4.

Theories About Emotional Development During Later Adulthood

Gerontologists have studied emotional development during later adulthood since the 1960s. Initial studies, which focused on institutionalized older adults, suggested that a blunting of emotions and an increase in negative affect occurred in older adulthood. In recent years, however, gerontologists emphasize that even though older adults experience more negative life events, the aging process does not compromise their emotional well-being (Kryla-Lighthall & Mather, 2009). Recent studies have found that older adults can develop compensatory mechanisms that help foster and maintain a strong sense of well-being, personal fulfillment, and high quality of life. These compensatory mechanisms include resilience, coping, optimization, spirituality, emotional vitality, and valuing of social ties involving reciprocal relationships (Young, Frick, & Phelan, 2009).

The theory of **selective optimization with compensation** has been proposed to explain successful aging based on a dynamic model of development as a continuous process of specialization and loss (Zarit, 2009). According to this theory, older adults *select* certain goals and tasks while disengaging from other goals; they *optimize* necessary resources to achieve these goals; and they *compensate* by establishing new resources to substitute for lowered or lost abilities and skills (Rohr & Lang, 2009). Morley (2009) describes the following examples of well-known people who illustrate this theory:

- Grandma Moses became a famous painter of miniatures after arthritis limited her ability to make quilts.
- Monet invented modern impressionism when his eyesight was clouded by cataracts.
- Renoir held his paintbrush in his clenched fist after he developed arthritis.
- Maurice Ravel composed his famous *Bolero* after he developed dementia.

Grove, Loeb, and Penrod (2009) described a nursing model based on this theory for developing health education programs for older adults in community settings.

The **socioemotional selectivity theory** has been proposed to explain emotional well-being during older adulthood. This theory proposes that in contrast to younger adults, who view time as unconstrained, older adults recognize that their time is limited, so they focus on emotional goals rather than on knowledge-seeking goals (Kryla-Lighthall & Mather, 2009). One study based on this theory suggests that health promotion messages may be more effective for older adults if they emphasize emotional goals, such as love and caring, rather than future-oriented or neutral goals (Zhang, Fung, & Ching, 2009). Studies using this theory to investigate interpersonal relationships in later life found that older adults experience less emotional distress, report fewer conflicts in daily interactions, perceive conflicts as less stressful, and are less likely to respond in an angry or confronting way than younger adults (Zarit, 2009).

Theories About Stress

Hans Selye, who proposed the first major theory about stress in the mid-1950s, defined **stress** as the sum of all the effects of factors that act on the body (Selye, 1956). According to Selye's theory, **stressors** include normal activities and disease states; and all factors, whether pleasant or unpleasant, are equally important. Moreover, people respond to stressors in three stages: alarm, resistance, and exhaustion. Limitations of this theory include the broad conceptualization of stress, the lack of distinction between pleasant and unpleasant stressors, and the failure to address the meaning of events for the person.

Holmes and Rahe (1967) proposed that stress was a mediator between a life event and adaptation to that event. They define life events as discrete and identifiable changes in life patterns that create stress and that can lead to negative health outcomes. According to this theory, stress causes physical and psychological harm that is in proportion to the intensity of the impact on and duration of a disruption in one's usual life pattern. Holmes and Rahe (1967) developed the Social Readjustment Rating Scale (SRRS) as a tool for measuring the duration and intensity of specific life events. The SRRS is a checklist of 43 life events, with relative weights assigned to each according to the usual amount of adaptive effort required by each event.

Because one of the criticisms of the SRRS is its assumption that life events always have a negative impact, researchers have developed variations of the SRRS that account for the meaning of life events for the person. Lazarus (1966), for instance, proposed a scale based on the cognitive appraisal approach. According to Lazarus, people initially appraise the significance of an event according to the way it actually or potentially affects their well-being. Secondarily, they appraise the event according to the personal and social resources that are available for coping, as well as the cost of these resources in relation to positive and negative outcomes. By using these concepts, Folkman and Lazarus (1980) proposed the Ways of Coping Checklist to measure individual thoughts, feelings, and actions in response to specific stressful situations.

Because most stress scales focus on life events of younger and middle-aged adults, they are not as applicable to older adults. In 1988, two nurses developed the Stokes/Gordon Stress Scale (SGSS), a 104-item checklist for use with older adults (Stokes & Gordon, 1988). The SGSS can be self-administered and scored to identify the level of stress that an older person is experiencing at a given time. Nurses identified the items included in this checklist through interviews with older adults, a literature review, and consultations with gerontological nurses. Nurses can address many of the significant stresses, such as decreasing eyesight and hearing, through interventions aimed at improving functional abilities. Other significant stresses, such as losses of, or changes in, relationships, can be addressed through the psychosocial interventions discussed in this chapter. Table 12-1 identifies some of the SGSS items and their corresponding relative weights.

In addition to addressing the impact of major life events (e.g., acute stress), studies address the impact of daily hassles (e.g., chronic stress). Gerontologists initially proposed that older adults experienced more stressors that are chronic; however, studies do not consistently support this. Rather, some recent studies suggest that older adults report less stress from daily hassles, such as those associated with chronic illness, which become stressful only when there is a flare-up or acute episode.

TABLE 12-1 Stokes/Gordon Stress Scale (SGSS): Selected Items		
Rank	**Event or Situation**	**Weight**
1	Death of a son or daughter (unexpected)	100
2	Decreasing eyesight	99
2	Death of a grandchild	99
3	Death of spouse (unexpected)	97
4	Loss of ability to get around	96
4	Death of son or daughter (expected, anticipated)	96
5	Fear of your home being invaded or robbed	93
5	Constant or recurring pain or discomfort	93
6	Illness or injury of close relative	92
7	Death of spouse (expected, anticipated)	90
7	Moving in with children or other family	90
7	Moving to an institution	90
8	Minor or major car accident	89
8	Needing to rely on cane, wheelchair, walker, hearing aid	89
8	Change in ability to do personal care	89
10	Loneliness or aloneness	87
11	Having an unexpected debt	86
11	Your own hospitalization (unplanned)	86
12	Decreasing hearing	85
13	Fear of abuse from others	84
13	Being judged legally incompetent	84
13	Not feeling needed or having a purpose in life	84
14	Decreasing mental abilities	84
15	Giving up long-cherished possessions	82
15	Wishing parts of your life had been different	82
16	Using your savings for living expenses	80
17	Change in behavior of family member	79
18	Taking a relative or friend into your home to live	78
19	Concern about elimination	77
19	Illness in public places	77
20	Feeling of remaining time being short	76
20	Giving up or losing driver's license	76
20	Change in your sleeping habits	76
21	Difficulty using public transportation system	75
23	Uncertainty about the future	73
25	Fear of your own or your spouse's driving	71
27	Concern for completing required forms	69
27	Death of a loved pet	69
29	Reaching a milestone year	67
32	Outstanding personal achievement	64
33	Retirement	63
35	Change in your sexual activity	59

Adapted with permission from Stokes, S. A. & Gordon, S. E. (1988). *User's manual, SGSS*. Pleasantville, NY: Pace University.

Theories About Coping

Theories about age-related differences in coping often address the following types of internal mechanisms that people use to deal with stressful situations: seeking information; maintaining a hopeful outlook; using stress reduction techniques; denying or minimizing the threat; channeling energy into physical activity; creating fantasies about various outcomes; finding reassurance and emotional support; identifying limited and realistic goals; identifying a positive purpose for the event; getting involved in other activities, such as work and family; and expressing oneself creatively, for example, through music, art, or writing. These coping styles are categorized as problem-focused (i.e., directed toward altering the source of stress) or emotion-focused (i.e., directed toward regulating one's response). Studies indicate that older adults are more likely to use coping mechanisms that involve management of thoughts and feelings, whereas younger adults are likely to take direct approaches to modify the events or challenging situations in their lives (Zarit, 2009).

Before the 1980s, gerontologists assumed that life events of older adulthood had negative effects on older adults. On the basis of this assumption, researchers tried, but failed, to identify specific changes that adversely affect older adults. There is now much agreement that both the meaning of the event to the individual and the coping resources available to the individual are the main determinants of whether the life event has a negative impact on health (George, 2006). Gerontologists have consistently identified social resources as a factor that affects coping, and there is much emphasis on the positive effects of strong social resources. Social resources include instrumental support (e.g., meals, transportation, personal care), informational support (e.g., information about resources and services), and emotional support (e.g., communication that provides comfort, companionship, and other evidence that the person is loved, valued, esteemed, and cared for). Studies show that older adults who have strong social supports as a coping resource experience a higher level of functioning; better mental and physical health; and better well-being, overall quality of life, and health-related quality of life (Cornwell & Waite, 2009; Drageset et al., 2009).

FACTORS THAT INFLUENCE PSYCHOSOCIAL FUNCTION IN OLDER ADULTS

Religion and Spirituality

Religion and spirituality are widely recognized as major coping resources that have a positive effect on many aspects of psychosocial function for older adults. Religion and spirituality are closely related but distinct concepts. Religion and religiosity, which have a strong social component, refer to an organized system of beliefs and behaviors that are shared by a group of people who are associated with a defined faith community. Examples of religious practices are rituals, prayers, meditation, worship services, attendance at church, and adherence to certain dietary practices and style of clothing. One intent of religion is to nurture spiritual development; however, spirituality is broader and less structured and does not necessarily include membership in a formal religious group. Elements of **spirituality** that are addressed in nursing references include the following (Burkhardt & Nagai-Jacobson, 2009; NANDA International, 2009):

- Connectedness to self: joy, love, surrender, serenity, self-forgiveness, and meaning and purpose in life
- Connectedness with others: service, compassion, loving sexuality, forgiveness of others, shared genuine presence, meaningful interactions with significant others, reciprocal giving and receiving

- Connectedness with power greater than self: awe, prayer, ritual, reverence, meditation, reconciliation, mystical experiences
- Engagement in creative activities: art, music, nature, poetry, writing, singing, spiritual literature.

Florence Nightingale viewed spirituality as intrinsic to human nature and emphasized that it was an individual's deepest and the most potent resource for healing. Definitions of spirituality generally include the following concepts: healing; wholeness; social justice; personal growth; interpersonal relationships; a sense of meaning and purpose to life; a transcendent relationship with a higher being; an association with reverence, mystery, and inspiration; connectedness with nature, other people, and the universe; and feelings of and behaviors arising from love, faith, hope, trust, and forgiveness.

Studies consistently find that religion becomes increasingly salient with age and that religiousness in older adults is associated with the following positive effects (Aldwin, Hofer, & McCammon, 2006; Idler, McLaughlin, & Kasl, 2009):

- Longer life expectancy
- Lower rates of cancer, alcoholism, hypertension, heart disease
- Better adaptation to medical illness
- Better immune system function
- Fewer hospitalizations and shorter hospital stays
- Greater well-being and life satisfaction
- Less anxiety and depression
- Lower rates of suicide
- Better adaptation to caregiving burden
- Faster recovery from depression
- Higher levels of hope and optimism
- Higher levels of participation in health promotion activities (e.g., increased exercise and smoking cessation).

Gerontologists conclude that the positive effects of participation in religious communities can be attributed in part to the social supports derived from these activities, whereas the positive effects of spirituality are associated with the developmental challenges of coming to terms with one's own mortality (Greenfield, Valliant, & Marks, 2009).

Some studies focus on particular aspects of religiosity and spirituality. For example, many studies focused on meditation, particularly mindfulness meditation, and found that it can strengthen neurologic circuits in the brain and increase brain activity associated with positive emotions (Bartol & Courts, 2009). Positive effects of meditation on psychosocial aspects of functioning that have been identified in studies include reduced anger, reduced anxiety, alleviation of depression, positive mood states, improved memory and cognitive function, and increased sense of well-being (Garland, Gaylord, & Park, 2009; Posadzki & Jaques, 2009). Studies that focused on meaning in life identified positive health effects, including increased longevity, for older adults who had a strong sense of purpose in life (Krause, 2009).

> ### ◆ Wellness Opportunity
>
> Nurses promote wellness by asking older adults about relationships that provide meaning in their lives.

Cultural Considerations

Cultural considerations are important for addressing many aspects of function, but they are especially important in relation to psychosocial function because a person's cultural background significantly influences the way a person defines and perceives all aspects of psychosocial function. In assessing psychosocial function in older adults, for example, it is essential to recognize that every society has standards of "normal" or "abnormal" behaviors, and these standards provide guidelines for determining whether behaviors are healthy or unhealthy. Many societies, however, do not have the rigid distinctions between health and illness that are part of Western cultures, and concepts, such as mental health, have little meaning in many non-Western societies (Kavanagh, 2008). Cultural perceptions determine all of the following aspects of psychosocial function:

- Definition of mental health and mental illness
- Belief about the causes of mental health and illness
- Expression of symptoms or clinical manifestations of mental health and illness
- Criteria for labeling or diagnosing someone as mentally ill
- Decisions concerning appropriate healer(s)
- Choice of treatment(s) to cure mental illness
- Determination that mental health has been restored after an illness episode
- Relative degree of tolerance for abnormal behavior by other members of society.

Cultural Considerations 12-1 identifies some of the cultural influences on psychosocial function and is particularly applicable to nursing care of older adults.

In some instances, people from diverse cultures may perceive or interpret physical symptoms and their interconnected

> ### A Student's Perspective
>
> *While I was caring for my client, she asked if she could tell me a story. She proceeded to tell me that a few nights earlier, she was lying in bed unable to sleep because of various health issues. All of a sudden, she heard this calm yet intense chant moving down the hall. One of the residents is Native American and recently received news that his nephew had passed away. He was performing a traditional chant in mourning for the loss of a loved one. My client said that the sound was peaceful and soothing as she lay awake in bed. She wished she could have recorded it to play every night. She felt it was special that this man was able to maintain his culture in a place far from home and that people respected his need to express himself in this way. She was very touched—and so was I—as she told me this story. I believe that maintaining one's culture is a part of the healing process and should be respected and upheld.*
>
> *Eliza T.*

psychological or emotional components in a manner that is unfamiliar to the nurse. For example, this is likely to occur with people who have a **culture-bound syndrome**, defined as a disorder that is "restricted to a particular culture or group of cultures because of certain psychosocial characteristics of those cultures" (Andrews, 2008a, p. 37). Because these conditions are unique to a particular culture, they may be unrecognized as a disease condition in the biomedical health care system and by professionals who do not share the same cultural background. More than 200 culture-bound syndromes are recognized, and some of these are listed as diagnoses in official diagnostic manuals, such as the American Psychiatric Association's *Diagnostic and Statistic Manual of Mental Disorders, Fourth Edition, Text Revision (DSM-IV-TR)* and the *International Classification of Mental Disorders (ICD-10)*. Table 12-2 lists selected culture-bound syndromes found in specific cultural groups.

Professionals and folk or indigenous healers with the same cultural background usually are knowledgeable about interventions for culture-bound syndromes. Older adults may be reluctant to discuss culture-bound syndromes or folk treatments with health care professionals, especially if the care provider has a different cultural background. The reasons for withholding such information are complex and may include fears that the nurse or other health care provider will disapprove, ridicule, or fail to understand their folk or indigenous healing system. Because of these factors, nurses may consider asking the person's permission to include folk or indigenous healers in discussions about health-related issues. These healers frequently have considerable insight into the cultural and psychosocial aspects of human behavior, and they may be remarkably successful in treating culture-bound syndromes and other disorders that have psychological and emotional components. Because herbal remedies that are sometimes used to treat culture-bound syndromes may interact with prescription or over-the-counter medications, nurses need to make every

CULTURAL CONSIDERATIONS 12-1

Cultural Influences on Psychosocial Function

Cultural Influences on Beliefs About the Cause of Mental Disorders

- In traditional Chinese culture, many diseases are attributed to an imbalance of yin and yang.
- Many Native American groups embrace a belief system in which balance and harmony are essential for mental and physical health.
- For some Hispanics, mental illness may be viewed as a punishment by a supreme being for past transgressions.
- Some African Americans, especially those of circum-Caribbean descent, may attribute the cause of mental illness to voodoo, sorcery, or other spiritual forces.

Cultural Influences on the Manifestations of Mental Illness

- Cultural norms determine whether behaviors such as any of the following are viewed as either normal or abnormal: dreams, fainting, visions, trances, sorcery, delusions, hallucinations, intoxication, suicide, speaking in tongues, communicating with spirits, and the use of certain substances (e.g., alcohol, tobacco, peyote, marijuana, and other drugs).
- Post-traumatic stress disorders are relatively common in immigrants and refugees.
- Hispanic older adults define mental health problems as alcohol and other drug abuse.
- Filipino Americans consider forgetfulness and anger to be mental health problems.

- Hispanic, Chinese, and other groups are likely to express psychological distress through physical symptoms.
- Although psychotic disorders (i.e., loss of contact with reality) occur in every society and are characterized by similar primary symptoms (e.g., insomnia, delusions, hallucinations, flat affect, and social or emotional withdrawal), the secondary features are highly influenced by cultural factors.
- In some groups, guilt and suicidal ideation do not accompany depression. For some peoples, suicide is an acceptable escape from problems.

Cultural Influences on Stress and Coping

- Cultural factors often create barriers to the use of formal support services by ethnic elders, and these barriers may increase the feelings of burden experienced by caregivers.
- African American families tend to use religion and spirituality to help them cope with caregiving stress, and religious organizations are a major source of social support for them.
- In Chinese families, cultural ideals promoting filial piety, family interdependence, veneration of elderly family members, and acceptance of family caregiving roles may affect the way families experience and cope with stress related to their roles as caregivers.

Source: Andrews, M. M., & Boyle, J. S., (2008). *Transcultural concepts in nursing care.* Philadelphia, PA: Wolters Kluwer/Lippincott Williams & Wilkins.

TABLE 12-2   Selected Culture-Bound Syndromes

Group	Disorder	Remarks
Blacks, Haitians	Blackout	Collapse, dizziness, inability to move
	Low blood	Not enough blood or weakness of the blood that is often treated with diet
	High blood	Blood that is too rich in certain things because of the ingestion of too much red meat or rich foods
	Thin blood	Occurs in women, children, and old people; renders the individual more susceptible to illness in general
	Diseases of hex, witchcraft, or conjuring	Sense of being doomed by spell; gastrointestinal symptoms, for example, vomiting; hallucinations; part of voodoo beliefs
Chinese, Southeast Asians	*Koro*	Intense anxiety that penis is retracting into body
Greeks	Hysteria	Bizarre complaints and behavior because the uterus leaves the pelvis for another part of the body
Hispanics	*Empacho*	Food forms into a ball and clings to the stomach or intestines, causing pain and cramping
	Fatigue	Asthma-like symptoms
	Mal ojo, "evil eye"	Fitful sleep, crying, diarrhea in children caused by a stranger's attention; sudden onset
	Pasmo	Paralysis-like symptoms of face or limbs; prevented or relieved by massage
	Susto	Anxiety, trembling, phobias from sudden fright
Japanese	*Wagamama*	Apathetic childish behavior with emotional outbursts
Koreans	*Hwa-byung*	Multiple somatic and psychological symptoms: "pushing up" sensation of chest, palpitations, flushing, headache, "epigastric mass," dysphoria, anxiety, irritability, and difficulty concentrating; mostly afflicts married women
Native Americans	Ghost	Terror, hallucinations, sense of danger
North Indians	Ghost	Death from fever and illness in children; convulsions, delirious speech (or incessant crying in infants); choking, difficulty breathing; based on Hindu religious beliefs and curing practices
Whites	Anorexia nervosa	Excessive preoccupation with thinness; self-imposed starvation
	Bulimia	Gross overeating and then vomiting or fasting

Source: Andrews, M. M. (2008). Cultural competence in the health history and physical examination [p. 40]. In M. M. Andrews & J. S. Boyle [Eds.], *Transcultural concepts in nursing care* [4th ed., pp. 34–65]. Philadelphia, PA: Lippincott Williams & Wilkins.

effort to elicit information about such remedies as part of an assessment (see Chapter 8).

The following case study is based on an example from Andrews and Boyle (2008).

Mrs. Y. is a 79-year-old native of the Philippines. She moved to an urban area in California to be near her four children, who live in the same state. She had lived in the same town in the Philippines for her entire adult life and had stayed there to care for her husband and her sister, who both required care for chronic conditions. Although she was a much-needed and highly esteemed member of her household in the Philippines, Mrs. Y., similar to many other immigrants, experienced role reversal when she lost her once-dominant position in the family and became financially dependent on her adult children after her relocation.

Similar to many older immigrants from the Philippines, Mrs. Y. had a more active social network before her relocation. She, similar to many of her peers, spoke a dialect and did not speak Tagalog, the language spoken by many younger residents of the Philippines. After her relocation to the United States, her communication and interaction with others became restricted to her extended family because she did not feel confident using her limited English and could not find other speakers of her dialect. To buffer the disequilibrium she felt as a result of her migration, Mrs. Y. sought comfort through prayer and regular attendance at the local Roman Catholic Church. She also began to regularly care for her two daughters' children.

You are the nurse at the local hospital who treated Mrs. Y. in the emergency department after she fractured her wrist. During your assessment, you noted that Mrs. Y.'s injury would place a strain on the family because they would temporarily be without their child care provider.

THINKING POINTS

- How would you involve the family members in the discharge plan for Mrs. Y. so that her recovery could be ensured, she would not lose respect, and she would not feel responsible to assume her usual duties until her injury healed and she felt better?
- What problems would you anticipate with communicating with Mrs. Y. in the emergency department? How would you handle these problems?
- What psychosocial repercussions did Mrs. Y.'s move to the United States have? Did she cope with these effectively? Would you have had any other suggestions for helping her to cope?
- How did Mrs. Y.'s culture influence her coping mechanisms?

RISK FACTORS THAT AFFECT PSYCHOSOCIAL FUNCTION

Theories about stress and coping and research about causes of impaired mental health in older adults provide information about risks that can affect psychosocial function. The following factors contribute to high levels of stress and poor coping in older adults:

- Poor physical health
- Impaired functional abilities
- Weak social supports
- Lack of economic resources
- An immature developmental level
- Narrow range of coping skills
- The occurrence of unanticipated events
- The occurrence of several daily hassles at the same time
- The occurrence of several major life events in a short duration
- High social status and feelings of high self-efficacy in situations that cannot be changed or in which control cannot be exerted over the environment.

In addition, because the ability to determine the potential for change influences one's response to a stressful situation, people who cannot realistically appraise a situation may have more difficulty coping effectively. This is particularly pertinent with regard to health and functioning because ageist attitudes and stereotypes may contribute to the false belief that health changes and functional decline are inevitable consequences of aging. Thus, nurses have important roles in teaching older adults about risk factors and potential interventions for health problems. For example, older adults who experience urinary incontinence or difficulties with sexual function may consider these changes to be inevitable consequences of age. On the basis of this appraisal, they are likely to use passive, emotion-focused coping mechanisms, trying simply to accept the situation. In addition, they are more likely to experience an unnecessary and unfortunate functional impairment and a diminished quality of life. By contrast, if the situation is appraised more accurately as a potentially treatable condition, more active, problem-focused coping mechanisms are likely to be used. Even when older adults accurately appraise health problems as changeable, they must identify health care professionals who understand the problem and who will attempt to find solutions. Thus, both older adults and health care professionals must accurately appraise the situation so they can initiate interventions and achieve wellness outcomes.

Older adults who normally have a sense of high self-efficacy may be particularly susceptible to disturbed self-esteem and feelings of powerlessness when they are in situations where they have little control over their environment. For example, studies have found that a sense of control over important aspects of one's life has positive effects on health and longevity, including improved general well-being and less depression (Angel, Angel, & Hill, 2009; Jang, Chiriboga, Lee, & Cho, 2009).

Learned helplessness is the experience of uncontrollable events that leads to expectations that future events will also be uncontrollable. Thus, actions that increase dependency or disempower older adults (e.g., providing assistance because this is more time-efficient rather than allowing the older person to function independently or with only a little assistance) are risk factors for diminished self-esteem and feelings of powerlessness. In addition, learned helplessness may contribute to depression, as discussed in Chapter 15.

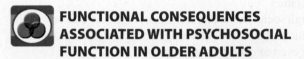

Wellness Opportunity

Nurses promote wellness by allowing older adults to function as independently as possible and providing the supports they need, even if this is not as time-efficient as doing things for them.

FUNCTIONAL CONSEQUENCES ASSOCIATED WITH PSYCHOSOCIAL FUNCTION IN OLDER ADULTS

Since the mid-1960s, many studies have used life event scales to measure the negative impact of stressful events, with particular emphasis on physical health effects. Although some studies have found an association between high stress and the occurrence of certain diseases (e.g., heart attacks), most people who experience life events do not become ill (George, 2006). Because the impact of life events on health is significantly affected by many interacting factors, older adults experience a wide range of both negative and positive functional consequences with regard to psychosocial function.

Negative functional consequences associated with psychosocial function in older adults include anxiety, loneliness, depression (refer to Chapter 15), and cognitive impairment (refer to Chapter 11). Up to 50% community-dwelling older adults report anxiety symptoms and epidemiologic studies report prevalence rates for anxiety disorders between 5.5% and 20% in community settings (Smith, Ingram, & Brighton, 2009). Anxiety in older adults is associated with increased illnesses, sleep disturbances, poor quality of life, increased use of services, and higher levels of disability (Weiss et al., 2009). Studies have found that anxiety is common in older adults who are disabled and is a significant predictor of progressing disability and admission to a nursing facility (Diefenbach, Tolin, Meunier, & Gilliam, 2009).

Older adults frequently experience feelings of loneliness, which is defined as a lack of satisfying human relationships, even when they are around other people. Common life events of older adulthood that can cause loneliness include retirement, widowhood, death of friends, social isolation because of health limitations, and moving to new environments. Studies have found that loneliness in older adults is associated with all the following functional consequences: disability, cognitive decline, higher depression scores, greater number

of chronic illnesses, increased use of health and social services, increased risk of being institutionalized, and increased mortality (Pitkala, Routasalo, Kautiainen, & Tilvis, 2009; Theeke, 2010).

In addition to focusing on anxiety, depression, and other negative emotions, gerontologists are also focusing on identifying the factors that affect emotional well-being and thereby improve health and the quality of life. The following characteristics of older adults are associated with emotional vitality and improved health (Aldwin, Hofer, & McCammon, 2006; Krause, 2006):

- Feeling happy, enjoying life
- Experiencing autonomy
- Experiencing personal growth
- Having a purpose in life
- Being extroverted and outgoing
- Feeling hopeful about the future
- Having positive relations with others
- Having a sense of self-acceptance
- Having a high sense of personal mastery
- Having a sense of hardiness and coherence
- Having low measures of anxiety and depression
- Having a sense of religious or spiritual connectedness
- Experiencing a sense of mastery over one's environment.

An important aspect of promoting psychosocial wellness for older adults is focusing at least some attention on strengths that can be supported rather than addressing only the negative functional consequences.

NURSING ASSESSMENT OF PSYCHOSOCIAL FUNCTION

Because psychosocial function encompasses a broad range of social, cognitive, and emotional aspects of functioning that are intertwined, the assessment of psychosocial function is addressed comprehensively in a separate chapter. Readers are directed to Chapter 13 for a thorough review of nursing assessment of psychosocial function.

NURSING DIAGNOSIS

The nursing diagnoses of Self-Esteem Disturbance or Situational Low Self-Esteem (or Risk for) are applicable in relation to some of the psychosocial adjustment issues of older adulthood. Situational Low Self-Esteem is defined as "development of a negative perception of self-worth in response to current situation (specify)" (NANDA International, 2009, p. 193). Related factors might be the internalization of ageist attitudes, the loss of roles or financial security, the need for a change to a more dependent living arrangement, and chronic illnesses that affect one's abilities and role identities.

If the nursing assessment identifies threats to the older person's sense of control, an appropriate nursing diagnosis is Powerlessness (or Risk for). This is defined as "perception that one's own action will not significantly affect an outcome; a perceived lack of control over a current situation or immediate happening" (NANDA International, 2009, p 190). Common related factors for older adults are forced retirement, loss of the ability to drive a vehicle, lack of involvement in decision making, chronic conditions that cause progressive functional declines (e.g., dementia), and institutional constraints, such as lack of privacy and the need to follow schedules that do not meet the needs of the individual.

Social Isolation is defined as "aloneness experienced by the individual and perceived as imposed by others and as a negative or threatening state" (NANDA International, 2009, p. 356). A closely related nursing diagnosis is Impaired Social Interaction, defined as "insufficient or excessive quantity or ineffective quality of social exchange" (NANDA International, 2009, p. 223). For example, nurses can use these diagnoses when they are making referrals for community resources to improve social supports for older adults.

Another nursing diagnosis that might be applied to the psychosocial needs of older adults is Ineffective Coping, which is defined as the "inability to form a valid appraisal of the stressors, inadequate choices of practiced responses, and/or inability to use available resources" (NANDA International, 2009, p. 254). Other nursing diagnoses that might be applicable with regard to specific aspects of psychosocial function include Relocation Stress Syndrome (or Risk for), Anxiety, Grieving, Chronic Sorrow, and Stress Overload.

Nurses can use any of the following diagnoses to address spiritual needs of older adults: Spiritual Distress (or Risk for) or Impaired Religiosity (or Risk for). In addition, nurses can use Readiness for Enhanced Spiritual Well-Being when they are addressing older adults' sense of meaning and purpose. This wellness diagnosis is defined as the "ability to experience and integrate meaning and purpose in life through connectedness with self, others, art, music, literature, nature, and/or a power greater than oneself that can be strengthened" (NANDA International, 2009, p. 292).

> **◆ Wellness Opportunity**
>
> Readiness for Enhanced Coping and Readiness for Enhanced Resilience are wellness nursing diagnoses that are applicable for many older adults who are experiencing psychosocial stress.

PLANNING FOR WELLNESS OUTCOMES

Wellness outcomes related to psychosocial function focus on stress reduction, enhanced coping skills, and improved quality of life. When planning wellness outcomes pertinent to Situational Low Self-Esteem (or Risk for) or Readiness for Enhanced Self-Concept, nurses can apply any of the following Nursing Outcomes Classification (NOC) terminology: Psychosocial Adjustment: Life Change; Self-Esteem; Adaptation to Physical Disability; Body Image; Grief Resolution; Personal Autonomy; Depression Level; and Quality of Life.

Outcomes for older adults who experience Powerlessness include Hope, Personal Autonomy, and Participation in Health Care Decisions. Outcomes related to the nursing diagnosis of Social Isolation include Loneliness Severity, Social Support, Social Involvement, Leisure Participation, and Personal Well-Being.

When nurses plan care for older adults with nursing diagnoses of Impaired Adjustment, Ineffective Coping, or Readiness for Enhanced Coping, any of the following NOC terminology might be pertinent: Psychosocial Adjustment: Life Change; Acceptance: Health Status; Adaptation to Physical Disability; Coping; Decision Making; Knowledge: Health Resources; Personal Well-Being; and Stress Level.

> **◆ Wellness Opportunity**
>
> Hope and Quality of Life would be appropriate NOC terminologies when nurses direct care toward improving psychosocial wellness.

 NURSING INTERVENTIONS TO PROMOTE HEALTHY PSYCHOSOCIAL FUNCTION

Nurses have many opportunities to promote healthy psychosocial function during the usual course of caring for older adults. For example, they can incorporate communication techniques and other interventions to enhance self-esteem, promote a sense of control, and address spiritual needs. They also can use **life review** and **reminiscence** interventions, especially in home and long-term care settings. In addition to incorporating interventions in usual care, nurses promote psychosocial wellness by facilitating referrals for social supports. In some settings, nurses can implement group interventions, such as healthy aging classes, to help older adults cope effectively with the life events of older adulthood.

The following Nursing Interventions Classification (NIC) terms relate to interventions discussed in this chapter: Active Listening; Anxiety Reduction; Caregiver Support; Coping Enhancement; Decision-Making Support; Emotional Support; Grief Work Facilitation; Hope Instillation; Presence; Religious Ritual Enhancement; Reminiscence Therapy; Resiliency Promotion; Role Enhancement; Self-Esteem Enhancement; Socialization Enhancement; Spiritual Growth Facilitation; Support System Enhancement; and Teaching: Group.

In addition to the interventions reviewed in this chapter, interventions that improve functional abilities promote psychosocial wellness because of the close relationship between physiologic and psychosocial aspects of health and function. Thus, interventions to improve functional abilities, which are discussed throughout this text, also promote psychosocial wellness. In addition to having physical benefits, participation in physical activity is beneficial for many aspects of psychosocial function, such as alleviation of anxiety and depression. A national longitudinal study of older adults in Canada concluded that physical activity interventions focused on improving mastery and fitness may have the greatest benefit in alleviating psychological distress (Cairney, Faulkner, Veldhuizen, & Wade, 2009). Other studies indicate that tai chi, qigong, and other meditative movement forms are especially beneficial for older adults (Rogers, Larkey, & Keller, 2009).

Enhancing Self-Esteem

Self-esteem enhancement is an essential component of nursing care for older adults because self-esteem is an important coping resource and a factor that influences well-being. Self-esteem refers to the feelings one has about one's self. It is the emotional component of self-concept and is based on one's perceptions of other people's opinions about oneself. Good self-esteem is a characteristic that is associated with being happier, healthier, less anxious, more independent, more self-confident, and more effective in meeting environmental demands than people with low self-esteem. Chapter 13 includes information on assessing self-esteem, whereas this chapter (12) focuses on nursing interventions that enhance self-esteem, with emphasis on addressing factors that threaten it (e.g., dependence, devaluation, depersonalization, and powerlessness).

Many factors that are threats to self-esteem are associated with staff and environments of institutional settings and can be addressed through relatively simple nursing interventions. This is particularly important in environments such as long-term care settings where the caregiving environment affects virtually every aspect of daily life for the residents. For instance, when older adults are admitted to institutional settings, nurses may be able to identify environmental or other factors that can quickly and easily be modified to promote a sense of control and minimize or eliminate a threat to self-esteem, as in the following examples:

- Ensuring easy access to their usual assistive devices (walkers, eyeglasses, hearing aids)
- Providing as much privacy as possible
- Asking about food preferences and ensuring as much choice as possible
- Asking open-ended questions, such as, "Is there anything that we can do to help you manage better while you're here?"
- Asking, "Is there anything you're worried about that I can help you with?"
- Ensuring that staff members address persons by their preferred names
- Involving older adults as much as possible in decisions that affect them.

Threats to self-esteem also arise when caregivers promote unnecessary dependence for their own convenience. For example, using incontinence products and telling a bedridden person to wet the bed because it is easier to change the disposable pad or brief than to assist with toileting is a tremendous blow to the person's self-esteem. Thus, interventions that improve independent function, which are discussed throughout this text, are important for enhancing self-esteem.

Because self-esteem depends to some extent on the perceived appraisal of significant others, nurses can use communication interventions to increase the older adult's perception of self-worth. Nurses must be aware of their ageist attitudes and avoid reflecting these attitudes in verbal statements. For example, even a remark such as "You certainly look good for 85 years old," although said with good intentions, can reinforce ageist attitudes. Hidden messages in this statement may be that it is better to look younger and that when you are old, you generally do not look good. Nurses can address ageism by avoiding even subtle messages that communicate negative attitudes. For instance, a statement, such as the following, might enhance an older person's self-esteem and challenge ageist attitudes: "At 85 years old, you must have a lot of wisdom. Can you share a bit of that wisdom with me?" Nonverbal communication may influence the person's perception of self-worth even more than verbal communication. For example, if a nurse walks past an older person sitting in a hallway without acknowledging his or her presence, this may be perceived as an indicator that the nurse does not value the older person. Even though the nurse may have been attending to responsibilities and had not intended to communicate a negative message, this action may adversely affect that older person's self-esteem. Thus, nurses must keep in mind that the perception of their actions is often more important than their intent, and they must use verbal and nonverbal messages to communicate feelings of positive regard whenever possible.

For dependent older adults, the negative impact of disability and functional impairments on self-esteem is heightened by behaviors of others that convey attitudes of **infantilization** (i.e., treating an adult in a way that is similar to the way infants are treated). For example, remarks, such as "He acts just like a baby" or "Now, now, dear, let's be a good girl," convey infantilization. Residents of nursing homes and assisted-living facilities view this kind of communication as being looked down upon by staff (Williams & Warren, 2009). The term **elderspeak**—also called "baby talk"—describes speech that is modified when addressed to older adults, usually by younger adults. Elderspeak is characterized by slowed speech, shortened sentences, elevated pitch and volume, simplistic vocabulary and grammar, and inappropriately intimate terms of endearment (Williams, Herman, Gajewsi, & Wilson, 2009). This type of communication is demeaning and patronizing, and it can have serious negative consequences. Researchers have found that elderspeak communication by nursing home staff caring for people with dementia was associated with increased resistance to care and with negative vocalizations (e.g., crying, screaming, yelling) (Herman & Williams, 2009; Williams et al., 2009). Moreover, it can reflect ageist attitudes or negative and inaccurate stereotypes. Thus, nurses need to monitor their communication with older adults to ensure that they avoid inappropriate terminology and elderspeak. Box 12-1 summarizes nursing interventions for enhancing self-esteem in older adults.

> **◆ Wellness Opportunity**
>
> Nurses can enhance self-esteem by pointing out an older adult's positive qualities during routine care activities.

Box 12-1 Nursing Interventions to Promote Self-Esteem

Communication Techniques

- Acknowledge person by using their preferred names and titles.
- When talking with older people, use the same tone of voice you use for your colleagues.
- Provide positive feedback for individual accomplishments, even in daily self-care tasks that require effort.
- Focus conversations on persons' strengths and positive attributes rather than on their limitations. (For example, for people who have physical impairments, focus on nonphysical attributes, such as personality characteristics or interpersonal relationships.)
- When negative functional consequences are attributed to old age, offer an alternative explanation and identify a contributing factor that is amenable to change. (For example, when older people attribute weakness "simply" to being old, remind them that they are recovering from hip surgery and should expect to improve with therapy.)
- Be cautious about communicating ageist attitudes, even inadvertently, in conversations.

Verbal Communication to Observe for and Avoid

- Do not use names or phrases that reflect ageist attitudes (e.g., "little old lady," "dirty old man"), even in jest.
- Do not raise your voice except when necessary to facilitate communication with someone who has impaired hearing.
- Do not use terms that are associated with babies (e.g., *diapers, baby food*).
- Do not use *we* or *us* unless the term is accurate. (For example, do not say "Let's take our medicine now.")
- Do not use the term *senile*.

Nonverbal Communication Techniques and Additional Nursing Actions

- When labeling clothing, put the person's name in an inconspicuous place.
- Use actions consciously to communicate positive regard (e.g., recognize the presence of someone as you walk past).

Promoting a Sense of Control

Perceived control is a factor that significantly affects psychosocial wellness because higher levels of perceived mastery are associated with enhanced levels of well-being, alleviation of depression, and increased participation in health promotion (Jang et al., 2009). Thus, nurses address psychosocial needs of older adults with interventions that promote a sense of control and that involve older adults in decisions. Nursing interventions to promote a sense of control for older adults include involving them as much as possible in organizing their schedule and providing information about their plan of care.

Many studies have confirmed the importance of modifying the way people perceive and explain events, shifting attention to factors that can be changed or controlled. In the classic study by Rodin and Langer (1980), whenever a nursing home resident attributed a problem to being old, the staff provided another explanation and identified a causative factor that was amenable to change. For instance, when residents

attributed feelings of fatigue to being old, they were reminded that they were awakened at 5:30 AM (Rodin & Langer, 1980). Nurses can listen for opportunities to challenge older adults' perceptions that promote a sense of hopelessness and rephrase the situation in a context that is empowering. For example, they can help older adults develop problem-focused coping mechanisms rather than passively, and sometimes inaccurately, accepting the negative functional consequences of aging.

Nursing interventions also address factors that can threaten perceived control, such as lack of privacy and loss of individuality, which commonly occur in institutional settings. Nurses can show respect for privacy by knocking on bedroom doors and asking permission before entering, by closing doors when privacy is desired, by asking permission before pulling bed curtains open, and by being careful about moving personal belongings without permission from the older person. Encouraging the person to have personal belongings and to arrange these belongings in whatever fashion is desired also shows concern for individuality.

Wellness Opportunity

Nurses show concern for individuality by asking an older adult about a family photograph or greeting card that is in view.

Involving Older Adults in Decision Making

Older people are frequently left out of the decision-making process, even for those decisions that most profoundly affect their lives, such as moving to a long-term care facility. This lack of involvement occurs for a variety of reasons, related both to the older adult and to the decision makers. Some of the barriers within the older adult may be dementia, depression, long-term passivity regarding decisions, or hearing impairments or other communication barriers. Some of the barriers within the decision makers that may thwart the decision-making process include stereotypes of older people as incompetent, perceptions that the older adult is not interested in or capable of making decisions, and an unwillingness to deal with the older person's anticipated resistance to the desired outcome.

Many of the reasons for excluding older adults from the decision-making process are related to the attitudes of the family and of professional caregivers, so one nursing intervention is to challenge these attitudes. For example, in acute care settings, nurses can facilitate communication between older patients and their primary care provider to ensure that the older person is included in decisions about medical treatment and discharge plans. In long-term care settings, nurses have numerous opportunities to involve older adults in decisions about their daily care, medical interventions, and discharge plans. In home settings, nurses can work with family members and older adults to ensure that the latter are involved in decisions about their care and that their rights are respected.

In any setting, nurses may have to remind health care professionals, as well as family members and other caregivers, that although people may gain rights by virtue of being a certain age, they do not lose their rights just because they reach a certain age. For additional discussion of nurses' role in decisions regarding long-term care for people with dementia, refer to Chapter 9.

Other aspects of decision making that can be addressed in nursing interventions are one's verbal interactions and choice of terminology. With regard to verbal communication, health care professionals often talk *about* older adults when in their presence rather than directing communication *to* them and focusing the conversation *on* them. This is especially common when family members or other caregivers are discussing situations with a nurse or other professional and the conversation takes place in the presence of the older person without directly involving him or her. In working with older adults, nurses need to pay particular attention to including older adults in conversations when the topic is directly related to them. When it is not appropriate to include the older adult in the conversation, the nurse can take steps to facilitate the conversation outside the presence of the older person. In these situations, the nurse can ask the older person's permission to discuss his or her situation with family member or caregivers and then report back to the older person, in language that the person can understand, about any discussions that take place or decisions that are made or pending.

With regard to terminology, the word "placement" often is used in reference to an older adult's admission to a nursing home. This term denotes passivity on the part of the older adult; it is closer to the terminology used when objects are placed on a shelf than to words normally used in reference to human beings. Nurses would communicate more positive feelings and a greater sense of control if they referred to an "admission" to a nursing home. The term admission suggests that certain criteria have been met and that an active decision has been made to determine whether the person meets these criteria. Even more important than using the correct terms, nurses must ensure that older adults are, in fact, actively involved in the decision-making process, rather than passively being "placed." Nurses can help older adults and their families with decisions about long-term care by helping them assess their situation and by correcting misinformation and providing accurate information about specific resources and the range of services available (as described in Chapter 6).

Addressing Role Loss

Meaningful roles (e.g., spouse, caregiver, volunteer) are important determinants of feelings of worth, efficacy, and self-esteem. Although role loss is a common occurrence in later adulthood, studies indicate that the development of new roles is an effective coping strategy for older adults (George, 2006). Participating in volunteer work is an excellent way of providing social interaction and a sense of purpose. Studies have found that volunteering is associated with many positive health effects, including reduced mortality, improved functioning, increased social interaction, reduced pain and depression, and increased life satisfaction and self-rated health (Morrow-Howell, Hong, & Tang, 2009; Schwingel, Niti, Tang, & Ng, 2009). The most important predictor of volunteering during older adulthood is participation in volunteer activities during earlier periods and it is also significantly associated with good physical health status (Mehrotra & Wagner, 2009).

Besides helping older adults develop new roles, nurses can focus on past and current achievements as an intervention for enhancing self-esteem, especially for older adults who must depend on others and have difficulty feeling a sense of accomplishment, or even a sense of basic usefulness. Nurses implement this intervention, which may be especially helpful for older adults who have difficulty identifying meaningful roles, in a group setting or on an individual basis.

> ### ◆ Wellness Opportunity
>
> Nurses can ask older adults about their accomplishments in areas, such as work and family, and give positive feedback about meaningful roles.

Encouraging Life Review and Reminiscence

Life review and reminiscence are two closely related processes that are used to promote psychosocial health in older adults. Butler (2001) describes life review as a progressive return to consciousness of past experiences, particularly unresolved conflicts, for reexamination and reintegration. If the reintegration process is successful, the process gives new significance and meaning to life and prepares the person for death by alleviating fear and anxiety (Butler, 2001). Positive effects of life review include accepting one's mortality, righting of old wrongs, taking pride in accomplishments, gaining a sense of serenity, and feeling that one has done one's best (Butler, 2001). Participants in a nursing study of life review in home settings reported that the intervention helped them integrate their lived experiences and was meaningful, pleasurable, and healing (Binder et al., 2009).

Reminiscence is based on the same theoretical framework as life review; however, it can be done outside the life review process, and it is more informal and less intense. Another difference is that life review addresses both pleasant and unpleasant issues of the past, whereas reminiscence focuses primarily on pleasant and positive experiences. Reminiscence therapy as a nursing intervention is the recall of past events, feelings, images, and memories that are associated with comfort, pleasure, and pleasant experiences. As a group therapy, the reminiscence group is one of the most widely used interventions for older adults, and it may be particularly effective for improving self-esteem, reducing social isolation, and improving depression and cognitive functioning (Hsu & Wang, 2009; Huang, Li, Yang, & Chen, 2009; Perese, Simon, & Ryan, 2008).

A Student's Perspective

Performing a life review on anyone from a time other than your own is an interesting experience. I found it to be an amazing opportunity to sit down with Mrs. B. and for her to open up to a 20-year-old girl that she had met only the week before. Within the first few minutes, she talked about her husband and I watched the tears roll down her face. This became the most significant part of our interview because I was able to understand how exposed she was allowing herself to be. It also made me realize how open the elderly can be in reminiscing about their lives and how important this topic is for them to share. It amazed me how just starting a conversation with an older person could bring so much emotion and joy at the exact same time.

The interview with Mrs. B. has affected my approach to older adults in clinical practice. I believe that a life review can be done on a daily basis while working with clients. This way, you can get to know each person on a personal level in order to provide individualized care. Each time you see a patient, you could continue the conversation and develop a relationship that benefits not only the client, but also yourself. I have learned that by showing interest in a person's life, you can allow them to discuss a significant part of who they have become, which is something they do not get to do on a daily basis.

Jillian B.

Fostering Social Supports

Nurses have many opportunities to foster the development of social networks for older adults, and this is an appropriate intervention for addressing social isolation. In some situations, particularly in home and long-term care settings, nurses are an integral part of the older person's social network. Social isolation is likely to occur because of any of the following factors that commonly occur in older adulthood:

- Hearing impairments and other communication barriers
- Chronic illnesses that limit activity or energy
- Lack of social opportunities because of caregiving responsibilities
- Mobility limitations, including the inability to drive a vehicle
- Mental or psychosocial impairments that interfere with relationships
- Loss of spouse, friends, or family through death, illness, or physical distance.

Thus, nursing interventions that address these risk factors (e.g., improved mobility or sensory function) are also likely to have the positive consequence of improved social supports.

In long-term care settings, nurses can foster positive social interactions in group settings, such as dining and activity rooms. Sometimes, a very simple intervention, such as positioning chairs (including wheelchairs) so that people can interact with each other, can significantly influence social contacts, either positively or negatively. Whenever possible, nurses should arrange room assignments to encourage opportunities for positive social interactions. In addition, nurses can facilitate referrals for social and therapeutic activities in long-term care facilities.

In home settings, nurses can identify community resources, such as volunteer friendly visitor and meal programs, to decrease social isolation. Support and education groups that primarily focus on coping with a chronic illness (e.g., stroke clubs, or better breathing groups) also provide excellent opportunities for social contact and the development of friendships with people who are in similar situations. For people who are socially isolated because of caregiving responsibility, caregiver support groups can enhance coping abilities and provide social support.

In any setting, nurses can encourage older adults to participate in structured group activities to enhance their well-being. A randomized control trial found that older adults who experienced loneliness showed significant health benefits from participation in weekly psychosocial groups for 3 months (Pitkala et al., 2009). In addition, one nursing study concluded that nurses have key roles in encouraging older women to make social connections because friendships are important in preventing loneliness, even when family members live nearby (Eshbaugh, 2009). Selected nursing interventions to promote psychosocial wellness are described in Box 12-2.

Wellness Opportunity

Nurses can talk with older adults about the benefits of support groups and provide a list of local resources that address specific needs of older adults and their caregivers.

Addressing Spiritual Needs

Addressing spiritual needs of patients is within the scope of nursing, as exemplified in the following interventions that are commonly included in nursing care:

- Intentionally communicating caring and compassion
- Facilitating reminiscence
- Honoring a person's integrity
- Providing active and passive listening
- Making referrals for spiritual care
- Caring for someone who feels hopeless
- Arranging for participation in religious services
- Encouraging or facilitating participation in activities such as prayer and meditation.

Nursing interventions to address the spiritual needs of older adults need to be individualized and offered only if the person is receptive to the interventions. In addition, nurses need to be nonjudgmental about religion and spirituality and avoid imposing their personal beliefs. Moreover, because cultural factors significantly influence a person's spirituality and religious beliefs, interventions must be culturally sensitive. Andrews (2008b) provides an excellent overview of specific cultural influences on religion and spirituality, including details about health-related beliefs and practices of selected religious groups in North America.

In addition to addressing spiritual needs as a routine part of psychosocial nursing care, nurses often address

Box 12-2 Nursing Interventions to Promote Psychosocial Wellness

Facilitating Maximum Independence

- Make sure that the person has access to all necessary assistive devices and personal accessories (e.g., wigs, canes, dentures, walkers, and hearing aids).
- Allow enough time for the person to perform tasks at her or his own pace, and avoid unnecessary dependence that results from an overemphasis on time efficiency.
- Make sure that the environment has been adapted as much as possible to compensate for sensory losses and other functional impairments.

Promoting a Sense of Control

- Make a conscious effort to involve older adults in decisions regarding their care, both in small daily matters and in major health care concerns.
- Ask about likes and dislikes and try to address personal preferences.
- Whenever possible, allow persons to choose between two alternatives, even if the options are in a very narrow range (e.g., "Would you prefer to wear the yellow sweater or the pink one today?").
- Ensure as much privacy, or perceived privacy, as possible.
- Knock on the door and ask for permission before entering a bedroom, even in institutional settings.
- Allow as much expression of individuality as possible in the personal environment (e.g., use personal furniture when possible and display family pictures in full view).
- Make sure that the call light is accessible for people who are confined.
- Do not talk about someone in his or her presence as if he or she does not exist.
- Avoid referring to nursing home *placement*. Refer instead to an *admission*, and include the person in the decision-making process.

Addressing Role Loss

- Identify new roles for people and acknowledge those past and present roles that are viewed positively.

- Encourage participation in reminiscence groups and other group therapies.
- Find opportunities to create meaningful roles, such as helper or assistant, by involving older adults in useful tasks, such as folding laundry.
- When older adults volunteer to assist others, acknowledge their contribution with a remark such as, "You certainly help us a lot when you help take Mrs. Smith to the dining room in her wheelchair."
- Acknowledge an older adult's nonphysical assets and attributes, such as family relationships or a good sense of humor.
- Focus on positive relationships by acknowledging or asking about the receipt of flowers, greeting cards, and other visible signs of concern expressed by others.
- Ask older adults about their responsibilities as parents, grandparents, or roommates and point out their positive contributions.
- Ask older adults about family photographs, initiate a discussion of positive relationships, and remind them that others care about them (e.g., encourage them to talk about their grandchildren and great-grandchildren).
- Ask older adults about accomplishments in areas such as work, family, hobbies, and volunteer activities.
- Respond with comments such as, "You must be proud of your children," or "You certainly have accomplished a lot."

Fostering Social Supports

- Use interventions to address hearing impairments and other communication barriers (see Chapter 16).
- Encourage participation in group activities.
- For people in wheelchairs, especially those who cannot move independently, position the chair in a way that promotes social interaction.
- For nursing home residents, plan table and room arrangements in a way that fosters social relationships.

spiritual needs during times of spiritual distress. For example, older adults are likely to express spiritual needs when they are coping with the loss of a significant relationship or dealing with news about a serious or terminal illness. Older adults who are caregivers for others, especially a spouse, are likely to express spiritual needs in relation to decisions about the care of the other person. For example, they may experience feelings of guilt about not being able to meet the needs of a dependent loved one or feelings of "playing God" with regard to decisions about mentally incompetent loved ones. In these circumstances, the provision of support, information, and reassurance from a nurse who has dealt with these decisions in professional experiences may be an effective counseling intervention. At times, information from the primary care provider may be helpful in alleviating spiritual distress associated with end-of-life decisions or decisions about long-term care. In these cases, the nurse may be able to

facilitate communication between the primary care provider and the family to alleviate the spiritual distress. Some nursing interventions that address spiritual needs of older adults are listed in Box 12-3.

Promoting Wellness Through Healthy Aging Classes

When older adults need assistance in coping with specific functional consequences or when they need education to clarify myths and misunderstandings about age-related changes, individual counseling may be the best intervention. When older adults need counseling about psychosocial adjustments, however, educational groups may be more effective. Nurses often are involved with establishing and leading support and educational groups for caregivers. Common themes that nurses can address in groups include use of resources, coping with losses, and promoting optimal functioning.

Box 12-3 Nursing Interventions to Address Spiritual Needs

Therapeutic Communication Interventions

- Use verbal and nonverbal communication to establish trust and convey empathic caring.
- Use active supportive listening.
- Convey nonjudgmental attitudes.
- Communicate respect for individuality.
- Provide a supportive presence.
- Be open to expressions of feelings such as fear, anger, loneliness, and powerlessness.
- Honor a person's integrity.
- Support the person in his or her feeling of being loved by others and by a higher power (e.g., God, Allah, Jehovah).
- Encourage verbalization of feelings about meaning of illness.
- Provide positive feedback about faith, courage, sense of humor, and other such feelings and experiences.
- Encourage discussion of events and relationships that provide spiritual support.

Actions to Foster Religious and Spiritual Activities

- Facilitate referrals for visits from religious care providers and sources of spiritual care (clergy, rabbis, church members, spiritual directors).

- Facilitate participation in religious services or activities (e.g., tapes, readings, videos, observations of "holy days").
- Assist with obtaining requested religious items (books, music, statues).
- Provide quiet and private time for individual spiritual or religious activities (e.g., prayer, reflection, meditation, guided imagery).
- Provide necessary support for religious rituals (e.g., lighting candles, receiving communion, praying the rosary).
- Encourage participation in relaxing and enjoyable activities (art, music, nature).

Interventions for Specific Circumstances

- Provide support and care during times of suffering.
- Assist in the process of dying.
- Assist a person who is fearful of the future.
- Provide care for the person who feels hopeless.
- Facilitate reconciliation among family members.
- Encourage participation in support groups.

An example of a nurse-led group intervention that allows for sharing of experiences among peers is the healthy aging class, developed by this author and used successfully during two decades in a variety of settings with older adults at various functional levels. This model is based on the belief that older adults who are beginning to recognize age-related physical and psychosocial changes or who are already dealing with such changes can benefit from sharing their experiences with their peers. Nurses can use this model, which is described in detail, to enhance the coping skills of older adults who are adjusting to any of the challenges of older adulthood.

Goals

Goals for older adults who participate in healthy aging classes are as follows:

- Recognize the impact of common age-related physical and psychosocial changes.
- Support and encourage any effective coping mechanisms already being used.
- Develop new skills that could be effective for coping with current stressors.
- Obtain information that will facilitate problem-focused coping mechanisms for stressful situations that are amenable to change.
- Provide an opportunity for the sharing of similar experiences with peers.

Setting

Nurses in any setting can initiate healthy aging classes, but long-term care institutions are perhaps the most conducive setting for the following reasons:

- Nurses have many opportunities to establish and lead groups.
- Residents of long-term care facilities provide a captive audience from which to select group members.
- Residents of long-term care institutions usually are not acutely ill, and they are dealing with psychosocial adjustments that are readily identified.
- Residents of long-term care settings have in common at least one major life event, which is a temporary or permanent move to a more dependent setting.

Community settings also are conducive to successful healthy aging classes, but nurses may have to be more creative in gathering the group members. Nurses who provide health services or education programs for senior centers or assisted-living facilities might be able to establish ongoing healthy aging classes as part of their responsibilities. In these settings, a healthy aging class may be an efficient, as well as effective, way of providing health education using a format that has the additional advantage of enhancing coping mechanisms.

In acute care settings, nurses usually do not plan and implement group therapies, but in rehabilitative settings, nurses may have the opportunity to initiate healthy aging classes. In psychiatric units, often there are enough older adults among the patients to warrant the implementation of healthy aging classes as a form of group therapy.

Membership Criteria

The primary criteria for group membership are that the person be willing to acknowledge age-related changes and be capable of acquiring insight into his or her adjustment to these changes. This author has led groups ranging from highly functional older adults in community settings to seriously impaired older adults in a hospital-based medical geropsychiatric unit. Group members may be coping with similar psychosocial stresses, but this is not necessarily a criterion for participation. For example, a healthy aging class can comprise older adults who all have some degree of depression or who are coping with a particular stressful event, such as widowhood. An ideal group includes members who are coping with various life events commonly associated with older adulthood and who are motivated to learn effective coping styles.

The group works best if the membership is stable and closed, but this is not always possible. A disadvantage of an open group is that it is very difficult to develop cohesiveness. If the membership is open and changing, the leader must be more directive, and the group as a whole will not be able to establish ongoing priorities for discussion topics. In addition, with changing membership, the leader has to focus more attention on the exchange of information about group members at the beginning of each session.

Size of Group and Length, Duration, and Frequency of Sessions

Although group size can range from 5 to 12 members, the ideal is about 8 members. Groups can be either ongoing or time-limited. When the membership is changing, such as in acute or rehabilitative settings, sessions can be an ongoing mode of therapy. In long-term care or community settings, it is best to schedule group meetings for a predetermined length of time, such as 8 to 10 weeks, and allow for changes in membership at the end of each period. One-hour sessions are held at weekly intervals, at a consistent time and place. In community settings, it can be helpful to convene the groups in conjunction with a meal program because participants will already have social relationships. As in institutional settings, a community center offers an audience from which to select the group members. Other potential community-based sites include assisted-living facilities and group settings, such as adult care homes (also called board-and-care homes).

Criteria for and Responsibilities of Group Leaders

One nurse can lead group sessions, but it is often helpful to have a coleader who has had social service training. An older adult who has made a positive psychosocial adjustment and who can serve as a role model also can be a good coleader. The nurse must be able to clarify myths and misunderstandings about age-related changes and be skilled in group dynamics. As with the reminiscence group, the healthy aging class is not an intense psychotherapy session; therefore, the group leader is not required to be specially trained in mental health. To lead a healthy aging class, however, a good understanding of both the physiologic and psychosocial aspects of aging is essential.

The primary responsibilities of the group leaders are to facilitate the discussion of psychosocial adjustments of older adulthood and to provide feedback and clarification to the members. As with other groups, the leader must ensure that all members have an opportunity to participate and that the members attend to the identified topic. The leaders also must ensure that the group reaches some conclusions before the end of each session so that members leave with a feeling of accomplishment relating to at least one psychosocial challenge of older adulthood.

Format

As in all educational groups, the leader begins with an explanation of the purpose of the group and an introduction of the leaders and members. The leader also reviews the details of the sessions, such as their length, the duration of the group, the role of the leader, and the expectations of the members. After addressing questions and introductory material, the leader introduces the concepts of life events and adjustments to the challenges of older adulthood. The leader can use a statement similar to the following: "Throughout life, certain events are likely to occur that affect us emotionally. These events may involve our health, our personal relationships, the place where we live, our job or career responsibilities and opportunities, or other events that require an adjustment on our part. These are called major life events, and they often occur at certain points of life. To begin our discussion today, let's look at some of the major life events that are likely to occur in younger adulthood, around the age of 20 to 30 years." The group then identifies various life events, such as finding a job, moving from the family home, finding a partner, and starting a family. The leader then asks members to identify life adjustments that are likely to occur between 30 and 50 years of age.

After the members have identified these life events, the leader emphasizes that one purpose of the healthy aging class is to identify effective ways of addressing the challenges inherent in the life events of older adulthood. The term *challenges* is used to communicate an active mode of addressing issues. The leader may want to discuss the phrase "challenges of older adulthood" and allow the group members to comment on what they see as challenges in their lives. As the members identify the life events of older adulthood, the leader writes the events on a board or paper so that all the members can see the list. The leader can then ask about life events that the members think they are likely to experience in the next few years. As events are identified, the members are also asked to identify the consequences of the events that require an adjustment. Examples of these life events and consequences have been discussed earlier in this chapter, and they are summarized in Figure 12-1. If group members do not identify all the life events, the leader may ask about a certain event, such as coping with one's own or a spouse's retirement. This discussion should continue until all the events and consequences in Figure 12-1 have been identified.

If the group is ongoing and has a stable membership, the leader may devote the majority of the first meeting to this discussion. The leader should emphasize that the rest of the meetings will be devoted to discussions of the identified issues, and that the first meeting will set the stage for future sessions. If the group is open and has a changing membership, the leader may need to be more directive during this first phase to limit the time spent on this topic. With changing membership, this initial identification of issues would be limited to the first 20 to 30 minutes. The group can then discuss coping mechanisms for one specific issue during the latter half of the meeting.

After the issues are identified, the leader summarizes the discussion, referring to the list of challenges written for the members to see. The members then share ideas about coping strategies that they have found to be helpful in adjusting to these changes. The leader may begin this part with a statement such as, "Now that we've identified the challenges of older adulthood, let's look at what things are helpful in responding to these challenges. I'd like each of you to share with the group one thing you do to help yourself face difficult challenges." After members have identified general coping mechanisms, the leader can suggest that the group choose one specific life event of older adulthood and discuss coping mechanisms that are helpful for addressing this challenge. Examples of coping strategies that might be discussed in relation to specific life events are summarized in Table 12-3. As these coping strategies are identified, they should be written on a board, and members should be encouraged to relate their personal experiences.

As the cohesiveness and trust level among members increase, particularly in closed groups, the sharing of experiences may become very open and revealing. The task of the leader, then, is to keep the discussion focused on appropriate coping mechanisms. In cohesive groups with highly functional members, the leader might have an opportunity to discuss the difference between emotion-focused and problem-focused mechanisms. The depth of discussion will depend on the degree of group cohesiveness and trust, the functional level of the members, and the comfort level and willingness of the leader to deal with the identified issues.

During the last 10 minutes of each session, the leader should attempt to bring the discussion to some closure on at least one issue. This may be accomplished by summarizing the issues and coping mechanisms that were identified. In open groups, the leader would end by encouraging those members who do not return to the group to look at coping mechanisms for their own specific issues, either by themselves or with a friend or confidant(e). For ongoing groups, the leader would end the session by facilitating agreement about the issues that will be discussed during the next session. The leader also can

TABLE 12-3 Coping Strategies for the Psychosocial Challenges of Older Adulthood

Psychosocial Adjustment	Coping Strategy
Ageist stereotypes	Develop a firm self-identity, challenge the myths, question any behaviors that are based on age-determined expectations
Retirement	Develop new skills, use time for hobbies and personal pursuits, become involved with meaningful volunteer activities
Reduced income	Take advantage of discounts for seniors
Declining physical health	Maintain good health practices (nutrition, exercise, rest)
Functional limitations	Adapt the environment to ensure safety and optimal functional status, take advantage of assistive devices and equipment, accept help when necessary
Changes in cognitive skills	Take advantage of educational opportunities, enroll in classes, keep mentally stimulated, join a discussion group, use the library, avoid dwelling on the things you cannot do and focus on your abilities, take advantage of increased potential for wisdom and creativity
Death of spouse, friends, and family members	Allow yourself to grieve appropriately, take advantage of opportunities for group or individual counseling and support, establish new relationships, renew old friendships, cherish the happy memories of the past, realize new freedoms
Relocation from family home	Look into the broad range of options for housing, appreciate the relief from the responsibilities of home ownership, take advantage of new services and opportunities for socialization
Other challenges to mental health	Maintain a sense of humor, use stress-reduction techniques, learn assertiveness skills, participate in support groups

encourage members to think about the identified issues in the interim.

EVALUATING THE EFFECTIVENESS OF NURSING INTERVENTIONS

Nurses evaluate the effectiveness of interventions for older adults with Self-Concept Disturbance by determining the extent to which older adults express positive views of themselves. Another measure of effective nursing care is that older adults no longer verbalize ageist attitudes. Nursing care of older adults who express a sense of Powerlessness is evaluated by the extent to which they become involved in decisions that affect them and the degree to which they express feelings of control over their lives. Nurses evaluate care for older adults with Ineffective Individual Coping by observing behaviors that reflect the use of a variety of coping strategies (see Table 12-3). For example, an older adult might learn to use problem-focused coping strategies for a situation he or she previously viewed as hopeless and unchangeable.

*M*r. P. is 86 years old and was recently admitted to a nursing facility for long-term care. His medical diagnoses are diabetes, glaucoma, retinopathy, and dementia of Alzheimer type. Mr. P. lived with his wife until 6 months ago, when she died after a brief illness. After her death, he needed help with all his activities of daily living, and his daughter arranged home care assistance for 6 hours a day. About 1 month ago, he started getting up and wandering outside at night. Once, he wandered off at 3:00 AM, and the police had to take him home. After this episode, he was afraid to be alone, and he agreed to go to a nursing facility because he could not afford to pay for 24-hour assistance at home.

During the first week in the nursing facility, Mr. P. was cooperative with the staff and sociable with the other residents. He was resistant to the morning schedule of getting up at 6:00 AM and eating breakfast in the dining room at 7:30 AM, but he passively complied when the staff firmly directed him. His daughter visited him daily and accompanied him to social and recreational activities with other residents. Mr. P. has been in the nursing facility for 10 days, and he is becoming very resistant to staff efforts to get him dressed for breakfast. When he attends group activities, he is disruptive, yelling about being a hostage in a monastery. Mr. P. tells other residents that he was tricked into coming to this place and that the only reason he has to stay is because his daughter has taken over his house and is living there with her family. He frequently paces up and down the corridors and says he has to find his daughter to take him home because his wife is sick and she needs him to take care of her. You walk with him in the hallway, and he says, "I don't know why they keep me locked up here. I can't do anything like I used to do at home. It's like a monastery where you have to get up in the middle of the night and they make you get cleaned up and eat breakfast when it's still dark out."

NURSING ASSESSMENT

Your nursing assessment shows that Mr. P. needs supervision in all activities of daily living because of poor vision and memory impairment. He needs some assistance with personal care, but he can dress himself if staff set his clothes out for him. When Mr. P. was admitted to the nursing facility, he was assigned to the "night-shift wakers" group, which means that the night shift is responsible for waking him and getting him ready for breakfast by 7:30 AM. The night-shift nursing assistants help him with showering, shaving, and dressing.

During the admission interview, Mr. P.'s daughter, Jane, said that his typical morning routine at home was to get up around 8:30 AM and get dressed independently, using the clothes that were set out for him by the home health aide. He

ate breakfast around 9:30 AM and then spent the day "working on his papers." Jane, who lives out of town, would call her father four times a week. When Jane talked with him on the phone, he always told her how busy he was working on his papers. Although Jane was paying all his bills from a joint bank account, Mr. P. would spend hours and hours with bill stubs, old bank statements, and an inactive checking account, thinking he was paying his bills.

Jane was staying at her father's house for the 2 weeks before his admission and for 1 week after admission to the nursing facility. She plans to return to town for a couple of days every other month and will visit her father at those times. The only nearby relative is a sister-in-law who comes to visit Mr. P. every 2 weeks.

NURSING DIAGNOSIS

You use the nursing diagnosis of Powerlessness related to relocation to a nursing facility and lack of control over activities of daily living. You select this diagnosis, rather than Impaired Adjustment or Ineffective Individual Coping,

because Mr. P. focuses on a theme of loss of control. Your assessment identifies several factors that contribute to his powerlessness, and you address these factors in your nursing care plan.

NURSING CARE PLAN FOR MR. P.

Expected Outcome	Nursing Interventions	Nursing Evaluation
Mr. P. will feel he has greater control over his morning schedule.	• Take Mr. P. off the "night-shift wakers" list and allow him to sleep until 8 AM. • Allow Mr. P. to wear his pajamas and robe to breakfast and to shower, bathe, and dress after breakfast.	• Mr. P. will no longer verbalize feelings of being locked up in a monastery or a prison.
Mr. P. will function as independently as possible.	• The staff will set out Mr. P.'s clothing and allow him to dress himself. • The staff will give Mr. P. positive feedback for dressing himself.	• Mr. P. will dress himself with minimal supervision. • Mr. P. will perform his personal care activities at a pace that is comfortable for him.
Mr. P. will engage in a familiar activity that gives him a meaningful role.	• Ask Jane to send a set of bill stubs, old bank statements, and the inactive checkbook so that Mr. P. can do his "work." • Encourage Mr. P. to "work with his papers" in the activity room, where he can interact with other residents. • Give Mr. P. positive feedback when he interacts with other residents. • Compliment Mr. P. about doing his paperwork.	• Mr. P. will resume his former routine of working with his papers and will interact with other residents.

Chapter Highlights

Life Events: The Age-Related Changes Affecting Psychosocial Function (Fig. 12-1)
• Retirement
• Relocation
• Chronic illness and functional impairments
• Decisions about driving a vehicle
• Widowhood
• Death of family and friends
• Ageist attitudes

Theories About Psychosocial Function in Older Adults
• Emotional development during later adulthood and theories about successful aging
• Stokes/Gordon Stress Scale (Table 12-1) can be used to identify stress level
• Older adults use problem-focused or emotion-focused coping styles depending on the type of stress
• Social supports are an important resource for coping.

Factors That Influence Psychosocial Function in Older Adults
• Religion and spirituality are increasingly important resources for older adults
• Cultural factors influence definitions perceptions of all aspects of psychosocial functioning (Cultural Considerations 12-1)
• Culture-bound syndromes: culturally specific disorders associated with psychosocial characteristics of a particular group (Table 12-2)

Risks Factors That Affect Psychosocial Wellness
• Physical, functional, and psychosocial health significantly affect coping skills
• The ability accurately to appraise a situation affects psychosocial function
• Learned helplessness results when uncontrollable events reinforce the idea that future events will also be uncontrollable.

Functional Consequences Associated With Psychosocial Function
• Negative functional consequences include anxiety, loneliness, depression, cognitive impairment.
• Older adults also experience emotional well-being (e.g., joy, happiness, satisfaction, purpose in life, sense of mastery).

Nursing Assessment of Psychosocial Function
• Refer to Chapter 13.

Nursing Diagnosis
• Self-Esteem Disturbance
• Situational Low Self-Esteem (or Risk for)
• Powerlessness
• Impaired Adjustment
• Social Isolation
• Readiness for Enhanced Coping
• Readiness for Enhanced Self-Concept

Planning for Wellness Outcomes
• Psychosocial Adjustment: Life Change
• Adaptation to Physical Disability

- Personal Autonomy
- Self-Esteem
- Quality of Life

Nursing Interventions for Psychosocial Wellness

- Enhancing self-esteem: improving functioning, using verbal and nonverbal communication, avoiding elderspeak
- Promoting a sense of control: providing information, rephrasing events, addressing threats such as lack of privacy and loss of individuality
- Involving older adults in decision making: challenging attitudes, facilitating communication, using verbal and nonverbal communication techniques
- Addressing role loss: identifying meaningful roles
- Encouraging life review and reminiscence
- Fostering social supports
- Addressing spiritual needs: communicating caring and compassion, instilling hope, referring for spiritual care, encouraging participation in religious activities
- Leading Healthy Aging classes

Evaluating Effectiveness of Nursing Interventions

- Positive self-perceptions
- Involvement in decisions
- Effective coping strategies

Critical Thinking Exercises

1. Take a sheet of paper and draw two vertical lines to make three equal columns. Think of someone you know in your personal life or professional practice who is 80 years old or older. In the left column, list three or more life events that this person has experienced in later adulthood. In the center column, describe the impact of the life event on the person's daily life. In the right column, list the coping mechanisms the person has used to deal with the life event. You can guess at the information, as needed, to complete the information in the center and right columns.

2. Think of a recent life event in your own life and answer the following questions: How close in time was the life event to other stressful events in your life? What impact did the life event have, and what were the manifestations of stress in your life (e.g., in your work, your health, your personal life, your relationships with other people)? What coping mechanisms did you use? Were the coping mechanisms effective? What coping mechanisms would you like to develop to prepare yourself for older adulthood?

3. You are asked to lead a 1-hour discussion titled "Mental Health and Aging" for a group of 10 people at a senior citizen center. Describe your approach to this topic. What would be your goals for the class? How would you involve the participants? What visual aids would you use?

Resources

For links to these resources and additional helpful internet resources related to this chapter, visit thePoint at http://thePoint. lww.com/Miller6e.

Clinical Tools

American Journal of Nursing and Hartford Institute for Geriatric Nursing
- *How to Try This,* article and video: Hyer, K. (2008). The Impact of Event Scale – Revised, *American Journal of Nursing, 108*(11), 60–68.
- *How to Try This,* article and video: Onega, L. L. (2008). Helping those who help others: The Modified Caregiver Strain Index, *American Journal of Nursing, 108*(9), 62–69.

Health Education

National Senior Service Corps

REFERENCES

Aldwin, D. F., Hofer, S. M., & McCammon, R. J. (2006). Modeling the effects of time: Integrating demographic and developmental perspectives. In R. H. Binstock & L. K. George (Eds.), *Handbook of aging and the social sciences* (6th ed., pp. 20–38). Boston: Academic Press.

Andrews, M. M. (2008a). Cultural competence in the health history and physical examination. In M. M. Andrews & J. S. Boyle (Eds.), *Transcultural concepts in nursing care* (5th ed., pp. 34–65). Philadelphia, PA: Lippincott Williams & Wilkins.

Andrews, M. M. (2008b). Religion, culture, and nursing. In M. M. Andrews & J. S. Boyle (Eds.), *Transcultural concepts in nursing care* (5th ed., pp. 355–407). Philadelphia, PA: Lippincott Williams & Wilkins.

Andrews, M. M., & Boyle, J. S. (2008). *Transcultural concepts in nursing care* (5th ed.). Philadelphia, PA: Wolters Kluwer/Lippincott Williams & Wilkins.

Angel, R. J., Angel, J. L., & Hill, T. D. (2009). Subjective control and health among Mexican-origin elders in Mexico and the United States: Structural considerations in comparative research. *Journal of Gerontology: Social Sciences, 64B,* 390–401.

Bartol, G. M., & Courts, N. F. (2009). The psychophysiology of body-mind healing. In B. M. Dossey & L. Keegan (Eds.), *Holistic nursing: A handbook for practice* (5th ed., pp. 601–615). Boston: Jones and Bartlett.

Binder, B. K., Mastel-Smith, B., Hersch, B., Symes, L., Malecha, A., & McFarlane, J. (2009). Community-dwelling, older women's perspectives on Therapeutic Life Review: A qualitative analysis. *Issues in Mental Health Nursing, 30,* 288–294.

Burkhardt, M. A., & Nagai-Jacobson, M. G. (2009). Spirituality and health. In B. M. Dossey & L. Keegan (Eds.), *Holistic nursing: A handbook for practice* (5th ed., pp. 617–645). Boston: Jones and Bartlett.

Butler, R. N. (2001). Life review. In M. D. Mezey (Ed.), *The encyclopedia of elder care* (pp. 401–402). New York: Springer Publishing Co.

Cairney, J., Faulkner, G., Veldhuizen, S., & Wade, T. J. (2009). Changes over time in physical activity and psychological distress among older adults. *Canadian Journal of Psychiatry, 54,* 160–169.

Cattell, M. G. (2009). Global perspectives on widowhood and aging. In J. Sokolovsky (Ed.), The cultural context of aging: Worldwide perspectives (3rd ed., Chapter 11, pp. 155–172). Santa Barbara, CA: Greenwood Press.

Cornwell, E. Y., & Waite, L. J. (2009). Social disconnectedness, perceived isolation, and health among older adults. *Journal of Health & Social Behavior, 50,* 31–48.

Diefenbach, G. J., Tolin, D. F., Meunier, S. A., & Gilliam, C. M. (2009). Assessment of anxiety in older home care recipients. *The Gerontologist, 49,* 141–153.

Drageset, J., Eide, G. E., Nygaard, H. A., Bondevik, M., Nortvedt, M. W., & Natvig, G. K. (2009). The impact of social support and sense of coherence on health-related quality of life among nursing home residents—a questionnaire survey in Bergen, Norway. *International Journal of Nursing Studies, 46,* 66–76.

Edwards, J. D., Perkins, M., Ross, L. A., & Reynolds, S. L. (2009). Driving status and three-year mortality among community-dwelling older adults. *Journal of Gerontology: Medical Sciences, 64A,* 300–305.

Eshbaugh, E. M. (2009). The role of friends in predicting loneliness among older women living alone. *Journal of Gerontological Nursing, 35*(5), 13–16.

Folkman, S., & Lazarus, R. S. (1980). An analysis of coping in a middle-aged community sample. *Journal of Health and Social Behavior, 21,* 219–239.

Garland, E., Gaylord, S., & Park, J. (2009). The role of mindfulness in positive reappraisal. *Explore, 5,* 37–44.

George, L. K. (2006). Perceived quality of life. In R. H. Binstock & L. K. George (Eds.), *Handbook of aging and the social sciences* (6th ed., pp. 320–336). San Diego, CA: Academic Press.

Greenfield, E. A., Valliant, G. E., & Marks, N. F. (2009). Do formal religious participation and spiritual perceptions have independent linkages with diverse dimensions of psychological well-being? *Journal of Health and Social Behaviors, 50,* 196–212.

Grove, L. J., Loeb S. J., & Penrod, J. (2009). Selective optimization with compensation: A model for elder health programming. *Clinical Nurse Specialist, 23,* 25–32.

Herman, R. E., & Williams, K. N. (2009). Elderspeak's influence on resistiveness to care: Focus on behavioral events. *American Journal of Alzheimer's Disease and Other Dementias, 24,* 417–423.

Holmes, T. H., & Rahe, R. H. (1967). The social readjustment rating scale. *Journal of Psychosomatic Research, 11,* 213–218.

Hsu, Y.-C., & Wang, J.-J. (2009). Physical, affective, and behavioral effects of group reminiscence on depressed institutionalized elders in Taiwan. *Nursing Research, 58,* 294–299.

Huang, S.-L., Li, C.-M., Yang, C.-Y., & Chen, J.-J. (2009). Application of reminiscence treatment on older people with dementia: A case study in Pintung, Taiwan. *Journal of Nursing Research, 17,* 112–118.

Idler, E. L., McLaughlin, J., & Kasl, S. (2009). Religion and the quality of life in the last year of life. *Journal of Gerontology: Social Sciences, 64B,* S28–S37.

Jang, Y., Chiriboga, D. A., Lee, J., & Cho, S. (2009). Determinants of a sense of mastery in Korean American elders: A longitudinal assessment. *Aging & Mental Health, 13,* 99–105.

Kang, S. K., & Chasteen, A. L. (2009). The development and validation of the age-based rejection sensitivity questionnaire. *The Gerontologist, 49,* 303–316.

Kavanagh, K. H. (2008). Transcultural perspectives in mental health nursing. In M. M. Andrews & J. S. Boyle (Eds.), *Transcultural concepts in nursing care* (5th ed., pp. 226–259). Philadelphia, PA: Lippincott Williams & Wilkins.

Kostyniuk, L. P., Molnar, L. J., & Eby, D. W. (2009). Safe mobility of older drivers: Concerns expressed by adult children. *Topics in Geriatric Rehabilitation, 25,* 24–32.

Krause, N. (2006). Religion and health in late life. In J. E. Birren & K. W. Schaie (Eds.), *Handbook of the psychology of aging* (6th ed., pp. 499–518). San Diego, CA: Academic Press.

Krause, N. (2009). Meaning in life and mortality. *Journal of Gerontology: Social Sciences, 64B,* 517–527.

Kryla-Lighthall, N., & Mather, M. (2009). The role of cognitive control in older adults' emotional well-being. In V. L. Bengston, M. Silverstein, N. M. Putney, & D. Gans (Eds.), *Handbook of theories of aging* (2nd ed., pp. 323–344). New York: Springer Publishing Co.

Lazarus, R. S. (1966). *Psychological stress and the coping process.* New York: McGraw-Hill.

Levy, B. R., & Leifheit-Limson, E. (2009). The stereotype-matching effect: Greater influence on functioning when age stereotypes correspond to outcomes. *Psychology and Aging, 24,* 230–233.

Mehrotra, C. M., & Wagner, L. S. (2009). Work, retirement, and leisure. In C. M. Mehrotra & L. S. Wagner. *Aging and diversity* (2nd ed., pp. 253–315). London: Taylor & Francis.

Morley, J. E. (2009). Successful aging or aging successfully. *Journal of the American Medical Directors Association, 10*(2) 85–86.

Morrow-Howell, N., Hong, S.-I., & Tang, F. (2009). Who benefits from volunteering? Variations in perceived benefits. *The Gerontologist, 49,* 91–102.

NANDA International. (2009). *Nursing diagnoses: Definitions and classification 2009–2011.* Oxford, England: Wiley-Blackwell.

Østbye, T., Krause, K. M., Norton, N. C., Tschanz, J., Sanders, L., Hayden, K., . . . Welsh-Bohmer, K. A. (2006). Ten dimensions of health and their relationship with overall self-reported health and survival in a predominantly religiously active elderly population: The Cache County Memory Study. *Journal of the American Geriatrics Society, 54,* 199–209.

Oxley, J., & Charlton, J. (2009). Attitudes to and mobility impacts of driving cessation: Differences between current and former drivers. *Topics in Geriatric Rehabilitation, 25,* 43–54.

Perese, E. F., Simon, M. R., & Ryan, E. (2008). Promoting positive student clinical experiences with older adults through use of group reminiscence therapy. *Journal of Gerontological Nursing, 34*(12), 46–51.

Pitkala, K. H., Routasalo, P., Kautiainen, H., & Tilvis, R. S. (2009). Effects of psychosocial group rehabilitation on health, use of health care services, and mortality of older persons suffering from loneliness: A randomized, controlled trial. *Journal of Gerontology: Medical Sciences, 64A,* 792–800.

Posadzki, P., & Jaques, S. (2009). Tai chi and meditation. *Journal of Holistic Nursing, 27,* 103–114.

Rodin, J., & Langer, E. (1980). Aging labels: The decline of control and the fall of self-esteem. *Journal of Social Issues, 36*(2), 12–29.

Rogers, C. E., Larkey, L. K., & Keller, C. (2009). A review of clinical trials of tai chi and qigong in older adults. *Western Journal of Nursing Research, 31,* 245–279.

Rohr, M. K., & Lang, F. R. (2009). Aging well together—A mini review. *Gerontology, 55,* 333–343.

Schwingel, A., Niti, M. M., Tang, C., & Ng, T. P. (2009). Continued work employment and volunteerism and mental well-being of older adults: Singapore longitudinal ageing studies. *Age Ageing, 38,* 531–537.

Selye, H. (1956). *The stress of life.* New York: McGraw-Hill.

Smith, M., Ingram, T., & Brighton, V. (2009). Evidence-based guideline: Detection and assessment of late-life anxiety. *Journal of Gerontological Nursing, 35*(7), 9–15.

Stokes, S. A., & Gordon, S. E. (1988). Development of an instrument to measure stress in the older adult. *Nursing Research, 37,* 16–19.

Stone, R. I. (2006). Emerging issues in long-term care. In R. H. Binstock & L. K. George (Eds.), *Handbook of aging and the social sciences* (6th ed., pp. 397–418). San Diego, CA: Academic Press.

Theeke, L. A. (2010). Sociodemographic and health-related risks for loneliness and outcome differences by loneliness status in a sample of U.S. older adults. *Research in Gerontological Nursing, 3,* 113–125.

Weiss, B. J., Calleo, J., Rhoades, H. M., Novy, D. M., Kunik, M. E., Lenze, E. J., & Stanley, M. A. (2009). The utility of the Generalized Anxiety Disorder Severity Scale (GADSS). *Depression & Anxiety, 26,* E10–E15.

Williams, K. N., & Warren, C. A. B. (2009). Communication in assisted living. *Journal of Aging Studies, 23,* 24–36.

Williams, K. N., Herman, R., Gajewsi, B., & Wilson, K. (2009). Elderspeak communication: Impact on dementia care. *American Journal of Alzheimer's Disease and Other Dementias<None>* 24, 11–20.

Young, H. M., & Cochrane, B. B. (2004). Healthy aging for older women. *Nursing Clinics of North America, 39,* 131–143.

Young, Y., Frick, K. D., & Phelan, E. A. (2009). Can successful aging and chronic illness coexist in the same individual? A multidimensional concept of successful aging. *Journal of American Medical Directors Association, 10,* 87–92.

Zarit, S. H. (2009). A good old age: Theories of mental health and aging. In V. L. Bengston, M. Silverstein, N. M. Putney, & D. Gans (Eds.), *Handbook of theories of aging* (2nd ed., pp. 675–691). New York: Springer Publishing Co.

Zhang, X., Fung, H., & Ching, B. H.-H. (2009). Age differences in goals: Implications for health promotion. *Aging and Mental Health, 13,* 336–348.

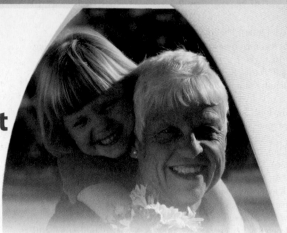

CHAPTER 13

Psychosocial Assessment

LEARNING OBJECTIVES

After reading this chapter, you will be able to:

1. Describe the purpose and scope of and procedure for a psychosocial assessment of older adults.

2. Describe communication techniques that are helpful for conducting a psychosocial assessment.

3. Describe how to assess each of the following specific components of mental status: physical appearance, motor function, social skills, response to the interview, orientation, alertness, memory, and speech and language characteristics.

4. Explain how to perform a nursing assessment of skills involved with decision-making and executive function in older adults.

5. Describe how to assess each of the following components of affective function: mood, anxiety, self-esteem, depression, happiness, and well-being.

6. Discuss distinguishing characteristics of delusions, hallucinations, and illusions as they relate to the underlying conditions common in older adults.

7. Explain how to perform a nursing assessment of the following aspects of social supports: social network, barriers to services, and economic resources.

8. Explain how to perform a nursing assessment of the spiritual needs of older adults including factors that cause spiritual distress as well as those that promote spiritual wellness.

KEY POINTS

abstract thinking	delusions
affect	executive dysfunction
circumstantiality	generalized anxiety
confabulation	disorder (GAD)
decision-making	hallucinations

illusions	Mini-Cog
insight	orientation
memory	social supports
mental status assessment	

Psychosocial assessment is a complex and challenging, but essential, aspect of nursing care for older adults. Although psychosocial impairments are often attributed to factors relating to normal aging or to untreatable conditions, a careful psychosocial assessment can identify the underlying cause(s) of mental changes, many of which can then be reversed or addressed through interventions. Thus, nurses can use assessment skills to improve quality of life for older adults by ensuring that psychosocial issues are identified and addressed. This chapter provides information on the assessment component of the nursing process related to cognitive and psychosocial function (Chapters 11 and 12). In addition, it supplements the assessment information in other chapters of this text, particularly the chapters on elder abuse (Chapter 10), dementia (Chapter 14), and depression (Chapter 15).

OVERVIEW OF PSYCHOSOCIAL ASSESSMENT OF OLDER ADULTS

In contrast to physical and functional assessment procedures, which are viewed as routine measures to identify the causes of troublesome symptoms, psychosocial assessment procedures are commonly perceived as formal psychological tests that analyze personality traits or identify the need for psychiatric treatment. Consequently, healthcare professionals may overlook the psychosocial component of assessment or relegate it to the realm of psychiatry. However, an assessment of psychosocial function is an essential component of holistic nursing care, which addresses the body–mind–spirit needs of older adults.

This chapter focuses on those aspects of psychosocial function that are pertinent to caring for older adults from a wellness perspective. This comprehensive perspective is like the emergency cart that is available in every hospital unit.

The cart stands ready at all times and is equipped with any items that would be needed to handle medical emergencies. When a serious medical problem arises, healthcare professionals quickly pull the cart to the patient's bedside and select the needed items. Similarly, nurses must have access to an array of skills for assessing psychosocial function as the need arises. In a few situations, their entire array of skills will be called into play, but in most situations, only a few of the examination tools will be necessary. Nurses can use the material in this chapter to "fill their **mental status assessment** carts," so they are prepared to select the appropriate tools for each situation.

The first sections of this chapter cover the purposes, procedures, and scope of a psychosocial assessment and are applicable to nursing care of all older adults. The second major section reviews unique aspects of communicating with older adults and applies the concepts to psychosocial assessment. Each of the following components, which nurses would selectively assess depending on the individual situation, are discussed in separate sections: mental status, **decision-making** and executive function, affective function, contact with reality, and **social supports**. Nurses can use the assessment boxes as a guide to observations and communication techniques pertinent to each aspect of psychosocial assessment.

Purposes of the Psychosocial Assessment Process

From a wellness perspective, the purposes of psychosocial assessment include the following:

- Detecting asymptomatic or unacknowledged health problems at an early stage
- Identifying signs or symptoms of psychosocial dysfunction (e.g., anxiety, depression, memory problems, depression, change in mental status)
- Identifying stressors and other risk factors (particularly those that are amenable to interventions) that affect cognitive, emotional, or social function
- Obtaining information about the person's usual personality, coping mechanisms, and cognitive abilities
- Identifying social supports and other coping resources that could be supported or strengthened
- Identifying the older adult's personal goals for psychosocial wellness.

As with other types of assessment, nurses use this information to plan interventions that are based on realistic expectations.

When the nursing assessment identifies mental changes in an older adult, a multidisciplinary approach is important for further assessment and implementation of effective interventions. A common mistake is to label the changes as "normal for the person's age." This is not only unfair to the older adult but can be detrimental, particularly if a treatable underlying condition is overlooked or appropriate interventions to improve functional abilities are neglected. As should be clear from the discussion of cognitive function in Chapter 11, age-related cognitive changes are rarely brought to the attention of healthcare professionals. For example, an older adult would be unlikely to make the following complaint: "I know I can learn new information, but I don't seem to be able to comprehend information as quickly as I used to." When mental changes are noted by other people or brought to the attention of healthcare professionals, it is more likely that they arise from pathologic processes than from age-related processes. Therefore, whenever changes in psychosocial function are identified, healthcare professionals must make every effort to identify the underlying cause and not attribute the changes to age.

Procedure for the Psychosocial Assessment

Nurses obtain psychosocial assessment information by interviewing older adults and their caregivers and by observing older adults in their environments. Opportunities for performing psychosocial assessments vary in different healthcare settings, and nurses obtain much of the assessment information informally during the course of their usual care. In acute care settings, nurses perform an assessment at the time of admission to establish a baseline for planning nursing care. Although the initial nursing assessment focuses on the patient's immediate needs, nurses should not overlook the psychosocial assessment, because it often provides clues to the causes of existing medical problems. Thus, as soon as the patient's condition is medically stable, the nurse should begin addressing psychosocial issues as an important component of holistic care and discharge planning. In long-term care settings, psychosocial assessment information is obtained as an ongoing part of care and is commonly addressed in team conferences. When nurses provide care in home and community settings, they can obtain valuable psychosocial assessment information by observing the interactions between older adults and their caregivers and environments.

In addition to interviewing and observing older adults, nurses obtain psychosocial assessment information from other sources. For example, when the older person's cognitive function is compromised, it is essential to obtain information from family members and others who can provide a reliable history of the mental changes. In long-term care settings, nursing assistants—the healthcare workers who spend the most time with residents—are an important source of psychosocial information. Nursing assistants are generally not included in team discussions when psychosocial problems are addressed, but nurses can obtain information from them and incorporate it in the care plans.

The tools for an effective psychosocial assessment are a trusting relationship, a listening ear, an intuitive mind, a sensitive heart, and good communication skills. Although nurses routinely provide patient care involving physically intimate activities such as bathing, they may be less confident about discussing psychosocial issues, particularly when the assessment involves concerns that would not normally be discussed with strangers. Moreover, older adults may feel threatened by psychosocial assessment questions, particularly if they are trying to cover up cognitive deficits. Thus, both the nurse and

Box 13-1 Self-Assessment of Attitudes About Psychosocial Aspects of Aging

What Is My Level of Comfort in Discussing Psychosocial Issues with Older Adults?
- How comfortable am I discussing emotional, cultural, spiritual, and psychosocial subjects?
- Are there certain topics with which I am uncomfortable (e.g., death, suicide, alcoholism, sexuality, spirituality, terminal illness, abusive relationships)?
- Does the person's age influence my degree of comfort (e.g., Am I more comfortable discussing issues with someone who is in their 60s than with someone who is in their 90s?)
- Does the person's gender influence my degree of comfort?
- To what groups of older adults do I find it easy or difficult to relate?
- How do I feel about older adults who are single, divorced, widowed, separated, or living together in a same-sex or heterosexual but unmarried relationship?

When I Was Growing Up . . .
- How were older adults in my family treated?
- What did I observe about the treatment of older adults in society?
- How were people with mental or emotional disorders viewed?
- What language was used to describe aging, old age, and older adults with disturbed mental function?
- What words did my family use, and what was the connotative meaning of the words used, to describe older adults? Was it positive, negative, or mixed?

What Experiences Have I Had with Older Adults . . .
- From different racial, ethnic, religious, and socioeconomic backgrounds?
- With functional impairments or mental, psychological, or emotional disorders?

personal information in conversations can facilitate the establishment of a trusting relationship. Offering a little information about their own pets or family, for instance, might encourage the older adult to share feelings that they might not mention otherwise and may help to establish a framework of mutual interest. Sharing information about ethnic background also can be an effective and nonthreatening way of obtaining information about possible cultural influences.

If formal mental status assessment tools are to be used, they can be introduced after the older adult is more comfortable with discussing psychosocial issues. Because questions about memory can be very threatening, the topic might be introduced as follows: "I notice you have a hard time remembering dates. Have you noticed any other problems with your memory? Is it okay with you if I ask some questions about your memory?" If no evidence of cognitive impairment is evident, but other people have expressed concern about the person's memory, a statement such as the following might be used: "Your daughter is concerned that you don't remember to keep appointments. Have you noticed any problems with your memory? Is it okay with you if I ask some questions about your memory?"

Scope of the Psychosocial Assessment

Nurses holistically address the psychosocial needs of older adults by identifying the unique meaning of events, with particular emphasis on the impact of health changes, for each older adult. Nurses can focus initial questions on events that occurred many years ago, because the person is likely to be quite comfortable discussing such topics. For example, a question such as, "What kind of work did you do?" may

the older adult may initially feel uncomfortable during a psychosocial assessment. Because increased awareness of one's own attitudes is an important first step in becoming comfortable with performing a psychosocial assessment, nurses can use a self-assessment guide (Box 13-1) to examine their own attitudes about older adults and identify areas of discomfort.

The nurse begins a psychosocial assessment by explaining the purpose of the questions with a statement like one of the following:
- "I'd like to get to know you better so we can make the best plans for follow-up after you leave the hospital."
- "I'd like to ask you some questions about your interests so we can plan for your care while you're here at the nursing facility."
- "I'd like to ask some questions about how you manage from day to day so we can identify any community services that might be helpful to you."

Nurses can ask initially about events of the remote past, such as where the person was born and grew up, as a nonthreatening way of leading into further questions about psychosocial function. Nurses may believe that it is unprofessional to talk about themselves, but incorporating some

A Student's Perspective

My experience interviewing Mr. M was an amazing one. I learned a lot about older adults and also about my interview technique. I think several of my techniques helped Mr. M. feel more comfortable and at ease. I told him if he felt uncomfortable answering any questions, he should feel free to pass and that did not happen once. I started asking him easy questions about his job and things like that. Then I moved into more personal questions related to his childhood and whether he thought it had been easy or difficult. I thought he might not remember a lot of that time in his life, but he told me many stories from when he was younger. He also had a lot of pride in the work that he did as a middle-aged adult when he was foreman in a factory.

Another technique I used was to allow him to wander away from the "path" of the question that I had asked him, because I didn't want him to feel conformed to answer the specific question. By using this technique, I learned much more about him than the scope of my original question, and it also gave him time to tell me things at his own pace. I could also tell what information he valued as important and what he found more private.

Erin H.

prompt a discussion of feelings about retirement. Because changes in living arrangements can precipitate feelings of loss, a nonthreatening question such as, "What were the circumstances of your moving here?" might lead to further discussion of the meaning of the living arrangement for that person. A question such as, "Do you ever think about moving from this house?" encourages a discussion of concerns about living arrangements. People who have experienced the loss of a pet may be reluctant to acknowledge the depth of their feelings. When an older person asks the nurse a question such as, "Do you have a dog?" he or she may be indirectly testing the nurse's feelings about pets. The astute nurse will use this opportunity to explore the person's feelings about the subject, perhaps responding, "No, but I have a cat. Have you ever had any pets?" Pets may be particularly significant for older adults and, indeed, may be one of the few meaningful relationships that are part of their daily life. In planning for hospital admissions and long-term care arrangements, consideration also must be given to the person's responsibilities for and relationship with pets. Therefore, even if the person does not initiate the topic, at least one question about pets is included in the psychosocial assessment of older adults.

> **DIVERSITY NOTE**
>
> Older adults from some Asian and African cultures may not approve of keeping dogs, cats, and other domestic animals indoors because they are considered unclean carriers of fleas, ticks, rabies, and other disease-causing organisms.

People are usually very receptive to discussing concerns about their health with a nurse, because they view the nurse as someone who is knowledgeable about health problems and committed to helping people deal with those problems. For the purposes of the psychosocial assessment, however, it is important to address not only the physical aspects of health problems but also to assess the meaning of medical conditions for the person, because adjusting to and coping with medical problems and functional limitations is a common and very challenging task for many older adults. Nurses also try to identify the person's concerns about the functional consequences that are likely to be associated with illness and disability, which may be more significant to the person than the immediate medical diagnosis. For example, older adults with diabetes may be less interested in knowing how the pancreas functions than in learning to cope with the attendant visual impairment or their fear of increasing dependence on others. Therefore, rather than focusing the assessment on medically labeled problems, the nurse begins with open-ended questions about the person's self-perceptions of health and function. Rather than asking specifically about the identified problem of diabetes, the nurse might begin with a question such as, "If you had to rate your health on a scale of 0% to 100%, what rating would you give it today?" After the person responds to this question, the nurse might ask additional questions, such

as, "What would have to be changed for you to feel 100% healthy?" or "What rating would you have given yourself a year ago?" Answers to these questions assist the nurse in assessing the impact of the illness on the person's life and in establishing realistic goals for interventions.

COMMUNICATION SKILLS FOR PSYCHOSOCIAL ASSESSMENT

Analogous to the use of a stethoscope and other tools for assessing physiologic function, nurses use skillful communication techniques as an essential tool for the psychosocial assessment. Good communication techniques are particularly important during a psychosocial assessment because of the sensitivity of the topics and the importance of establishing a trusting relationship. When caring for older adults, however, nurses encounter many communication barriers that make it more difficult to discuss personal information, such as feelings and life events. Thus, to perform an effective psychosocial assessment, nurses need to identify and address the barriers that commonly affect communication with older adults (as discussed in the following sections). In addition, techniques for communicating with people who have dementia are discussed in Chapter 14.

Identifying Communication Barriers

Nonverbal communication techniques are particularly important when discussing sensitive issues, but visual impairments can interfere with the older adult's ability to perceive nonverbal messages. Similarly, hearing impairment can be a source of uneasiness for both the nurse and the older adult if they need to speak loudly about sensitive topics or emotional issues.

External and internal distractions can interfere with the ability to focus on the conversation, particularly for older adults who are cognitively impaired. These barriers can occur in any of the following circumstances:

- Too much information being requested at one time (e.g., responding to questions about social background, cognitive abilities, and emotional function during a single interview)
- Too many people trying to communicate at one time (e.g., family members, caregivers, or more than one professional)
- Environmental noise, particularly for people who use hearing aids, which usually magnify background noises
- Physical discomfort (e.g., pain, thirst, hunger, fatigue, bladder fullness, or uncomfortable temperatures).

Communication barriers can also arise from pathologic disorders and adverse medication effects. For example, neurologic conditions (e.g., aphasia from strokes) often affect language and verbal skills, and cognitive impairments can interfere with a person's ability to listen, remember, and respond to questions. Similarly, people who are actively delusional or hallucinatory or who are not fully in touch with reality for any reason may have difficulty attending to the conversation. Adverse medication effects that can interfere with communication include mental changes and physical effects (e.g., dry mouth and tardive dyskinesia) as discussed in Chapter 8.

Sometimes nurses inadvertently use communication methods that are perceived as insensitive, uncaring, offensive, or condescending, as in the following examples:

- Giving false reassurances (e.g., "Everything's going to be okay") when the person is facing overwhelming circumstances
- Offering trite responses (e.g., "Why cry over spilled milk?") when the person is seriously depressed
- Changing the subject to avoid sensitive issues
- Jumping to conclusions
- Giving unwanted advice
- Minimizing the person's feelings
- Addressing older adults by any title other than their preferred name (e.g., using generic titles such as "dear," "honey," or "grandma")

These communication methods may interfere with the ability to develop the sense of trust that is necessary for discussing psychosocial issues.

Other verbal barriers include rapid or inarticulate speech and obstructive mannerisms, such as covering one's mouth or turning one's head away while talking. In institutional settings, much verbal communication takes place while nurses are walking down the hall, pushing a wheelchair, assisting with personal care, or performing other activities. During these activities, nurses can listen and engage in social conversation, but these are not the best times for asking personal questions or giving important information. Not only are the activities a distraction, but also they interfere with the face-to-face positioning that may be essential for effective communication (e.g., with people who are hearing impaired).

Cultural differences can create communication barriers that are difficult, and sometimes impossible, to overcome. For example, it is difficult to establish a trusting relationship when either the older adult or the nurse holds stereotypes or prejudices about the other person. Foreign-born people who have a condition that drains their energy or affects their cognitive function may revert to their native language, even if they previously spoke English well. In these situations, family members may be able to facilitate communication, or it may be appropriate to use interpreters, as discussed in Chapter 2. However, the nurse should consider the impact of the older adult's relationship with the interpreter on his or her willingness to discuss psychosocial issues openly.

Enhancing Communication With Older Adults

Because the initial tone of conversations influences further communication, nurses can use a simple introduction, which can establish rapport if it is done effectively. A verbal introduction is particularly important for patients who have difficulty reading name tags or remembering names and for those who need assistance, because it is easier to ask for help when they can address someone by name. Although checking a wristband or other identifier is an efficient and reliable way of confirming a patient's identity, it is not a substitute for exchanging names because people sometimes feel at a disadvantage if someone else knows their name when they do not know the other person's name. Rather, a more personal approach is to introduce yourself, explain your role, and then ask the person his or her preferred name, and use the wristband to confirm information. The following example illustrates this kind of introduction: "Good morning, my name is Carol Miller, and I'm the charge nurse today. Are you Senor Juan Garcia? You can call me Carol. What do you like to be called? I have your morning pills for you to take. Do you mind if I check your wristband first?" This approach is more likely to foster a trusting relationship than a scenario in which the nurse walks into a room, silently checks the wristband to confirm that the person is Juan Garcia, and says, "Here are your morning pills."

Touch is widely recognized as an important communication tool and is an intervention for many nursing diagnoses that are applicable to older adults including Hopelessness, Relocation Stress Syndrome, and Sensory/Perceptual Alterations: Kinesthetic. Although older adults are generally quite receptive to touch, particularly by a nurse whose responsibilities naturally entail much physical contact, cultural and gender factors can influence perceptions of touch. Thus, before touching a patient, nurses need to identify personal boundaries and assess the person's receptivity to being touched. Nurses can do this by asking questions such as, "Would it be helpful if I held your hand for a moment?"

Hand massage and other modes of touch can be effective tools for promoting comfort and facilitating communication. Nursing studies identify intentional touch as an important holistic nursing intervention that transforms the relationship between nurses and patients (Connor & Howett, 2009). In home and community settings, nurses can purposefully use a handshake to facilitate communication, particularly during an initial interaction with older adults. Although not all people are receptive to this form of nonverbal communication, no harm is done as long as a response has not been forced. In addition, a handshake or similar form of touch can provide assessment information about skin temperature, the presence or absence of tremors, and other characteristics of one upper extremity. It also can provide clues about the person's social skills and awareness of others.

Attentive listening is an important communication skill, and it can be particularly effective as a psychosocial assessment tool and to communicate respect and caring. Usually, the best communication occurs when the nurse is verbally quiet and nonverbally responsive. Asking open-ended questions and nonverbally responding to indicate interest in what the person is saying is usually effective in obtaining important information. Nonverbal responses, such as sustained eye contact, and short verbal responses such as, "And then what happened?" will encourage the person to elaborate on the information considered most important.

A Student's Perspective

The life review interview with Mrs. R. enlightened me for one very simple reason: she loves the life she lived. She has no regrets about her life and said she would change nothing. She is a very positive person, and hearing her outlook at life really got me thinking about the way I want to continue to live my life. It was inspiring to hear her views, and it takes away some of my fears of growing older.

The most significant point in the life review interview is actually the same as the most difficult part. We were discussing family, and I wasn't sure if I should ask about her late husband because I didn't know how to bring him up. I finally found a way to ask about him and immediately her eyes filled with tears. She began to describe him and the things they used to do together. It was sad; yet hearing about how much she loved him was touching. She continued to cry as she said he was the best person she ever knew. Without even thinking, I grabbed her hand. As she squeezed my hand, I saw her become more at ease. With just that little action, I feel like I made her feel better. I had no idea that holding someone's hand could have such a powerful effect.

Molly D.

Nurses have many opportunities to identify psychosocial issues by listening for pertinent concerns and asking appropriate questions to obtain further information. For example, consider the case of Mrs. P. who, during an admission interview, gave the following response to a question about where she lives:

I moved to Sunnybrook Retirement Village after my last stroke. I couldn't stay in my own home, because the bedrooms were on the second floor. The doctor told me I had to live where I could get help, and my daughter didn't want me with her. Now that I've fallen and broken my wrist, I'm not sure what the doctor will tell me. My daughter doesn't want to be bothered with me.

This response gives clues to several potential issues, which the nurse can explore with any of the following questions:
- "What do you miss most since you moved?"
- "You mentioned that your daughter didn't want you living with her. Is that something you had hoped you could do?"
- "Do you worry that the doctor will suggest that you go to a nursing home?"
- "Do you see your daughter as often as you'd like?"

Answers to these questions might uncover psychosocial concerns that need to be addressed as a part of discharge planning.

When communicating about psychosocial issues, it is important to periodically clarify the messages. One clarification technique is to repeat part of a prior answer when asking further questions. For example, saying to Mrs. P., "You mentioned that your daughter doesn't want you living with her . . ." gives feedback about what the nurse heard and leads into further questions about underlying feelings. Feedback can also be helpful when discrepancies between verbal and nonverbal

communication are observed. For example, Mrs. P. might begin to cry and clench her fists as she says, "My daughter has her own life to worry about. I can take care of myself. It doesn't bother me that I can't live with her." A statement such as, "You look awfully sad. Are you sure it doesn't bother you?" might lead to an acknowledgment of feelings such as anger, rejection, and loneliness.

When communicating with older adults, nurses might hear information that is contrary to their own values or cultural expectations, such as the following examples:
- Expressions of racial prejudice, including use of derogatory labels
- Attitudes of extreme passivity about decisions involving the patient's care
- Situations in which older adults are abused or exploited by friends, family, or others
- Attitudes about women or other groups that are judgmental or not in accordance with the nurse's beliefs.

When dealing with these kinds of experiences, it is helpful to be aware of one's own feelings and to address them accordingly. For example, during the psychosocial assessment, nurses must communicate a nonjudgmental attitude, but afterwards they can share their feelings with colleagues. In some situations, however, it is appropriate for nurses to acknowledge their feelings or opinions during the assessment. For instance, if the person describes an episode of extreme exploitation and expresses feelings of anger about the situation, the nurse can show empathy and understanding with a statement such as, "That sounds like a terrible situation to have been in." Nurses also need to consider that some of the information they obtain during a psychosocial assessment may involve legal or ethical issues and that, even though this information is beyond the original intent of the assessment, nurses may be required to take further action. For example, information about recent or ongoing abuse or exploitation may necessitate a referral for further investigation, discussed in Chapter 10.

Creating an Environment That Supports Good Communication

Face-to-face positioning facilitates verbal as well as nonverbal communication and is particularly important when visual or hearing impairments interfere with communication. Moreover, people usually feel more comfortable talking with others when they are at the same level of eye contact. Therefore, when conversing with someone in a bed or wheelchair, the nurse should sit in a chair. If possible, remove any physical barrier that interferes with direct face-to-face contact. For example, putting side rails down when talking with someone confined to bed or moving a walker that is in the line of vision can improve face-to-face communication. Before moving walkers or side rails, however, ask the older person's permission to do so; this demonstrates respect for the wishes of the individual. Nurses also need to consider safety considerations with regard to moving side rails or walkers by ensuring that these are left in the correct position before the nurse leaves.

Each person has his or her own "comfort zone" for communication, which is the physical space required for the person to feel at ease when communicating with others. This space varies according to the type of interactions and has been conceptualized as follows:

- Intimate distance is 0 to 18 inches.
- Personal distance is 1.5 to 4 feet.
- Social distance is 4 to 12 feet.

The provision of nursing care often requires that interactions take place in the intimate or personal zones even though the relationship would normally dictate that interactions take place in the social distance zone. Thus, nurses need to be aware of the influence of personal space on the comfort level of the older person and consider this during communication interactions. Because cultural factors strongly influence perception of appropriate distance zones and many other aspects of nonverbal communication (e.g., touch, eye contact), it is essential to be sensitive to cultural differences that may affect communication. Cultural Considerations 13-1 identifies some cultural influences on expressions of nonverbal communication.

During conversations with older adults, particularly when discussing psychosocial issues, nurses must provide as much privacy as possible. This may be difficult in institutional settings, particularly when patients or residents share rooms with others. Even in these situations, however, closing the door and pulling the bed curtain will increase the perception of privacy. In addition, nurses can take advantage of times when the roommate is out of the room, or it may be appropriate for the nurse to ask the roommate to allow private use of the room. Eliminating distracting noises is also essential for establishing an environment that supports good communication. In institutional settings, closing a door to bedrooms not only increases privacy but also eliminates noises from the hallway. Before closing a door or bed curtains, however, the nurse should ask permission from the older person. Asking permission shows respect for the person's territory and may be particularly important when talking with people who become anxious when they are in closed spaces. Likewise, if a radio or television is on, the nurse can ask permission to turn it off.

All the environmental modifications related to improving hearing and vision (discussed in Chapters 16 and 17, respectively) may be appropriate interventions for enhancing communication during a psychosocial assessment. One particularly easy and important consideration is the avoidance of background glare. In hospital or long-term care settings, people often stand in front of a window when talking to a patient/resident in a bed near the window. When the sun is shining or lights are reflected in the window, the background glare may interfere with the older person's ability to see the person in front of the window. In these situations, simply closing the window curtains or sitting on the other side of the bed may significantly improve communication. In home settings, lack of lighting is a more common problem than glare. Asking the person's permission to turn on lights can be a very effective and easy way of improving communication. After finishing the conversation, the nurse must remember to ask whether the person wants the environment returned to the way it was before. Turning on radios and televisions, replacing walkers and side rails, and leaving bed curtains and doors the way they were found shows respect

CULTURAL CONSIDERATIONS 13 - 1

Cultural Influences on Communication

Greetings

- Cultural groups that prefer to be greeted formally (e.g., Mr., Mrs., Ms.) include African Americans, Bosnians, Chinese, Filipino, Greeks, Haitians, Italians, Japanese, Koreans, Puerto Ricans, Russians, Turks.

Perception of Personal Space

- Cultural groups that are likely to have a closer range for personal distance include Arabs, Hispanics, Greeks, Japanese, Iranians, East Indian, Latin Americans, and Middle Easterners.
- British, Canadians, Irish, and European North Americans are likely to require the most personal space.
- Men usually like to have larger personal space than women.

Touch

- Cultural groups that are likely to be most comfortable with physical touch are Jews, French, Spanish, Italians, Indonesian, and Latin Americans.
- Cultural groups that are likely to be uncomfortable with touch are British, Chinese, Germans, Hindus, and North Americans.
- Asians may believe that it is disrespectful to touch the head, because it is thought to be a source of the person's strength.
- Vietnamese view the human head as the seat of life and highly personal; they may feel anxious if touched on their head or shoulders; if any orifice of the head is invaded, they may fear these procedures could provide an escape for the essence of life.
- Mexican Americans and Native Americans may view touch as a means for healing, preventing harm, or removing an evil spell.

Touch Between Men and Women

- Cultural groups that do not allow physical touch between men and women outside the home include Bosnians, Mexicans, Middle Easterners, Somalis.
- In many Hispanic and Middle Eastern cultures, male healthcare providers may be prohibited from touching or examining part or all of the female body.
- In some Asian cultures, touching between persons of the same sex (but not between those of the opposite sex) is common and acceptable.

Hand Shaking

- It is appropriate to greet Amish clients with a smile and a handshake.
- Middle Eastern women may not shake hands with men.
- Asian women may not shake hands with each other or with men.
- Native Americans may interpret vigorous handshaking as an aggressive action and are offended by a firm, lengthy handshake.

Eye Contact

- People from some Asian, Hispanic, Hindi, Hmong, Indochinese, Appalachian, Middle Eastern, and African American cultures may consider direct eye contact impolite, immodest, or aggressive, and they may avert their eyes when talking with healthcare professionals or, if female, when talking with men.
- Native Americans may direct their eye contact to the floor during conversations as an indication that they are paying close attention to the speaker.
- Hispanic cultures dictate appropriate deferential behavior in the form of downcast eyes toward others on the basis of age, sex, social position, economic status, and position of authority (e.g., elders expect respect from younger people).
- Cultural groups that are likely to maintain steady eye contact during conversations include Arabs, European Americans, Greeks, and Turks.
- Some cultural groups (e.g., Bosnians) maintain eye contact between women but not between men and women.

Facial Expression

- Italians, Jews, Hispanics, and African Americans smile readily and use many facial expressions along with words and gestures to communicate pain, happiness, or displeasure.
- Irish, English, and northern Europeans generally do not use facial expressions or other nonverbal expressions.

Source: Andrews, M. M., & Boyle, J. S. (2008). *Transcultural concepts in nursing care* (5th ed.). Philadelphia: Lippincott Williams & Wilkins; Purnell, L. D. (2009). *Guide to Culturally Competent Health Care* (2nd ed.). Philadelphia: F. A. Davis.

---

for the person's preferences. Box 13-2 summarizes verbal and nonverbal strategies to enhance communication with older adults and includes some strategies that are specific to communication during a psychosocial assessment.

 MENTAL STATUS ASSESSMENT

A mental status assessment is an organized approach to collecting data about a person's psychosocial function. The mental status assessment is very broad in scope, so this section focuses on cognitive abilities, and other aspects of psychosocial function (i.e., affective function, contact with reality, and social supports) are discussed in the following sections. Indicators of psychosocial function that are addressed in this section on a mental status assessment are physical appearance, psychomotor behavior, social skills, **orientation**, alertness, memory, and speech characteristics. Mental status assessments are performed by various healthcare professionals, with each discipline specializing in various components. For example, psychiatrists are skilled in assessing affective and cognitive components, whereas social workers are skilled in assessing family relationship components. In the framework of this text, nurses assess the aspects of psychosocial function that most directly influence the day-to-day activities of older adults.

The Mini-Mental State Examination (MMSE) has been widely used since the 1970s as a screening tool for cognitive impairment, but it takes at least 10 minutes to administer, and the formal tool must be purchased for use in clinical settings. Another concern about the MMSE is that it does not detect early stages of cognitive impairment, and scores are significantly influenced by factors such as education and social class (Pinto & Peters, 2009). In recent years, healthcare professionals have recognized the need for an evidence-based screening tool that is widely available and easy to administer. Thus, the

Box 13-2 Strategies to Enhance Communication With Older Adults

General Strategies

- Arrange for face-to-face positioning whenever possible.
- Ensure as much privacy as possible.
- Provide good lighting, and avoid background glare.
- Eliminate as much background noise as possible.
- Compensate as much as possible for vision or hearing impairments (e.g., make sure the person is using eyeglasses and hearing aid if appropriate).
- Begin contact with an exchange of names and, if appropriate, a handshake.
- Use culturally appropriate titles of respect, such as Señor, Señora, Señorita, Mr., Mrs., Ms., Dr., Reverend, Elder, Bishop, and so forth.
- Before calling a person by his or her first name, obtain permission or wait until you have been invited to use this familiar form of address. In some cultures, it is considered inappropriate or disrespectful for anyone but family or close friends to use first names.
- Be sure to pronounce names correctly. When in doubt, ask the older adult to say his or her name. Names that are difficult to pronounce may be written phonetically on the chart for later reference.
- Be aware of subtle linguistic messages that may convey bias or inequality (e.g., using Mr. and the surname to call a white man but addressing an African American woman by her first name).
- Avoid slang expressions, such as "Pop," "Grandma," "dear," "chief," or similar terms, unless the older adult suggests that you do so.
- Never use slang, pejorative, or derogatory terms to refer to ethnic, racial, religious, or any other group (e.g., gays or lesbians).
- Use touch purposefully—provided that the person is open to this—to reinforce verbal messages and as a primary method of nonverbal communication.
- In all interactions, be aware of cultural differences that influence the perception and interpretation of verbal and nonverbal communication.

Strategies Specific to a Psychosocial Assessment

- Explain the purpose of the psychosocial assessment in relation to a nursing goal; then, begin with questions about remote, nonthreatening topics.
- Use open-ended questions and learn to use silence effectively and comfortably.
- Periodically clarify the messages.
- Maintain good eye contact, use attentive listening, and encourage the person to elaborate on information.
- Remain nonjudgmental in your responses, but show appropriate empathy.
- Ask formal mental status questions, or the most threatening questions, toward the end of the interview.
- Gain the person's permission before asking formal assessment questions regarding memory and other cognitive abilities.

Mini-Cog, which consists of a three-item recall test and a simple clock-drawing test, is now widely used as a reliable and valid screening tool for cognitive impairment (Doerflinger, 2007). The Resources section at the end of this chapter includes materials that can be used to demonstrate the use of screening tools for assessing cognition and executive function/dysfunction. In addition, Chapters 12, 14, and 15 address the nursing assessment of other aspects of mental status. See also Web Re-

sources provided on thePoint, for more information. Screening tools are useful for identifying indicators of altered mental status, but they do not provide a broad or in-depth perspective on psychosocial function, as is presented in this chapter.

Physical Appearance

Physical appearance is readily observed and reveals many aspects of psychosocial function. Clothing, grooming, cosmetics, and hygiene provide many clues to psychological function, but they are only clues, and questions must be asked before any conclusions are drawn. For example, the presence of body odor, poor hygiene, and tattered clothing may be associated with any of the following conditions: depression, incontinence, impaired cognitive abilities, limited financial resources, overwhelming caregiving responsibilities, impaired vision or sense of smell, or lack of access to or inability to use bathing facilities.

Observations about how clothing fits provide clues to weight changes (e.g., if clothing is too tight or loose, particularly in the waist). A history of weight loss may provide clues to depression, cognitive impairment, medical status, or other barriers to adequate nutrition.

Observations about grooming practices, such as a woman's hair being dyed, can suggest any of the following questions about psychosocial function: Is this a reflection of positive or negative self-esteem? Does she want to appear younger than her age because she believes that old age is not as socially acceptable as youth? Does she want to deny her age because she associates old age with negative images? Similarly, an older woman's preference for wearing high-heeled shoes may be an indicator of self-image and of a desire to appear youthful. This is an important assessment issue because of the potential risk for falls and fractures.

Motor Function and Psychomotor Behaviors

Assessment of motor function, which includes posture, movement, and body language, can provide clues to broader aspects of psychosocial function. For example, stooped posture may be a clue to depression, whereas erect posture may indicate positive self-esteem. A shuffling, staggering, or uncoordinated gait could indicate neurologic deficits secondary to a disease process or adverse effects from alcohol or medications. Gait disturbances, as well as other abnormal movements, are possible signs of tardive dyskinesia or extrapyramidal symptoms. Evidence of tardive dyskinesia raises the question of past or present use of psychotropic medications (discussed in Chapter 8) and may give clues to psychiatric history.

Body language also provides clues to affective illnesses. Slouching and head hanging are common manifestations of withdrawal and depression. Poor eye contact, particularly looking at the floor, may be indicative of depression or the inability to answer questions, but nurses assess this in relation to cultural factors that influence the type and amount of eye contact considered to be appropriate. Depression is usually associated with slowed psychomotor function, but excessive activity can be a clue to agitated depression. Agitation can be symptomatic of cognitive, affective, or other psychiatric disturbances; it may also be an adverse medication effect or an indicator of a physiologic disturbance (e.g., dehydration, electrolyte imbalance) or a pathologic condition (e.g., pneumonia, urinary tract infection), particularly in older adults with dementia.

Similarly, psychomotor behaviors are part of the mental status assessment, because the ability to purposefully carry out simple motor skills is highly influenced by cognitive status. For example, observations of how someone navigates and avoids obstacles in the environment provide clues to the person's judgment and awareness of the environment. Nurses can assess psychomotor behaviors by asking the person to perform a simple activity of daily living (e.g., combing hair) and observing the person's ability to comprehend and perform the request.

Social Skills

Assessment of social skills provides information about many aspects of psychosocial function. For example, friendly and cooperative people with good conversational skills may use social skills to hide their cognitive deficits, particularly if they are motivated to do so. By contrast, people with long-standing patterns of hostility, social isolation, poor social skills, and a lack of ambition may be less motivated to perform well. In addition, people sometimes use the following social skills to cover up cognitive deficits: humor, evasiveness, leading the conversation, and making up answers to questions. Some older adults with dementia maintain very good social skills, even in the later stages of dementia when other skills have long since declined. Nurses also need to be aware of cultural factors that influence social skills and consider the cultural context of the relationship between the interviewer and the interviewee.

Response to the Interview

The older adult's initial response to the interview, as well as changes that occur during the interview, can provide important assessment information. For example, an older adult may initially be very receptive to the questions but may become defensive or sarcastic when he or she is uncomfortable with the line of questioning. In addition, nurses assess the amount of time and effort expended in answering questions. This is particularly important when trying to differentiate between dementia and depression because cognitively impaired people may exert great effort in responding to questions, but depressed people may lack energy or motivation to answer correctly. Thus, two people may score the same on a formal mental status questionnaire, but one may miss the questions because of dementia and the other may miss them because of depression. When nurses suspect that lack of motivation is a reason for incorrect or missing answers, they might clarify this by asking, "Is it that you don't know the answers or that you just don't feel like answering the questions?"

Nurses are likely to encounter attitudes of hostility, resistance, and defensiveness during the interview for a variety of reasons. A person who is depressed may be apathetic and may not want to expend the energy to answer the questions. A cognitively impaired person may be angry, hostile, or defensive, particularly if he or she is trying to hide or deny cognitive deficits. A person who has always been reclusive or suspicious may be unwilling to answer questions or may feel very defensive. Assessing the person's underlying attitude is as important as assessing the accuracy of responses to questions.

Assessing for **confabulation**, which is the process of making up information, is difficult when the nurse does not know the correct information. For example, questions about the person's place of birth or childhood experiences are not effective for assessing cognitive function unless the accuracy of the answers can be confirmed. **Circumstantiality**—another cover-up technique—involves the use of excessive details and roundabout answers in responding to questions.

Finally, nurses assess all information in relation to the person's usual personality traits. For example, highly sociable people might always use humor, whereas talkative people might naturally use circumstantiality. The use of humor and circumstantiality by people who are normally quiet and serious might indicate a great effort to cover up cognitive deficits. On the other hand, people who are normally quiet and withdrawn may be perceived falsely as being depressed. Finding out about the usual personality of an individual is difficult; however, nurses can ask a question such as, "Would you describe what you were like when you were 40 years old?" Family members and caregivers who have known the person for a long time are good sources of information about lifelong personality characteristics. Box 13-3 summarizes guidelines for assessing physical appearance, motor function, social skills, and responses to the interview in relation to the person's psychosocial function.

Orientation

Orientation to person, place, and time is the indicator of mental status that is most frequently assessed and documented. Often, however, orientation is viewed as the primary indicator of cognitive function, rather than as one small piece of a larger picture. For example, the following questions are the gold standard for assessing orientation: "What is your name?" "Where are you?" and "What time is it?" Based on the accuracy of each answer, the person is then labeled as "oriented times one," "oriented times two," or "oriented times three." The superficial use of orientation questions and the subsequent labeling of the person as oriented times one, two, or three, ignores important considerations, such as,

- Are any environmental clues available to the person to orient him to the time or place?
- Has the person been at the institution long enough to have learned its name?
- If the person cannot state the exact name of the facility, can she describe the type of facility it is or its general location?
- Do sociocultural factors influence the person's response to these questions?

Box 13-3   Guidelines for Assessing Physical Appearance, Motor Function, Social Skills, and Response to the Interview

Observations Regarding Physical Appearance and Motor Function

- What is the person's apparent age in relation to his or her chronologic age?
- How do the following factors reflect psychological function: hygiene, grooming, clothing, cosmetics?
- Does the person's physical appearance provide clues to dementia or depression or to other impairments of psychosocial function?
- What do the person's gait, posture, and body language indicate about his or her psychological function?
- Is there any evidence of tardive dyskinesia or other adverse medication effects?
- How does the person maneuver in the environment, and what does this reflect regarding judgment, vision, and other skills?

Observations Regarding Social Skills and Response to the Interview

- What are the person's lifelong patterns of social skills, and how do these influence the assessment process?
- How do the person's social skills influence the interviewer's interpretation of other aspects of psychosocial function?
- Is the person motivated to answer questions?
- What is the person's attitude about the interview?
- If the person does not answer the questions, or gives incorrect answers, is it because of inability, cultural factors, or lack of motivation?
- Does the person use any of the following in an attempt to hide possible cognitive deficits: humor, sarcasm, avoidance, evasiveness, confabulation, circumstantiality, or leading the conversation?
- Does the person manifest any of the following characteristics: anger, hostility, resistance, defensiveness, or suspiciousness?
- Do the person's underlying attitudes reflect his or her usual personality, or are they manifestations of cognitive or affective disturbances?

- Can the person name familiar people, such as a spouse or children, even if he cannot state his own name?
- If the person cannot give specific names of other people, can he describe the correct role of the other person?
- If the person cannot state the exact time, can she give the general time of day?
- Does the person have medical problems that interfere with cognition?
- Is the person taking medications that can influence mental function?

A good assessment extends beyond the three classic questions and describes levels of orientation that are meaningful for the person in a particular setting. For example, the following description is far more useful than simply noting that the person is "oriented times one":

> *Mrs. S. could state her name but did not remember the name of this hospital. She could not give her daughter's name but was able to introduce her daughter to me without stating her*

name. She thought that the month was December because of the Chanukah decorations in her room. She could not state the time because she did not have her watch with her, but she thought that it was afternoon because lunch had recently been served.

If the nurse had used only the standard questions of "What is your name?" "Where are you?" and "What time is it?" Mrs. S. would be judged to be "oriented times one." Most healthcare providers, after reading the results of that assessment, would have assumed that Mrs. S. had serious cognitive impairment, particularly if she were 85 years of age or older. Mrs. S.'s actual responses, however, reflected various cognitive skills involved in organizing information, making associations, and using judgment. The more detailed description shows that Mrs. S. is probably quite a logical person who has not yet learned the name of the hospital and who might have some temporary memory impairment because of anxiety, medications, or acute medical problems.

Alertness and Attention

Besides orientation, level of alertness is the mental status indicator that healthcare providers most frequently assess and document. Level of alertness is measured along a continuum, which includes stupor, drowsiness, somnolence, intermittent alertness/drowsiness, and hyperalertness. An important aspect of assessing the person's level of alertness is the identification of any factors that can either increase or decrease alertness, with particular attention to those factors that can be addressed. For example, excessive daytime drowsiness can be associated with any of the following factors: medical problems, electrolyte imbalances, adverse medication effects (e.g., narcotics, anticholinergics, psychoactive medications), depression, dementia, excessive alcohol intake, or lack of sleep at night because of a variety of reasons (e.g., caregiver responsibilities).

In addition to assessing level of alertness, nurses also assess attention, which includes the ability to focus on a task and filter out distractions. Nurses can assess this mental status indicator by noting the older adult's ability to follow directions or respond appropriately to questions. When assessing responses, however, nurses need to also consider that information-processing skills may be affected not only by attention but also by other conditions such as cognitive or sensory impairments.

Memory

Formal **memory** testing assesses the person's memory of remote events, recent past events, and immediate memory, which is further divided into retention, recall, and recognition. Nurses can assess memory during regular conversations because all verbal communication depends to some degree on memory function. Nurses pay particular attention to assessing memory in relation to activities that are important in daily life, such as remembering to pay bills, take medications, and shop for groceries. This assessment is made in relation to the expectations and demands of the person's usual environment. For example, if the person lives alone and manages finances independently, the ability to pay bills is quite important. By contrast, if the person lives with a daughter and her family, remembering the birth dates of grandchildren may be an important memory task.

Assessment of memory is particularly challenging because memory complaints are common among older adults, but they are not necessarily based on actual deficits in memory function. For example, people who are depressed may perceive their memory skills as disproportionately impaired and may even exaggerate their deficits. In contrast to this situation, older adults with dementia may have little or no awareness of their memory deficits, or they may deny memory problems as a self-protective response. Thus, the question, "Do you ever have trouble remembering things?" may elicit a positive response, but the response is likely to tell you more about the person's perception of memory than about his or her actual memory function. Although this question may be quite useful in identifying any concerns that the older adult might have, it is not very useful in assessing memory function.

In addition to assessing memory directly, the nurse assesses the person's use of memory aids by posing a question such as, "Is there anything you do to help you remember appointments or other things?" Assessment of the extent to which the person depends on memory aids is useful in setting goals and planning for improved memory function. For example, if the person's memory function is barely adequate and is based heavily on memory aids, then the potential for further improvement is minimal. By contrast, if the person has some memory deficits but does not use any memory aids, then the potential for improvement increases. Observations about the use of memory aids also may provide clues to unacknowledged memory deficits. For example, if the person denies problems with memory, but repeatedly refers to written notes during an interview, then he or she may be compensating for an impaired memory. In this situation, the person is quite willing to use memory aids but is unwilling to acknowledge the need for such aids. Box 13-4 summarizes guidelines for nursing assessment of orientation, alertness, and memory and includes examples of appropriate questions for assessing the different types of memory.

Speech and Language Characteristics

Speech and language characteristics provide important information about many aspects of psychosocial function, such as the ability to organize and communicate thoughts. In addition, a good assessment of language skills helps the nurse to identify words and language patterns that are most appropriate for use with an older person. Because speech and language skills are highly dependent on cultural, educational, and socioeconomic factors, it is important to consider these influences, particularly when assessing foreign-born older adults.

During any verbal interaction, nurses can assess all of the following speech and language characteristics: pace, tone, volume, articulation, ability to organize and communicate

Box 13-4 Guidelines for Assessing Orientation, Alertness, and Memory

Interview Questions to Assess Orientation

Note: Examples of direct questions are identified by quotation marks to distinguish them from the questions that are answered indirectly through observations.

- *Person:* "What is your name?" "What is your wife's name?" If names can't be given, can the person describe roles?
- *Place:* "What is your address?" "What is the name of this place?" "What kind of place is this?" "What is the name of this city?" "What is the name of this state?"
- *Time:* "What time is it?" "What day of the week is today?" "What month and date is it today?" "What season is it?"

Observations to Assess Alertness

- What is the person's level of alertness on the following continuum: hyperalert, alert, drowsy, somnolent, stuporous?
- Does the person's level of alertness fluctuate? If so, is there any pattern to the fluctuations?
- Are there physiologic factors that might influence the person's level of alertness, such as medical conditions or effects of chemicals or medications?
- Are there psychosocial factors that might influence the person's level of alertness, such as anxiety, depression, nighttime caregiving responsibilities, or any other factor that might disrupt nighttime sleep?

Interview Questions to Assess Memory

- *Remote events:* "Where were you born?" "Where did you go to grade school?" "What was your first job?" "When were you married?"
- *Recent past events:* "Do you live with anyone?" "Do you have any grandchildren?" "What are the names of your grandchildren?" "When was the last time you went to the doctor?"
- *Immediate memory, retention:* State three unrelated words and ask the person to repeat the information, both immediately and again after 5 minutes.
- *Immediate memory, general grasp and recall:* Ask the person to read a short story and then to summarize the information presented in the story.
- *Immediate memory, recognition:* Ask a multiple-choice question and then ask the person to choose the correct answer.

thoughts, and any abnormal speech or language characteristics. The following examples describe some common speech variations and associated conditions:

- Rapid pace: anxiety, agitation, or mental illness
- Slow-paced or excessively brief verbal communication: depression, cognitive impairment, or simple cautiousness
- Tone of voice: indirectly expressed feelings such as anger, hostility, and resentment
- Hypophonia (i.e., abnormally low speech volume): depression, physical illness, low self-esteem, or long-standing speech habits
- Abnormally loud volume: impaired hearing or long-term experience communicating with someone who is hearing impaired
- Poor articulation or slurred speech: hearing impairment, ill-fitting dentures, lack of teeth or dentures, nervous system disorder, effects of alcohol or medications

- Phonemic errors (i.e., incorrect pronunciation): hearing impairment, cognitive deficits, educational and cultural influences
- Semantic errors (i.e., misinterpretation of the meaning of words): hearing impairment, cognitive deficits
- Neologisms (i.e., self-created and meaningless words): dementia, psychotic disorder (e.g., schizophrenia), repetition of a word that was not heard accurately
- Incoherent speech: dementia, aphasia, psychiatric disorders, alcohol or medication effects
- Perseveration (i.e., a repetitive or stuttering pattern of verbal or written communication) and agnosia (i.e., difficulty finding the correct words or the inability to name an object accurately, particularly if it is unfamiliar): dementia

Aphasia is a communication disorder that is associated with neurologic conditions such as stroke or vascular dementia. Expressive aphasia occurs when comprehension abilities are not affected but word retrieval or word-finding abilities are impaired. Receptive aphasia occurs when verbal and comprehension abilities are impaired but some language skills are retained. Global aphasia, which is a combination of receptive and expressive aphasia, results from more extensive neurologic damage and is manifested by inconsistent and poorly controlled language skills.

Higher Language Skills

Reading, writing, spelling, and arithmetic are calculation and higher language skills that are assessed as indicators of cognition. As with assessments of other indicators, the person's education, occupation, and other influencing factors must be considered. Nurses can informally assess these skills in relation to how the person performs important daily activities. For example, for an older adult who lives alone, an assessment of the ability to pay utility bills and use money to purchase groceries is more valuable than a measurement of mathematical skills using a psychometric test. Likewise, a person's ability to read the daily newspaper or the markings on a thermostat may be a more valid gauge of functional ability than a score on a formal reading test.

Nurses can use written health education materials to assess reading and comprehension skills informally, and this method serves a practical purpose. For example, when collecting a urine sample, the nurse can give the person a list of instructions and ask him or her to read the instructions aloud. An observation of how well the person comprehends the instructions provides an assessment of reading skills that are important in daily life. Another opportunity for assessing reading comprehension may arise if the nurse observes that an older adult has a newspaper nearby. A nonthreatening question such as, "What's new in the paper today?" can provide information about the person's interests in outside events and his or her ability to comprehend and remember written information.

Nurses can assess writing and other higher language skills by observing older adults during interactions that pertain to their care. For example, nurses can observe the way an older

Box 13-5 Guidelines for Assessing Speech Characteristics, and Calculation and Higher Language Skills

Observations to Assess Speech Characteristics
- Is the pace of speech normal, slow, or fast?
- Is the tone of voice suggestive of underlying feelings, such as anger, hostility, or resentment?
- Is the volume abnormally soft or loud?
- Do the sentences flow coherently and smoothly?
- Is there evidence of any problem with integrating speech sounds into words (e.g., neologisms, or phonemic or semantic errors)?
- Do any of the following factors affect the person's speech: dry mouth, poorly fitting dentures, absence of teeth or dentures, alcohol or medication effects, or neurologic or other pathologic processes?
- Does the person exhibit any of the following: agnosia; perseveration; or expressive, receptive, or global aphasia?

Observations to Assess Calculation and Higher Language Skills
- What is the person's ability to comprehend written materials encountered in the course of routine activities, such as the daily newspaper or instructions for medications?
- What is the quality of the person's handwriting (e.g., his or her signature)?
- Is the person able to perform mathematical computations necessary for daily activities?

adult signs his or her name on documents such as permission forms. Nurses can also observe the older adult during the performance of more complex tasks such as compiling a written medication list or a list of questions to discuss with the primary care provider. Difficulty with writing skills is a common sign of early stages of dementia. Of all the higher language skills, spelling is the least important in terms of daily function, but it is a good indicator of changes in mental abilities.

With traditional psychometric testing, calculation is measured with the "7s" test: the person is asked to subtract 7 from 100 and to continue subtracting 7s. Because this test is highly influenced by level of education, it is not necessarily the most appropriate test for older adults. It may be better to ask the older person to add 3 plus 3 and to continue adding 3s. Older adults who are depressed may not answer correctly because they do not want to expend the energy to calculate serial sevens. Older adults who have dementia may be able to perform well on this task if they try hard and if they previously had highly developed mathematical skills. Box 13-5 summarizes the considerations that are important in assessing speech characteristics and calculation and higher language skills.

DECISION-MAKING AND EXECUTIVE FUNCTION

Decision-making—one of the most important and complex of all cognitive abilities—is an important aspect of psychosocial function because all legally competent older adults, including those with dementia, have the right to be involved in decisions about their care. Determination of competency is a complex issue with many implications not only for older adults and their families and caregivers but also for healthcare professionals (as discussed in Chapter 9). As an integral part of psychosocial nursing care, nurses assess cognitive skills—including **insight**, learning, memory, reasoning, judgment, problem-solving, and **abstract thinking**—that are involved with decision-making. Although no one assessment tool focuses specifically on decision-making, nurses assess this aspect of psychosocial function by observing the abilities of older adults to solve problems during the course of daily activities and by asking pertinent assessment questions.

Abstract thinking is difficult to assess because it is strongly influenced by other factors such as education, personality, and affective state. People who are very anxious or depressed may lack the attention or motivation required to respond to the questions typically used for the assessment of abstract thinking patterns. Similarity questions such as, "How are apples and oranges alike?" or "How are a table and chair alike?" are used to assess the person's ability to think abstractly.

During an interview, opportunities for assessing abstract thinking may arise, and the nurse listens for clues to the person's level of abstract versus concrete thinking. The following exchange is an example of an unsolicited opportunity that this author had to assess one older adult's concrete thinking pattern:

Nurse: How did you feel about having to move from your home in Texas to live with your daughter and her family here in Ohio?

Mr. L.: I don't know; how would you feel?

Nurse: I'm not sure how I'd feel; that's never happened to me. I'm not in your shoes.

Mr. L.: Well, here, put them on (stated emphatically while taking off his shoes to give to the nurse).

One interpretation of Mr. L.'s response is that his thinking pattern is very concrete, rather than abstract.

Nurses assess problem-solving abilities through observations about how older adults meet their needs in a particular situation. For instance, the nurse observes the way older adults use call lights to meet their needs when confined to a bed or the way in which they deal with complex decisions related to discharge planning. Similarly, a very important problem-solving task for an older adult who lives alone may be meeting basic safety needs. Therefore, questions such as, "What would you do if you fell at home and could not get up?" or "What would you do if you woke up and smelled smoke?" might be an appropriate way of assessing judgment related to safety. For an older adult who lives in a nursing home, a very important but complex problem-solving task may involve dealing with a disruptive roommate. In this situation, the answer to a question such as, "What would you do if your roommate started taking your belongings?" might provide the most pertinent information for assessing problem-solving skills.

Insight is the ability to understand the significance of the present situation. This skill is an important component of the problem-solving process, because it establishes a basis for planning care. Insight is influenced by psychosocial factors such as feelings, personality, and coping mechanisms. Denial is a defense mechanism that is often used to protect oneself from unpleasant realities; the stronger the denial is, the more limited the insight is. It is important to assess for denial because, if the person refuses to acknowledge that he or she has a condition, it will be very difficult to plan interventions. Nursing assessment of insight concentrates on those areas of function that are pertinent to the care plan. For example, in assessing the insight of an older adult who has been brought to the hospital with malnutrition and uncontrolled hypertension, the nurse may ask questions such as the following:

- Why did your daughter bring you to the hospital?
- How do you manage with grocery shopping and getting your meals?
- Do you take any medications?
- What are the medications for?
- What kinds of things does your daughter do for you?
- What kind of help do you think you might need when you leave the hospital?

Answers to questions such as these facilitate care planning because they help the nurse assess the person's understanding of the present situation.

When the person has little or no understanding of his or her health situation, the nurse tries to identify the factors that interfere with insight. In the example just described, insight may be absent or limited because of depression and feelings of hopelessness, lack of information about the medication regimen, denial of a reality that is too threatening, inability to remember information, or fear of losing independence. An essential component of discharge planning is identifying both the level of insight and the factors that interfere with insight. In addition, the nurse attempts to identify factors that may improve the person's insight. If insight is lacking because of denial that stems from exaggerated fears, then alleviating the fears may facilitate insight.

In recent years, healthcare professionals have recognized the importance of assessing executive function abilities in conjunction with determining a patient's capacity to safely and reliably plan and carry out activities related to daily living. Essential elements of executive function are abstract thinking and planning, initiating, sequencing, monitoring, and stopping complex behavior (Kennedy & Smyth, 2008). Cognitive abilities that are associated with executive function include insight, judgment, reasoning, attention, concept formation, cognitive flexibility, problem-solving, abstraction, and self-evaluation.

Executive dysfunction (also called executive function deficits) begins during the earliest stages of dementia and can be present even before memory problems are evident, particularly when the pathologic processes affect the frontal lobes. Indicators of executive function deficits include diminished mental flexibility, limited ability to think abstractly, difficulty with problem-solving, decline in ability to conceptualize, diminished ability to adapt to new situations, and difficulty shifting thought processes from one idea to another. People with executive cognitive dysfunction may perform well on the MMSE but still not be able to perform essential daily activities safely and independently. Kennedy and Smyth (2008) have described and demonstrated the use of easy-to-use and evidence-based screening tools for executive dysfunction in article and video form (see "Resources" for information on accessing these online tools).

Because it is important to assess executive skills in relation to a previous level of function, it may be necessary to ask family members or the person being assessed if they have noticed changes in these abilities in recent years. When families or healthcare providers have serious questions about the decision-making abilities of an older person, or when a major decision must be made and there is disagreement about it, a more comprehensive assessment using neuropsychological tests may be warranted. For example, if a cognitively impaired older person expresses a strong desire to live alone but family members question the person's ability to function safely, a comprehensive geriatric assessment with emphasis on decision-making and executive function skills will provide useful information.

AFFECTIVE FUNCTION

A person's **affect** refers to his or her mood, emotions, and expressions of emotions. Happiness and sadness are feelings commonly associated with affective states, but all of the following have been identified as *primary affects* (also called *discrete emotions*): joy, awe, hope, fear, pain, rage, pride, guilt, shame, anger, regret, relief, hatred, surprise, interest, boredom, elation, confusion, jealousy, depression, suspicion, frustration, anxiety, bewilderment, amorousness, and lack of feelings.

The components of affective state that are reviewed in this section are general mood, anxiety, self-esteem, depression, and happiness. These five aspects were selected for the following reasons:

- An assessment of general mood assists the nurse in determining appropriate goals based on the person's usual affective state.
- Anxiety is a common factor in older adults that can often be alleviated or minimized through nursing interventions.
- Self-esteem is a major determinant of feelings, particularly depression and happiness.
- Self-esteem is particularly important because older adults face many conditions that threaten their self-esteem.
- Depression and happiness are two primary affects that have been the target of much of the research regarding affective states in older people.

Nursing interventions are directed toward all of these affective components to improve the quality of life of older adults.

Guidelines for Assessing Affective Function

Affective function is assessed both quantitatively and qualitatively in relation to expectations about acceptable expressions of emotions. For example, people are expected to show some expression of sadness when talking about sad events. When the person's expression of feelings is not consistent with the external event, however, the affect is considered inappropriate. Affect is also assessed in relation to the personal meaning and the nearness in time of an event. People are expected to show greater feelings of sadness in response to tragic news than in response to neutral events. Likewise, people are expected to show a deeper affective response soon after experiencing a sad event than they would years after the event occurred.

The depth and duration of affect, which are important considerations in differentiating between dementia and depression in older adults, are also assessed. The affect of depressed people is generally sad and negativistic and is not influenced by external circumstances. By contrast, the affect of people who have dementia fluctuates more and changes in response to distractions. Emotional lability (i.e., emotional instability or fluctuation) is a characteristic of vascular dementia that is common in people who have had strokes.

Nonverbal behaviors, such as those indicating anxiety, sadness, and happiness, provide important information about a person's affective state that the person may not offer verbally. For example, despite a person's denial of feeling sad, he or she may exhibit the following nonverbal cues: crying, slouching over, looking at the ground, and having a mournful facial expression. The nurse uses this information as the basis for a leading comment such as, "You look like you're feeling sad."

Expressions of emotions are strongly determined by cultural norms and personality characteristics. In most Western societies, crying is more acceptable for women and children than for men and older boys, and showing anger and rage is more acceptable for men than for women. Cultural expectations also influence the way a person expresses feelings in certain circumstances. For example, a person may be expected to cry and loudly proclaim mournful feelings at a funeral but may be prohibited from expressing any feelings in front of strangers or in a public place such as a hospital. Because some emotions, such as anger or depression, are viewed as less acceptable than others, such as happiness, people learn to deny and hide feelings that may be judged as unacceptable. Older adults, particularly, may have learned that certain feelings should not be expressed directly or verbally. Thus, it is particularly important to observe for any indirect or nonverbal clues of anger, depression, and other less socially acceptable feelings.

In assessing the affective state of older adults, it is important to identify the terminology that is most acceptable. Many people will not admit to feeling anxious or depressed because they associate these terms with a serious mental illness or with a socially unacceptable state. Therefore, the nurse begins the assessment of affective state by focusing on feelings that are viewed positively or neutrally. If the person initiates the topic of feeling anxious or depressed, the nurse responds to those feelings and pursues a related line of questioning. In most circumstances, however, it is best to begin with open-ended questions. A simple question such as, "How are you feeling today?" when asked with sincerity, is a familiar and comfortable way of eliciting information.

Mood

Mood is closely associated with emotions but differs from them in that it is more pervasive, less intense, and longer lasting. People are usually quite comfortable describing their mood as either bad or good and are more likely to offer information about their mood than their emotions. Thus, during a mental status examination, a question such as, "How would you describe your usual mood?" may be perceived as less threatening than the question, "How do you feel most of the time?" Nonverbal behaviors provide many clues about a person's mood and may be more accurate than verbal responses as an indicator of affective state. Joy, anger, anxiety, sadness, happiness, and depression are examples of moods that are expressed in nonverbal behaviors in everyday life by most people.

Anxiety

Anxiety is defined as a feeling of distress, subjectively experienced as fear or worry and objectively expressed through autonomic and central nervous system responses. Moderate anxiety is beneficial because it motivates protective behaviors, but extreme anxiety is detrimental because it channels personal energy into defensive behaviors. Therefore, it is important to assess the degree of anxiety and the extent to which the anxiety is beneficial or detrimental. In recent years, increasing attention has been given to **generalized anxiety disorder (GAD)**, which has a significant negative impact on health, functioning, and quality of life for many older adults. GAD is characterized by persistent, excessive, and uncontrollable worry accompanied by physiologic symptoms including fatigue, irritability, restlessness, sleep disturbances, difficulty concentrating, and pervasive cognitive dysfunction (Allgulander, 2009). Despite the strong correlation between physical symptoms and emotional distress, older adults may not recognize the connection, and GAD is often unrecognized by healthcare providers (Calleo et al., 2009).

In assessing anxiety, nurses must identify the terminology that is most acceptable to the older adult. Words like "worries" and "concerns" are readily understood and usually elicit responses about sources of anxiety. Older adults also often use the phrases "nerve trouble" or "trouble with my nerves" in reference to anxiety states. Asking questions such as, "Do you ever have nerve trouble?" or "What kinds of things give you trouble with your nerves?" may elicit a response filled with information about sources of anxiety.

Nurses observe for nonverbal manifestations of anxiety to supplement the information obtained from verbal communication. In any adult, anxiety may be manifested in the following nonverbal ways: pacing, shakiness, restlessness, irritability, fidgeting, diaphoresis, tachycardia, hyperventilation, dry mouth, voice changes, smoking habits, urinary frequency, increased muscle tension, poor eye contact, poor attention span, inability to sit still, changes in eating patterns, rapid or disconnected speech, or repetitive motions of facial muscles or any extremities. Although any of these indicators may be observed in older adults, the presence of mobility limitations or pathologic conditions can interfere with some of them. For example, older adults who are confined to bed cannot pace but may experience subtle changes in eating or sleeping patterns because of anxiety. Older adults may be reluctant to report that they are worried or anxious; instead, they may focus on physiologic symptoms (e.g., pain, fatigue, anorexia, insomnia, or stomach distress).

Because anxiety is always a response to real or perceived threats, the nurse tries to identify sources of anxiety, even though they may not be readily apparent. Potential sources of anxiety (i.e., real or perceived threats) include health, assets, values, environment, self-concept, role function, needs fulfillment, goal achievement, personal relationships, and sense of security. People do not always recognize the source of their anxiety because it may arise from unconscious conflicts, unacknowledged fears, maturational crises, or developmental challenges. Even when people recognize the source of anxiety, they may be reluctant to discuss it, or they may refer to the threat only indirectly. For example, an older adult may have the perception that other people have the power to "put him away" in a nursing home simply because of a slight memory impairment. If the person knows other older adults who have been admitted unwillingly to a nursing home, this fear may be exacerbated. Further anxiety may arise from the person's fear of discussing the subject because of the perception that initiating the topic might precipitate actions leading to nursing home admission. Rather than directly talking about the fears, the person may provide vague clues, for instance: "I felt so sorry for Mildred when her son put her in the nursing home."

Nurses must phrase questions aimed at identifying sources of anxiety in the least threatening way possible. When older adults express concerns about other older people, it may be appropriate to ask questions aimed at determining whether they have the same worries about themselves. For example, in response to the statement, "I felt so sorry for Mildred," the nurse might ask, "Do you ever worry that you'll have to go to a nursing home?" Nurses use open-ended questions that allow for a wide range of answers to identify sources of anxiety that might not otherwise be revealed. For example, nurses in institutional settings can ask, "What is your biggest worry about going home?" or "Do you have any worries about how you'll manage at home after you leave here?" In home settings, the nurse might ask an even broader question such as, "Do you have any concerns about the future?" or "What kinds of things do you worry about?" Answers to these questions are usually filled with clues to sources of anxiety and lead to many additional questions.

Anxiety can be caused or exacerbated by physiologic conditions arising from disease processes or the adverse effects of bioactive substances, as in the following examples:

- Herbs, caffeine, nicotine, and medications (both prescription and over-the-counter) can cause physiologic anxiety reactions.

- Anxiety may be associated with withdrawal from nicotine or alcohol.
- Pathologic processes that diminish cerebral oxygen, such as pulmonary or cardiovascular diseases, can cause anxiety reactions.
- Endocrine disorders, such as hyperthyroidism, may be manifested primarily by anxiety or other psychosocial symptoms.
- People with dementia may show signs of excessive anxiety when they are experiencing pain or physical discomfort, particularly if their verbal communication skills are impaired.
- Pacing is a commonly observed manifestation of anxiety in ambulatory older adults who have dementia.

Therefore, information about medical conditions and the person's use of herbs, caffeine, and medications is an essential component of the anxiety assessment.

Medications that affect the central or autonomic nervous systems may precipitate or exacerbate anxiety. *Akathisia* is a frequently reported extrapyramidal effect of some neuroleptics that may subjectively or objectively be interpreted as anxiety. Akathisia is defined as an inner sense of restlessness that is worsened by inactivity and is manifested by motor restlessness. It is more common in women and older adults, and it can occur any time during the course of treatment with psychotropic medications. Therefore, if an older adult who is taking neuroleptics complains of certain feelings, such as "shaking on the inside," the possibility of adverse medication effects must be considered as a cause.

In addition to identifying sources and manifestations of anxiety, it is important to identify appropriate methods for reducing anxiety. Even if the sources of anxiety are not identified or cannot be changed, the experience of anxiety can be addressed through self-care interventions that improve coping. To this end, the nurse asks questions about usual coping methods. Questions such as, "What do you do when you have trouble with your nerves?" or "What do you find helpful when your nerves are bad?" can pave the way for a discussion about coping with anxiety. If the person cannot identify effective coping mechanisms, the nurse offers suggestions in a nonjudgmental way and assesses the person's response to them. For example, nurses can ask any of the following questions:

- "Does it help to talk to someone about your worries?"
- "Have you ever tried any relaxation methods when you're nervous?"
- "Do you find that taking a walk helps you when your nerves are bad?"

Evidence-based Practice box 13-1 summarizes guidelines on detection and assessment of late-life anxiety published by the University of Iowa, College of Nursing.

Self-Esteem

Self-esteem cannot be measured numerically, but nurses can observe for verbal and nonverbal indicators. For example, a statement such as, "You're wasting your time on me; you have more important things to do" is a clue to poor self-esteem. Nonverbal indicators of self-esteem include the way people dress, care for themselves, and present themselves to others. Although interpreting behaviors in relation to self-esteem must be done with caution, the following behaviors may be associated with low self-esteem: rigidity, procrastination, unnecessary apologies, lack of confidence, expectations of failure, exaggeration of deficits, disappointment in self, self-destructive behaviors, constant approval-seeking, overemphasis on weaknesses, inability to accept compliments, minimizing personal capabilities, disregarding one's own opinions,

---

Evidence-Based Practice   13-1

Detection and Assessment of Late-Life Anxiety

Statement of the Problem

- Anxiety, defined as apprehensive expectation and excessive worry, ranges from normal reactions to everyday stress to disabling levels, which are categorized as anxiety disorders.
- More than half of community-dwelling older adults report anxiety symptoms.
- Accurate assessment, referral, and treatment are necessary because anxiety is associated with functional disability, reduced quality of life, lower life satisfactions, impaired physical and social function, and feelings of worthlessness.
- The following factors can interfere with recognition of anxiety in older adults: (1) stigma associated with mental illness, (2) older adults may focus on somatic symptoms and complaints, (3) manifestations may be considered normal consequences of aging, (4) underreporting and denial of problems are common among older adults; (5) inability to determine the degree to which worry is associated with realistic concerns.
- Factors consistently associated with increased risk of late life anxiety include physical illness, psychosocial stress, depression, cognitive impair-

ment, and personal characteristics (i.e., female gender, advanced age, lower socioeconomic status, external locus of control, family history of anxiety disorder, alcohol or drug use, Latino ethnicity).

Recommendations for Nursing Assessment

- Nurses should assess for anxiety in any older adult who expresses worry or fear and who is at risk due to physical illness, recent psychosocial stress, depression, cognitive impairment, or somatic complaints that are not associated with an identifiable underlying cause.
- Nurses can use a screening tool, such as the Geriatric Anxiety Inventory, Short Anxiety Screening Test, Hospital Anxiety and Depression Scale, or the Rating Anxiety in Dementia Scale.

Adapted from *Evidence-Based Practice Guideline: Detection and Assessment of Late-Life Anxiety*. (2008). M. Smith, T. Ingram, V. Brighton. (2008). University of Iowa Gerontological Nursing Interventions Research Center. Available at National Guideline Clearinghouse, www.guideline.gov

inability to form close relationships, inability to accept help from others, and inability to say "no" when appropriate. It may be acceptable to ask some questions, however, particularly about the person's perception of positive qualities.

In addition to observing for indicators of self-esteem, nurses can ask questions that give insight into the older adult's self-perceptions. For example, a question such as, "What is the quality in yourself that other people admire the most?" is nonthreatening. Moreover, this kind of question helps identify strengths that can be supported, and it provides clues to self-esteem. Nursing assessment is also directed toward identifying actual and potential threats to self-esteem, so they can be addressed through interventions, as discussed in Chapter 12.

Because self-esteem is influenced by the person's perception of the opinions held by significant others, it is important to identify who the significant others are for any particular person (e.g., peers; spouse or partner; authority figures; and people in the work, church, and social environments). Culture often defines who adopts the role of the significant other. Some Chinese American older adults, for example, expect their oldest son to look after their affairs and make key decisions about their health and well-being. Widows in some Middle Eastern and African cultures expect one of their husband's brothers to take care of them—an arrangement that fosters social and economic security for women who have lost a spouse. Being cared for by a family member (rather than by strangers) enhances self-esteem for older adults from all cultural backgrounds and increases the likelihood that their needs will be met as they age.

Depression

Depression is discussed as a general component of a psychosocial assessment in this chapter, and it is covered more comprehensively as an aspect of impaired psychosocial function in Chapter 15. Nurses can apply information in this chapter when assessing all older adults and use the information in Chapter 15 as a guide to assessing and caring for older adults who are depressed.

Nurses assess for depression by identifying verbal and nonverbal cues. Direct questions such as, "Are you depressed?" are usually not effective in eliciting information because people may associate the word "depressed" with states of overwhelming grief. Older adults may be more comfortable responding to questions about whether they feel "sad," "blue," or "down in the dumps." Therefore, unless the older adult uses the term "depressed" to describe his or her feelings, other terminology is more likely to elicit an accurate response. As with other aspects of the mental status assessment, it is best to start with open-ended questions, such as, "How are you feeling right now?" or "How have you been feeling this week?"

One of the purposes of an assessment of depression is to identify the person's usual patterns of coping with losses. For this reason, the nurse encourages older adults to express their feelings about significant changes in their lives. For instance, when an older adult talks about a change that might be experienced as a loss, nurses can ask nonthreatening questions that might lead to a discussion of feelings, such as: "What's it like to live alone after 50 years of being married?" "How is life different since your friend moved away?" "Are there people you miss seeing since you retired?" "Are there any activities you miss doing since you no longer drive?" If the questions do not elicit information about feelings, the nurse can comment on specific feelings that the person is likely to be experiencing. For example, a remark such as, "It seems like it would be pretty sad and lonely being here all by yourself after 55 years of marriage" allows the person to agree, disagree, or offer an alternative to the suggested feelings. Be aware that, for older adults from some Asian, Native American, and other cultures, expressing one's emotions overtly or discussing them with a stranger may be considered inappropriate.

Happiness and Well-Being

Happiness in relation to aging is often equated with morale, wellness, contentment, well-being, life satisfaction, successful aging, quality of life, and "the good life." A recent literature review identified the following dimensions of well-being that can be addressed by healthcare professionals in relation to aging (Kiefer, 2008):

- Staying active
- Interacting with peers
- Feeling financially secure
- Having a sense of personal autonomy
- Setting personal goals and challenges
- Having positive social interactions
- Developing effective coping strategies
- Participating in exercise and sports activities
- Actively contributing to society through paid or volunteer work.

Although nurses cannot address all these dimensions in a psychosocial assessment, they can include a few questions about happiness and well-being so they can identify ways of promoting wellness through nursing interventions. Psychologists sometimes use the following question to assess happiness: "Taking all things together, how would you say things are today—would you say you're very happy, pretty happy, or not too happy these days?" Nurses can ask a similar question such as, "If you had to rate your present level of happiness on a scale of 0% to 100%, what rating would you give it?" Nurses can use the person's response as a base for additional questions such as, "What would have to change to increase the rating by 10%?" "What kinds of things interfere with your happiness?" "If you could change one thing to be happier, what would it be?" Older adults will usually respond to these questions in a realistic manner, and their answers will provide information for establishing appropriate goals. Box 13-6 summarizes the considerations involved in assessing affective function in older adults.

Box 13-6 Guidelines for Assessing Affective Function

General Affective Function

- Are the quantity and quality of emotions appropriate for the objective reality?
- What is the depth and duration of emotions regarding a particular event?
- What are the nonverbal cues to the person's affective state?
- How do sociocultural or environmental factors influence the person's expression of emotions?
- What terminology is acceptable to this person, particularly with regard to feelings such as anger, anxiety, and depression?
- Does the person have any pets, or has he or she lost any pets?

Observations and Questions to Assess Mood

- What is the person's usual affective state?
- What are the nonverbal indicators of the person's mood?

Observations and Questions to Assess Anxiety

- What are the nonverbal indicators of anxiety?
- What real or perceived threats are present that might be sources of anxiety for the person?
- Might any of the following factors be contributing to the person's anxiety: caffeine, pathologic conditions, medications, herbs, or interventions by folk or indigenous healers that act on the central or autonomic nervous systems?
- What methods of coping has the person tried, and what have been the effects of these interventions?
- "What kinds of things do you worry about?"
- "Do you have any worries that you'd be willing to discuss with me?"
- "Do you ever have trouble with your nerves?"

Observations and Questions to Assess Self-Esteem

- What verbal and nonverbal clues to self-esteem can be detected?
- What are the factors that influence self-esteem for this person?
- Does the environment present any real or potential threat to self-esteem?
- How are my actions as a nurse influencing the self-esteem of the older adults to whom I relate?
- Are caregiver attitudes, such as infantilization or the promotion of unnecessary dependence, affecting the person's self-esteem?

Observations and Questions to Assess Depression

- What are the verbal and nonverbal clues to depression?
- "Do you ever feel blue or down in the dumps?"
- "How has your life changed since your husband died?"
- "What do you miss the most since you moved from your family home?"

Observations and Questions to Assess Happiness and Life Satisfaction

- How is the person's happiness and life satisfaction influenced by the following: functional abilities, personal relationships, and socioeconomic resources?
- "On a scale of 0% to 100%, how happy would you say you are right now?"
- "If you could change one thing to increase your happiness rating, what would it be?"

CONTACT WITH REALITY

Although a certain amount of fantasy is acceptable in everyday patterns of thinking, people are expected to remain in contact with the world around them and to respond appropriately to the same realities that others perceive. People lose contact with reality for numerous reasons including dementia, delirium, psychotic disorders, and a transient denial of a threatening reality. Many of these underlying conditions are treatable; however, when older adults lose contact with reality, they are likely to be labeled as "senile." Thus, because of stereotypes about older people, as well as the broad array of potential causes for loss of contact with reality, the assessment of an older person's contact with reality is particularly challenging.

Loss of contact with reality includes a wide range of behaviors ranging from simple and harmless misperceptions of reality to unyielding **delusions** or disturbing **hallucinations**. For example, people who are in the early stages of dementia may actively conceal or refuse to acknowledge memory deficits and those in later stages of dementia may experience delusions that lead to behaviors that are inappropriate or even dangerous. For instance, if someone believes that his belongings have been stolen, he may report the theft to the police or insist on going out to look for the robber. Three types of loss of contact with reality are delusions, hallucinations, and **illusions**, which are defined as follows:

- **Delusions:** Fixed false beliefs that have little or no basis in reality and cannot be corrected by appealing to reason.
- **Hallucinations:** Sensory experiences that have no basis in an external stimulus. Visual and auditory hallucinations are most common, but tactile, olfactory, and gustatory hallucinations also occur.
- **Illusions:** Misperceptions of an external stimulus. They may be mistaken for hallucinations, but differ in having some basis in reality, whereas hallucinations do not.

Just as a fever is one manifestation of a physical illness, loss of contact with reality is one manifestation of a psychiatric imbalance. For example, common manifestations of loss of contact with reality in people with dementia include delusions, hallucinations, misidentification, and false accusations. Certain characteristics of delusions, hallucinations, and illusions are associated with specific conditions such as delirium, dementia, and depression. In addition, loss of contact with reality typically occurs in combination with other manifestations of an underlying condition. Thus, an astute nursing assessment of contact with reality can provide essential information for identifying underlying causes. Table 13-1 shows distinguishing features of delusions, hallucinations, and illusions, and the following sections address these in relation to associated conditions that are most common in older adults.

Delusions

Delusions are a psychological mechanism that helps people preserve their egos, maintain control over threatening situations, and organize information that is difficult to process. Paranoia—defined as an extreme degree of suspiciousness—is one of the

TABLE 13-1 Distinguishing Features of Delusions, Hallucinations, and Illusions

Underlying Cause	Accompanying Manifestations	Characteristics
Delirium	Diminished attention, a clouded state of consciousness, and other typical manifestations of delirium; metabolic disturbance, adverse medication effect, or other underlying cause.	*Delusions:* poorly organized, persecutory *Hallucinations:* vivid, visual, colorful, threatening; accusatory auditory hallucinations induced by alcohol withdrawal. *Illusions:* brief, poorly organized.
Dementia	Cognitive impairment (particularly memory deficits); alert level of consciousness. Agitation, anxiety, or wandering may be associated with loss of contact with reality. Neurologic manifestations may accompany hallucinations, particularly when the underlying cause is vascular dementia.	*Delusions:* not fixed, loosely organized, readily changed or forgotten. Themes may include theft, fears, misidentification of places or people, and spousal infidelity. *Illusions:* occur more commonly than hallucinations; may be partially attributable to environmental factors. *Hallucinations:* more often visual than auditory; may be partially attributable to environmental factors.
Depression	Typical depressive symptoms including anorexia, lack of energy, sleep disturbances, and weight loss.	*Delusions:* Themes may include death, guilt, money, illnesses, self-reproach, gloomy foreboding, diminished self-esteem, and feelings of worthlessness. There may be some basis in reality, but perceptions are exaggerated. *Hallucinations:* typically auditory and derogatory.
Paranoid disorder	Absence of cognitive deficits or affective disorders; long-term social isolation or suspicious personality; may be well-hidden for years.	*Delusions:* fixed and well-organized; may subside temporarily in different environments. Themes usually involve plots, noises, threats, obscenities, or sexual assaults. *Hallucinations:* If present, these are related to the delusional themes.

most common types of delusions in older adults. The following are typical paranoid complaints or behaviors of older adults:

- The accusation that others are stealing their money or belongings
- The perception that they are being cheated, observed, attacked, persecuted, or sexually harassed
- The accusation that others are coming in and taking things, or messing up their belongings
- The belief that they have been injured by medical interventions, such as pills or radiation

Although the terms *paranoia* and *delusions* are sometimes used interchangeably in geriatric practice and references, this is inaccurate because there are many types of delusions.

In older adults, delusions can arise from pathologic conditions such as delirium, dementia, depression, and paranoid disorder. Delusions associated with each of these disorders are characterized in unique ways and occur in combination with other manifestations of the underlying condition, as discussed in the following sections.

Delusions Associated with Delirium and Physiologic Conditions

Delusions arising from delirium—also referred to as an *acute confusional state*—are only one manifestation of a complex pathologic process that is further characterized by physiologic disturbances, diminished attention, a clouded state of consciousness, and possibly hallucinations. Assessment of such delusions is relatively easy because they are commonly accompanied by other manifestations of delirium and subside once the delirium resolves. Another characteristic of delusions associated with delirium is that they are likely to be

poorly organized and persecutory in nature. Delusions as a manifestation of delirium are not unique to older adults, and they often accompany delirium in people of any age. Older adults, however, are more susceptible to delirium because the older brain is less able to adapt to metabolic disturbances, and the older person is more likely to have risk factors such as dementia, physiologic disturbances, and adverse reactions to medication.

In addition to being associated with delirium, delusions may be caused by pathologic conditions such as strokes, thyroid disorders, or infectious processes. Delusions may be an adverse effect of medications or they can be caused by abuse of or withdrawal from alcohol or drugs. Some of the physiologic disorders that are likely to cause delusions or hallucinations in older adults are listed in Table 13-2.

TABLE 13-2 Physiologic Disorders Causing Delusions or Hallucinations

Type of Disorder	Specific Examples
Metabolic disorders	Uremia, dehydration, electrolyte imbalance
Endocrine disorders	Hypoglycemia, thyroid disorders
Neurologic disorders	Stroke, cerebral trauma, cortical ischemia
Deficiency states	Vitamin deficiencies (B_{12}, folate, niacin, thiamine)
Infections	Septicemia, pneumonia, urinary tract infections, subacute bacterial endocarditis
Adverse medication effects	Anticholinergics, anticonvulsants, antidepressants, anti-Parkinson agents, benzodiazepines, corticosteroids, digitalis toxicity, narcotics
Drug or alcohol abuse or withdrawal	Alcohol, barbiturates, meprobamate

Delusions Associated with Dementia

Delusions occur in up to 73% of people with dementia, with paranoid delusions being the most common type (Shaji, Bose, & Kuriakose, 2009). Delusions associated with dementia may be caused by impaired memory and an inability to integrate information. During the early stages of dementia, delusions may not be recognized as manifestations of structural brain disease, and they may be attributed to other psychiatric conditions (Omar et al., 2009). The psychiatric literature usually does not differentiate between delusions that are typical of people with dementia and those that are characteristic of people with psychotic disorders without dementia. Despite the lack of published studies, however, nurses and other professionals who care for people who have dementia can describe many examples of delusions that are not typical psychotic delusions. In contrast to delusions arising from psychotic states, delusions arising from dementia are not fixed and well-organized and are readily changed or forgotten. Common themes of delusions associated with dementia are fearfulness, theft of property, and belief that one's house is not one's own. Nurses may be reluctant to label these behaviors as delusions because they are probably misinterpretations of reality rather than fixed false beliefs. Until the geropsychiatric literature suggests a better term, however, delusion is the most accurate label.

It is important to recognize that communication techniques differ for people with psychosis or dementia. For example, a typical psychiatric nursing approach for dealing with delusions in people who are psychotic is to talk with the client about the delusional thoughts as a problem in his or her life. In contrast, for people with dementia, it is more appropriate to avoid arguing and to provide reassurance and distractions.

Delusions regarding theft of personal belongings are one of the most common behavioral manifestations of dementia and are particularly problematic in home and long-term care settings. These delusions occur because the person with dementia forgets where an article is kept or was placed; then, in an attempt to deny the memory impairment or as a defense against acknowledging the deficit to others, he or she comes to believe that the article has been stolen and accuses someone of stealing it. Caregivers, roommates, and family members are often the targets of such accusations when they live with the person suffering from delusions. For people living alone, the accusations may be directed at "strangers who come in when I'm gone." In these situations, nurses often deal not only with the delusional person but also with the family, caregivers, and nursing staff who are the target of the accusations.

Delusions associated with dementia commonly involve misidentification of, or false beliefs about, people or environments. These misidentifications arise from the person's inability to match his or her perceptions with the memory or recognition of people or environments that were once familiar. This type of delusion can lead to behaviors that are quite challenging. For example, in home settings, this false belief is particularly problematic when a spouse or other devoted caregiver is accused of being a stranger intent on harming the person. Another common misidentification delusion is the belief that the person is not in his or her own home. These delusions can lead to troublesome behaviors such as wandering and agitation, with the person insisting on going out to "find my home." Another delusion associated with dementia is the belief that deceased parents or other close relatives are still alive. Delusions such as this precipitate agitation and searching behavior, typified by the person who insists that he or she "has to go take care of Mother." Another common type of delusion that is similar to the misidentification type is a false belief about spousal infidelity. In these situations, the person with dementia may firmly believe that his or her spouse is having sexual relationships with other people.

People with dementia will readily talk about delusions, whereas those who do not have dementia typically withhold or are secretive about information. The challenge in assessing these delusions, however, is to identify the possible reality of the situation. Nurses cannot assume that all accusations are unfounded just because people have serious cognitive impairments. Thus, nurses must be sure that there is no basis in reality before labeling the thoughts as delusional, because even the most bizarre-sounding assertions may be based partially or entirely on reality.

Delusions Associated with Depression

Persecutory and other delusions can be a manifestation of a major depression, but they are often overlooked or attributed to other factors, particularly in older adults living in community or long-term care settings. For example, when dementia and depression coexist, the delusions may be attributed to the dementia rather than considered as possible indicators of a treatable affective disorder. Likewise, when a person with a paranoid personality becomes depressed, the delusions may be falsely attributed to the personality, particularly if the delusions are persecutory in nature. When delusions arise from depression, other manifestations of depression are usually identified in a thorough depression assessment, as discussed in Chapter 15.

Delusional themes may provide clues to an affective disorder, particularly if the focus is on a recent loss. Therefore, carefully listening to the content of the delusions is essential to an accurate assessment. In depressed older adults, delusional themes often revolve around an exaggerated emphasis on guilt, money, illnesses, self-reproach, gloomy foreboding, diminished self-esteem, or feelings of worthlessness. Although some basis may exist in reality, the feelings of being persecuted and deserving of punishment are grossly exaggerated. The following are some examples of delusions arising from depression:

- Mrs. N. believes that she is responsible for her husband's death; therefore, she believes she does not deserve help for her own illness.
- Mr. A. believes that his Medicare insurance has been canceled as punishment for his not cashing his Social Security

check and insists that he cannot go to a doctor because he has no insurance.

- Ms. K. has an unshakable belief that she has undiagnosed cancer and begins to plan for her funeral, even though numerous doctors have not found any disease process.
- Mr. M., who recently had surgery for prostate cancer, is convinced that his house is going to explode from a gas leak and repeatedly calls the gas company to come check it.

Delusions Associated with Paranoid Disorder

Paranoid disorder—also called *paranoid ideation*—refers to a delusional disorder that is not associated with schizophrenia and is characterized by the tendency to view individuals or agencies with suspicion or as having harmful intentions. Factors associated with an increased risk for developing a late-life paranoid disorder include depression, social isolation, pathologic conditions, sensory impairment, and sense of loss of control over the environment. Common themes of paranoid delusions include spies, noises, threats, obscenities, lethal gases, bodily harm, stolen belongings, sexual infidelity or molestation, poisoned food or water, and having people enter living quarters by mysterious means at night. The delusions may occur more often when the person is socially isolated or in a particular environment, such as the home. If the person takes action based on the delusions, such as moving to another apartment or living with a family member, the delusions may subside temporarily.

Many people who have a paranoid disorder function well in the community, with the exception of one or two functional areas that are influenced by the delusions. Sometimes, a delusional state that was previously well-hidden may surface when the person is admitted to a long-term care facility, and the staff may think that the problem is new. In other situations, nurses will identify a paranoid disorder on making a home visit or interviewing an older person who has been admitted to the hospital. If the person also suffers from dementia, the delusions may be interpreted mistakenly as evidence of advancing dementia. When this occurs, a recommendation for long-term institutional care may be made when other recommendations might be more appropriate.

Identifying a paranoid disorder in the psychosocial assessment is important so that the symptoms can be alleviated with appropriate interventions. When left unattended or written off as eccentricities, these disorders may progress to a point at which they seriously disrupt functional abilities. Therefore, when delusions and cognitive impairments coexist, it is essential to determine whether the delusions existed before the dementia and to what extent, if any, they interfered with daily activities. If the delusions are part of a long-term pattern that has not interfered with the person's ability to function in daily life, the person may be able to remain in the community with support services and treatment directed toward the cognitive impairment. When delusions interfere with daily activities, however, medical intervention (e.g., psychotropic medications) may be effective in eliminating the delusions or minimizing their effects so that the person can maintain an independent level of function. When interventions are directed toward both the delusions and the cognitive impairment, the older person may be able to remain independent.

Hallucinations and Illusions

In older adults, hallucinations and illusions are associated most often with dementia, depression, social isolation, sensory impairment, and physiologic disturbances including adverse medication effects. Visual hallucinations are common in people with Parkinson's disease and may be related not only to the disease but also to the medications used to treat it (Ecker, Unrath, Kassubek, & Sabolek, 2009).

People experiencing hallucinations may know that their behavior is not socially acceptable. They may not offer information about hallucinations; in fact, they may try to hide their hallucinatory experiences. Older adults who are socially isolated are particularly successful in hiding hallucinatory experiences. As with delusions, it is important to identify the underlying cause of hallucinations and illusions, because the selection of appropriate interventions depends on an accurate assessment.

Nurses assess hallucinations by making astute observations and asking nonthreatening questions. Although older adults usually do not know they are having hallucinations, they are sometimes aware of it, particularly if the hallucinations are caused by the adverse effects of medications (e.g., anticholinergics) or a chronic condition such as Parkinson's disease. Any of the following behaviors are clues to auditory or visual hallucinations:

- Reaching out for objects that are not there
- Stepping over objects on the ground that are not visible to others
- Conversing with people who are not there
- Reporting noises, such as knocking or ringing sounds, which have no environmental source.

An appropriate assessment technique is to elicit information from family and caregivers with a statement such as, "Sometimes people see or hear things that others don't perceive. Do you notice any evidence of that happening to your father?"

Because hallucinations and illusions are abnormal sensory experiences, it is essential to assess for environmental influences and to make sure that sensory deficits are compensated for as much as possible. For example, an older adult with visual impairment may look at a chair and misperceive it as someone sitting. In this case, it would be inaccurate to label this person as having hallucinations or illusions, and it would be more effective to ensure that he or she is wearing eyeglasses if indicated.

Hallucinations Associated with Delirium and Other Conditions

As with delusions associated with delirium, hallucinations and illusions arising from delirium are assessed within the context of other manifestations of a complex process. In addition to being accompanied by other signs and symptoms, hallucinations arising from delirium are brief, vivid, visual, colorful, threatening, and poorly organized. Occasionally, hallucinations or illusions are the earliest sign of delirium, and they may be overlooked or attributed to another condition (e.g., dementia). Visual hallucinations also occur in people with age-related macular degeneration, with the most commonly experienced images being of people or geometric patterns (Khan, Shahid, Thurlby, Yates, & Moore, 2008).

Hallucinations arising from drug or alcohol withdrawal may occur during the first days of admission to an acute care setting or in any circumstance in which the person suddenly does not have access to their usual drugs or alcohol. Auditory hallucinations associated with alcohol withdrawal are typically accusatory and threatening, and they are sometimes organized into a complete paranoid system. The detection of alcohol-induced delirium is particularly important in acute care settings because people who are dependent on alcohol are more likely to acknowledge the problem and agree to appropriate interventions when they are in a crisis. The following example illustrates such a situation.

> Mr. K. is 73 years old and has been caring for his wife, who has Alzheimer's disease, for several years. He is a very proud man who has difficulty accepting help. One morning, Mr. K. begins vomiting coffee-ground emesis and is admitted to an acute care setting with the diagnosis of gastrointestinal bleeding. On admission, Mr. K. is very pleasant and expresses concern about his wife's care. The next morning, Mr. K. complains angrily to the nurses about the bars on the windows and is belligerent about the fact that he has been put in jail. He develops additional manifestations of delirium and is treated for alcohol withdrawal.
>
> When the delirium has subsided, the nurse initiates a conversation about the care of his wife and asks him how he copes with the responsibility. Mr. K. admits that he has difficulty coping with his and his wife's declining health and his increasing loneliness and responsibilities. He has always been a social drinker, but he has gradually increased his consumption of alcohol to three six-packs of beer a day. As part of the discharge plan, Mr. K. agrees to talk with a sponsor from Alcoholics Anonymous.

Table 13-1 (page 243) summarizes the physiologic disorders, including some adverse medication effects, which are most likely to cause hallucinations.

Hallucinations and Illusions Associated with Dementia

Hallucinations and illusions may occur at any time in the course of a dementing illness and are also likely to occur during a transient ischemic attack—a condition associated with vascular dementia. Visual hallucinations are the most common type, followed by auditory hallucinations (Shaji et al., 2009). Visual hallucinations are strongly associated with diagnoses of Parkinson's disease and Lewy body dementia (Tsuang et al., 2009). When illusions occur, they are often related to environmental conditions that can be modified. For example, poor lighting or reflections from glass or mirrors

can cause visual illusions, and background noise can contribute to auditory illusions, particularly for people with hearing aids.

Psychiatric literature usually addresses illusions only with regard to misperceptions of visual or auditory stimuli, whereas an illusion, by definition, is a misinterpretation of any external stimulus. Nurses who care for people with dementia can cite numerous examples of behaviors that fit this broader definition of an illusion, such as the following:

- Mistaking the identity of caregivers, family members, or other familiar people
- Perceiving an object as something other than what it really is
- Taking an object under the mistaken belief that it belongs to them
- Refusing to believe that they are in their home when they really are.

These experiences might be labeled as delusions or disorientation, but they are more accurately defined as illusions because they involve a misinterpretation of reality rather than a false perception that has no base in reality.

Hallucinations Associated with Depression

Severely depressed older adults are more likely to experience delusions rather than hallucinations, but visual and auditory hallucinations of deceased loved ones commonly occur during periods of bereavement. Hallucinations associated with depression are likely to be auditory and derogatory, or they may involve visual perceptions of dead people. The following examples are typical of hallucinations arising from depression:

- Ms. C. reports that at night she hears the people in the next apartment saying that she has cancer.
- Mr. T. reports hearing younger men say that he is sexually impotent and that he was not a good provider to his wife (who died within the past year).
- Ms. F. looks down from her second-floor window and sees a man, dressed in black, lying injured on the sidewalk.
- Mr. S. insists that there is a pervasive smell of skunk coming from his basement, and he believes he will be contaminated if he goes downstairs.

Hallucinations Associated with Paranoid Disorder

If hallucinations are a symptom of paranoid disorder, they are likely to be closely related to the theme of the delusions. The following examples are characteristic of hallucinations arising from paranoid states:

- Mr. F. says that he hears people in the next apartment talking about him. These are the same people whom he believes will come in and steal things when he leaves the apartment.
- Ms. J. reports seeing men observing her when she undresses or takes a bath. Moreover, when she goes to the grocery store, the man at the checkout always offers her money in exchange for sexual favors.

Table 13-2 (page 243) summarizes the characteristics that distinguish delusions, hallucinations, and illusions according to their underlying causes.

Special Considerations for Assessing Contact With Reality in Older Adults

Assessment of contact with reality presents a special assessment challenge for nurses for a variety of reasons:

- People often try to conceal delusions and hallucinations.
- When delusions and hallucinations arise from social isolation, opportunities for assessment are extremely limited.
- To determine whether a reported experience is delusional, the nurse needs information about the reality, which is difficult to obtain if a reliable and objective observer is not available.
- Even after delusions or hallucinations are identified as such, the underlying factors may be difficult to identify.
- Older adults often have more than one underlying condition, such as a delirium superimposed on a dementia.

Delusions are usually more readily acknowledged than hallucinations, and the most effective tools for assessing delusions are asking leading questions and listening attentively. Most older adults will confide their delusions to a nurse who they perceive as interested, sympathetic, and nonjudgmental, particularly if a trusting relationship has been established. Difficulty arises, however, when nurses hear information that may be interpreted as delusional but, in fact, is based wholly or partially in reality. For example, financial exploitation, violation of rights, and other aspects of elder abuse are not uncommon, particularly in older adults who are cognitively impaired or who live with family members who are psychosocially impaired. When older adults who have cognitive impairments or a lifelong suspicious personality describe abusive or exploitative situations, they are likely to be considered delusional or not to be taken seriously. In these situations, the assessment challenge is to determine what is real, what is distorted, and what is not based at all in reality.

Nurses also consider the potential effects of environmental and interpersonal factors in contributing to delusions, illusions, or hallucinations. For example, the reflection of fluorescent lights on a highly polished floor can produce the illusion of water on the floor, and an older adult might walk around the reflection. Stressful interpersonal relationships may contribute to the development of paranoid ideations, particularly in the context of past or present exploitation or abuse. Another important assessment consideration is whether a lack of assistive devices, such as eyeglasses and hearing aids, is contributing to altered perceptions. For example, if someone usually depends on eyeglasses, contact lenses, or a hearing aid for adequate visual or auditory function, the absence of these items may contribute to the development of illusions or hallucinations.

During the assessment, nurses consider cultural factors that are likely to influence perceptions of reality and manifestations of mental illness, as discussed in Chapter 12. Religious

---

 Box 13-7 Guidelines for Assessing Contact With Reality

General Principles

- In assessing any loss of contact with reality, the effects of alcohol, medications, and physiologic disturbances must always be considered as potential causative influences.
- People who are not cognitively impaired are usually more reluctant to talk about delusions and hallucinations than people who have dementia.
- When people talk about things that might be delusional, it is important to determine, through information provided by a reliable and objective observer, whether their perceptions have any basis in reality.
- When delusions are initially identified, it is important to determine whether they are of recent onset or have been longstanding but only recently discovered.
- When delusions are identified in someone who has dementia, it is particularly important to consider the influence of treatable causative factors, such as depression or physiologic disturbances.
- People who have dementia are likely to have illusions rather than hallucinations.
- People who are socially isolated are usually quite successful in concealing hallucinations.
- In assessing hallucinations and illusions, it is particularly important to consider the influence of the environment.

Interview Questions to Assess Delusions, Hallucinations, and Illusions

- "Do you have any thoughts that you can't seem to get rid of?"
- "People sometimes have thoughts that they're afraid to talk about because they believe others will think they're 'crazy.' Do you ever have thoughts like that?"
- "Do you sometimes hear voices when you're alone?"
- "Do you sometimes think you see things that other people don't see?"

Nonverbal Clues to Hallucinations

- Extreme withdrawal and isolation
- Contentment with social isolation, particularly if the person previously had many social contacts
- Gestures and other actions that normally occur in response to perceived stimuli

---

background is a common cultural factor that can influence the content of delusions or hallucinations. For example, delusions and hallucinations in Irish Catholics are likely to focus on Jesus, a saint, or the Virgin Mary. Similarly, Muslims with African, Near Eastern, or Middle Eastern cultural heritage may focus on the Prophet Mohammed. Box 13-7 summarizes guidelines for assessing an individual's contact with reality.

SOCIAL SUPPORTS

Social supports, which are categorized as *informal* and *formal*, refer to the services provided to address functional and psychosocial needs. Although even the most independent people receive social supports (e.g., emotional support from family and friends), social supports are usually discussed in relation to meeting the needs of people who depend on others in some way for assistance. While friends, family, clergy, neighbors, or coworkers provide informal social support, workers who are paid by the older person or their family or by health and social service agencies or institutions provide formal social support.

Social supports significantly influence psychosocial function in older adults because they affect one's ability to cope with stressful life experiences by buffering them against harmful effects and improving one's physical and emotional well-being. Because the importance of social supports increases in relation to the degree of impairment of the older adult, it is essential to assess the social supports for any older adults who have conditions that affect their functional abilities. Nursing assessment of social supports identifies not only the resources that are needed, available, or being used to support the highest level of functioning but also the barriers to the use of appropriate resources. Specific aspects of social supports that nurses assess include social network, economic resources, and religion and spirituality. Box 13-8 summarizes important questions and considerations involved in assessing social supports.

Box 13-8 Guidelines for Assessing Social Supports

Interview Questions to Assess Social Supports

- "On whom do you rely for help?"
- "Is there anyone who helps you with grocery shopping? Getting to doctor appointments? Getting prescriptions filled? Managing your money and paying bills?"
- "Is there anyone you can talk to when you have worries or difficulties?"
- "Is there anything you would like help with that you don't have help with now?"
- "Is there anyone in the family who could help with grocery shopping?"
- "Have you ever received information about the transportation services (or meals, or other services) that are available through the senior center?"

Potential Barriers to the Use of Formal Supports

- Unwillingness to acknowledge, or lack of insight to recognize, the need for services
- Expectation that family members will provide the needed care
- Unwillingness to admit that family members cannot or will not provide the needed care
- Lack of financial resources to purchase services or unwillingness to spend money for services
- Perceived correlation between formal services and "welfare"
- Lack of transportation to access services
- Mistrust of service providers or an unwillingness to allow outsiders into the home
- Bad experiences with service providers or hearsay about the bad experiences of others
- Fear that the home situation will be judged as socially unacceptable, or embarrassment because it is socially unacceptable
- Fear that having outsiders in the house will lead to admission to a nursing home
- Lack of time, energy, or problem-solving ability to obtain information about and select the appropriate services
- Fear that the service will be provided by someone about whom the care recipient holds prejudices
- Language and cultural barriers

Interview Questions to Assess Financial Resources

- "Do you have any money worries?"
- "Do you have any concerns about paying for services that you might need?"
- "Would you like to talk to someone about any financial concerns?"
- "Do you think you can afford the kind of help that your doctor recommended?"
- "Have you received any advice about financial planning for nursing home care?"

Interview Questions to Assess Religious Affiliation

- "Do you belong to any church, synagogue, or mosque?"
- "Are you aware of any programs available at your church, synagogue, or mosque that might be helpful to you?"

DIVERSITY NOTE

A barrier to accepting social supports that is unique to American Indians is their cultural backdrop of historical trauma and intergenerational grief associated with their involuntary colonization experiences in the United States (Korn et al., 2009).

Social Network

Nursing assessment of the social network addresses the social supports that are important for day-to-day functioning as well as those that affect the person's quality of life. The nurse can initiate the assessment by asking a broad question such as, "Whom do you rely on for help?" The nurse can then ask more specific questions about how the person accomplishes tasks that are most important for day-to-day function. For example, in discussing a follow-up appointment for medical care, the nurse may ask, "How do you get to your doctor appointments?" Because a relationship with a confidant(e) is a significant predictor of quality of life for older adults, at least one question relating to this factor should be posed, such as, "Is there anyone you can talk to about your worries?" The answer to this question may also be important if the nurse or healthcare team is assisting the older adult with a decision about long-term care because the older adult may want the confidant(e) to be involved in the decision-making process. In addition, the response to this question may provide important information about whether the older person has recently experienced a loss, or change in the availability, of a confidant(e).

After identifying existing social networks, the nurse identifies the resources that might be helpful in addressing unmet needs. Such questions as "Do you have any grandchildren or neighbors who could help with shoveling the snow?" are aimed at identifying informal supports that are available but are not currently being used. A question such as, "Are you aware that the senior center has a van that takes people to doctor appointments?" is aimed at identifying the person's awareness of formal supports that may not be in use.

Barriers to Obtaining Social Supports

In addition to assessing the number and types of social supports available, nurses try to identify the barriers that interfere with the use of social supports. Many older adults who are eligible for service programs do not use these resources because they view them as costly, impersonal, overly structured, and hard to arrange. Because older adults prefer to receive help from family and friends, negative attitudes about the use of formal social supports may be a source of resistance to their use. Without adequate informal supports, or when conflicts exist between older adults and their informal supports, an increase in dependence can trigger less effective coping mechanisms. The following example is typical of such a situation:

> Mr. and Mrs. S. always expected their children to care for them, but the children moved to other cities and visit several times a year. Mr. and Mrs. S. refuse to accept any of the formal services that are available because of their cost, and also because they expect their children to provide the services out of filial responsibility. Furthermore, Mrs. S. cared for her parents when they were old, so she expects her daughter to do the same for her.
>
> Mr. and Mrs. S. frequently call their daughter and son-in-law to complain about their inability to get groceries and go to doctors' appointments. Rather than making use of transportation or other services available from the community, they neglect themselves. During the children's visit over the Christmas holiday, they find that their parents have not been eating adequately and are not taking their prescribed medications. When they mention these observations to their parents, Mr. and Mrs. S. tell their children, "If you loved us, you'd be taking care of us, and this wouldn't be happening."

In addition to some older people's preference for obtaining services from families rather than outside agencies, there are many other barriers to the use of formal services. Fears about outsiders coming into the home rank high among the barriers to the provision of in-home services. Financial barriers also often exist, either because of an inability or an unwillingness to pay for services. Additional barriers include unwillingness to accept help, lack of knowledge about types of services available, and not knowing where to go for specific services. The identification of these barriers is essential because counseling and educational interventions (e.g., providing information about services that are available) can address many of these issues. Issues that are not amenable to intervention may represent impenetrable barriers to the provision of social supports.

Assessing barriers to support services is particularly challenging because direct questions about these issues often are inappropriate and usually are very threatening. Rather, identification of these barriers is best accomplished by carefully listening to older people and their caregivers and by asking nonthreatening questions. For example, a caregiver might talk about a friend who had a home health aide who did nothing but watch television all day and got paid $18 an hour. In response to this, the nurse might ask, "Do you think that might happen if we arrange for a home health aide to care for your father?" Other attitudinal barriers, such as prejudices, may be identified through statements made by the caregiver about prior experiences.

Economic Resources

Financial issues are generally within the purview of social workers, and nurses usually prefer to avoid discussing money with older adults or their families. In planning for formal services for older adults, however, some assessment of financial assets is necessary, and the nurse is often the healthcare professional who obtains this information, particularly in home or other community settings. If no long-term care or community-based services are needed, the nurse can forego the financial assessment.

Many older adults and their families are shocked to find out that Medicare does not cover the costs of long-term care, with the exception of skilled care. In addition, people are often appalled by the restrictive definition of skilled care as well as many other restrictions that are applied to determine eligibility for services. Even if a social worker has explained these facts, it is usually the nurse who deals with the related anxiety and other emotional reactions of the older adults and their families. Because nurses are in a position to help older adults and their families address and cope with the financial issues of long-term care, they frequently become involved in assessing the financial resources of the person and family.

It is not always necessary to ask details about monthly income or the exact amount of savings and assets, but questions must be asked about the resources available for the purchase of services. Asking a question such as, "Do you have any money worries?" might reveal some anxieties that can be dealt with or allayed through counseling or the provision of accurate information. When the nurse reviews with the older adult or caregiver the services that are available, information also can be provided about the cost of these services, at which time a question such as, "Do you think you could afford this kind of help?" can be posed.

RELIGION AND SPIRITUALITY

As discussed in Chapter 12, religion and spirituality become more important in older adulthood, and they are resources that should be identified as a part of a comprehensive psychosocial assessment. The person's religious affiliation is assessed as a component of his or her social supports, whereas spirituality is assessed as a separate component of the psychosocial assessment. It is important to recognize that spirituality is an integral component of all humans but not all people identify with a religious affiliation.

Identification of religious affiliation is a simple but important part of the psychosocial assessment, because available religion-based programs for older adults may be perceived as more acceptable than those provided by a public or nonreligious agency. For example, an older Jewish person might be willing to go to the Jewish Community Center for a senior meal program, and an older Roman Catholic adult might be willing to accept mental health services from Catholic Social Services, but these people might refuse to avail themselves of the same kinds of services when they are offered by another organization. Often, religion-based services are viewed by the older adult as services that they deserve as a reward for years of attendance at or service to a church or synagogue. Although most religion-based programs serve older adults regardless of their religious affiliations, the programs are often perceived as more appropriate if the person is of the same faith.

In addition to being perceived as more appropriate, some religion-based services are not available elsewhere, and they are often provided by trained volunteers free of charge. Examples of programs or services that may be available to members of a particular church, synagogue, or mosque include transportation, respite care, peer counseling, chore assistance, friendly visiting, and telephone reassurance. Older adults can also take advantage of any church-, synagogue-, or mosque-based program that is available for people of all ages. The Stephen Ministries, founded in 1975, is an example of a volunteer program that is available in many Christian denominations throughout the United States. This program offers peer counseling and other services, provided by volunteers with special training in ministering to older, depressed, shut-in, and grieving persons.

Identification of a specific place of worship is also important because attendance at religious services may be a significant factor in the older adult's social life. For many older adults, particularly those with limited mobility or those who have full-time caregiving responsibilities, attendance at religious services is their only opportunity for social interaction and personal support. Most people who are unable to attend religious services can arrange for home visits by a clergy person or lay minister; indeed, these visits may be the only source of outside contact and emotional support that is acceptable to a home-bound older adult. Moreover, for people who are socially isolated, a visitor from their place of worship may be the only person monitoring the home situation. In these situations, health professionals who are concerned about home-bound older adults may be able to monitor their status through these visitors, as in the following example:

Mr. S. was admitted to the hospital after a syncopal episode that resulted in a minor car accident. On admission, Mr. S. was slightly unkempt and showed some memory deficits, but his self-care abilities improved during his 2-day hospitalization. The nurse suggested that Mr. S. consider home-delivered meals and the use of other community resources, but he refused these services. His situation did not warrant a report to a protective services agency.

The nurse was concerned because Mr. S. lived alone and had no outside contacts other than Ms. C., a lay minister who had visited weekly for 2 years. The nurse asked for and received permission from Mr. S. to contact Ms. C. to inform her of available community services. Ms. C. was grateful for the information and said that she would contact the appropriate agencies if Mr. S.'s condition declined or if he agreed to accept help.

In this situation, information about the church affiliation enabled the nurse to implement a discharge plan that otherwise would not have been possible.

Although nurses do not always include spiritual needs as a routine part of the assessment, there are many times when a nursing assessment of the spiritual needs of older adults is warranted. When an older person provides clues about spiritual distress or discomfort, the nurse must be willing to respond to the older person rather than simply ignore the clues, as discussed in Chapter 12. Moreover, when a nurse is addressing quality-of-life issues, it is important to include questions about spirituality. For example, when planning long-term care, it is particularly important to assess and address spiritual needs. Assessment of spiritual needs focuses on a discussion of sources of strength and meaning in the older person's life and is not intended to evaluate whether a person is more or less spiritual. As with all aspects of care, nurses need to be particularly aware of cultural influences on religious practices and expressions of spirituality. At the same time, however, they need to be cautious about generalizations with regard to any cultural group.

Nurses, like many people, may not be comfortable discussing spirituality, but they can increase their comfort level by recognizing their own feelings and acknowledging that spirituality is a universal human need. Nurses might avoid discussion of spiritual needs because they believe that they are not skilled in meeting these needs. However, nurses routinely identify many needs that they are not trained to meet directly. If nurses view the assessment of spiritual needs as an essential part of holistic care, they may become comfortable with addressing the spiritual needs of the older adults to whom they provide care. As with other broad health problems, nurses address the nursing aspects of those problems and refer the person to the appropriate resource for interventions that address the non-nursing aspects. In addition to providing direct nursing interventions to address spiritual needs, nurses suggest referrals to appropriate clergy or spiritual practitioners. Involvement with support groups can also be effective in dealing with spiritual distress when it arises from feelings of guilt, anger, or inadequacy.

Box 13-9 presents guidelines for assessing spiritual needs. Assessment of spiritual needs includes not only the factors that cause spiritual distress but also the factors that are essential to spiritual growth, even in the absence of spiritual distress.

Box 13-9 Guidelines for Assessing Spiritual Needs

Guidelines for Nursing Assessment

- Be aware of your own feelings about spirituality, so that you can recognize and respond to the spiritual needs of others.
- Recognize that spiritual needs are a universal human phenomenon. Although not all people experience spiritual distress, all people have spiritual needs and the potential for spiritual growth.
- Recognize that it is within the realm of holistic nursing care to identify and plan interventions for spiritual growth as well as for spiritual distress.
- Convey a nonjudgmental, open-minded attitude when eliciting information about a person's spirituality and religious beliefs.

Questions to Assess Spiritual Health

- "What in your life is meaningful and important?"
- "What do you hope to accomplish in your life?"
- "What do you do that gives you pleasure and satisfaction?"
- "Who are the people you can turn to when you need someone to listen to you or to help you?"
- "Do you believe in a higher being?" (examples: God, Goddess, Divinity) "How do you describe this being?"
- "Do you participate in any activities (rituals) that foster a connection with a higher being?" (examples: prayer or other religious activities)
- "What activities are helpful in bringing you inner peace and relieving stress?" (examples: meditation, walking in the woods)
- "What are your beliefs about death?"
- "Do you see a connection between your body, your mind, your emotions, and your soul?"
- "Is there anything you need or would like to have to support your beliefs and your spiritual needs?" (example: Bible, sacred or revered object)
- "Would you like to arrange a visit from a spiritual leader?"
- "Are there any health practices that you would like to consider, even though our society may not consider them to be conventional?" (examples: therapeutic touch, guided imagery)

Observations/Questions to Assess Spiritual Distress

- During the psychosocial interview, listen for clues to spiritual distress, such as the following: suicidal ideation; anger toward God; inability to forgive others; feelings of hopelessness, uselessness, or abandonment; questions about the meaning of life, losses, or suffering.
- "Are there any conflicts between your beliefs or values and actions that you feel you should be taking?" (example: feeling entitled to some time to oneself, which may be in conflict with the demands of caregiving for a spouse)
- "Are there any conflicts between what you believe in and what society or healthcare professionals are encouraging or suggesting you do?" (example: questioning the wisdom of using a feeding tube for a spouse who is chronically and severely impaired and unable to participate in the decision)
- "Do you have any special religious considerations that are not being addressed?" (examples: dietary practices, observance of religious holidays)
- *For people in institutional settings:* "Is there anything here that interferes with your spiritual needs?" (examples: noisy environment, lack of privacy)

Chapter Highlights

Overview of Psychosocial Assessment of Older Adults

- Psychosocial assessment is a complex process that involves the use of good communication skills, appropriate interview questions, purposeful observations, and relevant assessment tools.
- Nurses can assess their own attitudes to increase their comfort level in performing a psychosocial assessment of older adults (Box 13-1).

Communication Skills for Psychosocial Assessment (Box 13-2, Culture Considerations Box 13-1)

- Barriers to communication include visual and hearing impairments, internal and external distractions, pathologic disorders, adverse medication effects, poor communication methods, and cultural differences.
- Establishing rapport, using touch, listening, asking questions, and giving feedback can enhance communication during psychosocial assessment.
- Nurses create an environment for effective communication by speaking face-to-face at eye level, respecting the person's comfort zone, ensuring privacy, eliminating distractions, and facilitating optimal vision and hearing functioning.

Mental Status Assessment (Boxes 13-3, 13-4, and 13-5)

- An assessment of mental status involves an assessment of all of the following: physical appearance, motor function, social skills, response to the interview, orientation, alertness and attention, memory, speech characteristics, and calculation and higher language skills.

Decision-Making and Executive Function

- Assessment of cognitive skills, such as executive function, is particularly important for determining the ability of the older adult to participate in decision-making.
- Insight, learning, memory, reasoning, judgment, problem solving, and abstract thinking are some of the cognitive skills that are involved with decision-making.

Affective Function (Evidence-Based Practice Box 13-1)

- An assessment of affective function includes consideration of mood, anxiety, self-esteem, depression, and happiness and well-being.

Contact with Reality (Box 13-7, Tables 13-1 and 13-2)

- Nurses assess contact with reality within the context of behavioral indicators to identify potential underlying causes of any loss of contact with reality.
- Three types of loss of contact with reality are delusions, hallucinations, and illusions.

Social Supports (Box 13-8)

- Psychosocial assessment identifies social supports and economic resources as well as barriers to obtaining services.

Religion and Spirituality (Box 13-9)

• A holistic nursing assessment addresses religious affiliation and spirituality.

Critical Thinking Exercises

1. Complete the psychosocial self-assessment in Box 13-1.
2. Think of several different situations in the past few weeks in which you worked with older adults and answer the following questions:
   • What aspects of psychosocial function did you observe?
   • What questions did you ask that would give you information about their psychosocial function?
   • What information did you obtain about their social supports?
3. Name at least three things you would observe or determine in order to assess each of the following when you are working with older adults: physical appearance, social skills, orientation, alertness and attention, memory, speech characteristics, calculation and higher language skills, decision-making skills, anxiety, self-esteem, depression, and contact with reality.
4. What questions would you ask an older adult to identify social supports and barriers to the use of services?
5. What approach would you use to assess an older adult's spiritual health and identify spiritual distress?

Resources

For links to these resources and additional helpful Internet resources related to this chapter, visit thePoint at http://thePoint. lww.com/Miller6e.

Clinical Tools

American Journal of Nursing and Hartford Institute for Geriatric Nursing
   • *How to Try This,* article and video: Kennedy, G. J., & Smyth, C. A. (2008). Screening older adults for executive dysfunction. *American Journal of Nursing, 108*(12), 62–72.
   • *How to Try This,* article and video: Doerflinger, D. M. C. (2007). The Mini-Cog, *American Journal of Nursing, 107*(12), 62–71.
Hartford Institute for Geriatric Nursing
   • *Try This: Best Practices in Nursing Care to Older Adults* Issue 3 (2007), Mental Status Assessment of Older Adults: The Mini-Cog
   Issue 3D (2007). Brief Evaluation of Executive Dysfunction: An Essential Refinement in the Assessment of Cognitive Impairment.

Evidence-Based Practice

Smith, M., Ingram, T., & Brighton, V. (2009). Evidence-based practice guideline: Detection and assessment of late-life anxiety. *Journal of Gerontological Nursing, 35*(7), 9–15.
National Guideline Clearinghouse
   • Detection and assessment of late life anxiety

REFERENCES

Allgulander, C. (2009). Generalized anxiety disorder: Between now and DSM-V. *Psychiatric Clinics of North America, 32*, 611–628.

Andrews, M. M., & Boyle, J. S. (2008). *Transcultural concepts in nursing care* (5th ed.). Philadelphia, PA: Lippincott Williams & Wilkins.

Calleo, J., Stanley, M. A., Greisinger, A., Wehmanen, O., Johnson, M., Novy, D., . . . Kunik, M. (2009). Generalized anxiety disorder in older medical patients: Diagnostic recognition, mental health management and service utilization. *Journal of Clinical Psychology in Medical Settings, 16*, 175–185.

Connor, A., & Howett, M. (2009). A conceptual model of intentional comfort touch. *Journal of Holistic Nursing, 27*, 127–135.

Doerflinger, D. M. C. (2007). *How to try this,* article and video: The Mini-Cog. *American Journal of Nursing, 107*(12), 62–71.

Ecker, D., Unrath, A., Kassubek, J., & Sabolek, M. (2009). Dopamine agonists and their risk to induce psychotic episodes in Parkinson's disease: A case-control study. *BMC Neurology, 9*(23), doi:10.1186/1471–2377-9–23.

Kennedy, G. J., & Smyth, C. A. (2008). Screening older adults for executive dysfunction. *American Journal of Nursing, 108*(12), 62–71.

Khan, J. C., Shahid, H., Thurlby, D. A., Yates, J. R., & Moore, A. T. (2008). Charles Bonnet syndrome in age-related macular degeneration. *Ophthalmic Epidemiology, 15*(3), 202–208.

Kiefer, R. A. (2008). An integrative review of the concept of well-being. *Holistic Nursing Practice, 22*, 244–252.

Korn, L., Logsdon, R. G., Polissar, N. L., Gomez-Beloz, A., Waters, T., & Ryser, R. (2009). A randomized trial of a CAM therapy for stress reduction in American Indian and Alaskan Native family caregivers. *The Gerontologist, 48*, 368–377.

Omar, R., Sampson, E. L., Loy, C. T., Mummery, C. J., Fox, N. C., Rossor, M. N., & Warren, J. D. (2009). Delusions in frontotemporal lobar degeneration. *Journal of Neurology, 256*, 600–607.

Pinto, E., & Peters, R. (2009). Literature review of the Clock Drawing Test as a tool for cognitive screening. *Dementia and Geriatric Cognitive Disorders, 27*, 201–213.

Purnell, L. D. (2009). *Guide to culturally competent health care* (2nd ed.). Philadelphia, PA: F. A. Davis Co.

Shaji, S., Bose, S., & Kuriakose, S. (2009). Behavioral and psychological symptoms of dementia: A study of symptomology. *Indian Journal of Psychiatry, 51*, 38–41.

Smith, M., Ingram, T., & Brighton, V. (2009). Evidence-based guideline: Detection and assessment of late-life anxiety. *Journal of Gerontological Nursing, 35*(7), 9–15.

Tsuang, D., Larson, E. B., Bolen, E., Thompson, M. L., Peskind, E., Bowen, J., . . . Leverenz, J. B. (2009). Visual hallucinations in dementia: A prospective community-based study with autopsy. *American Journal of Geriatric Psychiatry, 17*(4), 317–323.

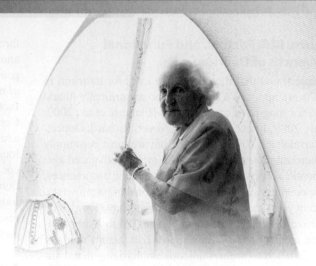

CHAPTER 14

Impaired Cognitive Function: Delirium and Dementia

LEARNING OBJECTIVES

After reading this chapter, you will be able to:

1. Describe delirium and discuss nursing assessment and interventions related to delirium.

2. Explain the appropriate use of terminology that describes impaired cognitive function in older adults.

3. Describe characteristics of Alzheimer's disease, vascular dementia, frontotemporal dementia, and dementia with Lewy bodies.

4. List the factors that affect the risk for development of dementia.

5. Discuss the functional consequences of impaired cognitive function.

6. Describe guidelines for initial and ongoing assessment of cognitively impaired older adults.

7. Identify nonpharmacologic interventions for addressing dementia-related behaviors, including environmental modifications and communication techniques.

8. Discuss medications for slowing the progression of dementia and for managing dementia-related behaviors.

K E Y   P O I N T S

Alzheimer's disease

behavioral and psychological symptoms of dementia (BPSD)

beta-amyloid

catastrophic reaction

cognitive reserve

delirium

dementia

excess disability

frontotemporal dementia

Lewy body dementia

mild cognitive impairment (MCI)

reality orientation

retained awareness

vascular dementia

Healthy older adults experience only minor changes in cognitive abilities (as described in Chapter 11), but as people age, they are increasingly likely to experience pathologic conditions that have a major impact on cognitive function. Nurses in all settings frequently care for older adults who have **dementia** or **delirium**, which are the two main causes of significant cognitive impairment in older adults. Nurses are responsible for identifying factors that contribute to impaired cognitive functioning in older adults. In addition, nurses and others who care for people with dementia must meet the challenge of preserving as much of the person's dignity and quality of life as possible, despite the serious and progressive losses the person with dementia experiences.

DELIRIUM

Overview and Types

Although delirium has been documented in patients for centuries, only in recent years have researchers and practitioners addressed delirium as a serious, preventable, treatable, commonly occurring, and often unrecognized condition that disproportionately affects older adults. Delirium is a syndrome characterized by acute onset, a fluctuating course, and disturbances in thought, memory, attention, behavior, perception, orientation, and consciousness. Three behavioral subtypes of delirium are hyperactive, hypoactive, and mixed. Clinical features of *hyperactive delirium* include restlessness, agitation, and increased psychomotor activity; whereas *hypoactive delirium* is characterized by slowed movement, paucity of speech, and unresponsiveness (Yang et al., 2009). Although hypoactive delirium is considered to be the less common type, recent studies indicate that this type is common but unrecognized among older adults and is associated with more serious consequences including increased mortality (Yang et al., 2009). Delirium develops over a short time (hours or days), fluctuates over the course of the day (usually affecting the sleep–wake cycle), and can persist for months.

Prevalence, Risk Factors, and Functional Consequences of Delirium

Studies have found that the prevalence rates for delirium in older adults are up to 89% for those who are critically ill and up to 70% for long-term care residents (Flaherty et al., 2009; Fong et al., 2009, Luetz et al., 2010; Voyer, Richard, Doucet, Cyr, & Carmichael, 2009b). Factors that are most commonly cited as increasing the risk for delirium include advanced age, pain, dementia, surgery, medications, physiologic disturbances, pathologic conditions, and impaired functional or cognitive status. In recent years, researchers and clinicians have focused on postoperative delirium, particularly in regard to using anticholinergic medications as a modifiable risk factor (Young & Flanagan, 2010). Researchers are also emphasizing that delirium is multifactorial and results from an interaction between predisposing factors that increase the person's baseline vulnerability and precipitating factors that account for the immediate

threat (Voyer, Richard, Doucet, & Carmichael, 2009a). Voyer and colleagues (2009b) identified dementia, functional dependency, pain, depression, behavioral disturbances, number of medications, dehydration, and malnutrition as predisposing factors among long-term care residents who had dementia. Common precipitating factors include surgery, infections, and acute medical conditions. Functional consequences include longer hospital stays, increased mortality, increased dependency, development of dementia, short- and long-term functional impairment, and higher rates of permanent residency in long-term care facilities. Table 14-1 summarizes some recent research findings related to the prevalence of, risk factors for, and consequences of delirium in older adults.

Nursing Assessment of Delirium

Frequent assessment and monitoring of mental status is imperative because delirium is often unrecognized in clinical

TABLE 14-1   Research Evidence: Delirium and Older Adults

Researchers	Setting	Findings
Alagiakrishnan et al., 2009	Hospital	Hospital-acquired delirium was associated with increased mortality, increased length of stay, and increased discharge to institutional setting
Ansaloni et al., 2010	Hospital	Independent variables for 351 patients with postoperative delirium: aged 75+, co-morbidity, preoperative cognitive impairment, psychopathology, poor glycemic control
Bjorkelund et al., 2010	Hospital	Use of multifactorial interventions for elderly hip fracture patients with no cognitive impairment on admission reduced the incidence of hospital-acquired delirium by 35%
Dasgupta & Hillier, 2010	Systemic review, 21 studies, various settings	Delirium is often persistent at discharge and beyond; persistence is associated with dementia, co-morbidity, delirium severity, hypoactive type, and hypoxic illness
Fong et al., 2009	Memory disorder clinic	Over 12 months, patients with dementia who become delirious experience the equivalent of an 18-month decline compared to those who do not experience delirium
von Guten & Mosimann, 2010	Long-term care	Lower cognitive function and depression were risk factors for delirium in residents on admission to a nursing facility
Han et al., 2009	Emergency department	Residing in a nursing home was an independent risk factor for delirium among emergency department patients aged 65+
Han et al., 2010	Emergency department	Delirium was an independent predictor of increased mortality at 6 months among emergency department patients aged 65+
Kiely et al., 2009	Skilled nursing facilities	One-third of 412 older adults who had delirium when discharged from acute care remained delirious at 6 months, and these subjects were 2.9 times more likely to die than those whose delirium resolved
McCaffrey, 2009	Hospital	During 3 days following hip or knee surgery, patients who had listened to music scored higher on the NEECHAM *acute confusion* than those in the control group
Pisani, Murphy, Araujo, & Van Ness, 2010	Medical ICU	Factors significantly associated with a longer duration of delirium were aged 75+, use of opioid doses greater than 54 mg/d, and haloperidol
Rudolph et al., 2010	Hospitals	Delirium occurred in 43% of patients after cardiac surgery and was independently associated with functional decline at 1 month
Silva, Jerussalmy, Farfel, Curiati, & Jacob-Filho, 2009	Hospital	Delirium was associated with higher in-hospital mortality in a group of 856 patients aged 60 to 104 years
Spronk, Riekerk, Hofhuis, & Rommes, 2009	ICU	Delirium occurred in 50% of patients but was poorly recognized by doctors and nurses
Voyer et al., 2009b	Nursing facilities	Use of physical restraints was the precipitating factor most strongly associated with delirium

settings, and delayed treatment is a major reason for increased morbidity and mortality (Flaherty et al., 2009). The Confusion Assessment Method (CAM) has been widely used as a screening tool since 1990 because of its ease of use and high degree of accuracy. A systematic review of literature found that this tool has high sensitivity (94%) and specificity (89%), has been translated into 10 languages, and has been adapted for use in ICU, emergency, and institutional settings (Wei, Fearing, Sternberg, & Inouye, 2008). The CAM follows a four-point algorithm, with the diagnosis of delirium being confirmed by the presence of features one and two and either three or four (Inouye et al., 1990). Flinn, Diehl, Seyfried, and Malani (2009) described the points in the algorithm with corresponding example questions:

1. Acute onset and fluctuating course: Is there evidence of acute change in mental status from baseline or abnormal behavior that tends to come and go or increase and decrease in severity?
2. Inattention: Does the patient have difficulty focusing or keeping track of what is being said? Is she or he easily distracted?
3. Disorganized thinking: Is the patient's thinking or conversation incoherent, disorganized, or illogical? Does he or she unpredictably switch topics?
4. Altered level of consciousness: What is the level of consciousness, and how does it change on the scale from alert, vigilant, lethargic, stupor, or coma?

The Hartford Institute for Geriatric Nursing recommends using CAM and a delirium algorithm for assessing and managing delirium (see Resources: Clinical Tools). Figure 14-1 illustrates a protocol for assessing and managing delirium in older adults, which was developed by the Hospital Elder Life Program (Sandhaus, Harrell, & Valenti, 2006).

Nursing Diagnosis and Outcomes

The nursing diagnosis of Acute Confusion is defined as an "abrupt onset of reversible disturbances of consciousness, attention, cognition, and perception that develop over a short period of time" (NANDA International, 2009, p. 164). Defining characteristics include fluctuation in cognition, consciousness, or psychomotor activity; hallucinations or misperceptions; increased restlessness or agitation; and lack of motivation to initiate or follow through with purposeful or goal-directed behavior.

To address this diagnosis, nurses can use the following Nursing Outcomes Classification (NOC) terms in their care plans: Anxiety Level, Cognition, Cognitive Orientation, Concentration, Distorted Thought Self-Control, Identity, Information Processing, Memory, Mood Equilibrium, Neurologic Status, Psychomotor Energy. In addition, the following NOC terms may be applicable to address causative factors: Electrolyte and Acid/Base Balance, Hydration, Infection Severity, Nutritional Status, Risk Control, and Sensory Function Status.

Wellness Opportunity

Nurses can use the NOC Comfort Level in their care plans to holistically address the needs of older adults with delirium.

Nursing Interventions for Delirium

Because of the complexity of delirium, it requires a multidisciplinary approach to management, with nurses having a key role in detection, ongoing assessment, and management. Models of management typically are multifactorial and include the following components: staff education; comprehensive geriatric assessment; interventions for all contributing factors (e.g., pain, medical conditions, sleep deprivation, adverse medication effects, fluid and electrolyte imbalances, vision or hearing impairments); orientation interventions; environmental modifications; physical and occupational therapies; nutritional interventions; measures for preventing complications (e.g., falls, injuries, sleep problems, pressure ulcers, aspiration); encouraging the presence of family and other support people; and comprehensive discharge planning (Flinn et al., 2009; Holroyd-Leduc, Khandwala, & Sink, 2010; Skrobik, 2009). The following are examples of specific interventions that nurses can include in care plans:

- Provision of aids to orientation (e.g., clock, watch, calendar) and aids to improve sensory function (e.g., eyeglasses, hearing aids)
- Frequent verbal orientation and reminders about daily events
- Environmental modification (e.g., noise reduction, familiar objects)
- Psychological support (e.g., cognitive and social stimulation)
- Identification of adverse medication effects and discussion of medication regimen with prescribing practitioners
- Promotion of physiologic stability (e.g., low-dose oxygenation, maintenance of fluid and electrolyte balance)
- Adequate pain management (refer to Chapter 28)
- Promotion of normal sleep-wake pattern (refer to Chapter 24)
- Maintenance of optimal bowel and bladder function (refer to Chapters 18 and 19)
- Physical activity (e.g., ambulation, physical therapy, occupational therapy)
- Provision of cognitively stimulating activities
- Encouragement of family and support people to be with the person

Figure 14-1 lists examples of research-based nursing interventions that address the physical needs of hospitalized older adults with delirium (Sandhaus et al., 2006).

The following Nursing Interventions Classification (NIC) terms are examples of interventions that can be used in care plans for acute confusion: Anxiety Reduction, Behavior Management, Cognitive Stimulation, Delirium Management, Energy Management, Environmental Management, Fluid/Electrolyte Management, Hallucination Management, Medication Management,

CARING FOR YOUR PATIENT WITH DELIRIUM

Features of delirium

- Acute onset of confusion with a fluctuating course
- Inattention: highly distractible, with difficulty focusing
- Disorganized thinking, altered level of consciousness, or both

Rule out physiologic causes

NEURO EVENT

- Check level of consciousness
- History of recent head injury
  (subdural hematoma)
- Neurologic check, noting motor deficit,
  pupil changes
- Diagnostic testing as ordered
- Lab studies (vitamin B_{12}, folate, blood chemistries,
  thyroid-stimulating hormone)

MEDICATION

- Check recent medication changes. Check drug levels.
  Avoid these medications: benzodiazepines, anticholinergics (diphenhydramine [Benadryl], oxybutynin [Ditropan], metoclopramide [Reglan]), steroids,
  histamine$_2$ blockers (famotidine [Pepcid], ranitidine
  HCl [Zantac]), drugs with high toxicity (digoxin [Lan-
  oxin], phenytoin sodium [Dilantin]), psychotropics

INFECTION

- Consider urinary tract infection or pneumonia
- Check temperature and vital signs
- Lab work
- Chest X-ray
- Urinalysis (culture and sensitivity)
- Blood culture
- Sputum culture

DEHYDRATION

- Monitor intake and output
- Check serum glucose
- Give I.V. fluid as needed
- Review lab work
- Ensure adequate nutrition and hydration
- Check for electrolyte imbalance

HYPOXIA

- Pulse oximetry
- Respiratory rate
- Sputum
- Arterial blood gases
- Chest X-ray

Address physical needs

SAFETY

- Glasses
- Hearing device
- Orientation or reorientation
- Gentle reassurance
- Family at bedside
- Early mobilization
- Fall-prevention protocol
- Consult physical therapy, occupational therapy

PAIN

- Provide comfort, supportive measures
- Give medication as ordered and assess pain control
- Avoid meperidine (Demerol) and
  propoxyphene/acetaminophen (Darvocet), which
  may cause seizures, delirium in elderly
- Use acetaminophen (Tylenol) around the clock
  as first-line analgesic
- Add a laxative to any opioid regimen

ELIMINATION

- Frequent toileting
- Bowel regimen
- Remove urinary drainage catheter as soon
  as possible
- Treat constipation

SLEEP

- Use comfort measures, back rub
- Allow for long intervals of uninterrupted sleep
- Avoid sedative-hypnotic medications

NUTRITION

- Assist or feed
- Give supplements as required
- Consult speech pathologist for swallow
  evaluation, nutritionist
- Skin assessment

SOURCE: Adapted from a delirium algorithm developed at
Moses Taylor Hospital.

FIGURE 14-1 Protocol for assessing and managing delirium in older adults published by the Hospital Elder Life Program. (Reprinted with permission from Sandhaus, S., Harrell, F., & Valenti, D. [2006]. Healthier aging: Here's help to prevent delirium in the hospital. *Nursing, 2006, 36*(7), 60–62.)

Mood Management, Nutrition Management, Pain Management, **Reality Orientation**, Sedation Management, and Surveillance: Safety.

Wellness Opportunity

Nursing interventions to holistically address the needs of older adults during confusional states include use of a Calming Technique, Emotional Support, Music Therapy, Presence, and Touch.

OVERVIEW OF DEMENTIA

Terminology to Describe Dementia

An understanding of impaired cognitive function is complicated by the many terms that are used interchangeably—and often inaccurately—to describe dementia. Recent evidence-based research has greatly improved the ability of clinicians to diagnose and treat different types of dementia, but it has also led to the proliferation of dementia-related terminology. Perhaps more than any other terms used in reference to older adults, those associated with cognitive impairments are the most misused, misunderstood, and emotionally charged. The following are some of the terms that healthcare professionals use in reference to cognitive impairment in older adults: confusion, dementia, senility, **Alzheimer's disease**, small strokes, memory problems, "old-timer's disease," organic brain syndrome, and hardening of the arteries. Different terms are more or less acceptable to different people and often the selection of a term is based on emotional preferences or lack of accurate information. Because cognitive impairment is an emotionally charged subject, nurses must understand the correct terminology, and then, choose the most appropriate term based on an understanding of the underlying causes for the impairment and an assessment of what term is most acceptable to the older adult and his or her caregivers.

By definition, *senility* means old age, and originally, it was a neutral term. Over the past two centuries, however, it became associated with infirmity, diseases, and feeblemindedness. Even today, the term *senile* is associated with conditions that occur simply because a person is old. Because of this long history of inaccurate and negative associations, healthcare professionals are advised never to use terms such as senile or senility.

During the early 1900s, the phrase *hardening of the arteries* was the common diagnostic label for cognitive impairment in older adults. This term suggested that there was a pathologic cause, but the condition was still viewed as an inevitable consequence of aging. This term is now considered outdated and is not used in reference to cognitive impairments.

By the 1950s, the phrase *organic brain syndrome (OBS)* was the commonly used term to describe a constellation of neurologic effects of underlying pathologic conditions. The term *acute organic brain syndrome* (also called *delirium*) referred to treatable conditions, whereas the term *chronic organic brain syndrome (COBS)* referred to an irreversible condition that was associated with vascular pathology. With the use of the terms OBS and COBS, cognitive impairments were no longer viewed as inevitable, but they were still considered untreatable.

In the 1960s, autopsy examination of brain specimens provided the first scientific evidence about the underlying causes of cognitive impairments. Based on these findings, researchers and practitioners concluded that as many as 25% of the changes previously attributed to COBS were actually manifestations of treatable conditions. During the 1970s, *pseudodementia* was used in reference to cognitive impairments caused by physiologic conditions, but this term is no longer used.

Dementia is the medical term that most accurately describes progressive declines in cognitive function. Dementia is a broad diagnostic term that includes a group of brain disorders characterized by a gradual decline in cognitive abilities (e.g., memory, understanding, judgment, decision-making, communication) and changes in personality and behavior. Unfortunately, this medical term is associated with the lay term "demented," which has a long history of pejorative use and is even more derogatory than the word "senile." Thus, nurses can use phrases such as "a person with dementia" or a "person with a dementing illness" to accurately refer to the medical syndrome of impaired cognitive function while avoiding pejorative connotations.

An additional point must be emphasized with regard to the term *dementia*. Dementia is not a single disease but a syndrome, and the term refers to a combination of manifestations that arise from different causes. Because Alzheimer's disease is the most common type of dementia, and the type with the longest history of recognition, *Alzheimer's disease* and *dementia* are often used interchangeably. Although knowledge about different types of dementia has increased significantly in recent decades, common usage of terms is not always accurate, even among healthcare professionals. In this chapter, theories about dementia are discussed in the following section, and the four most widely recognized types of dementia are described in the section on Types of Dementia. The term *dementia* is used throughout the chapter except when the information is pertinent to a particular type. The text refers to Alzheimer's disease when a source used that term; however, readers need to recognize that many of the citations in the literature on Alzheimer's disease refer to dementia in the broader sense.

Theories to Explain Dementia

The evolution of dementia terminology is indicative of the significant developments in our understanding of this syndrome during the past century. In recent decades, major progress was made in identifying pathologic changes, risk factors, and manifestations that characterize different types of dementia. However, despite more than 100 years of research on causes of impaired cognitive function in older adults, theories to explain dementia are still evolving and many questions remain unanswered.

During the 1800s, European physicians discovered neuritic plaques in the brains of older adults and identified these changes as the cause of senility or senile dementia. Around that same time, medical scientists discovered that arteries throughout the body lose their elasticity and grow hardened during later adulthood, and they theorized that this was the underlying cause of the brain changes in older adults. In 1906, Alois Alzheimer—a German physician—discovered that neuritic plaques in the autopsied brain specimens from a woman who was 55 years old at the time of her death had initially manifested cognitive and behavior changes around the age of 50 years. Based on these findings, physicians and researchers concluded that neuritic plaques caused presenile dementia, hardening of the arteries caused senile dementia, and Alzheimer's disease and senile dementia were distinct diseases differentiated by age at onset. Simply stated, if the onset of the cognitive impairment occurred before the age of 65 years, it was called Alzheimer's disease, whereas if the onset took place after the age of 65 years, it was called senility or a hardening of the arteries.

This chronologic distinction between senile and presenile dementia was not challenged until the 1960s, when autopsy studies found no association between the degree of atherosclerotic brain changes and the clinical manifestations of dementia during the person's lifetime. These landmark studies by Tomlinson, Blessed, and Roth (1968, 1970) led to the conclusion that the neuropathologic changes of Alzheimer's disease represent a single disease process, regardless of the age at onset. In 1974, another landmark study by Hachinski, Lassen, and Marshall found that cerebral atherosclerosis was both a major cause of cognitive impairments and the most common medical *mis*diagnosis. Moreover, these scientists denounced the use of the phrase "hardening of the arteries" and introduced the term "multi-infarct dementia" to describe dementias of cerebrovascular origin. Their rationale was that dementia was not caused by atherosclerosis or chronic ischemia but by the occurrence of multiple cerebral infarcts. Recent research indicates that both these terms are outdated and inaccurate, and the term **vascular dementia** is more appropriate, as discussed in the section on Types of Dementia.

Since the 1990s, theories about dementia have expanded, largely due to the development of brain imaging techniques that can provide information about different aspects of brain function. For example, computed tomography (CT) and magnetic resonance imaging (MRI) provide information about structural brain changes and lesions that can cause cognitive impairment. Single photon emission computed tomography (SPECT) and positron emission tomography (PET) scans provide specific information about metabolism rates for glucose and oxygen in the brain. Researchers currently use information from imaging techniques to supplement information from autopsies, clinical records, mental status tests, and other sources. In addition, many longitudinal studies provide valuable information about lifestyle patterns and cognitive function during adulthood, and some studies are designed to evaluate this information in relation to autopsy findings.

Diagnosing Dementia

Even with current advances in technology, the diagnosis of dementia is as much of an art as a science and pathologic brain changes can be clearly identified only on autopsy. The current approach to diagnosing dementia can be likened to the approach taken to diagnosing an infection. An infection is a generic diagnosis indicating the presence of a constellation of signs and symptoms (e.g., malaise, elevated temperature), but it does not indicate the causative factor. As additional information is collected, the specific type of infection is identified (e.g., pneumonia, urinary tract infection, bacterial, viral), and sometimes, more than one infection is discovered. Until the specific causative agent is identified, generic measures are taken (e.g., antipyretics, broad-spectrum antibiotics). After the specific causative agent is identified (e.g., through culture and sensitivity tests), the infection is treated with very specific antimicrobial agents. At all stages, comfort measures are used. Analogously, dementia is a generic diagnosis indicating a constellation of signs and symptoms (e.g., memory impairment, personality changes), but there are no clear indicators during early stages of most types of dementia. As the condition progresses and further information develops, one or more causative factors is likely to be identified. However, there is no diagnostic equivalent of a "culture and sensitivity" test for dementia, so it is difficult to distinguish between the different types of dementia. Thus, diagnosis of specific types of dementia is based on clinical observations, history of risk factors, and information from brain imaging and other available diagnostic data.

TYPES OF DEMENTIA

This chapter reviews current information about the four most commonly recognized types of dementia. It is important to realize that research is evolving, and there are significant overlaps in manifestations of the different types of dementia. Another complicating factor is that two (or more) types of dementia can—and often do—coexist in the same person; as the pathologic processes progress, it becomes more difficult to distinguish one type of dementia from another. Autopsy studies of older people who have died with dementia find that mixed pathologies account for most cases of dementia and that multiple neuropathologies are particularly common among those over the age of 80 years (Flicker, 2010; Jellinger & Attems, 2010). This chapter presents information that is clinically important in relation to each of the four most common types of dementia; however, information about functional consequences, assessment, and interventions applies to all types. Table 14-2 describes the distinguishing features of the four most common types of dementia: Alzheimer's disease, vascular dementia, **Lewy body dementia**, and **frontotemporal dementia**.

TABLE 14-2 Distinguishing Features of Common Types of Dementia

Type	Onset and Course	Typical Manifestations
Alzheimer's disease	Insidious onset; diagnosis often made retrospectively; slowly progressive over 5 to 10 years	Initial memory loss followed by gradual loss of other cognitive and communication abilities (e.g., confusion, disorientation, executive dysfunction); behavior and personality changes (e.g., depression, irritability, agitation, indifference)
Vascular dementia	Abrupt onset; stepwise decline over 5 years; history of vascular risks (e.g., stroke, hypertension)	Manifestations consistent with area of brain that is affected:, aphasia, memory impairment, apathy, depression, emotional lability, and sensory-motor deficits (e.g., hemiparesis, gait disturbances, hemisensory loss, urinary incontinence)
Lewy body dementia	Insidious onset with a progressive decline in cognitive, behavioral, and motor symptoms	Significant cognitive impairment; fluctuating levels of cognition; parkinsonism; hallucinations; sleep disturbances; loss of postural stability; highly sensitive to neuroleptic medications
Frontotemporal dementia	Gradual onset between the ages of 45 and 65; family history common; progressive decline in functioning	Early and progressive personality changes; language impairment (with or without impaired comprehension); behavioral disturbances (e.g., disinhibition, impulsivity, loss of empathy, apathy, repetitive behaviors)

Alzheimer's Disease

Various figures on the prevalence of Alzheimer's disease have been quoted, with many estimates indicating that 50% of people aged 85 years or older and up to 80% of nursing home residents have Alzheimer's disease. Although findings about the rates of Alzheimer's disease at specific ages vary, increased age is considered a major risk factor with the incidence and prevalence doubling every 5 years between the ages of 65 and 90 years (Jellinger & Attems, 2010; Kamat, Kamat, & Grossberg, 2010).

Pathologic Changes Associated With Alzheimer's Disease

The hallmark pathologic criterion for Alzheimer's disease is the presence of neuritic plaques and neurofibrillary tangles, as identified by Alzheimer in the early 1900s and confirmed by numerous autopsy studies performed since the 1960s. Although these pathologic alterations also occur in normal aging and other neurodegenerative diseases, the combination of a higher density in specific regions (e.g., the neocortex and hippocampus) and a clinical history consistent with Alzheimer's disease confirms the diagnosis of Alzheimer's disease. Loss or degeneration of neurons and synapses in these same regions is another central feature of Alzheimer's disease pathology. In addition, Alzheimer's disease is associated with a marked reduction in brain weight, as illustrated in Figure 14-2.

Alzheimer first described **beta-amyloid** as a "peculiar substance" in 1907, but this substance was not named or defined until 1984. By the early 1990s, scientists had identified beta-amyloid in the plaques and blood vessels as another pathologic hallmark of Alzheimer's disease. The discovery that beta-amyloid was a normal substance produced by many cells in the body laid the groundwork for much of the current research on the role of beta-amyloid and its precursor protein. Scientists now know that beta-amyloid is a tiny, insoluble protein fragment of a much larger protein called the *amyloid precursor protein*. The exact functions of the amyloid precursor protein have not been identified, but researchers recognize that this protein has multiple essential roles in cells throughout the body. What is known is that excessive amounts of beta-amyloid are found in the neuritic plaques and in the walls of the blood vessels in the brains of people with Alzheimer's disease and Down syndrome. Current research indicates that abnormal processing of beta-amyloid is the initiating event in Alzheimer's disease pathology and that this process does not immediately affect cognitive function (Jack et al., 2010).

Pathologic brain changes of Alzheimer's disease trigger changes in neurotransmitters that lead to the degeneration of healthy neurons and, eventually, to cell death. Specific effects on neurotransmitters include the loss of serotonin receptors and decreased production of acetylcholine, acetylcholinesterase, and choline acetyltransferase. The greatest reduction in transmitters

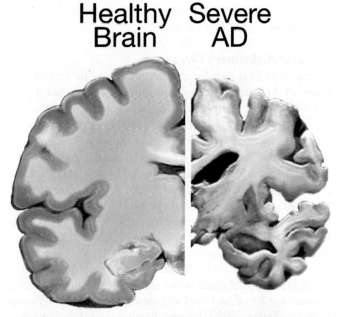

FIGURE 14-2 Pathologic brain changes cause significant atrophy. (Courtesy of the National Institute on Aging/National Institutes of Health.)

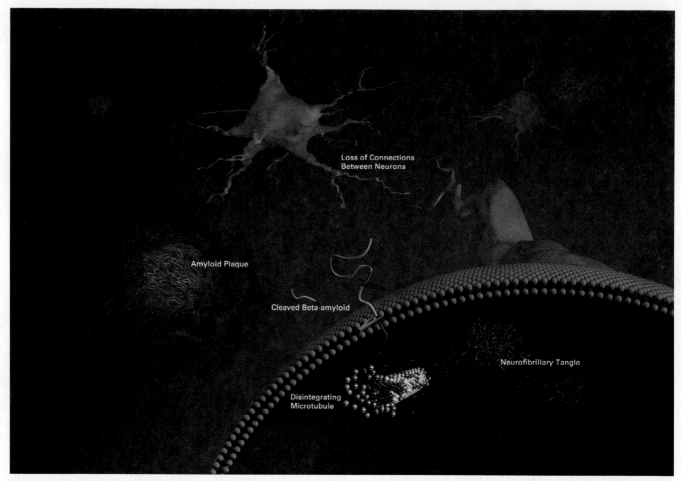

Loss of Connections
Between Neurons

Amyloid Plaque

Cleaved Beta-amyloid

Neurofibrillary Tangle

Disintegrating
Microtubule

FIGURE 14-3 Hallmark neuropathologic changes in Alzheimer's disease. (Courtesy of the National Institute on Aging/National Institutes of Health.)

occurs in the areas most affected by plaques and tangles, and these changes cause both cognitive and behavioral symptoms. Figure 14-3 illustrates the pathologic processes that are characteristic of Alzheimer's disease.

Risks for Alzheimer's Disease

Researchers first raised questions about genetic factors as a cause of Alzheimer's disease in the mid-1930s, but it was not until the late 1970s that the phrase "familial Alzheimer's disease" appeared in the literature. Familial (also called *early onset*) Alzheimer's disease refers to families in which two or more members—usually in more than one generation—have Alzheimer's disease. Onset for this type of Alzheimer's disease is typically before age 65 and often before age 55. Children of affected parents have a 25% to 50% chance of having Alzheimer's disease, and the risk is higher if the disease occurs in more than one generation and when the disease onset is before age 65 (Kamat et al., 2010). Abnormalities on chromosomes 1, 14, and 21 are associated with early onset familial Alzheimer's disease, but these abnormalities account for less than 1% of all types of Alzheimer's disease (Ertekin-Taner, 2010). Recent discoveries related to beta-amyloid, chromosomal mutations, and the amyloid precursor

protein form the basis for much genetics research. For example, people with Down syndrome have an extra chromosome 21 where the amyloid precursor protein gene is located, and they inevitably show Alzheimer's disease–like brain changes at around age 40 years. In addition, risk of Down syndrome increases in families of individuals with Alzheimer's disease.

Researchers are particularly interested in genetic factors associated with the later onset type of Alzheimer's disease, which constitutes between 90% and 95% of cases. Since the mid-1990s, a major focus of this research is on elucidating the role of the APOE genotype on chromosome 19. The three variants of the APOE genotype are designated as APOE-$_E$2, APOE-$_E$3, and APOE-$_E$4. Each person inherits one APOE gene from each parent, so there are six possible combinations (2/2, 2/3, 2/4, 3/3, 3/4, and 4/4). The inherited combination may be at least partially predictive of the risk for Alzheimer's disease, particularly with regard to APOE-$_E$4 (Tan & Seshadri, 2010). For example, APOE-$_E$3 genotype carriers have two to four times the risk of developing Alzheimer's disease than someone with APOE-$_E$3/$_E$3, and the odds increase to between 6 and 30 times for carriers of APOE-$_E$4/$_E$4 (Ertekin-Taner, 2010). By contrast, APOE-$_E$2 is associated with both a decreased risk for Alzheimer's disease and a later age at onset if the disease does develop.

Another area of intense research is the potential link between neuroinflammatory processes and Alzheimer's disease. Recent studies indicate that neuroinflammation could play a critical role in triggering the formation of neurofibrillary tangles that are characteristic of Alzheimer's disease (Metcalfe & Figueiredo-Pereira, 2010). Oxidative stress and immune dysregulation are two mechanisms that lead to these neuroinflammatory processes (Ciaramella et al., 2010; McNaull, Todd, McGuinness, & Passmore, 2010). This evolving area of research has potential for leading to promising interventions involving immunizations or drugs (DiBona et al., 2010; Tabira, 2010; von Bernhardi, 2010).

In addition to research on genetic factors and inflammatory processes, researchers are focusing on the following modifiable risks: depression, hypertension, diabetes, hyperlipidemia, smoking, obesity, heart failure, atrial fibrillation, low levels of mental and physical activity, and high dietary intake of total fat, saturated fat, and total cholesterol (de Toledo Ferraz Alves, Ferreira, Wajngarten, & Busatto, 2010; Kamat et al., 2010). Researchers are also investigating the potential role of conditions that occur during earlier years, which can increase the risk for developing dementia during later adulthood. For example, studies have found a dose-dependent relationship between moderate or severe head trauma and Alzheimer's disease (Kumar & Kinsella, 2010). Studies also show an association between brain damage and some heavy metals (e.g., lead, mercury, aluminum, manganese) and many environmental toxins (e.g., solvents, carbon monoxide). However, studies to date have not determined any direct link between these conditions and dementia (Kumar & Kinsella, 2010).

Preclinical Alzheimer's Disease

In recent years, longitudinal studies involving clinical studies during life and autopsy studies have confirmed that pathologic changes affect the brain years before symptoms are obvious. Thus, the concept of asymptomatic or preclinical Alzheimer's disease has emerged, and researchers and practitioners are trying to identify the factors that protect some people with pathologic changes from experiencing symptoms (Iacono et al., 2009). Currently, longitudinal studies are investigating the trajectory of people with **mild cognitive impairment (MCI)**, which is a transitional stage between normal cognitive aging and diagnosable dementia (Kelley & Minagar, 2009). People with MCI have short-term memory impairment, some difficulty with complex cognitive skills (e.g., written arithmetic), and more difficulty with daily activities. Longitudinal studies have consistently found that MCI is associated with a higher risk for Alzheimer's disease, a more rapid decline, and higher mortality (Knopman, 2010). Pathologic brain changes can be correlated with stages of disease as illustrated in Figure 14-4. Cognitive and behavioral changes associated with each of these stages are discussed in the section on Functional Consequences.

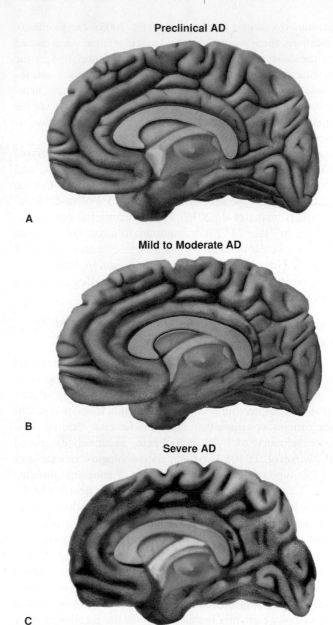

Preclinical AD

A

Mild to Moderate AD

B

Severe AD

C

FIGURE 14-4 **(A)** During preclinical Alzheimer's disease, subtle degenerative changes begin to occur, and the person develops mild cognitive impairment. **(B)** In mild to moderate stages of Alzheimer's disease, pathologic changes affect the areas of the brain that control memory, language, and reasoning. **(C)** In the severe stage of Alzheimer's disease, pathologic changes cause significant atrophy in many areas. (Courtesy of the National Institute on Aging/National Institutes of Health.)

Vascular Dementia

Vascular dementia has been identified as a common and distinct type of dementia for several decades. However, recent studies, particularly those based on autopsies, indicate that cerebrovascular damage most often occurs concurrently with the neuropathologic changes of other dementias. One study found that only 3% of 382 autopsied brains showed pure vascular dementia, and another study found that vascular lesions coexisted with Alzheimer's pathology in 77% of the cases of presumed vascular dementia (Morris, 2005). Despite these questions, there is agreement that vascular dementia is caused by the death of nerve cells in the regions nourished by the diseased vessels. Underlying pathologic processes can include infarctions from occlusion of large blood vessels, hemorrhage of large or small blood vessels, lacunar strokes of the small arteries, and Binswanger's disease involving diffuse lesions of the white matter (Cherubini et al., 2010).

Cardiovascular risk factors that are strongly associated with vascular dementia include stroke, hypertension, and atrial fibrillation. In addition, recent studies indicate that the APOE-ε4 genotype accounts for almost 25% of vascular dementia (Chuang et al., 2010). Typical manifestations are described in Table 14-2. It is important to recognize that even though vascular dementia is characterized by an abrupt onset and a stepwise progression, when it occurs in combination with other types of dementia—which it often does—the onset and progression appear to be gradual.

Lewy Body Dementia

Although **Lewy body dementia** is often cited as the second most prevalent type of dementia, it is often misdiagnosed as a movement disorder or Alzheimer's disease. A study of caregivers of people with Lewy body dementia found that half of the patients saw more than 3 doctors for more than 10 visits over the course of 1 year before being accurately diagnosed (Galvin et al., 2010). Two hallmark pathologic characteristics of this type of dementia are deposits of abnormal proteins (i.e., Lewy bodies) and formation of Lewy neurites in the brain. Because these same pathologic changes also occur in Parkinson's disease, scientists have described Lewy body dementia and Parkinson's disease as two sides of the same coin in a continuum of Lewy body diseases (Klein et al., 2010). Also, because autopsy studies found these pathologic changes in 14% to 24% of the brains of older adults who had no clinical manifestations of dementia, gerontologists suspect that Lewy body dementia has an asymptomatic preclinical stage (Frigerio et al., 2009; Markesbery, Jicha, Liu, & Schmitt, 2009). Researchers have not identified specific risks for this type of dementia; however, a family history of dementia is present in one quarter of people with Lewy body dementia (Farina et al., 2009).

Table 14-2 lists distinguishing features of Lewy body dementia. Nurses and primary care practitioners need to be alert to the clinical implications of the increased neuroleptic sensitivity that is characteristic of Lewy body dementia. People with this type of dementia are likely to have extreme, idiosyncratic, or fatal reactions to even low doses of cholinergic-type medications such as antipsychotics. For example, sedatives or antipsychotics may cause hallucinations, agitation, or extreme somnolence. Thus, anticholinergic medications, including over-the-counter products, should be avoided, and if they are used, doses should be minimal, and patients should be observed carefully for adverse effects. Another clinically important characteristic is that people with Lewy body dementia may decompensate rapidly and significantly when they have a medical condition (e.g., minor infection) or when their environment is changed. Also cognitive fluctuations commonly occur over minutes, hours, or days. Because of the serious clinical implications of this type of dementia and because it is often unrecognized, nurses need to be alert to the possibility that someone with Lewy body dementia may be misdiagnosed with another type of dementia or with Parkinson's disease.

Frontotemporal Dementia

Frontotemporal dementia describes a group of neurodegenerative conditions associated with disorders of tau (a type of protein in neurons) that cause atrophy in the frontal and temporal lobes. Frontotemporal dementia accounts for 30% to 50% of cases of dementia in people younger than 65 years of age, with the average age of onset being 54 years (Kertesz, 2010). Pick's disease was first identified as a type of frontotemporal dementia in 1892, and in recent years, scientists have classified frontotemporal dementia according to clinical presentations as behavioral or language (also called semantic) variants (Arvanitakis, 2010; Gordon et al., 2010). Researchers have linked frontotemporal dementia to abnormalities of at least 5 genes, and 30% to 50% of people with this type of dementia have a family history of early onset dementia (Riedijk, Niermeijer, Dooijes, & Tibben, 2009). Clinical manifestations of frontotemporal dementia (described in Table 14-2) differ significantly from those of other types of dementia during early stages. However, during middle and later stages, neuropsychiatric behaviors (e.g., apathy, irritability) are similar to, but more intense than, behaviors in other dementias (Grochmal-Bach et al., 2009).

FACTORS ASSOCIATED WITH DEMENTIA

From a wellness perspective, it is important to recognize not only the factors that increase the risk for dementia (as discussed in the section on types of dementia) but also those that protect against cognitive impairment. A state-of-the-science conference statement released by the National Institutes of Health (Daviglus et al., 2010) concluded that firm evidence-based recommendations cannot be drawn about the association of modifiable risk factors associated with cognitive decline. However, the consensus panel did recommend ongoing studies of interventions such as antihypertensive medications, omega-3 fatty acid, physical activity, and cognitive engagement. Table 14-3 summarizes some recent research findings related to strategies to prevent cognitive decline. One consistent finding is that many of the behaviors that have positive outcomes for overall wellness, including physical activity and healthy dietary practices, also have a positive effect on preventing cognitive decline.

As discussed in Chapter 11, there is increasing interest in the concept of **cognitive reserve**, which is the capacity to continue to function at an adequate cognitive level despite

TABLE 14-3 Research Evidence: Studies of Strategies to Prevent Cognitive Impairment

Researchers	Results
Duron & Hanon, 2010	Review of seven randomized double-blind, placebo-controlled trials of antihypertensives: Positive results, in terms of preventing dementia, were found in three of the trials, nonsignificant results were noted in four of the trials.
Eskelinen & Kivipelto, 2010	Review of longitudinal epidemiologic studies: Three of five found that coffee had favorable effects against cognitive decline; two other studies found positive effects on cognitive function from combined coffee and tea drinking.
Hamaguchi, Ono, & Yamada, 2010	In vitro studies indicate that curcumin may be one of the most promising compounds for prevention and treatment of dementia; however, two of four ongoing clinical trials have reported no significant benefits.
Kim, Lee, & Lee, 2010	Animal and laboratory studies indicate that curcumin, resveratrol, and green tea (naturally occurring phytochemicals) have potential for preventing Alzheimer's disease.
McGuinness & Passmore, 2010	Some clinical studies have found that Alzheimer's disease was substantially reduced in people who took statin medications, but randomized trials have not yet demonstrated preventive effects.
Morley, 2010	Epidemiologic and animal studies indicate that vitamin D, DHA (an omega-3 fatty acid), lutein, and alpha-lipoic acid have the best chance of proving to be clinically useful for improving cognitive function.
Radak et al., 2010	Regular physical activity is beneficial in preventing Alzheimer's disease and other neurodegenerative disorders.
Robinson, Ijioma, & Harris, 2010	Epidemiologic studies found a protective association between omega-3 fatty acids and prevention of cognitive decline.
Rolland, van Kan, & Vellas, 2010	Biologic and epidemiologic studies and short-term randomized controlled trials in nondemented participants indicate that physical activity improves cognitive function in older adults.
Scarmeas et al., 2009	Physical activity and a Mediterranean-type diet are independently associated with a reduced risk for Alzheimer's disease.
Sofi, Macchi, Abbate, Gensini, & Casini, 2010	Greater adherence to a Mediterranean diet is associated with decreased risk for Alzheimer's disease and other chronic degenerative diseases.
Weinmann, Roll, Schwarzbach, Vauth, & Willich, 2010	A meta-analysis of nine trials found a statistically significant advantage for people using standardized extract of ginkgo biloba compared to placebo for improving cognition.

brain pathology. One gerontologist commented that the final decade of the 1900s was called the Decade of the Brain, and the first decade of the 2000s could be designated as the Decade of Brain Fitness because of the current focus on improving and sustaining human cognitive function to the end of life (LaRue, 2010). Nurses have suggested that interventions to enhance cognitive reserve in people with early stage dementia may also be interventions to prevent delirium (Fick, Kolanowski, Beattie, & McCrow, 2009). Specific preventive strategies suggested by Fick and colleagues include physical activity, social interaction, challenging mental activities, and avoidance of inappropriate medications.

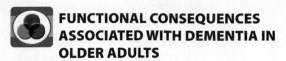

Wellness Opportunity

Nurses can teach all adults that engaging in social, mental, and physical activity is a risk-free way of promoting cognitive wellness and may also prevent dementia.

FUNCTIONAL CONSEQUENCES ASSOCIATED WITH DEMENTIA IN OLDER ADULTS

Functional consequences of dementia are discussed primarily in reference to Alzheimer's disease because these have been studied since the 1950s, and gerontologists are just beginning to identify the unique manifestations of different dementias. Moreover, many functional consequences are common to all of the dementias, and as pathologic processes progress, manifestations of all types of dementia become more similar. It is important to recognize, however, that during all stages and in all types of dementia, functional consequences vary tremendously among individuals because of unique personality characteristics, coexisting conditions (e.g., depression, functional impairments), and other influences. It also is imperative to acknowledge that the personhood of each individual who has dementia is always present and needs to be addressed in every interaction. In this and the following sections of this chapter, the experiences of people with dementia are included to illustrate the unique ways in which dementia affects individuals and their care partners. In addition to the functional consequences that directly affect the person with dementia, caregivers and families of people with dementia also experience significant consequences, and these are discussed in Chapter 27 of this text.

Stages of Dementia

In the mid-1980s, an American psychiatrist, Reisberg, proposed a seven-stage model for describing the functional consequences of Alzheimer's disease. Reisberg's staging schema, which has been updated and refined, is referred to as the Global Deterioration Scale/Functional Assessment Staging, or GDS/FAST. This staging system is widely used and has been found to be valid and reliable for staging Alzheimer's disease in diverse settings (Sabbagh et al., 2009). Table 14-4 summarizes the functional consequences associated with each of the seven stages of the GDS/FAST. According to this framework, the diagnosis of Alzheimer's disease is made retrospectively because it is based on a progression of manifestations.

Gerontologists, clinicians, people with dementia, and families and caregivers are intensely interested in identifying factors that influence not only the course of the disease but the person's survival time. One review of 48 studies that evaluated dementia prognosis and survival found that increased age, male gender, decreased functional status, and medical comorbidities were associated with a higher mortality rate in

TABLE 14-4 Global Deterioration Scale/Functional Assessment Staging (GDS/FAST) of Alzheimer's Disease

Stage	Effects on Functioning
1: Normal adult	No deficits or complaints
2: Age-associated memory impairment	Deficits consistent with normal aging (i.e., no objective findings, difficulty with word finding, forgets location of objects)
3: Mild cognitive impairment	Some deficits in performing complex tasks, particularly in demanding social and employment settings; diminished organizational skills; deficits noted by others for the first time
4: Mild dementia	Diminished ability to perform complex tasks (e.g., meal planning, financial management); decreased knowledge of current and recent events; flattened affect and withdrawal from challenging situations
5: Moderate dementia	Obvious cognitive deficits; unable to manage complex daily tasks without some supervision or assistance; difficulty remembering names of familiar people
6: Moderately severe dementia	Increasingly obvious cognitive deficits (e.g., disorientation, significant short-term memory impairment); personality and emotional changes (e.g., anxiety, delusions) Loss of abilities in the following order: (a) Difficulty putting clothing on properly without assistance (b) Unable to bathe independently (c) Unable to handle all aspects of toileting (e.g., does not wipe properly) (d) Occasional or frequent urinary incontinence (e) Occasional or frequent fecal incontinence
7: Severe dementia	Progressive loss of all verbal and psychomotor abilities: (a) Verbal abilities limited to six or fewer different words (b) Verbal abilities limited to a single intelligible word (c) Unable to walk without assistance (d) Unable to sit without assistance (e) Unable to smile (f) Unable to hold up head independently

Source: Reisberg, B. (1986). Dementia: A systematic approach to identifying reversible causes. *Geriatrics, 41*(4), 30–46.

people with dementia (Lee & Chodosh, 2009). Because dementia is strongly associated with shortened life expectancy, it is widely recognized as a terminal illness with death being the ultimate functional consequence. Thus, in recent years, there has been increasing recognition of the need to provide hospice and palliative care services during late-stage dementia.

Self-awareness of People With Dementia

One of the myths associated with dementia is that people with dementia deny their symptoms or have no awareness of their deficits. Unfortunately, this fallacy has led to serious misunderstandings on the part of some healthcare professionals as exemplified by statements such as, "If they can ask if they have Alzheimer's disease, then they don't have it." In recent years, this perception of a high prevalence of so-called denial in people with dementia has diminished, and gerontologists are researching insight and self-awareness through all stages of dementia. Lack of awareness of cognitive deficit, called *anosognosia,* is now recognized as a core diagnostic feature of frontotemporal dementia; it also occurs with Alzheimer's dementia when the frontal cortex is affected (Salmon et al., 2008; Shibata, Narumoto, Kitabayashi, Ushijima, & Fukui, 2008). However, increasing evidence shows that even when people with dementia have anosognosia, they maintain self-awareness of their needs and feelings, called **retained awareness**, from early stages to later stages (Bossen, Specht, & McKenzie, 2009). Studies also find that retained awareness is relevant to the identification of needs, particularly with regard to personal control, education and support, protection of self-esteem, and managing responses to the disease (Specht, Taylor, & Bossen, 2009). Even in later stages, the personhood—defined as the quality of being a person—of people with dementia is increasingly changed and hidden but not lost (Edvardsson, Winbad, & Sandman, 2008). Programs emphasizing the provision of person-centered care through all stages of dementia are based on these research findings. Studies of the feelings and experiences of individuals with dementia provide important insight into the awareness they retain, as described in boxes throughout this chapter with direct quotes from people with dementia. Box 14-1 summarizes statements of people with dementia about how they are perceived by others.

Personal Experiences of Dementia

During the early stages, only the individual with dementia and people who live, work, or have close contact with the person notice the initial changes, such as impaired judgment and short-term memory. When the changes are noticed, numerous explanations may be applicable, and the deficits may be attributed to such factors as depression or the occurrence of a major life event (e.g., retirement, widowhood). People in the early stages of dementia may withdraw from complex tasks as a way of protecting themselves from the effects of diminishing cognitive abilities. For example, employed people may retire without acknowledging cognitive impairments as the reason. People who do not have to perform complex intellectual or psychomotor tasks may be able to conceal or compensate for the cognitive losses until the deficits seriously interfere with activities of daily living (ADLs). As the disease progresses, however, the person with dementia is less able to cover up the changes, and people with less intimate contact will begin to question the underlying cause of the deficits.

Many first-person accounts of the lived experiences of people with dementia have been published since the 1990s. Although most of these memoirs describe dementia as an overwhelming challenge to be struggled with, defeated by, or succumbed to, some personal narratives reflect positive themes such as resiliency, a strong sense of self, striving for normalcy. Thus, it is important that healthcare practitioners recognize that the extent to which dementia is viewed as problematic varies. A study by Hulko (2009) suggested that people who are "more privileged" are more likely to view

Box 14-1   Lived Experiences: How People With Dementia Feel About Other's Perceptions

- It would be nice if a lot of people had more understanding and appreciate what you have got. I was in town, and this other lady started laughing because of the way I was trying to struggle to talk and that started to make me feel uncomfortable; I thought if only she understood, then perhaps she wouldn't stand there and laugh.
- If you say to someone, "Can you wait a couple of minutes; I've got dementia and I want to explain," they look at you and think there is nothing wrong with you; you should not be able to talk. Then again, you get some who say "HOW-ARE-YOU?" and you think, "Grr, I'm not that bad."
- It's as though that's it, you are dribbling and nodding, and that's the picture of Alzheimer's. But we are all sitting here and talking perfectly normally. We have got Alzheimer's of some form; we are not nodding and dribbling.
- The stigma is far more than cancer, far more . . . and people still do not talk about dementia; they still try to avoid it.
- I'm trying to guard that I don't get looked down on. I don't want the feeling of being back in first grade or whatever . . . of going in the other direction, of decreasing instead of improving, and I have inward anger.
- Everybody I have met has been absolutely amazed that (a) I can still talk and still think, and (b) that I have a diagnosis of dementia. They do not understand it.

- How another person reacts to you can make you very unhappy.
- No one really understands how hard it is to live life like this, so people tend to trivialize how you feel, patronize you, and make out that they feel the same way.
- Written off as being devoid of feelings and needs . . . It was clear to me that my dementia negated the things that I said. It was very painful.
- It has been proven by thousands of early stage people with dementia to be capable and intelligent beings just moving a little slower.
- My family members' relationships with me changed as soon as they found out that I was "no longer competent." The things that I say seem to be a lot more subject to question than they used to be. It's as if I can't possibly know anything anymore. At least that's the way I feel.
- Nobody thought to consider my background; nobody wanted to know about that. "Oh no, that doesn't matter, let's just look at you now." I think the difficulty is that you need a snapshot of how you were to compare it to how you are. They have no interest in that.

Sources: Alzheimer's Society (2008); Alzheimer's Society (2010a); Alzheimer's Society (2010b); Beard & Fox (2008); Beard, Knauss, & Moyer (2009); Clare, Rowlands, & Quin (2008).

dementia negatively and those who are more "marginalized" will dismiss the significance of dementia and resist being viewed as the sum of their symptoms (Hulko, 2009). Box 14-2 describes the experiences and feelings of people with dementia about the earliest changes and their diagnoses.

Common emotions and behaviors of people with dementia include loss, fear, shame, anger, sadness, anxiety, frustration, loneliness, depression, uncertainty, sense of uselessness, self-blame, diminished affect, and withdrawal from challenging activities. A major focus of emotional responses, particularly

Box 14-2   Lived Experiences: Feelings About Earliest Dementia Changes

- I knew my brain wasn't what it used to be because I've always remembered that I gave birth to my girls and one time I thought, "I can't remember what their birthday is."
- To sing a song that I have sung 100 times before to music I have heard 100 times before and I'm standing there thinking, "What the hell am I doing here and what am I going to sing?" This started to happen more and more, and when you are out on the stage on your own and you don't know what you are doing, it is a terrifying prospect.
- If I was getting dressed in the morning, I would put my clothes on, and I would guarantee you there was at least a pair of trousers, a shirt, or a hat and coat—and it had all gone on upside down, back to front.
- I was struggling at work. I became disorganized and was losing control of the class, which is something I had never done.
- I'm still the same person I've always been. It's just that now I'm *me* with Alzheimer's. I am still loving and caring, and I still have feelings, and I would like to think that I haven't changed in myself.
- Although I was expecting it by then, the words were still devastating to hear.
- I feel like I still have enough intelligence to be a person and not just someone you pat on the head as you go by . . . It's devastating, and it takes away your sense of self. I feel like I'm still a person and my wants and desires should at least be considered before decisions are made.

- I felt I had a shock. I just thought it can't be. I said it's for other people.
- The angst and anger that I went through during the diagnostic process. I could have actually gone and thumped people.
- It was as if the thunderclouds had been taken away because they had given an answer to me why I was treating my family so like a louse that I was.
- I was relieved really that what I was trying to convince people had been verified.
- I think the word Alzheimer's puts like a fear in you, like cancer does.
- I still have a memory so that's the good part. I forget that I have got dementia.
- It is a really frightening thing when no one can tell you how fast you will deteriorate. It is hard to get across how that feels, but it gnaws at you continually, and each day you wonder what faculty will be lost next.
- It is quite strange because dementia seems to hit people in very different ways. There are little threads of commonality in it, but everyone is affected in a slightly different way.
- I think I have a very different view about how long I'll be around, or when life will come to an end, or when I'll be incompetent than I did before the diagnosis. No question.
- I certainly think that it's important to let family be aware of one's problems. Not to the extent of complaining and complaining, but this is what it is, and I have to deal with that. I wouldn't deny it ever.

Sources: Alzheimer's Society (2008); Alzheimer's Society (2010a); Alzheimer's Society (2010b); Beard & Fox (2008); Beard, Knauss, & Moyer (2009); Clare, Rowlands, & Quin (2008).

during the early stages, is on readjusting one's self-concept, trying to maintain a sense of normalcy, and developing cognitive, social, and behavioral strategies to improve confidence (Cotter, 2009). Even during the later stages of dementia when cognitive abilities are severely impaired, emotional responses are directed toward preserving a sense of self. Dominant emotions during later stages of dementia include feelings of loss, anger, frustration, uncertainty, and lack of control or self-determination (Clare, Rowlands, & Quin, 2008). It is imperative to recognize that emotional responses of people with dementia may be blunted or altered, but they are never absent. As dementia progresses, the person is likely to express emotions nonverbally and behaviorally. Thus, two important responsibilities of caregivers are to encourage and interpret nonverbal communication, which becomes the primary mode of communication during later stages of dementia.

✦ Wellness Opportunity

Nurses holistically address psychosocial needs by recognizing that individuals vary significantly in their emotional responses, but people with dementia never lose the ability to respond to others.

Behavioral and Psychological Symptoms of Dementia

People with dementia exhibit a wide range of behaviors that are superimposed on their cognitive impairments. Gerontologists and clinicians commonly refer to these as **behavioral and psychological symptoms of dementia (BPSD)**, and studies have found prevalence rates between 58% and 97%, with higher prevalence being associated with an increasing severity of dementia (Shaji, George, Prince, & Jacob, 2009; Thompson, Brodaty, Trollor, & Sachdev, 2010). The common occurrence of BPSD has serious implications because it is strongly associated with increased functional limitations, increased use of medications, and decreased quality of life for people with dementia and their caregivers (Ishii, Weintraub, & Mervis, 2009; Okura et al., 2010).

The following manifestations are considered BPSD:

- Agitation, defined as inappropriate verbal, vocal, or motor activity that is not directly explained by needs or confusion (e.g., aggression, screaming)
- Psychiatric symptoms (e.g., delusions, hallucinations)
- Personality changes, inappropriate sexual behavior, disinhibition
- Mood disturbances (e.g., apathy, depression, euphoria, emotional lability)
- Aberrant motor movements (e.g., pacing, rummaging, wandering)
- Neurovegetative changes (e.g., appetite changes, sleep disturbances).

Aggressive behaviors are particularly problematic for caregivers in any setting. A systematic literature review found that

---

A Student's Perspective

There is a woman at my nursing home who has severe dementia, to the point where she often is not very kind to the nurses, PTs, OTs, and other staff. For most of our clinical rotation, I only heard reports of her being angry and sometimes insulting. This can be comical at times, and we all know not to take it personally because we know her attitude is a result of her disease. Understanding the chance I was taking, I went to talk to her during breakfast because she was just staring off into space. Kneeling at her eye level and placing my hand on her shoulder, I began by asking how her morning was. She complained about the cold weather and about how aggressive the OTs were in dressing her. I let her vent, I made some positive remarks, and I complimented her on how beautiful she looked that day.

As I rose to my feet to leave her a few minutes later, she reached for my arm and said, "You're such a sweetheart; you're so kind." My first internal reaction was to be blown away! I had never heard of this woman delivering compliments! But throughout the rest of the day, I couldn't keep the smile off my face. This encounter helped me realize that this woman's beautiful personality is still with her and will always be a part of her. Yes, right now it's being masked most of the time by her dementia, but she still has feelings of kindness and a desire for happiness that fight past her disease every once in a while. I'm just glad I got to be part of that moment and discover that she's still there and needs to be treated like it always. One day she'll have the opportunity and power to express her thanks for those who showed her love and patience.

Shannon H.

---

caregivers in nursing homes encountered a broad range of aggressive behaviors, including verbal (e.g., threats and insults) and physical (kicking and biting) aggression, particularly during personal care activities when the residents' personal space was violated (Zeller et al., 2009). Hypersexual behavior (i.e., inappropriate talk or actions) occurs in up to 30% of cognitively impaired older adults and may be associated with delirium or depression (Wallace & Safer, 2009).

Not all behavioral changes are problematic for caregivers, but the geriatric literature tends to focus on those behaviors that cause management problems. This emphasis reinforces fears and anxieties about the functional consequences of dementia that may never occur. Remarks such as, "I know he doesn't have Alzheimer's disease because he doesn't hallucinate," or "I know she doesn't have Alzheimer's disease because she's not violent," reflect a false belief that certain difficult behaviors are an inevitable consequence of dementia. A family caregiver was heard to ask, "Can you tell me if my mother will be the 'nice kind' or the 'mean kind' as her Alzheimer's gets worse?" This question at least acknowledges that not all people with dementia are difficult, but it reflects another negative and false belief about categorical types of behaviors in people with dementia. Environmental influences are one factor that determines whether behaviors are problematic. For example, in a locked institutional unit, wandering behaviors might not be problematic, whereas in a home setting, wandering may be both unsafe and otherwise problematic. Likewise, nighttime restlessness creates more problems for a spouse who is the sole caregiver than for nursing staff who are paid to provide 24-hour care.

The term **catastrophic reaction** has been used for several decades in reference to a wide range of behaviors that occur in people with brain damage and are disproportionate to the reactions that would normally be expected in a situation (Mace & Rabins, 2006). These behaviors involve a sudden and exaggerated response to a situation that the person with dementia perceives as threatening. The onset of a catastrophic reaction may be signaled by a sudden change in mood, increased restlessness, stubbornness, or wandering. In addition, any of the following behaviors may be a component of the catastrophic reaction: anger, crying, shouting, anxiety, irritability, combativeness, and physical or verbal aggression. Caregivers may interpret the overreaction as intentional and think the person is being obstinate, critical, or overly emotional. Caregivers sometimes can identify specific precipitants of these episodes (e.g., assistance during bathing), but at other times, they may be unable to identify any precipitating factor. Catastrophic reactions resolve when the perceived threat is removed or when the person with dementia again feels safe and secure.

NURSING ASSESSMENT OF DEMENTIA IN OLDER ADULTS

Dementia is a complex syndrome that usually involves a long course of manifestations and intermittent fluctuations. Thus, assessment is an ongoing process that focuses on identifying contributing and treatable conditions and negative consequences that develop during the course of dementia. It also is important to identify and address conditions that interfere with the assessment of dementia.

Factors That Interfere With the Assessment of Dementia

Attitudes, myths, and lack of information are risk factors that interfere with an appropriate assessment of, and interventions for, dementia. In recent years, tremendous progress has been made in understanding and identifying causes of impaired cognitive function; however, many older adults and their families and caregivers still view serious cognitive impairments as an expected and normal concomitant of aging. When this happens, treatable conditions are likely to be overlooked, and older adults are denied the appropriate interventions to treat or manage their conditions. Even in the absence of curative treatments, many interventions are effective in delaying the progression of the condition, managing symptoms, and assisting with long-term planning.

Cultural factors that influence perceptions about aging and illness can significantly affect both the evaluation and treatment of dementia. For example, some cultural groups accept cognitive impairment as "normal aging," whereas others view dementia-related behaviors as shameful. Gerontologists are just beginning to study various aspects of cultural influences on perception of mental changes and acceptance of interventions.

Initial Assessment

With the exception of delirium and poststroke dementia, impaired cognitive function is a slowly progressive process that requires careful assessment to correctly identify underlying causes. Often, the changes occur slowly over a period of years, and an assessment is delayed until the changes significantly interfere with normal functioning. The assessment process usually takes place over weeks or months and involves the compilation of information about both medical and psychosocial functioning. Because progressive cognitive impairment is a very complex phenomenon, the assessment process generally is multidisciplinary, requiring input from primary care providers, psychiatrists, nurses, social workers, and rehabilitation therapists. Members of the assessment team must work with the family and other caregivers to obtain information and determine the appropriate level of involvement of the cognitively impaired person with regard to discussing assessment results and planning care. The major nursing focus is to determine the person's level of function, to identify the factors that affect the person's level of function, and to identify the person's response to his or her illness. Frequently, the nurse serves as the team leader and is responsible for coordinating information and facilitating communication among team members and with the older adult and his or her family or other caregivers. Nurses can use Box 14-3 as a guide for assessing progressive cognitive impairments in older adults.

Ongoing Assessment of Consequences

Because dementia is a progressive condition that commonly coexists with other conditions, all people with dementia require ongoing assessment of all of the following:

- Changes in cognitive and psychosocial function related to the dementia (e.g., a decline in cognitive abilities, the onset of anxiety or depression)
- Changes in mental status related to concurrent conditions (e.g., delirium due to a medical condition or adverse medication effects)
- Changes in functional abilities
- Causes of behavioral changes related to treatable conditions (e.g., anxiety, physical discomfort, environmental factors).

Box 14-3 Assessing Progressive Cognitive Impairment in Older Adults

General Principles
- Assessment of impaired cognitive function usually takes place during several visits, and it might include a home assessment.
- The person with impaired cognitive function may not be a reliable reporter, but his or her perceptions should be an integral part of the assessment and the accuracy of information should be validated.
- Healthcare professionals must respect the person's rights and ask permission before obtaining information from others, including family members.
- Do not assume that the family has drawn accurate conclusions about events of the past (e.g., family members may state that the person retired and then showed cognitive deficits when, in reality, the person retired because of an inability to cope with job demands).

Focus of the Assessment
- The primary purpose of the assessment is to identify the causes of the cognitive impairment.
- An assessment of a person with impaired cognitive function is multidisciplinary and includes the following components: complete medical history and physical examination including a review of all medications; a functional assessment; a comprehensive psychosocial and formal mental status assessment; and an assessment of environmental and caregiver influences, with particular emphasis on those factors that affect safety and functional abilities.

- The assessment includes an interview with caregivers, family members, and other people who can describe the progression of the manifestations of impairment.
- Information about lifelong patterns of personality, coping, and performance characteristics is considered in relation to the person's current functional level.
- It may be necessary to ask probing questions to help family members recognize clues to cognitive deficits retrospectively.

Considerations in Assessing Risk Factors Contributing to Impaired Cognitive Function
- Never assume that all cognitive impairments and behavioral manifestations stem from a dementing illness.
- Because risk factors can either cause the initial cognitive impairments or develop later, causing additional impairments, they must be reassessed periodically.
- The following categories of risk factors must be assessed, both initially and on an ongoing basis: depression, physiologic alterations, functional impairments, adverse medication effects, and environmental and psychosocial influences.
- Early in the assessment, ensure that vision and hearing impairments are compensated for as much as possible and that the environment does not interfere with the person's performance (e.g., as possible, make sure the person is using eyeglasses and a hearing aid if needed, and make sure the lighting is optimal).
- A priority is to identify and treat those factors that are reversible before deciding on a long-term management plan.

A major goal of ongoing assessment is to identify factors that interfere with the person's level of functioning or quality of life, so that interventions can be initiated to alleviate these contributing factors. Even though dementia is a progressive condition that gradually affects all levels of functioning, some of the changes that occur are caused by concurrent conditions rather than by the dementia itself. Thus, ongoing assessment to identify all factors that affect level of functioning is essential. Another goal of ongoing assessment is to identify the person's strengths and limitations in order to plan individualized interventions to improve the person's functioning and quality of life. Because of the progressive and fluctuating nature of impaired cognitive function, the person's strengths and limitations will change periodically; so care plans must be updated frequently. One way of assessing strengths and weaknesses is to inquire about the ways in which dementia has affected daily living and how the person has coped with, or adjusted to, these changes. Box 14-4 summarizes some statements of people with dementia about ways of coping and daily living.

Nurses can use Table 14-4 as a guide to assessing the progression of dementia from early to later stages. The following guides in this text are pertinent for ongoing assessment of the many aspects of functional consequences associated with the progression of dementia: functioning and safety (Chapter 7), psychosocial function and depression (Chapters 12 and 15), hearing and vision (Chapters 16 and 17), urinary function (Chapter 19), fall risks (Chapter 22), and sleep and rest (Chapter 24). Nurses also can use the assessment tools in the

chapters on medications (Chapter 8) and pain (Chapter 28) to address those aspects of care that are particularly important for people with dementia. In addition, the assessment tools available from the Hartford Institute for Geriatric Nursing that are listed in the Clinical Tools section of this and other chapters are applicable to assessing aspects of functioning and care for people with dementia.

Wellness Opportunity

Nurses promote wellness by identifying factors that support optimal functioning rather than focusing only on those that are problematic.

NURSING DIAGNOSIS

A nursing diagnosis commonly used for people with dementia is Chronic Confusion, defined as "irreversible, long-standing, and/or progressive deterioration of intellect and personality characterized by decreased ability to interpret environmental stimuli; decreased capacity of intellectual thought processes; and manifested by disturbances of memory, orientation, and behavior" (NANDA International, 2009, p. 167). Additional nursing diagnoses that are applicable to functional consequences associated with psychosocial responses to dementia include Fear, Anxiety, Hopelessness, Impaired Memory, Social Isolation, Self-Esteem Disturbance, and Ineffective Individual Coping. During the later stages when dementia affects the

---

Box 14-4 Lived Experiences: Coping and Daily Living with Dementia

About Ways of Coping

- I think it is alright to allow yourself a bit of time to focus on the pain and fear. That is only human; but it is important to move away from the sad focus and not let it consume you.
- I try to be more patient with myself and forgive myself.
- Staying busy doing what I love to do really keeps me going and gets me through. I'm in two support groups; I have weekly mandolin lessons; I do a weekly men's meditation class with daily homework; I'm reading about consciousness and healing that supports my living in the now and taking care of my spirit.
- I try to do something that I can still do—not as well as before—but something that I can still do.
- It's very important to laugh and enjoy a joke or pleasantries with people.
- We have this problem and we can't change that, but we can improve our lives by not letting it just bring us unhappiness 24 hours a day.
- Usually I just slow down, and reset my expectations. Expecting that you can be who you used to be is just a recipe for pain and sadness.
- I need to have the knowledge that I'm doing what I can. Because oftentimes it's so subtle, and I curse it every now and then and that helps.
- I ask people not to expect me to remember to do things.

- Ahh! I have a great lack of ease with not remembering things. Oh God, it drives me crazy . . . but we have to accept what we cannot change.
- Going to church; I sing . . . makes me happy.

About Day-to-Day Living

- Tomorrow I'll have little memory of today, and this makes living today like pushing the rock up the hill knowing it will roll back.
- Inertia is a serious problem with me, and sometimes I seem glued to my chair. Likely it's just that it's so much effort to get myself organized to do things, that I'm mentally exhausted before I even start.
- I streamline everything and get rid of everything I don't use very often. Keeping the house clutter-free helps to minimize the time necessary to find misplaced items.
- I try to find ways to compensate. For example, I now use a GPS to help me from getting lost when I drive.
- My brother-in-law removed all my cabinet doors in my kitchen so I can see all my food in my pantry when I walk into my kitchen.
- I think it would be better if I did not drive; and actually mentally, it is much better that I make that decision than somebody makes that decision for me. Psychologically, it is very good that I am actually in a position where they said, "OK you can drive," and just left it at that, and I turned around and said, "Well, thanks very much, but I am actually not going to drive."

Sources: Alzheimer's Society (2008); Alzheimer's Society (2010b); Beard & Fox (2008); Beard, Knauss, & Moyer (2009); Clare, Rowlands, & Quin (2008).

---

person's functional abilities, applicable nursing diagnoses include Wandering, Imbalanced Nutrition, Urinary Incontinence, Self-Care Deficit, Impaired Verbal Vommunication, Risk for Falls, Risk for Injury, Disturbed Sensory Perception, and Disturbed Sleep Pattern. If cognitive deficits interfere with the person's ability to accurately take medications, the nurse might apply the diagnosis of Ineffective Therapeutic Regimen Management.

Nursing diagnoses also address the needs of caregivers because much of the care of people with dementia focuses on helping the family and other caregivers address the day-to-day needs and issues of the person with dementia. Nursing diagnoses that might be used to address caregiver needs include Family Coping and Caregiver Role Strain (or Risk for Caregiver Role Strain). During the later stages of dementia, the nursing diagnosis Anticipatory Grieving may be appropriate, particularly for spousal caregivers.

cation, Coping, Leisure Participation, Memory, Mood Equilibrium, Nutritional Status, Quality of Life, Self-Care Status, Sleep, Social Interaction Skills, and Symptom Control.

When friends, family members, or paid caregivers care for the person with dementia, nurses plan outcomes to promote caregiver wellness. In the early stages of dementia, the caregiver's foremost need might be for information about the disease and about resources that address the changing needs of the person with dementia and the caregiver's own needs. As the dementia progresses, caregivers are likely to need emotional support and practical assistance. Some NOC terms that are pertinent to caregivers include Anxiety Level, Cognition, Cognitive Orientation, Comfort Level, Communication, Coping, Leisure Participation, Memory, Mood Equilibrium, Nutritional Status, Quality of Life, Self-Care Status, Sleep, Social Interaction Skills, and Symptom Control..

Wellness Opportunity

Readiness for Enhanced Coping is a wellness nursing diagnosis that nurses can apply for people with dementia as well as their caregivers.

Wellness Opportunity

Hope is a NOC that would be applicable when nurses plan wellness outcomes to address body–mind–spirit needs of both people with dementia and their caregivers.

PLANNING FOR WELLNESS OUTCOMES

During all stages of dementia, nursing care is directed toward promoting the highest level of functioning, while also supporting the highest quality of life. Nurses can apply the following Nursing Outcomes Classification (NOC) terminology to address the needs of people with dementia: Anxiety Level, Cognition, Cognitive Orientation, Comfort Level, Communi-

 ## NURSING INTERVENTIONS TO ADDRESS DEMENTIA

Information about interventions to address dementia is evolving at a rapid pace, and research by nurses and other healthcare professionals is shedding light on appropriate interventions for treating the disease and managing the functional consequences. Many interventions are applicable to all people with dementia and are individualized according to specific manifestations (e.g., reassurance for anxiety and confusion, redirection for unsafe or inappropriate behaviors). Similarly, health promotion interventions (e.g., exercise and nutrition) are applicable for primary and secondary prevention.

As anyone who has cared for a person with dementia knows, interventions must be highly individualized and frequently modified. An intervention that works for one person may not work for others, and interventions that are effective one day will not necessarily be effective the next day. A dominant theme of research and practice is the implementation of person-centered interventions that are based on a comprehensive and ongoing assessment of the person's unique and changing needs. Thus, caring for people with dementia is a creative and challenging process.

A comprehensive discussion of interventions for specific behaviors associated with dementia is beyond the scope of this chapter, but there are many practical references available on the management of dementia. Table 14-5 lists examples of nursing studies of nonpharmacologic interventions for dementia-related behaviors. In addition to professional nursing references, numerous books have been written by highly qualified and experienced caregivers that are excellent references for any nurse caring for people with dementia. The Alzheimer's Association and other resources (refer to thePoint) provide health education materials and additional reliable information about interventions for people with dementia and their caregivers. This text addresses nursing interventions by reviewing theoretical frameworks, applying general principles in different clinical settings, and giving an overview of nursing interventions that are applicable in all settings.

Examples of Nursing Interventions Classification (NIC) terminology that may be applicable to caring for people with dementia include Active Listening, Activity Therapy, Anxiety Reduction, Behavior Management, Calming Technique, Dementia Management, Elopement Management, Emotional Support, Environmental Management, Exercise Promotion, Fall Prevention, Humor, Memory Training, Milieu Therapy, Mood Management, Music Therapy, Presence, Reality Orientation, Reminiscence Therapy, Self-Care Assistance, Spiritual Support, and Touch. Nurses can use the following NIC terms when they address caregiver needs: Anticipatory Guidance, Caregiver Support, Consultation, Coping Enhancement, Counseling, Decision-Making Support, Humor, Referral, Respite Care, Simple Relaxation Therapy, Spiritual Growth Facilitation, and Teaching.

TABLE 14-5 Research Evidence: Interventions for Dementia-Related Behaviors

Reference	Intervention	Results
Aman & Thomas, 2009	Structured exercise program for 30 minutes three times a week for 3 weeks	Improvement in agitation score and 6-meter walk times
Chenoweth et al., 2009	Person-centered care and dementia-care mapping	Models of person-centered care and dementia-care mapping are effective in reducing agitation, compared with usual care models
Deudon et al., 2009	8-week staff education and training program	Reduced BPSD in intervention group of residents with severe dementia
Fritsch et al., 2009	Storytelling groups of 10 to 12 residents once weekly for 1 hour for 10 weeks	Positive outcomes for staff and residents (compared with control group): increased alertness and interactions, improved staff perception of residents
Gitlin et al., 2009	Purposeful use of pleasurable and engaging activities in home settings	Improved quality of life for person with dementia and caregivers
Holliday-Welsch, Gessert, & Renier, 2009	10 to 15 minutes of massage therapy on 6 days during a 2-week period during time of usually high levels of agitation	Decreased level of agitation, immediately and at 1 and 2 weeks following the intervention
Palese, Menegazzo, Baulino, Pistrino, & Papparotto, 2009	Nursing interventions to manage disruptive vocalizations	Effective strategies for disruptive vocalizations were using multiple strategies, administering analgesics, managing physical needs
Riley-Doucet, 2009	Visual, auditory, tactile, and olfactory stimulation in home settings	Use of a multisensory environment helped those with dementia attend more to their immediate surrounds and improved family relationships
Park & Specht, 2009	Individualized music for 30 minutes prior to usual peak agitation time, twice weekly for 2 weeks, followed by no music for 2 weeks	Mean agitation levels were significantly lower while and after listening to preferred music, compared with before listening
Tappen & Williams, 2009	30-minutes sessions of therapeutic conversation three times a week for 16 weeks	Increased positive mood and decreased negative mood in treatment group, same level or decline in control group
Testad, Ballard, Bronnick, & Aarsland, 2010	2-day educational seminar for staff and monthly group guidance for 6 months	Improved quality of care as measured by reduced use of restraints and less agitation in intervention group compared with control group
Woods, Beck, & Sinha, 2009	Therapeutic touch with contact on the neck and shoulders twice daily for 3 days, during two separate treatment periods	Restlessness significantly decreased in experimental group, compared with control group

Promoting Wellness for People With Dementia

One way in which nurses promote wellness for people with dementia is by addressing concerns that improve quality of life. The consequences of dementia significantly affect all aspects of a person's life—most often in undesirable ways—but achieving quality of life is still possible. A review of studies identified the following key domains of quality of life for people with dementia: health, independence, self-determination, social interaction, financial security, psychological well-being, security and privacy, religion and spirituality, and being of use or giving meaning to life (Alzheimer's Society, 2010b). An essential intervention for promoting wellness is to pay careful attention to the verbal and nonverbal ways in which the person with dementia communicates his or her needs and feelings. Box 14-5 provides statements of people with dementia about their needs and quality of life.

Box 14-5 Lived Experiences: Needs and Quality of Life

About Needs

- Just explain it a bit more, like when he said, "I will refer you to the memory clinic," you know, another two or three sentences. I just want to put you in the picture as to what will go on there, what it's for, what the set up is.
- To be taken seriously.
- As you have been diagnosed, there should be a follow up with information on what you have got, how do you cope with it, what to look for, what's gonna happen.

About Quality of Life

- Quality of life is living with your family—your circle of friends and family.
- Friendship is good. Very important to have friends.
- Oh there's nothing better than peace and quiet to be happy and comfortable, but if you ain't got peace, you're upset, and when you've got peace and quiet, you don't have anything in the mind.
- To feel safe. I've lived here for about 2 years and feel secure and safe. No accidents. This is important.
- I want to keep my own environment . . . because I am familiarized with it.
- It's not just the environment in the house, it's when you go out . . . in the bank, environment in the shops you go into, or restaurants is another environment, which you have got to overcome.
- I think your physical health is very important because even though I've got problems in myself, with my brain through my vascular dementia, I feel that if you have got your physical fitness then it still gives you that form of independence that you can still do things. Like I can still go to the bathroom and shave, where if you haven't got good health and you start having problems as well, it must be horrendous.

Sources: Alzheimer's Society (2008); Alzheimer's Society (2010b).

Another way of promoting wellness for people with dementia is through interventions that support the person's strengths and individuality during all stages of dementia by providing person-centered care, as described in the following sections. Nurses also promote wellness through interventions that support optimal levels of functioning. For example, at least some of the functional decline associated with dementia can be categorized as **excess disability**, which is defined as limitations that are beyond what is to be expected. One study found that over half of the walking disability among nursing home residents with moderate dementia was potentially preventable through interventions (Slaughter, Eliasziw, Morgan, & Drummond, 2010).

Theoretical Frameworks for Nursing Interventions

Healthcare professionals increasingly recognize that dementia-related behaviors reflect an attempt to communicate needs that the person may not consciously recognize and cannot express verbally. Thus, nurses must direct their interventions toward the underlying needs of the person with dementia. Hall and Buckwalter (1987) proposed a theoretical framework for addressing dementia-related behaviors called the *progressively lowered stress threshold* (PLST) model. Briefly stated, this model posits that dysfunctional behaviors indicate a progressive lowering of the stress threshold, which in turn, interferes with the person's functioning and ability to interact with the environment. Common stressors associated with dysfunctional episodes are fatigue; change of environment, routine, or caregiver; misleading stimuli or inappropriate stimulus levels; internal or external demands that exceed functional capacity; physical stressors (e.g., pain, illness, depression); and affective response to loss. The goal of nursing care, then, is to maximize the person's function by relieving stressors that cause excess disability. The choice of interventions is based on an ongoing assessment of anxiety "as a barometer to determine how much activity and stimuli the anxious person can tolerate at any point during their illness. As anxious behaviors occur, activities and environmental stimuli are modified and simplified until the anxiety disappears" (Hall & Buckwalter, 1987, p. 403). This approach (summarized in Box 14-6) is highly individualized; from a nursing perspective, it is analogous to adjusting insulin doses for people with diabetes according to serum glucose levels. The PLST model has been widely used for research and can also be applied to teaching caregivers about effective interventions for coping with behaviors (Lindsey & Buckwalter, 2009).

General Principles of Nursing Interventions in Different Settings

Long-Term Residential Settings

In recent years, there has been increasing implementation of multifaceted models of care for people with dementia in long-term care settings, including assisted living and nursing facilities. Many nursing facilities have specially designed

Box 14-6 Nursing Interventions for People With Dementia Based on the Progressively Lowered Stress Threshold Model (PLST)

- Maximize safety by modifying the environment to compensate for cognitive losses.
- Control any factors that increase stress, such as fatigue; physical stressors; competing or overwhelming stimuli; changes in routine, caregiver, or environment; and activities or demands that exceed the person's functional ability.
- Plan and maintain a consistent routine.
- Implement regular rest periods to compensate for fatigue and loss of reserve energy.
- Provide unconditional positive regard.
- Remain nonjudgmental about the appropriateness of all behaviors except those that present threats to safety.
- Recognize individual expressions of fatigue, anxiety, and increasing stress, and intervene to reduce stressors as soon as possible.
- Modify reality orientation and other therapeutic interventions to incorporate only that information needed for safe function.
- Use reassuring forms of therapy, such as music and reminiscence.

Source: Hall, G. R., & Buckwalter, K. C. (1987). Progressively lowered stress threshold: A conceptual model for care of adults with Alzheimer's disease. *Archives of Psychiatric Nursing, 1,* 399–406.

special care units (SCUs) for people with dementia, and some assisted living facilities are designed specifically for the care of people with dementia. Essential features of these units for cognitively impaired residents include environmental modifications, family involvement, individualized care plans, dementia-specific activity programs, and specially trained and selected staff. Many long-term care facilities incorporate these features into all nursing care units and address the

individualized needs of the residents, as discussed in Chapter 6. Long-term residential facilities typically address the needs of people who are in moderate to severe stages of dementia, although some residents are in the early stages. Box 14-7 summarizes statements of people with moderate to severe dementia in a residential care home about their experiences.

Acute Care Settings

Older adults are rarely hospitalized for an initial evaluation of dementia, but they are frequently admitted to acute care settings for evaluation and treatment of medical problems that are superimposed on the dementia. Consequently, nurses in hospital settings usually deal not only with the acute illness but also with the dementia-related behaviors, which are exacerbated by the medical problem, the hospital environment, the unfamiliar caregivers, and the change in routines. Thus, nurses in acute care settings face a tremendous challenge in caring for people with dementia.

One of the most important initial interventions is to involve at least one of the older adult's usual caregivers in planning and implementing care for the cognitively impaired person. Although the person with dementia is likely to exhibit different behaviors in the hospital than at home, nurses must begin by identifying any interventions that were effective in the home environment. During the admission process, nurses may save a lot of time and frustration by interviewing the caregivers about specific methods that help or hinder care. For example, if nurses know that the person eats only sandwiches or needs assistance with a specific toileting routine, they can incorporate appropriate interventions in their care

---

Box 14-7 Lived Experiences: People With Moderate to Severe Dementia in Residential Care Homes

I Still Am Somebody

- I can remember all those things, and they come back. And I know I can't do them now, but if I think about them, I'm sort of living them again, so that's really nice.
- Well, I ebb and flow a bit because I'm older and I've had heart trouble for years, so I think, really, I do ever so well. I've got no complaints at all.
- I used to do a lot. I may get back to it, and particularly if we get a nice Spring sort of thing, it might be better for me.
- I'm thankful for what I can do, you know what I mean? I won't give in.

Nothing's Right Now

- Don't lose me, will you? Please don't lose me.
- Things you like to remember, you can't remember, and things that you can remember easily drift away in front of you.
- I don't know what's the matter with me and why people don't talk to me much. I feel to be an outsider.
- I don't know whether I'm stuck here for the rest of my life or what's happening really.
- I'm frightened; please help me to know.
- Nobody wants me. I mean, that's the case, nobody does. If I was wanted by anybody, I could be quite useful. But nobody knows that I want a job.

I'm All Right; I'll Manage

- I wouldn't say it was as good as home at a place like this. You're just one of a number—group—who are pretty well in a similar position, but you do your best and give as much help. I've been sorting books out all morning.
- It's not as nice as I'd like it to be, but I have to be satisfied with small things these days.
- I haven't got to do any shopping, I haven't got to cook any meals, and that's a lot, isn't it? You've gotta get used to it, haven't you?
- I never thought I'd come to a place like this, but I'm quite happy.
- I've got a pal; she helps me out.

It Drives Me Mad

- I'd rather be doing something, yes, although there's not a lot I can do . . . I'm capable of doing.
- I get bored here. They go to sleep and I feel like throwing something at them, because they . . . nobody talking or nobody goes walking. You've gotta do something, haven't you, to help you go through? Because it wasn't the things I've been used to. They just sit here; it drives me mad.
- I want to be free . . . or die. I don't mind dying, but I don't want to be coddled here.

Sources: Clare, Rowlands, Bruce, Surr, & Downs (2008); Clare, Rowlands, & Quin (2008).

plans. Because many people with dementia have lost the ability to express their needs verbally, nurses need to obtain information from family caregivers who understand how the person expresses needs.

In addition to obtaining information from a usual caregiver, nurses may consider involving the caregiver in the person's care or asking him or her to provide a familiar presence during the hospitalization. Despite a need for respite from caregiving responsibilities, family and other caregivers may be willing to provide assistance and guidance. This may be particularly helpful during the first few days of hospitalization, and with patients who are particularly difficult to manage. Nurses can find assessment and intervention tools for addressing the needs of hospitalized people with dementia, including cost-free videos demonstrating the application of these tools, at http://consultgerirn.org/resources or at www.nursingcenter.com.

Community Settings

In community settings, a major role of nurses is to work with family members or paid caregivers to provide appropriate interventions that focus on improving functioning for the person with dementia, alleviating the burden for the caregivers, and improving quality of life for all. An intervention that might be most effective, as well as efficient, is to encourage caregivers' participation in educational or support groups, which often are led or co-led by nurses. The number of groups addressing the needs of caregivers is increasing rapidly, and information about these groups is available from the Alzheimer's Association or local hospitals. Nurses also can encourage caregivers to purchase one of the many caregiver guides that are available in bookstores or through the Internet and other resources.

In addition to educating caregivers about specific management problems, nurses in community settings must be ready to discuss resources for medical care, home services, and other community-based services for people with dementia and their caregivers. As the number and range of services increase, it is becoming more and more difficult to keep up-to-date on the resources in one's own community. Although nurses cannot be expected to know all the details about all available community services, they should know generally about the services available. In addition, they must be able to suggest at least one information and referral resource from which caregivers can obtain specific information. A good rule of thumb is to suggest that caregivers call the local area agency on aging because this type of organization serves every part of the United States. Information about these services can be obtained from the national Alzheimer's Association and the Eldercare Locator (see Health Education; see also thePoint.).

Another major focus of community-based programs is health promotion for people with early-stage dementia. Findings from research reviews and focus groups indicate the need for support programs, health promotion programs, and activities to help the person manage the disease and to "nor-malize" life (e.g., exercise programs, fall prevention, cognitive stimulation) (Burgener, Buettner, Beattie, & Rose, 2009). One nursing study of people who had early stage dementia, and who participated in a 12-week health promotion course, showed significant improvements in measures of cognition and depression (Buettner & Fitzsimmons, 2009). There also is increasing evidence that cognitive training and memory rehabilitation programs can effectively improve functioning and quality of life during early stage dementia (Nomura et al., 2009; Yu et al., 2009). Nurses have important roles in referring people with dementia to support groups and other community-based resources. Box 14-8 summarizes statements of people with dementia about their lived experiences related to needing help from others and being part of a support group.

Improving Safety and Function Through Environmental Modifications

Environmental modifications are important interventions for people with dementia because environmental factors profoundly affect their safety, functioning, and quality of life. During the 1960s, gerontologists initially emphasized the importance of cognitive stimulation and suggested that reality orientation programs be widely implemented, particularly in nursing homes and other residential care settings. Reality orientation involves the repeated use of verbal and nonverbal indicators of time, place, and person in the context of the individual, group, and environment. Reality orientation interventions include frequent verbal reminders about the time of day from all staff and "reality orientation boards" that display information in large print about the day, date, and weather. Improving the person's self-esteem and sense of control and reducing confusion, anxiety, and disorientation are the goals. Reality orientation may be effective for some people with dementia, particularly when combined with other strategies, but this intervention must be tailored to individual needs rather than universally applied.

Currently, gerontologists emphasize the important role of the total physical and psychosocial environment as an intervention not only for safety and independent functioning but also for quality of life of people with dementia (Kiser & Zasler, 2009). In addition, environmental interventions are essential for preventing and addressing problematic behaviors such as wandering. A review of studies related to the therapeutic effects of music emphasizes that music improves cognition, communication, and quality of life in many ways for people with dementia (Foster, 2009). Examples of environmental factors that significantly affect the safety, functioning, behaviors, and well-being of people with dementia are

- Noise
- Music
- Floor surfaces
- Colors and color contrast
- Lighting (e.g., glare, shadows, brightness)
- Design and placement of exits and bathrooms
- Living things (e.g., plants, birds, fish, pets)

Box 14-8   Lived Experiences: Interventions, Experiences, and Feelings

About Needing Help from Others

- When the day comes that I have got to start asking for help and if that independence is taken away, then I would like to think that I could still be consulted and still have some say in my independence.
- It is very beneficial, when I am unable to verbalize what I want, for my wife to display multiple options and allow me to choose one.
- If all else fails, I rely on my partner and my family to come up with solutions I cannot solve.
- I think it would be nice if people gave you the courtesy of time to finish what you are trying to say.
- You can't do what you want. You have to ask. So you have to adjust your schedule to someone else's. I guess the best word for it is that it is somewhat humiliating to be in that position when you're used to running your own life.
- I had somebody helping me cook for a while and that really bothered me. It makes me feel "less than myself."
- Before I'd take a walk around the block rather than blow my stack. By the time I got back, my feet hurt so much that I quit worrying about what I was mad about. Now my husband will go with me, and that doesn't do it.

About Being Part of a Support Group

- Since it is difficult to maintain my old social networks, I reach out to others online through e-mail groups and chat rooms for people with dementia. These can be real life-savers some days.

- It is that bit of extra that you know these people are having the same problems and *really* understand.
- I commiserate with my friends going through the same things.
- When I've gotten real down, it seems as though my failure in things I do is exaggerated many times. I feel as though my power has been lost to do anything about it. I feel hopeless and helpless. Thank God for my chat group sticking with me to crawl out.
- I participate in the group in hopes that people with dementia will begin to be treated with more respect and dignity and to help others recognize how much coping we must do to accomplish even simple things throughout a normal day.
- I have always been a person who has wanted to make a difference in the world, and through the group, I feel I have been able to change a small part of the way some people think about early-stage dementia.
- Let's work together to change paradigms about what persons with dementia can and can't do. Don't limit us—help us push the envelopes of our new abilities.
- The benefits to me personally are so important, as I can still feel that I am a valuable contributing member of society, even though I'm "cognitively disabled."
- Today I have met people who are in very much the same boat as I am with things they can and can't do, so for me it's a relief to find that there are others in the same boat.

Sources: Alzheimer's Society (2010b); Beard & Fox (2008); Beard, Knauss, & Moyer (2009); Clare, Rowlands, & Quin (2008).

- Furniture (seating, placement, heights of tables and chairs)
- Safety devices (e.g., rails, grab bars)
- Provisions for privacy and social interaction
- Items that improve comfort and hominess (e.g., decorative items, textured items, meaningful personal belongings)
- Absence of potentially harmful items (e.g., clutter, obstacles, sharp knives, cleaning solutions and other potentially toxic products).

Box 14-9 summarizes environmental interventions and techniques to address safety and independence in ADLs.

Wellness Opportunity

Nurses promote emotional wellness by encouraging older adults with dementia to talk about happy memories of earlier years and by affirming the pleasant feelings the person experiences when recalling these events.

Communicating With Older Adults With Dementia

Verbal and nonverbal communication techniques are widely recognized as essential interventions for people with dementia throughout the entire course of the disease. Nurses need to pay particular attention to the effects of touch, facial expressions, tone of voice, and body language on communication. Box 14-10 summarizes techniques for facilitating communication with people with dementia. These techniques are general

guidelines, and it is important to adapt communication to the particular needs of each person with dementia. An assessment and intervention tool for addressing communication needs of people with dementia, including a cost-free video demonstrating the application of this tool, is available from the Hartford Foundation for Geriatric Nursing at http://consultgerirn.org/resources or at www.nursingcenter.com.

Teaching About Pharmacologic Interventions

Nurses have important roles in teaching caregivers about medications for dementia. Medications are becoming increasingly important in treating dementia because recent studies and guidelines support and encourage certain medications to slow the progress of the disease. In addition, many types of medications are being investigated for treating dementia, and some over-the-counter products are being promoted both for preventing and treating dementia. Moreover, nurses are frequently involved with decisions about medications for managing dementia-related symptoms.

Medications for Slowing the Progression of Dementia

In 1993, tacrine (Cognex) was approved as the first medication for the treatment of Alzheimer's disease; by 2001, the U.S. Food and Drug Administration (FDA) had approved three additional cholinesterase inhibitors. Although tacrine is still available, the other three medications—donepezil (Aricept), rivastigmine (Exelon), and galantamine (Razadyne, formerly

Box 14-9 Environmental Adaptations and Techniques for Improving Safety and Functioning in People With Dementia

General Environmental Modifications

- Modify the environment to compensate as much as possible for sensory deficits and other functional impairments. (Refer to interventions in Chapters 16 through 19 and 22).
- Use clocks, calendars, daily newspapers, and simple written cues for orientation (e.g., day, date, names, place, and events).
- Use simple pictures, written cues, or color codes for identifying items and places (e.g., toilet, bedroom).
- Use simple written cues to clarify directions for operating radios, televisions, appliances, and thermostats (e.g., on, off, directional arrows).
- Place pictures of familiar people in highly visible places, but use nonglossy pictures and nonglare glass in picture frames.
- Turn lights on as soon as or before it gets dark.
- Use nightlights, or leave dim lights on during the night.
- Provide adequate environmental stimuli while avoiding overstimulation.

Techniques to Ensure Safety

- Make sure the person carries some form of identification, along with the phone number of someone to call.
- Adapt the environment for safety (e.g., use alarm devices on doors to prevent wandering).
- Keep the environment uncluttered.
- Keep medications, cleaning solutions, and any poisonous chemicals in inaccessible places.

- Enroll the person in a protective program, such as the Safe Return program sponsored by the Alzheimer's Association.

Techniques to Facilitate Independent Performance of ADLs

- Keep all activities as simple and routine as possible.
- Establish routines that allow for maximum independence and the least amount of frustration.
- While keeping the routines as consistent as possible, recognize that they will have to be changed as the person's level of function changes.
- Lay out one set of clothing in the order in which the items are to be donned.
- If the person needs assistance with hygiene, use matter-of-fact statements such as "It's time for your bath."
- Arrange personal care items, such as grooming and hygiene aids, in a visible and uncluttered place, in the order in which the items are to be used.
- Leave a toothbrush on the bathroom sink with toothpaste already on it.
- Establish an individualized toileting plan that allows for maximum independence but minimal risk for incontinence episodes.
- Offer finger foods and nutritious snacks if the person will not sit at the table to eat a meal.

Box 14-10 Facilitating Communication With People Who Have Dementia

Verbal Communication

- Adapt your level of communication to the abilities of the person with dementia.
- Use very simple sentences.
- Present only one idea at a time.
- Allow enough time for processing.
- Avoid infantilization (e.g., do not talk baby talk or use a demeaning or condescending tone of voice).
- Assist with word finding (e.g., supply missing words, repeat the person's sentence with the correct word).
- Avoid shaming the person (e.g., do not emphasize deficits).
- Paraphrase what the person says, and ask for clarification about the meaning.
- If the person does not understand a statement, repeat the statement using the same words, or simplify the wording.
- Do not argue with the person, unless it is a matter of safety.
- Avoid complex or sarcastic humor.
- Use positive statements (i.e., avoid using statements containing the word "don't" or other negative commands).
- Involve the person with decisions to the best of his or her ability by offering simple and concrete choices (e.g., "Do you want chicken or steak?" rather than "What do you want to eat?").
- Do not ask questions that you know the person cannot answer correctly.
- Do not test the person's memory unnecessarily.

- Listen to the feelings the person is trying to express and respond to the feelings, rather than the statement.
- When discussing activities of daily living (ADLs), avoid statements, such as "You need a bath now," which may be interpreted as judgmental.

Nonverbal Communication

- Attract and maintain the person's attention (e.g., through eye contact, pleasant facial expressions).
- Use a relaxed and smiling approach.
- Reinforce verbal communication with appropriate nonverbal communication (e.g., demonstrate what you are asking the person to do).
- Use simple pictures rather than written cues.
- Use appropriate touch for communication (e.g., to gain the person's attention or reinforce feelings of concern), unless the person responds negatively to touch.
- Be aware of your own nonverbal communication.
- Keep in mind that your nonverbal cues will probably communicate more than your spoken words and will not necessarily be interpreted correctly.
- Closely observe all nonverbal cues exhibited by the person, particularly those that express feelings.
- Assume that all nonverbal expressions of the person with dementia are attempts to communicate needs or feelings.

called Reminyl)—are the standards for mild to moderate Alzheimer's disease because they have fewer adverse effects. Reviews of studies consistently find that these medications exert modest positive effects in improving or delaying the progression of functional decline and cognitive and behavioral symptoms (e.g., Prvulovic, Hampel, & Pantel, 2010; Seltzer, 2010). In 2003, memantine (Namenda) became the first medication approved for treatment of moderate to severe Alzheimer's disease. The physiologic action of this medication, which differs from that of cholinesterase inhibitors, blocks the neural toxicity associated with excess release of glutamate. Studies consistently show that memantine reduces symptoms and slows the rate of decline in patients in moderate to later stages of Alzheimer's disease (Thomas & Grossberg, 2009).

The usual pharmacologic approach is to begin a cholinesterase inhibitor before or during the moderate stage of dementia and to add memantine during the moderate or later stages. These drugs are usually started at a low dose, which is increased gradually if it is well-tolerated. The most common adverse effects of cholinesterase inhibitors are nausea, vomiting, diarrhea, weight loss, and loss of appetite. Adverse effects of memantine include dizziness, headache, constipation, and increased confusion.

Medications for Managing Dementia-Related Symptoms

Although psychotropic medications are used for dementia-related disruptive behaviors, decisions about the use of these medications are complex for several reasons. First, because difficult behaviors are often precipitated by modifiable factors, including medical conditions, environmental influences, and adverse medication effects (e.g., anticholinergic medications), initial interventions should always address any contributing factors. For example, if behaviors are due to the adverse effects of medications, initial interventions should focus on eliminating or reducing the dose. Second, there is always a risk that medications will further interfere with function and perhaps even cause serious harm. A third consideration is whether the behaviors justify the risks associated with medications. Bothersome or socially inappropriate behaviors may best be ignored or tolerated than treated with medications. However, if the behavior is unsafe, uncomfortable, or interferes with the function of the person with dementia or the rights or safety of others, then pharmaceutical intervention may be appropriate, but only if other interventions are not successful. In any situation, healthcare professionals should view behavior-modifying medications as one component of a comprehensive management plan that addresses the complex nature of dementia-related behaviors. Nurses can use information in Box 14-11 to guide decisions about behavior-modifying medications for people with dementia.

Antipsychotics are the most commonly used type of medication for BPSD (e.g., agitation, delusions, hallucinations, and physical aggression), and many studies focus on both the beneficial and adverse effects of this approach. In recent years, concern about the adverse effects of the older antipsychotics

---

 Box 14-11　Guidelines for Decisions About Behavior-Modifying Medications for People With Dementia

Considerations Regarding Behavior-Modifying Medications

- Identify contributing factors (e.g., environmental conditions; psychosocial factors, such as anxiety or depression; or physiologic factors, such as pain, discomfort, or medical disorders). If any of these factors are implicated, interventions should be directed at the causative factor.
- Explore whether the behaviors are caused by adverse medication effects? In this case, the appropriate intervention might be to reduce the dose of or discontinue a medication, rather than begin a new medication.
- Use medications only after nonpharmacologic measures have been implemented.
- Determine whether the behaviors truly justify the use of medications, or are the caregivers requesting medications for their own comfort and convenience?

Considerations Regarding the Choice and Dose of Medications

- Be sure the specific goals of and expectations for the medication interventions are clear to all caregivers.
- If the person is depressed, explain that antidepressants may be effective in treating the depression and that some functional improvement may occur, as the depression is alleviated.
- Don't assume that, just because medications are necessary and appropriate during one stage of dementia, they will be necessary and appropriate on an ongoing basis.

- Reevaluate medication regimens as the dementia progresses or as other conditions, such as medical disorders, affect the person's functional level.
- Select a particular medication based on current manifestations as well as prior experiences with medications because people with dementia exhibit a wide range of responses to various medications.
- Remember that some people with dementia, particularly those with dementia with Lewy bodies, are highly sensitive to even minute doses of psychotropic medications.
- Keep in mind that any behavior-modifying medication is likely to interfere with cognitive function and that the type of behavior-modifying medication should be appropriate for the type of behavioral manifestations (e.g., antipsychotics for delusions and hallucination, antianxiety agents for anxiety).
- When introducing an initial dose of medication, give one-half to one-third the normal adult dose.
- Increase dosage gradually until therapeutic effects are achieved; all the while, observe the person for adverse effects.
- Consider the half-life of a medication when determining the frequency of doses. Avoid medications with long half-lives (e.g., flurazepam, diazepam, chlordiazepoxide).

(e.g., haloperidol) led to increased use of the so-called atypical antipsychotics, including olanzapine (Zyprexa), quetiapine (Seroquel), and risperidone (Risperdal). However, studies found that serious adverse effects, including strokes, hip fractures, and death, are associated with all types of antipsychotics in people with dementia, particularly those aged 85 and over (Jalbert, Eaton, Miller, & Lapane, 2010; Pariente et al., 2010; Sacchetti, Turrina, & Valsecchi, 2010). Because no medication is both safe and consistently more effective than nonpharmacologic interventions for BPSD, there is much support for nonpharmacologic approaches (as already discussed).

> ### ✦ Wellness Opportunity
>
> Nurses holistically address behavioral symptoms by trying to identify nonpharmacologic interventions that improve quality of life for the person with dementia and his or her caregivers.

EVALUATING THE EFFECTIVENESS OF NURSING INTERVENTIONS

Nurses can evaluate the care of people with dementia according to the extent to which they receive necessary supports and maintain their dignity and quality of life. Because a decline in function is an inherent part of dementia, nursing care is evaluated on an ongoing basis as the person's condition changes and in relation to appropriate and changing goals. Nurses evaluate the degree to which quality of life is maintained by obtaining feedback about life satisfaction, which people in the early and middle stages of dementia usually can express verbally or nonverbally. For example, nurses can evaluate the extent to which the person enjoys or participates in meaningful activities and interactions. As dementia progresses, it becomes more difficult to obtain this kind of information, and nurses rely more on feedback from caregivers and their own judgment. During the later stages of dementia, measures of quality of life focus more on comfort and basic physical needs. Throughout the dementia course, care can be evaluated by the extent to which the person is free from pain, fear, and anxiety.

Another evaluation consideration is the extent to which the needs of caregivers are met. One evaluation criterion is whether caregivers express satisfaction with their own quality of life, despite the demands of the situation. Other criteria may be a caregiver's attendance at support groups and his or her use of resources to assist with or guide care.

---

*M*rs. D. is 85 years old and lives with her 86-year-old husband in a high-rise apartment for the elderly. Two years ago, Mrs. D. was diagnosed with Alzheimer's disease, but she was able to participate in her usual activities until the past year. Now she is neglecting her personal care and is unsafe during meal preparation.

When she wakes up several times nightly to go to the bathroom, she sometimes goes to the apartment door rather than returning to the bedroom. Mr. D. worries that she will leave in the middle of the night. This disrupts his sleep because he maintains a state of constant vigilance. Mr. D. has called a home care agency requesting home health aide assistance, and you are the nurse responsible for the initial assessment and for working with the home health aides.

NURSING ASSESSMENT

During your initial assessment, you find that Mrs. D. is pleasant and receptive but has little insight into her need for help. She acknowledges that her doctor told her she has "a memory problem" but reports that this problem doesn't affect her daily life, except that her husband has to remind her about things like turning the stove off after cooking meals. She acknowledges being lonely and says she misses being able to read books and talk to people. Mrs. D. takes donepezil (Aricept) and vitamin E and is otherwise physically healthy.

With regard to ADLs, Mrs. D. has not taken a bath or shower in several months, and she gets very angry if Mr. D. suggests that she take one. She gets confused about her clothing and sometimes wears her underwear over her regular clothes or wears a skirt and slacks at the same time. She insists on doing the meal preparation, but she is not safe while using the stove and gets confused about ingredients in recipes (e.g., she has used salt instead of sugar). Mrs. D. has always done the laundry and housekeeping, but in the past months, she "made a lot of mistakes," such as using powdered milk for laundry detergent.

Mr. D. reports feeling very stressed about the full-time responsibilities of caring for his wife. This stress has escalated in the past month because he no longer feels he can leave her alone. Mrs. D. "shadows" him and feels very insecure if he is out of her sight for more than a few minutes. Mr. D. took her everywhere with him for the past year, but in the last few months, this has become increasingly difficult. For example, when they are grocery shopping, Mrs. D. gets very impatient and pushes the cart into other people. Then, while they are

(case study continues on page 280)

waiting in the checkout line, she insists on taking one of each of the nearby tabloids and magazines, and she creates a scene if Mr. D. doesn't buy them for her.

Mr. D. confides that he expected to be able to care for his wife at home "until the end," but now he has doubts about his ability to keep her at home. He perceives her as "senile" and feels he should be able to meet her needs. There are no nearby family members who can help with her care,

but his son and daughter have offered to help pay for some services. Mr. D. is aware of support groups offered by the Alzheimer's Association, but he has not attended any because he cannot leave his wife alone. When asked about his health, Mr. D. says, "I see the doctor for my arthritis and heart problems, but I get along OK, except that I'm supposed to have cataract surgery, and I don't know how I'll manage to get that done."

NURSING DIAGNOSIS

Your nursing diagnosis for Mrs. D. is Altered Thought Processes related to the effects of dementia. You use the nursing diagnosis of Caregiver Role Strain for Mr. D. because you recognize the need to address Mr. D.'s problems. Your immediate goal is to arrange for supportive services and assistance with Mrs. D.'s

care because this will improve the quality of life for both Mr. and Mrs. D., and it will alleviate some of the caregiver stress for Mr. D. A long-term goal is to arrange for respite services, so Mr. D. can undergo cataract surgery. You also recognize the need for educational and support services for Mr. D.

NURSING CARE PLAN FOR MR. AND MRS. D.

Expected Outcome	Nursing Interventions	Nursing Evaluation
Mrs. D. will function at her highest level of independence.	• Work with Mr. D. to identify ways to improve Mrs. D.'s ability to function safely and independently in performing activities of daily living (ADLs). (For instance, Mr. D. can involve Mrs. D. in selecting an outfit to wear and can set out the clothing in the order in which it should be donned.) • Arrange for a home health aide (HHA) to work with Mrs. D. and assist her with complex tasks such as laundry, housekeeping, and meal preparation. • Teach the HHA to assume an "assistant" and "friend" role by providing only subtle supervision and minimal direct help with activities such as laundry.	• Mrs. D. will perform ADLs and instrumental activities of daily living (IADLs) with minimal assistance.
Mrs. D.'s quality of life will be maintained.	• Work with Mr. D. and the HHA to identify activities that are interesting, satisfying, and intellectually stimulating (e.g., "word find" games). • Explore the possibility of Mrs. D.'s attending an adult day care program for group activities. • Support Mrs. D. in carrying out familiar roles and meaningful activities.	• Mrs. D. will continue to engage in activities that are satisfying.
Mr. D. will use sources of support to alleviate caregiver-related stress.	• Arrange the HHA's schedule to enable Mr. D. to attend caregiver support groups and educational programs. • Help Mr. D. in identifying one activity per week that he could do to promote his own well-being (e.g., going to lunch with a friend). • Provide HHA assistance for 4-hour periods to allow Mr. D. time for grocery shopping and pursuing his own interests. • Provide Mr. D. with information about the "Caregiver Connection Hot Line" at the Alzheimer's Association, and suggest that he join this telephone support network.	• Mr. D. will verbalize feelings of being able to cope effectively with caregiver responsibilities. • Mr. D. will participate in one activity per week focused on his own needs and interests.

THINKING POINTS

- Use the GDS/FAST in Table 14-4 to assess Mrs. D.'s stage of dementia.
- What would you identify as Mr. D.'s needs as a caregiver?
- What health education information would you plan for Mr. D.?
- What approaches would you suggest for Mr. D. and home care workers for communicating with Mrs. D.?
- What challenges would you anticipate having to address as you provide ongoing supervision of the HHA and continue to work with Mr. and Mrs. D.?

Chapter Highlights

Delirium

- Characteristics: acute onset; fluctuating course; disturbances in thought, memory, attention, behavior, perception, orientation, and consciousness.
- Hyperactive delirium is easily recognized, and hypoactive delirium, which is common but unrecognized in older adults.
- Risk factors include advanced age, pain, dementia, surgery, medications, physiologic disturbances, and pathologic conditions
- Functional consequences include decline in functioning, increased mortality, and permanent residency in long-term care facilities (Table 14-1)
- Nursing assessment: Confusion Assessment Method (CAM)
- Nursing Diagnosis: Acute Confusion
- Nursing Outcomes: Cognition, Concentration, Information Processing, Memory
- Nursing Interventions: addressing risk factors (Fig. 14-1)

Overview of Dementia

- Terminology (senility, hardening of the arteries, organic brain syndrome) reflects complexity of causes and types of dementia
- Dementia is a syndrome of impaired cognition caused by brain dysfunction
- Theories to explain dementia are still evolving
- Diagnosis of specific types of dementia is based on clinical observations, history, and available diagnostic data

Types of Dementia

- Four main types of dementia have been identified (Table 14-2)
- Alzheimer's disease (Figs. 14-2, 14-3, and 14-4)
- Vascular dementia
- Lewy body dementia
- Frontotemporal dementia

Risk Factors Associated With Dementia

- Factors that increase the risk for dementia include genetic factors, lifestyle factors, and health status
- Factors under investigation for protecting against dementia include physical exercise, omega-3 fatty acids, and engaging in socially and cognitively stimulating and meaningful activities (Table 14-3)

Functional Consequences Associated With Dementia

- Stages of progression (Table 14-4)
- Self-awareness, common emotions and behaviors (Boxes 14-1 and 14-2)
- Behavioral and psychological symptoms of dementia and catastrophic reactions

Nursing Assessment of Dementia

- Initial assessment: multidisciplinary, focus on level of function, response to illness (Box 14-3)
- Ongoing assessment of consequences (Box 14-4, Table 14-1, assessment guides in other chapters, and Clinical Tools)

Nursing Diagnosis

- Wellness nursing diagnosis for person with dementia and caregivers: Readiness for Enhanced Coping
- Person with dementia: Chronic Confusion, Anxiety, Impaired Memory, Risk for Injury, Self-Care Deficit, Disturbed Sleep Pattern, Imbalanced Nutrition, Wandering, Urinary Incontinence
- Caregivers: Family Coping and Caregiver Role Strain (or Risk for), Anticipatory Grieving.

Planning for Wellness Outcomes

- Person with dementia: Anxiety Level, Cognition, Cognitive Orientation, Comfort Level, Communication, Memory, Mood Equilibrium, Nutritional Status, Self-Care Status, Sleep, Symptom Control
- Caregivers: Caregiver Emotional or Physical Health, Caregiver Stressors, Caregiving Endurance Potential
- For both the person with dementia and his or her caregivers: Coping, Quality of life

Nursing Interventions to Address Dementia

- Nursing studies of nonpharmacologic interventions for dementia-related behaviors (Table 14-5)
- Addressing quality of life (Box 14-5)
- Theoretical frameworks for nursing interventions: progressively lowered stress threshold (PLST) model (Box 14-6)
- General principles in long-term residential settings, acute care (Clinical Tools from Hartford Institute for Geriatric Nursing), and community settings (Boxes 14-7 and 14-8)
- Improving safety and functioning through environmental modifications (Box 14-9)

- Communicating with older adults who have dementia (Box 14-10, Clinical Tools)
- Teaching about medications for slowing the progression of dementia
- Teaching about medications for managing dementia-related symptoms (Box 14-11)

Evaluating the Effectiveness of Nursing Interventions
- Maintenance of dignity and quality of life for the person with dementia
- Extent to which needs of caregivers are met

Critical Thinking Exercises

1. Define each of the following terms, and describe the relevance of each term according to our current understanding of impaired cognitive function: senility, organic brain syndrome, hardening of the arteries, delirium, dementia, and Alzheimer's disease.
2. Describe the distinguishing features of each of the following types of dementia: Alzheimer's disease, vascular dementia, Lewy body dementia, and frontotemporal dementia.
3. You are working in a nursing clinic at a senior center. How would you respond to the following questions, posed by a 74-year-old woman: "I've been having memory problems lately, but I know it's not Alzheimer's, because I haven't done anything really stupid. What do you think I should do? My friend says ginkgo helps her a lot, and I was thinking of trying that. Do you know how much of it I should take?"
4. You are planning an inservice program to nursing home staff about medications used in the treatment of dementia and the management of dementia-related behaviors. What information would you present?

Resources

For links to these resources and additional helpful Internet resources related to this chapter, visit thePoint at http://thePoint. lww.com/Miller6e.

Clinical Tools

American Journal of Nursing and Hartford Institute for Geriatric Nursing
How to Try This, articles and videos:
- Bradway, C., & Hirschman, K. B. (2008). How to try this: Working with families of hospitalized older adults with dementia. *American Journal of Nursing, 108*(10), 52–60.
- Evans, L. K., & Cotter, V. T. (2008). Avoiding restraints in patients with dementia: Understanding, prevention, and management are the keys. *American Journal of Nursing, 108*(3), 40–49.
- Fick, D. M., & Mion, L. C. (2008). How to try this: Delirium superimposed on dementia. *American Journal of Nursing, 108*(1), 52–60.
- Horgas, A., & Miller, L. (2008). How to try this: Pain assessment in people with dementia. *American Journal of Nursing, 108*(7), 62–70.
- Kennedy, G. J., & Smyth, C. A. (2008). How to try this: Screening older adults for executive dysfunction. *American Journal of Nursing, 108*(12), 62–71.

- Maslow, K., & Mezey, M. (2008). How to try this: Recognition of dementia in hospitalized older adults. *American Journal of Nursing, 108*(1), 40–49.
- Messecar, D., Powers, B. A., & Nagel, C. L. (2008). How to try this: The Family Preference Index: Helping family members who want to participate in care of the hospitalized older adult. *American Journal of Nursing, 108*(9), 52–59.
- Miller, C. A. (2008). How to try this: Communication difficulties in hospitalized older adults with dementia. *American Journal of Nursing, 108*(3), 58–66.
- Rowe, M. (2008). How to try this: Wandering in hospitalized older adults. *American Journal of Nursing, 108*(10), 62–70.
- Stockdell, R., & Amella, E. J. (2008). How to try this: The Edinburgh Feeding Evaluation in Dementia Scale: Determining how much help people with dementia need. *American Journal of Nursing, 108*(8), 46–54.
- Waszyniski, C. (2007). How to try this: Detecting delirium. *American Journal of Nursing, 107*(12), 50–59.

Hartford Institute for Geriatric Nursing
Try This: Best Practices in Nursing Care to Older Adults
- Issue 13 (2007), Confusion Assessment Method (CAM)
- Issue 22 (2007), Assessing Family Preferences for Participation in Care in Hospitalized Older Adults
- Issue D1 (2007), Avoiding Restraints in Older Adults with Dementia
- Issue D2 (2007), Assessing Pain in Older Adults with Dementia
- Issue D3 (2007), Brief Evaluation Of Executive Dysfunction: An Essential Refinement In The Assessment Of Cognitive Impairment
- Issue D4 (2007), Therapeutic Activity Kits
- Issue D5 (2007), Recognition of Dementia in Hospitalized Older Adults
- Issue D6 (2007), Wandering in the Hospitalized Older Adult
- Issue D7 (2007), Communication Difficulties: Assessment and Interventions in Hospitalized Older Adults with Dementia
- Issue D8 (2007), Assessing and Managing Delirium in Older Adults with Dementia
- Issue D9 (2007), Decision-Making and Dementia
- Issue D10 (2007), Working with Families of Hospitalized Older Adults with Dementia
- Issue D 11.1 (2007), Eating and Feeding Issues in Older Adults with Dementia, Part I: Assessment
- Issue D 11.2 (2007), Eating and Feeding Issues in Older Adults with Dementia, Part II: Interventions

Evidence-Based Practice

Fletcher, K. (2008). Dementia. In E. Capezuti, D. Zwicker, M. Mezey, & T. Fulmer (Eds.), *Evidence-Based Geriatric Nursing Protocols for Best Practice* (3rd ed., pp. 83–109). New York: Springer Publishing Co.

Tullmann, D. F., Mion, L. C., Fletcher, K., & Foreman, M. D. (2008). Delirium: Prevention, early recognition, and treatment. In E. Capezuti, D. Zwicker, M. Mezey, & T. Fulmer (Eds.), *Evidence-Based Geriatric Nursing Protocols for Best Practice* (3rd ed., pp. 111–125). New York: Springer Publishing Co.

National Guideline Clearinghouse
- Delirium
- Dementia
- Caregivers

Health Education

Alzheimer's Association
Alzheimer's Disease Education and Referral (ADEAR) Center
Alzheimer's Society of Canada
Dementia Advocacy and Support Network (DASN) International
Family Caregiver Alliance
National Institute on Aging (NIA)
National Institute of Neurological Disorders and Stroke

REFERENCES

Alagiakrishnan, K., Marrie, T., Rolfson, D., Coke, W., Camicioli, R., Duggan, D., . . . Wiens, C. (2009). Gaps in patient care practices to prevent hospital-acquired delirium. *Canadian Family Physician, 55*(10), e41–e46.

Alzheimer's Society. (2008). *Dementia: Out of the shadows.* London: Alzheimer's Society.

Alzheimer's Society. (2010a). *My name is not dementia: People with dementia discuss quality of life.* London: Alzheimer's Society.

Alzheimer's Society. (2010b). *My name is not dementia: Literature review.* London: Alzheimer's Society.

Aman, E., & Thomas, D. R. (2009). Supervised exercise to reduce agitation in severely cognitively impaired persons. *Journal of American Medical Directors Association, 10,* 271–276.

Ansaloni, L., Catena, F., Chattat, R., Fortuna, D., Franceschi, C., Macitti, P., & Melotti, R. M. (2010). Risk factors and incidence of postoperative delirium in elderly patients after elective and emergency surgery. *British Journal of Surgery, 97,* 273–280.

Arvanitakis, Z. (2010). Update on frontotemporal dementia. *Neurologist, 16*(1), 16–22.

Beard, R. L., & Fox, P. J. (2008). Resisting social disenfranchisement: Negotiating collective identities and everyday life with memory loss. *Social Science & Medicine, 66,* 1509–1520.

Beard, R. L., Knauss, J., & Moyer, D. (2009). Managing disability and enjoying life: How we reframe dementia through personal narratives. *Journal of Aging Studies, 23*(2009), 227–235.

Bjorkelund, K. B., Hommel, A., Thorngren, K. G., Gustafson, L., Larsson, S., & Lundberg, D. (2010). Reducing delirium in elderly patients with hip fracture: A multifactorial intervention study [published online ahead of print March 15, 2010]. *Acta Anaesthesiologica Scandinavica,* doi:10.1111/j.1399-6576.2010.02232.x.

Bossen, A. L., Specht, J. K. P., & McKenzie, S. E. (2009). Needs of people with early-stage Alzheimer's disease. *Journal of Gerontological Nursing, 35*(3f), 8–14.

Buettner, L. L., & Fitzsimmons, S. (2009). Promoting health in early-stage dementia, evaluation of a 12-week course. *Journal of Gerontological Nursing, 35*(3), 39–49.

Burgener, S. C., Buettner, L. L., Beattie, E., & Rose, K. M. (2009). Effectiveness of community-based, nonpharmacological interventions for early-stage dementia, conclusions and recommendations. *Journal of Gerontological Nursing, 35*(3), 48–58.

Chenoweth, L. King, M. T., Jeon, Y. H., Brodaty, H., Stein-Parbury, J., Norman, R., . . . Luscombe, G. (2009). Caring for Aged Dementia Care Residents Study (CADRES) of person-centered care, dementia-care mapping, and usual care in dementia: A cluster-randomised trial. *Lancet Neurology, 8*(4), 317–325.

Cherubini, A., Lowenthal, D. T., Paran, E., Mecocci, P., Williams, L. S., & Sein, U. (2010). Hypertension and cognitive function in the elderly. *Disease of the Month, 56,* 106–147.

Chuang, Y. F., Hayden, K. M., Norton, M. C., Tschanz, J., Breitner, J. C., Welsh-Bohmer, K. A., & Zandi, P. P. (2010). Association between APOE epsilon4 allele and vascular dementia: The Cache County study. *Dementia and Geriatric Cognitive Disorders, 29*(3), 248–253.

Ciaramella, A., Bizzoni, F., Salani, F., Vanni, D., Spalletta, G., Sanarico, N., . . . Bossù P. (2010). Increased pro-inflammatory response by dendritic cells from patients with Alzheimer's Disease. *Journal of Alzheimer's Disease, 19*(2), 559–572.

Clare, L., Rowlands, J., Bruce, E., Surr, C., & Downs, M. (2008). The experience of living with dementia in residential care: An interpretative phenomenological analysis. *The Gerontologist, 48*(6), 711–720.

Clare, L., Rowlands, J. M., & Quin, R. (2008). Collective strength: The impact of developing a shared social identity in early-stage dementia. *Dementia, 7*(1), 9–30.

Cotter, V. T. (2009). Hope in early-stage dementia: A concept analysis. *Holistic Nursing Practice, 23*(5), 297–301.

Dasgupta, M., & Hillier, L. M. (2010). Factors associated with prolonged delirium: A systematic review. *International Psychogeriatrics, 22*(3), 373–394.

Daviglus, M. L., Bell, C. C., Berrettini, W., Bowen, P. E., Connolly, E., Cox, N. J., . . . Trevisan, M. (2010). NIH state-of-the-science conference statement: Preventing Alzheimer's disease and cognitive decline [published online ahead of print June 14, 2010]. *NIH Consensus State of Science Statements,* doi:10.1059/0003-4819-153-3-201008030-00258.

De Toledo Ferraz Alves, T. C., Ferreira, L. K., Wajngarten, M., & Busatto, G. F. (2010). Cardiac disorders as risk factors for Alzheimer's disease [published online ahead of print April, 2010]. *Journal of Alzheimer's Disease,* doi:10.3233/JAD-2010-091561.

Deudon, A., Maubourguet, N., Gervais, X., Leone, E., Brocker, P., Carcaillion, L., . . . Robert, P. H. (2009). Non-pharmacological management of behavioural symptoms in nursing homes. *International Journal of Geriatric Psychiatry, 24*(12), 1386–1395.

DiBona, D., Scapagnini, G., Candore, G., Castiglia, L., Colonna-Romano, G., Duron, G., . . . Vasto, S. (2010). Immune-inflammatory responses and oxidative stress in Alzheimer's disease: Therapeutic implications. *Current Pharmaceutical Design, 16*(6), 684–691.

Duron, E., & Hanon, O. (2010). Antihypertensive treatments, cognitive decline, and dementia [published online ahead of print February 2010]. *Journal of Alzheimer's Disease,* doi:10.1136/bmj.b5409.

Edvardsson, D., Winblad, B., & Sandman, P. O. (2008). Person-centered care of people with severe Alzheimer's disease: Current status and ways forward. *Lancet Neurology, 7,* 362–367.

Ertekin-Taner, N. (2010). Genetics of Alzheimer disease in the pre-and post-GWAS era. *Alzheimer's Research & Therapy, 2,* 3–7.

Eskelinen, M. H., & Kivipelto, M. (2010). Caffeine as a protective factor in dementia and Alzheimer's disease [published online ahead of print February 24, 2010]. *Journal of Alzheimer's Disease,* doi:10.3233/JAD-2010-1404.

Farina, E., Baglio, F., Caffarra, P. l., Magnani, G., Scarpini, E., Appollonio, I., . . . Castiglioni, S. (2009). Frequency and clinical features of Lewy Body Dementia in Italian Memory Clinics. *Acta Biomed, 80,* 57–64.

Fick, D. M., Kolanowski, A., Beattie, E., & McCrow, J. (2009). Delirium in early-stage Alzheimer's disease. *Journal of Gerontological Nursing, 35*(3), 30–38.

Flaherty, J. H., Shay, K., Weir, C., Kamholz, B., Boockvar, K. S., Shaughnessy, M., . . . Rudolph, J. L. (2009). The development of a mental status vital sign for use across the spectrum of care. *Journal of American Medical Directors Association,* doi:10.1016/j.jamda.2009.04.001.

Flicker, L. (2010). Cardiovascular risk factors, cerebrovascular disease burden, and healthy brain aging. *The Clinics in geriatric Medicine, 26,* 17–27.

Flinn, D. R., Diehl, K. M., Seyfried, L. S., & Malani, P. N. (2009). Prevention, diagnosis, and management of postoperative delirium in older adults. *Journal of the American College of Surgeons, 209*(2), 261–268.

Fong, T. G., Jones, R. N., Shi, P., Marcantonio, E. R., Yap, L., Rudolph, J. L., . . . Inouye, S. K. (2009). Delirium accelerates cognitive decline in Alzheimer disease. *Neurology, 72,* 1570–1575.

Foster, B. (2009). Music for life's journey: The capacity of music in dementia care. *Alzheimer's Care Today, 10*(1), 42–49.

Frigerio, R., Fujishiro, H., Maraganore, D. M., Klos, K. J., DelleDonne, A., Heckman, M. G., . . . Ahlskog, J. E. (2009). Is incidental Lewy Body Disease related to Parkinson Disease? Comparison of risk factor profiles. *Archives of Neurology, 66*(9), 1114–1118.

Fritsch, T., Kwak, J., Grant, S., Lang, J., Montgomery, R. R., & Basting, A. D. (2009). Impact of TimeSlips, a creative expression intervention program, on nursing home residents with dementia and their caregivers. *The Gerontologist, 49*(1), 117–127.

Galvin, J. E., Duda, J. E., Kaufer, D. I., Lippa, C. F., Taylor, A., & Zarit, S. H. (2010). Lewy body dementia: The caregiver experience of clinical care [published online ahead of print April 29, 2010]. *Parkinsonism Related Disorders,* doi:10.1016/j.parkreldis.2010.03.007.

Gitlin, L. N., Winter, L., Earland, T. V., Herge, E. A., Chernett, N. L., Piersol, C. V., & Burke, J. P. (2009). The tailored activity program to reduce behavioral symptoms in individuals with dementia: Feasibility, acceptability, and replication potential. *The Gerontologist, 49*(3), 428–439.

Gordon, E., Rohrer, J. D., Kim, L. G., Omar, R., Rossor, M. N., Fox, N. C., & Warren, J. D. (2010). Measuring disease progression in frontotemporal lobar degeneration. *Neurology, 74,* 666–673.

Grochmal-Bach, B., Bidzan, L., Pachalska, M., Bidzan, M., Lukaszwska, B., & Pufal, A. (2009). Aggressive and impulsive behaviors in Frontotemporal dementia and Alzheimer's disease. *Medical Science Monitor, 15*(5), CR248–CR253.

Hachinski, V. C., Lassen, N. A., & Marshall, J. (1974). Multi-infarct dementia: A cause of mental deterioration in elderly. *Lancet, 2,* 207–209.

Hall, G. R., & Buckwalter, K. C. (1987). Progressively lowered threshold: A conceptual model for care of adults with Alzheimer's disease. *Archives of Psychiatric Nursing, 1,* 399–406.

Hamaguchi, T., Ono, K., & Yamada, M. (2010). Curcumin and Alzheimer's disease [published online ahead of print April 12, 2010]. *CNS Neuroscience and Therapeutics.*

Han, J. H., Morandi, A., Ely, E. W., Callison, C., Zhou, C., Storrow, A. B., . . . Schnelle, J. (2009). Delirium in the nursing home patients seen in the emergency department. *Journal of the American Geriatric Society, 57*(5), 889–894.

Han, J. H. Shintani, A., Eden, S., Morand, A., Solberg, L. M., Schnelle, J., . . . Ely, E. W. (2010). Delirium in the emergency department: An independent predictor of death within 6 months [published online ahead of print April 02, 2010]. *Annals of Emergency Medicine,* doi:10.1016/j.annemergmed.2010.03.003.

Holliday-Welsch, D. M., Gessert, C. E., & Renier, C. M. (2009). Massage in the management of agitation in nursing home residents with cognitive impairment. *Geriatric Nursing, 30*(2), 108–116.

Holroyd-Leduc, J. M., Khandwala, F., & Sink, K. M. (2010). How can delirium best be prevented and managed in older patients in hospital? *Canadian Medical Association Journal, 182*(5), 465–470.

Hulko, W. (2009). From 'not a big deal' to 'hellish': Experiences of older people with dementia. *Journal of Aging Studies, 23,* 131–144.

Iacono, D., Markesbery, W. R., Gross, M., Pletnikova, O., Rudow, G., Zandi, P., & Troncoso, J. C. (2009). The Nun Study: Clinically silent AD, neuronal hypertrophy, and linguistic skills in early life. *Neurology, 73,* 665–673.

Inouye, S. K., van dyck, C. H., Alessi, C. A., Balkin, S., Siegal, A. P., & Horwitz, R. I. (1990). Clarifying confusion: The confusion assessment method. A new method for detection of delirium. *Annals of Internal Medicine, 113*(12), 941–948.

Ishii, S., Weintraub, N., & Mervis, J. R. (2009). Apathy: A common psychiatric syndrome in the elderly. *Journal of American Medical Directors Association, 10,* 381–393.

Jack, C. R. Jr., Knopman, D. S., Jagust, W. J., Shaw, L. M., Aisen, P. S., Weiner, M. W., . . . Trojanowski J. Q. (2010). Hypothetical model of dynamic biomarkers of the Alzheimer's pathological cascade. *Lancet Neurology, 9*(1), 119–123.

Jalbert, J. J., Eaton, C. B., Miller, S. C., & Lapane, K. L. (2010). Antipsychotic use and the risk of hip fracture among older adults afflicted with dementia. *Journal of American Medical Directors Association, 11*(2), 120–127.

Jellinger, K. A., & Attems, J. (2010). Prevalence of dementia disorders in the oldest-old: An autopsy study. *Acta Neuropathologica, 119*(4), 421–433.

Kamat, S. M., Kamat, A. S., & Grossberg, G. T. (2010). Dementia risk prediction: Are we there yet? *Clinics in Geriatric Medicine, 26,* 113–123.

Kelley, R. E., & Minagar, K. A. (2009). Memory complaints and dementia. *Medical Clinics of North America, 93,* 389–406.

Kertesz, A. (2010). Frontotemporal dementia, Pick's disease. *Ideggyogy Sz Journal, 63*(1–2), 4–12.

Kiely, D. K., Marcantonio, E. R., Inouye, S. K., Shaffer, M. L., Bergmann, M. A., Yang, F. M., . . . Jones, R. N. (2009). Persistent delirium predicts increased mortality. *Journal of the American Geriatric Society, 57*(1), 55–61.

Kim, J., Lee, H. J., & Lee, K. W. (2010). Naturally occurring phytochemicals for the prevention of Alzheimer's disease. *Journal of Neurochemistry, 112,* 115–140.

Kiser, L., & Zasler, N. (2009). Residential design for real life rehabilitation. *NeuroRehabilitation, 25,* 219–227.

Klein, J. C., Eggers, C., Kalbe, E., Weisenbach, S., Hohmann, C., Vollmar, S., . . . Hilker, R. (2010). Neurotransmitter changes in dementia with Lewy bodies and Parkinson disease dementia in vivo. *Neurology, 74,* 885–892.

Knopman, D. S. (2010). Mild cognitive impairment and on to dementia. Down the slippery slope but faster. *Neurology, 74,* 942–944.

Kumar, V., & Kinsella, L. J. (2010). Healthy brain aging: Effect of head injury, alcohol and environmental toxins. *Clinics in Geriatric Medicine, 26,* 29–44.

La Rue, A. (2010). Healthy brain aging: Role of cognitive reserve, cognitive stimulation, and cognitive exercises. *Clinics in Geriatric Medicine, 26,* 99–111.

Lee, M., & Chodosh, J. (2009). Dementia and life expectancy: What do we know? *Journal of the American Medical Directors Association,* doi:10.1016/j.jamda.2009.03.014.

Lindsey, P. L., & Buckwalter, K. C. (2009). Psychotic events in Alzheimer's disease: Application of the PLST model. *Journal of Gerontological Nursing, 35*(8), 20–27.

Luetz, A., Heymann, A., Radtke, F. M., Chenitir, C., Neuhaus, U., Nachtigall, I., . . . Spies, C. D. (2010). Different assessment tools for intensive care unit delirium: Which score to use? *Critical Care Medicine, 38*(2), 409–418.

Mace, N. L., & Rabins, P. V. (2006). *The 36-hour day* (4th ed.). Baltimore: The Johns Hopkins University Press.

Markesbery, W. R., Jicha, G. A., Liu, H., & Schmitt, F. A. (2009). Lewy body pathology in normal elderly subjects. *Journal of Neuropathology and Experimental Neurology, 68*(7), 816–822.

McCaffrey, R. (2009). The effect of music on acute confusion in older adults after hip or knee surgery. *Applied Nursing Research, 22*(2), 107–112.

McGuinness, B., & Passmore, P. (2010). Can statins prevent or help treat Alzheimer's disease? [published online ahead of print February 2010] *Journal of Alzheimer's Disease,* doi:10.3233/JAD-2010-091570.

McNaull, B. B. A., Todd, S., McGuinness, B., & Passmore, A. P. (2010). Inflammation and anti-inflammatory strategies for Alzheimer's disease-a mini-review. *Gerontology, 53,* 3–14.

Metcalfe, M. J., & Figueiredo-Pereira, M. E. (2010). Relationship between Tau pathology and neuroinflammation in Alzheimer's disease. *Mount Sinai Journal of Medicine, 77,* 50–58.

Morley, J. E. (2010). Nutrition and the brain. *Clinics in Geriatric Medicine, 26,* 89–98.

Morris, J. C. (2005). Dementia update 2005. *Alzheimer Disease and Associated Disorders, 19,* 100–116.

NANDA International (2009). *Nursing diagnoses: Definitions and classification 2009–2011.* Oxford: Wiley-Blackwell.

Nomura, M., Makimoto, K., Kato, M., Shiba, T., Matsuura, C., Shigenobu, K., . . . Ikeda, M. (2009). Empowering older people with early dementia and family caregivers: A participatory action research study. *International Journal of Nursing Studies, 46*(4), 431–441.

Okura, T., Plassman, B. L., Steffens, D. C., Llewellyn, D. J., Potter, G. G., & Langa, K. M. (2010). Prevalence of neuropsychiatric symptoms and the association with functional limitations in older adults in the United States: The aging, demographics, and memory study. *Journal of the American Geriatric Society, 58*, 330–337.

Palese, A., Menegazzo, E., Baulino, F., Pistrino, R., & Papparotto, C. (2009). The effectiveness of multistrategies on disruptive vocalization of people with dementia in institutions: A multicentered observational study. *American Association of Neuroscience Nurses, 41*(4), 191–200.

Pariente, A., Sanctussy, D. J., Miremont-Salame, B. G., Moore, N., Haramburu, F., & Fourrier-Reglat, A. (2010). Factors associated with serious adverse reactions to cholinesterase inhibitors: A study of spontaneous reporting. *CNS Drugs, 24*(1), 55–63.

Park, H., & Specht, J. K. P. (2009). Effect of individualized music on agitation in individuals with dementia who live at home. *Journal of Gerontological Nursing, 35*(8), 47–55.

Pisani, M. A., Murphy, T. E., Araujo, K. L., & Van Ness, P. H. (2010). Factors associated with persistent delirium after intensive care unit admission in an older medical patient population [published online ahead of print April 2010]. *Journal of Critical Care,* doi:10.1016/j.jcrc.2010.02.009.

Prvulovic, D., Hampel, H., & Pantel, J. (2010). Galatamine for Alzheimer's disease. *Expert Opinion on Drug Metabolism and Toxicology, 6*(3), 345–354.

Radak, Z., Hart, N., Sarga, L., Koltai, E., Atalay, M., Ohno, H., & Boldogh, I. (2010). Exercise plays a preventive role against Alzheimer's disease [published online ahead of print February 24, 2010]. *Journal of Alzheimer's Disease*, doi:10.3233/JAD-2010-091531.

Reisberg, B. (1986). Dementia: A systematic approach to identifying reversible causes. *Geriatrics, 41*(4), 30–46.

Riedijk, S. R., Niermeijer, M. F. N., Dooijes, D., & Tibben, A. (2009). A decade of genetic counseling in frontotemporal dementia affect families: Few counseling requests and much familial opposition to testing. *Journal of Genetic Counseling, 18*, 350–356.

Riley-Doucet, C. K. (2009). Use of multisensory environments in the home for people with dementia. *Journal of Gerontological Nursing, 35*(5), 42–52.

Robinson, J. G., Ijioma, N., & Harris, W. (2010). Omega-3 fatty acids and cognitive function in women. *Women's Health, 6*(1), 119–134.

Rolland, Y., van Kan, G. A., & Vellas, B. (2010). Healthy brain aging: Role of exercise and physical activity. *Clinics in Geriatric Medicine, 26*, 75–87.

Rudolph, J. L., Inouye, S. K., Jones, R. N., Yang, F. M., Fong, T. G., Levkoff, S. E., & Marcantonio E. R. (2010). Delirium: An independent predictor of functional decline after cardiac surgery. *Journal of American Geriatric Society, 58*(4), 643–649.

Sabbagh, M. N., Cooper, K., DeLange, J., Stoehr, J. D., Thind, K., Lahti, T., . . . Beach, T. G. (2009). Functional, global and cognitive decline correlates to accumulation of Alzheimer's pathology in MCI and AD [published online ahead of print December 1, 2009]. *Current Alzheimer's Research*, doi:10.2174/156720510791162340.

Sacchetti, E., Turrina, C., & Valsecchi, P. (2010). Cerebrovascular accidents in elderly people treated with antipsychotic drugs: A systematic review. *Drug Safety, 33*(4), 273–288.

Salmon, E., Perani, D., Collette, F., Feyers, D., Kalbe, E., Holthoff, V., . . . Herholz, K. (2008). A comparison of unawareness in frontotemporal dementia and Alzheimer's disease. *Journal of Neurology, Neurosurgery, and Psychiatry, 79*(2), 176–179.

Sandhaus, S., Harrell, F., & Valenti, D. (2006). Healthier aging: Here's help to prevent delirium in the hospital. *Nursing, 36*(7), 60–62.

Scarmeas, N., Luchsinger, J. A., Schupf, N., Brickman, A. M., Cosentino, S., Tang, M. X., & Stern, Y. (2009). Physical activity, diet, and risk of Alzheimer disease. *Journal of the American Medical Association, 302*(6), 627–637.

Seltzer, B. (2010). Galantamine-ER for the treatment of mild-to-moderate Alzheimer's disease. *Clinical Intervention in Aging, 5*, 1–6.

Shaji, K. S., George, R. K., Prince, M. J., & Jacob, K. S. (2009). Behavioral symptoms and caregiver burden in dementia. *Indian Journal of Psychiatry, 51*(1), 45–49.

Shibata, K., Narumoto, J., Kitabayashi, Y., Ushijima, Y., & Fukui, K. (2008). Correlation between anosognosia and regional cerebral blood flow in Alzheimer's disease. *Neuroscience Letters, 435*(1), 7–10.

Silva, T. J. A., Jerussalmy, C. S., Farfel, J. M., Curiati, J. A. E., & Jacob-Filho, W. (2009). Predictors of in-hospital mortality among older patients. *Clinics, 64*(7), 613–618.

Skrobik, Y. (2009). Delirium prevention and treatment. *Critical Care Clinics, 25*, 585–591.

Slaughter, S. E., Eliasziw, M., Morgan, D., & Drummond, N. (2010). Incidence and predictors of excess disability in walking among nursing home residents with middle-stage dementia: A prospective cohort study. *International Psychogeriatric, 4*, 1–11.

Sofi, F., Macchi, C., Abbate, R., Gensini, G. F., & Casini, A. (2010). Effectiveness of the Mediterranean diet: Can it help delay or prevent Alzheimer's disease? [published online ahead of print February 2010] *Journal of Alzheimer's Disease*, doi:10.3233/JAD-2010-1418.

Specht, J. K. P., Taylor, R., & Bossen, A. L. (2009). Partnering for care: The evidence and the expert. *Journal of Gerontological Nursing, 35*(3), 16–22.

Spronk, P. E., Riekerk, B., Hofhuis, J., & Rommes, J. H. (2009). Occurrence of delirium is severely underestimated in the ICU during daily care. *Intensive Care Medicine, 35*(7), 1276–1280.

Tabira, T. (2010). Immunization therapy for Alzheimer disease: A comprehensive review of active immunization strategies. *The Journal of Experimental Medicine, 220*, 95–106.

Tan, Z., & Sehadri, S. (2010). Inflammation in the Alzheimer's disease cascade: Culprit or innocent bystander? *Alzheimer's Research and Therapy, 2*, 6–9.

Tappen, R. M., & Williams, C. L. (2009). Therapeutic conversation to improve mood in nursing home residents with Alzheimer's disease. *Research in Gerontological Nursing, 2*(4), 267–276.

Testad, I., Ballard, C., Bronnick, K., & Aarsland, D. (2010). The effect of staff training on agitation and use of restraint in nursing home residents with dementia: A single-blind, randomized controlled trial. *Journal of Clinical Psychiatry, 71*(1), 80–86.

Thomas, S. J., & Grossberg, G. T. (2009). Memantine: A review of studies into its safety and efficacy in treating Alzheimer's disease and other dementias. *Clinical Interventions in Aging, 4*, 367–377.

Thompson, C., Brodaty, H., Trollor, J., & Sachdev, P. (2010). Behavioral and psychological symptoms associated with dementia subtype and severity. *International Psychogeriatric, 22*(2), 300–305.

Tomlinson, B. E., Blessed, G., & Roth, M. (1968). Observations on the brains of non-demented old people. *Journal of Neurological Science, 7*, 331–356.

Tomlinson, B. E., Blessed, G., & Roth, M. (1970). Observation on the brains of demented old people. *Journal of Neurological Science, 11*, 205–242.

Von Bernhardi, R. (2010). Immunotherapy in Alzheimer's disease: Where do we stand? Where should we go? *Journal of Alzheimer's Disease, 19*(2), 405–421.

Von Gunten, A., & Mosimann, U. P. (2010). Delirium upon admission to Swiss nursing homes: A cross-sectional study. *Swiss Medical Weekly, 140*(25–26), 376–381.

Voyer, P., Richard, S., Doucet, L., & Carmichael, P. H. (2009a). Predisposing factors associated with delirium among demented long-term care residents. *Clinical Nursing Research, 18*(2), 153–157.

Voyer, P., Richard, S., Doucet, L., Cyr, N., & Carmichael, P. H. (2009b). Precipitating factors associated with delirium among long-term care residents with dementia. *Applied Nursing Research*, doi:10.1016/j.apnr.2009.07.001.

Wallace, M., & Safer, M. (2009). Hypersexuality among cognitively impaired older adults. *Geriatric Nursing, 30*(4), 230–236.

Wei, L. A., Fearing, M. A., Sternberg, E. J., & Inouye, S. K. (2008). The confusion assessment method (CAM): A systematic review of current usage. *Journal of American Geriatric Society, 56*(5), 823–830.

Weinmann, S., Roll, S., Schwarzbach, C., Vauth, C., & Willich, S. N. (2010). Effects of Ginkgo biloba in dementia: A systemic review and meta-analysis. *Bio Med Central Geriatrics,* doi:10.1186/1471–2318-10–14.

Woods, D. L., Beck, C., & Sinha, K. (2009). The effect of therapeutic touch on behavioral symptoms and cortisol in persons with dementia. *Forschende Komplemenamedizin/Research in Complementary Medicine, 16*(3), 181–189.

Yang, F. M., Marcantonio, E. R., Inouye, S. K., Kiely, D. K., Rudolph, J. L., Fearing, M. A., & Jones, R. N. (2009). Phenomenological subtypes of delirium in older persons: Patterns, prevalence, and prognosis. *Psychosomatics, 50*(3), 248–254.

Young, C. C., & Flanagan, E. M. (2010). Delirium: The struggle to vanquish an ancient foe. *Critical Care Medicine, 38*(2), 693–694.

Yu, F., Rose, K. M., Burgener, S. C., Cunningham, C., Buettner, L. L., Beattie, E., . . . McKenzie, S. E. (2009). Cognitive training for early-stage Alzheimer's disease and dementia. *Journal of Gerontological Nursing, 35*(3), 23–28.

Zeller, A., Hahn, S., Needham, I., Kok, G., Dassen, T., & Halfens, R. J. G. (2009). Aggressive behavior of nursing home residents toward caregivers: A systematic literature review. *Geriatric Nursing, 30*(3), 174–187.

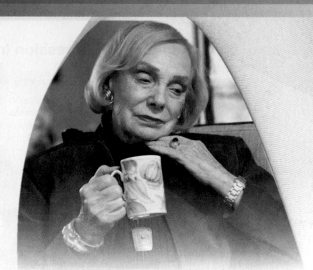

CHAPTER 15

Impaired Affective Function: Depression

LEARNING OBJECTIVES

After reading this chapter, you will be able to:

1. Describe theories that explain late-life depression.
2. Examine risk factors that cause or contribute to depression in older adults.
3. Discuss the functional consequences of late-life depression.
4. Describe the following aspects of nursing assessment: unique manifestations of late-life depression, depression in cognitively impaired older adults, cultural factors related to depression, and use of screening tools.
5. Identify interventions for addressing risk factors, improving psychosocial function, and teaching about antidepressants, psychosocial therapies, and complementary and alternative modalities.
6. Discuss nursing responsibilities related to assessing and preventing suicide in older adults.

KEY POINTS

antidepressants
bright-light therapy
cognitive triad theory
depression
depression in Alzheimer's disease
electroconvulsive therapy (ECT)
Geriatric Depression Scale-Short Form (GDS-SF)
late-life depression
learned helplessness theory

poststroke depression
psychomotor agitation
psychomotor retardation
psychosocial therapies
selective serotonin reuptake inhibitors (SSRIs)
serotonin and norepinephrine reuptake inhibitors (SNRIs)
St. John's wort
suicide
vascular depression

Despite the common occurrence of **depression** as an impairment of psychosocial function in older adulthood, it is often undetected and untreated. The term depression is difficult to define because it is considered a mood, a complaint, a syndrome, and a disease. Gerontological references, however, commonly use the term *depressive symptoms* to describe a constellation of symptoms that profoundly affect the quality of life of a significant number of older adults. Gerontologists have developed theories to explain depression in older adults, which is often called **late-life depression**, and healthcare practitioners have developed assessment tools to identify depression in older adults. Nurses have important roles in addressing depression because there is a range of nursing interventions that can have a significant positive impact on the quality of life of older adults.

THEORIES ABOUT LATE-LIFE DEPRESSION

Late-life depression is a multifaceted condition, which is caused by complex relationships and numerous other factors that commonly occur in older adults. Although no single theory can explain why older adults are likely to become depressed, some of the more common psychosocial, cognitive, and biologic theories explain causative factors from various perspectives. A major focus of recent research is the relationship between dementia and depression, and studies are just beginning to address questions about the very common co-occurrence of these two conditions.

Psychosocial Theories

Psychosocial theories focus on the impact of loss as well as the buffering effects of social supports and the social network in protecting against depression. Blazer (2002) reviewed psychosocial theories related to late-life depression and identified the following potential contributing factors:

- Ageism, loss of social roles, and lower socioeconomic status
- Early experiences including impoverishment and childhood trauma

Addressing Depression in Older Adults

Nursing Assessment

- Risk factors for depression or suicide
- Manifestations of depression
- Depression with cognitive impairment
- Geriatric Depression Scale: Short Form

Age-related changes

- Decreased cerebral blood flow
- Changes in neuroendocrine system
- Disruptions of circadian rhythm

Negative functional consequences

- Feelings of sadness, anxiety, decreased self-esteem
- Absence of life satisfaction
- Anorexia, sleep disturbances, lack of energy
- Increased morbidity and mortality
- Increased risk for suicide

Risk factors

- Psychosocial stressors (e.g., losses, role changes)
- Medical conditions
- Functional impairments
- Adverse medication effects
- Lack of social supports

Nursing Interventions

- Improving functional abilities and independence
- Strengthening social supports and fostering meaningful relationships
- Encouraging physical activity and good nutrition
- Teaching about preventing, identifying, and treating depression
- Facilitating referrals for mental health services

Wellness Outcomes

- Improved functioning
- Increased quality of life
- Prevention of suicide

- Recent social stressors including stressful life events
- Inadequate social network (e.g., no spouse/partner, few friends, small family network)
- Diminished social interaction
- Poor social integration (e.g., unstable environment, lack of strong religious affiliation)
- A combination of the preceding factors

The **learned helplessness theory** has also been used to explain late-life depression. A cognitively oriented formulation of this theory describes depression as a deficit in the following four areas: cognitive, motivational, self-esteem, and affective-somatic (Seligman, 1981). Depression occurs when people expect bad things to happen, believe they can do nothing to prevent them, and perceive that the events result from internal, stable, and global factors (Seligman, 1981). This theory would explain the occurrence of depression in older adults who are in situations over which they have little control. The learned helplessness theory supports the use of nursing interventions directed toward improving self-efficacy and a sense of control over one's environment.

Cognitive Triad Theory

Beck proposed the **cognitive triad theory** as a way of explaining depression in general, and late-life depression in particular (Beck, Rush, Shaw, & Emery, 1979). According to this theory, people appraise themselves by the "cognitive triad" of their self-image, their environment or experiences, and their future. Depressed people judge these three realms as lacking some features that are necessary for happiness. Examples of negative appraisals are feelings of worthlessness, interpretations of neutral events as bad, and unrealistic feelings of hopelessness. Beck postulates that depression is caused not by adverse events but by distorted perceptions, which impair one's ability to appraise oneself and the event in a constructive manner. The second element of Beck's theory involves schemas, or consistent cognitive patterns. Schemas are assumptions, or unarticulated rules, that influence thoughts, feelings, and behaviors. Depressed people typically hold negative assumptions that lead to faulty conclusions. For instance, a depressed person might believe, "I must not be important because the nurse didn't stop to see me." The third component of Beck's theory is the existence of certain logical errors such as personalization, minimization, magnification, and overgeneralization. This theory is supported by studies that have found a relationship between late-life depression and cognitive distortions or negative cognitions (Blazer, 2002).

Biologic and Genetic Theories

Biologic theories about late-life depression investigate the relationships among aging, depression, and changes in the brain, nervous system, and neuroendocrine system. Many theories have addressed the role of neurotransmitters, with particular emphasis on serotonin, dopamine, acetylcholine, and norepinephrine as causative or contributing factors. In addition, the following changes in the neuroendocrine system are associated with depression: elevated plasma cortisol levels, altered growth hormone secretion, altered response of thyroid hormones, and increased activity in the hypothalamic-pituitary-adrenal axis. Other biologic theories address anatomic changes (e.g., lesions in white or deep gray matter), neurophysiologic brain changes (e.g., decreased cerebral blood flow), and disruption of the circadian rhythms (e.g., sleep patterns). A longitudinal study of 110 dementia-free older adults found that depressive symptoms, over time, were associated with a loss of brain volume in several areas (Dotson, Davatzikos, Kraut, & Resnick, 2009). A neuroimaging study using positron emission tomography (PET) found that older depressed subjects had unique patterns of glucose metabolism compared to demographically matched controls and compared to changes observed in normal aging or in dementia (Smith et al., 2009). Gerontologists are also focusing on the relationship between cerebrovascular changes and depression, as discussed in the section on depression and dementia.

A major focus of investigation is the relationship between the age-related changes and the biologic changes associated with depression. Because many of these changes are similar, the risk for development of a depressive disorder that is associated with biologic changes increases with age (Blazer, 2002). Researchers have not been able to draw clear conclusions about cause–effect relationships among aging, depression, and biologic changes; however, there is undisputed evidence that "the more severe depressive disorders are strongly influenced by psychobiologic changes" (Blazer, 2002, p. 117).

Researchers have also focused on the interrelationship between biologic and genetic variables. For example, one focus of current theories is on variations in genes that can affect the release of neurotransmitters, particularly under stressful conditions. Studies are also addressing a potential link between specific genetic variations and an increased risk for suicidal behaviors (Huang, Oquendo, Currier, & Mann, 2009). A recent review of studies concluded that major depressive disorder is caused by the complex interplay of multiple inherited genetic factors and lifelong exposure to a wide range of environmental and psychosocial factors (Rot, Mathew, & Charney, 2009).

Theories About Depression and Dementia

Gerontologists recognize a high correlation between depression and dementia, with many studies finding that depression occurs in 30% to 50% of people with Alzheimer's disease and in 30% to 60% of people with vascular dementia (Blazer, 2002). There also is a stronger correlation between memory impairment and other cognitive changes in depressed older adults than in depressed younger people (Wilkins, Mathews, & Sheline, 2009). Studies also found that each new episode of depression increases the risk for dementia (Kessig, Sondergard, Forman, & Andersen, 2009).

Although dementia and depression share some common neuropathologic changes and manifestations (e.g., loss of interest, diminished cognitive function, and **psychomotor agitation** or retardation), researchers have not identified a specific cause–effect relationship. Research reviews have identified the following hypotheses about the relationship between depression and cognitive changes: (1) depression is a precursor or early manifestation of dementia; (2) depression occurs early in the course of dementia as a psychological reaction to eroding cognitive abilities; (3) depression and cognitive decline are manifestations of a common underlying central nervous system disorder; and (4) depression causes neurologic and neuroendocrine changes that cause cognitive decline (Bhalla et al., 2009; Brommelhoff, 2009; Dillon et al., 2009; Korczyn & Halperin, 2009).

Theories about **vascular depression** (also called **post-stroke depression**) propose that depression can arise in late life from cerebrovascular damage caused by ischemic or hemorrhagic strokes. Studies show that vascular depression is a common complication of stroke, with prevalence rates ranging from 19% to 79% (Carod-Artal, Ferreira, Trizotto, & Menezes, 2009; Hadidi, Treat-Jacobson, & Lindquist, 2009;

Skinner, Georgiou, Thorton, & Rothwell, 2009). Studies indicate that comorbidities, physical severity, cognitive impairment, and stroke severity are more important than stroke location as risks for depression (Christensen, Mayer, Ferran, & Kissela., 2009; Elkind, 2009). Characteristics of vascular depression include poor insight, less agitation, increased disability, more cognitive impairment, more **psychomotor retardation**, and less depressive ideation (e.g., feelings of guilt).

CLASSIFICATION OF DEPRESSION

Three of the mood disorders defined in the *Diagnostic and Statistical Manual of Mental Disorders, 4th Edition, Text Revision* (*DSM-IV-TR*) are bipolar disorders, major depressive disorder, and dysthymic disorder (American Psychiatric Association, 2000). In addition, the *DSM-IV-TR* lists criteria for bereavement and adjustment disorder with a depressed mood, which are closely associated with late-life depression. The majority of older adults who are admitted to hospitals for mood disorders are diagnosed with major depressive disorder, but dysthymic disorder and bereavement are much more common in community settings (Blazer, 2002).

Because most early studies of mood disorders of later life focused primarily on major depression, which affects less than 3% of older adults, depression is likely to be unrecognized and untreated in the majority of older adults who have other types of depression. Terms such as *minor, subthreshold, subclinical*, and *subsyndromal depression* more accurately reflect depressive symptoms that occur on a continuum, ranging from no depression to major depression. Characteristics that most commonly occur, with varying degrees of severity, in any type of depression in older adults are discussed in the Functional Consequences section of this chapter.

Since the early 2000s, gerontologists have used the term *late-life depression* to describe depression occurring in people over the age of 65. Studies indicate that more than half of the cases of depression have their first onset in later life (Fiske, Wetherell, & Gatz, 2009). Compared to adults with depression earlier in life, adults with late-life depression are more likely to have cognitive impairment, cardiovascular diseases, and other significant comorbidities, and they are less likely to have a family history of depression (Dillon et al., 2009; Wilkins et al., 2009). One study of depression in younger and older adults found that late-life depression subjects were more impaired in memory, verbal learning, and motor speed, and this could not be attributed to aging alone (Thomas, 2009). Researchers are also identifying the unique characteristics of late-life anxious depression as a common and severe subtype of late-life depression (Licht-Strunk, Beekman, de Haan, van Marwijk, 2009a). One preliminary study suggests that late-life anxious depression is not just a more severe form of depression but may have distinct neurobiological characteristics associated with vascular and degenerative changes in the brain (Andreescu et al., 2009).

Another trend in classifying depression in older adults is to identify the unique characteristics of depression with cognitive impairment. In the early 2000s, the National Institutes of Health assembled a panel of researchers and clinicians with extensive experience related to both late-life depression and Alzheimer's disease, who proposed the diagnostic criteria for **depression in Alzheimer's disease** (Olin et al., 2002). The main points of the criteria for depression in Alzheimer's disease include all criteria for the diagnosis of dementia of the Alzheimer's type (discussed in Chapter 14); three or more symptoms of depression (e.g., anorexia, hopelessness, depressed mood, psychomotor changes, disruptions in sleep, recurrent thoughts of death); presence of irritability, social isolation, or withdrawal; decreased positive affect or pleasure in response to social contact and usual activities; and the occurrence of symptoms during a 2-week period (Tagariello, Girardi, & Amore, 2009).

Gerontologists are also studying late-onset bipolar disorder because studies have found that 8% and 9% of patients with bipolar disorder were diagnosed after ages 65 and 60, respectively (Oostervink, Boomsma, Nolen, & The EMBLEM Advisory Board, 2009). Characteristics of bipolar disorder that initially occur during older adulthood include more frequent episodes of depression, fewer and milder mania episodes, and longer intervals between episodes of mania (Oostervink et al., 2009).

Wellness Opportunity

From a holistic nursing perspective, it is important to recognize that there are many types of depression, and in older adults particularly, depression is complex and likely to occur concomitantly with dementia and other conditions.

 ## RISK FACTORS FOR DEPRESSION IN OLDER ADULTS

Risk factors that are likely to cause or contribute to depression in older adults include demographic factors and psychosocial influences, medical conditions and functional impairments, and effects of medications and alcohol. Although these factors can increase the risk for depression in people of any age, older adults are more likely than younger people to have one or more of these variables. The following sections discuss each category of risk in relation to older adults. Additional risk factors for depression include cognitive impairments and dementia, as discussed in other sections of this chapter.

Demographic Factors and Psychosocial Influences

Demographic factors and psychosocial influences that are associated with depression in older adults include
- Female sex
- Personal or family history of depression

- Bereavement, loss of significant relationships
- Loneliness
- Chronic stress
- Recent social stressors
- Stressful social environment
- Loss of meaningful social interaction
- Lack of social supports
- Loss of significant roles
- Current or previous experiences of abuse or neglect
- Being a caregiver (including assuming primary care of a grandchild).

Although losses and stress can be risk factors for depression, social supports (e.g., having at least one close relationship) and effective coping mechanisms can protect older adults from depression. Thus, the stressors alone are not the primary risk factor for depression; rather, it is the combination of stressors and the absence of social supports that increases the risk for depression. In addition to causing the onset of depression, psychosocial factors can affect the duration of depression.

DIVERSITY NOTE

Russell and Taylor (2009) found that living alone is associated with higher levels of depression among Hispanics but not among non-Hispanics.

Medical Conditions and Functional Impairments

Medical conditions that are considered causative factors for depression are listed in Box 15-1. Some of these conditions are related to electrolyte imbalances or nutritional deficiencies, which can be easily identified and treated. For example, recent studies show that low levels of serum 25(OH)D (vitamin D) are associated with increased depression in older adults; supplemental vitamin D is associated with reduced depressive symptoms in women (Shipowick, Moores, & Corbett, 2009).

The relationships between medical conditions, functional impairments, and depression is complex and interactive, with depression contributing to medical illness and disability and medical illness and disability contributing to depression. Examples of interrelationships between depression and medical conditions or functional impairments include the following:

- Depression in medically ill older adults is associated with increased mortality, longer hospitalizations, and extended recovery time.
- Medical illnesses can threaten survival, independence, self-concept, role functions, economic resources, and sense of well-being.
- Disability leads to depression because it causes social isolation, low self-esteem, restricted social activity, strained interpersonal relationships, and loss of perceived control.
- Depression in medically ill older adults can lead to other health problems such as hip fractures and increased susceptibility to infection.

Box 15-1 Medical Conditions That Can Cause Depression

Central Nervous System Disorders
Parkinson's disease
Dementia
Strokes
Hemorrhage or hematoma
Tumors
Neurosyphilis
Normal-pressure hydrocephalus

Nutritional Deficiencies
Folate or vitamin B_{12} deficiency
Pernicious anemia
Iron deficiency
Vitamin D deficiency

Cardiovascular Disturbances
Myocardial infarction
Congestive heart failure
Coronary artery bypass surgery

Miscellaneous
Rheumatoid arthritis
Cancer, particularly of the pancreas or intestinal tract
Tuberculosis
Hip fracture

Metabolic and Endocrine Disorders
Diabetes
Hypothyroidism/hyperthyroidism
Hypoglycemia/hyperglycemia
Parathyroid disorders
Adrenal diseases
Hepatic or renal disease

Fluid and Electrolyte Disturbances
Hypercalcemia
Hypokalemia
Hyponatremia

Infections
Meningitis
Viral pneumonia
Hepatitis
Urinary tract infections

- Chronic pain is a common cause of depression, and it is sometimes a symptom of depression.
- Depression worsens pain, and pain worsens depression.
- Functional impairment is associated with depression as both a contributing factor and a consequence.
- Depression is a common cause of nutritional deficits in older adults and nutritional deficiencies can be a risk factor for depression.

Gerontologists emphasize that depression is a treatable component of medical conditions that has a significant negative effect on health-related quality of life for older adults (Gallegos-Carrillo et al., 2009). One study found that depression was more burdensome than physical symptoms in people with Parkinson's disease (Jones, Pohar, & Patten, 2009). Studies that address depression in people with diabetes, cardiovascular disease, chronic obstructive pulmonary disease, and chronic kidney disease consistently emphasize that depression occurs commonly with these conditions, is an independent risk for poorer outcomes, and should be identified and treated (de Voogd et al., 2009; Hedayati, Minhauddin, Toto, Morris, & Rush, 2009; Lin et al., 2009; Omachi et al., 2009; Subramaniam et al., 2009). Studies also found that improvement in depression can lead to improved functioning and have a meaningful effect on the ability to live at home (Li & Conwell, 2009).

Another risk factor is that depression often goes unrecognized as a concomitant condition in older adults with medical conditions. For example, depression in nursing home residents is often overlooked as a treatable condition (Thakur & Blazer, 2008). Although this is not a risk factor for causing depression, it is a risk factor for the progression of depression, subsequent functional decline, and increased morbidity and mortality.

Effects of Medications and Alcohol

People of any age may experience depression as an adverse medication effect, but older adults are at higher risk because they take more medications. Medications may be risk factors for depression in the following ways:

- Adverse medication effects can cause a depressive syndrome that improves or disappears when the medication is stopped.
- Adverse medication effects can induce a depression that does not remit when the medications are stopped.
- Adverse medication effects can simulate a depressive syndrome by causing lethargy, insomnia, and irritability.
- The withdrawal of certain medications, such as psychostimulants, can cause a depressive syndrome.

Depression as an adverse effect of medications is usually related to the use of medications, such as those listed in Box 15-2, that are prescribed for chronic conditions. However, depression can also be an adverse effect of alcohol or drugs that are abused (e.g., benzodiazepines). Moreover, although people of any age may experience adverse effects from alcohol, older people are more sensitive to these adverse effects because of age-related changes. Alcohol and depression have a synergistic relationship: alcohol causes depression and depression leads to alcohol abuse, which in turn exacerbates the depression.

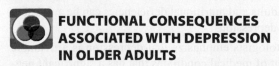

FUNCTIONAL CONSEQUENCES ASSOCIATED WITH DEPRESSION IN OLDER ADULTS

Depression has serious functional consequences for people of any age, but for frail and seriously depressed older adults, the effects can be life-threatening. Functional consequences

---

Box 15-2 Examples of Medications That Can Cause Depression

Analgesics
indomethacin
narcotics
propoxyphene

Antihypertensives and Cardiovascular Agents
beta blockers
clonidine
digitalis
guanethidine
hydralazine
methyldopa
reserpine

Antiparkinsonian Agents
levodopa

Central Nervous System Agents
alcohol
barbiturates
benzodiazepines
fluphenazine
haloperidol
meprobamate

Histamine Blockers
cimetidine

Steroids
corticosteroids
estrogen

Anti-Cancer (chemotherapeutic) agents

---

range from a negative impact on well-being and quality of life to the most serious consequence, which is **suicide**. These negative functional consequences are associated not only with major depression but also with minor and subclinical depression in older adults; these consequences often progress if treatment is not initiated (Lyness, Chapman, McGriff, Drayer, & Duberstein, 2009). This section discusses the wide range of functional consequences that are associated with depression. Suicide is addressed as a separate topic at the end of this chapter because nurses need to address it not only as the most serious consequence of depression but also as an entity in itself.

Physical Health and Functioning

A decline in physical functioning is one of the most consistently identified functional consequences of depression in older adults, particularly in those who are also cognitively impaired (Hybels, Pieper, & Blazer, 2009; Steffens, 2009). Additional functional consequences that affect health and functioning are a high number of physical complaints, perception of worse health, and inability to carry out important life functions such as managing money or medications (Licht-Strunk et al., 2009b). Many studies in a variety of settings

Box 15-3 Functional Consequences of Late-Life Depression

Impact on Physical Function
- Loss of appetite
- Weight loss
- Digestive system complaints, particularly dysphagia, flatulence, constipation, stomach distress, or early satiety
- Insomnia, hypersomnia, frequent awakening, early-morning awakening, and other sleep disturbances
- Fatigue, loss of energy
- Pain, discomfort, dyspnea, general malaise
- Slowed or increased psychomotor activities
- Loss of libido or other problems with sexual function

Impact on Psychosocial Function
- Affect: sad, low, "blue," worried, unhappy, "down in the dumps"
- Absence of feelings; feeling numb or empty
- Diminished life satisfaction
- Low self-esteem
- Loss of interest or pleasure
- Passivity, lack of motivation to do things
- Inattention to personal appearance
- Feelings of guilt, hopelessness, self-blame, unworthiness, uselessness, helplessness
- Anxiety, worry, irritability
- Slowed thinking, poor memory, inability to concentrate, poor attention span, inability to make decisions, exaggeration of any mental deficits
- Rumination about past and present problems and failures

found that depression is an independent risk for excess morbidity and mortality (Barca, Engedal, Laks, & Selbaek, 2009; Schoevers et al., 2009; Wolinsky et al., 2009). It is important to recognize that some of these consequences, such as the inability to manage money or medications, may be a central factor in preventing the person from living independently. Box 15-3 lists ways in which depression affects physical health and functioning.

Appetite disturbances, particularly anorexia, are among the most common physical complaints of depressed older adults. Sometimes, the depressed person does not complain of anorexia and may even deny the problem, but a caregiver or family member may note that the person is not interested in food and is losing weight. Other gastrointestinal complaints that may be functional consequences of depression include flatulence, constipation, early satiety, and attention to bowels. Any of these disturbances may be attributed to or caused by other factors such as medical conditions or adverse medication effects; however, depression must be considered as a possible underlying factor. Chronic fatigue and diminished energy are additional functional consequences of late-life depression that are likely to be attributed to or caused by other conditions.

Like weight loss and diminished appetite, sleep changes commonly occur in older adults, and they may or may not be caused by depression. Waking up more frequently during the night and early morning awakening are two changes in sleep

patterns that are characteristic of depression. One study of 5,109 community-dwelling adults between the ages of 58 and 100 years found that those subjects who slept more than 9 or less than 6 hours nightly were more likely to have a depressive disorder (van den Berg et al., 2009).

Older adults, like seriously depressed people of any age, are likely to experience psychomotor agitation or retardation. Psychomotor retardation is manifested as slowed body movements and slowed verbal responses, sometimes to the point of muteness. A monotonous or whispering tone of voice might also be an indicator of psychomotor retardation. Affected people often complain of feeling extremely fatigued and having little or no energy. In contrast to people with psychomotor retardation, people with psychomotor agitation present an atypical picture of depression. These people manifest high levels of activity such as pacing and hand wringing. They may be unable to sit still and may have verbal outbursts, such as shouting. Another activity associated with psychomotor agitation is compulsive behavior such as frequent toileting or handwashing.

Psychosocial Function and Quality of Life

Depression is inherently characterized by a depressed mood or sad affect, but older adults may not perceive or acknowledge these mood disturbances in themselves. Rather than acknowledging that they are depressed, older adults are more likely to talk about being "blue" or "down in the dumps." Depressed older people may feel like crying but may not be able to cry or identify the underlying reason for their sadness. Another psychosocial consequence of depression is the absence of life satisfaction even when the person has reasons to feel satisfied.

Anxiety, irritability, diminished self-esteem, and negative feelings about self are some of the more generalized affective consequences of depression. Studies indicate that the co-occurrence of anxiety and depression is associated with increased cognitive impairment (Beaudreau & O'Hara, 2009). The absence of feelings, or a feeling of emptiness, can also be a functional consequence of depression. A loss of interest in social activities may be the depression-related psychosocial change that is most obvious to others. Similarly, other people are likely to observe that the depressed older person has little or no concern about personal appearance. In addition, the depressed person may be overly or unrealistically worried about illnesses, financial affairs, and family issues.

Cognitive impairments can occur because of depression, and in older adults, these deficits are likely to be viewed as a primary problem rather than as a consequence of another problem. Depressed older adults may, in fact, exaggerate cognitive deficits and make statements about global deficits, such as, "I can't remember anything at all." In particular, they may emphasize memory deficits and attribute these to normal aging when the underlying problem is actually a depression-related difficulty in concentrating. See Box 15-3 for a list of functional consequences of depression that affect psychosocial function.

Depression has a major negative impact on quality of life. For example, depressed older adults report unsatisfactory social functioning, lower levels of life satisfaction, and poor perceptions of physical and mental health. In addition, many of the symptoms of depression (e.g., worry, fatigue, sad affect, sleep disturbances, loss of interest) directly interfere with well-being and quality of life. Moreover, depressed older adults often feel a sense of hopelessness. One study of community-living older adults found that feelings of sadness, irritability, worries about the future, and lack of positive affect were significant characteristics of older adults with subclinical depression (Adams & Moon, 2009).

Wellness Opportunity

Because people who are depressed tend to have very low self-esteem, nurses can point out concrete examples of positive qualities that they see in the person.

NURSING ASSESSMENT OF DEPRESSION IN OLDER ADULTS

Whereas Chapter 13 addressed all aspects of psychosocial assessment, this section focuses on the following specific aspects of late-life depression: identifying the unique manifestations of depression in older adults, identifying depression in people with dementia, and using screening tools to identify late-life depression. Assessing the suicide risk in older adults is discussed in the section on Suicide. The assessment information in Chapter 13, particularly Box 13-7, can be used with the information in the following sections as a guide for assessing depression in older adults.

Wellness Opportunity

Nurses can ask a depressed older adult, "Can you think of one thing that we can do to improve your quality of life today?"

TABLE 15-1 Comparison of Depression in Younger and Older Adults

Depressed Younger Adults	Depressed Older Adults
More likely to report emotional symptoms	Report more cognitive and physical symptoms
Sense of hopelessness, uselessness, and helplessness	Apathy; exaggeration of personal helplessness
Negative feelings toward self	Sense of emptiness, loss of interest, withdrawal from social activities
Insomnia	Hypersomnia; early morning awakening
Eating disorders	Anorexia, weight loss
More verbal expressions of suicidal ideation than successful attempts; more passive means of suicide	Less talk about suicide, but more successful attempts and more violent means of suicide

Identifying the Unique Manifestations of Depression

Assessment of late-life depression is complicated by a wide array of possible manifestations, as reviewed in the Functional Consequences section. Moreover, manifestations of depression in older adults may differ from those in younger adults. One study found that older adults are less likely to show affective symptoms and are more likely to have cognitive changes, physical complaints, and a loss of interest than younger adults (Fiske, Wetherell, & Gatz, 2009). Although it is difficult to generalize about manifestations of depression according to age categories, some conclusions about the differences in younger and older adults are summarized in Table 15-1.

In assessing depression in any cognitively impaired older adult, it is often difficult to distinguish between manifestations of depression and dementia. Table 15-2, which identifies specific features that are most likely to be associated with either dementia or depression, can be used as a guide for nursing assessment to differentiate between these two conditions.

TABLE 15-2 Distinguishing Features of Dementia and Depression

Parameter	Dementia	Depression
Onset of symptoms	Gradual onset, recognized only by hindsight	Abrupt onset, possibly involving a triggering event
Presentation of symptoms	Unawareness of symptoms, or attribution to nonpathologic causes	Exaggeration of memory problems and other cognitive deficits
Memory and attention	Impaired memory, particularly for recent events; poor attention; strong attempts to perform well	Memory and attention deficits attributable to lack of motivation and inability to concentrate
Emotions	Labile affect that changes in response to suggestions; possible apathy owing to cognitive impairments	Consistent feelings of sadness and being "down in the dumps"; unresponsive to suggestions
Response to questions	Evasive, angry, sarcastic; use of humor, confabulation, or social skills to cover up deficits	Slowed, apathetic, frequent response of "I don't know," with no effort expended
Personal appearance	Inappropriate dress and actions owing to impaired perceptions and thought processes	Little or no concern about appearance because of lack of motivation or diminished self-esteem
Physical complaints	Vague fatigue and weakness; complaints are inconsistent and easily forgotten	Anorexia, weight loss, constipation, insomnia, decreased energy
Neurologic features	Aphasia, agnosia, agraphia, apraxia, perseveration	Complaints of dysphagia without any physical basis
Contact with reality	Denial of reality; illusions more predominant than hallucinations; if present, delusions are aimed at explaining deficits	Exaggerated sense of gloom; possible auditory hallucinations or self-derogatory delusions

It is important to keep in mind that older adults frequently have both depression and dementia, so manifestations will not always be clearly distinguishable.

Cultural factors can influence one's perception of depression, and nurses must consider these, particularly during their assessments. Nurses can use the information in Cultural Considerations 15-1 to identify some of the cultural variations in expressions of depression. In addition, nurses need to be aware of and sensitive to the fact that many cultural groups attach a strong stigma to depression and other forms of mental illness. Thus, they need to use appropriate communication techniques when assessing for depression and discussing interventions with older adults and their caregivers.

Wellness Opportunity

Nurses respect individual preferences by listening carefully to identify acceptable terminology in older adults who do not want to acknowledge being "depressed."

Using Screening Tools

Concerns about depression being unrecognized and undertreated in older people have stimulated the development of very brief screening tools that healthcare professionals can use in a variety of settings. The U.S. Preventive Services Task Force (USPSTF) recommends depression screening for adults in settings where support staff, such as a screening nurse, is available to facilitate interventions (U.S. Preventive Services Task Force, 2009). The Patient Health Questionnaire (PHQ-2) is a two-item screening tool that is recommended for use in assisted living facilities and other community-based settings because of its brevity, sensitivity, and ease of use (Watson, Zimmerman, Cohen, & Dominik, 2009). The two screening questions recommended by the USPSTF and the PHQ-2 are (1) During the past 2 weeks (or month), have you felt down, depressed, or hopeless? and (2) During the past 2 weeks (or month), have you felt little interest or pleasure in doing things? A positive response to either of these two questions warrants further assessment with a formal depression scale.

The **Geriatric Depression Scale-Short Form (GDS-SF** or GDS-15) is a 15-question screening tool that is widely used across healthcare settings for older adults and can be administered in 5 to 7 minutes. Studies have found that the GDS-SF is reliable, effective, and easily used to detect depression in older adults, including those with cognitive impairment (Greenberg, 2007; Kurlowicz & Harvath, 2008). Another advantage is that the tool and scoring form can be downloaded for free in English and more than 30 other languages from www.stanford.edu/~yesavage/GDS.html. The Hartford Institute for Geriatric Nursing recommends the GDS-SF (Figure 15-1) as an evidence-based screening tool for late-life depression (Greenberg, 2007). The Clinical Tools at the end of this chapter provide information about a demonstration video and additional information about the GDS-SF.

CULTURAL CONSIDERATIONS 15-1

Cultural Variations in Expressions of Depression

Cultural Group	Common Expressions of Depression
African Americans	Fatigue and somatic complaints. "I sure have a lot of troubles." "I know God won't give me more than I can handle."
Alaskan Natives/ Native Americans	Feeling "heavy" or "out of harmony"; may complain of heart problems
Bosnians	Express emotional distress in somatic symptoms such as gastrointestinal or respiratory complaints
Caribbean blacks	Stress from a weakness or deficiency in character; influenced by fear of being ostracized by peers
Chinese Americans	Shameful to discuss; may be called "neurasthenia" (i.e., symptoms produced by social stressors)
Cubans	Attribute symptoms to "nerves," anxiety, or extreme stress; shameful
Filipinos	Shameful to discuss; may refer to *Lungknot* (i.e., sadness)
Greeks	Emotional distress is likely to present with somatic complaints such as dizziness and paresthesias
Haitians	The concept of *voudun* attributes depression to being possessed by malevolent spirits or punishment for not honoring protective spirits; depression can be viewed as a hex placed by a jealous or envious individual
Hindus	Psychological distress is expressed through physical symptoms such as headaches, burning sensation in feet or forehead, and tingling pain in lower extremities
Japanese Americans	Because of shame and stigma, emotional distress may be expressed through physical symptoms and may become severe before help is sought
Koreans	Emotions are expressed as physical complaints, including headaches, insomnia, anorexia, lack of energy
Mexican Americans	Sign of weakness, shameful to discuss, common response to stress
Puerto Ricans	Use *depression* to convey sadness, grief, or anguish; use *nervioso* (nervousness) or *ataque de nervios* (attack of nerves) to describe depressive symptoms
South Asians	References to *Dil uddas hona*, associated with spiritual unhappiness
White British	Associate depression with genetic predisposition, traumatic childhood, or poor relationship with mother
People from countries with a recent history of war, violence, or political upheaval	May be associated with post-traumatic stress disorder; feelings of helplessness; memories of war-related brutalities; may be at increased risk for suicide

Sources: Andrews, M. M., & Boyle, J. S. (2008). *Transcultural concepts in nursing care* (5th ed.). Philadelphia, PA: Lippincott Williams & Wilkins; Lawrence, V., Murray, J., Banerjee, S., Turner, S., Sangha, K., Byng, R., . . . Macdonald, A. (2006). Concepts and causation of depression: A cross-cultural study of the beliefs of older adults. *The Gerontologist, 46,* 23–32; Lipson, J. G., & Dibble, S. L. (2005). *Culture and clinical care.* San Francisco: UCSF Nursing Press; and Purnell, L. D. (2009). *Guide to culturally competent health care* (2nd ed.). Philadelphia: F.A. Davis Co.

Geriatric Depression Scale (Short Form)

	Yes	No
1. Are you basically satisfied with your life?	Yes	No
2. Have you dropped many of your activities and interests?	Yes	No
3. Do you feel that your life is empty?	Yes	No
4. Do you often get bored?	Yes	No
5. Are you in good spririts most of the time?	Yes	No
6. Are you afraid that something bad is going to happen to you?	Yes	No
7. Do you feel happy most of the time?	Yes	No
8. Do you often feel helpless?	Yes	No
9. Do you prefer to stay at home rather than go out and do new things?	Yes	No
10. Do you feel you have more problems with memory than most?	Yes	No
11. Do you think it is wonderful to be alive now?	Yes	No
12. Do you feel pretty worthless the way you are now?	Yes	No
13. Do you feel full of energy?	Yes	No
14. Do you feel that your situation is hopeless?	Yes	No
15. Do you think that most people are better off than you are?	Yes	No

Score: ___/15   One point for "No" to questions 1, 5, 7, 11, 13

One point for "Yes" to other questions

Normal	3 ± 2
Mildly depressed	7 ± 3
Very depressed	12 ± 2

FIGURE 15-1 Geriatric Depression Scale (short form). (From Yesavage, J. A., Brink, T. L., Rose, T. L., Lum, O., Huang, V., Adey, M., et al. [1983]. Development and validation of a geriatric depression screening scale: A preliminary report. *Journal of Psychiatric Research, 17,* 37–49. (Available at ww.stanford.edu/~yesavage/GDS.html.)

NURSING DIAGNOSIS

Because there is no specific nursing diagnosis for depression, the following nursing diagnoses may be applicable: Ineffective Coping, Hopelessness, Chronic Low Self-Esteem, Social Isolation, Powerlessness, Caregiver Role Strain, Risk for Imbalanced Nutrition, and Adult Failure to Thrive. Related factors commonly found in older adults are relocation, ageist attitudes, financial concerns, social isolation, caregiving responsibilities, multiple social stressors, loss of significant roles or relationships, functional impairments (including cognitive deficits), and increased dependence (e.g., owing to the loss of the ability to drive). Risk For Compromised Resilience is a new nursing diagnosis for the 2011–2012 edition of NANDA-I taxonomy.

> **Wellness Opportunity**
>
> Nurses can use the wellness nursing diagnosis of Readiness For Enhanced Coping for older adults who are interested in improving their coping skills to address depressive symptoms that are not severe.

PLANNING FOR WELLNESS OUTCOMES

When caring for older adults who are depressed, nurses identify outcomes as an essential part of the planning process. The following Nursing Outcomes Classification (NOC) terminology is applicable to depressed older adults: Coping, Hope, Self-Esteem, Social Support, Social Involvement, Role Performance, Caregiver Emotional Health, and Caregiver. Specific interventions to achieve outcomes related to depression and suicide are discussed in the following sections.

> **Wellness Opportunity**
>
> Quality of life is a wellness outcome that is achieved by addressing the functional and psychosocial consequences of depression.

NURSING INTERVENTIONS TO ADDRESS DEPRESSION

Although all nurses are responsible for addressing depression in older adults, those who work in community-based and long-term care settings have the most ongoing opportunities to identify manifestations of depression and to request further evaluation and treatment. In recent years, primary care physicians and nurse practitioners have been the healthcare professionals evaluating and managing depression, and referrals to psychiatrists and other mental health professionals for depression have become less common. This trend is due to the emphasis on cost-effectiveness and the availability of safer and more effective antidepressant medications. Nursing protocols for depression in elderly patients emphasize the important responsibility of nurses in reducing the negative consequences of depression through early recognition, intervention, and referral of patients with depression (Kurlowicz & Harvath, 2008).

Nursing Interventions Classification (NIC) terminology pertinent to interventions for older adults who are depressed include the following: Caregiver Support, Coping Enhancement, Counseling, Crisis Intervention, Emotional Support, Eexercise Promotion, Grief Work Facilitation, Hope Instillation, Mood Management, Music Therapy, Role Enhancement, Self-Esteem Enhancement, Suicide Prevention, and Teaching: Individual.

The next sections review the role of the nurse in planning and implementing interventions for late-life depression.

Alleviating Risk Factors

Nurses promote wellness for depressed older adults by addressing the many risk factors that are well within the realm of nursing, such as functional impairments, adverse medication effects, and excess alcohol use. Many nursing interventions that improve the level of functioning are also effective for alleviating or preventing depression. For example, dementia, sensory impairments, urinary incontinence, and mobility impairments are examples of conditions that can contribute to depression and will respond to nursing interventions (refer to Chapters 14, 16, 17, 19, and 22).

> ### ✦ Wellness Opportunity
>
> Nurses promote wellness by challenging ageist stereotypes that falsely attribute functional impairments to inevitable consequences of aging.

If adverse medication effects are a risk factor for depression, nurses can educate the person about this potential relationship and identify problem-solving strategies to address the adverse effects. One such strategy, particularly for older adults who are unaccustomed to raising questions about their medications, is to teach them about communicating with the prescribing healthcare provider (as discussed in Chapter 8). For example, if the older person understands that there is a wide array of antihypertensive medications and that not all of them will cause depression, the person can use this information in discussing the problem with his or her primary care provider. Nurses can also reassure the older adult that it is acceptable to initiate this kind of problem-solving discussion with healthcare practitioners. When the nurse, rather than the patient, is the one who communicates with the primary care provider, the nurse can raise appropriate questions about depression as an adverse medication effect. This problem-solving approach is particularly important when the primary care provider is considering adding an antidepressant medication to a regimen that includes a depression-inducing medication. In these situations, the solution may be to change medications rather than to add another medication and increase the risk for adverse effects.

If excess alcohol use is a risk factor for depression, individual and group interventions can be effective, particularly when the alcohol abuse is a reaction to recent losses. Alcoholics Anonymous (AA) is the most widely used group program for alcoholics of any age, and in some areas, age-homogeneous groups have been established, including some for older adults. Nurses can encourage older adults to initiate contact with AA, or they might directly facilitate the referral if the person agrees to this. Individual and family counseling may also be effective, and nurses can suggest or facilitate referrals for these mental health services.

Improving Psychosocial Function

Nurses can use health promotion interventions, such as the ones discussed in Chapter 12, for addressing risk factors for and symptoms of depression. In any clinical setting, nurses can focus on interventions to promote autonomy, personal control, self-efficacy, and decision-making about daily care as an intervention for depression (Kurlowicz & Harvath, 2008).

Interventions to strengthen social supports and foster meaningful roles are particularly pertinent and relatively easy to implement. Nurses have many opportunities to encourage participation in group meal or social programs. Most communities in the United States have some social programs for older adults, and many provide transportation. Many churches and religious organizations also have programs designed to meet the social needs of isolated older adults. Volunteer visitor or phone call programs, for example, are sometimes available to address the needs of people who have difficulty with getting out of the house. Other programs such as pet therapy or "Adopt-a-Grandparent" are available in some home, community-based, and long-term care settings, and they can be helpful in alleviating loneliness and depression. Nurses can also encourage older adults to maintain social contacts through simple measures such as phone calls.

Involvement in volunteer activities can enhance self-esteem and provide meaningful roles for older adults who are mildly depressed. Nurses can suggest that older adults explore opportunities for volunteer activities through organizations such as the National Senior Service Corps (previously called the Retired Senior Volunteer Program), which is one of many programs in the United States that assist older adults in becoming involved in volunteer activities.

> ### ✦ Wellness Opportunity
>
> Nurses promote quality of life by encouraging an older adult to engage in activities that are pleasant and meaningful to that person.

Promoting Health Through Physical Activity and Nutrition

The beneficial effects of exercise with regard to preventing and alleviating anxiety, depression, and other psychosocial impairments are widely recognized. Studies consistently find that participation in physical exercise is one of the interventions that protects older adults from becoming depressed (Hong, Hasche, & Boland, 2009). One study found that breaking 1 hour of walking per week into shorter periods on 3 to 5 days was more effective in alleviating depression than a single 1-hour session weekly (Legrand & Mille, 2009). Older adults, however, may not view exercise as important, or they may be reluctant to participate in exercise programs because of chronic illnesses such as arthritis. If older adults understand the benefits of exercise for both their physical and mental health, and if an individually tailored program is developed for them, they may be more willing to become involved in exercise programs. In community and long-term care settings, nurses can facilitate the establishment of group exercise programs and encourage depressed older adults to participate in them. In addition to encouraging participation in exercise programs, nurses can encourage participation in many other forms of physical activity. Even in hospital settings, nurses can facilitate referrals to physical, occupational, and recreational therapists as a psychosocial nursing intervention (Kurlowicz & Harvath, 2008).

Nutrition is an important consideration as an intervention for depression for three reasons. First, depression often negatively affects nutritional status, and this can cause additional negative consequences. Second, good nutrition has a positive effect on mental health and cognitive function. Third, constipation is both a consequence of depression and an adverse effect of some antidepressant medications, and nutritional interventions can be effective in alleviating it. During phases of serious depression, malnutrition can lead to medical problems, which may progress to the point of being life-threatening. Nutritional supplements, hyperalimentation, or tube feedings may be necessary interventions when depression seriously interferes with eating. When depression is severe enough to lead to malnutrition, the older person must be evaluated for in-patient psychiatric care. Interventions for less severely depressed older people are aimed at maintaining adequate hydration and nutrition and preventing or managing constipation (as discussed in Chapter 18).

✦ Wellness Opportunity

Nurses address the body–mind–spirit interrelationship by incorporating interventions for optimal nutrition as an essential component of care for depressed older adults.

Providing Education and Counseling

Many types of individual and group **psychosocial therapies** are effective interventions for late-life depression. For example, when multiple stressors challenge the person's coping abilities and contribute to depression, individual or group therapy can be an important intervention for improving the person's psychosocial health and alleviating depression. Nurses can provide counseling and emotional support for all depressed older adults, and in some situations, they can provide specific psychosocial therapies. Some examples of holistic interventions that are within the scope of nursing include the following (Helming & Jackson, 2009):

- Helping older adults identify nonverbalized fears and provide reality-based information to help them evaluate the fear
- Assisting older adults to verbalize emotions by identifying and labeling them so they can communicate more effectively about their emotions and fear
- Providing counseling based on basic psychological theories and concepts

- Encouraging "storytelling" and helping older adults to acknowledge their strengths as well as weaknesses through the power of storytelling
- Facilitating referrals to appropriate mental health services.

Nurses need to be sufficiently familiar with psychosocial therapies that are commonly used for depressed older adults, so they can encourage or facilitate referrals for these interventions. Evidence-based guidelines identify the following therapies as effective for depression in older adults (Blazer, 2002; Institute for Clinical Systems Improvement, 2008):

- Behavior therapy (e.g., problem solving, practicing assertiveness, setting up a daily schedule)
- Cognitive therapy (e.g., conscious restructuring of negative thought processes)
- Interpersonal therapy (e.g., modification of relationships or expectations about relationships)
- Supportive therapy (e.g., evaluating the person's strengths and weaknesses and facilitating choices that improve coping abilities)
- Dynamic psychotherapy (e.g., resolution of intrapsychic conflicts)
- Bibliotherapy (e.g., readings and exercises to assist the person in identifying and reducing dysfunctional thought processes)

In addition to these types of "talking therapies," self-care interventions that address the body–mind connection can alleviate symptoms of depression. One study found that an 8-week mindfulness-based psychoeducational intervention was effective in reducing anxiety and depression in adults who had chronic heart failure (Sullivan, 2009).

In recent years, group therapies have been recognized as an effective and efficient intervention for depressed older adults. Group therapy is effective for depressed older adults because it imparts information, improves self-esteem, enhances social interaction, encourages attitudinal changes, and facilitates personal development (Blazer, 2002). Support and self-help groups are two commonly used types of interventions to improve psychosocial function and alleviate depression in older adults who are coping with life events such as caregiving, widowhood, or grief reactions; nurses can educate older adults about the availability of such groups. Other group models used as interventions for late-life depression include reminiscence, relaxation, art therapy, focused imagery, creative movement, and cognitive–behavioral strategies. In addition to groups specifically targeted for depression, groups such as the "Healthy Aging Class" (described in Chapter 12), which are directed at developing coping skills, may be effective in alleviating depression.

Although adult daycare programs are not primarily a group therapy for depressed older adults, they are a commonly available resource for providing structured social and therapeutic activities. Similarly, many community-based senior programs provide opportunities for group meals, exercise, and social interaction, and these can be quite effective in alleviating mild to moderate depression in older adults. Information about these and other group programs for older adults can be obtained from local offices on aging, and nurses can encourage older adults or their caregivers to seek out and take advantage of these programs.

Facilitating Referrals for Psychosocial Therapies

Nurses have important roles in facilitating referrals for appropriate psychosocial therapies, particularly for older adults who are seriously depressed. In addition to facilitating referrals for mental health services, nurses often have opportunities to initiate discussion of psychosocial therapies during the course of their usual work with older adults. Interdisciplinary geropsychiatric and geriatric assessment offer assessment and treatment of late-life depression, and some community mental health centers have programs for depressed older adults. Nurses can either suggest or directly facilitate referrals to these programs.

A major consideration with regard to referrals for depression interventions is that there is compelling evidence to support the effectiveness of many psychosocial therapies as well as the use of antidepressant medications, either alone or in combination (Institute for Clinical Systems Improvement, 2008; Chatwin et al., 2009; Kurlowicz & Harvath, 2008). Researchers also emphasize the need to persist with the treatment of depression and to try different treatments if the first or second approaches are not effective (Kok, Nolen, & Heeren, 2009).

> ✦ **Wellness Opportunity**
>
> Nurses promote wellness when they convince an older person that depression is not a necessary consequence of aging but is a condition that can respond to treatment.

Teaching About and Managing Antidepressant Medications

Types of Antidepressant Medications

Nurses need to understand the types of **antidepressants** available in order to educate older adults about their medications. Biochemical theories of depression have guided the development of various antidepressant medications. For example, the observation that depression was a common adverse effect of drugs that deplete the brain of catecholamine led to the development of tricyclic and other cyclic antidepressants, which block the reuptake of chemical messengers at neuronal synapses in the brain. As scientists have discovered more information about brain function and neurotransmitters, pharmaceutical companies have made major advances in developing safe and effective antidepressants. Major types of antidepressants are monoamine oxidase inhibitors, cyclic antidepressants, selective serotonin reuptake inhibitors, serotonin and norepinephrine inhibitors, and atypical antidepressants (i.e., those that do not fit any other category).

Monoamine oxidase inhibitors (MAOIs) were the first medications used as antidepressants. After their use became widespread in the 1960s, it was discovered that medications in this category can cause dangerous and even fatal adverse effects (e.g., hypertensive crisis) when they interact with numerous other medications and with certain types of food. Another disadvantage of using MAOIs is the common occurrence of confusion, restlessness, agitation, and paranoid ideation in older adults who are cognitively impaired (Blazer, 2002). Because there are so many contraindications to the use of MAOIs in older adults, they are used with extreme caution and only when other therapies have been ineffective. Thus, older adults who are taking an MAOI are usually very closely supervised and evaluated by a psychiatrist or other primary care practitioner. Examples of MAOIs are phenelzine, isocarboxazid, and tranylcypromine.

Cyclic antidepressants—used widely since the late 1950s—are considered particularly effective in alleviating the following depression-related symptoms: loss of libido, sleep and appetite disturbances, and loss of interest and pleasure in activities. Cyclic antidepressants are usually categorized as tricyclic antidepressants (which were the first ones developed) and second-generation agents (which have been widely used since the mid-1980s). Cyclic antidepressants differ more in their potential for adverse effects than in their therapeutic effects. Because cyclic antidepressants affect several neurotransmitters, they are associated with a variety of anticholinergic and other detrimental effects. Two particular areas of concern in geriatric care are the potential for adverse cardiovascular and anticholinergic effects. The most likely cardiovascular effects are orthostatic hypotension and altered cardiac rate and rhythm. Serious anticholinergic effects include blurred vision, urinary retention, and cognitive impairments. Additional common side effects are sedation, constipation, dry mouth, and weight gain. Because of these side effects, people with glaucoma, prostatic hyperplasia, or cardiac conduction abnormalities should not take cyclic antidepressants. In addition, cyclic antidepressants should be avoided in people with dementia or Parkinson's disease because of the potential adverse effect of cognitive impairment. Anticholinergic potency varies among the tricyclic antidepressants, with amitriptyline having the strongest anticholinergic effects and desipramine having the weakest. As a rule of thumb for older adults, cyclic agents with weaker anticholinergic effects should be prescribed over those with stronger anticholinergic effects.

During the late 1980s, pharmaceutical companies developed two classes of antidepressants that were chemically unrelated to and more selective in their action than the cyclic antidepressants. **Selective serotonin reuptake inhibitors (SSRIs)** relieve symptoms of depression by blocking the reuptake of serotonin, so the level of this neurotransmitter is increased in the brain cells. **Serotonin and norepinephrine reuptake inhibitors (SNRIs)** increase the levels of both serotonin and norepinephrine by inhibiting the reuptake of these neurotransmitters in the brain cells. This type of antidepressant is also called dual reuptake inhibitors. The therapeutic effectiveness of SSRIs and SNRIs is similar to that of cyclic antidepressants, but they have minimal cholinergic, histaminic, dopaminergic, and noradrenergic effects. SSRIs are currently considered the first-line medications for depression because they are effective for most people and their adverse effects are more tolerable and less dangerous (Blazer, 2002; Institute for Clinical Systems Improvement, 2008). For example, an important consideration for older adults is that SSRIs are less likely than cyclics to cause orthostatic hypotension and anticholinergic effects. This is particularly important for older adults who have cognitive impairments and for those who are at high risk for falls.

Although SSRIs are safer than other types of antidepressants, nurses need to be aware of important adverse effects and drug interactions. For example, because SSRIs are metabolized in the liver and some of them are highly bound to plasma protein, SSRIs may interact with other drugs that are metabolized in the liver or are highly protein-bound. Nurses also need to know that hyponatremia is an adverse effect that occurs in up to 32% of older adults who take SSRIs (Bowen, 2009). In addition, nurses need to observe for potential interactions between SSRIs and nicotine, alcohol, and other medications (including some over-the-counter products). For example, the risk for gastrointestinal bleeding is increased when SSRIs are used concurrently with nonsteroidal anti-inflammatory drugs or low-dose aspirin. Also, serious adverse effects can occur when an SSRI is taken with another drug or dietary supplement that increases serotonin levels in the brain (e.g., meperidine, dextromethorphan, L-tryptophan, St. John's wort). Drug interactions may occur even after an SSRI with a long half-life (e.g., fluoxetine) has been discontinued. Common adverse effects of SSRIs include nausea, vomiting, diarrhea, headache, nervousness, insomnia, tremor, dry mouth, and sexual dysfunction. Withdrawal effects of SSRIs include nausea, tremor, anxiety, dizziness, palpitations, and paresthesias.

A meta-analysis of randomized controlled trials comparing 12 commonly prescribed antidepressants identified mirtazapine, escitalopram, venlafaxine, and sertraline as the most efficacious medications, with escitalopram and sertraline having the most favorable results with regard to both efficacy and acceptability (Cipriani et al., 2009). Desvenlafaxine is a newer SNRI antidepressant (related to venlafaxine) that is both efficacious and well-tolerated but has not been compared with other antidepressants in long-term trials (Perry, 2009; Soares, 2009; Thase et al., 2009).

Antidepressants that are commonly used for older adults are listed in Table 15-3 according to their classifications. Special considerations in the use of some of these antidepressants are as follows: venlafaxine may cause an increase in blood pressure; mirtazapine can be helpful for stimulating appetite, but it also can be sedating; trazodone and nefazodone are very sedating and may be useful in the treatment of depression with sleep disturbances; bupropion has a stimulating effect, which can sometimes be therapeutic but is contraindicated in people with a seizure disorder; bupropion and mirtazapine have the lowest rate of sexual side effects. Also, it is

TABLE 15-3 Antidepressants Commonly Used for Older Adults

Category	Examples	Trade Names
Selective serotonin reuptake inhibitors (SSRIs)	Citalopram	Celexa
	Escitalopram	Lexapro
	Fluvoxamine	Luvox
	Paroxetine	Paxil
	Sertraline	Zoloft
Serotonin and norepinephrine reuptake inhibitors (SNRIs)	Desvenlafaxine	Pristiq
	Duloxetine	Cymbalta
	Venlafaxine	Effexor
Serotonin modulators	Nefazodone	Serzone
	Trazodone	Desyrel
Dopamine reuptake inhibitors	Bupropion	Wellbutrin
Cyclic antidepressants	Amoxapine	Asendin
	Desipramine	Norpramin
	Imipramine	Tofranil
	Nortriptyline	Pamelor
Tetracyclic antidepressants	Mirtazapine	Remeron

important to monitor serum sodium levels initially and periodically for older adults who are taking SSRIs.

Nurses also need to be aware of that the following antidepressants that are contraindicated in older adults due to their adverse effects: amitriptyline (Elavil), doxepine (Sinequan), and fluoxetine daily dose (Prozac). Psychomotor stimulants (e.g., methylphenidate) have been used for decades for certain types of depression, but they are not commonly used for older adults.

DIVERSITY NOTE

African Americans with coronary heart disease are less likely than whites to be treated with antidepressants, despite having similar levels of depression (Waldman et al., 2009).

Nursing Responsibilities Regarding Antidepressants

An important nursing responsibility regarding antidepressants is to educate older adults about the primary purpose of these medications, which is to alleviate depressive symptoms so that the person is able to respond to additional interventions such as psychosocial therapy. For older adults who have both depression and dementia, antidepressant medications may improve the affective symptoms so that overall abilities are improved and the person is able to function more effectively and independently.

Nursing responsibilities regarding antidepressant medication therapy include observing for both adverse and therapeutic effects and educating the older adult about the unique aspects of these medication therapies. Another important responsibility is educating older adults about the need for ongoing evaluation and treatment of depression including the monitoring of antidepressant medication use. Older adults who have been diagnosed with major depressive disorder are at high risk of recurrence, and this risk is increased if antidepressant medications are not maintained for at least 6 months. Older adults often want to discontinue medications when

Box 15-4 Health Education About Antidepressant Medications

Information to Be Shared With the Older Adult
- Immediate improvement will not be evident, but a fair trial must be given to the medication as long as serious adverse effects are not noticed.
- The fair trial may take as long as 12 weeks, but some positive effects should be noticed within 2 to 4 weeks.
- If one type of antidepressant is not effective, another type may be effective.
- Antidepressants cannot be used on an "as needed" basis.
- Antidepressants should be viewed as part of a comprehensive approach to treating depression, and psychosocial therapies should be considered along with antidepressants.
- Antidepressants can interact with alcohol, nicotine, and other medications, including over-the-counter medications, possibly altering the effects of the medication or increasing the potential for adverse effects.
- The prescribing health care practitioner should be asked about potential adverse effects and drug–drug or food–drug interactions.
- The prescribing healthcare practitioner should be consulted before discontinuing an antidepressant.
- If postural hypotension occurs, the effects can be minimized through such interventions as changing position slowly and maintaining adequate fluid intake.
- If monoamine oxidase inhibitors (MAOIs) are prescribed, certain medications must be avoided, and a low-tyramine diet must be followed (i.e., avoidance of beer, yogurt, red wine, fermented cheese, and pickled foods, as well as excessive amounts of caffeine and chocolate).

Principles Regarding Dosage and Length of Treatment
- Older adults should be started at one-half to one-third the normal adult dose.
- Dosages can be increased gradually until maximal therapeutic levels are reached, while observing for adverse effects.
- Age-related changes may increase the time needed for medication to reach maximal effectiveness.
- A once-daily regimen usually is effective.
- Bedtime administration of an antidepressant may facilitate sleep as a result of the drug's hypnotic effects, but some antidepressants (e.g., fluoxetine) may be better taken in the morning because of side effects such as agitation.
- The length of treatment is usually 6 months for a first-time depression, 1 to 2 years for people with a history of a prior depressive episode, and lifetime maintenance for people with a history of three or more depressive episodes.

their depressive symptoms resolve, and nurses need to teach them about the importance of ongoing antidepressant therapy and periodic reevaluations after medications are discontinued. This is particularly important because a patient's beliefs about the use of medications affect adherence; therefore, beliefs need to be explored before and during medication therapy. Box 15-4 summarizes guidelines for the nursing responsibilities regarding antidepressant medications.

Teaching About Electroconvulsive Therapy

Electroconvulsive therapy (ECT) is a treatment that has a high efficacy rate and is the most effective treatment available for severe depressive episodes (Payne & Prudic, 2009). Studies have found that ECT is at least as effective, and perhaps more effective, as medications for older depressed patients, and it can be life-saving for seriously depressed older adults (Kennedy et al., 2009; Little, 2009). Evidence-based guidelines have identified the following factors that indicate consideration for ECT treatment (Institute for Clinical Systems Improvement, 2008):
- Geriatric depression
- When antidepressants are ineffective, not tolerated, or pose significant medical risk
- When any of the following conditions exist: catatonia, severe risk of suicide, depression with psychosis, predominance of melancholic symptoms
- When the patient's health is significantly compromised due to depression (e.g. not eating, functional impairment)
- Combination of depression and Parkinson's disease.

ECT is contraindicated in certain medical conditions such as serious arrhythmias, acute myocardial infarction, uncompensated congestive heart failure, and increased intracranial pressure (Greenberg & Kellner, 2005). The efficacy of ECT is substantially increased when antidepressant medications are prescribed to prevent a relapse (Sackeim et al., 2009).

Prevalent negative attitudes about ECT are attributable, in part, to the alleged inhumane use of this procedure when it was first developed a half-century ago. In recent years, however, the technique for administering ECT has been refined, and the risks, discomfort, and side effects are now quite minimal. Most adverse effects—such as headache, nausea, bradycardia, memory impairment, and muscle pain—are transient. Occasionally, however, the adverse cognitive effects may be more extensive or even permanent, particularly after several courses of ECT. Adverse cognitive effects can be described as follows (Greenberg & Kellner, 2005):
- Acute confusional state (disorientation), lasting for less than an hour and occurring after each treatment
- Anterograde amnesia (impaired ability to retain new memories), lasting for several weeks and occurring after a course of treatment
- Retrograde amnesia (forgetting events immediately before the treatment), lasting for several months and occurring after a course of treatment

With the exception of psychiatric settings, nurses will not be involved with the care of people who are undergoing ECT. Nurses caring for depressed people in any setting, however, need to maintain an open mind about this therapy. In addition, nurses may be in a position to encourage older adults or their caregivers to seek advice about ECT from knowledgeable professionals.

Teaching About Complementary and Alternative Interventions

There has been increasing interest in the use of herbs and other natural remedies for depression. **St. John's wort** (*Hypericum perforatum*) is widely used in Europe and is the most commonly used antidepressant in Germany. Since 1998, the National Institutes of Health Office of Alternative Medicine has sponsored randomized, controlled, double-blinded studies in the United States to compare placebo, St. John's wort, and prescription antidepressants. A comprehensive review of recent studies concluded that St. John's wort is an effective treatment for some types of depression (e.g., minor depression), but it also has adverse effects and interactions that nurses need to be aware of (Carpenter, Crigger, Kugler, & Loya, 2008). Common side effects include fatigue, headache, restlessness, anorgasmia, polyuria, hypothyroidism, pruritus, photosensitivity, dry mouth, and gastrointestinal effects. Drug interactions identified in studies include antidepressants, carbamazepine, digoxin, simvastatin, theophylline, and warfarin. St. John's wort is widely available and relatively inexpensive, but products are not standardized or regulated for quality (see Chapter 8 for further considerations regarding herbs).

Bright-light therapy is an evidence-based treatment of some types of depression, including those with seasonal patterns, both as a stand-alone intervention and to enhance the effects of antidepressants (Institute for Clinical Systems Improvement, 2008; Howland, 2009). Bright-light therapy involves exposure to 5,000 to 10,000 lux of bright light for 30 to 60 minutes daily. Nurses can use Box 15-5 as a guide to teaching older adults about interventions that may be helpful for preventing or alleviating depression.

Box 15-5 Interventions Commonly Used for Preventing or Alleviating Depression

Health Promotion Interventions
- Participate in enjoyable exercise for a minimum of 30 minutes five times weekly.
- Seek individual or group counseling to address stressful situations.
- If symptoms of depression affect daily functioning or quality of life, seek evaluation and treatment from a primary care practitioner.

Nutritional Considerations
- Ensure adequate intake of (or use supplements of) the following nutrients: vitamins B, C, and D; magnesium; selenium.

Complementary and Alternative Therapies
- St. John's wort, 300 mg three times daily, may be effective in reducing the symptoms of mild to moderate depression; however, do not take this with an antidepressant, and be sure to talk with your primary care practitioner about using it. Observe for interactions with other medications.
- Bright-light therapy for a half hour, daily
- Art, dance, music, drama, yoga, t'ai chi, qigong, massage, imagery, meditation, relaxation, stress management, spiritual healing

EVALUATING THE EFFECTIVENESS OF NURSING INTERVENTIONS

Nurses evaluate their care of depressed older adults by documenting improved coping skills and diminished manifestations of depression. For example, the person may report diminished feelings of hopelessness and improved appetite and sleep. Another measure reflecting improved quality of life would be the older adult's interest and participation in meaningful activities. Effectiveness of nursing interventions may also be evaluated by whether the older adult has begun taking antidepressant medications and participating in individual or group therapies. Evidence-based Guidelines 15-1 summarizes guidelines for nursing assessment and interventions related to depression in older adults.

SUICIDE

Although suicide is the most serious functional consequence of late-life depression, nurses and other healthcare workers tend to overlook this risk. This tendency is partially attributable to the fact that old age is associated with passivity and nonviolence, whereas suicide is associated with aggressiveness and violence. The following statistics draw attention to the seriousness of this issue (Centers for Disease Control and Prevention, 2007; Centers for Disease Control and Prevention, 2009):

- Adults aged 65 years and older constitute 13% of the population in the United States, but they commit 18% of all suicides.
- Despite the high death rate for suicide among younger age groups, death rates for suicide are consistently highest among older adults; 16.4 suicides occurred per 100,000 population among people aged 75 years or older, compared with 12.6 suicides per100,000 population among those aged between 20 and 34 years.
- The ratio of suicide attempts to completed suicides is highest among adults aged 65 years and older (4:1) in contrast to a ratio of 200:1 among those aged between 15 and 24 years.
- Almost three-quarters of older adults who were treated in emergency rooms for suicide attempts had a history of depression.
- The most common mechanism for suicide among older adults is the use of a firearm, except for older Asian/Pacific Islanders, in which case suffocation accounted for 53% of suicides.

Suicide rates and mechanisms vary significantly by sex and ethnicity, as illustrated in Figures 15-2 and 15-3.

Official data about suicide do not include information about suicidal events that are unreported for reasons such as family efforts to conceal evidence and difficulty determining the true cause of death in medically ill people. Nor do these rates reflect the unrecognized suicidal acts that older adults

Evidence-Based Practice   15-1
Depression in Older Adults

Statement of the Problem

- Depression is highly prevalent in older adults and is not a natural part of aging.
- Depressive symptoms are associated with higher morbidity and mortality rates in older adults; specific consequences of depression include heightened pain and disability, delayed recovery from illness or surgery, worsening of medical conditions, and suicide.
- Depressive symptoms are more common in older adults who have dementia or more severe or chronic disabling conditions.
- Nurses are at the front line in the early recognition of depression and the facilitation of mental health services.

Recommendations for Nursing Assessment

- Depression may range in severity from mild symptoms to more severe forms, both of which can persist over longer periods and have serious negative consequences for the older adult.
- Depression can occur for the first time in late life or it can be part of a long standing affective disorder.
- Recognition of depression in older adults is hindered by the coexistence of medical illnesses, disability, cognitive dysfunction, and psychosocial adversity in older adults.
- The nursing standard of practice for depression in older adults includes the following assessment parameters: identifying risk factors and high-risk groups, using GDS-SF for screening, performing a focused depression assessment on all high-risk groups, obtaining and reviewing medical history and physical/neurologic examination, assessing for medications and medical conditions that may contribute to depression, assessing cognitive function and level of functioning.

- Risks for late-life suicide include depressive symptoms, perceived health status, sleep quality, absence of a confidant, disruption of social support, family conflict, loneliness.

Recommendations for Care

- For severe depression (e.g., GDS 11 or greater), refer for psychiatric evaluation and treatment with medication, psychosocial therapies, hospitalization, or ECT.
- For less severe depression (e.g., GDS score between 6 and 10), refer to mental health services for psychosocial therapies and determination whether antidepressant therapy is warranted.
- For all levels of depression, develop an individualized plan integrating nursing interventions that address issues such as safety, nutrition, risk factors, health education, social support, pleasant reminiscence, and relaxation therapies.

Recommendations for Patient Teaching

Teach older adults and caregivers about the following:
- Depression is common, treatable, and not the depressed person's fault.
- Adherence to the prescribed treatment regimen, including medications, is imperative to prevent recurrence.
- It is important to be aware of the therapeutic and adverse effects of the prescribed antidepressant.

SOURCE: Kurlowicz, L. H., & Harvath, T. A. (2008). Depression. In E. Capezuti, D. Zwicker, M. Mezey, & T. Fulmer (Eds.), *Evidence-based geriatric nursing protocols for best practice* (3rd ed., pp. 57–82). New York: Springer Publishing Co.

indirectly or subtly use to take their own lives such as refusal to eat, failure to take medically necessary medications, and other means of self-neglect.

Assessing the Risks for Suicide

Nursing assessment of suicide risk is particularly important because most older people give clues, sometimes to many people, about potential suicide. These clues, however, may be subtle, and the person who hears them may not associate them with suicide risk, particularly in older adults. By identifying risk factors, nurses can initiate interventions to prevent suicide. This is particularly important because three-quarters of older people who commit suicide visit their primary care provider within 1 month before the act, but they are not likely to directly express suicidal ideation. Thus, healthcare providers need to assess for risks and identify those older adults who may be contemplating suicide. The following are some of the more commonly identified risks for suicide in

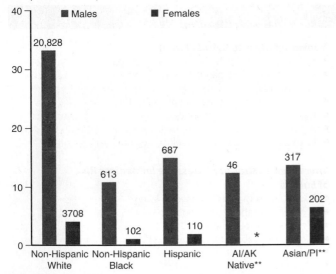

Rate per 100,000 Population

FIGURE 15-2 Suicide rates for people 65+ years in the United States according to race/ethnicity and sex, 2002–2006. Numbers shown are suicide deaths per 100,000 population. *All rates are age specific. Rates based on <20 deaths are not shown as they are statistically unreliable. **AI/AK Native: American Indian/Alaskan Native, PI: Pacific Islander. (*Source:* Centers for Disease Control and Prevention. [2009]. Atlanta, GA.)

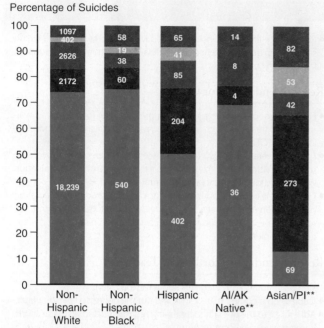

FIGURE 15-3 Percentage of suicides among people 65+ years in the United States, by race/ethnicity and mechanism, 2002–2006. Numbers shown are suicide deaths per 100,000 population. (*Source:* Centers for Disease Control and Prevention. [2009]. Atlanta, GA.)

older adults (Cukrowicz et al., 2009; Hicks & Woods, 2009; Liu & Chiu, 2009; Mitty & Flores, 2008):

- Depression, which may be masked by excessive focus on physical complaints

- Personal or family history of depression
- Past suicide attempts
- Loneliness, limited social support
- Family discord
- Feelings of abandonment
- Recent bereavement
- Presence of chronic or severe pain

Because depression is the factor most consistently identified across studies as a risk factor for suicide, it is important to assess for suicidal ideation in any depressed older adult. In addition to these factors that alert the nurse to risk for suicide, the factors that are most strongly predictive of actual suicide are a history of previous attempts and current suicide ideation that includes a plan or evidence of preparation of a plan.

When risk factors or clues to potential suicide are identified, the nurse must further assess the actual risk for a suicide attempt. This assessment is multilevel, with each level of questions depending on the response to the previous level. Nurses begin the assessment with level 1 questions to determine the presence or absence of suicidal thoughts. Although healthcare professionals may be reluctant to initiate questions about suicide because they fear that this line of questioning may "put ideas in the person's head," this fear is unfounded. People who do not have suicidal thoughts usually respect the necessity of the questions but do not begin thinking about suicide just because the topic was broached. Even so, rather than beginning with a blunt question such as, "Do you ever think about committing suicide?" the nurse can phrase the question in such a way that the person will give clues to his or her intent if it exists but will not be offended by the question if it does not (see Box 15-6 for examples).

 Box 15-6 Guidelines for Assessing Suicide Risk

Risk Factors for Suicide in Older Adults
- Demographic factors: white race, male gender
- Depression, particularly when accompanied by insomnia, agitation, and self-neglect
- Chronic illness with increasing dependence and helplessness; diagnosis of cancer or a terminal illness
- Poor social supports; social isolation, particularly recent isolation
- History of psychiatric illness, particularly major depression
- Onset of major depression within the past year
- Family history of suicide; personal or family history of suicide attempts
- Patterns of impulsive behavior
- Alcohol abuse
- Poor communication skills

Verbal Clues to Suicide Intent
- "Pretty soon you won't have to worry about me."
- "I would be better off dead."
- "I'll make sure I won't be a burden to others."
- Expressions of hopelessness
- Remarks about life being unbearable
- Reflections on the worthlessness of life

Nonverbal Clues to Suicide Intent
- Making a will; giving belongings away; preparing for own funeral
- Serious self-neglect, particularly in people who have no cognitive impairments
- Frequent visits to primary care provider(s)
- Excessive use of medications or alcohol
- Accumulation of prescription medications
- Unusual preoccupation with self and withdrawal from others

Interview Questions to Assess the Immediate Risk of Suicide
- "Do you think that life is not worth living?"
- "Do you think about escaping from your problems?"
- "Do you wish you were dead?"
- "Do you think about harming yourself?"
- "Do you think about ending your life?"
- "Do you have a plan?"
- "What would you do to take your life?"
- "Have you ever started to act on a plan to harm yourself?"
- "Under what circumstances would you act on that plan?"
- "What prevents you from acting on the plan?"

Nurses need to recognize that older adults may express a loss of interest in living and may even state that they wish they were dead, but these verbalizations are not necessarily associated with suicidal thoughts. Many times these expressions arise from feelings of being overwhelmed with an illness or stressful situation, and they are not indicators of a desire to take one's own life. These expressions may also be related to dementia or an inability to express one's feelings accurately, which sometimes occurs after strokes. In these situations, nurses need to further assess for depression and identify stressful conditions that can be addressed through interventions.

If suicidal thoughts are suspected or identified at level 1, nurses ask level 2 questions, which are aimed at determining the presence or absence of thoughts about self-harm. If the answer to any of these questions is positive, nurses ask level 3 questions, which are very direct and specific because this information is crucial to assessing the immediate risk for suicide. If the person describes a detailed plan and has access to all the necessary implements, the potential for suicide is extremely high. By contrast, if the person has a plan that is vague or that cannot possibly be carried out, the immediate potential for suicide is lower. For example, if the plan involves a gun, but the person does not have a gun and cannot get out of the house, then the chance of a successful suicide is low. By contrast, if the person threatens to consume the bottle of barbiturates that is readily available in the medicine cabinet, then the chance of a successful suicide is quite high. Nurses proceed to level 4 questions to assess the immediacy of the risk when the person has described a plan. When answers to levels 3 or 4 are positive, the nurse must plan immediate interventions to deal with the suicide risk. An essential nursing responsibility with regard to level 4 questions is to ask what prevents the person from carrying out the plan because this information provides a base for supporting important patient-identified reasons for living.

Nursing Diagnosis and Outcomes

If the nursing assessment identifies risk factors for suicide, an applicable nursing diagnosis would be Risk for Suicide, defined as "at risk for self-inflicted, life-threatening injury" (NANDA International, 2009, p. 330). Related factors would include any risk factors and verbal and nonverbal clues to suicide. An example is an 85-year-old widower who says his life is no longer worthwhile and who makes frequent visits to his doctor for complaints of weight loss and sleep disturbance. Outcomes for older adults at risk for suicide include Suicide Self-Restraint and Personal Safety Behavior.

Nursing Interventions for Preventing Suicide

Nurses do not routinely encounter suicidal older adults, but they need to be prepared to implement immediate interventions whenever they identify a patient at risk. The most important intervention is to seek psychiatric resources and activate referrals to the appropriate protective service agency rather than attempting to deal with potentially suicidal people without the help of specialized resources. One study found that the provision of care management services significantly reduced suicidal ideation in depressed older adults (Alexopoulos, 2009). All communities have some emergency psychiatric resources, and nurses can follow institutional policies regarding referrals for appropriate services. In any situation, nurses use appropriate communication techniques to address potentially suicidal older adults. Some guidelines for working with people who are potentially suicidal are listed in Box 15-7.

Evaluating the Effectiveness of Nursing Interventions

Nursing care of older adults who are at high risk for self-harm are evaluated by the prevention of harm. Another measure is the degree to which the older adult develops coping skills to deal with the issues that underlie his or her suicidal thoughts. Nurses can also find out whether the older adult obtained suggested mental health services and determine the effectiveness of any referrals that were made.

 Box 15-7 Nursing Interventions for People Who Are Potentially Suicidal

Communicating With Someone Who Is Potentially Suicidal
- Be direct and honest; do not be afraid to ask direct questions, such as, "Are you thinking of hurting yourself?"
- Express feelings of concern and confidence.
- Acknowledge the person's feelings of helplessness and hopelessness.
- Encourage the person to talk about the precipitating event, if there is one.
- Emphasize that suicide is only one of several options; then explore other options.
- Emphasize positive relationships; talk about the negative impact of suicide on survivors.
- Maintain a nonjudgmental attitude.

- Make a contract: ask the person to agree to do certain things for limited amounts of time and to call for help if he or she cannot keep the agreement.
- Discuss reasons that the person identifies for not carrying out a suicide plan and find ways to support and strengthen these.
- Discuss the problems openly with the family and caregivers.

Crisis Intervention
- Focus on the immediate precipitating event.
- Reduce the immediate danger by removing the implements, interfering with the plan, and providing constant supervision.
- Obtain psychiatric help; call a suicide hot line or activate emergency psychiatric services if necessary.

*M*rs. D. is 81 years old. Recently, she was diagnosed with vascular dementia. She lives with her husband, who has diabetes, macular degeneration, and severe arthritis. Mrs. D. had managed all household and financial responsibilities until approximately 1 year ago, when she began having trouble with her memory. Mrs. D. was evaluated at the geriatric assessment program where you work, and she was advised to stop driving and to arrange for some help with complex tasks such as bill paying and grocery shopping. Two months after the initial evaluation, Mrs. D. returns for follow-up and informs you that she limits her driving to short, daytime trips in familiar areas. When asked about getting help with complex tasks, she states, "I just don't have any energy to make all those calls you suggested. Besides, I don't want anyone else looking at my finances or going to the store for me."

NURSING ASSESSMENT

A mental status assessment indicates that Mrs. D.'s level of cognitive impairment is unchanged since her initial evaluation. She has some deficits in calculation, short-term memory, abstract thinking, problem-solving, and language skills. Your psychosocial assessment reveals that Mrs. D. has a very sad affect and low self-esteem, and she expresses feelings of hopelessness and helplessness. She admits to being overwhelmed with feelings of responsibility for herself and her husband, and she says she feels "paralyzed because there's no light at the end of the tunnel." She scored 11 on the GDS-15.

When you ask about her daily life, Mrs. D. says she spends most of her time at home because she does not have the energy to go out. She admits that she has difficulty falling asleep at night, and she wakes up at around 4 AM and is unable to return to sleep. She naps for a couple of hours in the

morning and in the afternoon because "I feel tired all the time, and I can't go out and do things anyway." Her appetite is poor, and in the past 2 months, her weight declined from 140 pounds to 126 pounds (her height is 5′6″). She complains of constipation and "heartburn."

When you ask about meaningful activities, she tells you she no longer goes to her weekly bowling club because it meets in the evening, and she does not want to drive at night. She has also given up her church activities (Thursday discussion club and Sunday service) because she does not want to inconvenience anyone by having them drive her. She feels it is "demeaning to have to tell my friends that I need a ride." She used to enjoy reading, but she has not felt like going to the library, and she is not interested in any of the books she has at home.

NURSING DIAGNOSIS

You use the nursing diagnosis of Ineffective Individual Coping, related to depression and declining cognitive abilities. Evidence comes from Mrs. D.'s sad affect, low self-esteem, loss of interest in activities, feelings of hopelessness and help-

lessness, inability to address her problems effectively, and a GDS-15 score indicative of depression. Physical manifestations are her poor appetite, weight loss, sleep disturbances, and complaints about constipation and heartburn.

NURSING CARE PLAN FOR MRS. D.

Expected Outcome	Nursing Interventions	Nursing Evaluation
Mrs. D. will be able to identify her coping patterns.	• Ask Mrs. D. to describe her prior experiences in dealing with her husband's illness. • Help Mrs. D. to identify coping strategies that have been helpful in the past.	• Mrs. D. will recognize and acknowledge the coping strategies that have been helpful in the past.
Mrs. D. will learn about depression and be encouraged to obtain further evaluation of her depression.	• Talk with Mrs. D. about her signs and symptoms of depression, emphasizing the fact that depression is a treatable condition. • Discuss the relationship between depression and the inability to cope effectively with stressful situations.	• Mrs. D. will follow through with an appointment with a geropsychiatrist or talk with her primary care practitioner.

Expected Outcome	Nursing Interventions	Nursing Evaluation
	• Ask Mrs. D. if she is willing to see a geropsychiatrist, or talk to her primary care practitioner for further evaluation and treatment.	
	• Explain that antidepressant medications can be very effective when combined with counseling.	
Effective coping strategies for addressing Mrs. D.'s declining abilities will be identified.	• Discuss with Mrs. D. several options for ongoing support and counseling to assist her in coping with her declining abilities (e.g., the "Something for You" support group for people with memory loss; or individual counseling sessions with the social worker who is affiliated with the geriatric assessment program).	• Mrs. D. will attend one support group on a trial basis and talk with you about the experience at her next appointment in 1 month.
	• Emphasize the importance of developing short-term goals that can be addressed through problem-solving (e.g., suggest that Mrs. D. begin to address her lack of meaningful activities by going to the library for reading material).	• Mrs. D. will make an appointment for counseling with the social worker. • Mrs. D. will participate in one meaningful activity each week for the next month.

THINKING POINTS

- What risk factors are likely contributing to Mrs. D.'s depression?
- What further assessment information would you obtain?
- What questions on the GDS-15 (Figure 15-1) do you think would be indicative of depression for Mrs. D.?
- What additional interventions would you suggest for Mrs. D.?

Chapter Highlights

Theories about Late-Life Depression
- Psychosocial (impact of losses, learned helplessness)
- Cognitive triad (negative appraisals cause distorted perceptions and lead to faulty conclusions)
- Biologic and genetic (changes in the nervous system, genetic variables)
- Depression and dementia (common neuropathologic changes, vascular depression)

Classification of Depression
- Major depression
- Subclinical depression
- Late-life depression
- Depression with cognitive impairment

Risk Factors for Depression in Older Adults
- Demographic and psychosocial
- Medical conditions and functional impairment (Box 15-1)
- Effects of alcohol and medications (Box 15-2)

Functional Consequences Associated With Depression in Older Adults (Box 15-3)
- Physical health and functioning
- Psychosocial function and quality of life

Nursing Assessment of Depression in Older Adults
- Unique manifestations in older versus younger adults (Table 15-1)
- Differentiating between dementia and depression (Table 15-2)
- Cultural variations in expressions of depression (Cultural Considerations 15-1)
- Screening tools (Figure 15-1)

Nursing Diagnosis
- Readiness for Enhanced Coping
- Ineffective Coping
- Hopelessness
- Caregiver Role Strain
- Risk for Imbalanced Nutrition
- Risk for Compromised Resilience

Planning for Wellness Outcomes
- Coping
- Hope
- Caregiver Emotional Health
- Nutritional Status
- Physical Well-Being

Nursing Interventions to Address Depression (Boxes 15-4 and 15-5)

- Alleviating risk factors (addressing functional limitations, teaching about adverse effects of medications and excessive alcohol)
- Improving psychosocial function (social supports, meaningful activities)
- Promoting health through physical activity and nutrition
- Providing education and counseling (individual and group psychosocial interventions)
- Facilitating referrals for psychosocial therapies
- Teaching about antidepressant medications (Table 15-3)
- Teaching about ECT
- Teaching about alternative care practices (e.g., St. John's wort, bright-light therapy)

Evaluating the Effectiveness of Nursing Interventions

- Improved coping skills
- Fewer manifestations of depression
- Expressed feelings of improved quality of life
- Effective use of appropriate mental health services

Suicide

- Suicide rates and mechanisms (Figures 15-2 and 15-2)
- Nursing assessment of suicide risk (Box 15-6)
- Nursing diagnosis and outcomes
- Nursing interventions for preventing suicide (Box 15-7)
- Evaluating effectiveness of interventions

Critical Thinking Exercises

1. Think of an older adult in your personal life or professional practice who is or has been depressed. What are (were) the risk factors in that person's situation that might play (have played) a part in the depression?
2. Describe at least four cultural variations in the way depression might be expressed.
3. What assessment observations would you make and what questions would you ask to differentiate between dementia and depression in older adults?
4. Make up a case example of someone who is potentially suicidal and who would require all four levels of suicide assessment. Describe how you would phrase the questions for each of the levels.
5. Describe a teaching plan for an 84-year-old woman for whom Paxil, 10 mg daily, has been prescribed.

Resources

For links to these resources and additional helpful Internet resources related to this chapter, visit thePoint at http://thePoint.lww. com/Miller6e.

Clinical Tools

American Journal of Nursing and Hartford Institute for Geriatric Nursing
- *How to Try This*, article and video: The Geriatric Depression Scale: Short Form, by S. A. Greenberg (2007), *American Journal of Nursing, 107*, 60–69.

Hartford Institute for Geriatric Nursing
- *Try This: Best Practices in Nursing Care to Older Adults* Issue 4 (2007), The Geriatric Depression Scale (GDS) (Updated)

Evidence-Based Practice

Kurlowicz, L. H., & Harvath, T. A. (2008). Depression. In E. Capezuti, D. Zwicker, M. Mezey, & T. Fulmer (Eds.), *Evidence-Based Geriatric Nursing Protocols for Best Practice* (3rd ed., pp. 57–82). New York: Springer Publishing Co.

National Guideline Clearinghouse
- Detection of depression in older adults with dementia
- Detection of depression in the cognitively intact older adult

Agency for Healthcare Research and Quality
- Screening for depression
- Post-myocardial infarction depression

Health Education

Depression and Bipolar Support Alliance
Geriatric Mental Health Foundation
National Institute of Mental Health, DEPRESSION Awareness, Recognition, and Treatment Program (D/ART)
Mental Health America
National Senior Service Corps

REFERENCES

Adams, K. B., & Moon, H. (2009). Subthreshold depression: characteristics and risk factors among vulnerable elders. *Aging & Mental Health, 13*(5), 682–692.

Alexopoulos, G. S. (2009). Reducing suicidal ideation and depression in older primary care patients: 24-month outcomes of the PROSPECT study. *American Journal of Psychiatry, 166*, 882–890.

American Psychiatric Association. (2000). *Diagnostic and statistical manual of mental disorders* (4th ed., text revision). Washington: American Psychiatric Association.

Andreescu, C., Butters, M., Lenze, E. J. Venkatraman, J. K., Nable, M., Reynolds, C. F., & Aizenstein. (2009). fMRI activation in late-life anxious depression: A potential biomarker. *International Journal of Geriatric Psychiatry, 24*(8), 820–828.

Andrews, M. M., & Boyle, J. S. (2008). *Transcultural concepts in nursing care* (5th ed). Philadelphia, PA: Lippincott Williams & Wilkins.

Barca, M. L., Engedal, K., Laks, J., & Selbaek, G. (2009). A 12 months follow-up study of depression among nursing-home patients in Norway. *Journal of Affective Disorders, 120*, 141–148.

Beaudreau, S. A., & O'Hara, R. (2009). The association of anxiety and depressive symptoms with cognitive performance in community-dwelling older adults. *Psychology and Aging, 24*, 507–512.

Beck, A. T., Rush, A. J., Shaw, B., & Emery, G. (1979). *Cognitive therapy of depression*. New York: Guilford Press.

Bhalla, R. K., Butters, M. A., Becker, J. T., Houck, M. S., Snitz, B. E., Lopez, O. L., . . . Reynolds, C. F. 3rd. (2009). Patterns of mild cognitive impairment after treatment of depression in the elderly. *American Journal of Geriatric Psychiatry, 17*, 308–316.

Blazer, D. G. (2002). *Depression in late life* (3rd ed.). New York: Springer.

Bowen, P. D. (2009). Use of selective serotonin reuptake inhibitors in the treatment of depression in older adults: Identifying and managing potential risk for hyponatremia. *Geriatric Nursing, 30*, 85–88.

Brommelhoff, J. A. (2009). Depression as a risk factor or prodromal feature for dementia: Findings in a population-based sample of Swedish twins. *Psychology and Aging, 24*, 373–384.

Carod-Artal, F. J., Ferreira, C. L., Trizotto, D. S., & Menezes, M. C. (2009). Poststroke depression: prevalence and determinants in Brazilian stroke patients. *Cerebrovascular Diseases, 28*, 157–162.

Carpenter, C., Crigger, N., Kugler, R., & Loya, A. (2008). *Hypericum* and nurses: A comprehensive literature review on the efficacy of St. John's work in the treatment of depression. *Journal of Holistic Nursing, 26*, 200–207.

Centers for Disease Control and Prevention. (2007). Nonfatal self-inflicted injuries among adults aged ≥65 years—United States, 2005. *MMWR. Morbidity and Mortality Weekly Report, 56*(38), 989–993.

Centers for Disease Control and Prevention. (2009). *Facts at a Glance: Suicide.* Available at: www.cdc/gov/violenceprevention.

Chatwin, J., Kendrick, T., Dowrick, C., Tylee, A., Moriss, R., Peveler, R., . . . Mann, A. (2009). Randomised controlled trial to determine the clinical effectiveness and cost-effectiveness of selective serotonin reuptake inhibitors plus supportive care, versus supportive care alone, for mild to moderate depression with somatic symptoms in primary care: The THREAD (THREshold for AntiDepressant response) study. *Evidence-based Mental Health, 12*(4), 109.

Christensen, M. C., Mayer, S. A., Ferran, J. M., & Kissela, B. (2009). Depressed mood after intracerebral hemorrhage: the FAST trial. *Cerebrovascular Diseases, 27*, 353–360.

Cipriani, A., Santilli, C., Furukawa, T. A., Signoretti, A., Nakagawa, A., McGuire, H., . . . Barbui, C. (2009). Escitalopram versus other antidepressive agents for depression. *Cochrane Database of Systematic Reviews*, (2):CD006532. doi:10.1002/14651858.CD006532.pub2.

Cukrowicz K. C., Duberstein P. R., Vannoy S. D., Lynch T. R., McQuoid, D. R., & Steffens, D. C. (2009). Course of suicide ideation and predictors of change in depressed older adults [published online ahead of print July 9, 2008]. *Journal of Affective Disorders, 113*(1–2), 30–36. doi:10.1016/j.jad.2008.05.012.

de Voogd, J. N., Wempe, J.B., Koeter, G. H., Postema, K., van Sonderen, E., Ranchor, A. V., . . . Sanderman, R. (2009). Depressive symptoms as predictors of mortality in patients with COPD. *Chest, 135*(3), 619–625.

Dillon, C., Allegri, R. F., Serrano, C. M., Iturry, M., Salgado, P., Glaser, F. B., Taragano, F. E. (2009). Late- versus early-onset geriatric depression in a memory research center. *Neuropsychiatric Disease and Treatment*, (Suppl. 5), S17–S26.

Dotson, V. M., Davatzikos, C., Kraut, M. A., & Resnick, S. M. (2009). Depressive symptoms and brain volumes in older adults: A longitudinal magnetic resonance imaging study. *Journal of Psychiatry and Neuroscience, 34*, 367–375.

Elkind, M. S. V. (2009). Outcomes after stroke: Risk of recurrent ischemic stroke and other events. *The American Journal of Medicine, 122*, S7–S13.

Fiske, A., Wetherell, J. L., & Gatz, M. (2009). Depression in older adults. *Annual Review of Clinical Psychology, 5*, 363–389.

Gallegos-Carrillo, K., Garcia-Pena, C., Mudgal, J., Romero, X., Duran-Arenas, L., & Salmeron, J. (2009). *Journal of Psychosomatic Research, 66*, 127–135.

Greenberg, R. M., & Kellner, C. H. (2005). Electroconvulsive therapy: A selected review. *American Journal of Geriatric Psychiatry, 13*, 268–280.

Greenberg, S. A. (2007). How to try this: The Geriatric Depression Scale: Short Form, *American Journal of Nursing, 207*(10), 60–69.

Hadidi, N., Treat-Jacobson, D. J., & Lindquist, R. (2009). Poststroke depression and functional outcome: a critical review of literature. *Heart & Lung, 38*, 151–162.

Hedayati, S. S., Minhauddin, A. T., Toto, R. D., Morris, D. W., & Rush, A. J. (2009). Prevalence of major depressive episode in CKD. *American Journal of Kidney Disease, 54*, 399–402.

Helming, M. B., & Jackson, C. (2009). Relationships. In B. M. Dossey & L. Keegan (Eds.), *Holistic nursing: A handbook for practice* (5th ed., pp. 367–391). Boston: Jones and Bartlett Publishers.

Hicks, L. E., & Woods, N. (2009). Depression and suicide risks in older adults: A case study. *Home Healthcare Nurse, 27*(8), 482–487.

Hong, S-I., Hasche, L., & Bowland, S. (2009). Structural relationships between social activities and longitudinal trajectories of depression among older adults. *The Gerontologist, 49*, 1–11.

Howland, R. H. (2009). Somatic therapies for seasonal affective disorder. *Journal of Psychosocial Nursing and Mental Health Services, 47*, 17–20.

Huang, G. H., Oquendo, M. A., Currier, D., & Mann, J. J. (2009). Increased risk of suicide attempt in mood disorders and TPH1 genotype. *Journal of Affective Disorders, 115*, 331–338.

Hybels, C. F., Pieper, C. F., & Blazer, D. G. (2009). The complex relationship between depressive symptoms and functional limitations in community-dwelling older adults: The impact of subthreshold depression. *Psychology and Medicine, 39*, 1677–1688.

Institute for Clinical Symptoms Improvement. (2008). *Major depression in adults in primary care.* National Guideline Clearinghouse (www.guideline.gov)

Jones, C. A., Pohar, S. L., & Patten, S. B. (2009). Major depression and health-related quality of life in Parkinson's disease. *General Hospital Psychiatry, 31*, 334–340.

Kennedy, S. H., Milev, R., Giacobbe, P., Ramasubbu, R., Lam, R. W., Parikh, S. V., . . . Ravindran, A. V. (2009). Canadian Network for Mood and Anxiety Treatments (CANMAT). Clinical guidelines for the management of major depressive disorders in adults. IV Neurostimulation therapies. *Journal of Affective Disorders, 117*, (Suppl. 1), S44–S53.

Kessig, L. V., Sondergard, L., Forman, J. L., & Andersen, P. K. (2009). Antidepressants and dementia. *Journal of Affective Disorders, 117*, 24–29.

Kok, R. M., Nolen, W. A., & Heeren, T. J. (2009). Outcome of late-life depression after 3 years of sequential treatment. *Acta Psychiatry Scandinavia, 119*, 274–281.

Korczyn, A. D., & Halperin, I. (2009). Depression and dementia. *Journal of the Neurological Sciences, 283*, 139–142.

Kurlowicz, L. H., & Harvath, T. A. (2008). Depression. In E. Capezuti, E. Zwicker, M. Mezey, & T. Fulmer (Eds.), *Evidence-based geriatric nursing protocols for best practice* (3rd ed., pp. 57–82). New York: Springer Publishing Co.

Lawrence, V., Murray, J., Banerjee, S., Turner, S., Sangha, K., Byng, R., . . . Macdonald, A. (2006). Concepts and causation of depression: A cross-cultural study of the beliefs of older adults. *The Gerontologist, 46*, 23–32.

Legrand, F. D., & Mille, C. R. (2009). The effects of 60 minutes of supervised weekly walking (in a single vs. 3–5 session format) on depressive symptoms among older women: Findings from a pilot randomized trial. *Mental Health and Physical Activity*, [article in press] doi:10.1016/j.mhpa.2009.09.002

Li, L. W., & Conwell, Y. (2009). Effects of changes in depressive symptoms and cognitive functioning on physical disability in home care elders. *Journal of Gerontology: Medical Sciences, 64A*, 230–236.

Licht-Strunk, E., Beekman, A. T., de Haan, M., & van Marwijk, H. W. (2009a). The prognosis of undetected depression in older general practice patients. A one year follow-up study. *Journal of Affective Disorders, 114*, 310–315.

Licht-Strunk, E., van Marwijk, H., Hoekstra, T., Twisk, J., De Haan, M., & Beekman, A. (2009b). Outcome of depression in later life in primary care: Longitudinal cohort study with three years' follow-up. *British Medical Journal, 338*, a3079. doi:10.1136/bmj.a3079.

Lin, E., Heckbert, S., Rutter, C., Katon, W., Ciechanowski, P., Ludman, E., . . . Korff, M. (2009). Depression and increased mortality in diabetes: Unexpected causes of death. *Annals of Family Medicine, 7*(5), 414–421.

Lipson, J. G., & Dibble, S. L. (2005). *Culture and clinical care.* San Francisco: UCSF Nursing Press.

Little, A. (2009). Treatment-resistant depression. *American Family Physician, 80*(2), 167–172.

Liu, I. C., & Chiu, C. H. (2009). Case-control study of suicide attempts in the elderly. *International Psychogeriatrics, 21*, 896–902.

Lyness, J. M., Chapman, B. P., McGriff, J., Drayer, R., & Duberstein, P. (2009). One-year outcomes of minor and subsyndromal depression in older primary care patients. *International Psychogeriatrics, 21*, 60–68.

Mittey, E., & Flores, S. (2008). Suicide in late life. *Geriatric Nursing, 29*, 160–165.

NANDA International. (2009). *Nursing diagnoses: Definitions and classification 2009–2011*. Oxford: Wiley-Blackwell.

Olin, J. T., Schneider, L. S., Katz, I. R., Meyers, B. S., Alexopoulos, G. S., Breitner, J. C., . . . Lebowitz B. D. (2002). Provisional diagnostic criteria for depression of Alzheimer disease. *American Journal of Geriatric Psychiatry, 10*, 125–128.

Omachi, T. A., Katz, P. P., Yelin, E. H., Gregorch, S. E., Iribarren, C., Blanc, P. D., & Eisner, M. D. (2009). Depression and health-related quality of life in chronic obstructive pulmonary disease. *The American Journal of Medicine, 122*(778), e9–e15.

Oostervink, F., Boomsma, M. M., Nolen, W. A., & the EMBLEM Advisory Board. (2009). Bipolar disorder in the elderly: Different effects of age and of age of onset. *Journal of Affective Disorders, 116*, 176–183.

Payne, N. A. & Prudic, J. (2009). A perspective on the evolution and current practice of ECT. *Journal of Psychiatric Practice, 15*(5), 346–368.

Perry, R. (2009). Desvenlafaxine: A serotonin-norepinephrine reuptake inhibitor for the treatment of adults with major depressive disorder. *Clinical Therapeutics, 31*(PT), 1374–1404.

Purnell, L. D. (2009). *Guide to culturally competent health care* (2nd ed). Philadelphia: F.A. Davis Co.

Rot, M., Mathew, S. J., & Charney, D. S. (2009). Neurobiological mechanisms in major depressive disorder. *Canadian Medical Association Journal, 180*(3), 305–312.

Russell, D. & Taylor, J. (2009). Living alone and depressive symptoms: The influence of gender, physical disability, and social support among Hispanic and non-Hispanic older adults. *Journal of Gerontology: Social Sciences, 64*(B), 95–104.

Sackeim, H. A., Dillingham, E.M., Prudic, J., Cooper, T., McCall, W. V., Rosenquist, P., . . . Haskett, R. F. (2009). Effect of concomitant pharmacotherapy on electroconvulsive therapy outcomes: short-term efficacy and adverse effects. *Archives of General Psychiatry, 66*(7), 729–737.

Schoevers, R. A., Geerlings, M.I., Deeg, D. J., Holwerda, T. J., Jonker, C., & Beekman, A. T. (2009). Depression and excess mortality: Evidence for a dose responsive relation in community living elderly. *International Journal of Geriatric Psychiatry, 24*(2), 169–176.

Seligman, M. E. P. (1981). A learned helplessness point of view. In L. P. Rehm (Ed.), *Behavior therapy for depression* (pp. 123–141). New York: Academic Press.

Shipowick, C. D., Moore, C. B., & Corbett, C. (2009). Vitamin D and depressive symptoms in women during the winter: A pilot study. *Applied Nursing Research, 22*, 221–225.

Skinner, R., Georgiou, R., Thorton, P., & Rothwell, N. (2009). Psychoneuroimmunology of stroke. *Immunology Allergy Clinics of North America, 29*(2009), 359–379.

Smith, G. S., Kramer, E., Ma, Y., Kingsley, P., Dhawan, V., Chaly, T., Eidelberg, D. (2009). The functional neuroanatomy of geriatric depression. *International Journal of Geriatric Psychiatry, 24*(8), 798–808.

Soares, C. N. (2009). Assessing the efficacy of desvenlafaxine for improving functioning and well-being outcome measures in patients with major depressive disorder: A pooled analysis of 9 double-blind, placebo-controlled, 8-week clinical trials. *The Journal of Clinical Psychiatry, 70*(10), 1365–1371.

Steffens, D. C. (2009). A multiplicity of approaches to characterize geriatric depression and its outcomes. *Current Opinion in Psychiatry, 22*(6), 522–526.

Subramaniam, M., Sum, C. F., Pek, E., Stahl, D., Verma, S., Liow, P. H., Chong, S. A. (2009). Comorbid depression and increased health care utilization in individuals with diabetes. *General Hospital Psychiatry, 31*(3), 220–224.

Sullivan, M. J. (2009). The support, education, and research in chronic heart failure study (SEARCH): A mindfulness-based psychoeducational intervention improves depression and clinical symptoms in patients with chronic heart failure. *American Heart Journal, 157*(1), 84–90.

Tagariello, P., Girardi, P., & Amore, M. (2009). Depression and apathy in dementia: Same syndrome or different constructs? A critical review. *Archives of Gerontology and Geriatrics, 49*, 246–249.

Thakur, M., & Blazer, D. G. (2008). Depression in long-term care. *Journal of the American Medical Directors Association, 9*(2), 82–87.

Thase, M. E., Kornstein, S. G., Germain, J. M., Jiang, Q., Guico-Pabia, C., & Ninan, P. T. (2009). An integrated analysis of the efficacy of desvenlafaxine compared with placebo in patients with major depressive disorder. *CNS Spectrums, 14*(3), 144–154.

Thomas, A. J. (2009). A comparison of neurocognitive impairment in younger and older adults with major depression. *Psychological Medicine, 39*(5), 725–733.

U.S. Preventive Services Task Force. (2009). Screening for depression in adults: U.S. Preventive Services Task Force recommendation statement. *Annals of Internal Medicine, 151*, 784–792.

Van Den Berg, J. F., Luijendijk, H. J., Tulen, J. H., Hofman, A., Neven, A. K., & Tiemeier, H. (2009). Sleep in depression and anxiety disorders: A population-based study of elderly persons. *Journal of Clinical Psychiatry, 70*, 1105–1113.

Waldman, S. V., Blumenthal, J. A., Babyak, M. A., Sherwood, A., Sketch, M., Davidson, J., & Watkins, L. L. (2009). Ethnic differences in the treatment of depression in patients with ischemic heart disease. *American Heart Journal, 157*, 77–83.

Watson, L. C., Zimmerman, S., Cohen, L. W., & Dominik, R. (2009). Practical depression screening in residential care assisted living: Five methods compared with gold standard diagnoses. *American Journal of Geriatric Psychiatry, 17*(7), 556–564.

Wilkins, C. H., Mathews, J., & Sheline, Y.I. (2009). Late life depression with cognitive impairment: Evaluation and treatment. *Clinical Interventions in Aging, 4*, 51–57.

Wolinsky, F. D., Mahncke, H. W., Vander Weg, M. W., Martin, R., Unverzagt, F. W., . . . Tennstedt, S. L. (2009). The ACTIVE cognitive training interventions and the onset of recovery from suspected clinical depression. *Journal of Gerontology: Psychological Sciences, 64B*(5), 577–585.

PART 4

Promoting Wellness in Physical Function

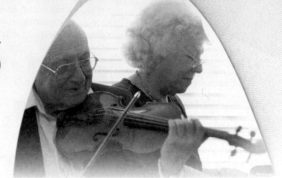

CHAPTER 16

Hearing

LEARNING OBJECTIVES

After reading this chapter, you will be able to:

1. Describe age-related changes that affect hearing.
2. Identify risk factors that affect hearing wellness.
3. Discuss the functional consequences that affect hearing wellness.
4. Conduct a nursing assessment of hearing, with emphasis on identifying opportunities for health promotion.
5. Identify nursing interventions to promote hearing wellness for older adults by addressing risk factors that interfere with hearing.

KEY POINTS

assistive listening device
cerumen
conductive hearing loss
hearing aid
mixed hearing loss
noise-induced hearing loss (NIHL)

otosclerosis
presbycusis
sensorineural hearing loss
tinnitus

Performance of many important daily activities—including communicating, protecting oneself from danger, and enjoying music, voices, and sounds—is highly dependent on good hearing. In older adults, age-related changes combine with risk factors to affect hearing wellness. Nurses promote wellness for older adults when they use health promotion interventions to improve hearing and communication. This chapter addresses the functional consequences associated with hearing in older adults and provides guides for nursing assessment and interventions.

 ## AGE-RELATED CHANGES THAT AFFECT HEARING

Auditory function depends on a sequence of processes, beginning in the three compartments of the ear and ending with the processing of information in the auditory cortex of the brain (see Table 16-1). Sounds are coded according to intensity and frequency. Intensity, or amplitude, reflects the loudness or softness of the sound and is measured in decibels (dB). Frequency, which is measured in cycles per second (cps) or hertz (Hz), determines whether the pitch is high or low. Sound intensity and frequency may be altered if certain risk factors come into play. Even in the absence of risk factors, normal age-related changes affect frequency, causing hearing problems for many older adults.

External Ear

Hearing begins in the external or outer ear, which consists of the pinna and the external auditory canal (Figure 16-1). These cartilaginous structures localize sounds so the person can identify the sources. The pinna undergoes changes in size, shape, flexibility, and hair growth with increasing age, but these changes do not affect the conduction of sound waves in healthy older adults. The auditory canal is covered by skin and lined with hair follicles and cerumen-producing glands. **Cerumen**, or earwax, is a natural substance that is genetically determined to be either dry (flaky and gray) or wet (moist and brown or tan). The function of cerumen is to cleanse, protect, and lubricate the ear canal. Cerumen is naturally expelled, but it can build up in older adults because of age-related changes,

Promoting Hearing Wellness in Older Adults

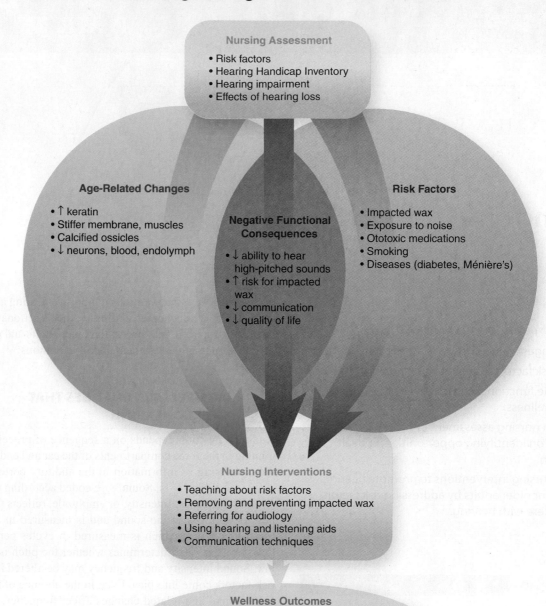

Nursing Assessment

- Risk factors
- Hearing Handicap Inventory
- Hearing impairment
- Effects of hearing loss

Age-Related Changes

- ↑ keratin
- Stiffer membrane, muscles
- Calcified ossicles
- ↓ neurons, blood, endolymph

Negative Functional Consequences

- ↓ ability to hear high-pitched sounds
- ↑ risk for impacted wax
- ↓ communication
- ↓ quality of life

Risk Factors

- Impacted wax
- Exposure to noise
- Ototoxic medications
- Smoking
- Diseases (diabetes, Ménière's)

Nursing Interventions

- Teaching about risk factors
- Removing and preventing impacted wax
- Referring for audiology
- Using hearing and listening aids
- Communication techniques

Wellness Outcomes

- Improved communication
- Increased social interaction
- Increased safety and functioning
- Better quality of life

such as an increased concentration of keratin, the growth of longer and thicker hair (especially in men), and thinning and drying of the skin lining the canal. An age-related diminution in sweat gland activity further increases the potential for cerumen to accumulate by making the wax drier and more difficult to remove. A prolapsed or collapsed ear canal is another age-related condition that can occur and affect localization and perception of high-frequency sounds.

DIVERSITY NOTE

Whites and African Americans are likely to have wet cerumen, whereas Asians and Native Americans are likely to have dry cerumen.

Middle Ear

The tympanic membrane is a transparent, pearl-gray, slightly cone-shaped layer of the flexible tissue separating the outer

TABLE 16-1 Functional Consequences of Age-Related Changes Affecting Hearing

	Change	Consequence
External Ear	• Longer, thicker hair • Thinner, drier skin • Increased keratin	Potential for impacted cerumen and subsequent impaired sound conduction
Middle ear	• Diminished resiliency of tympanic membrane • Calcified, hardened ossicles • Weakened and stiff muscles and ligaments	Impaired sound conduction
Inner ear and nervous system	• Diminished neurons, endolymph, hair cells, and blood supply • Degeneration of spiral ganglion and arterial blood vessels • Decreased flexibility of basilar membrane • Degeneration of central processing systems	*Presbycusis:* diminished ability to hear high-pitched sounds, especially in the presence of background noise

and middle ear. Its primary functions are to transmit sound energy and protect the middle and inner ear. With increased age, collagenous tissue replaces the elastic tissue, resulting in a thinner and stiffer eardrum. Sound vibrations pass through the tympanic membrane to the three auditory ossicles: the malleus, incus, and stapes. These bones are connected to each other but move independently, acting as a lever to amplify sound. Their primary function is to transmit vibrations across the air-filled middle ear, through the oval window, and into the fluid-filled inner ear. Transmission of sound is influenced by the frequency of each sound and is the most effective in the middle-frequency range of normal voices and the least effective at the lowest and highest frequencies. Age-related calcification of the ossicular bones can interfere with

the transfer of sound vibrations from the tympanic membrane to the oval window.

The middle ear muscles and ligaments contract in response to loud noises, stimulating the acoustic reflex, which protects the delicate inner ear and filters out auditory distractions originating from one's own voice and body movements. With increased age, the middle ear muscles and ligaments become weaker and stiffer and have a detrimental effect on the acoustic reflex. In addition, these degenerative changes diminish the resiliency of the tympanic membrane.

Inner Ear

In the inner ear, vibrations are transmitted to the cochlea, where they are converted to nerve impulses and coded for

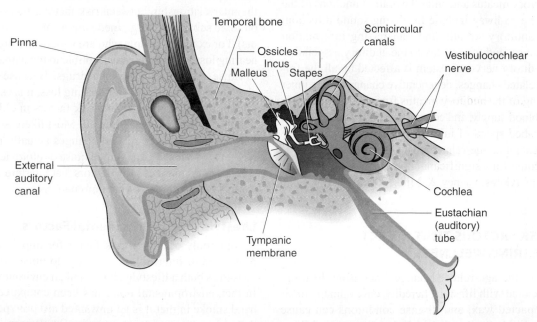

FIGURE 16-1 The ear. Age-related changes in structures of the ear can affect hearing in older adults.

intensity and frequency. Nerve impulses stimulate fibers of the eighth cranial nerve and send the auditory message to the brain. This process transpires primarily in the sensory hair cells of the organ of Corti in the cochlea.

Age-related changes of the inner ear include loss of hair cells, reduction of blood supply, diminution of endolymph production, decreased basilar membrane flexibility, degeneration of spiral ganglion cells, and loss of neurons in the cochlear nuclei. These inner ear changes result in the degenerative hearing impairment termed **presbycusis**. One classification system for presbycusis is based on the specific structural source of the impairment as follows:

- *Sensory presbycusis* is associated with degenerative changes of the hair cells and the organ of Corti and is characterized by a sharp hearing loss at high frequencies.
- *Neural presbycusis*, which is caused by degeneration of nerve fibers in the cochlea and spiral ganglion, is characterized by reduced speech discrimination.
- *Metabolic presbycusis* is caused by degenerative changes in the stria vascularis and a subsequent interruption in essential nutrient supply. Initially, these changes reduce the sensitivity to all sound frequencies; eventually, they interfere with speech discrimination.
- *Mechanical presbycusis* results from mechanical changes in the inner ear structures and is characterized by a hearing loss that initially involves lower frequencies and gradually spreads to higher frequencies and interferes with speech discrimination.

Although useful for explaining the physiologic basis for various types of presbycusis, in reality, presbycusis usually involves several age-related processes.

Auditory Nervous System

From the inner ear, the auditory nerve fibers pass through the internal auditory meatus and enter the brain. Functions of the auditory nerve pathway include localizing sound direction, fine-tuning auditory stimuli, and transferring information from the primary auditory cortex to the auditory association area. The auditory nervous system is affected by all the following age-related changes: degenerative changes in the inner ear, narrowing of the auditory meatus from bone apposition, diminished blood supply, and central nervous system changes (e.g., diminished speed of information processing). Recent studies indicate that age-related changes in central auditory function account for a significant component of hearing loss in older adults (Gates, Feeney, & Mills, 2008).

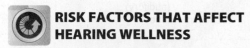

RISK FACTORS THAT AFFECT HEARING WELLNESS

In addition to the age-related changes that affect hearing, factors associated with lifestyle, heredity, environment, medications, impacted wax, and disease conditions can cause hearing loss. Evidence-based guidelines identify the follow-

---

Box 16-1 Risk Factors for Impaired Hearing

Genetic predisposition
Increased age
Recreational or occupational exposure to noise
Cigarette smoking
Ototoxic medications
    Aminoglycosides
    Aspirin and other salicylates
    Cisplatin
    Erythromycin
    Ibuprofen
    Imipramine
    Indomethacin
    Loop diuretics
    Quinidine
    Quinine
Ototoxic environmental chemicals
    Carbon monoxide
    Fuels
    Lead
    Mercury
    Organophosphates
    Styrene
    Toluene

---

ing risk factors for hearing impairment (Adams-Wendling & Pimple, 2008):

- Age 65 years or older
- Residence in a nursing facility
- Cognitive or visual impairments
- Exposure to excessive noise
- Use of ototoxic medications
- Male gender

Much of the research on risk factors focuses on modifiable risk factors, such as noise, that can be addressed through health promotion interventions. Research is also focusing on the interrelationship between risk factors, such as noise and ototoxic substances (e.g., medications or environmental toxins). For example, people who are genetically predisposed to hearing loss may be more susceptible to the damaging effects of noise exposure or ototoxic drugs. Because age-related changes increase the risk for hearing loss, it is especially important to identify modifiable risk factors in older adults so that those risks can be addressed. Most likely, some hearing loss attributed to age-related changes actually results from risk factors, such as exposure to noise or ototoxic substances. Box 16-1 summarizes some factors that interfere with hearing wellness, either alone or in combinations.

Lifestyle and Environmental Factors

A commonly occurring risk factor for impaired hearing is prolonged or intermittent exposure to noise, which can be viewed as both a lifestyle choice and an environmental factor. In fact, environmental noise has been compared to second-hand smoke in that it is an unwanted airborne pollutant produced by others without consent and at times, places, and

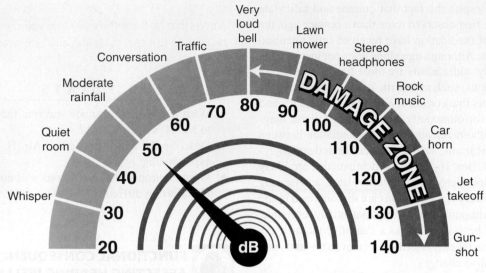

FIGURE 16-2 Noise levels associated with common activities are measured in decibels (dB). Sounds louder than 80 dB are potentially harmful to ears.

volumes over which bystanders have no control (Tompkins, 2009). Studies indicate that although age-related changes account for a greater amount of hearing loss than occupational noise exposure, **noise-induced hearing loss (NIHL)** is still the most important preventable cause of hearing loss in the United States (Dobie, 2008). Occupations associated with an increased risk for NIHL include farmers, musicians, truck drivers, armed services members, and aviation workers (Jansen, Hellerman, Dreschler, & deLaat, 2009; Helfer et al., 2010; Karimi, Nasiri, Kazerooni, & Oliaei, 2010; McCullagh & Robertson, 2009; Wagstaff, 2009). Use of headphones and earphones with personal music players is recreational activity that increases the risk of NIHL (Kim, Hong, Shim, Cha, & Yeo, 2009; Vogel, Verschuure, van der Ploeg, Brug, & Raat, 2010).

Some older adults may have worked in occupational settings before noise level recommendations were enforced by the National Institute for Occupational Safety and Health. For instance, older people who were once employed as weavers or textile workers are likely to have been exposed to detrimentally noisy environments during their work years. Because the effects of NIHL and age-related changes are cumulative, the hearing loss may not be noticed until later adulthood.

Exposure to toxic chemicals in the workplace or the environment is another risk factor for hearing loss that has been under investigation since the 1990s, with current research focusing on metals, solvents, asphyxiants, and pesticides/herbicides. Cigarette smoking, as well as living in a household with a smoker, is another factor being investigated both as an independent risk and as a condition that potentiates the effects of noise to cause hearing loss.

Hunting, woodworking, and other leisure-time activities can also contribute to NIHL, especially if people engaging in these activities do not use protective ear devices. Other activities that are likely to cause sensorineural damage unless protective mechanisms are used include listening to loud music; operating tractors, chain saws, or leaf blowers; and riding motorcycles, airplanes, snowmobiles, or motorboats. Figure 16-2 illustrates the noise levels of various activities. Sounds louder than 80 dB are considered potentially ototoxic.

> **DIVERSITY NOTE**
>
> Moderate to severe age-related hearing loss in women is strongly associated with a maternal family history of hearing loss and in men is significantly, but less strongly, associated with a paternal family history (McMahon, Kifley, Rochtchina, Bewall, & Mitchell, 2008).

Impacted Cerumen

Impacted cerumen is common in older adults as a leading cause of hearing loss. Age-related changes, which make the cerumen dryer, harder, and coarse, increase the risk of impaction. The use of hearing aids also increases the possibility of impacted wax, which can damage or interfere with the function of the hearing aid. In addition to causing a hearing loss, impacted cerumen can cause pain, infection, tinnitus, dizziness, or chronic coughing (due to stimulation of a branch of the vagus nerve) (McCarter, Courtney, & Pollart, 2007; University of Texas School of Nursing, 2007). Cerumen accumulation is preventable and treatable and, most important, it is readily amenable to nursing interventions, as discussed later in this chapter. Studies indicate that up to 57% of older nursing home residents have impacted cerumen (Roland et al., 2008). Moreover, studies of hospitalized older adults indicate that 75% of those who had earwax removed had improved hearing (McCarter et al., 2007).

Medication Effects

Medications can cause or contribute to hearing impairments by damaging the cochlear and vestibular divisions of the auditory nerve. Despite the fact that quinine and salicylate ototoxicities were first observed more than a century ago, the ototoxic effects of medication have received little attention in clinical settings. Although age alone does not increase the risk for ototoxicity, older adults are more likely to be taking ototoxic medications, such as aspirin and furosemide. Other contributing factors that commonly occur in older adults and increase the risk for ototoxicity include renal failure, long-term use of ototoxic medications, and potentiation between two ototoxic medications, such as furosemide and aminoglycoside antibiotics. Box 16-1 lists medications that are likely to be ototoxic. Ototoxicity is often dose related, and hearing loss may be temporary if medications are discontinued or the dose is reduced. Although ototoxicity is potentially reversible, medications may be overlooked as a causative factor if the hearing loss is mistakenly ascribed to inevitable and irreversible degenerative changes.

Disease Processes

Otosclerosis is a hereditary disease of the auditory ossicles that causes ankylosis of the footplate of the stapes to the oval window. Otosclerosis usually begins in youth or early adulthood, but the hearing loss may not be detected until middle or later adulthood, when age-related middle ear changes compound the disease-related changes. Otosclerosis primarily causes a conductive hearing loss, but some sensorineural loss also may occur. Initially, it is difficult to hear soft and low-pitched sounds; as the hearing loss worsens, the person is likely to experience dizziness, tinnitus, or balance problems.

Ménière disease and acoustic neuromas are auditory system diseases that commonly cause hearing impairment. Studies have found that diabetes is an independent risk factor for hearing impairment (Bainbridge, Hoffman, & Cowie, 2008). Other conditions and systemic diseases that can cause or contribute to hearing impairment include syphilis, myxedema, hypertension, meningitis, hypothyroidism, head trauma, high fevers, Paget disease, radiation for head and neck cancers, and viral infections (e.g., measles and mumps).

✦ Wellness Opportunity

Modifiable and preventable risk factors for hearing loss include noise, medications, and impacted cerumen.

---

*M*r. H. is 60 years old and owns a small home-remodeling business. He has been a carpenter for 38 years, but in the past 9 years, he has spent most of his time in the office, managing his business. He enjoys hunting and fishing on weekends. He has smoked two packs of cigarettes a day since he was 16 years old. His wife has been telling him she thinks he hears only what he wants to hear. Mr. H.

admits that he turns the television volume up louder than he used to but denies having any "real hearing problem."

THINKING POINTS

- What age-related changes and risk factors contribute to Mr. H.'s hearing loss?
- Describe the hearing loss that Mr. H. is likely to be experiencing.
- What environmental conditions will contribute to Mr. H.'s hearing difficulty?

FUNCTIONAL CONSEQUENCES AFFECTING HEARING WELLNESS

In 2006, 32% of people between the ages of 65 and 74 years, 46% of those between the ages of 75 and 84 years, and 62% of those aged 85 years and older had a hearing loss (Federal Interagency Forum on Aging-Related Statistics, 2008). Hearing impairment is most likely to occur in men, people of low economic status, and people exposed to prolonged job-related or recreational noise. Poor health is also associated with a higher risk for impaired hearing, as is a family history of otosclerosis.

DIVERSITY NOTE

Whites are twice as likely as African Americans or Hispanic Americans to be deaf or hearing impaired. Men are more likely than women to experience hearing loss.

Hearing losses are categorized according to the site of the impairment. Abnormalities of the external and middle ear impair the sound conduction mechanism and are classified as **conductive hearing losses**. Abnormalities of the inner ear interfere with the sensory and neural structures and are classified as **sensorineural hearing losses**. Sensorineural hearing loss often is age related or noise induced. A hearing loss that involves both conductive and sensorineural impairments is called a **mixed hearing loss**.

Effects on Communication

Accurate comprehension of speech depends on speech pace, sound frequencies, environmental noise, and internal auditory function. Hearing acuity for high-frequency tones begins to decline in early adulthood, and by the age of 30 years for men and 50 years for women, there is some decline in hearing sensitivity at all frequencies.

DIVERSITY NOTE

In addition to having an earlier age of onset for hearing loss, hearing levels decline more rapidly in men, so the cumulative effects are usually noticed by men in their 50s and women in their 60s.

Box 16-2 Guidelines for Assessing Hearing

Questions to Identify Risk Factors for Hearing Loss

- Do you have a family history of hearing loss or deafness?
- Have you been exposed to loud noises in your job or leisure activities?
- Do you have a history of any of the following: diabetes, hypothyroidism, Ménière disease, or Paget disease?
- What medications do you take? (Refer to Box 16-1 to identify potentially ototoxic medications.)
- Have you ever had impacted wax in your ears?

Questions to Assess Awareness and Presence of Hearing Deficit

- Do you have any trouble with your hearing?
- Have you noticed any change in your ability to understand conversations or hear words?
- Are you bothered by any noises in your ears, such as ringing or buzzing?

Questions to Ask if Hearing Loss Is Acknowledged

- How long have you noticed a hearing loss?
- Do you notice differences in hearing in your left ear, versus your right ear?
- Has there been a progressive loss, or did the hearing problem begin suddenly?
- Describe your hearing difficulty.
- Are there any conditions, such as noisy environments or particular voices or sounds, that especially interfere with your hearing?
- Does your hearing loss interfere with your ability to communicate with others, either individually or in groups?
- Are there any activities that you would like to do but feel you cannot because of hearing problems?

discernment of a hearing deficit. If the older adult denies having a hearing problem but shows behavioral cues indicative of a hearing deficit, the nurse elicits further information by asking leading questions such as "I notice you turn your left ear toward me. Is your hearing better in that ear?"

Nurses ask questions about changes in the older adult's social activities to identify psychosocial consequences of hearing impairment that can be addressed through interventions. If no hearing impairment is present, questions about lifestyle do not necessarily have to be included as part of the hearing assessment. When a person acknowledges the existence of a hearing impairment, however, the nurse then asks about any associated changes in social and occupational activities.

Wellness Opportunity

Nurses address the whole person by including questions about the impact of a hearing loss on his or her quality of life.

The nurse assesses the older person's attitudes toward hearing loss, hearing aids, and assistive listening devices because these attitudes influence his or her acceptance of interventions. This is an important aspect of promoting hearing wellness, because more than one-third of older adults could

Speech comprehension is most directly influenced by the frequency of *phonemes*, the smallest units of sound. Each phoneme in a word has a different frequency; generally, vowels have lower frequencies and consonants have higher frequencies. Although most word phonemes have lower-range frequencies, sibilant consonants (those that have a whistling quality, such as *ch, f, g, s, sh, t, th,* and *z*) have higher-range frequencies. Because the earliest and most universal age-related changes affect one's ability to code higher-frequency sounds, words rich in sibilants will be most affected by age-related changes of the auditory system.

Presbycusis, as mentioned earlier, is the sensorineural hearing loss associated with an age-related degeneration of the auditory structures. Presbycusis usually occurs in both ears, but the degree of impairment in each ear can vary. An early functional consequence of presbycusis is the loss of ability to hear high-pitched sounds and sibilant consonants. When high-pitched sounds are filtered out, words become distorted and jumbled, and sentences become incoherent. For example, someone with presbycusis might interpret a sentence like "I think she should go to the store" as "I wish we could go to the show." This characteristic, known as *diminished speech discrimination*, is influenced by the speaker's rate of speech: rapid, slow, or slurred speech patterns make it increasingly difficult for the older person to discern words. As the hearing loss progresses, explosive consonants, such as *b, d, k, p,* and *t,* also become distorted.

Background noise and environmental conditions, such as echoing or poor acoustics, compound the effects of sensorineural hearing loss and can interfere with the ability to recognize words, even in the absence of a significant hearing loss. Thus, older adults in a hospital or long-term care facility, for example, may be particularly sensitive to background noises to which the staff may have become accustomed. One nursing study identified the following sources of noise that were most bothersome to patients: voices, carts, foot traffic, overhead pages, and alarms from monitoring devices (Dube et al., 2008). People with sensorineural hearing loss are sometimes hypersensitive to high-frequency sounds, causing a very narrow range in which sound is heard adequately and comfortably.

A conductive hearing loss is characterized by a reduced intensity of sounds and difficulty hearing vowels and low-pitched tones. In contrast to presbycusis, all frequencies of sounds are heard equally once the sound threshold is reached, and background noise does not interfere as much with speech comprehension. Often there is a history of otosclerosis, perforated eardrum, or other ear disease. In older adults, impacted cerumen is a common contributing factor. Depending on the causative factor, conductive hearing loss occurs in one or both ears. See Table 16-1 for a summary of the functional consequences of age-related changes affecting hearing.

Effects of Hearing Loss on Overall Wellness

Because it is a primary component of communication, hearing enables people to enjoy humor, appreciate music, obtain

information, relate to others, and respond to threats. Thus, hearing deficits inevitably affect usual daily activities and have a variety of impacts on the quality of life, safety, and functioning. Because hearing impairment involves many associated losses, people experiencing a progressive hearing loss may go through the following stages of acceptance (Kozak & Grundfast, 2009):

- Denial: "I can hear fine, but other people don't speak as clearly as they used to."
- Anger: "Why don't people just speak up and look at me when they are speaking?"
- Bargaining: "I would like to get by without a hearing aid just a little longer."
- Depression: "I am never going to have a normal life again."
- Acceptance: "I will manage and do what I can to regain some normalcy."

Hearing loss can interfere with performance on mental status examinations because of the concomitant reduction of sensory stimuli. In addition, people who cannot discriminate words may be reluctant to respond to questions and may refrain from answering rather than risk feeling foolish. Poor performance on tests of cognitive abilities can mistakenly lead to a perception that the person has cognitive impairments or dementia when, in fact, the person simply has a hearing loss. Additional psychosocial consequences of hearing loss include fear, boredom, apathy, anxiety, depression, social isolation, and low self-esteem. When hearing loss interferes with one's ability to perceive reality accurately, it can lead to suspiciousness, paranoia, and loss of contact with the reality. When only parts of a conversation are heard, a person is likely to believe that the conversation is about him or her, and persecutory delusions can develop.

The extent of psychosocial consequences of hearing impairment depends to some degree on the lifestyle of the person affected. For example, hearing impairments are relatively more detrimental for people whose occupations or interests are highly dependent on good hearing. By contrast, hearing loss is less likely to have detrimental effects for people who have few social relationships and who do not depend on hearing for occupational or leisure activities.

DIVERSITY NOTE

Hearing loss may have a greater social impact on older men and a greater emotional impact on older women. Thus, men may withdraw from social interactions and women may continue to be active but worry about how well they can participate (Taylor & Jurma, 2003).

In addition to having a negative influence on the quality of life, hearing deficits can affect the safety and functioning of older adults. For example, people with hearing impairments are likely to be less responsive when warning signals are sounded for fires, ambulances, and other emergencies. Besides creating actual safety hazards, the hearing deficit can lead to fear and anxiety about personal safety. Even mild hearing impairment in older adults is associated with [...] tional decline and increased dependency in daily activ[...]

Negative societal attitudes about aging and hearing l[...] result in a doubly negative effect on the person who is [...] well as hard of hearing. The older person may be reluc[...] acknowledge a hearing deficit, choosing to limit opport[...] for communication rather than face the stigma associate[...] hearing impairments. These attitudes and accompanyi[...] haviors can cause other psychosocial consequences s[...] loneliness, social isolation, and even a more rapid progr[...] of the hearing loss. Geropsychologists who studied th[...] tionship between age stereotypes and hearing loss fou[...] negative perceptions of aging—particularly those rel[...] physical appearance—were associated with a greater [...] in hearing over a 3-year period (Levy, Slade, & Gill, [...] Moreover, Levy and colleagues (2006) found that age [...] types had a greater influence on hearing loss than oth[...] factors such as age, sex, depression, or smoking histor[...]

Wellness Opportunity

Nurses can initiate conversations that reflect positive and nonjudg[...] tal attitudes about aging and hearing loss.

*M*r. H. is now 69 years old and has been retire[...] several years. He spends several days a week hunting [...] fishing seasonally. He also spends time in his baser[...] making small pieces of furniture and doing other w[...] working. He continues to smoke but has cut down t[...] pack per day. His wife and he attend the weekly "L[...] Bunch" group at the local senior center where you a[...] nurse. They make an appointment to talk with you be[...] Mrs. H. is concerned about her husband's hearing. M[...] who blames his problem on "old age," refuses to hav[...] evaluation for a hearing aid because he does not thi[...] aid would do any good and "besides, it would stick ou[...] a sore thumb."

THINKING POINTS

- What factors contribute to Mr. H.'s hearing loss?[...]
- What environmental and other conditions might [...] the hearing loss worse?
- What myths or misunderstandings are likely to [...] ence Mr. H.'s perception of his hearing problem[...] potential interventions for it?

PATHOLOGIC CONDITION AFFECTING HEARING: TINNITUS

Tinnitus is the persistent sensation of ringing, roaring[...] ing, buzzing, or other types of noise that do not origi[...] the external environment. Tinnitus is a common path[...]

ITEM	YES (4 pts)	SOMETIMES (2 pts)	NO (0 pts)
Does a hearing problem cause you to feel embarrassed when you meet new people?	_____	_____	_____
Does a hearing problem cause you to feel frustrated when talking to members of your family?	_____	_____	_____
Do you have difficulty hearing when someone speaks in a whisper?	_____	_____	_____
Do you feel handicapped by a hearing problem?	_____	_____	_____
Does a hearing problem cause you difficulty when visiting friends, relatives, or neighbors?	_____	_____	_____
Does a hearing problem cause you to attend religious services less often than you would like?	_____	_____	_____
Does a hearing problem cause you to have arguments with family members?	_____	_____	_____
Does a hearing problem cause you difficulty when listening to TV or radio?	_____	_____	_____
Do you feel that any difficulty with your hearing limits or hampers your personal or social life?	_____	_____	_____
Does a hearing problem cause you difficulty when in a restaurant with relatives or friends?	_____	_____	_____

RAW SCORE_____ (sum of the points assigned each of the items)

INTERPRETING THE RAW SCORE
0 to 8 = 13% probability of hearing impairment (no handicap/no referral)
10 to 24 = 50% probability of hearing impairment (mild-moderate handicap/refer)
26 to 40 = 84% probability of hearing impairment (severe handicap/refer)

FIGURE 16-3 The screening version of the Hearing Handicap Inventory for the Elderly (HHIE-S). (Reprinted with permission from Ventry, I., & Weinstein, B. [1983]. *Identification of elderly people with hearing problems* [pp. 37–42]. Rockville, MD: American Speech-Language-Hearing Association. Copyright, American Speech-Language-Hearing Association.)

recommended by the Hartford Institute for Geriatric Nursing.

Wellness Opportunity

Nurses promote self-care by asking an older adult to use the HHIE-S and then reviewing the results of this assessment to identify goals.

Observing Behavioral Cues

Behavioral cues related to hearing loss provide important information about the presence of a hearing impairment, the psychosocial consequences of any such impairment, and the person's attitudes about assistive devices. If the older adult denies a hearing deficit that has been noticed by others, behavioral cues can be an important source of assessment information. Denial of a hearing deficit can be rooted in lack of awareness of the impairment because of gradual onset or, if the older person is socially isolated, can be caused by a paucity of opportunities for communication. Feelings of embarrassment or misconceptions that the hearing loss is an inevitable and untreatable consequence of aging can also contribute to denial. Box 16-3 lists behavioral cues that the nurse should observe as part of the hearing assessment.

Using Hearing Assessment Tools

Nurses assess hearing by using an otoscope to examine the ear and a tuning fork to check hearing. The purpose of the otoscopic examination is to identify impacted wax and other factors that can interfere with hearing, whereas the purpose of the tuning fork test is to detect hearing impairments and to differentiate between conductive and sensorineural losses. Box 16-4 describes the procedure for performing a nursing assessment of hearing using the otoscope and tuning fork. A handheld audioscope is another assessment tool that is recommended in nursing guidelines; however, this tool is not as widely available as an otoscope

Box 16-3 Guidelines for Assessing Behavioral Cues Related to Hearing

Behavioral Cues to a Hearing Deficit
- Inappropriate or no response to questions, especially in the absence of opportunities for lip reading
- Inability to follow verbal directions without cues
- Short attention span, easy distractibility
- Frequent requests for repetition or clarification of verbal communication
- Intense observation of the speaker
- Mouthing of words spoken by the speaker
- Turning of one ear toward the speaker
- Unusual physical proximity to the speaker
- Lack of response to loud environmental noises
- Speech that is too loud or inarticulate
- Abnormal voice characteristics, such as monotony
- Misperception that others are talking about him or her

Behavioral Cues About Psychosocial Consequences
- Uncharacteristic avoidance of group settings
- Lack of interest in social activities, especially those requiring verbal communication or those that the person enjoyed in the past (e.g., bingo, card games)

Behavioral Cues About Assistive Devices
- Not using a hearing aid that has been purchased
- Failure to obtain batteries for a hearing aid
- Expression of embarrassment about using assistive devices

or tuning fork. When a hearing deficit is identified, the nurse can recommend that further evaluation be conducted at a speech and hearing center or by a specialized physician, such as an otolaryngologist.

*R*ecall that Mr. H. is a 69-year-old participant in activities at the local senior center where you are the nurse. You are meeting with Mr. and Mrs. H. to discuss Mrs. H.'s concerns about her husband's hearing problem.

THINKING POINTS
- Which of the questions and considerations in Boxes 16-2 and 16-3 would you use in assessing Mr. H.?
- Would you involve Mrs. H. in any part of the assessment? If so, how would you involve her?
- What health promotion advice would you give Mr. H. at this time?

NURSING DIAGNOSIS

On the basis of the nursing assessment, the nurse might identify an actual hearing deficit or risk factors for impaired hearing. An appropriate nursing diagnosis for an older adult with a hearing impairment would be Disturbed Sensory Perception: Auditory. This diagnosis is defined as a "change in the amount or patterning of incoming stimuli accompanied by a diminished, exaggerated, distorted, or impaired response to such stimuli" (NANDA International, 2009, p. 163). When nurses focus on promoting wellness, they can use the diagnosis of Readiness for Enhanced Communication, defined as "a pattern of exchanging information and ideas that is sufficient for

Box 16-4 Guidelines for Otoscopic and Tuning Fork Assessment

Using the Otoscope to Assess Factors That Could Interfere With Hearing
- Hold the otoscope upside down, resting your hand on the person's head to stabilize the instrument.
- Before inserting the speculum, pull the pinna upward and backward, while tilting the person's head slightly back and toward the opposite shoulder.
- If cerumen has accumulated to the point of interfering with the examination or occluding the canal, follow the cerumen removal procedure described in the section on Nursing Interventions.
- Normal otoscopic findings in older adults include the following:
  Small amount of cerumen
  Pinkish-white epithelial lining, no redness or lesions
  Pearl-gray tympanic membrane, which is less translucent than in younger adults
  Light reflex anteroinferiorly from the umbo
  Visible landmarks

Using the Tuning Fork to Detect Hearing Impairment
- Use a tuning fork with frequencies of 512 to 1024 cps (Hz).
- Hold the tuning fork firmly at the stem.
- Strike the fork against the palm of your hand, or strike the fork with a rubber reflex hammer, to set it in motion.

Weber Test
Procedure: Place the tip of a vibrating tuning fork at the center of the person's forehead. Ask where they hear the sound and whether it is louder in one ear than in the other.
Normal finding: The sound from the tuning fork is heard equally in both ears.
Abnormal finding: The sound from the tuning fork is heard better in one ear, indicating a possible hearing loss.

Rinne Test
Procedure: Mask one ear, then place a vibrating tuning fork on the mastoid process of the opposite ear until the person indicates that the sound from the vibrations can no longer be heard. Then, quickly place the tuning fork in front of the ear canal with the top near the ear canal.
Normal finding: The duration the tuning fork vibrations can be heard over the ear canal is approximately twice as long as the time it can be heard over the mastoid bone.
Abnormal finding: The length of time the tuning fork vibrations are heard in front of the ear is shorter than twice as long as the time it can be heard when placed on the mastoid process. In such a case, the person should undergo further tests for impaired hearing.

meeting one's needs and life's goals, and can be strengthened" (NANDA International, 2009, p. 180).

If psychosocial consequences are identified, other pertinent nursing diagnoses might include Anxiety, Impaired Social Interaction, and Ineffective Coping. When the hearing impairment is severe and uncompensated to the point that the person does not function safely, then Risk for Injury might be an applicable nursing diagnosis.

> **Wellness Opportunity**
>
> Nurses can use the wellness nursing diagnosis of Readiness for Enhanced Communication for older adults who are willing to explore possibilities for improving their hearing through health promotion interventions.

PLANNING FOR WELLNESS OUTCOMES

When older adults experience impaired hearing or when risk factors threaten hearing wellness, nurses identify wellness outcomes as an essential part of the planning process. Nursing Outcomes Classifications (NOCs) that most directly relate to interventions to improve hearing for an older adult are Hearing Compensation Behavior and Sensory Function: Hearing. In addition, any of the following nursing-sensitive outcomes are applicable to describe the effectiveness of interventions to improve hearing: Loneliness Severity, Communication Ability, Risk Control: Hearing Impairment, Social Involvement, Social Interaction Skills, and Personal Safety Behavior. Specific interventions to achieve these outcomes are discussed in the following section.

> **Wellness Opportunity**
>
> Quality of Life is a wellness outcome that is achieved through nursing interventions that improve communication for older adults with impaired hearing.

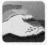

NURSING INTERVENTIONS FOR HEARING WELLNESS

Nursing interventions aim to promote hearing wellness through preventing hearing loss, assisting older adults to compensate for hearing deficits, and using communication methods that facilitate optimal communication. Specific interventions to achieve these goals are discussed in detail in the following sections. Nurses can use any of the following examples of pertinent Nursing Interventions Classification (NIC) terminologies in care plans: Communication Enhancement: Hearing Deficit, Ear Care, Environmental Management, Environmental Management: Safety, Health Education, Health Screening, Health System Guidance, and Risk Identification.

> **Wellness Opportunity**
>
> Nurses can emphasize that even though interventions to prevent hearing loss ideally begin early in life, it is never too late to begin protecting ears from noise.

Promoting Hearing Wellness for All Older Adults

For all older adults, nurses can challenge the perception that hearing loss is an inevitable consequence of growing older by teaching about interventions to protect hearing, with emphasis on NIHL. Many older adults engage in recreational or occupational activities that can cause NIHL and may not realize that age-related changes increase their susceptibility to development of hearing loss. Nurses can also teach about the importance of having a hearing screening done by self-assessment (e.g., using the HHIE-S) or by audiometry. Nurses can use Box 16-5 and resources listed at the end of this chapter to teach older adults about health promotion actions they can take to prevent or address hearing loss.

For older adults with modifiable risk factors, such as smoking and the use of ototoxic medication, nurses can focus their health education on alleviating the risks. For example, nurses can teach older adults and their caregivers about the potential ototoxicity of the medications listed in Box 16-1. This information is particularly important for older adults who have additional risk factors for impaired hearing. When effective medication alternatives are available, or when the older adult is experiencing hearing difficulties, efforts should be made to avoid the use of these medications. As with other questions about medication, older adults and their caregivers

Box 16-5   Health Promotion Teaching About Hearing

Prevention of Hearing Loss
- Because exposure to loud noise is a major contributing factor to hearing loss, it is important to limit your exposure or use ear protectors that are appropriate to the task (e.g., when mowing the lawn, using equipment with gas or electric motors).
- Because smoking increases the risk of hearing loss, consider this as another reason to quit smoking.

Early Detection and Treatment of Hearing Loss
- Because some medications and medical conditions can cause hearing problems, ask your primary care practitioner to thoroughly evaluate for these conditions.
- Have your ears checked for impacted wax and talk with your primary health practitioner about preventing impacted wax if this has been a problem for you.
- Obtain evaluation at a speech and hearing center for a hearing aid, assistive hearing device, or aural rehabilitation services.
- Consider using amplifying devices (e.g., for phones, radios, doorbells) or sound substitution devices (e.g., flashing lights, closed-captioned television) as needed for safety and improved quality of life.
- Take advantage of available assistive listening devices in public places (e.g., churches, theaters, government buildings).

should be advised to discuss their concerns about ototoxic medications with the prescribing health care practitioner.

Nurses can also teach about interacting effects of two or more risk factors, such as smoking and age-related changes, or medication effects and a genetic predisposition to ototoxicity. People who already experience a mild hearing impairment may be motivated to protect their hearing by avoiding hazardous noise and protecting their ears when they are exposed to noise. Similarly, if they are experiencing a hearing loss and recognize that nicotine can be ototoxic, they may be more motivated to stop smoking.

Whenever a nursing assessment identifies a hearing impairment, nursing interventions should focus on a referral for medical and audiology evaluations. Sometimes the nursing interventions also need to address barriers to obtaining a hearing aid, as discussed in the section on hearing aids. Nurses in community or residential settings for older adults may be able to find an audiologist who is willing to provide screening programs at little or no cost. As long as the sponsors of these programs do not have a vested interest in promoting a particular type of hearing aid, they may be effective resources for screening programs.

Preventing and Alleviating Impacted Cerumen

Nurses can promote hearing wellness through interventions and health education aimed at alleviating or preventing hearing impairment caused by impacted wax. Types and examples of over-the-counter eardrop solutions that can be used to soften cerumen are as follows:

- Water-based: water, saline, docusate sodium, hydrogen peroxide, acetic acid, sodium bicarbonate
- Oil-based: almond oil, olive oil, mineral oil
- Non-water-, non-oil-based: carbamide peroxide (Debrox), choline salicylate, and glycerol (Audax).

The liquid form of docusate sodium (but not syrup forms) is effective, inexpensive, and readily available as a ceruminolytic agent. This solution is inexpensive and readily available in many settings where older adults receive care. The schedule for instillation of otic drops varies from semiweekly to monthly.

When an ear canal is impacted with cerumen, the nurse must determine whether there are any contraindications to irrigating, such as pain, swelling, a recent ear infection, or a history of ruptured tympanic membrane. If any condition is identified, the nurse instructs the person to seek medical care from an otolaryngologist or other qualified professional.

If there are no contraindications, the following procedure should clear the canal of cerumen:

1. Soften the cerumen with a ceruminolytic agent, instilled for at least 15 minutes prior to the irrigation.
2. Irrigate the canal with body-temperature tap water by using an ear syringe and gentle pressure.
3. Aim water at the sides of the canal, and allow drainage from the ear to collect in a basin.
4. Drain excessive fluid from the ear by tilting the head toward the affected side.

5. If the cerumen is difficult to remove, instill a softening preparation twice daily for several days, and then attempt irrigation again.

After the built-up wax has been removed, teach the person to prevent the recurrence of impacted cerumen by using a ceruminolytic agent, as discussed earlier in this section. See Evidence-based Guidelines 16-1 (page 322) for information on removing impacted cerumen.

Compensating for Hearing Deficits

Interventions for hearing-impaired people should be considered only after a medical evaluation is performed to identify treatable causes of the hearing loss. An audiologist can then evaluate and more thoroughly determine the best approach for facilitating communication. People who have irreversible hearing deficits and who are interested in corrective measures can be encouraged to participate in an aural rehabilitation program. Individualized aural rehabilitation programs consist of counseling, together with any or all of the following services: amplification devices, auditory training, lip reading, and speech skills. These programs are available at speech and hearing centers, which are often affiliated with hospitals, medical centers, or universities. Internet resources, such as the National Association for Hearing and Speech Action Web site and others can provide information about local resources for the evaluation and treatment of hearing disorders. Nurses play an important role in suggesting referrals for aural rehabilitation, discussing such programs with older adults and their caregivers, and facilitating or encouraging the use of recommended sound amplification devices.

Sound amplification is generally achieved by using hearing aids or assistive listening devices. Hearing aids are individually prescribed and require audiology services, whereas assistive listening devices are not individualized and are available without professional assistance or recommendation. These two types of sound amplification are discussed in the following sections.

Surgical implantation of an electronic device, such as a cochlear implant, may be indicated to compensate for damaged or nonfunctional parts of the inner ear. Adults who have lost all or most of their hearing later in life are candidates for this type of surgery, but extensive evaluation of the person is necessary to determine the appropriateness of the procedure. As this procedure becomes more common, nurses will be caring for more older adults who have had cochlear implants. One nursing implication is that the implanted devices are not compatible with magnetic resonance imaging (MRI), so nurses need to make sure that MRIs are not ordered for people with cochlear implants.

Assistive Listening Devices

Any device that amplifies or replaces sounds for individual or group communication without being individualized is categorized as an **assistive listening device** (also called a *personal listening system*). A stethoscope is an assistive listening

Statement of the Problem

- Cerumen is normally expelled from the ear canal by a self-cleaning mechanism, but excessive or impacted cerumen occurs in high-risk populations, which include older adults, people who are cognitively impaired, and people who use hearing aids.
- Impacted cerumen, which affects between 19% and 65% of patients aged 65+ years, is underdiagnosed and undertreated.
- Impacted cerumen can cause hearing loss (ranging from 5 dB to 40 dB); diminished cognitive function; and symptoms such as pain, itching, tinnitus, cough, dizziness, and sensation of fullness.
- Cerumen impaction may interfere with hearing aid performance by reducing the intensity of sound, changing the resonance properties of the ears, or causing feedback and poor fitting.
- Cerumen impaction is the cause of damage to 60% to 70% of hearing aids that are sent for repair.
- There are strong data indicating that removal of impacted cerumen can improve hearing.
- Older patients are often unaware that they have a cerumen impaction potentially impairing their hearing or that removal of the impaction may improve their hearing; they may even rate their hearing ability as good or fair.

Recommendations for Nursing Assessment

- Arrange for or perform an otoscopic examination whenever any of the following manifestations occur: hearing loss, ear pain, tinnitus, cough, or vertigo.
- Arrange for or perform an otoscopic examination at intervals of 3–12 months for older adults who use hearing aids.

Recommendations for Patient Teaching

Teach older adults and caregivers about the following measures:
- Use the following measures to reduce the risk of developing impacted cerumen: instill ceruminolytic agents prophylactically and have the ear canal irrigated by a health care professional.
- Do not insert cotton-tipped applicators or any other foreign object in ear canals.
- Make sure that hearing aids are properly cleaned and cared for.
- If you have an increased risk for cerumen impaction, have your ears cleaned and checked by a qualified health care practitioner every 6–12 months.

Recommendations for Care

Ceruminolytic Agents

- Ceruminolytics are wax-softening agents that disperse the cerumen and reduce the need for other interventions.
- Three types of ceruminolytics are water-based (e.g., water, saline, docusate sodium, hydrogen peroxide, sodium bicarbonate); oil-based (e.g., almond oil, mineral oil, olive oil); and non-water-, non-oil-based (e.g., Debrox, Audax).
- Studies comparing two or more ceruminolytic agents indicate that any type of ceruminolytic is better than no treatment, but no particular agent is more effective than others.

Aural Irrigation

- Irrigating the ear canal with a stream of water is effective in removing impacted cerumen.
- Instillation of ceruminolytic agents 15 minutes or for several days prior to the irrigation improves the success of the treatment.
- Irrigation can be done with an ear syringe or an electronic jet irrigator; oral/dental jet irrigators can be equipped with specially designed tips to prevent overinsertion and direct the water away from the tympanic membrane (e.g., OtoClear system).
- Physicians often delegate the task of aural irrigation to nurses.
- Ear irrigation should not be performed on patients with a history of ear surgery or those who have any abnormality of the ear canal or a nonintact tympanic membrane; it should be used cautiously in patients with diabetes.

Manual Removal

- Manual removal is the use of an instrument (e.g., ear curettes or probes) by a skilled practitioner to remove the impacted cerumen.

Potentially Harmful Interventions

- Cotton-tipped swabs should not be used because they can cause further impaction and other complications.
- Home use of oral jet irrigators and cotton-tipped swabs are associated with increased risk of damage to the ear canal.
- Ear candling (also called *ear coning* or *thermo-auricular therapy*) is a commonly used alternative practice for cerumen removal. Research indicates that ear candling is not effective and is associated with considerable risks.

SOURCE: Roland, P. S., Smith, T. L., Schwartz, S. R., Rosenfeld, R. M., Ballachanda, B., Earll, J. M., . . . Wetmore, S. (2008). Clinical practice guideline: Cerumen impaction. *Otolaryngology—Head and Neck Surgery, 139*, S1–S21.

device commonly used by health care workers, and megaphones and microphones are examples of amplification devices used for group communication. Closed-captioned television is an assistive device that substitutes visual cues for auditory cues. Nurses can encourage older adults and their caregivers to obtain information from the resources listed at thePoint at http://thePoint.lww.com/Miller6e.

Assistive listening devices, which consist of a small, battery-powered amplifier and headphones, can be used easily in any setting to improve communication temporarily. Advantages of assistive listening devices over hearing aids include lower cost and the fact that several people can share the device. In addition, most of these devices do not require as much manual dexterity as hearing aids, and some of them are more effective than hearing aids in filtering out background

noise. Assistive listening devices can be used alone or with hearing aids. Figure 16-4 shows several examples of devices that can be used to enhance communication with someone who is hard of hearing.

Assistive listening devices are available for home use to amplify specific sounds, such as those from the radio, doorbell, television, or telephone. Telephone receivers with an amplifying device, called a T-coil, can be used with the "T" position on a hearing aid. Other devices serve as substitutes for sound when amplification is impractical or ineffective: flashing lights for doorbells or doormats and alarm clocks that vibrate the pillow or flash a light, for example. People with more serious hearing impairments but with adequate vision may benefit from closed-captioned television, which provides subscripts for many programs. Since 1990, all

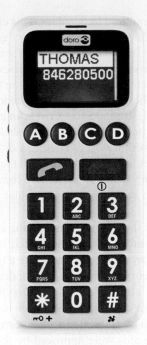

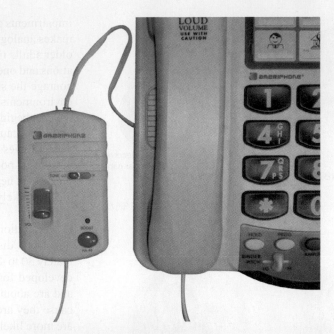

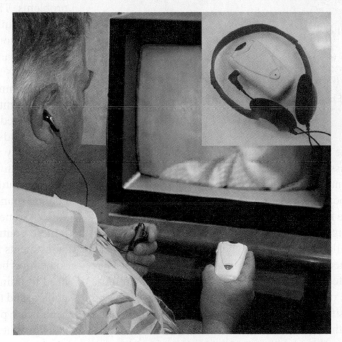

FIGURE 16-4 (A) Cell phone with amplification, large keypad, two-way speakerphone, and vibrating ringer alert. **(B)** Easy-to-use in-line phone amplifier. **(C)** Personal sound amplifier with volume control, swiveling microphone, and lightweight earbud headphones. (Courtesy of ActiveForever.com)

televisions with screens 13 in or larger are required to include a closed-captioned option.

Portable assistive listening devices are available for use in public places. Churches, theaters, and government buildings sometimes equip their facilities with assistive devices to amplify sound, and hearing-impaired people can ask about arrangements for using these devices. Small, hand-sized amplifiers can be attached temporarily to any telephone, and special devices are also available for mobile phones. In residential and institutional settings for older adults, having an assistive listening device available may be useful for nurses, especially when they are providing health education interventions.

Hearing Aids

A **hearing aid** is a battery-operated device that consists of an amplifier, a microphone, and a receiver. Hearing aids can be classified by size, location worn, and technology. The largest are approximately of the size of a deck of cards and are worn on the body, whereas the new, smaller types fit completely in the ear canal. These smaller types can be seen only with close inspection of the ear and have a nylon string attached for insertion and removal. Preferred hearing aid locations include in-the-ear, in-the-canal, and completely-in-the-canal (Figure 16-5). Body-worn and behind-the-ear hearing aids have become much less popular in recent years

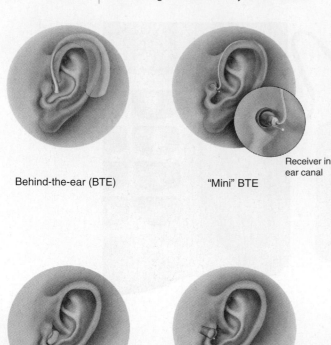

Behind-the-ear (BTE)   "Mini" BTE

Receiver in ear canal

In-the-ear (ITE)   Completely-in-canal (CIC)

FIGURE 16-5 Examples of four types of hearing aids.

because of the availability of smaller, more powerful hearing aids made possible by newer technology.

Until recently, the amplifying power of a hearing aid was strongly associated with its size because most hearing aids used the same type of technology, and severely impaired people needed larger, body-worn aids. New technology, however, has made available a variety of types of hearing aids that can be programmed and adjusted for individual differences. Currently, the effectiveness of a hearing aid is associated more with the type of technology used than with its size. Hearing aids are classified by whether they are analog or digital and according to the degree of individualized adjustments or programming possible. As discussed later, the cost of hearing aids increases as the programming becomes more adjustable and individualized.

Conventional, or traditional, hearing aids use analog technology to amplify sound but they do not correct distortions. These aids are the simplest type and are adjusted by the manufacturer on the basis of an evaluation by an audiologist. Although the person wearing the aid can adjust its volume and the audiologist can make some minor adjustments, the aid becomes less effective as the person's hearing changes and may need to be replaced if the hearing loss progresses. Because analog aids amplify all sounds equally, they tend to be unsatisfactory for people who have only a mild high-frequency hearing loss and may be more beneficial to people with

impairments at multiple frequencies. This characteristic also makes analog aids difficult to use in noisy environments, but older adults may find that they are satisfactory in quiet situations and one-on-one conversations. Nurses may need to encourage the selective use of analog aids in their appropriate environments. These aids are the least expensive type, with the cost beginning around $400. Cost is an important consideration because only the most comprehensive health insurance policies cover the cost of hearing aids and most people pay out-of-pocket for hearing aids. Until the cost of more sophisticated hearing aids decreases, these conventional hearing aids are likely to remain the most popular choice for older adults.

A variation of the conventional hearing aid is the recently developed disposable hearing aid, which lasts for approximately 30 to 40 days and costs approximately $40. They were developed for people with a mild to moderate hearing loss and are about as effective as other analog hearing aids. Because they are not customized, they may not fit as well and are more likely to be associated with discomfort or feedback problems. These aids were approved by the U.S. Food and Drug Administration in 2000 and cannot be obtained without a prescription from a qualified hearing specialist. If these disposable hearing aids become more popular, it is likely that choices in size and amplification will increase.

Programmable analog hearing aids are more advanced than conventional hearing aids because they are selectively programmed to meet the needs of a hearing-impaired person. A major advantage of these hearing aids is that they are acoustically superior to conventional models and can be adjusted for different listening situations. Some programmable aids can automatically adjust their volume to the level of incoming sound by making soft sounds louder and loud sounds softer. Some programmable aids are equipped with a tiny remote control device, so the user can conveniently make adjustments for different environments. Remote devices are sometimes built into a wristwatch. Disadvantages include the need to train the wearer, the cost of up to several thousand dollars, and the need for frequent adjustments by the hearing health care professional.

Digital hearing aids use the most advanced technology and are the most flexible for individual needs because the audiologist uses a computer to program the aid to amplify specific frequencies for each person's hearing loss. The digital technology examines the incoming sounds and adapts the amplification without adding noise or distortion. In addition, some of these aids have directional microphones, enabling them to collect sounds from two directions and allowing the wearer to adjust the directionality. These aids can be programmed for different listening environments, and the wearer can use a remote control device to adjust the aid for various listening situations. The only disadvantage of these aids is their high cost, which is at least several thousand dollars.

Despite the major improvements in hearing aids in the last decade, only approximately 20% of people who could benefit from a hearing aid actually use one. Nurses can address negative attitudes and have a positive effect on the use of hearing aids by helping older adults to explore the many options for amplification and by encouraging them to obtain accurate information from audiologists and reputable organizations listed in the Resource section at the end of this chapter.

Nurses can encourage older adults and their families to obtain initial information about hearing aids from consumer and health care organizations, rather than primarily from a hearing aid dealer who sells only one kind of device. Many Web sites provide objective information about the various types of hearing aids. The International Hearing Society, for example, distributes a Hearing Aid Helpline consumer kit free of charge, and the Better Business Bureau provides information about local hearing aid dealers.

If financial or transportation limitations are problematic for an older person who is otherwise receptive to obtaining a hearing aid, nursing interventions can be aimed at identifying community resources to address these concerns. For example, the AUDIENT program is a national nonprofit hearing care alliance that provides access to quality hearing aids and audiology care for people with limited incomes.

In addition to the high cost of hearing aids, common barriers to obtaining and using them are the high levels of manual dexterity, fine motor movement, and good vision required to adjust the volume and other controls and to change batteries. Many of these barriers can be addressed by selecting the most appropriate hearing aid and by working closely with the audiologist to identify ways of simplifying the process.

Nurses who work with older adults in residential or other institutional settings can teach about the most effective use of hearing aids in different circumstances. For example, the older adult can be encouraged to use the aid for one-on-one conversations but to remove it in the dining area or other large social areas where there is a lot of background noise. Nurses promote realistic expectations with regard to hearing aids by explaining that hearing aids do not restore normal hearing but do improve communication and the quality of life. Nurses also need to work with caregivers to provide additional support during the initial adjustment period.

Although it is impossible to know about all the available hearing aids, nurses need to keep up to date on various types and their implications for older adults. For example, it is important for nurses to know whether a person has an analog or a digital hearing aid, because the person with an analog aid may not be willing to use it in settings where background noise is problematic. It is also important for nurses to know whether the person has a remote control device for the hearing aid, so the nurse can assist with adjusting the settings and give special attention to keeping track of the device.

Nurses must be familiar enough with hearing aids to assist older adults and their caregivers with their use and care. Although nurses can expect that initial hearing aid use and care instructions will be provided by the hearing aid provider,

Box 16-6 Use and Care of Hearing Aids

Guidelines for Insertion and Use
- With the volume of the device turned off and the canal portion pointing into the ear, insert the hearing aid.
- Make sure the aid fits snugly in the ear canal.
- The M, T, and O settings designate microphone, telephone, and off, respectively.
- Turn the M-T-O switch to M.
- Turn the volume up slowly, beginning at one-third to one-half volume, until a comfortable level is reached.
- If whistling (feedback) occurs, check the position of the device in the ear and the volume. The aid may not fit snugly enough, or the volume may be too high.
- Begin wearing the aid for short periods, in a familiar and quiet environment and in one-on-one conversations.
- Gradually increase the duration the aid is worn, the variety of environments, and the number of people included in conversations.
- Allow several months before expecting to feel totally comfortable with the hearing aid.
- Avoid noisy environments and eliminate background noise when possible (e.g., turn off televisions and radios; close doors to rooms).
- Use the appropriate setting (T) for telephone calls.
- Understand that hearing aids do not restore hearing to normal, but rather amplify sound, including all environmental noises.

Guidelines for Care and Maintenance
- Keep a fresh battery available (batteries can be expected to last for 70–85 hours), but do not purchase batteries more than 1 month in advance.
- Turn off the hearing aid before changing the battery.
- Remove the battery or turn off the aid when not in use.
- Clean the aid weekly, using warm, soapy water for the earmold and a toothpick or pipe cleaner for the channel.
- Never use alcohol on the earmold because this will cause drying and cracking.
- Check the earmold for cracks or scratches.
- Avoid extreme heat, cold, or moisture (e.g., do not leave the hearing aid near the stove, do not wear it while using a hair dryer, and do not wear it outside in rainy or extremely cold weather unless it is protected well).
- Avoid exposure to chemicals, such as hairspray or permanent solutions.
- Avoid dropping the aid on a hard surface; when handling it, keep it over a soft or padded surface.

these instructions may have to be reviewed or revamped as dependency needs and caregiver roles change. Older adults who normally depend on family members for assistance with their hearing aid may not be able to use and care for it properly when they are in a hospital or nursing home. Likewise, nurses in home settings may have to teach caregivers about hearing aids if the older adult needs assistance that was not previously provided by that caregiver. This situation is likely to arise if the caregiver changes or if the older adult becomes more dependent because of increased functional impairment. Box 16-6 summarizes the teaching points related to the use and care of hearing aids.

Communicating With Hearing-Impaired Older Adults

Good communication techniques are essential in assisting older adults to compensate for hearing deficits. The primary functional consequence of presbycusis is a diminished acuity for high-frequency sounds, which is exacerbated by fast-paced speech and environmental noise. Therefore, communication interventions are directed toward improving the clarity of words, slowing the rate of speech, and eliminating environmental noise and distractions. Verbal techniques that enhance auditory communication should be augmented by nonverbal techniques, such as body language and written communication, as described in Box 16-7. Nurses can apply these techniques and use this box for teaching caregivers how to improve communication with hearing-impaired people. In recent years, increased attention has been directed toward planning or modifying environments to diminish background noise and to improve the ability of people to hear. Although some noise control modifications, such as using window draperies, are

relatively simple and can be applied to many settings, other measures, such as selection of building materials, need to be implemented while environments are being designed.

Box 16-7 Techniques for Communicating With Hearing-Impaired People

- Stand or sit directly in front of, and close to, the person.
- Talk toward the better ear, but make sure your lips can be seen.
- Make sure the person pays attention and looks at your face.
- Address the person by name, pause, and then begin talking.
- Speak distinctly, slowly, and directly to the person.
- Do not exaggerate lip movements because this will interfere with lip reading.
- Avoid chewing gum, covering your mouth, or turning your head away.
- If the person does not understand, repeat the message by using different words.
- Avoid or eliminate any background noise.
- Do not raise the volume of your voice; rather, try to lower the tone while still speaking in a moderately loud voice.
- Keep all instructions simple and ask for feedback to assess what the person heard.
- Avoid questions that elicit simple yes or no answers.
- Keep sentences short.
- Use body language that is congruent with what you are trying to communicate.
- Demonstrate what you are saying.
- Use large-print written communication and pictures to supplement verbal communication.
- Make sure only one person talks at a time; arrange for one-on-one communication whenever possible.
- If eyeglasses normally are worn to improve vision, make sure they are clean.
- Provide adequate lighting so that the person can see your lips; avoid settings in which there is glare behind or around you.

*M*r. H. is now 83 years old and has been a widower for 1 year. He has given up hunting and woodworking because he developed Parkinson disease 11 years ago and cannot manage the necessary fine motor movements. He continues to fish seasonally, play poker monthly, and smoke one pack of cigarettes per day. In addition to Parkinson disease, he has hypertension and coronary artery disease. He still lives in his own home and attends the local senior center for meals and social activities three times a week. His hearing loss has progressed to the point that he has difficulty with phone conversations and has to turn the television up loud. He cannot hear the doorbell. At the senior center, participants avoid conversations with him because he has difficulty hearing.

You are the nurse at the senior center, and you see him during the weekly "Wellness Clinic" for blood pressure checks. One week, he tells you that his daughter is upset with him because he never answers his phone when she calls, and she cannot have a decent phone conversation with him. She lives in another state and worries about him. She has offered to pay for a hearing aid evaluation for him, but he has told her "those things stick out like a sore thumb and they don't do any good anyway. I can hear anything I want to hear and there's a lot I don't care to hear so why should you spend a lot of money for something that I won't use." He asks your opinion about this and is wondering whether he should at least get a checkup to pacify his daughter. He expects he will be told that nothing can be done and that his daughter will have to be satisfied with the situation.

THINKING POINTS

- Which information in Box 16-2 would be most pertinent to obtain at this time?
- What myths and misunderstandings influence Mr. H.?
- What nursing diagnosis would you apply to Mr. H.?
- Which information in Box 16-5 would be pertinent to this situation?
- What health promotion teaching would you do to address Mr. H.'s resistance to having his hearing evaluated?
- What additional health promotion advice would you give?
- Because you usually see Mr. H. weekly, you can develop a long-term teaching plan. How would you establish priorities for immediate and long-term goals?

EVALUATING EFFECTIVENESS OF NURSING INTERVENTIONS

Nurses observe compensatory behaviors of hearing-impaired older adults to evaluate the effectiveness of interventions for the nursing diagnosis of Disturbed Sensory Perception: Auditory. The following are indicators of successful interventions:

- Improved ability to communicate
- Effective use of hearing aids and amplification devices
- Increased participation in social activities
- Environmental modifications to eliminate background noise
- Appropriate participation in aural rehabilitation program.

Evaluation of effectiveness of interventions varies in different health care settings. For example, nurses in short-term settings provide health education as part of a discharge plan that includes information about resources for hearing evaluations. Evaluation of the effectiveness of this intervention is based on the patient's positive response to the nurse's suggestions, but the nurse is not likely to know whether the person followed through with the referral and had beneficial outcomes. In home, community, and long-term care settings, nurses address long-term goals by facilitating referrals for audiology services. In these settings, the evaluation of interventions is based on the person's use of additional resources to improve communication abilities.

*M*r. H. is an 89-year-old widower who has had Parkinson disease for 17 years. Presbycusis is listed as an additional diagnosis on his medical record. He is being admitted to a nursing home because his condition has declined to the point that his daughter, Ms. D., can no longer manage his care in her home, where he has lived for several years. He is medically stable but needs assistance in all activities of daily living.

NURSING ASSESSMENT

During the admission interview, you notice that Mr. H. has difficulty hearing your questions and that he frequently asks his daughter to give the requested information. He shows no significant cognitive deficits, but he seems to have difficulty understanding verbal communication. When you ask about any hearing impairment, Ms. D. tells you that her father has used hearing aids for 5 years and has been reevaluated periodically at a speech and hearing center. Two months ago, he obtained new hearing aids, but wears them only for one-on-one conversations with her. Because of Mr. H.'s tremors and difficulty with fine motor movements, Ms. D. cares for his hearing aids and assists with their insertion and removal.

Ms. D. has encouraged her father to wear his hearing aids during family gatherings, but he says the noise from small children is too annoying. Except for family gatherings, Mr. H. has very few opportunities for social interaction, and he has become more and more withdrawn. He used to enjoy playing poker, but has not played in several years because all of his friends have died. Now he spends much of his time watching closed-captioned television programs. Ms. D. hopes that her father will respond to the opportunities for social interaction provided at the nursing home and that his quality of life will improve.

NURSING DIAGNOSIS

In addition to nursing diagnoses related to Mr. H.'s chronic illness and self-care deficits, you identify a nursing diagnosis of Impaired Social Interaction related to the effects of hearing loss. You select this rather than Disturbed Sensory Perception:

Auditory as a nursing diagnosis because Mr. H.'s hearing impairment has already been evaluated and sound amplification devices are available to him.

NURSING CARE PLAN FOR MR. H.

In your care plan, you address the psychosocial consequences of Mr. H.'s hearing impairment. Your nursing care is directed toward improving his social interaction through the use of

available devices and through other communication techniques that will enhance his social interaction skills.

Expected Outcome	Nursing Interventions	Nursing Evaluation
Mr. H. will develop effective communication techniques for resident-staff interactions.	• During the initial interview, talk with Mr. H. and Ms. D. about the importance of good verbal communication with staff; emphasize the need for the staff to get to know Mr. H so his needs can be addressed.	• Mr. H. will wear his hearing aids during all one-on-one conversations with staff. • Mr. H. will report satisfactory verbal interactions with the staff.

(case study continues on page 330)

Expected Outcome	Nursing Interventions	Nursing Evaluation
	• Ask Mr. H. to wear his hearing aids during all one-on-one interactions with staff.	• Mr. H.'s hearing aids will be maintained in good operating condition.
	• Use good communication techniques when talking with Mr. H (as in Box 16-7).	
	• Make sure all staff members provide appropriate assistance with insertion and removal of Mr. H.'s hearing aids.	
	• Include hearing aid maintenance as part of the daily responsibilities of the nursing aide.	
Mr. H. will engage in social interaction with one other resident.	• During the initial care plan conference, identify several other residents who might converse with Mr. H.	• Mr. H. will wear his hearing aids at least once daily for a conversation with one other resident.
	• Ask the staff to encourage one-on-one conversations between Mr. H. and the selected resident (e.g., suggest that they watch closed-captioned television programs together).	
	• Ask Mr. H. to wear his hearing aids during one-on-one interactions with residents.	
	• Provide assistance with inserting and removing hearing aids as needed.	
	• Provide a quiet environment for one-on-one conversations with other residents.	
Mr. H. will engage in small group activities with other residents.	• During the first monthly care review conference, ask the activities staff to invite Mr. H. to a poker game with three other residents in the small-group room.	• By the second month in this facility, Mr. H. will participate in weekly poker games with three other residents.
	• Make sure that environmental noise is controlled as much as possible.	

THINKING POINTS

- What nursing responsibilities would you have with regard to addressing Mr. H.'s hearing impairment? How would you work with other staff to implement the care plan described in the concluding case example?
- What are some of the advantages and disadvantages of hearing aids in a long-term care setting? How would you address the disadvantages?

- How would you involve Ms. D. in the care plan to address Mr. H.'s hearing impairment?
- If Mr. H. were in an acute care setting, how would you address his hearing problem?

Chapter Highlights

Age-Related Changes That Affect Hearing (Figure 16-1, Table 16-1)

- External ear: thicker hair, thinner skin, increased keratin
- Middle ear: less resilient tympanic membrane, calcified ossicles, stiffer muscles and ligaments
- Inner ear and auditory nervous system: fewer neurons and hair cells, diminished blood supply, degeneration of spiral ganglion and central processing systems

Risk Factors That Affect Hearing Wellness (Figure 16-2, Box 16-1)

- Lifestyle and environmental factors: smoking, background noise, exposure to noise or toxic chemicals
- Genetic predisposition to otosclerosis
- Impacted cerumen
- Ototoxic medications: aminoglycosides, aspirin, loop diuretics, quinine
- Disease processes: diabetes, Paget disease, Ménière disease

Functional Consequences Affecting Hearing Wellness (Table 16-1)

- Presbycusis: diminished ability to hear high-pitched sounds, especially in the presence of background noise
- Predisposition to impacted cerumen
- Psychosocial consequences: depression, social isolation, declines in cognitive function, diminished quality of life

Pathologic Condition Affecting Hearing

- Tinnitus: persistent sensation of noises that do not originate in the external environment

Nursing Assessment of Hearing (Figure 16-3; Boxes 16-2, 16-3, and 16-4)

- Screening tool: The Hearing Handicap Inventory for the Elderly
- Past and present risk factors (e.g., use of ototoxic medications, noise exposure, family history of otosclerosis)
- Attitudes about hearing aids if impairment is present
- Impact of hearing impairment on communication and quality of life
- Behavioral cues to impaired hearing
- Otoscopic examination for impacted cerumen
- Tuning fork tests for hearing

Nursing Diagnosis

- Readiness for Enhanced Communication
- Disturbed Sensory Perception: Auditory
- Additional diagnoses that address the functional consequences of impaired hearing are as follows: Impaired Communication, Anxiety, Impaired Adjustment, Impaired Social Interaction, Ineffective Individual Coping, and Risk for Injury

Planning for Wellness Outcomes

- Improved communication
- Increased social interactions
- Improved quality of life
- Increased safety and functioning

Nursing Interventions for Hearing Wellness (Figures 16-4 and 16-5; Boxes 16-5, 16-6, and 16-7)

- Teaching about interventions to address modifiable risk factors: smoking, exposure to noise, use of ototoxic medications
- Removing and preventing impacted cerumen
- Promoting referrals for audiology services
- Using assistive listening devices
- Teaching about the use and care of a hearing aid
- Communicating with hearing-impaired older adults
- Compensating for hearing deficits by using hearing devices and hearing aids

Evaluating Effectiveness of Nursing Interventions

- Improved communication
- Use of appropriate amplification aids
- Appropriate environmental modifications
- Increased participation in social activities

Critical Thinking Exercises

1. Describe presbycusis and explain the functional consequences of this condition as it affects the everyday life of an older adult.
2. What risk factors would you consider in an 83-year-old person who complains of recent problems with hearing?
3. What advice would you give to someone who asks you about a brochure she received from a hearing aid company that offers free hearing screenings describing a new high-powered hearing aid? The person has trouble hearing but has never had an evaluation.
4. Describe at least 10 ways in which you can adapt your communication for a hearing-impaired person.
5. Find at least one resource (*not* a hearing aid dealer) in your community that you could recommend to an older adult who needs a hearing evaluation.
6. Visit at least three Internet sites that provide educational materials about hearing impairment, and choose the one you think would be best for obtaining health information brochures.

Resources

For links to these resources and additional helpful Internet resources related to this chapter, visit thePoint. at http://thePoint.lww. com/Miller6e.

Clinical Tools

Hartford Institute for Geriatric Nursing
- *Try This: Best Practices in Nursing Care to Older Adults* Issue Number 12 (2007), Hearing Screening in Older Adults: A Brief Hearing Loss Screener

Evidence-Based Practice

Adams-Wendling, L., & Pimple, C. (2008). Evidence-based guideline: Nursing management of hearing impairment in nursing facility residents. *Journal of Gerontological Nursing, 34*(11), 9–17.

Cacchione, P. Z. (2008). Sensory changes. In E. Capezuti, D. Zwicker, M. Mezey, & T. Fulmer (Eds.), *Evidence-Based Geriatric Nursing Protocols for Best Practice* (3rd ed., pp. 477–502). New York: Springer Publishing Co.

National Guideline Clearinghouse
- Hearing impairment in nursing facility residents
- Evaluation and management of obstructing cerumen

Health Education

American Speech-Language-Hearing Association
American Tinnitus Association
AUDIENT, alliance for accessible hearing care
Better Hearing Institute
Canadian Hard of Hearing Association
International Hearing Society
Hearing Loss Association of America (formerly Self Help for Hard of Hearing People)
National Campaign to Prevent Noise-Induced Hearing Loss
National Institute on Deafness and Other Communication Disorders

REFERENCES

Adams-Wendling, L., & Pimple, C. (2008). Evidence-based guideline: Nursing management of hearing impairment in nursing facility residents. *Journal of Gerontological Nursing, 34*(11), 9–17.

Bainbridge, K. E., Hoffman, H. J., & Cowie, C. C. (2008). Diabetes and hearing impairment in the United States: Audiometric evidence from the National Health and Nutrition Examination Survey, 1999–2004. *Annals of Internal Medicine, 149*(1), 1–10.

Dobie, R. A. (2008). The burden of age-related and occupational noise-induced hearing loss in the United States. *Ear and Hearing, 29*(4), 565–577.

Dube, J. A., Barth, M. M., Cmiel, C. A., Cutshall, S. M., Olson, S. M., Sulla, S. J., . . . Holland, D. E. (2008). Environmental noise sources and interventions to minimize them: A tale of 2 hospitals. *Journal of Nursing Care Quarterly, 23*(3), 216–224.

Federal Interagency Forum on Aging-Related Statistics. (2008). Indicator 17: Sensory impairments and oral health. In *Older Americans 2008: Key indicators of well-being*. Washington, DC: Government Printing Office.

Gates, G. A., Feeney, M. P., & Mills, D. (2008). Cross-sectional age-changes of hearing in the elderly. *Ear and Hearing, 29*(6), 865–874.

Helfer, T. M., Canham-Chervak, M., Canada, S., & Michener, T. A. (2010). Epidemiology of hearing impairment and noise-induced hearing injury among U.S. military personnel, 2003–2005. *American journal of preventive medicine, 38*(Suppl. 1), S71–S77.

Hidalgo, J. L.-T., Gras, C. B., Lapeira, J. T., Verdejo, M.-A. L., del Campo del Campo, J. M., Rabadán, F. E. (2009). Functional status of elderly people with hearing loss. *Archives of Gerontology and Geriatrics, 49*, 88–92.

Jansen, E. J., Hellerman, H. W., Dreschler, W. A., & deLaat, J. A. (2009). Noise induced hearing loss and other hearing complaints among musicians of symphony orchestras. *International Archives of Occupational and Environmental Health, 82*(2), 153–164.

Karimi, A., Nasiri, S., Kazerooni, F. K., & Oliaei, M. (2010). Noise induced hearing loss risk assessment in truck drivers. *Noise and Health, 12*(46), 49–55.

Kim, M. G., Hong, S. M., Shim, H. J., Cha, C. I., & Yeo, S. G. (2009). Hearing threshold of Korean adolescents associated with the use of personal music players. *Yonsei Medical Journal, 50*(6), 771–776.

Kozak, A. T., & Grundfast, K. M. (2009). Hearing loss. *Otolaryngology Clinics of North America, 42*, 79–85.

Levy, B. R., Slade, M. D., & Gill, T. M. (2006). Hearing decline predicted by elders' stereotypes. *Journals of Gerontology: Series B, Psychological Sciences and Social Sciences, 61*, P82–P87.

McCarter, D. F., Courtney, A. U., & Pollart, S. M. (2007). Cerumen impaction. *American Academy of Family Physicians, 75*, 1523–1528, 1530.

McMahon, C. M., Kifley, A., Rochtchina, E., Bewall, P., & Mitchell, P. (2008). The contribution of family history of hearing loss in an older population. *Ear and Hearing, 29*(4), 578–584.

McCullagh, M., & Robertson, C. (2009). Too late smart: farmers' adoption of self-protective behaviors in response to exposure to hazardous noise. *American Association of Occupational Health Nurses Journal, 57*(3), 99–105.

Montano, J. (2007). An advocate for self-assessment: Barbara Weinstein. *The ASHA Leader, 12*(14), 42–43.

Muluk, N. B., & Oguztürk, O. (2008). Occupational noise-induced tinnitus: Does it affect workers' quality of life? *Journal of Otolaryngology: Head and Neck Surgery, 37*(1), 65–71.

NANDA International. (2009). *Nursing diagnoses: Definitions and classification 2009–2011*. Oxford, England: Wiley-Blackwell.

Roland, P. S., Smith, T. L., Schwartz, S. R., Rosenfeld, R. M., Ballachanda, B., Earll, J. M., . . . Wetmore, S. (2008). Clinical practice guideline: Cerumen impaction. *Otolaryngology—Head and Neck Surgery, 139*, S1–S21.

Shulman, A., & Goldstein, B. (2009). Subjective idiopathic tinnitus and palliative care: A plan for diagnosis and treatment. *Otolaryngological Clinics of North America, 42*, 15–37.

Taylor, K. S., & Jurma, W. E. (2003, November 3). Gender-specific audiologic rehabilitation programs and self-perception of handicap in the elderly. *Audiology Online*. Available at www.Audiologyonline.com/articles/article_detail.asp?article_id=509.

Tompkins, O. S. (2009). Secondhand noise and stress. *American Association of Occupational Health Nurses Journal, 57*(10), 436.

University of Texas School of Nursing. (2007). *Evaluation and management of obstructing cerumen*. National Guideline Clearinghouse. Available at www.guideline.gov.

Vogel, I., Verschuure, H., van der Ploeg, C. P., Brug, J., & Raat, H. (2010). Estimating adolescent risk for hearing loss based on data from a large school-based survey. *American Journal of Public Health, 100*(6), 1095–1100.

Wagstaff, A. S. (2009). Hearing loss in civilian airline and helicopter pilots compared to air traffic control personnel. *Aviation, Space, and Environmental Medicine, 80*(10), 857–861.

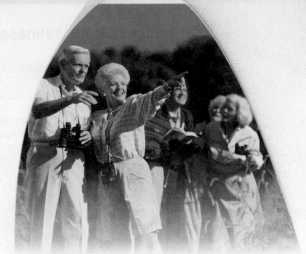

CHAPTER 17

Vision

LEARNING OBJECTIVES

After reading this chapter, you will be able to:

1. Describe age-related changes that affect vision.

2. Identify risk factors that can affect visual wellness.

3. Discuss the functional consequences that affect visual wellness.

4. Describe three pathologic conditions that cause vision impairments in older adults.

5. Conduct a nursing assessment of vision, with emphasis on identifying opportunities for health promotion.

6. Identify nursing interventions to facilitate visual wellness in older adults by addressing risk factors that interfere with vision.

KEY POINTS

accommodation	enophthalmos
acuity	entropion
age-related macular	glare
degeneration (AMD)	glaucoma
arcus senilis	low-vision aids
blepharochalasis	ophthalmologist
cataracts	optician
color perception	optometrist
critical flicker fusion	presbyopia
dark adaptation	visual field
depth perception	visual impairment
ectropion	

Because important daily activities—including communicating, enjoying visual images, and maneuvering in the environment—are highly dependent on eyesight, visual impairments can profoundly affect a person's safety, functioning, and quality of life. Although age-related changes and

risk factors affect visual wellness, nurses have an array of interventions to assist older adults in maintaining optimal visual function. This chapter addresses functional consequences affecting vision in older adults and focuses on the role of nurses in assessing vision and helping older adults to achieve visual wellness.

AGE-RELATED CHANGES THAT AFFECT VISION

Visual function depends on a sequence of processes, beginning with the perception of an external stimulus and ending with the processing of neural impulses in the cerebral cortex. Age-related changes affect all of the structures involved in visual function; however, in the absence of disease processes, these gradual changes have only a subtle impact on the daily activities of the older person.

Eye Appearance and Tear Ducts

Age-related changes in the appearance of the eye and eyelids usually do not affect vision, but they can affect wellness by causing anxiety and discomfort. Changes in the eyelids and surrounding skin include loss of orbital fat, development of wrinkles, decreased elasticity of the eyelid muscles, and accumulation of dark pigment around the eyes. These changes contribute to the overall appearance of sunken eyes, called **enophthalmos**. Loss of orbital fat and muscle elasticity can progress to the point of causing an eyelid fold and impairing vision. This condition, termed **blepharochalasis**, can be surgically treated. Relaxation of the lower eyelid muscles to an extreme degree results in the age-related conditions of ectropion or entropion. In **ectropion**, the lower eyelid falls away from the conjunctiva, blocking the flow of tears through the lower punctum and decreasing lubrication of the conjunctiva. In **entropion**, the lower eyelid becomes inverted and the eyelashes irritate the cornea, eventually leading to infection.

Arcus senilis, also called *corneal arcus*, is another noticeable age-related change in appearance of the eye that can be observed in most eyes by the age of 80 or 90 years. Arcus senilis is the development of a yellow or gray—white ring

Promoting Visual Wellness in Older Adults

Nursing Assessment
- Risk factors
- Environmental conditions (glare, lighting)
- Effects on daily activities
- Health behaviors (eye exams, protective measures)

Age-Related Changes
- ↓ elasticity in eyelids
- ↓ tear production
- ↑ corneal opacity
- Degenerative changes in all structures involved in visual function

Negative Functional Consequences
- ↓ ability to focus on near objects
- ↑ sensitivity to glare
- Need for ↑ illumination
- Dry eyes
- Difficulty driving at night

Risk Factors
- Glare, poor lighting
- Exposure to ultraviolet rays
- Smoking
- Nutrient deficiencies
- Adverse medication effects
- Diseases (diabetes, hypertension)

Nursing Interventions
- Addressing risk factors
- Modifying environments
- Suggesting aids to improve vision
- Referring for eye care
- Teaching about dry eyes

Wellness Outcomes
- Improved vision
- ↑ safety and functioning
- Better quality of life

between the iris and the sclera, which occurs because of the accumulation of lipids in the outer part of the cornea. Studies show an association between arcus senilis and the following conditions: diabetes, hypertension, hypercholesterolemia, cigarette smoking, and coronary heart disease (Fernandez, Sorokin, & Thompson, 2007). Other changes in the eye's appearance include diminished corneal translucency, yellowing of the sclera, and fading of the pigment in the iris.

Age-related changes in the tear ducts reduce the production of tears and can lead to dry eye syndrome and complaints of dryness, burning, or photosensitivity. Subsequent irritation and rubbing of the cornea can lead to infections. Contrary to what might be expected, dry eye syndrome can cause excessive tearing because the lack of normal lubricating tears stimulates the production of reflex tears. Nurses can promote wellness by teaching older adults about comfort measures to relieve bothersome symptoms, as discussed later in this chapter.

The Eye

Age-related changes in the eye itself also affect visual wellness. Specific structures of the eye that change with age include the cornea, lens, iris and pupil, ciliary body, vitreous, and retina (Figure 17-1).

The *cornea* is a translucent covering over the eye that refracts light rays and provides 65% to 75% of the focusing power of the eye. As the eye ages, the cornea becomes opaque and yellow, interfering with the passage of light, especially ultraviolet (UV) rays, to the retina. Other corneal changes, such as the accumulation of lipid deposits, can cause an increased scattering of light rays and have a blurring effect on vision. In addition, age-related changes in the curvature of the cornea influence the refractive ability.

The *lens* consists of concentric and avascular layers of clear, crystalline protein. The lens has no blood supply, so it depends on the aqueous humor for metabolic and support functions. The transparent lens fibers are continually forming new layers without shedding old layers. As new layers form peripherally, the old layers are compressed inward toward the center, where they eventually become absorbed into the nucleus. This process gradually increases the size and density of the lens, causing a tripling of its mass by 70 years of age. Thus, the lens gradually becomes stiffer, denser, and more opaque.

Because of these age-related changes, the lens moves forward in the eye and is less responsive to the ciliary muscle. These changes also interfere with the transmission of light rays, diffusing the rays that pass through the lens and reducing the amount of light reaching the retina. These changes do not affect all wavelengths equally; rather, the most detrimental effect occurs with the shorter blue and violet wavelengths.

The *iris* is a pigmented sphincter muscle that dilates and contracts to control pupillary size and regulate the amount of light reaching the retina. With increasing age, the iris becomes sclerotic and rigid and the *pupil* becomes smaller. These changes interfere with the ability to respond to low levels of light and reduce the amount of light that reaches the retina.

The *ciliary body* is a mass of muscles, connective tissue, and blood vessels surrounding the lens. These muscles regulate the passage of light rays through the lens by changing the shape of the lens. The ciliary body is responsible for **accommodation**, a process that controls one's ability to focus on near objects. In addition, the ciliary body produces aqueous fluid. Because of age-related changes, muscle cells are replaced with connective tissue, and the ciliary body gradually becomes smaller, stiffer, and less functional. With advanced age, diminished secretion of aqueous humor interferes with the nourishment and cleansing of the lens and cornea.

The *vitreous* is a clear, gelatinous mass that forms the inner substance and maintains the spherical shape of the eye. Age-related changes cause the gelatinous substance to shrink and a proportionate increase in the liquid portion. Because of these changes, the vitreous body pulls away from the retina, resulting in symptoms such as floaters, blurred vision, distorted images, or light flashes. In addition, these changes can cause light to scatter more diffusely through the vitreous, reducing the amount of light reaching the retina.

The process of transforming visual stimuli into neural impulses begins in the rods and cones, which are pigment-producing photoreceptor cells in the *retina*. Rods do not perceive colors, but they are responsible for vision under low light. Cones require high levels of light to function effectively, and they are responsible for **color perception** and **acuity**, which is the ability to detect details and discern objects. Rods

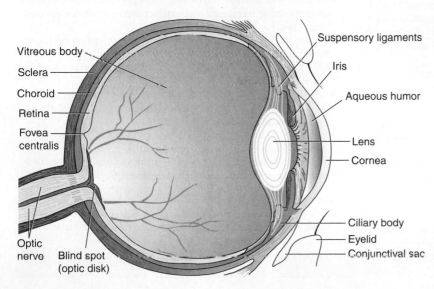

FIGURE 17-1 The eye. Age-related changes in structures of the eye can affect vision in older adults.

are distributed throughout the peripheral retina and cones are concentrated in the central and most sensitive part of the macula, called the *fovea*. Although both the rods and cones diminish with increasing age, the impact of these changes is minimal because loss of cones occurs primarily in the periphery of the retina, with only a minimal loss in the fovea. Also, although the number of rods declines in the central retina, the remaining rods increase in size and maintain their ability to capture light. Additional age-related changes in retinal structures include accumulation of lipofuscin and thinning and sclerosis of the blood vessels and pigment epithelium.

The Retinal–Neural Pathway

Photoreceptor cells converge in the ganglion cells of the optic nerve. Neurosensory information is passed from the optic nerve, through the thalamus, to the visual cortex. Age-related changes affecting these neurons, as well as other central nervous system changes that affect cognitive function, can interfere with visual function in older adults.

EFFECTS OF AGE-RELATED CHANGES ON VISION

Best-corrected visual acuity begins to decrease in adults, regardless of race, sex, ethnicity, or socioeconomic status, after age 50, even in the absence of any risk factors. Even the exceptional persons who have 20/20 visual acuity at the age of 90 years experience subtle changes in overall vision and optical quality. However, despite the universal prevalence of age-related vision changes, most older adults can perform their usual activities by using low-vision aids and modifying their environment. **Visual impairment**, which is defined as vision loss that cannot be corrected by eyeglasses or contact lenses alone, ranges from mild impairment to blindness. Mild visual impairments are caused by normal age-related changes, but they are significantly exacerbated by environmental conditions such as glare and poor lighting. Compensatory interventions for the effects of age-related vision changes are quite effective for promoting visual wellness. For example, people who use reading glasses and bright but nonglaring light to

---

Evidence-Based Practice   17-1
Vision Changes

Statement of the Problem

- Older adults experience the following age-related changes and functional outcomes affecting vision:
  Decreased dark adaptation, increasing the safety risk when environmental lighting changes
  Pupils become smaller, diminishing the ability to adjust to glare and changes in lighting conditions
  Decreased upward gaze, which decreases the field of vision
  Smaller visual field, which increases the safety risk for driving and maneuvering in the environment
  Decreased sensitivity of the cornea, resulting in delayed recognition of injury
  Decreased production of tears, leading to dryness and irritation.
- Presbyopia, which is due to normal age-related loss of elasticity of the lens, leads to a decrease in the eyes' ability to focus on near objects and adapt to light.
- In addition to the effects of age-related vision changes, there is a high prevalence of visual impairment among older adults resulting from the following conditions: cataracts, macular degeneration, glaucoma, diabetic retinopathy, hypertensive retinopathy, temporal arteritis, and detached retina.
- Older adults account for 30% of all visually impaired people.
- Studies have found a prevalence rate of visual impairment of 40% to 50% of older adults in long-term care settings.

Recommendations for Nursing Assessment

Assess all the following parameters in relation to vision:
- Health history of any conditions that predispose older adults to visual impairment (e.g., diabetes, hypertension)
- Specific questions related to visual health (e.g., last eye examination, usual eyesight, changes in vision, use of eye drops, history of trauma or surgery, family history of eye problems)
- Medications that may exacerbate sensory problems (e.g., anticholinergics)
- External structures to identify eyelid lag or lens cloudiness
- Older adult's interest in receiving treatment for visual impairment.

- Use screening tests for distance and near vision, contrast sensitivity, and visual fields.

Recommendations for Patient Teaching

Teach older adults and caregivers about the following measures:
- Obtain an annual eye examination with either an optometrist or an ophthalmologist.
- Add color contrast to fixtures in the home (e.g., light switches, faucets) to create a safer and more functional environment.

Recommendations for Care

- Be aware of the impact of vision changes on safety and quality of life: increased risk of falls, difficulty or inability to read (including medication labels), difficulty driving, difficulty navigating environments (especially stairs or curbs), diminished ability to remain independent.
- Obtain a medical history and develop a care plan that ensures continuation of ongoing therapeutic regimens for people with chronic eye conditions (e.g., eye drops for glaucoma).
- Provide adequate nonglare lighting and identify the lighting that is best for each individual.
- Encourage the use of the person's eyeglasses and additional magnification if appropriate.
- Add color contrast to fixtures and electronics in the room if appropriate.
- For patients with diabetes or hypertension, schedule an annual dilated-eye examination by an ophthalmologist.
- In long-term care settings, initiate a mechanism to trigger a reminder about annual eye examinations for residents.
- When vision is worse than 20/125, refer patients to a low-vision specialist to provide training in the use of visual assistive devices.

SOURCE: Cacchione, P. Z. (2008). Sensory changes. In E. Capezuti, D. Zwicker, M. Mezey, & T. Fulmer (Eds.), *Evidence-based geriatric nursing protocols for best practice* (3rd ed., pp. 477–502). New York: Springer. Modified version is available online at: http://consultgerirn.org

improve their ability to read are compensating for mild visual impairment. These mild visual impairments are discussed in the following sections, and consequences of more significant visual impairments are discussed in the Pathologic Conditions Affecting Vision section.

Loss of Accommodation

Presbyopia is the loss of accommodation, which is the ability to focus clearly and quickly on objects at various distances. Presbyopia is an initial and universal age-related vision change, which begins in early adulthood and affects all humans to some degree by their mid-50s (Ferrer-Blasco, Gonzalez-Meijome, & Montes-Mico, 2008). This vision change is caused by degenerative changes in the lens and the ciliary body. Functionally, accommodative changes gradually extend the near point of vision, which is the closest point at which a small object can be seen clearly. A typical example of the effects of presbyopia is the need to hold reading materials farther from the eye to focus clearly on the print.

Diminished Acuity

Visual acuity is customarily assessed by using a Snellen chart, and it is measured against a normal value of 20/20. Visual acuity is best around age 30, after which it gradually declines. Diminished acuity results from age-related ocular changes, including decreased pupillary size, scatter of light in the cornea and lens, opacification of the lens and vitreous, and loss of photoreceptor cells in the retina. These changes interfere with the passage of light to the retina, causing a threefold reduction in retinal illumination between the ages 20 and 60.

Acuity is also influenced by conditions, such as size and movement of the object and the amount of light reflected off an object. Because poor illumination compounds the effects of age-related ocular changes with regard to visual acuity, older people require more illumination to see objects clearly. In addition, because visual acuity is more impaired for moving objects than for stationary objects, it becomes more impaired with increasing speed of the object. These changes in visual acuity can particularly affect night driving competence.

Delayed Dark and Light Adaptation

The ability to respond to dim light, called **dark adaptation**, begins to decline around the age of 20 years and diminishes more markedly after age 60. This decline is associated with decreased retinal illumination and age-related changes in the retina and retinal–neural pathways. As a result, the older adult requires more time to adapt to dim lighting when moving from a brighter to a darker environment. For instance, when entering a darkened movie theater, an older person needs extra time to adapt to the changes in lighting before proceeding to a seat.

Age-related changes in the lens and pupil interfere with the response to bright lights because they reduce the amount of light reaching the retina. In practical terms, this means that an older person responds more slowly to lights, such as car or bus headlights and requires more time to recover from exposure to glare and bright lights.

Increased Glare Sensitivity

Glare occurs when scattered light in the optic media reduces the clarity of visual images. Glare is experienced when light is reflected from shiny surfaces, when the light is excessively bright or inappropriately focused, or when bright light originates from several sources at once. Glare is classified according to three types: veiling, dazzling, and scotomatic. *Veiling glare* is caused by the scattering of light over the retinal surface and results in diminished contrast of the viewed object. Veiling glare occurs, for example, when bright fluorescent lights in a grocery store reflect on the clear plastic covering over food products in a white case. *Dazzling glare*, which is caused by bright visual displays, interferes with the ability to discern details. Glass-covered directories in brightly lit shopping malls produce a dazzling glare that interferes with a person's ability to read the words in the directory, particularly if there is poor contrast between the letters and the background. *Scotomatic glare* is a blinding glare caused by loss of retinal sensitivity and overstimulation of retinal pigments during exposure to bright lights. For example, sunshine can create scotomatic glare, especially at sunrise or sunset.

Beginning in the fifth decade, age-related changes increase a person's sensitivity to glare and the time required to recover from glare. Glare sensitivity is influenced primarily by opacification of the lens; however, it is affected also by age-related changes in the pupil and vitreous. Functionally, these changes can significantly affect the person's ability to read signs, see objects, drive at night, and maneuver safely in bright environments. In many modern buildings and shopping malls, the bright lights, large windows, and highly reflective floors generate glare that can lead to accidents and inaccurate perceptions.

Reduced Visual Field

A **visual field** is an oval-shaped area encompassing the total view that people perceive while looking at a fixed point straight ahead. The scope of the visual field narrows slightly between the ages of 40 and 50 years and then declines steadily. Functionally, the visual field is important when people engage in tasks that require a broad perception of the environment and moving objects. Walking in crowded places and driving a vehicle are examples of activities that depend on the field of vision.

Diminished Depth Perception

Depth perception is the visual skill responsible for locating objects in three-dimensional space, judging differences in the depth of objects, and observing relationships among objects in space. Functionally, depth perception enables people to use objects effectively and to maneuver safely in the environment.

TABLE 17-1 Age-Related Changes Affecting Vision

Change	Consequences
Appearance and Comfort • Decreased elasticity of the eyelid muscles • Enophthalmos • Decreased tears	• Potential for ectropion, entropion, blepharochalasis • Potential for dry eye syndrome • **Presbyopia:** diminished ability to focus on near objects
Structures • Corneal yellowing and increased opacity • Changes in the corneal curvature • Increase in lens size and density • Sclerosis and rigidity of the iris • Decrease in pupillary size • Atrophy of the ciliary muscle • Shrinkage of gelatinous substance in the vitreous • Atrophy of photoreceptor cells • Thinning and sclerosis of retinal blood vessels • Degeneration of neurons in the visual cortex	• Diminished accommodation • Diminished acuity • Slower response to changes in illumination • Increased sensitivity to glare • Narrowing of the visual field • Diminished depth perception • Altered color perception • Distorted perception of flashing lights • Slower processing of visual information

Stereopsis, or the disparity between retinal images that is caused by the separation of the two eyes, is the primary ocular characteristic that affects depth perception. Additional factors that influence depth perception include prior perceptual experiences of the observer; movement of the observer's head or body; and characteristics of the object, such as size, height, distance, texture, brightness, and shading. Although depth perception declines with increasing age, studies indicate that despite age-related changes in stereopsis, older adults are able to discriminate depth differences in a manner that is similar to younger adults (Norman et al., 2008).

Altered Color Vision

Pigments in the retinal cones absorb light in the red, blue, or yellow ranges of the spectrum. As with many other visual functions, color perception is influenced by the type and quantity of light waves reaching the retina. Consequently, any age-related changes that interfere with retinal illumination—including lens opacification, pupillary miosis, retinal or retinal–neural changes—can interfere with accurate color perception. Opacification and yellowing of the lens interferes most directly with shorter wavelengths, causing an altered perception of blues, greens, and violets. Low levels of illumination and other environmental factors also interfere with color perception.

Functionally, altered color perception is manifested as a relative darkening of blue objects and a yellowed perception of white light. Accurate color perception is not essential in all daily activities, but it is important, for instance, in differentiating between medications that are similar in color or tone, especially those in the blue–green and yellow–white ranges. In addition, altered color perception can interfere with the detection of spoiled food.

Diminished Critical Flicker Fusion

Critical flicker fusion is the point at which an intermittent light source is perceived as a continuous, rather than flashing, light. The ability to perceive flashing lights accurately is a function

of the retinal receptors and is influenced by extraocular factors, such as the size, color, and luminance of the object. Age-related changes in the retina and retinal–neural pathway, as well as changes that decrease retinal illumination, interfere with critical flicker fusion. Low levels of illumination further exacerbate the effects of these changes. Functionally, diminished critical flicker fusion distorts the perception of a flashing light, making it appear to be a continuous light. Thus, diminished critical flicker fusion can interfere with the discernment of emergency vehicles and road construction lights, especially at night.

Slower Visual Information Processing

Age-related changes of the retinal–neural pathway affect the accuracy and efficiency of visual information processing. Thus, older adults generally need more time to process visual information, but the effects are minimal or negligible when tasks are familiar. Table 17-1 summarizes age-related vision changes and their effects on vision.

RISK FACTORS THAT AFFECT VISUAL WELLNESS

Lifestyle, nutritional, and environmental factors—including both immediate and long-term conditions—exacerbate age-related vision changes and interfere with visual wellness. For example, long-term exposure to UV light (i.e., sunlight) is associated with the development of **cataracts** (age-related changes in the lens) and loss of photoreceptor cells, particularly the cones. Furthermore, older adults are more vulnerable to eye damage from sunlight because age-related changes alter the protective response to harmful UV light. Warmer environmental temperatures are associated with an earlier age of onset for presbyopia (i.e., loss of near vision). Dry eyes can be caused by environmental conditions such as wind, sunlight, low humidity, and secondhand smoke. Other environmental influences on visual wellness include glare, dim lighting, and poor color contrast. Studies found that poor nutrition increased the risk for age-related macular degeneration (AMD) (Montgomery et al., 2010). Cigarette smoking is a lifestyle factor that increases the risk for cataracts and macular degeneration. One study found that smoking was associated with approximately four times higher odds of visual impairment (Jin & Wong, 2008).

Wellness Opportunity

Poor lighting and exposure to sunlight are risk factors that can readily be addressed through simple self-care practices.

Chronic conditions can adversely affect visual function in various ways. Vision impairments commonly occur in people with Alzheimer or Parkinson disease, even during the early stages. Dementia with Lewy bodies is commonly characterized by visual hallucinations and impairments of visuospatial skills (Hamilton et al., 2008). People with diabetes are at increased risk for developing cataracts, glaucoma, and diabetic retinopathy. People with hypertension or hypercholesterolemia are at higher risk for AMD. Malnutrition has been associated with cataract development, and vitamin A deficiency has been associated with dry eyes from reduced tear production.

Medications that are associated with adverse effects on vision include aspirin, haloperidol, nonsteroidal anti-inflammatory agents, tricyclic antidepressants, digitalis, anticholinergics, phenothiazines, isoniazid, tamoxifen, amiodarone, sildenafil, and oral or inhaled corticosteroids. Cataracts are common in people with glaucoma because of the anticholinesterase drugs used in glaucoma treatment. Medications that can cause or contribute to dry eyes include estrogen, diuretics, antihistamines, anticholinergics, phenothiazines, beta-blockers, and antiparkinson agents. Systemic anticoagulants can precipitate intraocular hemorrhage in people with preexisting macular degeneration.

---

*M*rs. F. is 60 years old and has used "readers" (reading glasses) for 15 years but has never needed glasses for anything other than reading and sewing. She recently noticed that she has trouble reading the glass-enclosed directory at the shopping mall. She works in an office building with an atrium that has skylights, and she has trouble reading the signs on the doors.

THINKING POINTS

- What age-related factors contribute to the vision changes that Mrs. F. notices?
- What environmental factors are likely to contribute to Mrs. F.'s difficulty when she is in the shopping mall or at work?
- When Mrs. F. is in her home environment, what tasks might be more difficult because of age-related vision changes?

FUNCTIONAL CONSEQUENCES AFFECTING VISUAL WELLNESS

The most serious visual impairments that affect older adults are associated with pathologic conditions, such as cataracts, glaucoma, or AMD, all of which are increasingly likely to occur with advanced age. Visual impairments are categorized as "functional" when acuity is 20/50 or worse, as "low vision" when it is between 20/70 and 20/200, and as "blindness" when it is 20/400 or worse. Trouble seeing, even with corrective lenses, affects 13.6% of people between ages 65 and 74 years, 20% of those who are between ages 75 and 84 years, and 26.5% of those 85 years and older (Federal Interagency Forum on Aging-Related Statistics, 2008). The following sections describe the functional consequences that are associated with the types of visual impairments that are most likely to occur in older adults.

DIVERSITY NOTE

Although 16.4% of older adults who are above the poverty level report trouble seeing, 25% of those who are below the poverty level report trouble seeing (Federal Interagency Forum on Aging-Related Statistics, 2008).

Effects on Safety and Function

Because visual impairments are associated with many aspects of safety and functioning, people who are visually impaired are likely to be more dependent in their activities of daily living. Age-related vision changes most directly influence the following activities:

- Getting outside
- Driving a vehicle
- Shopping for groceries
- Going up and down stairs
- Getting in and out of bed or a chair
- Maneuvering safely in dark or unfamiliar environments
- Seeing markings on clocks, radios, thermostats, appliances, and televisions
- Reading newspapers, directories, small-print signs and posters, and labels on food items and medication containers.

Most of these activities are affected not only by alterations in visual skills but also by environmental conditions, such as glare and lighting.

Visual impairments threaten safe functioning because they can affect gait, balance, and postural stability. They also increase the risk of falls, fractures, and other serious injury secondary to falling. Studies have found an association between impaired vision and an increased risk of all the following: falls, mortality, hip fractures, medication noncompliance, automobile accidents, and decreased quality of life (Kalinowski, 2008). Specific age-related vision changes that increase the risk for falls include diminished acuity, reduced visual field, diminished depth perception, impaired contrast sensitivity, and increased sensitivity to glare. One recent study found a strong correlation between diminished contrast sensitivity and gait change and postural instability (Wood et al., 2009). In addition, delayed processing of visual information can interfere with the quick responses necessary for avoiding falls.

Effects on Quality of Life

Age-related vision changes develop gradually and often go unnoticed for many years. As the changes progress and interfere with usual activities, older adults may withdraw from activities rather than acknowledge a vision problem or adjust to the changes. Studies have found that visual impairments are associated with anxiety, depression, and lower levels of psychological well-being (Mabuchi et al., 2008). One study found that vision loss was a strong predictor of both onset and persistence of depression (Chou, 2008).

Of course, a person's usual lifestyle influences the extent of any psychosocial impact related to vision changes. If the preferred leisure activities require good visual skills, the older adult is likely to become bored and even depressed when vision changes interfere with endeavors, such as reading, sewing, or needlework. Similarly, when artistic pursuits and entertainment events are important activities, diminished visual function can interfere with the person's quality of life. By contrast, the effect of vision impairment on lifestyle may be minimal for people who prefer music or other activities that are less dependent on visual skills.

One's living environment and support systems are other determinants of the psychosocial consequences of vision changes. Good visual skills are more important for people who live alone or who provide care for others than they are for people who live with, or have frequent contact with, others who have good vision. Also, if visually impaired people can modify their living environment to compensate for the impairments, the psychosocial consequences will be minimized. By contrast, people who live in institutional settings may experience relatively greater negative consequences because of their inability to alter environmental conditions.

Some older adults who notice declines in vision develop fears that negatively affect their quality of life. For example, people may mistakenly fear going blind if they think they have a serious and progressive disease when, in reality, they have a treatable condition. Fear of blindness may be based on myths, inaccurate information, or the experiences of friends who have serious visual impairments. Negative or hopeless attitudes about vision changes can deter the older person from acknowledging the problem or seeking help. Fear of falling is another source of anxiety associated with impaired vision. Inaccurate depth perception can lead to frequent bumping into objects, and the older adult may feel insecure and unsafe, even in familiar environments. If the person has experienced falls or tripping, or knows someone who suffered a fracture as a result of falling, the fears may be magnified.

Wellness Opportunity

Nurses assess the impact of vision impairment on the whole person so they can address fears, anxieties, and other responses that affect quality of life.

Effects on Driving

Vision changes can significantly affect driving skills and exert a profound impact on older adults, their families, and the society. Because driving is associated with considerable safety and independence concerns for drivers and their families—and because unsafe drivers place others at risk—there has been intense and increasing interest in the effects of vision changes on the driving skills of older adults. Visual dimensions that influence driving abilities are near vision, visual search, dynamic vision, contrast sensitivity, and visual processing speed. Consequences of visual impairment with regard to driving include the following:

- Slower dark and light adaptation creates problems when driving in and out of tunnels and when driving at night on streets with variable lighting.
- Decreased peripheral vision interferes with the wide visual field that is important for avoiding collisions.
- Decreased acuity interferes with the perception of moving objects, especially fast-moving vehicles.
- Diminished accommodation and acuity create problems when the older adult tries to read dashboard indicators after focusing on the road.
- Glare interferes with the perception of objects and is heightened by rainy, snowy, or sunny conditions.
- Bright sunlight shortly after sunrise or before sunset can significantly interfere with the perception of red and green traffic lights because of increased sensitivity to glare.
- If the car has tinted windows, the diminished illumination further interferes with visual skills.

In recent years, gerontologists and clinicians are focusing attention on identifying variables that affect driving in older adults, and many studies address visual skills as an important factor. For example, Baldock, Berndt, and Mathias (2008) found that drivers with deficits in contrast sensitivity are likely to approach points on a road at which a maneuver is required (e.g., an intersection) too quickly. Studies have also found an association between driving cessation and all the following visual function measures: cataracts, glaucoma, contrast sensitivity, baseline visual acuity, and peripheral visual field deficits (Ackerman, Edwards, Ross, Ball, & Lunsman, 2008; Ramulu, West, Munoz, Jampel, & Friedman, 2009).

Wellness Opportunity

Nurses need to be aware of the far-reaching implications of the ability to drive not only on safety of the individual and others but also on independence and the quality of life.

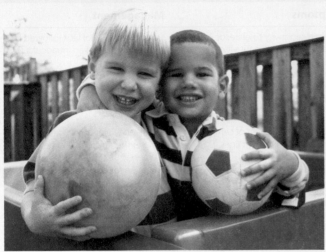

Normal vision

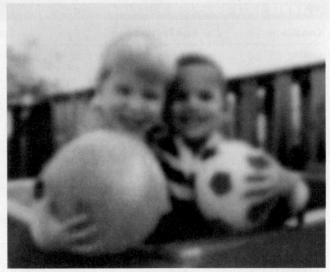

Cataracts

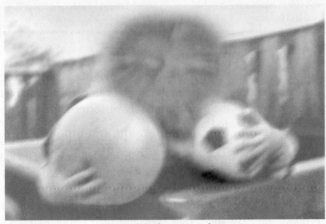

Macular degeneration

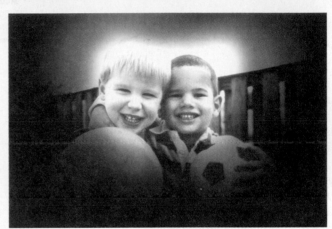

Glaucoma

FIGURE 17-2 Examples of normal vision, vision with cataracts, vision with age-related macular degeneration, and vision with glaucoma. (Courtesy of the National Eye Institute, National Institutes of Health.)

PATHOLOGIC CONDITIONS AFFECTING VISION

Chronic conditions that interfere with visual wellness occur very commonly in older adults, so nurses have important roles in detecting and managing these conditions. Health promotion interventions are particularly important with conditions such as glaucoma because interventions can prevent vision impairment. However, this condition is often undiagnosed so the interventions are not implemented in a timely manner. Among older adults, the three most common pathologic eye conditions are cataracts, AMD, and glaucoma (Figure 17-2, Table 17-2).

DIVERSITY NOTE

Worldwide, women account for nearly two-thirds of people who are blind; most of these women are older than 60 years, and 90% of them live in poverty (Gilbert & Bassett, 2007).

Cataracts

Cataracts are a leading and reversible cause of visual impairment, affecting approximately 50% of people aged 80 years and older. Cataracts are caused by the progression of age-related changes in the lens that begins around age 40 and eventually can progress to total opacification. As cataracts develop, the normally transparent lens becomes cloudy, transmission of light to the retina is diminished, and vision is impaired. In addition to being caused by age-related changes, risk factors include systemic disease, medications, and environmental factors, as summarized in Table 17-2. Also, cataracts are likely to occur more commonly after glaucoma surgery or other types of eye surgery. The most modifiable and preventable risk factors for cataracts are cigarette smoking and exposure to sunlight.

Cataracts usually occur in both eyes, but they do not necessarily progress bilaterally at the same rate. Cataracts are classified according to their location: *cortical* cataracts occur

TABLE 17-2 Common Disease Conditions Affecting Vision

Condition	Risk Factors	Symptoms	Management
Cataract	Advanced age, exposure to sunlight, smoking, diabetes, malnutrition, trauma or radiation to the eye or head, medications (corticosteroids, phenothiazines, amiodarone, benzodiazepines, anticholinesterases)	Increased sensitivity to glare, decreased contrast sensitivity, blurred vision, distorted images, double vision, diminished color perception, frequent eyeglass prescription changes	Surgical removal of lens followed by implantation of an intraocular lens
Age-related macular degeneration (AMD)	Advanced age, non-Hispanic white ethnicity, family history of AMD, smoking, hypertension, hyperlipidemia, medications (tamoxifen, phenothiazines, chloroquine)	Gradual progressive loss of central vision, distorted straight lines, blurred vision	Visual rehabilitation programs, argon laser therapy for wet type, experimental treatments under investigation for both types
Glaucoma	Advanced age, African American race, family history of glaucoma, diabetes, medications (anticholinergics, corticosteroids)	**Chronic:** Slow onset, diminished vision in dim light, increased sensitivity to glare, decreased contrast sensitivity, diminished peripheral vision **Acute:** sudden onset, intense pain, blurred vision, halos around lights, nausea, and vomiting	**Chronic:** Medical therapy with miotics, adrenergic agonists, carbonic anhydrase inhibitors, beta-blockers, and prostaglandins (administered as eye drops) **Acute:** immediate treatment with medications to reduce pressure, followed by laser surgery

in the cortex, *nuclear* cataracts occur in the nucleus, and *posterior subcapsular* cataracts occur on the back of the membrane that surrounds the lens. The location of cataracts significantly influences their impact, with nuclear cataracts interfering the most with vision.

In their early stages, cataracts do not necessarily affect visual acuity, but as they progress, they cause difficulty performing activities such as reading and night driving (see Figure 17-2). People with cataracts are likely to experience any of the following vision changes:

- Dimmed or blurred vision
- Distorted or double images
- Frequent changes in corrective lenses
- An increased sensitivity to glare
- A need for more light when reading
- The perception of a "film" over the eye
- A diminished ability to discern contrast
- The perception of halos around bright lights
- Distorted or diminished color perception (e.g., blue appears dulled, and red, yellow, and orange appear brighter).

Cataracts cannot be treated with medication, but in the early stages, they are managed by the prescription of stronger eyeglasses or contact lenses. When visual acuity declines to the point that it affects the person's safety or the quality of life and provides a reasonable likelihood of improved vision, cataract surgery is usually recommended. When surgery is required for both eyes, the procedure is usually done on one eye at a time, with the second surgery being done after the first one heals completely. However, a recent study of immediate versus delayed sequential cataract surgery found that subjects who had cataract surgery on both eyes in one session experienced greater improvements and a more rapid visual rehabilitation (Nassiri, Nassiri, Sadeghi Yarandi, & Rahnavardi,

2009). An optometrist or ophthalmologist can diagnose cataracts, but only an ophthalmologist can perform cataract surgery, which is the most commonly performed operation in the United States today.

Surgeons typically remove the affected lens through a process called *phacoemulsification*, in which they break up the clouded lens with ultrasound waves and then aspirate the tiny particles with a suction device. After the cataract is removed, the surgeon implants an intraocular lens. The surgical procedure is done with local anesthesia, takes less than 1 hour, and has a very low rate of complications. If the person needed corrective lenses before the surgery, the surgeon can insert an intraocular lens that mimics the natural focusing ability of the eye and results in improved vision, with little or no need for additional correction. One drawback of the intraocular lens is that some patients report continued difficulty with glare and halos.

Nurses have an important role in dispelling myths that might interfere with older adults obtaining surgical treatment for cataracts. For example, older adults might think that cataract surgery is riskier or more complicated than it actually is because they are familiar with experiences of friends or relatives who had cataract surgery many years ago. Nurses can emphasize that advances in surgical techniques for cataract surgery have significantly improved both the process and the outcomes of cataract surgery for older adults in recent years. In addition, nurses can emphasize that there are many benefits, especially when the vision impairment interferes with safety and the quality of life.

DIVERSITY NOTE

African Americans are less likely than whites to undergo cataract surgery (National Eye Institute, 2007).

Although nurses need not be thoroughly familiar with the surgical techniques, they can emphasize that the cataract surgery today is much simpler and has an extremely high success rate in significantly improving safety, functioning, and the quality of life. Moreover, nurses can encourage older adults to seek reliable information and periodic evaluations from eye care professionals, rather than simply tolerating a loss of vision because of cataracts.

Wellness Opportunity

Nurses promote responsible decision making by encouraging older adults and their caregivers to explore risks and benefits of cataract surgery.

Age-Related Macular Degeneration

Age-related macular degeneration (AMD) is the leading cause of severe vision loss and blindness in people older than 55 years in the United States and other developed countries (Coleman, Chan, Ferris, & Chew, 2008). AMD, in various stages, affects 18% of people between ages 70 and 74 years, and 47% of people aged 85 years and older. AMD is associated with the risk factors summarized in Table 17-2. Longitudinal studies found that AMD is significantly associated with serious function consequences, including higher rates of blindness, depression, hip fracture, and residence in long-term care facilities (Wysong, Lee, & Sloan, 2010). Prevention of AMD focuses on control of modifiable risk factors, such as smoking, and the use of a nutritional supplement that contains all of the following: vitamin C 500 mg, vitamin E 400 IU, beta-carotene 15 mg, zinc oxide 80 mg, and cupric oxide 2 mg (Coleman et al., 2008).

DIVERSITY NOTE

AMD is more common in white individuals than in people of any other ethnic origin; in people 75 years and older, female gender may be a risk factor (Coleman et al., 2008).

Early in the disease, deposits of yellow by-products of retinal pigment, called *drusen*, build up in the macula, which is the area in the middle of the retina where visual acuity is the best. As the disease progresses, it is classified either as *dry type*, which accounts for 80% to 90% of cases, or *wet (exudative) type*. In the dry type, damage is caused by the death of the photoreceptors, which is seen on funduscopy as tiny areas of atrophy of the retinal pigment epithelium. The dry type of AMD usually progresses slowly and does not cause total blindness; however, if the wet type develops, visual loss can be rapid and severe. In the wet type, the damage is caused by the formation of new blood vessels in the choroid, a process called *choroidal neovascularization*, followed by hemorrhage into the subretinal space.

In the early stage of AMD, the person experiences blurred vision and has difficulty reading, especially in dim light.

Similar to most other eye conditions, AMD occurs in both eyes, but it can appear initially in only one eye, and its course may differ in each eye. As AMD progresses, it affects central vision and significantly interferes with activities such as reading, driving, watching television, recognizing people, and performing many self-care activities (see Figure 17-2). The primary treatment goal for patients with either type of AMD is to reduce the risk of further vision loss.

Laser photocoagulation and photodynamic therapy are two interventions that are used for treating the choroidal neovascularization that occurs in the wet type of AMD for people who meet the medical criteria for these two treatments. A disadvantage of these treatments is that many patients do not experience significant long-term effects. Some progress is being made with regard to biologic or pharmacologic agents that halt the disease process, so nurses can encourage anyone with AMD to obtain information about clinical trials and new developments through sources such as the National Eye Institute and other reliable organizations. Nurses can serve in support roles for people with AMD by encouraging them to participate in vision rehabilitation programs so they can learn the most effective ways of compensating for declining vision. People with AMD are usually taught to test their eyes daily by using the Amsler grid (Figure 17-3) so they will be aware of sudden changes. In long-term care settings and for older adults with memory problems, nurses may have to provide daily reminders or assistance with performing this task. Nurses also need to encourage people with AMD to receive ongoing evaluation by eye care practitioners to detect treatable aspects of this disease.

Wellness Opportunity

Nurses holistically address needs of people with AMD by encouraging them to explore support groups and educational services associated with a sight center.

Glaucoma

The term **glaucoma** refers to a group of eye diseases in which the ganglion cells of the optic nerve are damaged by an abnormal build-up of aqueous humor in the eye. *Aqueous humor* is a clear fluid that is produced in the anterior chamber of the eye and normally maintains eye pressure between 10 and 20 mm Hg. If the fluid cannot flow out of the anterior chamber of the eye through the channel between the iris and the cornea, it accumulates and pushes the optic nerve into a cupped or concave shape. The resulting damage to the optic nerve causes a loss of peripheral vision. If left untreated, the damage can progress to blindness.

DIVERSITY NOTE

African Americans have an earlier age of onset of glaucoma than do whites (National Eye Institute, 2007).

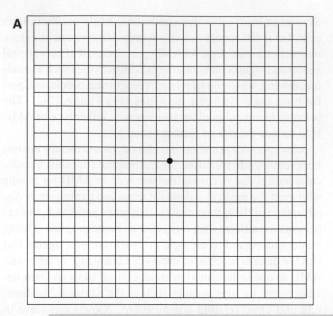

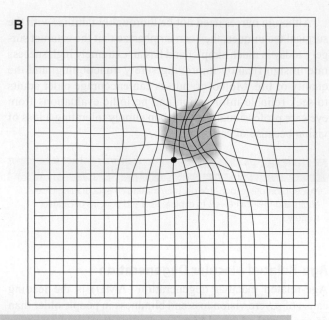

Instructions for Use

1. Tape this page at eye level where light is consistent and without glare.

2. Put on your reading glasses and cover one eye.

3. Fix your gaze on the center black dot.

4. Keeping your gaze fixed, try to see if any lines are distorted or missing.

5. Mark the defect on the chart.

6. TEST EACH EYE SEPARATELY.

7. If the distortion is new or has worsened, arrange to see your ophthalmologist at once.

8. **Always** keep the Amsler grid the **same distance** from your eyes each time you test.

FIGURE 17-3 Amsler grid. **(A)** People with age-related macular degeneration (AMD) use the Amsler grid to perform a simple daily test for sudden changes in their condition. **(B)** This is what the Amsler grid might look like to someone with AMD. (*Part A:* Reprinted with permission from American Macular Degeneration Foundation, 888-MACULAR, www.macular.org.)

Chronic (open-angle) glaucoma, which accounts for as much as 90% of cases of glaucoma in the United States, occurs when the drainage canals become clogged. This condition has an insidious onset and affects vision when the optic nerve becomes damaged. Early signs include increased intraocular pressure, poor vision in dim lighting, and increased sensitivity to glare. If the condition progresses, manifestations include headaches, "tired eyes," impaired peripheral vision, a fixed and dilated pupil, the perception of halos around lights, and frequent changes in the prescription for corrective lenses. Chronic glaucoma usually occurs in both eyes, but it can begin in only one eye and does not necessarily progress at the same rate in both eyes. Because chronic glaucoma progresses slowly and causes little or no visual impairment in the early stage, annual assessments of intraocular pressure are necessary to detect the condition before visual impairments occur. Chronic glaucoma is most commonly managed with medications, but surgical treatment options include laser surgery and other types of eye surgery. Medication management commonly includes one or more of the following types of eye drops: miotics, prostaglandins, beta-blockers, adrenergic agonists, and carbonic anhydrase inhibitors.

Normal-tension glaucoma is another type of glaucoma that occurs in older adults. With this type of glaucoma, the intraocular pressure is within the normal range, but the optic nerve is damaged and the visual field is narrowed (see Figure 17-2). This condition is often managed with the same medications and surgical approaches that are used for chronic glaucoma.

Acute (closed-angle) glaucoma is caused by a sudden complete blockage of the flow of aqueous humor. This condition has an abrupt onset in one or both eyes and should be considered a medical emergency. People with acute glaucoma present with increased intraocular pressure, severe eye pain, clouded or blurred vision, dilation of the pupil, and nausea and vomiting. This condition can be precipitated by medications that cause pupil dilation, such as anticholinergics. Immediate treatment with medications is usually effective for acute attacks, but surgical intervention is often needed.

Health education for older adults with glaucoma focuses on the importance of adhering to ongoing medication routines and regularly being evaluated by their eye care practitioner. If older adults with glaucoma are admitted for institutional care, nurses need to ensure that prescribed eye drops are administered as ordered. In home care situations, nurses may need to develop a plan for administering eye drops on a daily or more frequent basis. If an older adult has memory problems, establishing a routine for administering eye drops can be quite challenging. Many times, complicated eye drop regimens can be simplified by working with the eye care practitioner to decrease the number of eye drops that are necessary or to prescribe a longer-acting medication that can be administered less frequently.

Wellness Opportunity

Nurses promote self-care by teaching people with glaucoma to be aware of prescription and over-the-counter medications that can exacerbate glaucoma.

---

*M*rs. F. is now 72 years old and has been retired for several years. You are the nurse at her local senior center, and she makes an appointment to see you. Mrs. F.'s medical history indicates that she has smoked a pack of cigarettes a day for 40 years and has been taking medications for hypertension and arthritis for 5 years. During a recent medical checkup, her doctor said he thought she had early cataracts, but he told Mrs. F. that he felt it was too early to do anything about them. She has never had an eye examination, other than what her regular doctor does periodically. When asked about her symptoms, Mrs. F. tells you that she sometimes feels like there is a film over her eyes and she has trouble seeing when she is outside on sunny days. Mrs. F. says that she never liked wearing sunglasses and hopes she will not have to start wearing them now. She has recently purchased stronger reading glasses, and these help a little with reading and sewing.

THINKING POINTS

- What factors likely contributed to the development of Mrs. F.'s cataracts?
- When Mrs. F. is driving during the day, what difficulties might she notice because of vision changes? Because of environmental conditions?
- When Mrs. F. is driving at night, what difficulties might she notice because of vision changes? Because of environmental conditions?
- When Mrs. F. is in her home, what changes in visual abilities might she notice because of cataracts?

 NURSING ASSESSMENT OF VISION

Nursing assessment of vision is aimed at identifying the following:
- Factors that interfere with visual wellness
- Vision problems

- The impact of vision changes on safety, independence, or the quality of life
- Opportunities for promoting visual wellness
- Barriers to implementing interventions.

Nursing assessment of visual function is not a substitute for an examination by an eye care specialist. Whereas the purpose of an examination by an eye care specialist is to detect and initiate appropriate treatment of vision problems, the goal of the nursing assessment is to assist the older adult in minimizing the negative consequences of vision changes. Nursing assessment also aims at identifying modifiable risk factors that can be addressed through health promotion. Nurses assess visual abilities by interviewing the older adult (or caregivers of dependent older adults), by observing the older adult's ability to perform activities of daily living, and by testing the older adult's visual skills.

Interviewing About Vision Changes

Nurses use interview questions to elicit the following information: past and present risk factors for vision impairment, the person's awareness of any vision changes, the impact of these changes on daily activities and the quality of life, and the person's attitudes about interventions (Box 17-1). The interview begins with direct questions about the person's awareness of any changes in vision. If the person acknowledges a visual impairment, nurses elicit additional details about the onset and progression of vision changes. Nurses also ask about symptoms that cause discomfort or that indicate the possible presence of disease processes.

Nurses then ask about the impact of vision changes on the person's usual or desired activities. If the person has acknowledged vision changes, nurses can ask specific questions about how these changes have influenced usual activities. If the person is not aware of vision changes, nurses inquire about any difficulties performing complex activities, such as driving, shopping, and meal preparation. Questions about leisure interests are incorporated into the interview to obtain information about the psychosocial consequences of vision impairments. Although the older adult may not associate lifestyle changes with vision impairments, questions about changes in hobbies and leisure activities can help nurses identify the need for interventions to improve visual wellness. Because poor vision increases the risk for falls, especially tripping-related falls, nurses ask about a history of tripping, falling, and near-falling.

Wellness Opportunity

Nurses assess the impact of vision changes on the person's relationships with other people as one aspect of the quality of life.

Identifying Opportunities for Health Promotion

Nurses identify opportunities for health promotion by asking about the person's usual eye care practices and about factors that can interfere with visual wellness. Information about the

Confrontation Test, which nurses can use to assess distance acuity and peripheral vision.

Nurses can informally test near acuity by asking the person to read a newspaper or other printed material of various type sizes. Another method is to ask the person to read a line or two of a form that needs to be signed and then observe the person's ability to find the signature line. Nurses can create additional opportunities for assessing acuity by providing written educational materials and asking the person to read a specific part, such as a phone number. Nurses can informally assess distance acuity by asking the person to look out a window or down a hallway and to describe certain details, such as the words on a sign.

> *R*ecall that you are the nurse at the senior center in Mrs. F.'s neighborhood. During a recent visit, the 72-year-old Mrs. F. told you that she feels like there is a "film" over her eyes, and she has trouble seeing when she is outside on sunny days. Several months ago, Mrs. F.'s doctor told her that she has "early cataracts," but she has not had any further evaluation.

THINKING POINTS

- Which questions from Box 17-1 would you ask Mrs. F. at this time?
- What sort of information might you be able to glean from behavioral or environmental cues about Mrs. F.'s ability to see? (See Box 17-2.)
- Would assessing Mrs. F.'s vision by using vision screening tests be appropriate? (See Box 17-3.) If so, which tests would you perform?
- What health promotion education would you give Mrs. F. at this time?

NURSING DIAGNOSIS

On the basis of the nursing assessment, the nurse might identify actual vision impairment or risk factors for impaired vision. An appropriate nursing diagnosis for an older adult with impaired vision would be Disturbed Sensory Perception: Visual. This is defined as a "change in the amount or patterning of incoming stimuli accompanied by a diminished, exaggerated, distorted, or impaired response to such stimuli" (NANDA International, 2009, p. 163). Related factors that commonly affect older adults include age-related vision changes (e.g., presbyopia), sensory organ alterations (e.g., glaucoma), and environmental factors (e.g., glare, dim lighting, or poor color contrast). The care plan at the end of this chapter is based on a nursing diagnosis of Disturbed Sensory Perception: Visual related to age-related changes, sensory

organ alterations, and environmental factors. Other nursing diagnoses might be addressed if the visual impairment interferes with the older adult's safety, quality of life, or performance of activities of daily living. Possible diagnoses to address these functional consequences include Anxiety, Ineffective Coping, Self-Care Deficit, Risk for Injury, Impaired Social Interaction, Readiness for Enhanced Coping, and Readiness for Enhanced Self-Care.

> **Wellness Opportunity**
>
> The wellness nursing diagnosis of Readiness for Enhanced Knowledge: Improved Vision would be applicable for older adults who are willing to explore interventions that improve their vision.

PLANNING FOR WELLNESS OUTCOMES

When older adults experience vision impairments or have risk factors that affect visual functioning, nurses identify wellness outcomes as an essential part of the planning process. The Nursing Outcomes Classifications (NOCs) that most directly relate to interventions to improve vision for older adults are Vision Compensation Behavior, and Sensory Function: Vision. In addition, nurses can use any of the following NOCs to describe the effectiveness of interventions to improve vision: Coping, Adaptation to Physical Disability, Self-Care: Activities of Daily Living, Stress Level, Knowledge: Personal Safety, Fall Prevention Behavior, and Risk Control: Visual Impairment. Specific interventions to achieve these outcomes are discussed in the following section.

> **Wellness Opportunity**
>
> Quality of Life is a wellness outcome that is achieved through nursing interventions that improve visual function.

NURSING INTERVENTIONS FOR VISUAL WELLNESS

Nurses promote visual wellness through interventions directed toward preventing vision loss, promoting comfort measures for dry eyes, and implementing or teaching about methods to foster optimal visual function. Interventions to achieve these goals are discussed in detail in the following sections. The following pertinent Nursing Interventions Classification (NIC) terminologies may be applicable to care plans: Communication Enhancement: Visual Deficit, Coping Enhancement, Eye Care, Environmental Management, Environmental Management: Safety, Health Education, Health Screening, Health System Guidance, Risk Identification, and Fall Prevention.

Health Promotion for Visual Wellness

Health promotion interventions focus on maintaining vision at an optimal level by compensating for any visual deficits

Box 17-4 Health Promotion Teaching About Visual Wellness

Prevention and Early Detection of Disease
- Minimize exposure to sunlight by using broad-brimmed hats and close-fitting sunglasses with UV-absorbing lenses.
- Have eyes examined annually or more frequently if you notice a change in vision; make sure the examination checks for glaucoma, cataracts, and retinal disease.
- Use the appropriate eye care practitioner (ophthalmologist, optometrist, and optician) as described in Box 17-5.
- Because smoking is a risk factor for many eye diseases, quit smoking.
- Because diabetes and hypertension are risk factors for eye disease, make sure these conditions are managed optimally.

Nutritional Considerations
- Include foods high in lutein, such as fruits, corn, spinach, green leafy vegetables, and egg yolks.
- Lutein supplements of 10 mg/d are safe and may be effective in preventing cataracts and age-related macular degeneration.
- People who have macular degeneration or risk factors for this conditions are encouraged to take a daily supplement containing the following: 500 mg vitamin C, 400 IU vitamin E, 15 mg beta-carotene, 80 mg zinc oxide, and 2 mg cupric oxide (copper). However, people who smoke are advised to avoid beta-carotene because it can increase the risk of developing lung cancer.

and identifying any treatable conditions at an early stage. Nurses can teach older adults about preserving optimal visual function by reducing or eliminating risk factors that can cause visual impairments. For example, the use of broad-brimmed

hats and close-fitting sunglasses with UV-B—absorbing lenses have the long-range effect of protecting the eyes from harmful rays and the immediate benefit of screening out sun glare that can interfere with visual function. In addition, nurses can teach about preventing eye disease through nutritional interventions. Studies confirm that consumption of foods high in lutein—a carotenoid found in corn, egg yolk, and green leafy vegetables—can improve vision and protect against cataracts and AMD (Najm & Lie, 2008). Health promotion teaching also emphasizes the importance of annual eye examinations and timely evaluation of any changes in vision. These teaching points are summarized in Box 17-4, which nurses can use for older adults or their caregivers.

In providing health education, it may be helpful to review the differences between opticians, optometrists, and ophthalmologists and provide information about health insurance coverage for these services, as detailed in Box 17-5. Educational materials describing the scope of services of these eye care providers are distributed by eye care professionals and organizations listed in the Resources section at the end of this chapter.

Older adults and their caregivers may also benefit from the many educational brochures that are available on the subjects of eye diseases, common vision problems, age-related eye changes, and low-vision aids. Nurses can use these publications to supplement and reinforce the health education components of their care plans. National and local sight centers and other organizations provide these materials at little or no cost, and some brochures are available in Spanish and other languages. In addition, much of the information can be obtained and printed directly from these organizations' Web

Box 17-5 Eye Care Practitioners

Practitioners

Ophthalmologists are licensed doctors of medicine (MD) or osteopathy (DO) who are trained to diagnose and treat diseases and conditions of the eye. Ophthalmologic services include the following:
- Comprehensive eye examinations
- Diagnosis of eye diseases and disorders of the eye
- Prescription medications for eye problems (e.g., glaucoma)
- Eye surgery and postoperative care (e.g., cataracts)
- Laser treatments (e.g., retinopathy)
- Prescriptions for eyeglasses and contact lenses
- Prescriptions for low-vision aids
- Referrals for low-vision aids and training
- Medical referrals for diseases of the body that affect the eyes

Optometrists are licensed doctors of optometry (OD), not physicians, who are trained to examine eyes, screen for common eye problems, and prescribe eye exercises or corrective lenses. Optometrists use diagnostic medications, and in more than half the states in America, they can prescribe certain therapeutic drugs for eye diseases. Optometric services include the following:
- Comprehensive eye examinations
- Eye refractions to determine the need for corrective lenses
- Prescriptions for eyeglasses, contact lenses, and low-vision aids

- Vision therapy to improve certain skills, such as tracking and focusing the eyes
- Referrals for low-vision aids and training
- Referrals to physicians for surgery, medication, or further evaluation
- Diagnosis of eye disorders (in some states)
- Postoperative care (in some states)

Opticians are eye care practitioners who are trained to fit, adjust, and dispense eyeglasses and contact lenses that have been prescribed by an optometrist or ophthalmologist. In many states, opticians are licensed. They do not perform eye examinations or refractions, and they cannot prescribe corrective lenses or medications.

Health Insurance Coverage

Medicare and other primary health insurance programs do not cover routine eye examinations, although some supplemental or managed care plans do provide coverage. However, Medicare will cover glaucoma screening once yearly for people who are at high risk for glaucoma and an eye examination when needed to diagnose potential vision problems. Medicare also covers ophthalmologic services for the treatment of eye diseases, including cataract surgery. Medicare covers eyeglasses and contact lenses only when they are part of postsurgical cataract care.

sites. The National Association for the Visually Handicapped (NAVH) is an excellent resource for information about interventions for older adults with visual impairments. In contrast to publications from organizations that focus primarily on blindness, materials from the NAVH are written for people with gradual and partial visual losses. The American Academy of Ophthalmology and the American Optometric Association also are good sources of free pamphlets about eye problems that commonly affect older adults. Do-it-yourself eye test kits are available from Prevent Blindness America. This kit enables people to determine whether they are seeing as well as they should and provides guidelines for obtaining further evaluation.

> **Wellness Opportunity**
>
> Nurses promote self-care by encouraging older adults and their families to obtain information from reliable resources.

Comfort Measures for Dry Eyes

If pertinent, simple measures to relieve dry eyes can be discussed. Use of over-the-counter artificial tears or ocular lubricants, especially before reading or engaging in other activities that require frequent eye movements, will usually relieve symptoms. People who use eye drops more frequently than every 3 hours should be advised to use preservative-free solutions to prevent any adverse effects from the preservatives. Other comfort measures, such as applying cold compresses or wearing wraparound glasses, are designed to prevent evaporation of tears. Maintenance of adequate environmental humidity, especially during the winter months or in dry climates, also decreases evaporation of eye moisture and adds to eye comfort. People who experience discomfort from dry eyes should avoid irritants, such as smoke and hairspray, and adverse environmental conditions, such as hot rooms and high wind. People who are bothered by dry eyes and are taking a medication that might exacerbate the discomfort should be encouraged to discuss the problem with their primary care practitioner.

Environmental Modifications

Simple environmental modifications can improve the older person's safe performance of activities of daily living, thereby reducing risks of falls and accidents. Because older adults require more light for adequate vision, proper nonglare lighting is the single most important—as well as the easiest and the least costly—intervention to improve visual function (Box 17-6). Optimal illumination depends on both the quality and the quantity of lighting. For example, selection of broad-spectrum fluorescent lights and daylight-simulating lamps may be particularly beneficial in compensating for age-related vision changes.

Another important consideration in adapting the environment for optimal visual function is color contrast. Appliances

Box 17-6 Considerations for Optimal Illumination

- Older adults need at least three times as much light as younger people do.
- Older adults function best in environments with bright, broad-spectrum, nonglaring, indirect sources of light.
- Sources of illumination should be placed 1 to 2 feet away from the object to be viewed.
- The amount of light decreases fourfold when the distance is doubled.
- Flickering light, such as that generated by a single fluorescent tube, will cause fatigue and decreased visual performance.
- Light bulbs should be kept clean.
- Increased illumination has a greater positive effect on impaired vision than it does on normal vision.
- A gradual decrease in illumination from foreground to background is better than sharp contrasts in lighting.
- Moderate overhead lighting can be used to enhance brighter foreground lighting and prevent sharp contrasts.
- To reduce glare from reading material, place the light source to the left side of right-handed readers and to the right side of left-handed readers.
- Avoid glossy paper for reading materials.

and other items, such as ovens, irons, radios, thermostats, and televisions, may be difficult to use because of poor color contrast around the control mechanisms. Modifications can easily be made to improve the older person's ability to use these items safely and accurately. For example, two dots of red nail polish can be used to mark a designated and commonly used temperature setting, and the older adult can be instructed to turn the dial above or below the matching dots for higher or lower settings.

Architectural designs and institutional constraints may limit the extent of environmental adaptations that nurses can implement, especially in institutional settings. In most settings, however, nurses can improve the visual abilities of older adults by using appropriate colors to enhance contrast, by using curtains to control light and glare, and by placing chairs in positions that enhance illumination and avoid glare. Nurses have many opportunities to teach older adults and their caregivers about the environmental modifications that are most effective for optimal visual function. Box 17-7 summarizes some environmental adaptations that can be used to compensate for deficits in visual skills and improve safety. All older adults can benefit from these environmental modifications, even in the absence of diagnosed eye disorders, because they are effective ways of improving vision for all people.

Low-Vision Aids

People with visual impairments can improve their safety and quality of life by using **low-vision aids** that improve focus, contrast, magnification, or illumination (Box 17-8). Low-vision aids are most beneficial when used in conjunction with environmental modifications. For example, magnifiers

Box 17-7 Environmental Adaptations for Improving Visual Performance

Illumination, Glare Control, and Dark/Light Adaptation
- Position a 60- or 75-watt soft-white light bulb above and close to the head of the older person.
- Use a clear plastic shower curtain, rather than solid colors or printed curtains, for the tub or shower.
- Use light-colored, sheer curtains to eliminate glare from windows.
- Place nightlights in hallways and bathrooms, or keep a high-intensity flashlight at the bedside.
- Use illuminated light switches.
- Provide good lighting in stairways and hallways.
- Use illuminated or magnifying mirrors.

Color Contrast
- Use brightly colored tape or paint on the edges of stairs, especially on the top and bottom steps.
- Use light-colored and dark-colored cutting boards to contrast with dark and light foods.
- Use contrasting, rather than matching, colors for china, placemats, and napkins.
- Use a toilet seat that contrasts with the bathroom walls and floor. Use colored bars of soap on white sinks and tubs.
- Use utensils with brightly colored handles.

- Place pillows of contrasting colors on stuffed furniture.
- Use decorative or lighted plates over light switches and wall sockets; avoid switch plates that blend in with the wallpaper or paint.
- Place decorative items of contrasting colors, such as plants and ceramics, on tables to provide cues to depth, especially on light-colored furniture that is in a room with light-colored walls.
- Use brightly colored grooming utensils, such as combs, brushes, and razors.
- Use pens with black ink rather than blue ink.

General Adaptive Measures and Environmental Modifications
- Do not rearrange furniture without informing or showing the older person.
- Advise older adults to pause in doorways when going from light to dark rooms (or vice versa) to allow time for their eyes to adjust to the light change.
- Teach older people to use their feet and hands as probes to feel for curbs, steps, edges of chairs, and the like.
- When walking with an older person, stop when necessary to allow a change in focus from near to far and from light to dark.

are most effective when combined with measures that improve illumination and control glare. Reading glasses and other optical aids that magnify an image for visual tasks are available with or without a prescription. Low-vision aids also can be used to enhance contrast, reduce glare, improve lighting, or enlarge the image. Printed and Internet catalogues with illustrations of low-vision aids are available through the NAVH and other organizations. Also, local sight centers are good sources of low-vision aids, as well as training related to their use.

Although special low-vision aids can be obtained through catalogues, Internet sites, or sight centers, everyday items, if used advantageously, can serve as low-vision aids. An example of a low-vision aid that may be available to nurses is a photocopy machine that can be used to convert regular-print materials into large-print materials. Likewise, household lamps placed in the correct position and equipped with the right wattage bulb can also serve as low-vision aids. Lighthouse International provides educational materials that illustrate examples of effective color contrast and effective ways of making text legible. These free materials, which can be obtained from Lighthouse International (listed in the Resources section at the end of this chapter) can be used as guides for developing more readable printed materials for signage, health education, and other purposes.

Nurses can teach about the appropriate use of low-vision aids so that the most effective outcomes are achieved. For example, if people understand that halving the distance of a light source increases illumination by fourfold, they are more likely to place lights in the most effective positions. As an

illustration of this principle, a light bulb that is 1 foot away from someone will provide four times as much illumination as one that is 2 feet away. Nurses can use information presented in Boxes 17-6 and 17-9 to teach about effective use of lights and magnification. Local sight centers provide detailed training in the use of low-vision aids, and the NAVH publishes a helpful guide regarding their use.

Wellness Opportunity

Nurses promote self-care for people who are visually impaired by facilitating referrals to local vision rehabilitation services and encouraging older adults and their families to use these resources.

Maintaining and Improving the Quality of Life

As discussed earlier, the psychosocial consequences of impaired vision can be quite significant for older adults. Many of the interventions that help older adults compensate for visual deficits and function at their highest level will also improve their quality of life and address the psychosocial consequences of impaired vision. The use of appropriate reading glasses and good environmental lighting may enable the older adult to read books, newspapers, and magazines. Subsequently, their quality of life may improve because they experience satisfying social interactions and increased intellectual stimulation. Nurses also encourage participation in support and educational groups because these interventions serve an important role in improving the quality of life for people with significant or progressive vision loss.

Box 17-8 Low-Vision Aids for Improving Visual Performance

Enlargement Aids
- Microscopic spectacles
- Handheld or standing magnifiers

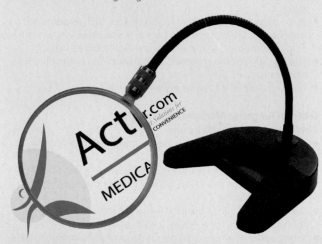

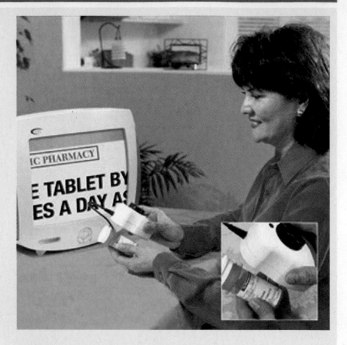

BOX FIGURE 17-8. Examples of low-vision aids. **(A)** A combination of high-intensity lamp and magnifier.

- Binoculars and handheld or spectacle-mounted telescopes
- Magnifying sheets
- Field expanders for diminished peripheral vision
- Large-print books, magazines, and newspapers
- Photocopy machines or printers to enlarge print
- Telephones with enlarged letters and numbers, or a pad with enlarged letters and numbers designed to fit over rotary-dial or push-button phones
- Large numbers on rulers, playing cards, and other items
- Thermometers with good color coding and enlarged numbers
- Large-eye sewing needles

Illumination Aids
- High-intensity lights
- Gooseneck lamps
- Floor or table lamps with three-way light bulbs

Contrast Aids
- Use of broad-tipped felt markers in dark, yet bright, colors and colored construction paper for making signs
- Red print on a yellow background or white letters on a green background
- Reading and signature guides (typoscopes)
- Clip-on yellow lenses

Glare Control Aids
- Sunglasses with UV-absorbing lenses
- Sun visors and broad-brimmed hats
- Nonglare (antireflective) coating on eyeglasses
- Yellow and pink acetate sheets
- Pinhole occluders

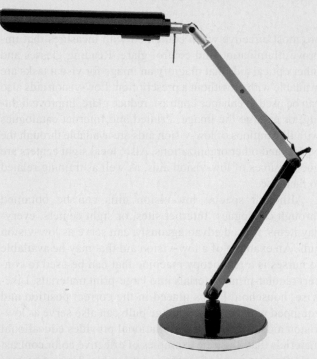

BOX FIGURE 17-8. **(B)** A handheld digital magnifier that works with any television to magnify print. **(C)** A versatile lamp that uses an energy-efficient high-definition tube bulb for good contrast and brightness. (Photographs courtesy of ActiveForever.com.)

Box 17-9 Guidelines for Using Magnifying Aids

Using a Handheld Magnifier
- Begin by holding the magnifier close to the reading material.
- Slowly move the magnifier toward the face until the image totally fills the lens.
- For optimal focus, move the magnifier back toward the print about a distance of 2 cm.

Using a Stand Magnifier
- Rest the stand flat against the reading material.
- Do not move the stand.

Using a Spectacle-Mounted Magnifier
- Begin with the reading material close to the nose.
- Slowly move the material away until it becomes clear.

*M*rs. F. is now 81 years old. She had cataract surgery and an intraocular lens implanted in her left eye when she was 76 years old, and in her right eye when she was 77. Her vision was good until a year ago, when she developed macular degeneration. She knows this condition will be progressive, but she continues to drive and live alone. Her current medical conditions are arthritis, hypertension, and coronary artery disease. She quit smoking several years ago after she was hospitalized for coronary artery disease. You are the nurse at the senior care center where Mrs. F. comes for lunch several times a week. During an appointment with you, Mrs. F. confides that she is terrified of becoming totally blind and of losing her independence. Her grandmother went blind several years before she died and she had to go to a long-term care facility.

T H I N K I N G   P O I N T S

- Which nursing diagnosis or diagnoses would you apply to Mrs. F. at this time?
- Which information in Boxes 17-4 through 17-9 might be appropriate for Mrs. F.?

- What health promotion advice would you give?
- Would you suggest any referrals for information or community resources?
- What interventions would address Mrs. F.'s fear of becoming blind and losing her independence?

EVALUATING EFFECTIVENESS OF NURSING INTERVENTIONS

Nurses observe compensatory behaviors of visually impaired older adults to evaluate the effectiveness of interventions for Disturbed Sensory Perception: Visual. The following are indicators of successful interventions:
- Use of corrective lenses and low-vision aids to achieve the best possible visual function
- Adaptations of the environment for safety and improved visual function (e.g., bright, nonglare lighting, good color contrast)
- Expressed feelings of safety in relation to visual function
- Maximum independence in activities such as dressing, personal care, using appliances, and managing medications
- Expressed feelings of improved quality of life, despite visual impairments.

Nurses evaluate the effectiveness of interventions to improve independence by assessing and reassessing the older adult's abilities before and after interventions. When interventions address the psychosocial impact of visual impairment, nurses observe the extent to which the person's quality of life and the ability to participate in enjoyable activities is improved. For example, better lighting and the use of audiobooks or large-print books may enable someone to enjoy reading again. Nurses evaluate the effectiveness of health education interventions according to the person's expressed intent to follow through with the recommended referral or course of action. In home, community, and long-term care settings, nurses may be able to facilitate referrals for vision screening or other vision care services. In these settings, nurses evaluate the effectiveness of interventions based on feedback from older adults or their caregivers about the actual use of suggested resources.

*M*rs. F. is now 86 years old and is recovering from a recent fractured hip, which occurred when she fell while getting out of bed to go to the bathroom at night. After a brief hospitalization for surgical repair of the fractured hip and a 2-week period of skilled rehabilitation, Mrs. F. was referred to a home care agency for therapy, assessment, monitoring of her medical status, and evaluation of her ability to manage at home.

(case study continues on page 354)

THINKING POINTS

- How would you address concerns about Mrs. F. living alone? What aspects of her safety and quality of life would you consider?
- How would you use any of the boxes in this chapter for health promotion teaching?
- What additional nursing diagnoses and outcomes would you identify for Mrs. F.?

- What additional interventions and referrals would you consider for Mrs. F.?
- Identify at least one resource in your community that might provide help or information for Mrs. F. Call that agency to obtain information about their services.

Chapter Highlights

Age-Related Changes That Affect Vision (Figure 17-1, Table 17-1)

- Changes in appearance include arcus senilis, loss of orbital fat, and diminished elasticity of eyelid muscles
- Diminished tear production
- Degenerative changes affect all structures of the eye, the retinal–neural pathway, and the visual cortex of the brain

Effects of Age-Related Changes on Vision

- Diminished ability to focus clearly on objects at various distances
- Diminished ability to detect details and discern objects
- Slower adaptive response to changes in lighting
- Increased sensitivity to glare
- Narrowed visual field
- Diminished depth perception
- Altered color perception so objects look darker and whites appear more yellowed
- Diminished ability to perceive flashing lights
- Slower processing of visual information

Risks Factors That Affect Visual Wellness

- Environmental factors: glare, sunlight, poor lighting, low humidity
- Lifestyle factors: poor nutrition, cigarette smoking
- Chronic conditions: diabetes, hypertension, Alzheimer or Parkinson disease
- Adverse medication effects: estrogen, corticosteroids, anticholinergics, beta-blockers, antiparkinson agents

Functional Consequences Affecting Visual Wellness

- Presbyopia (diminished ability to focus on near objects)
- Need for three to five times more light than previously
- Difficulty with night driving
- Increased risk for unsafe mobility and falls
- Increased difficulty in performing usual activities

Pathologic Conditions Affecting Vision (Figures 17-2 and 17-3, Table 17-2)

- Cataracts
- AMD
- Glaucoma

Nursing Assessment of Vision (Boxes 17-1 through 17-3)

- Vision screening tests
- Risk factors that affect vision
- Influence of vision changes on performance of activities of daily living
- Attitudes about eye examinations and preventive measures
- Attitudes regarding use of low-vision aids

Nursing Diagnosis

- Readiness for Enhanced Knowledge: Improved Vision
- Disturbed Sensory Perception: Visual
- Additional diagnoses that address the functional consequences of visual impairment include the following: Anxiety, Ineffective Coping, Self-Care Deficit, Risk for Injury, Impaired Social Interaction, Readiness for Enhanced Coping, and Readiness for Enhanced Self-Care

Planning for Wellness Outcomes

- Improved visual function
- Increased safety
- Improved independence in activities of daily living
- Improved quality of life

Nursing Interventions for Visual Wellness (Boxes 17-4 through 17-9)

- Prevention and detection of eye disease
- Comfort measures for dry eyes
- Environmental modifications (e.g., optimal illumination)
- Low-vision aids

Evaluating Effectiveness of Nursing Interventions

- Use of corrective lenses and other aids that improve vision
- Environmental adaptations for optimal safety and visual function
- Improved independence in daily activities
- Expressed feelings of improved quality of life in relation to visual function

Critical Thinking Exercises

1. Describe presbyopia and explain the functional consequences of this condition in the everyday life of an older adult.

2. What environmental factors are likely to interfere with the visual function of older adults?

3. Describe the specific effects of glaucoma, cataracts, or AMD on one's ability to see a television program.

4. How would you assess the visual abilities of an older adult?

5. Explain the differences between opticians, optometrists, and ophthalmologists.

6. List at least 10 adaptations that might be implemented to improve the visual function of older adults.

Resources

For links to these resources and additional helpful Internet resources related to this chapter, visit thePoint at http://thePoint.lww.com/Miller6e.

Evidence-Based Practice

Cacchione, P. Z. (2008). Sensory changes. In E. Capezuti, D. Zwicker, M. Mezey, & T. Fulmer (Eds.), *Evidence-based geriatric nursing protocols for best practices* (3rd ed., pp. 477–502). New York: Springer.
National Guideline Clearinghouse
  • Age-related macular degeneration
  • Cataract in the adult eye
  • Dry eye syndrome
  • Glaucoma
  • Vision rehabilitation for adults

Health Education

American Academy of Ophthalmology
American Foundation for the Blind
American Optometric Association
Canadian National Institute for the Blind
Lighthouse International
Lions Clubs International
National Association for Visually Handicapped
National Eye Institute
Prevent Blindness America
The Glaucoma Foundation

REFERENCES

Ackerman, M. L., Edwards, J. D., Ross, L. A., Ball, K. K., & Lunsman, M. (2008). Examination of cognitive and instrumental functional performance as indicators for driving cessation risk across 3 years. *Gerontologist, 48*(6), 802–810.

Baldock, M. R. J., Berndt, A., & Mathias, J. L. (2008). The functional correlates of older drivers' on-road driving test errors. *Topics in Geriatric Rehabilitation, 24*(3), 204–223.

Chou, K.-L. (2008). Combined effect of vision and hearing impairment on depression on older adults: Evidence from the English Longitudinal Study of Ageing. *Journal of Affective Disorders, 106,* 191–196.

Coleman, H. R., Chan, C. C., Ferris, F. L., III, & Chew, E. Y. (2008). Age-related macular degeneration. *The Lancet, 372,* 1835–1844.

Federal Interagency Forum on Aging-Related Statistics. (2008). *Older Americans 2008: Key indicators of well-being.* Washington, DC: Government Printing Office.

Fernandez, A., Sorokin, A., & Thompson, P. D. (2007). Corneal arcus as coronary disease risk factor. *Atherosclerosis, 193*(2), 235–240.

Ferrer-Blasco, T., Gonzalez-Meijome, J. M., & Montes-Mico, R. (2008). Age-related changes in the human visual system and prevalence of refractive conditions in patients attending an eye clinic. *Journal of Cataract Refractive Surgery, 34,* 424–432.

Gilbert, S. S., & Bassett, K. (2007, January). Bridging the gender gap. *Cataract & Refractive Surgery Today,* 65–67.

Hamilton, J. M., Salmon, D. P., Galasko, D., Raman, R., Emond, J., Hansen, L. A., . . . Thal, L. J. (2008). Visuospatial deficits predict rate of cognitive decline in autopsy-verified dementia with Lewy bodies. *Neuropsychology, 22*(6), 729–737.

Jin, Y. P., & Wong, D. T. (2008). Self-reported visual impairment in elderly Canadians and its impact on healthy living. *Canadian Journal of Ophthalmology, 43*(4), 407–413.

Kalinowski, M. A. (2008). "Eye"dentifying vision impairment in the geriatric patient. *Geriatric Nursing, 29*(2), 125–132.

Mabuchi, F., Yoshimura, K., Kashiwagi, K., Shioe, K., Yamagata, Z., Kanba, S., . . . Tsukahara, S. (2008). High prevalence of anxiety and depression in patients with primary open-angle glaucoma. *Journal of Glaucoma, 17*(7), 552–557.

Montgomery, M. P., Kamel, F., Pericak-Vance, M. A., Postel, E. A., Agarwal, A., Richards, M., . . . Schmidt, S. (2010). Overall diet quality and age-related macular degeneration. *Ophthalmic Epidemiology, 17,* 58–65.

Najm, W., & Lie, D. (2008). Dietary supplements commonly used for prevention. *Primary Care Clinics and Office Practice, 35,* 749–767.

NANDA International. (2009). *Nursing diagnoses: Definitions and classification 2009–2011.* Oxford, England: Wiley-Blackwell.

Nassiri, N., Nassiri, N., Sadeghi Yarandi, S. H., & Rahnavardi, M. (2009). Immediate vs delayed sequential cataract surgery: A comparative study. *Eye, 23*(1), 89–95.

National Eye Institute. (2007). *Report of the ocular epidemiology strategic planning panel.* Retrieved from www.nei.nih/gov/strategicplanning. finalreport.asp

Norman, J. F., Norman, H. F., Craft, A. E., Walton, C. L., Bartholomew, A. N., Burton, C. L., . . . Crabtree, C. E. (2008). Stereopsis and aging. *Vision Research, 48,* 2456–2465.

Ramulu, P. Y., West, S. J., Munoz, G., Jampel, H. D., & Friedman, D. S. (2009). Driving cessation and driving limitation in glaucoma: the Salisbury Eye Evaluation Project. *Ophthalmology, 116,* 1846–1853.

Wood, J. M., Lacherez, P. F., Black, A. A., Cole, M. H., Boon, M. Y., & Kerr, G. K. (2009). Postural stability and gait among older adults with age-related maculopathy. *Investigative Ophthalmology & Visual Science, 50*(1), 482–487.

Wysong, A., Lee, P. P., & Sloan, F. A. (2010). Longitudinal incidence of adverse outcomes of age-relate macular degeneration. *Archives of Ophthalmology, 127,* 320–327.

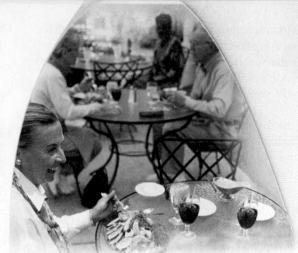

CHAPTER 18

Digestion and Nutrition

LEARNING OBJECTIVES

After reading this chapter, you will be able to:

1. Describe age-related changes that affect eating patterns and digestive processes.
2. List age-related changes in nutritional requirements.
3. Identify risk factors that affect the digestion and nutrition of older adults.
4. Explain the effects of age-related changes and risk factors on digestion and nutrition.
5. Assess aspects of nutrition, digestion, behaviors that affect eating and food preparation, and oral care pertinent to care of older adults.
6. Identify nursing interventions to promote optimal nutrition, digestion, and oral care.

K E Y   P O I N T S

body mass index (BMI)
cholelithiasis
constipation
dietary fiber
Dietary Reference Intakes
 (DRIs)
dysphagia

Mini Nutritional
 Assessment (MNA)
olfaction
protein-energy
 undernutrition
xerostomia

Digestion of food and maintenance of nutrition are influenced to a small degree by age-related gastrointestinal changes and to a large degree by risk factors that commonly occur in older adulthood. Although older adults can easily compensate for age-related changes in the digestive tract, they have more difficulty compensating for the many factors that interfere with their ability to obtain, prepare, and enjoy food. This chapter discusses age-related changes and functional consequences in relation to digestion, eating patterns, and nutritional requirements.

 AGE-RELATED CHANGES THAT AFFECT DIGESTION AND EATING PATTERNS

Age-related changes affect the senses of smell and taste and all the organs of the digestive tract. These changes have very few functional consequences for healthy older adults, but they increase the vulnerability of older adults to risk factors.

Smell and Taste

Both senses, taste and smell, affect food enjoyment, and both these senses decline in older adults because of a combination of age-related changes and risk factors. The ability to smell depends on the perception of odorants by the sensory cells in the olfactory mucosa and on central nervous system processing of that information. The ability to detect and identify odors is best between the ages of 30 and 40 years, after which it gradually declines. Even in healthy older adults, age-related changes affect all structures involved in **olfaction** (i.e., the ability to smell odors), which begins in the nose and ends in the brain (Lafreniere & Mann, 2009). Additional conditions that can interfere with olfaction include smoking or chewing tobacco, viruses, neurodegenerative diseases, poor oral health, periodontal disease, nasal sinus disease, trauma, and medications. Researchers are currently focusing on diminished sense of smell as one of the earliest clinical signs of dementia, Parkinson disease, and other neurodegenerative conditions (Doty, 2009; Welge-Lussen, 2009).

The ability to taste depends primarily on receptor cells in the taste buds, which are located on the tongue, palate, and tonsils. Characteristics of taste sensation are measured according to the ability to perceive the intensity of taste, which diminishes with aging, and the ability to identify different tastes. Although results of studies are inconsistent, with at least one study finding that taste cells can regenerate, the sense of taste probably declines with age (Visvanathan & Chapman, 2009). Older adults who smoke, are malnourished, wear dentures, take medications, or have medical conditions (e.g., diabetes) are likely to experience significant difficulty in detecting flavors.

Promoting Digestive and Nutritional Wellness in Older Adults

Nursing Assessment

- Usual nutrient intake
- Oral health
- Usual eating patterns
- Risks that affect food preparation, intake, and enjoyment
- Measures of nutritional status

Age-Related Changes

- Less efficient chewing
- ↓ senses of smell and taste
- ↓ saliva secretion
- Slower motility
- Degenerative changes affecting digestion
- Daily intake: need fewer but higher quality calories

Negative Functional Consequences

- Difficulty procuring and preparing food
- ↓ enjoyment of food
- ↓ absorption of nutrients
- ↑ tendency to develop constipation

Risk Factors

- Conditions that affect ability to obtain, prepare, consume, or enjoy food
- Poor oral care
- Effects of medications
- Cultural and socioeconomic factors
- Environmental factors

Nursing Interventions

- Teaching about nutrition and digestion
- Preventing/addressing constipation
- Promoting oral and dental care
- Referring for home-delivered meals and group meal progams

Wellness Outcomes

- Improved nutritional status
- Improved oral hygiene
- Elimination of risk factors
- ↑ sense of well-being

Oral Cavity

Digestion begins when food enters the mouth and is acted on by the teeth, saliva, and neuromuscular structures responsible for mastication. Age-related changes in the teeth and support structures influence digestive processes and food enjoyment. With increased age, the tooth enamel becomes harder and more brittle, the dentin becomes more fibrous, and the nerve chambers become shorter and narrower. Because of these age-related changes, the teeth are less sensitive to stimuli and

more susceptible to fractures. These changes, along with decades of abrasive and erosive action, also cause a gradual flattening of the chewing cusps. The bones supporting the teeth of older adults diminish in height and density, and teeth may loosen or fall out, particularly in the presence of pathologic conditions (e.g., periodontal disease).

Saliva and the oral mucosa play important roles in digestion. Saliva is essential for promoting chewing and swallowing and for maintaining a moist oral mucosa. Saliva facilitates digestion by supplying digestive enzymes, regulating oral flora, remineralizing the teeth, cleansing the taste buds, lubricating the soft tissue, and preparing food for chewing. Healthy older adults do not experience any significant decreases in salivary flow; however, approximately 30% of people 65 years and older experience **xerostomia** (dry mouth) because of medications and diseases (Turner & Ship, 2007). Medications that are most likely to cause xerostomia are anticholinergics, antidepressants, antipsychotics, antiemetics, analgesics, antihypertensives, and antihistamines (Lam, Kiyak, Gossett, & McCormick, 2009; Ney, Weiss, Kind, & Robinson, 2009; Uher et al., 2009). Other common causes are dehydration, diabetes, and radiation therapy to the head and neck (Visvanathan & Nix, 2010).

Age-related changes of the oral mucosa include loss of elasticity, atrophy of epithelial cells, and diminished blood supply to the connective tissue. These changes can be exacerbated by conditions common in older adults (e.g., xerostomia, vitamin deficiencies), making the oral mucosa more friable and susceptible to infection and ulceration.

Age-related neuromuscular changes that can affect mastication and swallowing include diminished muscle strength and reduced tongue pressure (Ney et al., 2009). Healthy older adults will not experience significant swallowing problems, unless there are additional risk factors, such as tooth loss or neurologic conditions (as discussed in the section on Risk Factors).

Esophagus and Stomach

The second phase of digestion occurs when a combination of propulsive and nonpropulsive waves propels food through the pharynx and esophagus into the stomach. In older adults, the esophagus stiffens and the peristaltic waves decrease (Gregersen, Pedersen, & Drewes, 2008). *Presbyphagia* refers to the slowed swallowing that is associated with age-related changes and can increase the risk for aspiration (Ney et al., 2009).

After passing through the esophageal sphincter, food enters the stomach, where gastric enzymes liquefy it and gastric action transforms it into chyme. Gastric emptying is slowed when the meal consists of more than 500 calories (Morley, 2007). Although some earlier studies indicated that diminished gastric secretion was an age-related change, more recent studies found that gastric acid and pepsinogen secretion increase with aging in healthy people (Morley, 2007).

Intestinal Tract

After the chyme passes into the small intestine, digestive enzymes from the small intestine, liver, and pancreas convert the food substances into nutrients. A process of segmentation moves the chyme backward and forward, facilitating the digestion of food and the absorption of nutrients through the villi in the walls of the small intestine. Age-related changes that occur in the small intestine include atrophy of muscle fibers and mucosal surfaces; reduction in the number of lymphatic follicles; gradual reduction in the weight of the small intestine; and

shortening and widening of the villi, which gradually form parallel ridges rather than finger-like projections. These structural changes do not significantly affect motility, permeability, or transit time in the intestinal tract; however, they may affect immune function and absorption of some nutrients, such as folate, calcium, and vitamins B_{12} and D.

After nutrients are absorbed in the small intestine, the chyme passes into the large intestine, where water and electrolytes are absorbed and waste products are expelled. Age-related changes in the large intestine include reduced secretion of mucus, decreased elasticity of the rectal wall, and diminished perception of rectal wall distention. Although these age-related changes have little or no impact on motility of feces through the bowel, they may predispose the older person to constipation.

Liver, Pancreas, and Gallbladder

The liver assists in digestion by producing and secreting bile, which is essential for the utilization of fats. It also plays an important role in the metabolism and storage of medications and nutrients. With increasing age, the liver becomes smaller and more fibrous, lipofuscin (a brown pigment) accumulates, and blood flow to the liver decreases by approximately one-third. However, some of these changes may be pathologic, rather than age-related, in origin. Despite any age-related or pathologic changes, the liver has an enormous regenerative and reserve capacity, which allows it to compensate for such changes without significantly affecting digestive function.

A primary digestive function of the pancreas is the secretion of enzymes essential for neutralizing acids in the chyme and breaking down fats, proteins, and carbohydrates in the small intestine. The pancreas also functions as an endocrine gland and produces insulin and glycogen, which are essential for glucose metabolism. Age-related changes in the pancreas include decreased weight, hyperplasia of the duct, fibrosis of the lobe, and decreased responsiveness of pancreatic B cells to glucose. These changes do not directly affect digestive functioning; however, the effects on glucose metabolism can increase the susceptibility of older adults to the development of type 2 diabetes.

Age-related changes that affect the gallbladder and biliary tract include diminished bile acid synthesis, widening of the common bile duct, and increased secretion of cholecystokinin, a peptide hormone that contracts the gallbladder and relaxes the biliary sphincter. These age-related changes can increase the susceptibility of older adults to the development of **cholelithiasis** (gallstones). In addition, a higher level of cholecystokinin can suppress the appetite.

 AGE-RELATED CHANGES IN NUTRITIONAL REQUIREMENTS

Since 1941, the Recommended Dietary Allowances (RDAs) had been the primary reference standard for measuring intake levels of essential nutrients that met the needs of healthy people. In 2001, the Food and Nutrition Board, the Institute of

Medicine, the National Academy of Sciences, and Health Canada jointly published a major revision of the RDAs, and recommended the use of Dietary Reference Intakes (DRIs). An advantage of the DRIs is that they establish standards for meeting the basic nutrient needs of healthy adults according to specific age groups (e.g., adults aged 51 to 70 years and those 70 years and older) rather than generalizing for all adults. In addition, the DRIs are applicable for health promotion because they include indicators for preventing chronic disease and avoiding the harmful effects of consuming too much of a nutrient. These standards need to be adjusted to compensate for people who have conditions such as nutrient deficiencies and medical conditions. In addition, adjustments for food and drug interactions may be necessary for people who take one or more medications. DRIs that increase with aging are calcium (1200 mg for those 50 years and older) and vitamin D (400 and 600 IU/day for those aged 51 to 70 years and those 70 years and older, respectively). The DRI for iron decreases to 8 mg/day in women 51 years and older as a result of menstruation cessation. Evidence accumulated since the publication of the DRIs indicate that the DRI for vitamin D should be increased to 1000 IU/day for all adults (Marra & Boyar, 2009).

Calories

The energy-producing potential of food is measured in units called *calories*. Caloric requirements are determined by a combination of factors, including height, weight, sex, body build, health–illness state, and the usual level of physical activity. Energy requirements gradually decrease throughout adulthood because of decreased physical activity and the decline in basal metabolic rate that is associated with diminished muscle mass. Thus, nutritional guidelines recommend a gradual reduction in calories beginning between the ages of 40 and 50 years. This decrease in caloric intake requires a proportionate increase in the quality of calories (nutritional density) to meet minimal nutritional requirements. Thus, nutritional deficiencies will occur unless a reduced caloric intake is accompanied by an increased intake of foods with a high nutritional value and a concomitant decrease in the intake of foods containing little or no nutrients.

DIVERSITY NOTE

Mean caloric intake for groups in the United States is highest in whites and lower in African Americans (Bowman, 2009).

Protein

Protein provides the essential components for new tissue growth in the human body. Age-related changes, such as decreased lean body mass and muscle tissue and decreased plasma albumin and total body albumin levels, may influence protein requirements in older adults. The RDA for daily protein intake for all adults 19 years and older is 0.8 g/kg of body weight. This can be achieved if approximately 10% to 20% of the daily caloric intake is derived from protein. Although national surveys indicate that most adults exceed the RDA for

protein, studies indicate that 11% of women 71 years and older have intake less than the RDA (Fulgoni, 2008). One review of studies concluded that the RDA for older adults should be increased to 1.0 to 1.2 g/kg protein for optimal muscle and bone health (Gaffney-Stomberg, Insogna, Rodriguez, & Kerstetter, 2009). Another study emphasized that a dietary plan of 25 to 30 g of high-quality protein at every meal would preserve muscle mass in older adults (Paddon-Jones & Rasmussen, 2009).

Carbohydrates and Fiber

Carbohydrates provide an essential source of energy and fiber. Without an adequate intake of carbohydrates, the body will derive energy from fat and protein, causing an increase in serum cholesterol and triglyceride levels and a depletion of water, electrolytes, and amino acids. **Dietary fiber** (i.e., the nondigestible carbohydrates and lignin in plants) has received much attention in recent years, primarily for its role in disease prevention, as an essential food component. The average daily intake of fiber for Americans is 10 to 15 g, which is significantly less than recommended amounts of the 25 to 38 g/day for adult women and men, respectively (Slavin, 2008). A review of studies found that dietary fiber intake from whole foods (12 to 33 g/day) or supplements (42.5 g/day) may lower blood pressure, improve serum lipid levels, and reduce indicators of inflammation. Studies found that dietary fiber may play a role in prevention and treatment of obesity, diabetes, cardiovascular disease, and colorectal cancer (Dahm et al., 2010; Du et al., 2010; Hopping et al., 2010; Maki et al., 2010). Dietary guidelines suggest a daily intake of five to nine servings of fruits and vegetables, with at least 55% of the total calories consumed derived from complex carbohydrates.

Fats

The primary functions of fat are to assist in temperature regulation, provide a reserve source of energy, facilitate the absorption of fat-soluble vitamins, and reduce acid secretion and muscular activity of the stomach. Fats are also useful in providing a feeling of satiety and improving the taste of foods. Fats are categorized according to their source. Saturated fats are derived from animals, whereas unsaturated fats are found in vegetables. Although either type of fat can meet nutritional needs, only the saturated fats are associated with the detrimental accumulation of serum cholesterol. Adults in most industrialized societies consume far more calories in fats than is healthy or necessary. Because excessive fat intake is associated with harmful effects, such as hyperlipidemia, fat should constitute no more than 10% to 30% of a person's daily caloric intake. Those fats that are consumed should be polyunsaturated and monounsaturated fatty acids, rather than cholesterol and saturated fats (see Chapter 20 for further discussion of types of fat).

Water

Water is so commonly available that it is often overlooked as a nutritional requirement. However, it is essential for all metabolic activities and must be consumed in adequate amounts for proper physiologic performance. The functions of water include regulating body temperature, maintaining a suitable metabolic environment, diluting water-soluble medications, and facilitating renal and bowel excretion. Potential consequences of reduced body water include decreased efficiency of thermoregulation, increased susceptibility to dehydration, and increased concentrations of water-soluble medications in the body.

Throughout life, the proportion of total body water as a percentage of body weight gradually decreases. Whereas water constitutes approximately 80% of a newborn infant's weight, it represents 60% of a younger adult's weight, and approximately 50% or less of an older adult's weight. This decrease in total body water is associated with a loss of lean body mass and is influenced by sex and the degree of leanness, with women and obese people having a lower percentage of body water than do men and lean, muscular people. In older adults, total body water may be further diminished by poor fluid intake. The recommended amount of water intake (in beverages, drinking water, and food) is the same for adults of all ages: 3.7 liters for men and 2.7 liters for women. Approximately 80% of total water intake comes from drinking water and beverages and 20% comes from food (Buyckx, 2009).

 ## RISK FACTORS THAT AFFECT DIGESTION AND NUTRITION

Certain behaviors and common disease processes are likely to interfere with nutrition and digestion in older adults. Some detrimental behaviors, such as limiting fluid intake and avoiding fresh fruit, may be based on myths and misconceptions. Although these conditions can create risks for people at any age, they occur more commonly in older adults, and the potential for harm is much greater than in other age groups because of the collective effects of risk factors and age-related changes. Risk factors affect every phase of digestion and nutrition, and they can significantly influence eating patterns and nutritional intake. Researchers identified the following factors associated with inadequate nutrition in community dwelling older adults: poverty, impaired cognition, functional impairment, medication usage, poor oral health, poor physical or mental health, and lack of social support or access to community resources (Locher et al., 2008). Risks that can cause specific nutrient deficiencies are listed in Table 18-1, along with the related functional consequences.

TABLE 18-1 Causes and Consequences of Nutrient Deficiencies

Nutrient	Possible Causes of Deficiency	Functional Consequences of Deficiency
Calories	Anorexia, depression, mental or physical impairments	Weight loss, lethargy, edema, anemia
Protein	Lack of teeth or dentures, anorexia, depression, dementia, high alcohol or carbohydrate consumption	Poor tissue healing, hypoalbuminemia, reduced protein binding of drugs
Fat	Neomycin, phenytoin, laxatives, alcohol, colchicine, cholestyramine	Inability to absorb vitamins A, D, E, and K
Vitamin A	Mineral oil, neomycin, alcohol, cholestyramine, aluminum antacids, liver disease	Dry skin and eyes, photophobia, night blindness, hyperkeratoses
Thiamine (B_1)	High consumption of alcohol or caffeinated tea, pernicious anemia, diuretics	Neuropathy, muscle weakness, heart disease, dementia, anorexia
Riboflavin (B_2)	Malabsorption syndromes, chronic diarrhea laxative abuse, alcoholism, liver disease	Cheilitis, glossitis, photophobia, blepharitis, conjunctivitis
Niacin (B_3)	Poor dietary habits, diarrhea, cirrhosis, alcoholism	Dermatitis, stomatitis, diarrhea, dementia, depression
Pyridoxine (B_6)	Diuretics, hydralazine	Dermatitis, neuropathy
Folate (B_9)	Anticonvulsants, triamterene, sulfonamides, alcohol, smoking	Macrocytic anemia, elevated levels of homocysteine
Vitamin B_{12}	Malabsorption syndrome, H_2-receptor blockers, proton pump inhibitors, colchicine, oral hypoglycemics, potassium supplements, vegetarian diet	Pernicious anemia, weakness, dyspnea, glossitis, numbness, dementia, depression
Vitamin C	Aspirin, tetracycline, lack of fruits and vegetables in diet	Lassitude, irritability, anemia, ecchymosis, impaired wound healing
Vitamin D	Phenytoin, mineral oil, phenobarbital, sunlight deprivation	Muscle weakness and atrophy, osteoporosis, fractures
Vitamin E	Malabsorption syndromes	Peripheral neuropathy, gait disturbance, retinopathy
Vitamin K	Mineral oil, warfarin sodium (Coumadin), antibiotics, cholestyramine, phenytoin	Ecchymosis; hemorrhage involving the gastrointestinal, urinary, or central nervous system
Calcium	Phenytoin, aluminum-based antacids, laxatives, tetracycline, corticosteroids, furosemide, high intake of fiber or caffeine	Osteoporosis, fractures, low back pain
Iron	Achlorhydria; neomycin; aspirin; antacids; low intake of animal protein; high consumption of fiber, caffeine, or tannic acid (contained in some teas)	Anemia, weakness, lassitude, pallor
Magnesium	Alcohol, diuretics, diarrhea, bulk-forming laxatives	Cardiac arrhythmias, neuromuscular and central nervous system irritability, disorientation
Zinc	Penicillamine, aluminum-based antacids, bulk-forming laxatives, high consumption of fiber	Poor wound healing, hair loss
Potassium	Laxatives, furosemide, antibiotics, corticosteroids, diarrhea	Weakness, cardiac arrhythmias, digitalis toxicity
Water	Diuretics, laxatives, immobility, incontinence, diarrhea	Dry skin and mouth, dehydration, constipation
Fiber	Poor dietary habits	Constipation, hemorrhoids

Box 18-1 Stats in Brief: Prevalence of Risks

Older Adults With No Natural Teeth		*Older Adults and Dental Care*	
Percentage of Older Adults With No Natural Teeth, by Age Group		*Percentage of Older Adults Who Had Dental Care During the Past Year (2006–2007), by Age Group*	
• Age 65–74 years	22.0	• Age 65–74 years	59.2
• Age 75–84 years	29.1	• Age 75–84 years	56.9
• Age 85+ years	35.6	• Age 85+ years	50.6
Percentage of Adults 65+ Years With No Natural Teeth, by Poverty Level		*Percentage of Adults 65+ Years Who Had Dental Care During Past Year (2006–2007), by Poverty Level*	
• Poor	39.5	• Poor	36.4
• Near poor	34.3	• Near poor	46.1
• Not poor	20.4	• Not poor	73.0
Percentage of Adults 65+ Years With No Natural Teeth, by Race and Hispanic Origin		*Percentage of Adults 65+ Years Who Had Dental Care During Past Year (2006–2007), by Race and Hispanic Origin*	
• White	25.3	• White	60.5
• Black	34.4	• Black	37.3
• Asian	20.7	• Asian	60.0
• Hispanic	26.0	• Hispanic	44.6

Source: National Health Statistics Reports. (July 2009). Washington, DC: U.S. Department of Health and Human Services.

Conditions Related to Oral Care

Oral health influences nutritional status because it affects chewing, eating, swallowing, speaking, and social interaction. Lack of teeth and inadequate dental care (see Box 18-1) are two conditions common in older adults that have detrimental effects on eating and nutrition. Some factors that contribute to inadequate dental care include low income, less education, lack of transportation, lack of dental insurance, high cost of dental services, more pressing health concerns, and inaccessibility of services as a result of distance or environmental barriers, such as stairs to dental offices. In addition, because preventive dental care is a recent trend, older adults may believe that they should visit a dentist only when a toothache does not respond to home remedies. Inadequate oral care is especially problematic for older adults in long-term care settings because many studies have documented the lack of oral health care for nursing home residents (Boczko, McKeon, & Sturkie, 2009; Haumschild & Haumschild, 2009; Jablonski et al., 2009). Adverse effects of poor oral health include malnutrition, dehydration, periodontal disease, respiratory infections (e.g., pneumonia and aspiration pneumonia), joint infections, cardiovascular disease, poor glycemic control in diabetes, and increased risk of stroke (Haumschild & Haumschild, 2009; O'Connor, 2008).

Until recently, tooth loss was so common among older people that it has been inaccurately viewed as a normal consequence of aging; but the oral health of older people has improved in the past few decades so that older adults today are less likely to be edentulous (without any teeth). Tooth loss in older adulthood is often attributable to inadequate dental care, periodontal disease, and other pathologic conditions that occur with increasing frequency in later years.

DIVERSITY NOTE

African Americans, Native Americans, and Alaska Natives are more likely than white Americans to have fewer natural teeth.

Wellness Opportunity

Nurses promote wellness by exploring reasons that older adults do not obtain dental care so they can address these barriers.

Functional Impairments and Disease Processes

Functional impairments are strongly associated with poor nutrition, particularly with regard to dependence on others for assistance with eating (Oliveira, Fogaca, & Leandro-Merhi, 2009). For example, mobility or visual impairments can interfere with the ability to procure and prepare food. In community settings, the extent to which functional impairments affect nutrition depends to a large degree on the availability of social supports, such as family, friends, or agencies that assist with providing food.

Dysphagia (difficulty swallowing) is a functional impairment that can significantly affect chewing, safe swallowing, and nutrition. More than half of nursing home residents have dysphagia, which most commonly is caused by neurologic and neuromuscular disorders. Because nurses caring for older

Statement of the Problem

- Dysphagia is defined as impairment of any part of the swallowing process.
- Prevalence of dysphagia ranges from 14% of community-residing older adults up to 60% of nursing home residents.
- Dysphagia is common in older adults with neurologic conditions, including stroke, dementia, multiple sclerosis, and Parkinson disease.
- In addition to neurologic conditions, the following factors can increase the risk of dysphagia: absence of teeth, decreased saliva production, poorly fitting dentures, decreased level of consciousness, certain medications (e.g., anesthesics, anticholinergics, sedatives, psychotropics, antihistamines, amiodarone).
- Dysphagia increases the risk of aspiration and aspiration pneumonia.
- Poor oral hygiene increases the risk for pneumonia.

Recommendations for Nursing Assessment

- Speech–language pathologists are responsible for performing comprehensive swallowing assessments, but nurses are responsible for identifying patients/residents who are at risk for dysphagia.
- Nursing assessment includes interview questions about difficulty with chewing or swallowing, avoidance of certain foods or beverages, sensation of food being stuck in throat, inability to handle secretions, voice changes, and so forth.
- A recommended three-step nursing assessment of swallowing is: (1) examine the level of consciousness, posture, voluntary cough, voice quality, and saliva control; (2) have the patient/resident drink 1 teaspoon of water; (3) if the teaspoon of water clears safely, have the patient/resident drink a small glass of water.

- Signs and symptoms of dysphagia include drooling, coughing during meals, hoarse voice following meals, gurgling sounds in the throat, upper respiratory tract infection, wet lung sounds, or packing food in the cheeks.
- Signs and symptoms of aspiration pneumonia include chills, cough, fever, elevated respiratory rate, pleuritic chest pain, rales, delirium.

Recommendations for Nursing Interventions

- Speech–language pathologists are the health care professionals who usually assume primary responsibility for recommendations, but nurses are responsible for initiating the referrals in a timely manner and implementing interventions.
- Interventions for prevention of aspiration during feeding of dysphagia individuals include the following: rest for 30 minutes before eating, sit upright, avoid rushing or forced feeding, alternate small amounts of solid and liquid foods, minimize distractions.
- Interventions for prevention of aspiration based on recommendations of speech–language pathologist include the following: nectar- or honey-thick liquids, chin-down position, head turned to one side, placement of food in one side of mouth, use of adaptive equipment, muscle strengthening exercises.
- Recognize that individuals with dysphagia require approximately 30 minutes for eating/assisted feeding.
- Good oral care is imperative for all patients with dysphagia because is it associated with a lower incidence of pneumonia.
- Referrals for regular and "as-needed" dental care
- Be prepared to perform the Heimlich maneuver.

SOURCES: Cook (2009); Ney et al. (2009); Palmer and Metheny (2008); Sandhaus, Zalon, Valenti, and Harrell (2009); Tanner (2010).

---

adults are responsible for assessment and interventions related to this common problem, the topic is addressed in the Evidence-Based Practice Box 18-1.

Disease processes also increase the risk for nutritional and digestive consequences. Vitamin B_{12} deficiency increases with increasing age and, in older adults, it is associated with malabsorption of foods resulting from atrophy of gastric mucosa (Allen, 2009). Other pathologic conditions interfere with appetite and enjoyment of food in many ways. For example, infections, hyperthyroidism, hypoadrenalism, and congestive heart failure are associated with anorexia, and rheumatoid conditions and chronic obstructive pulmonary disease (COPD) are associated with both decreased appetite and increased energy expenditure. Dementia and other neurodegenerative disorders often have serious negative effects on eating and nutrition related to procuring and preparing food, remembering to eat, and chewing and swallowing food.

Medication Effects

Medications can create risk factors for impaired digestion and inadequate nutrition through their effects on digestion, eating patterns, and utilization of nutrients. Adverse medication effects are more likely to occur in older adults because of the increased use of medications. Table 18-2 lists examples of medications and the related adverse effects on digestion and nutrition.

Medications can affect nutrition by interfering with the absorption and excretion of nutrients, as in the following examples:

- Broad-spectrum antibiotics can alter intestinal flora and impair nutrient synthesis.
- Medications and vitamins that are similar in chemical structure may compete at sites of action, thus altering their excretion pattern.
- Some medications bind to particular ions and form compounds that cannot be absorbed (e.g., tetracycline can bind to iron and calcium).
- Diuretics can interfere with the transport of water, sodium, glucose, and amino acids.
- Nutritional supplements and herbal preparations also can affect nutrients (e.g., long-term use of beta-carotene supplements can cause a vitamin E deficiency).

Additional food, herb, and medication interactions are discussed in Chapter 8.

Lifestyle Factors

Alcohol and smoking can alter an older person's nutritional status in several ways. Alcohol has a high caloric content but low nutrient value, so it provides empty calories. In addition, it interferes with the absorption of the B-complex vitamins and vitamin C. Alcoholism is often unrecognized

TABLE 18-2 Potential Effects of Medications on Digestion and Nutrition

Medication Examples	Potential Effect on Digestion and Nutrition
Digoxin, theophylline, fluoxetine, antihistamines	Anorexia
Anticholinergics, narcotics, calcium channel blockers, iron, aluminum- and calcium-based antacids	Constipation
Cimetidine, laxatives, antibiotics, cardiovascular drugs, cholinesterase inhibitors	Diarrhea, nausea, vomiting
Nonsteroidal anti-inflammatory drugs (NSAIDs), aspirin, corticosteroids	Gastric irritation
Phenytoin, nifedipine, diltiazem, cyclosporine	Gum hyperplasia
Anticholinergics, potassium-depleting medications	Paralytic ileus
Bulk-forming agents when taken before meals, anticholinergics	Early satiety
Potassium supplements, NSAIDs, bisphosphonates, prednisone	Dysphagia
Antihistamines, salicylates, hypoglycemics, antiparkinson drugs, psychoactive drugs	Altered smell and taste sensations
Mineral oil, cholestyramine	Diminished absorption of vitamins A, D, E, and K
Anticonvulsants	Diminished storage of vitamin K, decreased absorption of calcium
Aluminum- or magnesium-based antacids	Diarrhea; decreased levels of calcium, fluoride, and phosphorus
Ampicillin, amoxicillin, cephalosporins, clindamycin	Clostridium difficile diarrhea
Products containing sodium bicarbonate	Sodium overload, water retention
Gentamicin and penicillin	Hypokalemia
Tetracyclines	Diminished absorption of zinc, iron, calcium, and magnesium
Neomycin	Diminished absorption of fat, iron, lactose, nitrogen, calcium, potassium, and vitamin B_{12}
Aspirin	Gastrointestinal bleeding; decreased levels of iron, folate, and vitamin C
Corticosteroids	Increased need for calcium, phosphorus, B vitamins, and vitamins C and D

and undertreated in older adults and may be a common contributing factor to nutritional disorders. Smoking diminishes the ability to smell and taste food and interferes with absorption of vitamin C and folic acid.

Psychosocial Factors

Psychosocial factors are likely to affect an older person's appetite and eating patterns. Any changes in mealtime companionship, as may occur through loss or disability of a spouse, are likely to have a negative impact on eating patterns. Eating alone is associated with poor nutritional status of older adults,

particularly men (Hsieh, Sung, & Wan, 2010). When older adults have established a long-term pattern of preparing meals for family and spouse, it may be especially difficult for the older adult to adjust to purchasing, preparing, and eating food for just one person. Similarly, older adults who have never participated in the purchase or preparation of foods may have great difficulty assuming these tasks after the loss of a spouse or other person who performed these tasks. If the older adult depends on others for assistance in procuring food, any factors that limit the availability of support resources may affect the older adult's ability to obtain food.

Wellness Opportunity

Nurses can work with older adults to identify ways of promoting positive social interaction during mealtimes.

Stress and anxiety affect digestive processes through their influence on the autonomic nervous system. Although stress-related effects on digestion are not unique to older adults, any alteration of the autonomic nervous system may compound age-related effects that otherwise would not have much effect. Older adults who are depressed are likely to experience anorexia and loss of interest in food. Confusion, memory problems, and other cognitive deficits may significantly interfere with eating patterns and the ability to prepare food. Studies indicate that cognitive impairment and depression are associated with poor nutritional status in older adults in community and long-term care settings (Grieger, Nowson, & Ackland, 2009; Johansson, Sidenvall, Malmberg, & Christensson, 2009; Sahyoun, Anyanwu, Sharkey, & Netterville, 2010).

Cultural and Socioeconomic Factors

Ethnic background, religious beliefs, and other cultural factors strongly influence the way people define, select, prepare, and eat food and beverages. Cultural factors also can influence eating patterns and selection of food in relation to health status. For example, some Asian and Hispanic people may classify foods, beverages, and medicines as hot or cold, and they may select a particular food on the basis of their belief that their illness would respond to warm, hot, cool, or cold types of remedies. According to this health belief model, illnesses are caused by an imbalance between hot and cold, and so must be treated with substances that have the opposite characteristics. The characteristics of "hot" and "cold" are not related to temperature of the food but are culturally defined by different groups.

Cultural dietary customs usually are not detrimental for healthy older adults, as long as the diet includes essential nutrients and avoids extremes. However, for older adults with medical conditions that require diet modification (e.g., diabetes or hypertension), cultural food patterns may aggravate the condition and create barriers to nutritional therapy. Cultural Considerations 18-1 summarizes some of the food habits that are associated with major cultural and religious

CULTURAL CONSIDERATIONS 18-1

Cultural Influences on Eating Patterns

African Americans

- "Soul food" is common, particularly in the southern United States.
- Common main courses: wild game, fried fish and poultry, pork and all parts of the pig
- Common vegetables and side dishes: corn, rice, okra, greens, legumes, tomatoes, hot breads, sweet potatoes
- Methods of food preparation: stewing, barbecuing, and frying with lard or salt pork
- Low consumption of milk (possibly owing to lactose intolerance)
- Low calcium dietary intake

Asian Americans

- Common foods: rice, wheat, pork, eggs, chicken, soybean products, and a variety of vegetables
- Methods of food preparation: stir-frying with lard, peanut oil, or sesame oil; seasoning with ginger, soy sauce, sesame seeds, and monosodium glutamate
- Beverages: green tea; rare use of milk products because lactose intolerance is common

Hispanic Americans

- Common main courses: eggs, tacos, chicken, corn tortillas, pinto or calico beans

- Common vegetables and side dishes: rice, corn, squash, bread, tomatoes
- Methods of food preparation: frying with lard; seasoning with garlic, onions, and chili powder
- Beverages: herbal teas, carbonated soda, milk in hot beverages

Native Americans

- May obtain foods from their natural environment (e.g., fish, roots, fruits, berries, wild greens, and wild game)
- May depend on commodity foods provided by the U.S. Department of Agriculture
- May be influenced by tribal culture
- May have limited use of dairy products because of lactose intolerance

Religious Influences

- Some groups of Jews follow prescribed rules for preparing and serving foods (e.g., they eat only kosher meat and poultry and do not eat shellfish or any pork products).
- Mormons do not drink tea, coffee, or alcohol.
- Hindus may be vegetarians.
- Seventh-Day Adventists may be lacto–ovovegetarians.
- Many Catholics do not eat meat on Ash Wednesday or Good Friday.

groups in the United States. Nurses should remember, though, that individual older adults vary in their eating patterns and may not adhere to the patterns of their cultural group. It is usually not necessary to try to change culturally influenced eating patterns, but it is important to recognize any cultural factors that may affect older adults' nutritional status.

Wellness Opportunity

Nurses address cultural needs by identifying food preferences and finding reasonable ways to provide these foods.

A person's past and present economic status also influences food choices. If nutrient intake has been inadequate because of long-standing financial limitations, the progressive effects of poor nutrition may precipitate new problems in older adults, especially in combination with age-related changes in nutrient intake and utilization. People of low socioeconomic status usually have a narrower selection of foods than do people of higher socioeconomic status. Lower socioeconomic status, including educational level, is associated also with lack of dental care and more tooth loss (Starr & Hall, 2010). Studies indicate that approximately 19% of all older Americans meet criteria for actual or marginal food insecurity due to financial constraints and 83% of older adults do not consume a good quality diet, with those in poverty having the lowest scores for healthy eating (Kamp, Wellman, & Russell, 2010; Lee, Fischer, & Johnson, 2010).

Environmental Factors

Environmental factors affect the enjoyment of food and the ability to obtain and prepare it. Many barriers to food enjoyment have been identified in the dining environments of long-term care facilities and other institutional settings. Older adults in congregate housing and long-term care facilities may find it difficult to adjust to unfamiliar environments. Moreover, they may not desire the mealtime social interaction that is part of the institutional environment. A noisy or crowded dining room may have a negative impact on food enjoyment and consumption. Such an environment may be particularly stressful for older adults who use hearing aid or who are accustomed to eating alone. The potential outcomes of a move to a new environment include poor nutrition and loss of interest in eating, particularly during the initial adjustment period.

Environmental influences, such as inclement weather conditions, particularly affect functionally impaired older adults who live in their own homes. For example, older persons who walk to the store or depend on public transportation may be unable or unwilling to obtain groceries in snowy or rainy weather. Likewise, older adults may not be able to tolerate hot or sultry conditions, especially if transportation is not readily available. People who depend on others for transportation or who have difficulty maneuvering in adverse weather conditions are likely to shop for groceries less frequently and to purchase their groceries at smaller convenience stores, where prices are higher and selection is limited. The additional cost and limited selection may interfere with food intake and lead to nutrient deficiencies. Finally, environmental conditions and packaging trends in the grocery store may create additional difficulties for older people, especially those who are functionally impaired. For example, the combined glare of fluorescent lights; highly polished floors; shiny, clear wrappers; and white freezer cases often make it extremely difficult, if not impossible, for older adults with vision changes to read labels, especially when the print is small and contrasts poorly against the background.

Behaviors Based on Myths and Misunderstandings

Myths and misunderstandings may be detrimental to a person's food intake and behaviors related to bowel function. For example, during the 1950s and 1960s, a widely held belief was that roughage and raw fruits or vegetables were harmful to the older person. It is now known that lack of roughage in the diet and consumption of only cooked fruits and vegetables are eating patterns that contribute to constipation by slowing the transit time of feces through the large intestine. Another commonly held belief is that a daily bowel movement is the norm for good digestive function. Rigid adherence to this standard may, in fact, lead to the unnecessary and detrimental use of laxatives. Advertisements have further reinforced this false belief by implying that daily bowel movements should be attained through medication. Although recent advertising trends emphasize the achievement of healthy bowel patterns through the ingestion of high-fiber food items, the negative impact of long-term beliefs may be difficult to overcome.

Misunderstandings about fluid intake may also interfere with digestion and nutrition. Many older adults reduce the amount of liquids they consume in an attempt to decrease the incidence of urinary incontinence. Fluid intake may also be restricted if functional limitations, such as impaired mobility or manual dexterity, interfere with either the ability to obtain liquids or the ease of urinary elimination. Reduced fluid intake can have a number of detrimental consequences, such as constipation, xerostomia, and diminished food enjoyment.

> **Wellness Opportunity**
>
> Nurses identify myths and misunderstandings about constipation and teach older adults about habits that promote healthy elimination patterns.

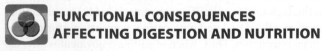 **FUNCTIONAL CONSEQUENCES AFFECTING DIGESTION AND NUTRITION**

Functional consequences affect the following aspects of digestion and nutrition of older adults:
- Procurement, preparation, and enjoyment of food
- Mastication and digestion of food
- Nutritional status
- Psychosocial function.

Negative functional consequences occur primarily because of the many risk factors that affect older adults, rather than because of age-related changes alone.

Ability to Procure, Prepare, and Enjoy Food

Activities involved in procuring, preparing, consuming, and enjoying food depend on the skills of cognition, balance, mobility, and manual dexterity, as well as on the five senses. Food procurement depends on getting to the grocery store, pushing a shopping cart, reaching for food items on high shelves, reading the small print on shelves and food packages for cost and nutrition information, and coping with the glare of bright lights, especially in the frozen-food sections. Age-related changes and conditions that may interfere with these activities include vision impairments and any illness, such as arthritis, that limits mobility, balance, or manual dexterity.

Food preparation activities that are likely to be more difficult for older adults include cutting food items, measuring ingredients accurately, carrying food and liquid without spilling, standing for long periods in the kitchen, reaching for items on high shelves and in cupboards, safely using the oven or stove, and reading the temperature controls correctly. Impairments of vision, balance, cognition, mobility, or manual dexterity are likely to cause difficulties in performing these tasks.

Diminished sensory function can affect food enjoyment in all the following ways:
- Inaccurate perception of color, taste, or smell can interfere with appetite and food appeal.
- Diminished gustatory and olfactory sensitivity may lead to excessive use of condiments and seasonings, such as salt and sugar.
- Visual and olfactory impairments may make it difficult to detect spoiled food.

Moreover, food choices are influenced by the condition of the oral cavity and teeth, as well as by the quantity and the quality of natural or replacement teeth.

> **Wellness Opportunity**
>
> Nurses promote wellness through interventions that improve the older adult's independence in procuring and preparing satisfying meals.

Changes in Oral Function

Digestive processes in healthy older adults are not significantly affected by age-related changes, but older adults often have digestive complaints (e.g., "heartburn," constipation) caused by commonly occurring risk factors. For example, many negative functional consequences are associated with medications (see Table 18-2). Xerostomia causes negative functional consequences because it can interfere with oral comfort, food enjoyment, and taste sensitivity. In addition, diminished saliva production makes it more difficult to chew food and increases the susceptibility of the teeth and tongue to bacterial action. Older adults with poor oral health are likely to avoid eating whole fruits, raw vegetables, and meat (Quandt et al., 2010). A review of studies identified the following consequences of impaired salivary function: gingivitis; oral lesions; dental caries; excessive plaque; periodontal disease; and impaired taste, speech, chewing, and swallowing (Turner & Ship, 2007). The functional consequences of being edentulous or using dentures include avoidance of certain foods, decreased chewing efficiency, and increased susceptibility to accidental choking from ineffective mastication. Because edentulous people tend to avoid meats, salads, fresh fruits, and raw vegetables, they may be at risk for nutritional deficiencies (Savoca et al., 2010; Tsakos, Herrick, Sheiham, & Watt, 2010).

Nutritional Status and Weight Changes

Because older adults need fewer calories, a deficiency of essential minerals or vitamins is likely to occur if the quantity of calories is reduced without a corresponding increase in the quality of the food consumed. In addition, risk factors (e.g., medications and pathologic processes) that commonly occur in older adults often cause nutrient deficiencies. For example, iron deficiency is associated with chronic diseases and low socioeconomic status. Other minerals and vitamins that commonly are deficient in older adults are zinc, calcium, most B vitamins, and vitamins D and E. See Table 18-1 for examples of nutrient deficiencies and associated risk factors and functional consequences that are likely to affect older adults.

Although studies related to specific nutritional deficits among older adults are clouded by a lack of common definitions, numerous studies conclude that dietary intake for most older adults does not meet recommended daily allowance standards. A review of studies concluded that the prevalence of undernutrition in older adults was 45% in the community, 50% to 84% in hospitals, and between 84% and 100% in residential care facilities (Visvanathan & Chapman, 2009). Specific nutrients that are likely to be deficient in older adults in the United States include fiber, calcium, magnesium, potassium, and vitamins C, D, E, and K (Burnett-Hartman, Fitzpatrick, Gao, Jackson, & Schreiner, 2009; Lichtenstein, Rasmussen, Yu, Epstein, & Russell, 2008).

A type of malnutrition that is common in frail older adults is **protein-energy malnutrition** (also called *protein-calorie malnutrition*), which occurs when the intake of calories and protein is less than the amount required to meet daily needs. This condition is associated with a high-carbohydrate, low-protein diet, which often results from one or several of the risk factors already discussed (e.g., depression, loss of appetite, pathologic conditions). Characteristics of mild or moderate protein-energy malnutrition include weakness, lethargy, unintentional weight loss, diminished muscle mass, marked decrease in subcutaneous fat, and impaired ability to respond to physiologic stresses (e.g., surgery, infection). If the condition progresses and becomes severe, it is characterized by edema and loss of visceral protein. In a study of patients between the ages of 65 and 99 years, negative consequences of protein-energy malnutrition included anemia, decreased

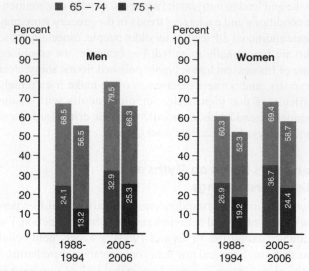

FIGURE 18-1 Percentage of people aged 65+ who are overweight and obese, by sex and age group, 1988 to 2006.

thyroid function, altered insulin production, anomalies in salt and water retention, loss of skeletal muscle mass, decreased glomerular filtration rate, decreased creatinine clearance, and increased risk of pneumonia (Price, 2008).

Age-related changes in body composition and carbohydrate metabolism contribute to gradual weight gains. The proportion of body fat to lean tissue begins to increase around 30 years of age and leads to disproportionately increased abdominal fat during later adulthood. This pattern of fat distribution is associated with increased risk for diabetes, cardiovascular disease, and other chronic conditions. The gradually increasing prevalence of obesity is a major public health concern for all population groups, but it is most prevalent among older adults between the ages of 65 and 74 years, as illustrated in Figure 18-1. Even though there is some evidence that the **body mass index (BMI)** standards should be increased for older adults, there continues to be strong evidence that abdominal obesity as measured by waist circumference is an independent risk factor for many serious chronic conditions (Houston, Nicklas, & Zizza, 2009).

Quality of Life

Good food and nutrition are important components of health-related quality of life in many ways. Food-related activities are often a focal point of celebrations, religious rituals, or gatherings to share significant events. In addition, mealtimes are typically associated with caring, comfort, nurturing, and social interaction. Thus, when mealtime enjoyment is affected in any way, the psychosocial aspects of eating are also affected. Older adults who enjoyed participating in family meals or eating in restaurants may withdraw from these activities if food is no longer enjoyable. Similarly, when these events are no longer part of life for older adults, they may lose interest in eating.

Perhaps even more detrimental than the psychosocial consequences of diminished food enjoyment are the psychosocial effects of inadequate nutrition. When fluid or nutrient intake is inadequate, older adults are likely to develop malnutrition and dehydration because of impaired homeostatic mechanisms. Changes in mental status, including memory impairment, are among the early signs of malnutrition, dehydration, and electrolyte imbalance in older adults. Sometimes these mental changes are attributed incorrectly to irreversible conditions (e.g., dementia) rather than to a treatable and reversible metabolic imbalance. For example, deficiencies of vitamins B_{12} or D are common nutritional causes of mental changes (Morley, 2010).

PATHOLOGIC CONDITIONS AFFECTING DIGESTIVE WELLNESS: CONSTIPATION

Constipation—defined as "decrease in normal frequency of defecation accompanied by difficult or incomplete passage of stool and/or passage of excessively hard, dry stool" (NANDA International, 2009, p. 102)—is one of the most common pathologic conditions associated with digestion. The normal frequency for bowel movements, which shows significant individual variation but does not necessarily change with aging, ranges from three times daily to once or twice weekly. Another characteristic is that persons experience a feeling of incomplete evacuation after a bowel movement. Approximately one-half of institutionalized older adults report problems with constipation and three-fourths use laxatives daily (Bouras & Tangalos, 2009). Prevalence rates are highest among women and increase gradually after the age of 50 years, with the largest increase after the age of 70 years (McCrea, Miaskowski, Stotts, Macera, & Varma, 2009).

Although constipation is a common complaint of older adults, it is caused by risk factors rather than age-related changes alone. Risk factors common in older adults include functional impairments (e.g., diminished mobility), pathologic conditions (e.g., hypothyroidism), adverse medication effects (including long-term laxative abuse), and poor dietary habits (e.g., inadequate intake of bulk, fiber, and fluid). Because constipation occurs so commonly in older adults, nurses assess for risk factors and initiate health promotion interventions, as discussed in the sections on Nursing Assessment and Nursing Interventions.

*M*r. and Mrs. D., who are 71 and 72 years old, respectively, attend the senior center where you provide monthly group health education sessions and weekly one-on-one "Counseling for Wellness" sessions. Mrs. D. makes an appointment to see you because her bowels get "bound up" and she always feels "bloated." When you ask

about her bowel patterns, she reports that she has a bowel movement "about every other day" and has to "sit on the commode for a good half-hour before anything happens." She has taken milk of magnesia every night for approximately 20 years, but "it doesn't seem to be any help anymore." She avoids fresh fruits and vegetables because her mother always told her that canned fruits and vegetables were easier to digest. She rarely eats cereal and uses white bread. Her weight is approximately 125% of her ideal body weight, and she does not walk often because of trouble with arthritis. She takes levothyroxine (Synthroid), 100 mcg once daily, and an over-the-counter generic calcium supplement that contains 500 mg calcium carbonate twice daily.

THINKING POINTS

- Identify at least five risk factors that are likely to contribute to Mrs. D.'s constipation.
- Describe how you would begin addressing one of these risk factors in health education.

NURSING ASSESSMENT OF DIGESTION AND NUTRITION

Nurses assess digestion and nutrition to identify (1) effects of age-related changes on digestion, nutrition, and eating patterns; (2) risk factors that interfere with optimal nutrition; (3) cultural factors that influence eating patterns; (4) nutritional status and usual eating patterns; and (5) negative functional consequences of altered digestion or inadequate nutrition. On the basis of this assessment information, nurses identify opportunities for health promotion interventions.

Interviewing About Digestion and Nutrition

Nurses use an assessment interview to identify opportunities for health promotion by asking about the following information:

- Usual eating patterns and nutrient intake
- Health behaviors associated with oral care
- Age-related changes and risk factors that affect nutritional needs or digestive processes
- Environmental or social support factors that affect the procurement, preparation, and enjoyment of food
- Symptoms of gastrointestinal dysfunction.

Nurses can assess the adequacy of nutrient intake by asking older adults to describe foods and beverages consumed during an average day. In addition, nurses follow a logical sequence for assessment questions by beginning with information about the oral cavity and ending with questions about bowel elimination. A major goal for assessing patterns of bowel elimination is to identify opportunities for health education about constipation. Box 18-2 summarizes interview questions for a nursing assessment of nutrition and digestion in older adults.

Wellness Opportunity

Nurses promote personal responsibility by asking older adults to keep a 7-day diary of food and beverage intake and eating patterns and reviewing this to identify strengths and weaknesses of their diet.

Observing Cues to Digestion and Nutrition

Nurses observe oral health indicators and eating patterns and environments for cues to digestion and nutrition. In addition, they consider social and cultural factors that influence eating and nutrition. Box 18-3 summarizes observations and cultural considerations that are pertinent to nursing assessment of digestion and nutrition.

The Hartford Institute for Geriatric Nursing recommends the use of the Kayser-Jones Brief Oral Health Status Examination as an evidence-based tool to evaluate oral health status of older adults in a variety of settings (Chen, 2007). Nurses in institutional settings can assess behavioral cues to

digestion and nutrition by observing older adults during meals. Nursing assessment of chewing and swallowing is especially important for older adults at risk for dysphagia, as described in the Evidence-Based Practice box 18-1.

Wellness Opportunity

Nurses observe environmental conditions to identify positive or negative effects on eating patterns.

Using Physical Assessment and Laboratory Information

Physical assessment and laboratory data provide important additional information for assessing the older adults' nutritional and hydration status. Height, weight, and BMI provide important clues to nutritional status. The BMI—a measure of body composition related to body fat—is commonly used as an indicator of malnutrition. Healthy BMI is between 18.5 and 24.9 lb/in^2 for adults. Although there is no benefit to severe obesity, reviews of studies indicate that the ideal BMI for older men and women is closer to 25 lb/in^2 and 35 lb/in^2, respectively (Flicker et al., 2010; Oreopoulos, Kalantar-Zadeh, Sharma, & Fonarow, 2009).

 Box 18-2 Guidelines for Assessing Digestion and Nutrition

Assessing Oral Comfort and Chewing Ability
- Do you have any difficulty with soreness or bleeding in your mouth?
- Do you have any teeth that hurt, are loose, or are sensitive to hot or cold temperatures?
- Do your gums bleed?
- Do you have any problems chewing or swallowing food or liquids? *If yes, ask about particular types of food or liquids that are problematic.*
- Are there foods you avoid because of problems with chewing or swallowing?
- Does your mouth or tongue ever feel dry?

Assessing Dental Habits and Attitudes Toward Dental Care
- How often do you see a dentist?
- When is the last time you had dental care?
- Where do you go for dental care?
- *If the person does not seek dental care at least once per year:* What prevents you from seeing the dentist?
- How do you care for your teeth?
- Do you use dental floss? *If yes:* How often? *If no* Have you ever been taught to use dental floss?

Assessing Nutritional Needs
- Do you have diabetes, heart disease, or any condition that requires dietary modifications?
- Do you have any food allergies?
- What medications do you take?
- What is your usual daily activity pattern?

Identifying Patterns of Food Procurement
- How do you get your grocery shopping done?

- Do you have any help getting to the store?
- Where and how often do you do your grocery shopping?
- What is your usual food budget?
- Do you have any difficulty getting food because of problems with vision, walking, or transportation?

Identifying Patterns of Food Preparation and Consumption
- Where do you eat your meals?
- With whom do you eat?
- Does anyone help you prepare your meals?
- Do you have any trouble fixing your meals (e.g., difficulty opening containers)?
- Do you have any difficulties getting around your kitchen, using appliances, or reaching the cupboards?
- Have there been recent changes in your eating or food preparation patterns (e.g., loss of eating companion or change in caregiver situation)?

Assessing Patterns of Bowel Elimination
- How often do you have a bowel movement?
- Have you noticed any recent changes in your pattern of bowel movements?
- Do you have any difficulty with your bowel movements? (e.g., Do you strain with bowel movements? or Is the stool hard, dry, or difficult to pass?)
- Do you ever have problems with loose stools or diarrhea?
- Do you take laxatives or any other products to help you move your bowels?
- Do you ever have pain or bleeding when you move your bowels?

Box 18-3 Behavioral Cues to Nutrition and Digestion

Observations to Assess Oral Health

- Condition of lips, teeth, gums, tongue, and oral mucous membrane
- Number of teeth and use of full or partial dentures
- Fit of dentures
- Oral care items: condition of toothbrush, type of toothbrush or denture cleaning supplies, use of floss

Observations to Assess Eating Patterns

- Does the person seem to enjoy eating meals with others, or does the presence of other people seem to interfere with mealtime enjoyment?
- If the person has dentures, are they worn at meals? If not, why not?
- What are the person's between-meal food and fluid consumption patterns?
- Are enjoyable noncaffeinated liquids readily available for between-meal fluid intake?
- What cultural influences affect the person's food preferences and preparation?

Observations to Assess the Eating Environment

- Do environmental or social influences negatively affect mealtime enjoyment (e.g., a noisy dining room or disruptive mealtime companions)?

- If the person eats alone, is this the best arrangement, or should consideration be given to providing mealtime social interaction?

Cultural Considerations That May Influence Nutrition and Eating Patterns

- What are the usual patterns of meals eaten (e.g., content, frequency, timing)? What is the usual social context of meals?
- Are there any culturally influenced food taboos or preferences? (Refer to Cultural Considerations 18-1.)
- Are there any special foods that are important because of religious or cultural factors? (If yes, are they accessible to the older adult?)
- Are certain foods or beverages avoided or preferred in relation to an illness or chronic condition (e.g., foods or beverages that are considered yin and yang foods)?
- Is there a preference for the temperature of beverages (e.g., use of iced or heated beverages)?
- Is the person's ethnic background likely to increase his or her chance of being lactose intolerant? (Prevalence is highest among Asians, American Indians, and African and American blacks; high among Hispanics; and lowest among whites of northern European descent.)

Nurses need to consider individual circumstances in relation to ideal body weight because standardized tables do not necessarily provide the most realistic or appropriate goal for older adults. Rather, for many older adults, maintenance of a stable weight may be more important because patterns of weight loss and gain are important indicators of overall health condition. Weight loss is considered in relation to percentage of loss, which is calculated by subtracting current weight from usual weight and dividing that by the usual weight—for example, (160 lb − 120 lb)/160 lb = 40 lb/160 lb, or a 25% weight loss. An unintentional weight loss of more than 5% of body weight in 1 month or more than 10% in 6 months is considered a significant indicator of poor nutrition (Kruizenga et al., 2010).

Although there are many indicators of dehydration, tongue dryness is strongly associated with poor hydration status (Vivanti, Harvey, & Ash, 2010). Assessment of skin turgor in older adults may be more accurate on the forehead and over the anterior chest wall because these areas are less affected by age-related skin changes. Orthostatic hypotension, oliguria or anuria, changes in mental status, and dry tongue and mucous membranes are common manifestations of dehydration in older adults. Urinalysis provides clues to the hydration status, with highly concentrated urine (i.e., specific gravity above 1.030) being an indicator of dehydration. Blood values that may be altered in dehydration include sodium, hematocrit, hemoglobin, creatinine, osmolality, and blood urea nitrogen, all of which may be elevated. In addition, a sudden loss of body weight might be an indicator of dehydration.

Laboratory data can provide clues to nutritional deficiencies, even before any clinical signs are evident; however, test results must be evaluated in relation to persons' overall health status. For instance, low serum albumin is an indicator of poor nutrition, but it also occurs with trauma, edema, infection, and neoplasm. Box 18-4 summarizes information about physical assessment indicators and laboratory values that are especially important in assessing the nutritional status of older adults. Additional indicators of nutrient deficiencies are listed in Table 18-2 in the column describing functional consequences.

Using Assessment Tools

Nutrition assessment tools are used for identifying people at risk for dehydration and nutritional problems so that preventive and therapeutic interventions can be implemented. The **Mini Nutritional Assessment (MNA)** is an evidence-based tool that has been widely used since 1990 in a variety of settings. Advantages of this tool include validation and reliability, ease of use, low cost, acceptability, effectiveness, and availability in many languages (Skates & Anthony, 2009). The MNA consists of 6 screening and 12 assessment questions and takes approximately 15 minutes to complete. The Hartford Institute for Geriatric Nursing recommends the use of this tool and provides additional information and a cost-free video in collaboration with the *American Journal of Nursing* at http://consultgerirn.org or www.nursingcenter.com (DiMaria-Ghalili & Guenter, 2008). Figure 18-2 illustrates a six-item short form, which can be administered in 5 minutes and has been validated as a first-step screening process for identifying older adults who should be assessed further for poor nutrition (Kaiser et al., 2009).

Box 18-4   Physical Assessment and Laboratory Data

Examination of the Oral Cavity
- Inspect the oral cavity by using a tongue depressor and a light.
- Observe for evidence of oral disease, including pain, lumps, soreness, bleeding, swelling, loose teeth, and abraded areas.
- Note the presence or absence of teeth, dentures, and partial bridges.

Normal Findings
- Lips: pink, moist, symmetrical
- Teeth: intact, without cavities or tartar
- Gums: pink, no bleeding
- Mucous membranes: pink, moist
- Tongue: pink, moist, presence of numerous varicosities on under-surface
- Pharynx: soft palate rises slightly when "ahh" is vocalized

Indicators of Nutritional Deficiency
- Lips: dry, fissured, cracked at corners
- Teeth: decayed or missing
- Gums: red, swollen, recessed, spongy or prone to bleeding
- Mucous membranes: dry, ulcerated, inflamed, bleeding, white patches
- Tongue: dry, swollen, reddened, or very smooth

Examination of the Abdomen and Rectum
- Examine the abdomen with the person lying comfortably in the supine position.
- Perform a rectal examination with the person in the side-lying position.

Normal Findings
- Symmetrical, soft abdomen that moves with respirations
- Audible bowel sounds (heard through the diaphragm of a stethoscope) occurring at irregular intervals (5 to 15 seconds apart)

- Smooth skin around anus; no evidence of hemorrhoids, fissures, inflammation, or rectal prolapse
- Soft, brown stool that tests negative for occult blood

Indicators of Nutritional Deficiency
- Swollen abdomen
- Stool that tests positive for occult blood

General Physical Assessment Indicators of Malnutrition
- Weight loss
- Lack of subcutaneous fat
- Diminished size and strength of muscles
- Skin that is dry, rough, or tissue thin
- Abnormal pulse or blood pressure
- Edema, especially in the face or lower extremities
- Hair that is dry, dull, thin, brittle, or sparse
- Dry or dull-looking eyes
- Listless, apathetic, or depressed mood
- Difficulty with walking or maintaining balance

Laboratory Data
- Biochemical data that will provide information about nutritional status: serum ferritin; serum or red blood cell folate and vitamin B_{12}; complete lipid profile; and serum albumin, glucose, sodium, and potassium levels
- Urinalysis results should be within the normal adult range, except for a slight decrease in the upper limit for specific gravity

Indicators of Nutritional Deficiency
- Anemia
- Lymphocytopenia
- Serum albumin level of less than 3.5 g/dL
- Cholesterol levels of less than 160 mg/dL
- Total iron-binding capacity less than 250 mcg/dL

---

*R*ecall that you are the nurse at the senior center attended by Mr. and Mrs. D., who now are 75 and 76 years old, respectively. During a "Counseling for Health" session, Mrs. D. asks your advice about her gradual unintended weight loss over the past few months. Although Mrs. D. continues to cook meals because her husband enjoys eating, she states that food no longer appeals to her. You notice that her mouth is very dry and her teeth are in poor condition. She had a stroke 2 years ago and recovered well except for some dysphagia and right-sided weakness. She takes an antidepressant and two blood pressure medications but does not know the names of the pills. She asks what she can do about the weight loss.

THINKING POINTS

- What risk factors are likely to be contributing to Mrs. D.'s weight loss?

- Make a list of assessment questions you would use with Mrs. D. Select applicable questions from Box 18-2 and list any additional questions that you would use for further assessment.
- What would you ask Mrs. D. to do to provide additional assessment information so that you can plan some teaching interventions?

NURSING DIAGNOSIS

The nursing assessment may identify problems related to nutrition, digestion, or oral health. If nutritional deficits are identified, a pertinent nursing diagnosis is Imbalanced Nutrition: Less than Body Requirements, defined as "intake of nutrients insufficient to meet metabolic needs (NANDA International, 2009, p. 74). Related factors that may affect older adults include medications, anorexia, depression, chewing or swallowing difficulties, social isolation, and inability to procure or prepare food.

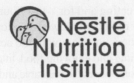

Mini Nutritional Assessment
MNA®

Last name:	First name:
Sex: Age: Weight, kg: Height, cm: Date:	

Complete the screen by filling in the boxes with the appropriate numbers. Total the numbers for the final screening score.

Screening

A Has food intake declined over the past 3 months due to loss of appetite, digestive problems, chewing or swallowing difficulties?
0 = severe decrease in food intake
1 = moderate decrease in food intake
2 = no decrease in food intake ☐

B Weight loss during the last 3 months
0 = weight loss greater than 3 kg (6.6 lbs)
1 = does not know
2 = weight loss between 1 and 3 kg (2.2 and 6.6 lbs)
3 = no weight loss ☐

C Mobility
0 = bed or chair bound
1 = able to get out of bed / chair but does not go out
2 = goes out ☐

D Has suffered psychological stress or acute disease in the past 3 months?
0 = yes   2 = no ☐

E Neuropsychological problems
0 = severe dementia or depression
1 = mild dementia
2 = no psychological problems ☐

F1 Body Mass Index (BMI) (weight in kg) / (height in m^2)
0 = BMI less than 19
1 = BMI 19 to less than 21
2 = BMI 21 to less than 23
3 = BMI 23 or greater ☐

IF BMI IS NOT AVAILABLE, REPLACE QUESTION F1 WITH QUESTION F2.
DO NOT ANSWER QUESTION F2 IF QUESTION F1 IS ALREADY COMPLETED.

F2 Calf circumference (CC) in cm
0 = CC less than 31
3 = CC 31 or greater ☐

Screening score ☐☐
(max. 14 points)

12-14 points: Normal nutritional status
8-11 points: At risk of malnutrition
0-7 points: Malnourished

For a more in-depth assessment, complete the full MNA® which is available at **www.mna-elderly.com**

Ref.   Vellas B, Villars H, Abellan G, et al. *Overview of the MNA® - Its History and Challenges*. J Nutr Health Aging 2006;10:456-465.
Rubenstein LZ, Harker JO, Salva A, Guigoz Y, Vellas B. *Screening for Undernutrition in Geriatric Practice: Developing the Short-Form Mini Nutritional Assessment (MNA-SF)*. J. Geront 2001;56A: M366-377.
Guigoz Y. *The Mini-Nutritional Assessment (MNA®) Review of the Literature - What does it tell us?* J Nutr Health Aging 2006; 10:466-487.
® Société des Produits Nestlé, S.A., Vevey, Switzerland, Trademark Owners
© Nestlé, 1994, Revision 2009. N67200 12/99 10M
For more information: www.mna-elderly.com

FIGURE 18-2 The Mini Nutritional Assessment-Short Form (MNA-SF). (From Nestlé Nutrition Services. Copyright Nestlé, 1994, Revision 2009. Available at www.mna-elderly.com.)

If the nursing assessment identifies constipation or risks for constipation, the applicable nursing diagnosis is Constipation. The nursing assessment may also identify certain oral health problems that are common in older adults. These include xerostomia, medication effects, chewing difficulties, periodontal disease, diminished taste sensation, ill-fitting dentures, inadequate oral hygiene, and broken or missing teeth. A relevant nursing diagnosis to address these problems would be Impaired Oral Mucous Membrane.

> **Wellness Opportunity**
>
> Nurses can use the wellness diagnosis of Readiness for Enhanced Nutrition for older adults who express an interest in improving nutritional patterns.

PLANNING FOR WELLNESS OUTCOMES

Nurses can apply the following Nursing Outcomes Classification (NOC) terms to address risk factors and promote improved nutrition in older adults: Appetite, Bowel Elimination, Knowledge: Diet, Nutritional Status, Oral Hygiene, Self-Care: Eating, Sensory Function: Taste and Smell, Swallowing Status, Weight: Body Mass. NOCs related to Constipation include Hydration, Bowel Elimination, Medication Response, and Symptom Control.

> **Wellness Opportunity**
>
> Knowledge: Health Promotion would be the NOC term for older adults who are ready to improve their nutrition to protect themselves from illness.

 ## NURSING INTERVENTIONS TO PROMOTE HEALTHY DIGESTION AND NUTRITION

Nurses can apply the following Nursing Interventions Classification (NIC) terminologies in care plans: Bowel Management, Environmental Management, Health Education, Nutrition Management, Nutritional Counseling, Oral Health Maintenance/Promotion, Referral, Self-Care Assistance, and Weight Management. Nursing interventions to promote healthy digestion and nutrition in older adults include health education about optimal nutrition and disease prevention and direct interventions to eliminate risk factors that interfere with digestion, nutrition, and oral health.

Addressing Risk Factors That Interfere With Digestion and Nutrition

Nursing interventions may be needed to address functional consequences of age-related changes even in healthy older adults. For example, if older adults experience early satiety during meals, they may benefit from eating five smaller meals a day, rather than the customary three meals a day. Similarly, nurses can encourage older adults to maintain a sitting or upright position during eating and for ½ to 1 hour after eating to compensate for any effects of slowed swallowing.

When functional limitations interfere with the activities involved in procuring, preparing, and enjoying food, interventions focus on improving the persons' access to palatable and nutritious meals. For the community-living older adults, this may involve identifying resources that offer assistance in obtaining food. Home-delivered meal programs may be available to older adults at minimal cost, and group meal programs are available in almost every community through the federally funded National Nutrition Program for the Elderly, established under the Older Americans Act. Studies found that formal meal programs are effective in reducing nutritional risk for community-living older adults (Kamp et al, 2010). In addition to providing inexpensive and nutritionally balanced meals, these programs provide opportunities for social interaction. Local offices on aging may provide assistance with transportation or grocery shopping and are an excellent source of information about group and home-delivered meal programs. When environmental barriers, such as high cupboards, interfere with older adults' ability to prepare meals safely, environmental modifications can be made. Nurses can apply many of the environmental adaptations suggested in the chapters on vision (see Chapter 17) and mobility (see Chapter 22) to improve the ability of older persons to prepare meals. When older adults have functional impairments nurses can suggest specially adapted items for improving independence in eating and food preparation, such as the ones illustrated in Figure 18-3.

In long-term care settings, nurses can use the following interventions to address risk factors:

- Plan seating arrangements in the dining area to improve social interaction and to minimize the negative effects of disruptive people.
- Use low- or no-sodium flavor enhancers (e.g., herbs and lemon).
- Provide good oral hygiene before meals.
- Provide easy access to fluids and nutritious snacks.

When older adults are misinformed about constipation, or when other risk factors (e.g., a low-fiber diet) interfere with good bowel function, nursing interventions are directed toward education. Daily use of bran cereals or bran mixed with other foods is a common and effective strategy for preventing constipation. Box 18-5 identifies some of the foods and other interventions that aid in preventing constipation.

> **Wellness Opportunity**
>
> Nurses try to find "teachable moments" so they can correct any myths or misconceptions associated with unhealthy eating patterns.

When medications affect nutrition and digestion, nurses, caregivers, or older adults can discuss this problem with prescribing health care practitioners to identify ways of alleviating this risk or addressing the consequences. If over-the-counter medications have a detrimental effect on nutrition or digestion, nurses educate older adults about medication–nutrient interactions and discuss ways of addressing the negative

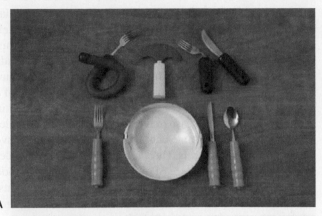

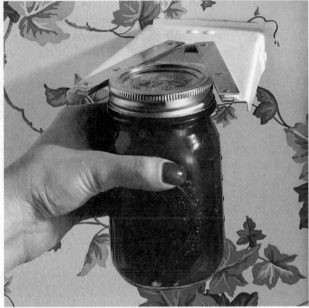

FIGURE 18-3 Examples of adapted equipment for improved independence in eating and food preparation: (**A**) Assistive feeding devices help to grasp and get food on the utensils. (**B**) Wall-mounted jar opener. (Courtesy of ActiveForever.com)

Box 18-5 Health Education Regarding Constipation

- A bowel movement every day is not necessarily the norm for every adult.
- Each adult has an individual pattern of bowel regularity, with the normal range varying from 3 times a day to 2 times a week.
- Include several portions of the following high-fiber foods in your daily diet: fresh, uncooked fruits and vegetables; bran and other cereal products made from whole grains.
- Drink 8 to 10 glasses of noncaffeinated liquid, including fruit juices, every day.
- Avoid laxatives and enemas.
- If medication is needed to promote bowel regularity, a bulk-forming agent (e.g., psyllium or methylcellulose) is least likely to have detrimental effects, especially if fluid intake is adequate.
- Do not ignore the urge to defecate; try to respond as soon as you feel the urge.
- Exercise regularly.

effects. Pharmacists help by suggesting interventions that will compensate for, or minimize, the effects of both prescription and over-the-counter medications on nutrition and digestion.

When alcohol consumption interferes with nutrition, interventions might address the potential problem of alcoholism, or they may be aimed at compensating for the detrimental effects on nutrition. Nurses can recommend vitamin supplementation for people with a history of alcoholism after a medical evaluation has been performed to identify any underlying conditions, such as pernicious anemia.

Promoting Oral and Dental Health

Nurses have important responsibilities in implementing interventions to promote oral and dental health. If older adults have avoided dental care because of resignation to poor oral health or a poor understanding of the need for preventive dental care, nurses attempt to change these attitudes through education. Nurses also emphasize the importance of obtaining dental care every 6 months and, if appropriate, facilitate referrals for dental care. For homebound older adults, home dental services are often available, especially in large urban communities. In addition, low-cost dental services and dentures may be available through schools of dentistry. Nurses need to be familiar with local resources, so that they can inform older adults and their caregivers about the dental services that are available in their community. In long-term care settings, nurses are usually responsible for facilitating referrals for dental care every 6 months. For older adults in any setting, if xerostomia interferes with digestion or nutrition, nurses may suggest or facilitate a referral for a medical evaluation to identify disease processes or medication effects that may be contributing factors.

Good oral care is an essential, but often overlooked, component of daily nursing care for dependent older adults. In institutional settings, staff education about oral care, including information about the myths related to oral health and aging, is imperative (O'Connor, 2008). The following evidence-based recommendations related to oral care:

- Use a toothbrush with soft nylon bristles.
- Use toothpaste with fluoride to reduce cavities and prevent periodontal disease.
- Plain foam swabs can be used for edentulous older adults; lemon glycerin swabs are detrimental and should never be used.
- If commercial mouth rinses are used, dilute them with equal amounts of water to diminish the drying effect of the alcohol contained in the mouthwash.
- Brush dentures before placing them in a denture cup, with complete denture care provided in the morning and before bedtime.
- People with gastrostomy tubes require mouth care every 4 hours; care includes clearing the tongue to prevent buildup of mucus.
- Chlorhexidine (e.g., Peridex) is recommended for debilitated patients at risk for oral fungal infections, dental decay, and gingivitis, but it is used only under the direction of a dentist.

For independent older adults, nurses provide health education about oral care, including alleviation of dry mouth if this is pertinent, as described in Box 18-6. Older adults who have any impairment of manual dexterity can adapt handles of toothbrushes for ease of use or obtain specially designed brushes to increase the self-care abilities. Nurses can also suggest the use of battery-operated brushes, which are effective, easy to use, and relatively inexpensive. Child-size toothbrushes (manual or automatic) may be easier to use for dependent older adults, especially if access to all their teeth is limited.

> ### ◆ Wellness Opportunity
>
> Nurses promote independence and self-care in oral hygiene by facilitating referrals for occupational therapy for older adults with functional impairments.

Promoting Optimal Nutrition and Preventing Disease

Therapeutic diets have long been recognized as essential interventions for diseases, such as diabetes and cardiovascular conditions, and in recent years, there is increasing recognition of the role nutrients play in preventing disease. Nutritional interventions for healthy aging emphasize the inclusion of foods containing antioxidants and other nutrients that may play a protective and preventive role. For example, there is strong support from longitudinal studies that a diet rich in antioxidants and omega-3 fatty acids prevents age-related macular degeneration (Montgomery et al., 2010; Raniga & Elder, 2009; Parekh et al., 2009). In analyzing information about nutrients as preventive interventions, distinctions must be made between nutrients obtained from foods and those that are found in supplements. For example, a high dietary intake of a particular nutrient (e.g., carotenoids) may be beneficial in health promotion or disease prevention, but a dietary supplement product with the same nutrient may not necessarily have the same beneficial effects. Thus, nurses need to educate older adults about the importance of obtaining nutrients from food sources rather than relying primarily on dietary supplements.

Nurses teach older adults about basic nutritional requirements, using easy-to-understand educational materials. Current recommendations for older adults, according to national dietary guidelines published by the Federal Interagency Forum on Aging-Related Statistics (2008), are that older adults need to:

- increase their intakes of whole grains, dried peas and beans, all types of fruits and vegetables (especially dark green and orange vegetables), and fat-free or low-fat milk and milk products;
- replace solid fats with oils, including those in fish, nuts, and seeds;
- consume less sodium and saturated fat; and
- consume less food and beverages with added sugar, solid fats, and alcohol.

 Box 18-6 Health Education Regarding Oral and Dental Care

Health Education Regarding Care of the Teeth and Gums

- Oral care should include daily use of dental floss and twice-daily brushing of all tooth surfaces.
- Use a soft-bristled toothbrush and fluoridated toothpaste.
- If you have any limitations that interfere with your ability to use a regular toothbrush, you may benefit from using an electric or battery-powered brush or a brush with a specially designed handle (available where medical supplies are sold).
- Easy-to-use floss aids are inexpensive and widely available for facilitating dental flossing; they are especially helpful for people with any limitations in manual strength or dexterity or limited range of motion in the upper extremities.
- Some mouth rinses have cleansing, antimicrobial, and moisturizing effect, but they are used in conjunction with, not instead of, brushing.
- Avoid using alcohol-containing mouthwashes because of their drying effect.
- Because sugar is a major contributing factor to tooth decay, it is important to limit the intake of sugary substances, especially substances that are kept in the mouth for long periods (e.g., gum, hard candy).
- After eating sugar-containing foods, rinse your mouth or brush your teeth.
- Visit a dentist every 6 months for regular oral care.
- If partial or complete dentures are worn, remove them at night, keep them in water, and clean them before placing them back in your mouth.

Health Education Regarding Dry Mouth

- Excessive dry mouth may be caused by medical conditions or medication effects and should be evaluated before symptomatic treatment is initiated.
- Drink at least 10 to 12 glasses of noncaffeinated fluid during the day, and drink sips of water at frequent intervals.
- Suck on xylitol-flavored fluoride tablets or sugar-free hard candies to stimulate saliva flow.
- Chew sugar-free gum with xylitol for 15 minutes after meals to stimulate saliva flow and promote oral hygiene.
- Try using one of the many brands of saliva substitutes available at drugstores, but avoid those that contain sorbitol because this can worsen the condition.
- Avoid sucking lozenges containing citric acid because of their detrimental effects on tooth enamel.
- Avoid alcohol, alcohol-containing mouthwashes, and highly acidic drinks (e.g., orange or grapefruit juice) because these tend to exacerbate the condition.
- Avoid smoking because this exacerbates the symptoms and further irritates the oral mucous membranes.
- Pay particular attention to oral hygiene because a dry mouth increases the risk for gum and dental diseases.
- Maintain optimal room humidity, especially at night.

Box 18-7 Guidelines for Daily Food Intake for Older Adults

- Because older adults need fewer calories but the same amount of nutrients, it is important to select a variety of high-quality foods and avoid "empty calories."
- Use salt, sugar, and sodium only in moderation.
- Avoid saturated fats and replace solid fats with oils, including those in fish, nuts, and seeds.
- Choose foods rich in fiber.
- Drink plenty of liquids without added sugars.
- Basic nutritional requirements will be met if the daily diet includes at least the minimum number of servings from each food group listed below and if it includes complex carbohydrates and high-fiber foods. Basic nutritional requirements are as follows:

Servings and Food Group

6–9	Bread, rice, pasta, and cereal
3–4	Vegetables
2–3	Fruits
2–3	Meat, fish, poultry, or legumes (dried peas and beans, lentils, nut butters, soy products)
2–3	Non-fat or low-fat milk, cheese, yogurt, and dairy desserts 8 or more 8-ounce glasses of water or other fluids that are low in added sugars

Healthy older adults generally maintain optimal nutritional status through the daily intake of the foods listed in Box 18-7 and illustrated in Figure 18-4. If older adults have any illness or take any medications or chemicals that interfere with homeostasis, digestion, or nutrition, the daily diet will have to be modified to compensate for these effects. If, for any reason, the food intake is inadequate to meet daily nutritional requirements, older adults can be encouraged to use a broad-spectrum vitamin and mineral supplement. Studies indicate that older adults who take multivitamin/mineral supplements are less likely to be deficient in the following nutrients: vitamins B_6 and C, folate, zinc, and magnesium (men and women); and vitamins A and E (men only) (Marra & Boyar, 2009).

Wellness Opportunity

Nurses promote personal responsibility by suggesting that older adults use the modified food guide pyramid shown in Figure 18-4 to identify beneficial and detrimental eating patterns.

Nutrition education can be provided on an individual basis or in group settings, perhaps with registered dietitians. In acute care settings, registered dietitians are usually available, but their services are often limited to people who have special dietary needs or an identified nutritional problem. In long-term care settings, a registered dietitian generally assesses the nutritional needs and usual eating patterns of older adults and establishes a plan of care aimed at attaining and maintaining optimal nutrition. In commu-

nity settings, nurses sometimes provide nutrition education to groups of older adults. Nurses making home visits include nutrition education in their health teaching, make referrals for registered dietitian assessment and recommendations, and use available community resources to supplement these interventions. Nurses can use the Transtheoretical Model (discussed in Chapter 5) as an effective approach to working with older adults toward improved nutrition and changes in eating patterns (Wright, Velicer, & Prochaska, 2009).

*M*rs. D. returns for a "Counseling for Health" follow-up session with a 7-day diet history and a list of her medications, as you requested. You review the diet history and find that in response to your previous health education about constipation, Mrs. D. now uses whole-wheat bread instead of white and eats more fresh fruits and vegetables. You assess that her daily intake is only approximately 800 calories, of which pastries account for a high percentage. She rarely eats meat, perhaps because of the poor condition of her teeth. Her medications include citalopram (Celexa) 20 mg daily; clonidine (Catapres) 0.2 mg daily; and triamterene 37.5 mg/hydrochlorothiazide 25 mg (Dyazide) daily.

THINKING POINTS

- What specific risk factors do you address in your health teaching interventions?
- What health teaching would you give about alleviating risk factors?
- What interventions would you suggest to improve Mrs. D.'s nutrition?
- What interventions would you suggest to address Mrs. D.'s dry mouth (which you noticed during Mrs. D.'s last visit)?
- What health teaching would you provide about oral and dental care?

EVALUATING EFFECTIVENESS OF NURSING INTERVENTIONS

Nursing care for older adults with Imbalanced Nutrition: Less than Body Requirements is evaluated by determining whether older adults have a daily nutrient intake that corresponds with metabolic needs and by older adults' achieving a body weight within 110% of their ideal body weight. For older adults with constipation, or risks for constipation, evaluation criteria would depend on their verbalizing accurate information about constipation, identifying the factors that contribute to constipation, and reporting that they pass soft stools on a regular basis without any straining or discomfort.

Modified MyPyramid for Older Adults

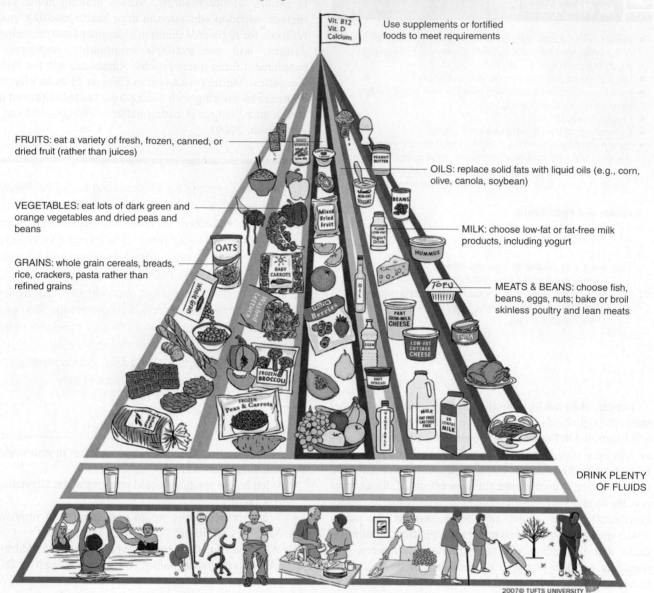

Vit. B12
Vit. D
Calcium

Use supplements or fortified
foods to meet requirements

FRUITS: eat a variety of fresh, frozen, canned, or
dried fruit (rather than juices)

OILS: replace solid fats with liquid oils (e.g., corn,
olive, canola, soybean)

VEGETABLES: eat lots of dark green and
orange vegetables and dried peas and
beans

MILK: choose low-fat or fat-free milk
products, including yogurt

GRAINS: whole grain cereals, breads,
rice, crackers, pasta rather than
refined grains

MEATS & BEANS: choose fish,
beans, eggs, nuts; bake or broil
skinless poultry and lean meats

DRINK PLENTY
OF FLUIDS

BE ACTIVE with lots of enjoyable physical activity: walk, dance, garden, play

2007© TUFTS UNIVERSITY

FIGURE 18-4 The modified food guide pyramid for people aged 70+ years. (Available at http://nutrition.tufts.edu. Courtesy of Tufts University.)

M r. D. is an 85-year-old widower who was referred for home care after a hospitalization in the Acute Care for the Elderly (ACE) unit for congestive heart failure. During the hospitalization, the geriatric assessment team diagnosed protein-energy undernutrition because Mr. D.'s weight (116 lb) is only 75% of his ideal body weight (155 lb). In addition, laboratory work revealed the following abnormal values: hemoglobin, 11%; hematocrit, 35%; and serum albumin, 3.2 g/dL. Mr. D.'s congestive heart failure is stable, and he ambulates with a walker but is very weak. In addition to orders pertaining to assessment and management of the newly diagnosed congestive heart failure, home care orders include nursing assessment of his home situation, nutrition education, and monitoring of weight. The geriatric assessment team in the ACE unit, which included a registered dietitian, recommended that Mr. D. have a daily intake of 1600 calories, including a minimum of 60 g of protein (240 calories). Mr. D. could meet this goal if his daily intake included the minimum number of servings from each food group as listed in Box 18-7.

NURSING ASSESSMENT

Mr. D. lives alone in a senior high-rise apartment and, until recently, participated in social activities and took advantage of van transportation to get to medical appointments and the grocery store. He used to prepare his own meals and shop for his groceries once a week but has not been out of his apartment in the past month because of gradually increasing weakness, shortness of breath, and swelling in his legs. After his health began declining, a neighbor began doing his grocery shopping. Typical meals are toast and coffee for breakfast; canned soup, a lunch meat sandwich, and cookies for lunch; and a Budget Gourmet entree for supper. Mr. D. says that he never really learned to cook very well but that he got along "well enough for a man my age." He says that he does not particularly enjoy the convenience foods that he eats but states, "They sure are easy to fix, even if they are boring."

Mr. D. acknowledges that he has thought about going to the daily noon meal offered at a nearby church but has not followed through because "the senior van doesn't go there, but it does go to the grocery store. Besides, I'm never very hungry because food just doesn't interest me the way it used to when I had Magda's good Hungarian cooking." Mr. D. reports a gradual weight loss of approximately 50 lb since his wife died 2 years ago. He says that he was too heavy when his wife used to do the cooking, so he is not concerned about his weight loss. He has full dentures but has not used them for the past year because they do not fit well anymore. He has not done anything about his dentures because he manages to chew the kinds of food he buys. In addition, his dentist retired 2 years ago, and he has not considered going to a new one.

NURSING DIAGNOSIS

One of the nursing diagnoses that you address in your home care plan is Altered Nutrition: Less than Body Requirements, related to social isolation, declining health, ill-fitting dentures, and lack of enjoyment of food. You also question whether depression may be a contributing factor. Evidence comes from his low body weight, laboratory data consistent with poor nutritional status, and his descriptions of his eating and food preparation patterns.

NURSING CARE PLAN FOR MR. D.

Expected Outcome	Nursing Interventions	Nursing Evaluation
Mr. D. will state what his daily needs are for each food group.	• Give Mr. D. a copy of Box 18-7 and use it as a basis for teaching about daily nutrient requirements.	• Mr. D. will describe an eating pattern that meets his daily nutritional needs.
Mr. D. will identify a method for meeting his nutrient needs.	• Gain Mr. D.'s permission to arrange for home health aide assistance three times weekly for meal preparation and grocery shopping.	• Mr. D. will describe an acceptable plan for meeting his nutritional needs.
	• Explore with Mr. D. various options for broadening his food selection to improve his nutritional intake (e.g., including dairy products and more fruits and vegetables).	• Mr. D. will gain between 0.5 and 1 lb weekly until he reaches the goal of 150 lb.
	• Develop a meal plan with Mr. D. that includes foods that he enjoys but are not currently part of his diet. Discuss the nutritional value of these foods and suggest that he add new food items in each of the food group categories in which he is deficient.	
Mr. D. will have his dentures evaluated and modified or replaced.	• Discuss with Mr. D. the importance of dentures in chewing efficiency and food enjoyment.	• Mr. D. will chew his food with dentures that fit properly.
	• Discuss the long-term detrimental effects of lack of dentures.	
	• Explore ways of obtaining a dental evaluation	

THINKING POINTS

- What risk factors are likely to be contributing to Mr. D.'s gradual weight loss during the past 2 years?

- What further assessment information would you want to have?

Chapter Highlights

Age-Related Changes That Affect Digestion and Eating Patterns
- Diminished senses of smell and taste
- Less efficient chewing
- Decreased saliva secretion
- Degenerative changes in all structures of the gastrointestinal tract

Age-Related Changes in Nutritional Requirements
- Calories: need less quantity, better quality
- Protein: minimum daily intake of 1.0 to 1.2 g/kg of body weight
- Fiber: 25 to 38 g/day
- Fat: no more than 10% to 30% of daily caloric intake

Risk Factors That Affect Digestion and Nutrition
- Poor oral care (Box 18-1)
- Conditions that can lead to nutritional deficiencies (Table 18-1)
- Functional impairments and disease processes
- Dysphagia (Evidence-Based Practice box)
- Effects of medications (Table 18-2)
- Psychosocial factors (e.g., dementia, depression, loneliness)
- Cultural and socioeconomic factors (Cultural Considerations Box 18-1)
- Environmental factors (e.g., noisy or unpleasant environment in institutional setting)
- Behaviors based on myths and misunderstandings (e.g., overuse of laxatives)

Functional Consequences Affecting Digestion and Nutrition
- Diminished ability to procure, prepare, and enjoy food
- Changes in oral function
- Changes in nutrition needs and weight changes (Figure 18-1)
- Effects on quality of life

Pathologic Condition Affecting Digestive Wellness
- Constipation: two or fewer bowel movements weekly, or hard, dry feces

Nursing Assessment of Digestion and Nutrition (Figure 18-2, Boxes 18-2 through 18-4)
- Usual nutrient intake and eating patterns
- Risks that interfere with any aspect of obtaining, preparing, eating, and enjoying food
- Physical examination and laboratory data regarding nutritional status
- The Mini Nutritional Assessment tool

Nursing Diagnosis
- Readiness for Enhanced Nutrition
- Altered Nutrition: Less than Body Requirements
- Constipation
- Impaired Oral Mucous Membrane

Planning for Wellness Outcomes
- Improved: appetite, nutritional status, oral hygiene, depression level
- Self-care: eating, oral hygiene
- Increased knowledge about diet, improved health beliefs about constipation

Nursing Interventions to Promote Healthy Digestion and Nutrition (Figures 18-2 and 18-4, Boxes 18-5 through 18-7)
- Teaching older adults about nutrition and digestion
- Applying daily food guide to older adults
- Promoting oral and dental health
- Referring for community resources (e.g., home-delivered meals, group meal programs)

Evaluating Effectiveness of Nursing Interventions
- Daily nutrient intake that corresponds to metabolic needs
- Achieving/maintaining body weight within 110% of ideal body weight for the individual
- Achieving/maintaining regular bowel elimination

Critical Thinking Exercises

1. Discuss specific ways in which each of the following conditions might influence the eating patterns of older adults: depression, medications, sensory changes, cognitive impairments, functional impairments, economic factors, social circumstances, and oral health factors.
2. Describe at least three characteristics of eating patterns for each of the following cultural groups: Native Americans, Hispanic Americans, African Americans, and Asian Americans.
3. How would you assess digestion and nutrition for an older adult in each of the following settings: home, long-term care facility, and acute care facility?
4. Outline a health education plan for teaching older adults about constipation. Include the following points: definition of constipation, risk factors for constipation, and interventions to prevent and address constipation.
5. Outline a health education plan for teaching older adults about oral and dental care.

Resources

For links to these resources and additional helpful Internet resources related to this chapter, visit the Point at http://thePoint.lww.com/Miller6e.

Clinical Tools

American Journal of Nursing and Hartford Institute for Geriatric Nursing, *How to Try This,* articles and videos
- Stockdell, R., & Amella, E. J. (2008). The Edinburgh Feeding Evaluation in Dementia Scale: Determining how much help people with dementia need at mealtime. *American Journal of Nursing, 108*(8), 46–54.
- DiMaria-Ghalili, R. A., & Guenter, P. A. (2008). The Mini Nutritional Assessment. *American Journal of Nursing, 108*(2), 50–59.

Hartford Institute for Geriatric Nursing, *Try This: Best Practices in Nursing Care to Older Adults*
- Issue 9 (2007), Assessing nutrition in older adults
- Issue 20 (2007), Preventing aspiration in older adults with dysphagia
- Issue D11.1 2007), Eating and feeding issues in older adults with dementia, Part I: Assessment
- Issue D 11.2 (2007), Eating and feeding issues in older adults with dementia: Part II: Interventions

Evidence-Based Practice

Amella, E. J. (2008). Mealtime difficulties. In E. Capezuti, D. Zwicker, M. Mezey, & T. Fulmer (Eds.), *Evidence-Based Geriatric Nursing Protocols for Best Practice* (3rd ed., pp. 337–351). New York: Springer Publishing Co.

DiMaria-Ghalili, R. A. (2008). Nutrition. In E. Capezuti, D. Zwicker, M. Mezey, & T. Fulmer (Eds.), *Evidence-Based Geriatric Nursing Protocols for Best Practice* (3rd ed., pp. 353–367). New York: Springer Publishing Co.

Mentes, J. C. (2008). Managing oral hydration. In E. Capezuti, D. Zwicker, M. Mezey, & T. Fulmer (Eds.), *Evidence-Based Geriatric Nursing Protocols for Best Practice* (3rd ed., pp. 369–390). New York: Springer Publishing Co.

O'Connor, L. J. (2008). Oral health care. In E. Capezuti, D. Zwicker, M. Mezey, & T. Fulmer (Eds.), *Evidence-Based Geriatric Nursing Protocols for Best Practice* (3rd ed., pp. 391–402). New York: Springer Publishing Co.

Health Education

American Dietetic Association
Canadian Council of Food and Nutrition
Food and Drug Administration
Food and Nutrition Information Center
Mini Nutritional Assessment
National Dairy Council
National Oral Health Information Clearinghouse

REFERENCES

Allen, L. H. (2009). How common is vitamin B-12 deficiency? *The American Journal of Clinical Nutrition, 89*(Suppl.), 693S–696S.

Boczko, F., McKeon, S., & Sturkie, D. (2009). Long-term care and oral health knowledge. *Journal of American Directors Association, 10,* 204–206.

Bouras, E. P., & Tangalos, E. G. (2009). Chronic constipation in the elderly. *Gastroenterological Clinics of North America, 38,* 463–480.

Bowman, S. A. (2009). Socioeconomic characteristics, dietary and lifestyle patterns, and health and weight status of older adults in NHANES, 1999–2002: A comparison of Caucasians and African Americans. *Journal of Nutrition and the Elderly, 28*(1), 30–46.

Burnett-Hartman, A. N., Fitzpatrick, A. L., Gao, K., Jackson, S. A., & Schreiner, P. J. (2009). Supplement use contributes to meeting recommended dietary intakes for calcium, magnesium, and vitamin C in four ethnicities of middle-aged and older Americans: The Multi-Ethnic Study of Atherosclerosis. *Journal of the American Dietetic Association, 109,* 422–429.

Buyckx, M. E. (2009). Hydration and human health: Critical issues update. *Nutrition Today, 44*(1), 6–7.

Chen, C. C.-H. (2007). The Kayser-Jones Brief Oral Health Status Examinations (BOHSE). *Try this: Best Practices in Nursing Care to Older Adults.* The Hartford Foundation for Geriatric Nursing. Retrieved from http:consultgerirn.org

Cook, I. J. (2009). Oropharyngeal dysphagia. *Gastroenterology Clinics of North America, 38,* 411–431.

Dahm, C. C., Keogh, R. H., Spencer, E. A., Greenwood, D. C., Key, T. J., Fentiman, I. S., . . . Rodwell Bingham, S. A. (2010). Dietary fiber and colorectal cancer risk: A nested case-control study using food diaries. *Journal of the National Cancer Institute, 102*(9), 614–626.

DiMaria-Ghalili, R. A., & Guenter, P. A. (2008). The Mini Nutritional Assessment. *American Journal of Nursing, 108*(2), 50–54.

Doty, R. L. (2009). The olfactory system and its disorders. *Seminars in Neurology, 29*(1), 74–81.

Du, H., Van Der A, D. L., Boshuizen, H. C., Forouhi, N. G., Wareham, N. J., Halkjaer, J., . . . Feskens, E. J. (2010). Dietary fiber and subsequent changes in body weight and waist circumference in European men and women. *American Journal of Clinical Nutrition, 91*(2), 329–336.

Federal Interagency Forum on Aging-Related Statistics. (2008). *Older Americans 2008: Key indicators of well-being.* Washington, DC: Government Printing Office.

Flicker, L., McCaul, K. A., Hankey, G. J., Jamrozik, K., Brown, W. J., Byles, J. E., & Almeida, O. P. (2010). Body mass index and survival in men and women aged 70 to 75. *Journal of the American Geriatrics Society, 58*(2), 234–241.

Fulgoni, V. L., III. (2008). Current protein intake in America: Analysis of the National Health and Nutrition Examination Survey, 2003–2004. *American Journal of Clinical Nutrition, 87*(Suppl.), 1554S–1557S.

Gaffney-Stomberg, E., Insogna, K. L., Rodriguez, N. R., & Kerstetter, J. E. (2009). Increasing dietary protein requirements in elderly people for optimal muscle and bone health. *Journal of the American Geriatrics Society, 57*(6), 1073–1079.

Gregersen, H., Pedersen, J., & Drewes, A. M. (2008). Deterioration of muscle function in the human esophagus with age. *Digestive Diseases and Sciences, 53*(12), 3065–3070.

Grieger, J. A., Nowson, C. A., & Ackland, L. M. (2009). Nutritional and functional status indicators in residents of a long-term care facility. *Journal of Nutrition and the Elderly, 28*(1), 47–60.

Haumschild, M. S., & Haumschild, R. J. (2009). The importance of oral health in long-term care. *Journal of American Medical Directors Association, 10,* 667–671.

Hopping, B. N., Erber, E., Grandinetti, A., Verheus, M., Kolonel, L. N., & Maskarinec, G. (2010). Dietary fiber, magnesium, and glycemic load alter risk of type 2 diabetes in a multiethnic cohort in Hawaii. *Journal of Nutrition, 140*(1), 68–74.

Houston, D. K., Nicklas, B. J., & Zizza, C. A. (2009). Weighty concerns: The growing prevalence of obesity among older adults. *Journal of the American Dietetic Association, 109,* 1886–1895.

Hsieh, Y. M., Sung, T. S., & Wan, K. S. (2010). A survey of nutrition and health status of solitary and non-solitary elders in Taiwan. *Journal of Nutrition and Health and Aging, 14*(1), 11–14.

Jablonski, R. A., Munro, C. L., Grap, M. J., Schubert, C. M., Ligon, M., & Spigelmyer, P. (2009). Mouth care in nursing homes: Knowledge, beliefs, and practices of nursing assistants. *Geriatric Nursing, 30*(2), 99–106.

Johansson, L., Sidenvall, B., Malmberg, B., & Christensson, L. (2009). Who will become malnourished? A prospective study of factors associated with malnutrition in older persons living at home. *Journal of Nutrition and Health and Aging, 13*(10), 855–861.

Kaiser, M. J., Bauer, J. M., Ramsch, C., Uter, W., Guigoz, Y., Cederholm, T., . . . Sieber, C. C. (2009). Validation of the mini nutritional assessment short-form (MNA-SF): A practical tool for identification of nutritional status. *Journal of Nutrition and Health and Aging, 13*(9), 782–788.

Kamp, B. J., Wellman, N. S., & Russell, C. (2010). Position of the American Dietetic Association, American Society for Nutrition, and Society for Nutrition education: Food and nutrition programs for community-residing older adults. *Journal of the American Dietetic Association, 110*(3), 463–472.

Kruizenga, H. M., de Vet, H. C., Van Marissing, C. M., Stassen, E. E., Strijk, J. E., Van Bokhorst-de Van Der Schueren, M. A., . . . Visser, M. (2010). The SNAQ(RC), an easy traffic light system as a first step in the recognition of undernutrition in residential care. *Journal of Nutrition and Health, and Aging, 14*(2), 83–89.

Lafreniere, D., & Mann, N. (2009). Anosmia: Loss of smell in the elderly. *Otolaryngology Clinics of North America, 42*, 123–131.

Lam, A., Kiyak, A., Gossett, A. M., & McCormick, L. (2009). Assessment of the use of xerogenic medications for chronic medical and dental conditions among adult day health participants. *The Consultant Pharmacist: The Journal of the American Society of Consultant Pharmacists, 24*(10), 755–764.

Lee, J. S., Fischer, J. G., & Johnson, M. A. (2010). Food insecurity, food and nutrition programs, and aging: Experiences from Georgia. *Journal of Nutrition for the Elderly, 29*(2), 116–149.

Lichtenstein, A. H., Rasmussen, H., Yu, W. W., Epstein, S. R., & Russell, R. M. (2008). Modified MyPyramid for older adults. *The Journal of Nutrition, 138*, 5–11.

Locher, J. L., Ritchie, C. S., Robinson, C. O., Roth, D. L., West, D. S., & Burgio, K. L. (2008). A multidimensional approach to understanding under-eating in homebound older adults: The importance of social factors. *Gerontologist, 48*(2), 223–234.

Maki, K. C., Beiseigel, J. M., Jonnalagadda, S. S., Gugger, C. K., Reeves, M. S., Farmer, M. V., . . . Rains, T. M. (2010). Whole-grain ready-to-eat oat cereal, as part of a dietary program for weight loss, reduces low-density lipoprotein cholesterol in adults with overweight and obesity more than a dietary program including low-fiber control foods. *Journal of the American Dietetic Association, 110*(2), 205–214.

Marra, M. V., & Boyar, A. P. (2009). Position of the American Dietetic Association: Nutrient supplementation. *Journal of the American Dietetic Association, 109*(12), 2073–2085.

McCrea, G. L., Miaskowski, C., Stotts, N. A., Macera, L., & Varma, M. G. (2009). A review of the literature on gender and age differences in the prevalence and characteristics of constipation in North America. *Journal of Pain and Symptom Management, 37*(4), 737–745.

Montgomery, M. P., Kamel, F., Pericak-Vance, M. A., Haines, J. L., Postel, E. A., & Agarwal, A. (2010). Overall diet quality and age-related macular degeneration. *Ophthalmic Epidemiology, 17*(1), 58–65.

Morley, J. E. (2007). The aging gut: Physiology. *Clinics in Geriatric Medicine, 23*, 757–767.

Morley, J. E. (2010). Nutrition and the brain. *Clinics in Geriatric Medicine, 26*, 89–98.

NANDA International. (2009). *Nursing diagnoses: Definitions and classification 2009–2011*. Oxford, England: Wiley-Blackwell.

Ney, D., Weiss, J., Kind, A., & Robinson, J. A. (2009). Senescent swallowing: Impact, strategies and interventions. *Nutrition in Clinical Practice, 24*(3), 395–413.

O'Connor, L. J. (2008). Oral health care. In E. Capezuti, D. Zwicker, M. Mezey, & T. Fulmer (Eds.), *Evidence-based geriatric nursing protocols for best practice* (3rd ed., pp. 391–402). New York: Springer Publishing Co.

Oliveira, M. R. M., Fogaca, K. C. P., & Leandro-Merhi, V. A. (2009). Nutritional status and functional capacity of hospitalized elderly. *Nutrition Journal, 8*(11), 54–62.

Oreopoulos, A., Kalantar-Zadeh, K., Sharma, A. M., & Fonarow, G. C. (2009). The obesity paradox in the elderly: Potential mechanisms and clinical implications. *Clinics in Geriatric Medicine, 25*, 643–659.

Paddon-Jones, D., & Rasmussen, B. B. (2009). Dietary protein recommendations and the prevention of sarcopenia: Protein, amino acid metabolism and therapy. *Current Opinion in Clinical Nutrition and Metabolic Care, 12*(1), 86–90.

Palmer, J. L., & Metheny, N. A. (2008). How to try this: Preventing aspiration in older adults with dysphagia. *American Journal of Nursing, 108*(2), 40–48.

Parekh, N., Voland, R. P., Moeller, S. M., Blodi, B. A., Ritenbaugh, C., Chappell, R. J., . . . Mares, J. A. (2009). Association between dietary fat intake and age-related macular degeneration in the Carotenoids in Age-Related Eye Disease Study (CAREDS): An ancillary study of the Women's Health Initiative. *Archives of Ophthalmology, 127*(11), 1483–1493.

Price, D. M. (2008). Protein-energy malnutrition among the elderly: Implications for nursing care. *Holistic Nursing Practice, 22*(6), 355–360.

Quandt, S. A., Chen, H., Bell, R. A., Savoca, M. R., Anderson, A. M., Leng, X., . . . Arcury, T. A. (2010). Food avoidance and food modification practices of older rural adults: Association with oral health status and implications for service provision. *The Gerontologist, 50*(1), 100–110.

Raniga, A., & Elder, M. J. (2009). Dietary supplement use in the prevention of age-related macular degeneration progression. *New Zealand Medical Journal, 122*(1299), 32–38.

Sahyoun, N. R., Anyanwu, U. O., Sharkey, J. R., & Netterville, L. (2010). Recently hospital-discharged older adults are vulnerable and may be underserved by the Older American Act Nutrition Program. *Journal of Nutrition for the Elderly, 29*(2), 227–240.

Sandhaus, S., Zalon, M., Valenti, D., & Harrell, F. (2009). Promoting evidence-based dysphagia assessment and management by nurses. *Journal of Gerontological Nursing, 35*(6), 20–27.

Savoca, M. R., Arcury, T. A., Leng, X., Bell, R. A., Anderson, A. M., Anderson, A. M., . . . Quandt, S. A. (2010). Severe tooth loss in older adults as a key indicator of compromised dietary quality. *Public Health Nutrition, 13*(4), 466–474.

Skates, J. J., & Anthony, P. (2009). The Mini Nutritional Assessment—An integral part of geriatric assessment. *Nutrition Today, 44*(1), 21–28.

Slavin, J. L. (2008). Position of the American Dietetic Association: Health implications of dietary fiber. *American Dietetic Association, 108*(10), 1761–1731.

Starr, J. M., & Hall, R. (2010). Predictors and correlates of edentulism in healthy older people. *Current Opinion in Clinical Nutrition and Metabolic Care, 13*(1), 19–23.

Tanner, D. C. (2010). Lessons from nursing home dysphagia malpractice litigation. *Journal of Gerontological Nursing, 36*(3), 41–46.

Tsakos, G., Herrick, K., Sheiham, A., & Watt, R. G. (2010). Edentulism and fruit and vegetable intake in low-income adults. *Journal of Dental Research, 89*(5), 462–467.

Turner, M. D., & Ship, J. A. (2007). Dry mouth and its effects on the oral health of elderly people. *Journal of the American Dental Association, 138*(9, Suppl.), 15S–20S.

Uher, R., Farmer, A., Henigsberg, N., Rietschel, M., Mors, O., Maier, W., . . . McGuffin, P. (2009). Adverse reactions to antidepressants. *British Journal of Psychiatry, 195*(3), 202–210.

Visvanathan, R., & Chapman, I. M. (2009). Undernutrition and anorexia in the older person. *Gastroenterology Clinics of North America, 38*, 393–409.

Visvanathan, V., & Nix, P. (2010). Managing the patient presenting with xerostomia: A review. *International Journal of Clinical Practice, 64*(3), 404–407.

Vivanti, A., Harvey, K., & Ash, S. (2010). Developing a quick and practical screen to improve the identification of poor hydration in geriatric and rehabilitative care. *Archives of Gerontology and Geriatrics, 50*(2), 156–164.

Welge-Lussen, A. (2009). Ageing, neurodegeneration, and olfactory and gustatory loss. *B-ENT, 5*(Suppl. 13), 129–132.

Wright, J. A., Velicer, W. F., & Prochaska, J. O. (2009). Testing the predictive power of the transtheoretical model of behavior change applied to dietary fat intake. *Health Education Research, 24*(2), 224–236.

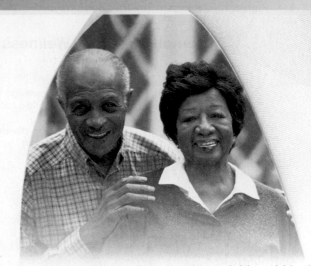

CHAPTER 19

Urinary Function

LEARNING OBJECTIVES

After reading this chapter, you will be able to:

1. List age-related changes that affect the complex processes involved in urinary elimination.

2. Describe risk factors that influence kidney function and urinary elimination.

3. Describe the functional consequences of age-related changes and risk factors related to each of the following aspects of urinary function: the elimination of medications and metabolic wastes, patterns of urinary elimination, and consequences of incontinence for older adults and their caregivers.

4. Define urge, stress, mixed, and functional incontinence.

5. Propose interview questions and describe observations and laboratory data that are used in the nursing assessment of urinary function in older adults.

6. Identify interventions for addressing risk factors that influence urinary elimination and for alleviating and managing incontinence.

KEY POINTS

benign prostatic
  hyperplasia
bladder diary
continence training
mixed urinary
  incontinence
nocturia
overactive bladder (OAB)

pelvic floor dysfunction
pelvic floor muscle training
  (PFMT)
prompted voiding
stress urinary incontinence
urge urinary
  incontinence
urinary incontinence

The primary function of urinary elimination is the excretion of water and chemical wastes, such as metabolic and pharmacologic byproducts, that would become toxic if allowed to accumulate. Efficient urinary excretion depends on renal blood flow, filtering activities within the kidneys, good functioning of the urinary tract muscles, and nervous system control over voluntary and involuntary mechanisms of elimination. Control of urinary elimination also depends on ambulatory and sensory abilities and on social, emotional, cognitive, and environmental factors.

Healthy older adults experience very few functional consequences affecting urinary elimination, but when risk factors are present, negative functional consequences, such as **urinary incontinence**, are common. Urinary incontinence is defined as any involuntary leakage of urine. An important risk factor—and one that can be alleviated through health education interventions—is the false belief that urinary incontinence is an inevitable part of aging. Nurses have many opportunities to improve quality of life for older adults by addressing the risk factors that contribute to urinary incontinence.

 ## AGE-RELATED CHANGES THAT AFFECT URINARY WELLNESS

Age-related changes in the kidneys, bladder, urethra, and control mechanisms in the nervous and other body systems affect the physiologic processes that control urinary elimination. In addition, any age-related change that interferes with the skills involved in socially appropriate urinary elimination can interfere with urinary control. Age-related changes that directly or indirectly affect urinary function and control are discussed in the next two sections.

Changes in the Kidneys

The complex process of urinary excretion begins in the kidneys with the filtering and removal of chemical wastes from the blood. Blood circulates through the glomeruli, where liquid wastes, called *glomerular filtrate*, pass through Bowman's capsule and the renal tubules to the collecting ducts. During this process, substances needed by the body (such as water, glucose, and sodium) are retained, and waste products are excreted in the urine. These functions are important for maintaining homeostasis and excreting many medications. Excretory function, which is measured by the glomerular

Promoting Urinary Wellness in Older Adults

Nursing Assessment

- Attitudes and knowledge
- Usual patterns of fluid intake and voiding
- Risk factors (drugs, diseases, functional limitations)
- Environmental barriers
- Signs and symptoms of urinary dysfunction

Age-Related Changes

- ↓ functioning nephrons
- ↓ renal blood flow
- ↓ elasticity in urinary tract muscles
- Degenerative changes in cerebral cortex

Negative Functional Consequences

- ↓ ability to maintain homeostasis
- ↓ clearance of some drugs
- ↓ bladder capacity
- Urgency
- Chronic residual urine
- Predisposition to urinary incontinence

Risk Factors

- Myths and misperceptions
- Functional impairments
- Environmental barriers
- Diseases (vaginitis, BPH, UTI)
- Medication effects (diuretics)

Nursing Interventions

- Teaching about normal urinary function
- Teaching about preventing and alleviating incontinence
- Managing incontinence

Wellness Outcomes

- Longer intervals of continence
- Self-care practices
- ↑ self-esteem
- Improved quality of life

filtration rate (GFR), depends on the number and efficiency of nephrons and on the amount and rate of renal blood flow.

The kidney increases in weight and mass from birth until early adulthood, when the number of functioning nephrons begins to decline, particularly in the cortex, where the glomeruli are located. This decline continues throughout life, resulting in an approximately 25% decrease in kidney mass by the age of 80 years. The remaining glomeruli undergo various age-related changes such as increased size, diminished lobulation, and thickened basement membrane. In addition, the proportion of sclerotic glomeruli increases from fewer than 5% at the age of 40 years to 35% by the age of 80 years. Beginning in the fourth decade, renal blood flow gradually diminishes, particularly in the cortex, at a rate of 10% per decade.

An average decline in renal function of 1% per year has been widely accepted since the 1970s as a hallmark of aging that begins between the ages of 30 and 40 years. Most studies indicate that a gradual decline in renal function is a normal age-related change and any *substantial* decline in renal function is associated with common pathologic conditions such as hypertension (Glassock & Winearls, 2009; Lerma, 2009).

Renal tubules regulate the dilution and concentration of urine, and subsequent excretion of water from the body, in a diurnal rhythm. The physiologic processes responsible for urine concentration and water excretion are influenced by the following factors:

- The amount of fluid in the body
- Resorption of water through, and transport of substances across, the tubular membrane
- Osmoreceptors in the hypothalamus, which regulate the level of circulating antidiuretic hormone (ADH) according to plasma–water concentration
- Substances and activities that influence ADH secretion, such as caffeine, medications, alcohol, pain, stress, and exercise
- The concentration of sodium in the glomerular filtrate.

Normally, production of ADH is stimulated by hemorrhage, dehydration, and other conditions that affect plasma volume or osmolality. This physiologic protective mechanism helps to maintain plasma volume and conserve fluid and sodium under conditions of water or sodium deprivation.

Many age-related changes affect the renal tubules and thereby affect the dilution and concentration of urine. These changes include fatty degeneration, diverticula, a loss of convoluted cells, and alterations in the composition of the basement membranes. Functionally, the renal tubules in older adults are less efficient in the exchange of substances, the conservation of water, and the suppression of ADH secretion in the presence of hypo-osmolality. Age-related changes also decrease the ability of the older kidney to conserve sodium in response to salt restriction. These age-related changes predispose healthy older adults to hyponatremia and other fluid and electrolyte imbalances, particularly in the presence of any condition that alters renal circulation, water or sodium balance, or plasma volume or osmolality.

Changes in the Bladder and Urinary Tract

After being filtered by the kidneys, liquid wastes pass through the ureters into the bladder for temporary storage. The bladder is a balloon-like structure composed of collagen, smooth muscle (called *detrusor*), and elastic tissue. Liquid wastes are eliminated from the bladder through a complex physiologic process involving the following mechanisms:

- The ability of the bladder to expand for adequate storage and to contract for complete expulsion of liquid wastes
- The maintenance of higher urethral pressure relative to intravesicular pressure
- Regulation of the lower urinary tract through autonomic and somatic nerves
- Voluntary control of urination (micturition) through the cerebral centers.

Age-related changes alter each of these mechanisms and affect urinary function in older adults.

In younger adults, the bladder stores 350 to 450 mL of urine before the person experiences sensations of fullness and discomfort. With increasing age, hypertrophy of the bladder muscle and thickening of the bladder wall interfere with the bladder's ability to expand, limiting the amount of urine that can be stored comfortably to approximately 200 to 300 mL.

As urine flows into the bladder, the smooth muscle expands without increasing intravesical pressure, and the urethral pressure increases to the point that it is slightly higher than the intravesical pressure. As long as the volume of urine does not rise above 500 to 600 mL, this balance can be maintained, and urination can be controlled voluntarily. If the volume rises above this level, or if the detrusor muscle contracts involuntarily, the intravesical pressure will exceed the urethral pressure, and leakage of urine is likely to occur. In addition to the amount of urine in the bladder, the following factors influence the balance between intravesical and urethral pressure:

- Abdominal pressure
- Thickness of the urethral mucosa
- Tone of the pelvic, detrusor, urethral, and bladder neck muscles
- Replacement of the smooth muscle tissue in the bladder and urethra with less elastic connective tissue.

Internal and external sphincters regulate urine storage and bladder emptying. The internal sphincter is part of the base of the bladder and is controlled by autonomic nerves. The external sphincter is part of the pelvic floor musculature and is controlled by the pudendal nerve. When urination takes place, the detrusor and abdominal muscles contract, and the perineal and external sphincter muscles relax. When necessary, the external sphincter contracts to inhibit or interrupt voiding and to compensate for sudden surges in abdominal pressure. Age-related changes involving the loss of smooth muscle in the urethra and the relaxation of the pelvic floor muscles reduce the urethral resistance and diminish the tone of the sphincters.

Changes in Control Mechanisms

Changes in the nervous system and other regulatory systems affect urinary function. For example, motor impulses in the spinal cord control urination, but higher centers in the brain are responsible for detecting the sensation of bladder fullness, for inhibiting bladder emptying when necessary, and for stimulating bladder contractions for complete emptying. As the bladder fills, sensory receptors in the bladder wall send a signal to the sacral spinal cord. In healthy older adults, degenerative changes in the cerebral cortex may alter both the sensation of bladder fullness and the ability to empty the bladder completely. In younger adults, a sensation of fullness begins when the bladder is about half full. This sensation occurs at a later point for older adults, so the interval between the initial perception of the urge to void and the actual need to empty the bladder is shortened, which may trigger an episode of incontinence.

Many structures involved in urination contain estrogen receptors and are affected by hormonal changes, particularly those that occur in menopausal women. For example, diminished estrogen causes a loss of tone, strength, and collagen support in the urogenital tissues and can contribute to a decrease in urethral closure pressure, which predisposes to urinary leakage problems. Also, because nerve endings depend on estrogen, diminished estrogen increases sensitivity to irritating stimuli, which leads to an increased urge to void. The decline in estrogen associated with menopause may partially account for the increased prevalence and earlier onset of incontinence in women.

Diminished thirst perception is another age-related change that can affect homeostasis and urinary function. Healthy older adults who are deprived of fluid do not sense thirst, experience discomfort from dry mouth, or drink enough water to rehydrate themselves. With conditions that place additional demands on fluid and electrolyte balance, such as fever or infection, diminished thirst sensation can interfere with the mechanisms that normally compensate for these physiologic stresses. Consequently, older people are likely to be at increased risk of dehydration because of inadequate fluid intake.

Changes Affecting Control Over Socially Appropriate Urinary Elimination

Control over urination depends not only on the functioning of the urinary tract and nervous system, but also on the factors that influence a person's capacity for socially appropriate urinary elimination. Some internal and external conditions that affect these skills are

- Cognition, balance, mobility, coordination, visual function, manual dexterity
- Identification of a designated receptacle in a private area
- Accessibility and acceptability of toilet facilities
- Ability to get to and use a suitable receptacle
- The interval between the perception of the urge to void and the actual need to empty the bladder
- Voluntary control over the urge to void from the time of its perception until the person is able to use an appropriate receptacle.

These factors are influenced by age-related changes that directly affect urinary elimination, as well as by those changes that affect the ability to identify and reach appropriate toilet facilities. For example, increased postural sway is an age-related change that can interfere with one's ability to stand still. With increasing postural sway, older men may find it more difficult to maintain a standing position for urination.

Standards for socially appropriate urinary elimination may vary according to different social environments. For example, an independent, community-living older adult is expected to remain free of urinary odors or wetness and to urinate in private, designated places; however, a dependent or institutionalized older adult may not be expected to adhere so strictly to these standards. In any setting, the attitudes and behaviors of caregivers can significantly influence patterns of urinary elimination, as discussed in the following section on risk factors.

 ## RISK FACTORS THAT AFFECT URINARY WELLNESS

As with many other areas of functioning, risk factors play a more significant role than age-related changes in causing negative functional consequences for urinary function. This is particularly true with regard to urinary incontinence, as discussed in that section. Factors that can significantly affect urinary function overall include behaviors based on myths and misunderstandings, functional impairments, disease processes, and environmental and lifestyle influences.

Behaviors Based on Myths and Misunderstandings

Attitudes based on myths or lack of knowledge about urinary function can have a detrimental effect on the behavior of older adults and their caregivers. For example, the perception of urinary incontinence as an inevitable consequence of aging deters older adults from seeking help from healthcare professionals. Primary care practitioners often reinforce these misperceptions and fail to ask about incontinence, even though approximately 80% of people with urinary incontinence can be cured or improved (Wound, Ostomy and Continence Nurses Society, 2009). Cultural factors may also influence perceptions and help-seeking behaviors. For example, one study found that older Korean American women do not seek help for urinary incontinence because they may see it as a family problem rather than an individual's problem (Kang & Crogan, 2008). Another study found that approximately 80% of women from a Middle Eastern culture did not seek help for incontinence because of embarrassment and because they assumed that this was a normal part of aging (El-Azab & Shaaban, 2010). Because of such attitudes of resignation, early signs and symptoms of urinary dysfunction may be managed inappropriately, and the problem may progress.

Attitudes, behaviors, and expectations of caregivers may also interfere with the approach to urinary incontinence in older adults. For instance, when episodes of incontinence are noted soon after the admission of the older adult to a long-term care facility, some nursing staff members are likely to view the resident as having chronic incontinence, and their subsequent behaviors may reinforce the expectation of incontinence. In reality, the episode of incontinence may have occurred because the toilet is too far away or the older adult could not readily locate it. When staff members assume that incontinence is the norm for that person, they might initiate use of absorbent products by the resident, giving the older adult the message that voluntary control over urination is not expected.

In acute and long-term care settings, staff attitudes and nursing procedures strongly influence the standards for urinary elimination. In acute care facilities, indwelling catheters are often inserted in the emergency room or during surgical procedures, and they often remain in place unnecessarily. One study found that a nursing protocol, which allowed nurses to discontinue the use of unnecessary indwelling catheters resulted in a 67.7% reduction of overall catheter days (from 136 to 44) (Voss, 2009). In recent years, the use of indwelling catheters in long-term care facilities has been reduced because of stricter federal regulations about this as a quality of care issue (Rogers et al., 2008). In any setting, caregivers or staff may encourage the use of pads or other incontinence products because this is easier and more convenient than assisting the older adult to get to the bathroom. In these situations, dependent older adults are likely to behave according to the expectations of the caregivers, and incontinence will be the inevitable consequence.

Limited fluid intake in response to the fear or onset of incontinence—or for any reason—is another behavior that can unintentionally exacerbate incontinence. If bladder fullness is not adequately achieved, as in states of dehydration or limited fluid intake, the neurologic mechanism that controls bladder emptying will not function effectively, and incontinence can occur because the person does not perceive the urge to void. Dehydration and inadequate hydration also cause increased bladder irritability, with subsequent uninhibited contractions and incontinence.

> **◆ Wellness Opportunity**
>
> Nurses should examine their own attitudes and behaviors about incontinence to be sure they are based on accurate information rather than on misperceptions or ageist perspectives that could blind them to opportunities to promote urinary wellness.

Functional Impairments

Functional impairments are a major risk factor for the development of incontinence because they can interfere with the ability to recognize and respond to the urge to void in a timely manner. With age-related changes that shorten the interval between the perception of the urge to void and the actual need to empty the bladder, any delay in reaching an appropriate receptacle can result in incontinence. Thus, dependency in performing activities of daily living (ADLs) for any reason is strongly associated with incontinence. Conditions such as arthritis or Parkinson's disease may slow the ambulation of older adults as well as their ability to manipulate clothing. Likewise, dementia and other conditions that impair cognitive abilities can interfere with the timely processing of information that is necessary for maintaining voluntary control over urination. Finally, restraints can cause significant functional limitations and increase the risk for developing incontinence.

Pathologic Conditions

Disease processes that commonly increase the risk of urinary incontinence in older adults include those that involve the urinary tract and supporting structures and those that affect other systems and cause incontinence through indirect effects. Most of the conditions that affect the urinary tract are gender-specific, whereas conditions that affect other systems can affect all older adults.

Conditions of the Genitourinary Tract

Pelvic floor dysfunction (i.e., weakening or stretching of pelvic floor muscles) in women can cause pelvic organ prolapse—a condition in which part of the vaginal wall bulges. Studies identified obesity, increased age, and a high number of vaginal births as risk factors for this condition (Sung & Hampton, 2009). Pelvic floor dysfunction can lead to urinary frequency and incontinence because it interferes with the complete emptying of the bladder, resulting in residual urine and an increased risk of bacteriuria. Pelvic floor muscles are also affected by degenerative changes associated with the age-related decrease in estrogen levels. This can cause atrophy of the vaginal and trigonal tissue with subsequent diminished resistance to pathogens. Vaginitis and trigonitis may develop and cause urinary urgency, frequency, and incontinence.

Benign prostatic hyperplasia (i.e., enlarged prostate) is a common cause of voiding problems in older men, while prostatic carcinoma is a less common cause. In its early stage, prostatic hyperplasia obstructs the vesical neck and compresses the urethra, causing a compensatory hypertrophy of the detrusor muscle and subsequent outlet obstruction. With progressive hypertrophy, the bladder wall loses its elasticity and becomes thinner. Subsequently, urine retention occurs, increasing the risk of bacteriuria and infection. Eventually, the ureter and kidney are affected, and hydroureter, hydronephrosis, diminished GFR, and uremia may develop. Men with prostatic hyperplasia may experience **nocturia** (excessive urination at night), decreased urine flow, incomplete bladder emptying, and urinary urgency and frequency.

Urinary tract infections are a common cause of incontinence in older adults, with an annual incidence of 10% (Mohsin & Siddiqui, 2010). Because indwelling catheters are a major cause of urinary tract infections and other complications, evidence-based practice emphasize the importance of on-going evaluations of the necessity of these devices (O'Donohue et al., 2010; Voss, 2009; Wilde et al., 2010). One study found that reducing the use of indwelling catheters eliminated catheter-associated urinary tract infections during the 6-month intervention period (Elpern et al., 2009). Manifestations of urinary tract infections in older adults may be very subtle; urinary incontinence may be the initial or primary sign. A change in behavior or level of functioning may be the presenting sign, particularly in people with dementia. Older adults are also likely to have chronic bacteriuria—a condition characterized as 10^5 or more colony-forming units without symptoms of urinary tract infection. The prevalence of chronic bacteriuria in nursing home residents is 25% to 50% of women and 15% to 40% of men (Nicolle, 2009).

> **DIVERSITY NOTE**
>
> Women are more likely than men to have a urinary tract infection.

Other Conditions That Cause Urinary Incontinence

Many pathologic conditions affecting either the central or peripheral nervous system increase the risk for developing incontinence. Although dementia is strongly associated with urinary incontinence, the relationship between these two conditions is complex, and incontinence should be viewed as preventable and treatable. For example, older adults with dementia may lack the perceptual abilities that are necessary for finding and using appropriate facilities, but they may be able to maintain continence when given appropriate cues and reminders.

Conditions of the gastrointestinal tract that can cause incontinence include gastroenteritis, constipation, and fecal impaction. The mass of stool that is present with constipation or fecal impaction places pressure on the bladder and diminishes its storage capacity. In turn, this causes urinary frequency, urgency, and incontinence. Fecal impaction can also obstruct the bladder outlet, causing bladder distention and urinary retention or incontinence.

Other conditions that are highly associated with incontinence are obesity, diabetes, alcoholism, multiple sclerosis, Parkinson's disease, cerebrovascular accident, and chronic obstructive pulmonary disease (COPD). Metabolic disturbances that induce diuresis, such as diabetes and hypercalcemia, can lead to incontinence. Conditions that affect mental status, such as delirium, may be manifested or accompanied by urinary incontinence. Likewise, many conditions that affect physiologic processes, such as acute illness, can cause or exacerbate incontinence. Any acute illness or surgical intervention that temporarily limits mobility or compromises mental abilities also represents a risk factor for urinary incontinence.

Wellness Opportunity

Nurses holistically assess older adults by recognizing that urinary incontinence can be an indicator of physiologic disturbances (e.g., urinary tract infection), psychosocial conditions (e.g., dementia or depression), or a combination of functional limitations and environmental barriers.

Medication Effects

Medications influence urinary function in a number of ways and are common risk factors in the development of urinary incontinence. For example, loop diuretics increase urinary output, placing additional demands on the urinary system and compounding the effects of an age-related decrease in bladder capacity. Older adults with other urinary tract conditions may be particularly susceptible to adverse medication effects. For example, men with prostatic hyperplasia are at increased risk for urinary retention when they take an adrenergic or anticholinergic agent. Some medications that are used to treat incontinence can also cause incontinence. For instance, terazosin, which is used for benign prostatic hyperplasia, can cause urethral relaxation and stress incontinence. Thus, it is imperative that causes of incontinence be identified accurately before treatment is initiated.

In addition to causing incontinence through their direct effects on the urinary tract, medications can cause incontinence through their effects on functional abilities. Anticholinergics (including those in over-the-counter agents) can cause cognitive and other functional impairments, which can interfere with voluntary control over urination. Many medications cause constipation, which is a causative factor for incontinence. This adverse effect may be particularly detrimental in the presence of prostatic hyperplasia or weakened pelvic floor muscles.

In addition to creating risk factors for incontinence, medications can increase ADH secretion, which may compound age-related effects that predispose older adults to hyponatremia. Medications that stimulate ADH secretion include aspirin, narcotics, acetaminophen, antidepressants, barbiturates, chlorpropamide, clofibrate, fluphenazine, and haloperidol. Table 19-1 presents some types and examples of medications that can cause incontinence in older adults.

Environmental Factors

Environmental factors may impede or prevent older adults—particularly those with mobility limitations—from reaching

TABLE 19-1 Medications That Can Cause Urinary Incontinence

Medication Type	Examples	Mechanism of Action
Diuretics	Furosemide, bumetanide	Increased diuresis can cause urinary urgency, frequency, and polyuria
Anticholinergic agents	Antihistamines, antipsychotics, antidepressants, antispasmodics, anti-Parkinsonian agents	Decreased bladder contractility and relaxed bladder muscle can cause urinary retention, frequency, and incontinence
Adrenergics (alpha-adrenergic agonists)	Decongestants	Decreased bladder contractility and increased sphincter tone can cause urinary retention, frequency, and incontinence
Alpha-adrenergic blockers	Prazosin, terazosin, doxazosin	Decreased urethral and internal sphincter tone can cause leakage and stress incontinence
Calcium channel blockers	Nifedipine, nicardipine, isradipine, felodipine, nimodipine	Decreased bladder contractility can cause urinary retention, frequency, nocturia, and incontinence
Angiotensin-converting enzyme inhibitors	Captopril, enalapril, lisinopril	Can cause chronic cough, which precipitates or exacerbates stress incontinence
Hypnotics and antianxiety agents	Benzodiazepines	Can interfere with voluntary control over urination by causing sedation, delirium, and cognitive impairments
Alcohol	Wine, beer, liquor	Can interfere with voluntary control over urination by causing sedation, delirium, increased diuresis, and cognitive impairments

Box 19-1 Environmental Factors That Can Contribute to Urinary Incontinence

- Stairways between the bathroom level and the living or sleeping areas
- A distance to the bathroom that is more than 40 feet
- Living arrangements where several or many people share a bathroom
- Small bathrooms and narrow doors and hallways that do not accommodate walkers or wheelchairs
- Chair designs and bed heights that hinder mobility
- Poor color contrast, as between a white toilet and seat and light-colored floor or walls
- Public settings with poorly visible or poorly color-contrasted signs designating gender-specific bathroom facilities
- Public settings with dim lighting and out-of-the-way bathroom facilities
- Very bright environments, where glare interferes with the perception of signs for bathrooms
- Mirrored walls, which reflect bright lights and create glare

and using the toilet in home, public, and institutional settings. Examples of environmental obstacles include stairs, an absence of grab bars and railings, and toilet seats that are not the appropriate height. Box 19-1 summarizes some environmental risk factors that may contribute to the incidence of incontinence in older adults.

FUNCTIONAL CONSEQUENCES AFFECTING URINARY WELLNESS

Despite the many age-related changes in the urinary tract, the elimination of wastes is not significantly affected in healthy, nonmedicated older adults. However, with any unusual physiologic demands, such as those that occur with medications or disease conditions, older adults are likely to experience functional consequences affecting homeostatic mechanisms and urinary control. Age-related changes and risk factors also cause functional consequences in patterns of urinary elimination and predispose older adults to incontinence. When incontinence occurs, additional functional consequences, particularly psychosocial effects, can be quite serious.

Effects on Homeostasis

Functional consequences related to renal function in healthy older adults include impaired absorption of calcium and a predisposition to hyponatremia and hyperkalemia. Age-related changes in the kidney and in aldosterone secretion interfere with compensatory mechanisms that maintain fluid and electrolyte balance, so older adults have a delayed and less effective response to variations in sodium intake than younger individuals. Similarly, diminished renal function lengthens the time needed for pH imbalances to be corrected in older adults. Even with normal states of hydration, a decrease in GFR delays water excretion and may lead to hyponatremia in healthy older adults. Likewise, even routine

daily activities can challenge the renal function of older adults because of diminished renal efficiency. For example, when older adults perspire during exercise, they may tire easily because of age-related delays in the mechanisms controlling water and sodium conservation.

With increasing age, the kidneys become less responsive to ADH and are less able to concentrate urine, causing a decrease in the maximal urinary concentration. Age-related changes also increase urine production at night in older adults compared with younger adults, even in the absence of pathologic factors.

Older adults who take certain medications or have medical conditions are likely to experience functional consequences such as the following:

- Diuretics are more likely to cause hypovolemia and dehydration in older adults than in younger people.
- Under conditions of physiologic stress (e.g., surgery, infection, or excessive fluid loss), older adults are likely to develop dehydration, volume depletion, and other fluid and electrolyte imbalances.
- Volume depletion may occur soon after the onset of fever-producing illnesses because of the inability to compensate for insensible fluid losses.
- Any condition or medication that stimulates ADH secretion, such as pneumonia or chlorpropamide, is likely to cause water intoxication and hyponatremia in older adults because of their diminished ability to compensate for excessive levels of ADH.

Diminished renal function contributes to the increased incidence of drug interactions and adverse medication reactions in older adults. These age-related changes are most likely to affect water-soluble medications that are highly dependent on GFR (e.g., digoxin, cimetidine, and aminoglycoside antibiotics) or renal tubular function (e.g., penicillin and procainamide). Unless medication doses are adjusted to account for age-related changes in GFR and renal tubular function, excretion may be delayed and toxic substances are likely to accumulate. These adverse medication effects can significantly impair physical and mental abilities and have profound functional consequences, as discussed in Chapter 8.

Effects on Voiding Patterns

Because of age-related changes, the bladder of the older adult has a smaller capacity, empties incompletely, and contracts during filling. Thus, older adults experience shorter intervals between voiding, and they have less time between the perception of the urge to void and the actual need to empty the bladder. Older adults often describe this by saying, "When you gotta go, you gotta go." Another consequence is that the bladder retains up to 50 mL of residual urine after voiding, causing symptomatic or asymptomatic bacteriuria and predisposing older adults to urinary tract infections.

Age-related changes in the diurnal production of urine in the kidneys cause a shift in voiding pattern to more urinary output at night than during the day. Pathologic conditions (e.g., hypothyroidism, heart failure, venous insufficiency) and certain medications (e.g., calcium channel blockers) are risk factors that lead to urinary frequency and nocturia associated with a supine position (Rahn & Roshanravan, 2009). In addition, an overactive bladder and pathologic conditions (e.g., pelvic floor dysfunction in women and benign prostatic enlargement in men) are common causes of nocturia in older adults (van Kerrebroeck, Hashim, Holm-Larsen, Robinson, & Stanley, 2010). Functional consequences of nocturia include disturbed sleep, increased risk for nighttime falls, and decreased quality of life (Bliwise et al., 2009; Endeshaw, 2009; Vaughan et al., 2010).

PATHOLOGIC CONDITION AFFECTING URINARY FUNCTION: URINARY INCONTINENCE

As stated, age-related changes alone do not cause urinary incontinence; they predispose older adults to it, making it the most commonly occurring pathologic condition associated with the urinary tract in older adults. The estimated prevalence of incontinence for older adults ranges from 38% for community-dwelling older adults to 60% for those in long-term care facilities and up to 90% for people with dementia (Dowling-Castronovo & Bradway, 2008; French Phelps, Pothula, & Mushkbar, 2009; Griebling, 2009). Studies identify all the following risk factors for urinary incontinence: increased age, functional limitations, impaired cognition, obesity, smoking, white race, constipation, vaginal delivery, low vitamin D levels, medications (e.g., oral estrogen, antipsychotics), and pathologic conditions (diabetes, stroke, arthritis, Parkinson's disease) (Amselem et al., 2010; Badalian & Rosenbaum, 2010; Byles, Millar, Sibbritt, & Chiarelli, 2009; Menezes, Hashimoto, & de Gouveia Santos, 2009). Studies also found a strong relationship between depression and urinary incontinence, but conclusions are not clear about whether depression is a risk for or consequence of urinary incontinence (Melville, Fan, Rau, Nygaard, & Katon, 2009).

Urinary incontinence is a focus of much attention among healthcare consumers and practitioners, particularly with regard to its effects on quality of life (Botlero, Bell, Urquhart, & Davis, 2010; Tennstedt et al., 2010). Urinary incontinence is categorized according to signs and symptoms as follows:

- **Stress urinary incontinence** is characterized by an involuntary leakage of urine as a result of an activity that increases abdominal pressure (e.g., lifting, coughing, sneezing, laughing, or exercise).
- **Urge urinary incontinence** is characterized by involuntary urinary leakage due to the inability to hold urine long enough to reach a toilet after perceiving the urge to void.
- **Mixed urinary incontinence** is characterized by leakage of urine with both the sensation of urgency and activities such as coughing, sneezing, or exertion.

When any type of urinary incontinence develops, a comprehensive assessment is warranted to identify the causes and risk factors that can be addressed through interventions, as discussed later in this chapter.

Overactive bladder (OAB) is a syndrome characterized by bothersome urgency, usually accompanied by nocturia and daytime frequency, and sometimes accompanied by urge urinary incontinence. In recent years, OAB has become widely recognized because of advertisements related to prescription medications for the treatment of this condition. By definition, OAB is not always accompanied by incontinence, but in reality, many people with this condition also experience incontinence. One study of 311 adults between the ages of 18 and 97 years found a prevalence of OAB in 60.5% of men and 48.3% of women, with 37% and 92% of the men and women, respectively, also experiencing incontinence (Cheung, Khan, Choi, Bluth, & Vincent, 2009). In this study, obesity was a major risk factor for OAB, particularly in premenopausal women. Other studies have found that diuretics, particularly loop diuretics, are associated with OAB (Ekundayo et al., 2009).

DIVERSITY NOTE

Prevalence rates for urinary incontinence in community-based women are highest for whites, lower for Asian Americans, and lowest for blacks (Townsend, Curhan, Resnick, & Grodstein, 2010).

Urinary incontinence can negatively affect an older adult's quality of life through both physical and psychosocial consequences. Physical consequences of incontinence include a predisposition to falls, fractures, pressure ulcers, skin infections or irritations, urinary tract infections, and limitation of functional status (Dowling-Castronovo & Bradway, 2008; Hasegawa, Kuzuya, & Iguchi, 2010). Psychosocial consequences associated with urinary incontinence include significantly decreased quality of life, shame or embarrassment, anxiety, depression, social isolation, and loss of self-confidence. Another consequence is that people who have experienced episodes of incontinence may become preoccupied with covering up any evidence of wetness or urinary odors, so they can avoid social stigma.

Psychosocial consequences also arise if caregivers have infantilizing attitudes and behaviors (e.g., unnecessarily using incontinence products rather than providing assistance with toileting) toward the older person who is incontinent. These attitudes and behaviors can have a devastating effect on the older adult's dignity and self-esteem. In addition, older adults who do not understand age-related changes may have exaggerated fears of progressive incontinence, triggered by the onset of urgency or frequency. Even in older adults who are not incontinent, the experience of urinary urgency and frequency can cause psychosocial consequences, such as anxiety, restricted activity, feelings of insecurity and powerlessness, and embarrassment about frequent trips to the bathroom.

For caregivers of dependent older adults in home settings, the onset of urinary incontinence may create additional stress, particularly if urinary incontinence is compounded by environmental barriers or functional limitations. Tasks related to incontinence are some of the most difficult, stressful, and time-consuming aspects of caregiving. Caregivers in home settings are likely to feel angry, guilty, frustrated, or inadequate

A Student's Perspective

One morning, I was caring for a client with a Foley catheter. While preparing her to go to breakfast, I noticed there was no cover on her catheter bag and asked her if she had one. My client explained she once had a cover, but the nurses did not know where it went. I decided to do some searching, which only required my asking the laundry lady, and I discovered that several covers were stored in the linen closet. When I came back to the client's room with the cover, my client was so grateful. She said she had been asking for a long time if she could get another one, but the nurses and aides never cared to search for one. She explained that she doesn't like everyone to be able to see her catheter bag as she rides around the nursing home in her wheelchair. My finding the cover for her catheter bag was a very simple act requiring very little effort, but it showed me the importance of putting a little extra time into the client's care. Although this seemed like a miniscule problem to the nurses, it was a real concern to my client. I hope that as we continue in our nursing careers we remember to do these simple acts, because a seemingly insignificant thing to us can mean the world to a client.

Katrina D.

he changes the subject. She says that he will not talk with his doctor about it because he "hears so much about prostate cancer, and he's afraid that he has an untreatable condition." She asks your advice about this and asks if you would talk with him when he comes to see you next week. Your next group health education session is entitled "Control of Urine: What's Normal With Aging?" and you plan to have separate group discussions for the men and women. Since Mr. and Mrs. U. usually attend these sessions, you see this as an opportunity to initiate health education about this sensitive topic.

THINKING POINTS

Decide what information you would include in the group session about each of the following topics:

- What can older men (women) expect of their urinary tract?
- What factors increase the risk of having problems with urinary control in older men (women)?

when dealing with incontinence on a daily basis. Lifelong attitudes about control over urination may contribute to feelings of disgust about the care demands, which may be further compounded by feelings of guilt about this initial reaction to caregiving tasks. If the caregiver perceives intentionality on the part of the dependent person in his or her failure to control urination, these feelings will likely be intensified. In institutional settings, nursing staff and other caregivers may experience these same feelings to a lesser degree.

Wellness Opportunity

Nurses address the person's relationships with others by being sensitive to the psychosocial responses of family caregivers who are dealing with incontinence.

*M*r. and Mrs. U., who are 69 and 68 years old, respectively, attend the senior center where you provide monthly group health education sessions, weekly blood pressure checks, and one-on-one "Counseling for Wellness" sessions. During a recent health counseling session, Mrs. U. confided that she does not know what to do about her husband's "smelly dribbling" and that she worries that he has prostate problems. She has perceived a strong odor of urine and has noticed yellow stains on his clothing when she does the laundry. Even their children have mentioned the odor to her, but when she tries to discuss it with her husband,

NURSING ASSESSMENT OF URINARY FUNCTION

Nurses can identify opportunities for health promotion interventions by assessing all of the following aspects of urinary function:

- Risk factors that influence overall urinary function
- Risk factors that increase the potential for incontinence
- Signs and symptoms of any dysfunction involving urinary elimination
- Fears and attitudes about urinary dysfunction
- Psychosocial consequences of incontinence

Nurses obtain most of this information by interviewing older adults and caregivers of dependent older adults. In addition, the nurse obtains objective data from laboratory tests and by observing behaviors, behavioral cues, and environmental influences.

Talking With Older Adults About Urinary Function

Because urinary elimination is associated with certain social expectations, discussion of this topic may be particularly influenced by a person's attitudes and feelings. Although nurses usually learn to discuss urinary elimination with relative ease, older adults may feel uncomfortable with the topic, particularly if there are gender or age differences between the older person and the nurse or if a communication barrier, such as a hearing impairment, exists. In addition, if older adults accept urinary leakage as an inevitable consequence of aging, they may not volunteer information.

Terminology related to urinary elimination presents further difficulties in interviewing older adults. In social settings, people commonly use euphemisms to avoid directly discussing urination (e.g., "I'm going to the powder room," "I'm going to take a leak," "I have to use the john"). Even the sounds associated with urinary elimination may be viewed as embarrassing, so people may run the faucet or flush the toilet to disguise the sound of urination when others are present. Because of this social context, successful interviewing about urinary elimination and incontinence depends on identifying the terms that are least embarrassing and most understandable to the older adult. If any hearing impairment is present, a term such as "urinate," which is not used in everyday social language or a one-syllable word like "pee" may be difficult to understand or may be misinterpreted. Although phrases like "use the toilet" and "go to the bathroom" are not specific to urinary elimination, they may prove to be acceptable, particularly if additional questions are asked in order to distinguish between urinary and bowel elimination. Similarly, the term "incontinence" may be problematic for people who may not be familiar with this term. Hearing impairments, if present, may further interfere with the comprehension of this word. Rather than referring to incontinence, it may be more acceptable to older adults to discuss "trouble holding their water." Older adults may tend to use words such as "accidents," "leaking," "weak kidneys," or "bladder trouble" to describe incontinent episodes.

The nurse can set the stage for direct questions about urinary elimination by focusing initial questions on risk factors. Nurses can indirectly assess the perception of and attitudes about urinary incontinence by observing responses to the interview questions. If the older adult acknowledges incontinence, the nurses asks about any actions the person has taken and what impact the incontinence has had on their daily activities and social life.

> **Wellness Opportunity**
>
> Nurses show respect for older adults by using terms such as "briefs" rather than terms such as diapers, which are associated with infants.

Identifying Opportunities for Health Promotion

Box 19-2 presents interview questions related to urinary elimination. If the information is already available from other

---

 Box 19-2 Guidelines for Assessing Urinary Elimination

Interview Questions to Assess Risk Factors Influencing Urinary Elimination
- (Men) Have you had any surgery for prostate or bladder problems?
- (Men) Have you ever been told you had prostate problems? (or Do you think you have prostate problems?)
- (Women) Have you had any children? (If yes, ask about the number of pregnancies and any problems with childbirth.)
- (Women) Have you had any surgery for pelvic, bladder, or uterine disorders?
- (Women) Have you had any infections in your vaginal area?
- Do you have any pain, burning, or discomfort when you urinate (pass water)?
- Have you had any urinary tract infections?
- Do you have any chronic illnesses?
- What medications do you take?
- Do you have any problems with your bowels?
- How much water and other liquids do you drink during the day? (Ask for details about timing and the amount of alcoholic, carbonated, and caffeinated beverages consumed.)

Interview Questions to Assess Risk Factors for Socially Appropriate Urinary Elimination
- Do you have any trouble walking or any difficulty with balance?
- Do you have any trouble reading signs or finding restrooms when you are in public places?

Interview Questions to Assess Signs and Symptoms of Urinary Dysfunction
- Do you ever leak urine?
- Do you ever wear pads or protective garments to protect your clothing from wetness?
- Do you ever have difficulty holding your urine (water) long enough to get to the toilet? (or How long can you hold your urine after you first feel the need to go to the bathroom?)

- Do you have trouble holding your urine (water) when you cough, laugh, or make sudden movements?
- Do you wake up at night because you have to go to the bathroom to urinate (pass water)? (If the response is affirmative, try to differentiate between this symptom and the habit of going to the bathroom after waking up for some other reason.)
- Immediately after urinating (passing your water), does it feel like you have not emptied your bladder completely?
- Do you have to exert pressure during urination to feel like your bladder is being completely emptied?
- (Men) When you urinate (pass water), do you have any difficulty starting the stream or keeping the stream going?

Interview Questions If Incontinence Has Been Acknowledged
- When did your incontinence begin?
- What have you done to manage the problem? (Have you cut down on the amount of liquids you drink? Do you empty your bladder at frequent intervals as a precautionary measure?)
- Are there certain things that make the problem worse or better?
- Does it happen all the time, or just at certain times?
- Do you have any pain when you urinate (pass water)?
- (Women) Do you feel any pressure in your pelvic area?

Interview Questions to Assess Fears, Attitudes, and Psychosocial Consequences of Incontinence
- Have you ever sought help or talked to a primary care provider or other healthcare professional about this problem?
- Have you changed any of your activities because you need to stay near a toilet?
- Do you avoid going to certain places because of difficulty holding your urine (water)?

parts of an assessment (e.g., medication use and medical history), the nurse incorporates it into the assessment of urinary elimination rather than repeat questions. Nurses supplement their assessment interview by obtaining information about the person's patterns of urinary elimination and by assessing environmental factors that may interfere with control over urinary elimination.

A **bladder diary**—also called a bladder record, incontinence chart, or voiding or urinary diary—is one method of obtaining information about patterns of urinary elimination (Figure 19-1). This widely recommended assessment tool is used to document information about fluid intake, the times of urinations, and other factors that can affect continence (Dowling-Castronovo & Specht, 2009). Nurses use information from the bladder diary to identify potential causes of and interventions for incontinence, particularly with regard to identifying opportunities for health education.

> **Wellness Opportunity**
>
> Nurses promote self-care by encouraging older adults to assess their patterns of urinary elimination in relation to factors such as food and fluid intake.

Older adults who are cognitively impaired or dependent on others for their care may not be able to keep a bladder diary. In these situations, or when incontinence is an unacknowledged problem, observations on patterns of urinary elimination are particularly important. In long-term care facilities and other institutional settings, nurses have many opportunities to observe behavioral cues to incontinence. In home settings, caregivers of dependent older adults may observe behavioral cues and provide valuable information about urinary elimination patterns. Box 19-3 summarizes specific observations that may yield important assessment information.

Home environments are assessed for barriers that might interfere with the quick performance of urinary elimination (refer to Box 19-1). Stairways, long hallways, poor lighting, and cluttered surroundings can lengthen the time needed to get to the toilet, particularly for people who have a functional impairment or use assistive devices, such as a walker. Also, it is important to assess the environment for safety and assistive devices or their potential benefit to the individual. For instance, an elevated toilet seat, grab bars near the toilet, and grab bars on the walls leading to the toilet may improve the person's ability to urinate safely. See Box 19-3 for specific environmental factors that can affect socially appropriate urinary elimination.

Using Laboratory Information

Data from urinalysis and blood chemistry tests contribute important information to the assessment of urinary elimination. A midstream or second-void specimen is the best type of sample for a urinalysis. At the age of 80 years, the normal upper limit for specific gravity is 1.024, and slight proteinuria is normal in older adults. Other than these two variations, the

Box 19-3 Guidelines for Assessing Behavioral Cues to and Environmental Influences on Incontinence

Behavioral Cues
- Does the older adult use disposable or washable pads or products?
- Is there an odor of urine on clothing, floor coverings, or furniture (particularly couches and stuffed chairs)?
- Has the older adult withdrawn from social activities, particularly those held away from home?

Environmental Influences
- Where are the bathroom facilities located in relation to the older adult's usual daytime and nighttime activities?
- Does the person have to go up or down stairs to use the toilet at night or during the day?
- Are there any grab bars or other aids in, near, or on the way to the bathroom?
- Would the person benefit from using an elevated toilet seat?
- Does the person use a urinal or other aid to cut down on the number of trips to the bathroom?
- How many people share the same bathroom facilities?
- Is privacy ensured?

urinalysis results should be within the normal range for healthy older adults.

Blood chemistry values that may be helpful in assessing renal function include the following: electrolyte level, creatinine level, creatinine clearance, nonprotein nitrogen level, and blood urea nitrogen level. In older adults, the serum creatinine may not be an accurate indicator of the GFR, but a 24-hour urine collection for creatinine clearance may have greater value as an indicator of renal functioning.

*R*ecall that you are the nurse at the senior center attended by Mr. and Mrs. U. After your class ("Control of Urine: What's Normal With Aging?"), Mr. U. schedules an appointment for a Counseling for Wellness session. He tells you that he has a "little dribbling" problem but has ignored it because it did not bother him very much. He has not talked with any doctor about this because he thought it was "to be expected," but now that he attended your session, he thinks that maybe he should have the problem evaluated and wants further information from you. During other health counseling sessions with Mr. U., he has told you that he is taking medications for hypertension and Parkinson's disease.

THINKING POINTS

- What risk factors are likely to be contributing to Mr. U.'s problems with urinary control?

Your Daily Bladder Diary

This diary will help you and your health care team figure out the causes of your bladder control trouble. The "sample" line shows you how to use the diary.

Your name: _____

Date: _____

Time	Drinks		Trips to the Bathroom		Accidental Leaks	Did you feel a strong urge to go?	What were you doing at the time?
	What kind?	How much?	How many times?	How much urine? (circle one)	How much? (circle one)	Circle one	Sneezing, exercising, having sex, lifting, etc.
Sample	Coffee	2 cups	✓✓	(sm) med lg	sm (med) lg	Yes (No)	Running
6–7 a.m.				sm med lg	sm med lg	Yes No	
7–8 a.m.				sm med lg	sm med lg	Yes No	
8–9 a.m.				sm med lg	sm med lg	Yes No	
9–10 a.m.				sm med lg	sm med lg	Yes No	
10–11 a.m.				sm med lg	sm med lg	Yes No	
11–12 noon				sm med lg	sm med lg	Yes No	
12–1 p.m.				sm med lg	sm med lg	Yes No	
1–2 p.m.				sm med lg	sm med lg	Yes No	
2–3 p.m.				sm med lg	sm med lg	Yes No	
3–4 p.m.				sm med lg	sm med lg	Yes No	
4–5 p.m.				sm med lg	sm med lg	Yes No	
5–6 p.m.				sm med lg	sm med lg	Yes No	
6–7 p.m.				sm med lg	sm med lg	Yes No	
7–8 p.m.				sm med lg	sm med lg	Yes No	
8–9 p.m.				sm med lg	sm med lg	Yes No	
9–10 p.m.				sm med lg	sm med lg	Yes No	
10–11 p.m.				sm med lg	sm med lg	Yes No	
11–12 midnight				sm med lg	sm med lg	Yes No	
12–1 p.m.				sm med lg	sm med lg	Yes No	
1–2 p.m.				sm med lg	sm med lg	Yes No	
2–3 a.m.				sm med lg	sm med lg	Yes No	
3–4 a.m.				sm med lg	sm med lg	Yes No	
4–5 a.m.				sm med lg	sm med lg	Yes No	
5–6 a.m.				sm med lg	sm med lg	Yes No	

FIGURE 19-1 Example of a bladder diary. (Courtesy of the National Association for Continence [NAFC]. Available at www.nafc.org/Uploads/OnlineUroLog.pdf.)

- Make a list of assessment questions that you would use with Mr. U. (Use applicable questions from Box 19-2 and any additional questions that might be appropriate.)
- What observations would you make as part of your assessment?
- What would you teach Mr. U. about filling out the voiding diary (see Figure 19-1)?

NURSING DIAGNOSIS

When the nursing assessment identifies any risk factors for incontinence or any complaints about or evidence of incontinence, an applicable nursing diagnosis would be Impaired Urinary Elimination, defined as "dysfunction in urinary elimination" (NANDA International, 2009, p. 98). Major defining characteristics commonly found in older adults include urgency, frequency, dribbling, nocturia, hesitancy, and incontinence. When nurses identify negative functional consequences related to urinary problems, the following nursing diagnoses might be applicable: Anxiety, Social Isolation, Disturbed Body Image, Disturbed Sleep Pattern, Impaired Skin Integrity, or Caregiver Role Strain (or Risk f or).

> **Wellness Opportunity**
>
> Nurses can use the wellness nursing diagnosis of Readiness For Enhanced Urinary Elimination for older adults who are interested in learning self-care practices such as pelvic floor muscle training.

PLANNING FOR WELLNESS OUTCOMES

Nursing care plans are directed toward preventing, minimizing, or compensating for the negative functional consequences that affect urinary elimination. Specific outcomes related to urinary elimination include Fluid Balance or Kidney Function (maintenance of homeostasis) and Risk Detection or Medication Response (prevention of adverse medication effects). Outcomes for older adults who have urinary incontinence include achieving continence and preventing negative consequences; initial outcomes focus on controlling and alleviating, rather than simply managing, incontinence.

The following NOC terminology is pertinent to older adults who experience urinary incontinence and related consequences: Urinary Continence; Urinary Elimination; Self-Care: Toileting; Depression Self-Control; Fear Level; Health Beliefs: Perceived Control; Immobility Consequences: Physiologic; and Tissue Integrity: Skin.

In addition, any of the following NOCs may be pertinent to caregivers, particularly family members, who are caring for someone with urinary incontinence: Caregiver Stressors; Caregiver Well-Being; Caregiver Performance: Direct Care; Caregiver Lifestyle Disruption; Caregiver Emotional Health; and Caregiver Endurance Potential.

> **Wellness Opportunity**
>
> Quality of life is an outcome that can be achieved for older adults and their caregivers through nursing interventions that are effective in alleviating or managing urinary incontinence.

 ## NURSING INTERVENTIONS TO PROMOTE HEALTHY URINARY FUNCTION

Nurses have numerous opportunities to promote wellness in relation to urinary function, particularly for older adults who have difficulty maintaining urinary control. For example, nurses can challenge myths about urinary incontinence, address attitudes of resignation, and teach self-care interventions. The following NIC terminology is pertinent to promoting urinary continence and addressing the associated psychosocial consequences: Biofeedback; Emotional Support; Environmental Management; Exercise Promotion; Fluid Management; Health Education; Pelvic Muscle Exercise; Perineal Care; Prompted Voiding; Referral; Self-Esteem Enhancement; Teaching: Individual; Urinary Bladder Training; Urinary Elimination Management; and Urinary Habit Training.

Teaching About Urinary Wellness

Healthy older adults are not significantly affected by age-related kidney changes during normal activities; however, under conditions of physiologic stress, such as exercise, homeostasis can be affected unless the older adult initiates compensatory actions. Thus, nurses teach older adults about functional consequences affecting homeostasis and inform them of self-care actions to prevent problems. For example, nurses can explain that exercising in a cool (rather than hot) environment and increasing one's fluid intake prior to exercise may compensate for the age-related diminished ability to conserve water and sodium. Nurses can also suggest that older adults take protective measures when they are in very hot and humid environments. Examples of appropriate protective measures are the use of fans and air conditioners; an increase in fluid intake; and avoidance of alcoholic, carbonated, and caffeinated beverages.

Older adults taking normal doses of water-soluble medications may experience adverse medication effects because of diminished renal function. Therefore, when water-soluble medications are prescribed for older adults, dose adjustments should be based on an accurate assessment of kidney function and serum drug levels. Nurses need to be aware of and teach older adults about the increased potential for adverse medication effects, particularly when the older adult is taking more than one medication. Further information about adverse medication effects and interventions for medication management is discussed in Chapter 8.

Perhaps the risk factor most amenable to nursing interventions is the false perception of incontinence as an inevitable effect of aging for which nothing can be done. Because this

Box 19-4   Health Education to Promote Urinary Wellness

Promoting Good Urinary Function
- Drink 8 to 10 glasses of noncaffeinated liquid every day.
- Do not depend on thirst sensation as an accurate indicator for adequate fluid intake—drink liquids even if you do not feel thirsty.
- Avoid excessive use of alcoholic, caffeinated, or carbonated beverages, particularly before bedtime.
- Avoid foods and beverages that can irritate the bladder (e.g., sugar, caffeine, alcohol, chocolate, artificial sweeteners, and spicy and acidic foods).
- Drink 1 or 2 glasses of fluid before, and every 15 minutes during, periods of sweat-producing exercise or activity.
- Avoid smoking.
- Maintain ideal body weight and good physical fitness.
- Take steps to prevent constipation (refer to Chapter 18, Box 18-5).
- Practice pelvic muscle exercises (refer to Box 19-6).
- Seek medical advice from a knowledgeable practitioner about any difficulties with urinary continence.

Understanding Why Incontinence May Occur
- If incontinence occurs, a pathologic condition or other influencing factor can usually be identified through a comprehensive evaluation.
- A requirement for voluntary control over urination is the signal of the need to void because of a full bladder. Restricting fluid intake interferes with this signal.
- Highly concentrated urine, from inadequate fluid intake, will stimulate involuntary bladder contractions and may lead to incontinence.
- Consistently emptying the bladder at intervals of less than 1 or 2 hours may contribute to problems with incontinence.

Correcting Myths About Incontinence
- Incontinence is not an inevitable age-related change.
- Normal age-related changes affecting urination include a shortened interval between the perception of the urge to void and the actual need to empty the bladder, an increased frequency of voiding, and the need to get up to urinate several times during the night.
- Nocturia, urgency, and frequency do not necessarily lead to total incontinence.

---

attitude is based on myths or a lack of information, it can be changed through education. Nurses can emphasize the need for a comprehensive evaluation of urinary incontinence so that risk factors can be alleviated. Teaching older adults the rationale for maintaining adequate fluid intake as a means of preventing incontinence and maintaining good urinary function is a simple but important intervention. Older adults may be more willing to consume adequate amounts of fluid if they understand that concentrated urine can cause incontinence by stimulating bladder contractions. Nurses can also explain that because older adults often do not experience a sensation of thirst, even in the presence of dehydration, their intake of liquids may be inadequate if they drink fluids only when thirsty. Interventions to promote adequate fluid intake include identifying nonalcoholic, noncaffeinated, and noncarbonated beverages that the older adult will drink at appropriate intervals, even in the absence of a thirst sensation. Teaching about normal age-related changes, such as a decreased sensation of thirst, can help to challenge ageist beliefs that negative functional consequences are inevitable. Health education about appropriate management strategies for urinary incontinence is an important nursing intervention because studies indicate that some modifying strategies are detrimental to health over the long-term (St. John, Wallis, Griffiths, & McKenzie, 2010).

When a risk factor contributes to incontinence or otherwise interferes with normal urinary elimination, interventions focus on optimal management of the precipitating factor. For example, if postmenopausal estrogen depletion leads to vaginitis and trigonitis, health education is directed toward encouraging the older woman to seek medical treatment for the underlying condition. When fecal impaction or chronic constipation are risk factors for urinary incontinence, interventions are aimed at attaining and maintaining good bowel function, as discussed in Chapter 18. **Pelvic floor muscle**

training (PFMT), as discussed in the next section, is another health promotion intervention that can be performed by men and women who are at increased risk of developing, or are already experiencing, urinary incontinence. Box 19-4 summarizes teaching points about self-care activities that promote optimal overall urinary function and help older adults maintain continence.

Wellness Opportunity

Nurses promote personal responsibility by encouraging older adults to talk with their primary care practitioner about identifying risk factors for urinary incontinence that can be addressed through self-care measures.

Promoting Continence and Alleviating Incontinence

If self-care interventions cannot alleviate urinary incontinence, a comprehensive evaluation must be done to determine the underlying cause of the incontinence. Nurses can facilitate referrals to specialty clinics, primary care practitioners, or a geriatric assessment program for an evaluation. Interventions also address contributing factors such as environmental conditions, resources and abilities of caregivers, functional and cognitive abilities of the older adult, and negative effects and social acceptability of the intervention. Evidence-based guidelines are available for the evaluation and management of urinary incontinence, but the scope of the guidelines varies, with some focusing on a specific target group, clinical setting, or professional group (e.g., women, acute care, nurses). Sources of guidelines are listed at the end of this chapter.

The following types of interventions are used, often in combination, for the control of incontinence: health education,

PFMT, biofeedback and stimulation devices, urinary control devices, **continence training**, environmental modifications, medications, and surgical and minimally invasive procedures. If incontinence cannot be alleviated, aids and equipment can be used to minimize its functional consequences.

Pelvic Floor Muscle Training

When weakening of the pelvic floor musculature contributes to incontinence, exercises to strengthen these muscles can cure or improve incontinence. A. H. Kegel, an American gynecologist for postpartum therapy, first advocated PFMT in the late 1940s. Since then, many variations of these exercises have been promoted, both for the control of incontinence and for the enhancement of sexual pleasure. Other terms used interchangeably with PFMT include Kegels, Kegel exercises, pelvic muscle exercises, pelvic floor training, and pelvic muscle rehabilitation. This intervention is sometimes used with biofeedback, behavioral training, or pelvic floor electrical stimulation for improved effectiveness. Studies support the effectiveness of PFMT as a first-line intervention for men and women with stress and mixed incontinence (Fritel et al., 2010; Hung, Hsiao, Chih, Lin, & Tsauo, 2010; Sari & Khorshid, 2009). A Cochrane review of 14 studies involving 836 women found that women who performed PFMT were more likely to report they were cured or improved and had better continence-specific quality of life. This review also found that PFMT helped with stress, urge, or mixed incontinence but was most effective for stress urinary incontinence alone as well as when performed in a supervised program for at least 3 months (Dumoulin & Hay-Smith, 2010). Although most of the studies have focused on PFMT in women, studies also support the effectiveness of this intervention for men. One controlled trial of 332 incontinent men following radical prostatectomy found that those enrolled in a pelvic muscle re-education program achieved continence earlier than those in the control group (Marchiori, Bertaccini, Manferrari, Ferri, & Martorana, 2010).

The goal of PFMT is the improvement of urethral resistance through active exercise of the pubococcygeal muscle. There are no contraindications to or negative effects of these exercises, which can be initiated by any motivated person who is able to learn the technique. A very important aspect of teaching about PFMT is to help the person accurately identify the pubococcygeal muscle. Once the pubococcygeal muscle is identified, the person must practice contracting and relaxing this muscle, gradually increasing the ability to hold the contraction. It is important to emphasize that improvement is very gradual, and full effects are not noticed until 3 to 6 months of regular exercise have been completed. Even after full effects are achieved, daily maintenance exercises must be continued. Box 19-5 summarizes the points to cover when teaching adults to do these exercises. In addition to teaching about PFMT, nurses can facilitate referrals to physical therapists who are skilled in teaching about these exercises.

In recent years, devices and equipment have become available as PFMT training aids, many of which are available without a prescription. Weighted vaginal cones can be used to gradually improve the strength of contractions. A pelvic floor muscle exerciser, consisting of a vaginal probe connected to a hand-held indicator, can be used to monitor the strength of contractions. Educational materials are available from the organizations listed in the Resources section of this chapter.

Biofeedback and Stimulation Devices

Biofeedback and various methods of nerve stimulation are sometimes used as interventions for stress, urge, or mixed

---

Box 19-5 Instructions for Performing Pelvic Muscle Exercises

Purpose: To prevent the involuntary loss of urine by strengthening the pelvic floor muscles

Frequency: Minimum of 3 sets of 10 contractions/relaxations daily, continued indefinitely

Position: Lying, sitting, walking, or standing with the muscles of your thighs, buttocks, and abdomen relaxed

Results: Most people begin to notice an improvement in urinary control after 3 to 6 weeks, but some will not notice the improvement until several months later

Techniques to Identify the Pubococcygeal Muscle

- Contract the muscle that stops the flow of urine. Do NOT do this regularly when urinating.
- (*Women*) Imagine that you are sitting on a marble and trying to suck it up into your vagina.
- (*Women*) Lie down and insert a finger about three quarters of the way up your vagina. Squeeze the vaginal wall so you feel pressure on your finger and a sensation in your vagina.
- (*Men*) Stand in front of a mirror and try to make the base of your penis move up and down without moving the rest of your body.

Additional information: You can ask your primary care practitioner for a referral to a physical therapist or continence advisor who can teach you to do these exercises.

- Biofeedback, weighted vaginal cones, or a perineometer (a balloon-like device that is placed in the vagina) can be used to assist in identifying the pubococcygeal muscle and in measuring the strength of the contraction.

Method

- Tighten your pubococcygeal muscle and hold for a period of at least 3 seconds; gradually increase the contraction time by 1 second per week until you can do a 10-second squeeze
- Relax this muscle for an equal period; rest and take deep breaths between contractions
- Do 10 sets of a contraction–relaxation cycle (one exercise) 3 times daily
- Breathe normally during these exercises and do NOT tighten other muscles at the same time. Be careful not to contract your legs, buttocks, or abdominal muscles while you are contracting your pubococcygeal muscle.
- For each of the daily sessions, vary your position (e.g., perform the exercise while lying down in the morning, standing in the afternoon, and sitting in the evening).

incontinence, either alone or with other treatments such as PFMT or bladder training. Studies indicate that these interventions are effective for improving urinary control, particularly for stress incontinence and after radial prostatectomy (Mariotti et al., 2009; Schmidt, Sanches, Silva, Ramos, & Nohama, 2009). Most nurses are not directly involved with administering these therapies, but they need to be familiar with the range of treatment options for incontinence, so they can facilitate appropriate referrals. Nurses can emphasize that many effective and noninvasive therapies are available, and they can encourage incontinent older adults to obtain information about these therapies from knowledgeable healthcare practitioners.

Biofeedback involves the use of monitoring devices to provide information about the physiologic activity involved in urination. Typically, a sensor is placed in the vagina of women or in or around the anus of men and connected to a computer that provides information about how the pelvic floor muscles are relaxing and contracting. The person uses this information to monitor the strength of muscle contractions to improve the effectiveness of PFMT.

Pelvic floor electrical stimulation, which can be done in office and home settings, uses an electrode to deliver small amounts of electrical stimulation to the nerves and muscles of the bladder and pelvic floor. This stimulation improves continence by increasing the sphincter tone and strengthening the levator and periurethral muscles. Devices that deliver pulsed magnetic fields to the pelvic floor muscles are also used as noninvasive methods of treating incontinence. Pulsed magnetic therapy is a passive treatment that does not depend on the person's ability to perform PFMT. Sacral nerve stimulation therapy is effective for urge incontinence and involves the surgical implantation of a neurostimulator under the abdominal skin. The neurostimulator, which is about the size of a stopwatch and can be adjusted nonsurgically, sends mild electrical pulses to the sacral nerves that control bladder function. This improves continence by inhibiting involuntary bladder contraction and promoting an increase in bladder volume.

Wellness Opportunity

Using biofeedback and other devices acknowledges the connection between the person's body and mind and may enhance self-care abilities.

Urinary Control Devices

A variety of intravaginal or intraurethral devices are available for resolving stress incontinence. Pessaries have been used for many decades to treat pelvic organ prolapse in women and are currently recommended as an inexpensive, simple, low-risk, conservative treatment (Atnip, 2009). These pelvic organ support devices are placed in the vagina to support the bladder, compress the urethra, or both. They are available in many sizes and shapes and are individually fitted by a primary care practitioner (Figure 19-2). Pessaries need to be removed and reinserted at intervals ranging from nightly to once every few months, depending on the type that is used.

In recent years, many urinary control devices have become available or are used in clinical trials for self-insertion into the urethra. For example, one type of device controls urination through the inflation and deflation of a small balloon that rests at the bladder neck. Other currently available devices for women include urethral plugs; intraurethral catheters with unidirectional valves; and external occlusive devices, which cover the external urinary meatus and provide a watertight seal to prevent leakage. For men, foam-cushioned penile

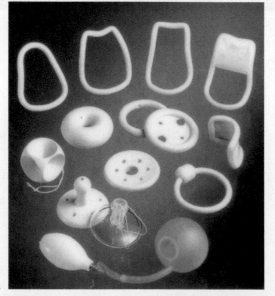

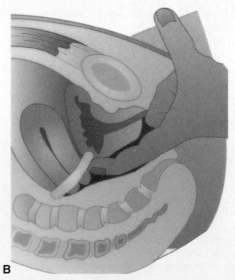

A   B

FIGURE 19-2 Examples of pessaries. Various shapes and sizes of pessaries available (**A**), insertion of one type of pessary (**B**). (From Smeltzer, S. C., Bare, B. G., Hinkle, J. E., & Cheever, K. [2008]. Brunner and Suddarth's textbook of medical-surgical nursing [11th ed.]. Philadelphia: Lippincott Williams & Wilkins.)

clamps with compression mechanisms are available. Because the options of urinary control devices for both men and women are rapidly evolving, nurses should encourage people with urinary incontinence to obtain current information from a qualified healthcare provider or from the National Association for Continence (listed in the Resources section at the end of this chapter).

Indwelling catheters have been widely used for decades as a urinary control device for incontinence. However, in recent years, their use has been questioned because of the high rate of associated urinary tract infections and other complications. Their use in long-term care facilities has come under particular scrutiny, and the number of residents who have indwelling catheters is viewed as an indicator of quality of care in long-term care facilities (with lower numbers of indwelling catheters being associated with better quality of care). The only acceptable indications for the use of internal catheters, according to the Centers for Medicare and Medicaid Services (CMS), are stage III or IV pressure sores when urine impedes healing, urinary retention that cannot be treated medically or surgically, or terminal illnesses with which position changes are painful. Intermittent clean catheterization is sometimes used as a self-care or caregiver-administered intervention for some types of incontinence.

Continence Training

Continence training can be categorized as (1) methods that are self-directed by motivated and cognitively intact people or (2) methods that are directed by motivated caregivers of cognitively impaired people. The goal of continence training is to achieve a continent interval of 2 to 4 hours between voiding. These intervals will not necessarily be equal and will usually be longer during the night. In self-directed programs, the person hopes to regain voluntary urinary control, whereas in caregiver-directed programs, the caregiver hopes to reduce the episodes of incontinence. Self-directed continence training, alone or in combination with biofeedback or medications, is most successful with urge incontinence. Continence training cannot be effective if the bladder capacity is less than 150 mL.

Although specific techniques vary, essential elements of any continence training program include motivation, an assessment of voiding patterns, an individualized and carefully timed intake of approximately 2000 mL of fluid per day, timed voiding in the most appropriate place, methods of reinforcing expected behaviors, and ongoing monitoring. During the initial assessment, diaries are used to record times and circumstances of toileting as well as times of and reasons for any episode of incontinence. After the usual voiding pattern is identified, the older adult is encouraged to resist the sensation of urgency and to postpone voiding rather than responding immediately to an urge.

With caregiver-directed methods—often referred to as prompted voiding programs—the caregiver uses the initial assessment of voiding patterns to establish a schedule for assisting with voiding. The caregiver gradually increases the

Box 19-6 Continence Training Programs

Goal of Programs: To achieve voluntary control over urination at intervals of 2 to 4 hours

Terminology
Terms used for self-directed programs: bladder drill, bladder training, bladder retraining, bladder exercise, bladder retention exercise
Terms used for caregiver-directed programs: scheduled toileting, routine toileting, prompted voiding, timed voiding, habit training

Method
Step 1: Identify the usual voiding pattern, noting the times of incontinence and information about fluid intake. During the first few days, keep a diary to record the following information at hourly intervals: dry or wet, amount voided, place of voiding, fluid intake, and sensation and awareness of need to void.
Step 2: Using information from the voiding diary, establish a schedule that allows for emptying of the bladder before incontinence is likely to occur.
Step 3: Provide the equipment and assistance necessary for optimal voiding at scheduled times.
Step 4: Provide 2000 mL of noncaffeinated liquids per day for liquid intake. Consume the largest amounts during the early part of the day, and limit fluid intake at about 2 to 4 hours before bedtime.
Step 5: Gradually increase the length of time between voidings until the interval is 2 to 4 hours long.

interval between voidings until the person can maintain continence for 2 to 4 hours. These methods are most successful when the timed intervals are flexible and are adjusted based on a good assessment of the person's needs and voiding patterns. A review of studies found that prompted voiding is effective for reducing urinary incontinence episodes in residents of long-term care facilities (Fink, Taylor, Tacklind, Rutks, & Wilt, 2008). Caregiver-directed programs include the use of behavior modification techniques, such as praising the person for staying dry between scheduled trips to the bathroom and self-initiating requests to use the toilet. Box 19-6 identifies some of the terms used for and the general principles of continence training programs.

Environmental Modifications

When incontinence is associated with the inability to reach an appropriate receptacle after perceiving the need to void, interventions are directed toward modifying the environment and improving functional abilities. If environmental adaptations cannot be made, as in public places, older adults are encouraged to become familiar with the location and arrangement of the bathroom facilities before the need to urinate is imminent. In home and institutional settings, the provision of bedside commodes and privacy can be an effective intervention. If space is limited or privacy cannot be assured, however, bedside commodes may not be acceptable. Box 19-7 lists environmental modifications that can be implemented to prevent incontinence when functional limitations are a

Box 19-7 Environmental Modifications for Preventing Incontinence

Modifications to Enhance Visibility of Facilities
- Use contrasting colors for the toilet seat and surroundings.
- Provide adequate lighting in and near toilet areas, but avoid creating glare.
- Use nightlights in the pathway between the bedroom and bathroom.

Modifications to Improve the Ability to Use the Toilet in Time
- Encourage the use of chairs or beds that are designed to help the person arise unaided after sitting or lying.
- Install handrails in the hallway(s) leading to the bathroom.
- Make sure the pathway to the bathroom is safe and uncluttered.

Modifications to Improve the Ability to Use the Toilet
- Place grab bars at appropriate places to facilitate getting on and off the toilet and to assist men in maintaining their balance when standing at the toilet.
- Use elevated toilet seats or an over-the-toilet chair to compensate for any functional limitations of the lower extremities.
- If the person has functional limitations involving the upper extremities, clothing for the lower body should feature easy-open closures such as Velcro or elastic waistbands.

contributing factor. Interventions discussed in chapters on vision (Chapter 17) and mobility (Chapter 22) can address functional limitations that can contribute to incontinence.

Wellness Opportunity

Nurses promote self-care by helping older adults to identify ways of improving their functional abilities that can affect urinary control.

Medications
Medications have varying degrees of success for treating incontinence, but their effectiveness depends greatly on identi-

fying and addressing the specific type of incontinence. Medications can also effectively treat an underlying condition that contributes to incontinence (e.g., vaginitis and benign prostatic hyperplasia). If medications are prescribed, nurses are responsible for knowing their expected positive effects as well as their potential adverse effects.

Medications that act on the autonomic nervous system are most often used for the control of incontinence. Alpha-adrenergic agents control stress incontinence by increasing bladder outlet resistance through stimulating receptors at the trigone and internal sphincter. Alpha-adrenergic blocking agents, used either alone or in combination with cholinergic agents, can treat incontinence by decreasing bladder outlet resistance. Antimuscarinic agents are used for urge urinary incontinence and OAB because they control the uninhibited or unstable bladder by blocking the transmission of nerve impulses.

In recent years, geriatricians have expressed concern about the adverse effects of antimuscarinic agents, which are used increasingly for the treatment of OAB. All antimuscarinic agents have the potential to cross the blood–brain barrier when the integrity of the barrier is compromised by conditions such as diabetes, dementia, stroke, and Parkinson's disease. In addition, antimuscarinic agents can have the same adverse effects as other anticholinergics, which is particularly problematic with regard to drug interactions and cumulative effects. A review of studies found that oxybutynin (Ditropan) is the antimuscarinic agent most strongly associated with cognitive impairment, and darifenacin (Enablex) is the agent with the most evidence for no cognitive impairment (Kay & Ebinger, 2008). In addition to darifenacin, antimuscarinic agents that have relatively few cognitive effects are transdermal oxybutynin, fesoterodine (Toviaz), tolterodine (Detrol), and solifenacin (Vesicare) (Saks & Arya, 2009). Nurses need to raise questions about a potential relationship between the onset and worsening of mental changes in anyone taking medications with antimuscarinic action, particularly if the person takes other anticholinergic agents. Table 19-2 lists types and examples of medications that are approved for treating urinary incontinence.

TABLE 19-2 Medications Approved for Treating Urinary Incontinence

Type of Urinary Incontinence	Type of Medication	Examples
Urge incontinence and overactive bladder syndrome	Anticholinergic action to relax the bladder and inhibit uncontrolled contractions	darifenacin (Enablex) fesoterodine fumarate (Toviaz) oxybutynin (Ditropan) oxybutynin transdermal patch (Oxytrol) or gel (Gelnique) solifenacin (Vesicare) tolterodine (Detrol) trospium (Sanctura)
Incontinence and retention associated with prostatic hyperplasia	Anti-adrenergic action to relax the smooth muscle of the urethra and prostatic capsule	Alfuzosin (Uroxatral) doxazosin (Cardura) dutasteride (Avodart) finasteride (Proscar) tamsulosin (Flomax) terazosin (Hytrin)
Urinary retention with incontinence	Cholinergic action stimulates bladder contractions	bethanechol (Urecholine)

Surgical and Minimally Invasive Procedures

Surgical procedures have been used for many decades to control incontinence when structural abnormalities, such as a cystocele, are identified as the underlying cause. For example, several types of bladder suspension surgery or "sling" procedures are used for stress incontinence. The goal of bladder suspension surgery is to reposition the urethra so that the pelvic floor muscles can squeeze it more effectively. When urinary incontinence is caused by a loss of sphincter control, it may be treated successfully by surgical implantation of an artificial urinary sphincter—a device with an inflatable cuff that is placed around the urethra to hold it closed. To operate the artificial urinary sphincter, men squeeze a pump in the scrotum, whereas women press a valve in the labia to deflate the cuff, which automatically reinflates after voiding is completed.

In recent years, several minimally invasive surgical procedures have been developed for treating incontinence. Periurethral injections of a bulking agent (e.g., collagen) are effective for long-term treatment of stress incontinence when it is caused by intrinsic sphincter deficiency (Ghoniem, Corcos, Comiter, Westney, & Herschorn, 2010). Minimally invasive procedures that are used include the tension-free vaginal tape system for women and visual laser ablation and transurethral needle ablation for benign prostatic hyperplasia. In addition, a wire mesh stent can be placed in the man's urethra to maintain the flow of urine through an enlarged prostate.

◆ **Wellness Opportunity**

Nurses promote self-care by encouraging older adults to seek further evaluation by qualified healthcare professionals rather than relying solely on the reported experiences of friends.

Managing Incontinence

When incontinence cannot be alleviated, it can be managed with the use of various aids and equipment, including disposable and washable incontinence products and collecting devices, such as urinals and commodes. When used in conjunction with environmental modifications to increase the accessibility of toilet facilities, such equipment usually has beneficial effects; however, when aids and equipment are used by caregivers as substitutes for other methods of promoting continence, they are beneficial only to the caregiver and are detrimental to the older adult. For example, if protective products are used to manage incontinence, the positive effect for the caregiver may be the ease of care; however, the negative effects for the older adult include the likelihood of skin breakdown and decreased self-esteem. Because continence aids can be beneficial as well as detrimental, they should be used only after careful evaluation of all contributing factors.

When an older adult depends on a caregiver for assistance with urinary elimination, the nurse who is planning interventions must consider the needs, limitations, and abilities of the caregiver. In institutional settings, staff is expected and trained to care for incontinent patients or residents using the most appropriate interventions. In home settings, the nurse must consider the total caregiving situation, and the needs of the caregiver may take precedence over the needs of the older adult, particularly if the caregiver has functional limitations.

Selection of the numerous products available for managing incontinence depends on factors such as cost, convenience, and effectiveness. Economic considerations are particularly important because disposable incontinence products can be quite expensive, particularly if used daily. The initial and periodic cost of reusable products also needs to be considered, as does the time and expense of laundering. Many types of products are designed specifically for either male or female incontinence. Products are also available according to degrees of absorbency, ranging from light to heavy protection. Absorbency of some disposable products is enhanced by the addition of gel or fiber materials. Often different products will be needed to address incontinence under particular circumstances. For example, a person may need a product with light protection during the day and heavy protection during the night. Ease of use is a major consideration, particularly for people who are able to manage incontinence with little or no supervision. "Pull-ups" now provide a convenient alternative to the products with tabs that cannot be easily removed before and reapplied after toileting. Box 19-8 lists factors to be considered in selecting and using various types of aids and equipment for managing urinary incontinence. Nurses can keep up-to-date on new developments in incontinence products by visiting the Internet sites listed in the Resources section of this chapter.

*M*r. and Mrs. U. are now 73 and 72 years old, respectively, and continue to attend the senior center where you are the nurse. Mr. U. has been under the care of a urologist for 3 years and has been taking terazosin for prostatic hyperplasia. Until recently, he was able to maintain urinary continence, but lately his Parkinson's has worsened. Then, 1 month ago he started taking 80 mg of furosemide daily for congestive heart failure. He makes an appointment to ask your advice about incontinence products that would be best for him because "it's just hopeless to get to the toilet on time because our only bathroom is upstairs, and I like to be downstairs during the day." He reports that he limits his fluid intake to 4 cups of liquid daily, which includes 2 cups of black coffee. Because of his Parkinson's disease, he has trouble standing at the toilet and usually sits down; however, he is "slow and clumsy" in managing his clothing. His son bought him some "jogging" outfits with elastic waists, but he does not wear them because he prefers to "dress up" when he goes to the senior center, so he wears trousers with belts.

THINKING POINTS WITH REGARD TO MR. U.

- What risk factors are likely to be contributing to Mr. U.'s incontinence, and which factors might be alleviated with interventions?
- What environmental modifications might be helpful in addressing the incontinence?
- What health education would you give about alleviating risk factors?
- What health education would you give about incontinence products?

*M*rs. U. also makes an appointment to see you to discuss her recent problem with incontinence. She tells you that for several years she has been wearing "light-days pads" because "I have trouble holding my water whenever I sneeze or cough." In the past few months, she notices that she has to go to the bathroom every hour or two and is reluctant to be away from her house for more than an hour at a time. Her health has been good overall, but her arthritis has been getting worse, and she is very slow in her mobility, particularly when she needs to go up and down stairs. She drinks about 6 cups of liquid daily, consisting mostly

of tea and coffee. She has heard some of her friends talking about "those Kegel exercises we had to do when we had our babies." One friend even talked about having some "cones she puts in to help her with exercises."

THINKING POINTS WITH REGARD TO MRS. U.

- What risk factors are likely to be contributing to Mrs. U.'s incontinence?
- What environmental modifications might be helpful in addressing the incontinence?
- What health education would you give about alleviating risk factors?
- What health education would you give about Kegel exercises?
- What health education would you give about incontinence products?

EVALUATING EFFECTIVENESS OF NURSING INTERVENTIONS

Nursing care for older adults with urinary incontinence is evaluated by measuring the extent to which the person can achieve periods of continence that are as long as possible. When older adults attribute incontinence to aging processes, nurses evaluate the effectiveness of their teaching by the degree to which the person verbalizes accurate information and understands the importance of identifying treatable causes. Another measure of the effectiveness of nursing interventions in such cases would be that the person seeks evaluation for

---

Box 19-8 Considerations Regarding Continence Aids and Equipment

Assessment Considerations

- What are the costs of various disposable and washable products, both initially and over a period of time? (Include the time and expense of laundry when considering costs of washable products.)
- What are the preferences of the incontinent person? (e.g., Is a "brief" or "pull-up" style garment more acceptable than a "diaper" style product? Also, how much noise a product makes when the person is walking or moving around in social settings may influence the acceptability of a product.)
- What level of absorbency is appropriate for different circumstances?
- What are the needs and abilities of the caregivers of dependent older adults in home settings? (Can the caregiver manage the tasks involved in toileting?)
- What are the secondary benefits of various aids? (For example, in home settings, if the care of an individual with an indwelling catheter is covered by Medicare as skilled care, will additional services, such as home health aide assistance, also be covered?)
- What are the consequences if the incontinence cannot be managed in the home setting? (For example, will the older adult need to be in a long-term care setting?)

Teaching Related to Aids and Equipment

- Many types of external collecting devices are available for men and women (e.g., male or female urinals, condom catheters, retracted penis pouches, and bedside urinals with attached drainage bags).
- An elevated toilet seat with rails can be used to increase safety and transfer mobility.
- Commodes are useful in diminishing the distance between the place of usual activities and toilet facilities.
- A variety of commodes are available and can be selected according to needs and preferences of the dependent person.
- If commodes are viewed as socially unacceptable, measures can be taken to ensure privacy and increase their social acceptability. Privacy can be ensured by placing an attractive screen around the commode.
- Commodes are now available that are attractively designed to resemble normal furniture items.
- A bedpan can be placed on a regular chair, particularly in the bedroom, and removed when not in use.

his or her incontinence, rather than accepting this condition as inevitable.

If incontinence cannot be resolved, nursing care is directed toward managing urinary elimination in such a way as to maintain the dignity of the older adult and to prevent negative consequences. In these situations, the effectiveness of nursing interventions might be measured by the extent to which the person maintains daily activities. For example, if older adults restrict their social activities because of incontinence, a measure of the success of nursing interventions might be that they begin using incontinence products to permit them to be away from their home for 4 hours at a time. For people with total incontinence, a measure of the effectiveness of nursing interventions would be the absence of skin irritation and breakdown.

Mrs. U., who is now 79 years old, is being transferred to a long-term care facility for rehabilitation after sustaining a hip fracture. An indwelling catheter was inserted before her hip surgery 7 days ago, and it was removed yesterday. She is ambulating with a walker but needs one-person assistance. The discharge summary describes her as incontinent of urine. Mrs. U. hopes to regain her independence in performing ADLs so that she can return to her own home, where she lives with her husband.

NURSING ASSESSMENT

During your functional assessment, Mrs. U. tells you she has had "trouble holding her water" since they removed the catheter yesterday. She is quite embarrassed about this and has not discussed it with any other healthcare practitioner. She says that she had too many other questions to discuss with her orthopedic surgeon and states that the nurses kept a large absorbent pad on her bed so that she would not have to walk to the bathroom. When she went to physical therapy, she used sanitary napkins, which her friend brought to her. She limited her fluid intake to a cup of coffee with each meal and a few sips of water with her pills.

Further assessment of Mrs. U's incontinence reveals that, for many years, she has had difficulty with "leaking," particularly when she coughs, sneezes, or exercises. Also, she gets up to urinate about four to five times nightly. It was during one of these trips to the bathroom that she tripped and fractured her hip. She says that she wakes up a lot during the night and goes to the bathroom because she is afraid of wetting the bed. She does not feel the need to urinate every time she wakes up but goes to the bathroom to prevent any leakage. She limits her fluid intake to 6 glasses per day and does not drink anything after 5 PM. A few years ago, a nurse taught her how to do "Kegels and they helped for a couple years, but I don't bother to do them anymore." She tearfully confides that she thinks that the orthopedic surgeon damaged a nerve in her bladder, which she believes is the reason she has such little control over urination since the surgery. She thinks that the hospital staff inserted the catheter because she has "weak kidneys." She states, "Before I had this fractured hip, I just had the usual problems holding water like all my friends have, but now it's really bad and I'll probably never be able to hold my water again. I wish you'd just put that tube back in me, so I can go home again and not worry about accidents."

NURSING DIAGNOSIS

In addition to the nursing diagnoses related to Mrs. U.'s impaired mobility, you address her problem with urinary incontinence. In deciding which type of urinary incontinence to include in your nursing diagnosis, you conclude that both Stress Incontinence and Functional Incontinence are appropriate because of the combination of long-term and recent factors that contribute to her incontinence. Your nursing diagnosis is Stress/Functional Incontinence related to limited mobility, recent indwelling catheter, and insufficient knowledge of normal urinary function and pelvic muscle exercises. Evidence for this diagnosis can be found in Mrs. U.'s statements reflecting misconceptions and lack of information and in her description of current and past problems with incontinence. Evidence is also derived from your observations that she needs one-person assistance for walking and that she uses sanitary napkins and bed pads for urinary incontinence.

(case study continues on page 404)

NURSING CARE PLAN FOR MRS. U.

Expected Outcome	Nursing Interventions	Nursing Evaluation
Mrs. U.'s knowledge of normal urinary function will increase.	• Discuss normal urinary function using a balloon partially filled with water and a simple illustration of the female urinary tract. • Emphasize the relationship between adequate fluid intake and continence.	• Mrs. U. will be able to describe normal urinary function and the mechanisms involved in maintaining continence.
Mrs. U.'s knowledge about causative factors for incontinence will increase.	• Describe age-related changes that contribute to incontinence using the information in Box 19-4. • Discuss the effects of frequent bladder emptying and limited fluid intake on the maintenance of continence. • Discuss the relationship between limited mobility and urinary incontinence.	• Mrs. U. will describe age-related changes that influence urinary elimination. • Mrs. U. will identify risk factors that contribute to her incontinence.
Mrs. U.'s misconceptions about her urinary incontinence will be corrected.	• Emphasize that as Mrs. U. regains her mobility, she will regain continence. • Emphasize that urinary incontinence is not an inevitable consequence of aging. • Explain that the orthopedic surgeon was not operating on or near her bladder or urinary tract. • Explain that the Foley catheter probably contributed to her current incontinence, but that this is a temporary situation that will resolve with proper interventions. • Emphasize that the nursing home staff will work with her to improve or alleviate her incontinence.	• Mrs. U. will state correct information about the relationship between her hip surgery and her incontinence. • Mrs. U. will express confidence in regaining urinary control.
The factors that contribute to Mrs. U.'s functional incontinence will be eliminated.	• Provide a bedside commode for Mrs. U.'s use until she is able to walk to the bathroom without assistance. • Work with the physical therapy staff to teach Mrs. U. a proper technique for independent transfer to the commode. • The nursing and dietary staff will provide 2000 mL of fluids per day taking into consideration Mrs. U.'s preferences. • The nursing and dietary staff will work with Mrs. U. to schedule her fluid intake at acceptable times of the day with minimal intake in the evening. • Talk with Mrs. U. about eliminating the bed pads as soon as she feels confident about maintaining continence.	• Mrs. U. will be continent of urine, except for stress incontinence.

Expected Outcome	Nursing Interventions	Nursing Evaluation
Mrs. U. will regain full control over urination.	• Suggest that Mrs. U. seek a comprehensive assessment of her urinary incontinence. • Give Mrs. U. a copy of Box 19-5 as a guide for performing PFMT. • Emphasize the need to perform PFMT on an ongoing basis for the alleviation of stress incontinence. • Give Mrs. U. information about health education that may be helpful for her.	• Mrs. U. will report a reduction in or elimination of her stress incontinence.

THINKING POINTS

- What myths and misunderstandings affect Mrs. U's attitude about urinary incontinence?
- What risk factors are contributing to Mrs. U's urinary incontinence?
- What additional assessment information would you want to obtain?

Chapter Highlights

Age-Related Changes That Affect Urinary Wellness
- Kidney: degenerative changes, decreased blood flow, decreased number of functioning nephrons
- Urinary tract muscles: hypertrophy of bladder muscle, replacement of smooth muscle with connective tissue, relaxation of pelvic floor muscles
- Voluntary control mechanisms: central nervous system, urinary tract, age-related changes of other systems (e.g., increased postural sway)

Risk Factors That Affect Urinary Wellness
- Misperceptions and attitudes (e.g., resignation, viewing urinary incontinence as "normal," staff and caregiver attitudes that interfere with maintaining continence)
- Functional impairments that affect control over socially appropriate urinary elimination (e.g., dependency in ADLs)
- Pathologic changes of the genitourinary tract (e.g., pelvic floor dysfunction, benign prostatic hyperplasia)
- Other pathologic conditions (e.g., dementia, Parkinson's, constipation)
- Medication effects (Table 19-1)
- Dietary and lifestyle factors (e.g., obesity, tobacco smoking, intake of caffeinated beverages)
- Environmental factors (Box 19-1)

Functional Consequences Affecting Urinary Wellness
- Effects on homeostasis: diminished ability to maintain electrolyte balance, changes in diurnal pattern of urine production
- Delayed excretion of water-soluble medications and increased risk of drug interactions and adverse effects
- Diminished bladder capacity; urinary urgency and frequency

- Decrease in the interval between the signal of the need to void and the actual need to empty the bladder

Pathologic Condition Affecting Urinary Function
- Urinary incontinence: stress urinary incontinence, urge urinary incontinence, mixed urinary incontinence, overactive bladder
- Diminished quality of life due to urinary incontinence
- Practical and psychosocial effects of urinary incontinence on the older adult and caregivers

Nursing Assessment of Urinary Function (Figure 19-1, Boxes 19-2 and 19-3)
- Talking with older adults about urinary function (finding appropriate terminology)
- Identifying usual voiding patterns and influencing factors (Figure 19-1)
- Identifying risk factors for urinary incontinence
- Identifying risk factors that influence renal function and homeostasis
- Identifying symptoms of impaired urinary elimination
- Being alert to misunderstandings about urinary elimination
- Psychosocial consequences of incontinence (e.g., anxiety, depression, social isolation)

Nursing Diagnosis
- Readiness for Enhanced Urinary Elimination
- Impaired Urinary Elimination
- Social Isolation
- Caregiver Role Strain (or Risk for)

Planning for Wellness Outcomes
- Urinary Continence
- Urinary Elimination
- Health Beliefs: Perceived Control
- Caregiver Stressors
- Caregiver Endurance Potential

Nursing Interventions to Promote Healthy Urinary Function (Table 19-2, Boxes 19-5 through 19-8)

- Teaching older adults about age-related changes and preventing urinary incontinence
- Promoting continence and alleviating incontinence (pelvic floor muscle training, urinary control devices, continence training, environmental modifications, medications, and surgical or minimally invasive procedures)
- Managing urinary incontinence

Evaluating Effectiveness of Nursing Interventions

- Longer intervals of continence
- Accurate understanding of normal urinary function and risks for incontinence
- Self-care practices to promote continence and urinary wellness
- Use of resources for further evaluation of incontinence when appropriate

Critical Thinking Exercises

1. Describe how each of the following age-related changes or risk factors might influence urinary function in older adults: medications; renal function; functional abilities; environmental conditions; altered thirst perception; changes in the urinary tract and nervous system; and myths and misunderstandings on the part of older adults, their caregivers, and healthcare professionals.
2. What are the psychosocial consequences of urinary incontinence for older adults and their caregivers?
3. Describe how you would address the following statement made by a 74-year-old woman: "Of course I have to wear pads all the time, just like when I was a teenager. I haven't talked to the doctor because I figured this was pretty normal at my age."
4. Describe the nursing assessment, with regard to urinary elimination, for a 75-year-old man and a 75-year-old woman.

Resources

For links to these resources and additional helpful Internet resources related to this chapter, visit thePoint at http://thePoint. lww.com/Miller6e.

Clinical Tools

American Journal of Nursing and Hartford Institute for Geriatric Nursing
- *How to Try This,* article and video: Dowling-Castronovo, A., & Specht, J. K. (2009). Assessment of transient incontinence in older adults. *American Journal of Nursing, 109*(2), 62–71.

Hartford Institute for Geriatric Nursing
- *Try This: Best Practices in Nursing Care to Older Adults* Issue 11.1 (2007), Urinary Incontinence Assessment in Older Adults, Part I: Transient Urinary Incontinence
  Issue 11.2 (2008), Urinary Incontinence Assessment in Older Adults, Part II: Established Urinary Incontinence

Evidence-Based Practice

Dowling-Castronovo, A., & Bradway, C. (2008). Urinary incontinence. In E. Capezuti, D. Zwicker, M. Mezey, & T. Fulmer (Eds.), *Evidence-Based Geriatric Nursing Protocols for Best Practice* (3rd ed., pp. 309–336). New York: Springer Publishing Co.
National Guideline Clearinghouse
  - Urinary incontinence in older adults admitted to acute care
  - Urinary incontinence in women
  - Prevention of fecal and urinary incontinence in adults

Health Education

International Continence Society
National Association for Continence (NAFC)
The American Geriatrics Society (AGS) Foundation for Health in Aging
The Canadian Continence Foundation
The Simon Foundation for Continence

REFERENCES

Amselem, C., Puigdollers, A., Azpiroz, F., Sala, C., Videla, S., Fernandez-Fraga, X., . . . Malagelada, J. (2010). Constipation: A potential cause of pelvic floor damage? *Neurogastroenterology and Motility: The Official Journal of the European Gastrointestinal Motility Society, 22*(2), 150–153.

Atnip, S. D. (2009). Pessary use and management for pelvic organ prolapse. *Obstetrics and Gynecology Clinics of North America, 36,* 541–563.

Badalian, S. S., & Rosenbaum, P. F. (2010). Vitamin D and pelvic floor disorders in women: Results from the National Health and Nutrition Examination Survey. *Obstetrics and Gynecology, 115*(4), 795–803.

Bliwise, D. L., Foley, D. J., Vitiello, M. V., Ansari, F. P., Ancoli-Israel, S., & Walsh, J. K. (2009). Nocturia and disturbed sleep in the elderly. *Sleep Medicine, 10*(5), 540–548.

Botlero, R., Bell, R. J., Urquhart, D. M., & Davis, S. R. (2010). Urinary incontinence is associated with lower psychological general well-being in community-dwelling women. *Menopause, 17*(2), 332–337.

Byles, J., Millar, C. J., Sibbritt, D. W., & Chiarelli, P. (2009). Living with urinary incontinence: A longitudinal study of older women. *Age and Ageing, 38,* 333–338.

Cheung, W. W., Khan, N. H., Choi, K. K., Bluth, M. H., & Vincent, M. T. (2009). Prevalence, evaluation and management of overactive bladder in primary care. *BMC Family Practice, 10*(8), 1–7. doi:10.1186/1471-2296-10-8.

Dowling-Castronovo, A., & Bradway, C. (2008). Urinary incontinence. In E. Capezuti, D. Zwicker, M. Mezey, & T. Fulmer (Eds.), *Evidence-based geriatric nursing protocols for best practice* (3rd ed., pp. 309–336). New York: Springer Publishing Co.

Dowling-Castronovo, A., & Specht, J. K. (2009). How to try this: Assessment of transient incontinence in older adults. *American Journal of Nursing, 109*(2), 62–71.

Dumoulin, C., & Hay-Smith, J. (2010). Pelvic floor muscle training versus no treatment, or inactive control treatments for urinary incontinence in women. *Cochrane Database of Systematic Reviews,* Issue I, article no. CD005654. doi:10.1002/14651858.CD005654.pub2.

Ekundayo, O. J., Markland, A., Lefante, C., Sui, X., Goode, P. S., Allman, R. M., . . . Ahmed, A. (2009). Association of diuretic use and overactive bladder syndrome in older adults: A propensity score analysis. *Archives of Gerontology and Geriatrics, 49*(1), 64–68.

El-Azab, A. S., & Shaaban, O. M. (2010). Measuring the barriers against seeking consultation for urinary incontinence among Middle Eastern women. *BMC Women's Health, 10*(3), 1–6.

Elpern, E. H., Killeen, K., Ketchem, A., Wiley, A., Patel, G., & Lateef, O. (2009). Reducing use of indwelling urinary catheters and associated urinary tract infections. *American Journal of Critical Care, 18*(6), 535–541.

Endeshaw, Y. (2009). Correlates of self-reported nocturia among community-dwelling older adults. *Journal of Gerontology: A Biological Sciences Medical Sciences, 64*A(1), 142–148.

Fink, H. A., Taylor, B. C., Tacklind, J. W., Rutks, I. R., & Wilt, T. J. (2008). Treatment interventions in nursing home residents with urinary incontinence: A systematic review of randomized trials. *Mayo Clinic Proceedings, 83*, 1332–1343.

French, L., Phelps, K., Pothula, N. R., & Mushkbar, S. (2009). Urinary problems in women. *Primary Care: Clinics in Office Practice, 36*, 53–71.

Fritel, X., Fauconnier, A., Bader, G., Cosson, M., Debodinance, P. L., Deffieux, X., . . . French College of Gynaecologists and Obstetricians. (2010). Diagnosis and management of adult female stress urinary incontinence: Guidelines for clinical practice from the French College of Gynecologists and Obstetricians. *European Journal of Obstetrics, Gynecology and Reproductive Biology, 151*(1), 14–19.

Ghoniem, G., Corcos, J., Comiter, C., Westney, O. L., & Herschorn, S. (2010). Durability of urethral bulking agent injection for female stress urinary incontinence: 2-year multicenter study results. *Journal of Urology, 183*(4), 1444–1449.

Glassock, R. J., & Winearls, C. (2009). Ageing and the glomerular filtration rate: Truths and consequences. *Transactions of the American Clinical and Climatological Association, 120*, 419–423.

Griebling, T. L. (2009). Urinary incontinence in the elderly. *Clinics in Geriatric Medicine, 25*, 445–457.

Hasegawa, J., Kuzuya, M., & Iguchi, A. (2010). Urinary incontinence and behavioral symptoms are independent risk factors for recurrent and injurious falls, respectively, among residents in long-term care facilities. *Archives of Gerontology and Geriatrics, 50*(1), 77–81.

Hung, H. C., Hsiao, S. M., Chih, S. Y., Lin, H. H., & Tsauo, J. Y. (2010). An alternative intervention for urinary incontinence: Retraining diaphragmatic, deep abdominal and pelvic floor muscle coordinated function. *Manual Therapy, 15*(3), 273–279.

Kang, Y., & Crogan, N. L. (2008). Social and cultural construction of urinary incontinence among Korean American elderly women. *Geriatric Nursing, 29*(2), 105–111.

Kay, G. G., & Ebinger, U. (2008). Preserving cognitive function for patients with overactive bladder: Evidence for a differential effect with darifenacin. *International Journal of Clinical Practice, 62*(11), 1792–1800.

Lerma, E. V. (2009). Anatomic and physiologic changes of the aging kidney. *Clinics in Geriatric Medicine, 25*, 325–329.

Marchiori, D., Bertaccini, A., Manferrari, F., Ferri, C., & Martorana, G. (2010). Pelvic floor rehabilitation for continence recovery after radical prostatectomy: Role of a personal training re-educational program. *Anticancer Research, 30*(2), 553–556.

Mariotti, G., Sciarra, A., Gentilucci, A., Salciccia, S., Alfarone, A., Pierro, G. D., & Gentile, V. (2009). Early recovery of urinary continence after radical prostatectomy using early pelvic floor electrical stimulation and biofeedback associated treatment. *Journal of Urology, 181*(4), 1788–1793.

Melville, J. L., Fan, M.-Y., Rau, H., Nygaard, I. E., & Katon, M. D. (2009). Major depression and urinary incontinence in women: Temporal associations in an epidemiologic sample. *American Journal of Obstetrics & Gynecology, 201*, 490.1.e1–490.1.e7.

Menezes, M. A. J., Hashimoto, S. Y., & de Gouveia Santos, V. L. C. (2009). Prevalence of urinary incontinence in a community sample from the city of Sao Paulo. *Journal of the Wound, Ostomy and Continence Nurses Society, 36*(4), 436–440.

Mohsin, R., & Siddiqui, K. M. (2010). Recurrent urinary tract infections in females. *The Journal of the Pakistan Medical Association, 60*(1), 55–59.

Nicolle, L. E. (2009). Urinary tract infections in the elderly. *Clinics in Geriatric Medicine, 25*, 423–436.

O'Donohue, D., Winsor, G., Gallagher, R., Maughan, J., Dooley, K., & Walsh, J. (2010). Issues for people living with long-term urinary catheters in the community. *British Journal of Community Nursing, 15*(2), 65–70.

Rahn, D. D., & Roshanravan, S. M. (2009). Pathophysiology of urinary incontinence, voiding dysfunction, and overactive bladder. *Obstetrics and Gynecology Clinics of North America, 36*, 463–474.

Rogers, M. A., Mody, L., Kaufman, S. R., Fries, B. E., McMahon, L. F. Jr., & Saint, S. (2008). Use of urinary collection devices in skilled nursing facilities in five states. *Journal of the American Geriatric Society, 56*(5), 854–861.

Saks, E. K., & Arya, L. A. (2009). Pharmacologic management of urinary incontinence, voiding dysfunction, and overactive bladder. *Obstetrics and Gynecology Clinics of North America, 36*, 493–507.

Sari, D., & Khorshid, L. (2009). The effects of pelvic floor muscle training on stress and mixed urinary incontinence and quality of life. *Journal of the Wound, Ostomy and Continence Nurses Society, 36*(4), 429–435.

Schmidt, A. P., Sanches, P. R., Silva, D. P. Jr., Ramos, J. G., & Nohama, P. (2009). A new pelvic muscle trainer for the treatment of urinary incontinence. *International Journal of Gynecology and Obstetrics, 105*(3), 218–222.

St. John, W., Wallis, M., Griffiths, S., & McKenzie, S. (2010). Daily-living management of urinary incontinence, a synthesis of the literature. *Journal of the Wound, Ostomy and Continence Nurses Society, 37*(1), 80–90.

Sung, V. W., & Hampton, B. S. (2009). Epidemiology of pelvic floor dysfunction. *Obstetrics and Gynecology Clinics of North America, 36*, 421–443.

Tennstedt, S. L., Chiu, G. R., Link, C. L., Litman, H. J., Kusek, J. W., & McKinlay, J. B. (2010). The effects of severity of urine leakage on quality of life in Hispanic, white, and black men and women: The Boston Community Health Survey. *Urology, 75*(1), 27–28.

Townsend, M. K., Curhan, G. C., Resnick, N. M., & Grodstein, F. (2010). The incidence of urinary incontinence across Asian, black, and white women in the United States. *American Journal of Obstetrics & Gynecology, 202*, 378.e1–378.e7.

van Kerrebroeck, P., Hashim, H., Holm-Larsen, T., Robinson, D., & Stanley, N. (2010). Thinking beyond the bladder: Antidiuretic treatment of nocturia. *The International Journal of Clinical Practice, 64*(6), 807–816.

Vaughan, C. P., Brown, C. J., Goode, P. S., Burgio, K. L., Allman, R. M., & Johnson, T. M. II. (2010). The association of nocturia with incident falls in an elderly community-dwelling cohort. *International Journal of Clinical Practice, 64*(5), 577–583.

Voss, A. M. B. (2009). Incidence and duration of urinary catheters in hospitalized older adults, before and after implementing a geriatric protocol. *Journal of Gerontological Nursing, 35*(6), 35–41.

Wilde, M. H., Brasch, J., Getliffe, K., Brown, K. A., McMahon, J. M., Smith, J. A., . . . Tu, X. (2010). Study on the use of long-term urinary catheters in community-dwelling individuals. *Journal of Wound, Ostomy, and Continence Nursing, 37*(3), 301–310.

Wound, Ostomy and Continence Nurses Society. (2009). Position statement: Role of the wound, ostomy continence nurse or continence care nurse in continence care. *Journal of Wound Ostomy Continence Nursing, 36*, 529–531.

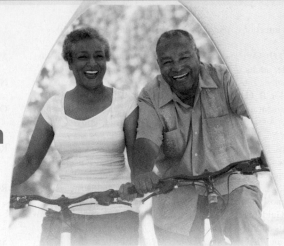

CHAPTER 20

Cardiovascular Function

LEARNING OBJECTIVES

After reading this chapter, you will be able to:

1. Describe age-related changes that affect cardiovascular function.

2. Identify risk factors for cardiovascular disease and orthostatic and postprandial hypotension.

3. Describe the functional consequences of age-related changes and risk factors related to cardiovascular function.

4. Assess cardiovascular function and risks for cardiovascular disease with emphasis on those that can be addressed through health promotion interventions.

5. Teach older adults and their caregivers about interventions to reduce the risk for cardiovascular disease.

KEY POINTS

abdominal obesity
adaptive response
atherosclerosis
atypical presentation
baroreflex mechanisms
cardiovascular disease
DASH dietary pattern
home blood pressure
 monitoring
hypertension
lipid disorders
Mediterranean dietary
 pattern

metabolic syndrome
obesity
orthostatic hypotension
physical inactivity
plaque
postprandial
 hypotension
pseudohypertension
stepped-care approach
systolic hypertension
white coat
 hypertension

The cardiovascular system helps maintain homeostasis by bringing oxygen and nutrients to organs and tissues and by transporting carbon dioxide and other waste products to other body systems for removal. Because the cardiovascular system has a tremendous adaptive capacity, healthy older adults will not experience any significant change in cardiovascular performance because of age-related changes alone. In the presence of risk factors, however, the cardiovascular system is less efficient in performing life-sustaining activities, and serious negative functional consequences can occur.

 ## AGE-RELATED CHANGES THAT AFFECT CARDIOVASCULAR FUNCTION

As with many aspects of physiologic function, it is difficult to determine whether cardiovascular changes are attributable to normal aging or other factors. Knowledge about distinct age- or disease-related changes in cardiovascular function is confounded by the fact that, until recently, there was no technology to detect asymptomatic pathologic cardiovascular processes, such as the occlusion of a major coronary artery. Thus, some conclusions from earlier studies may have attributed pathologic changes to normal aging. Studies using newer diagnostic techniques found that 36% and 39% of men and women, respectively, have subclinical coronary heart disease and only 12.6% of people aged 85 years or older have neither clinical nor subclinical disease (Cademartiri, LaGrutta, de Feyter, & Kresstin, 2008). Currently, many studies of age-related changes are longitudinal and include subjects who have been carefully screened for asymptomatic **cardiovascular disease**.

In addition, because sociocultural factors affect cardiovascular function, it is difficult to draw conclusions about lifestyle factors that affect entire societies. Systolic blood pressure, for example, increases gradually in adults who live in Western societies but not in those from less industrialized societies. Therefore, changes that have been attributed to increased age may, in fact, be related to lifestyle, sociocultural factors, or pathologic conditions. Cross-cultural studies are now being used to identify the effects of lifestyle and other sociocultural factors that affect cardiovascular function. A major focus of research is on identifying those risk factors that are most amenable to interventions so that evidence-based interventions can be recommended.

Promoting Cardiovascular Wellness in Older Adults

Nursing Assessment
- Usual heart rate, sounds, rhythm
- Blood pressure, including hypotension
- Risks for cardiovascular disease
- Signs and symptoms of cardiovascular disease
- Knowledge about cardiovascular disease

Age-Related Changes
- Myocardial degenerative changes
- Arterial stiffening
- ↑ peripheral resistance
- Altered baroreflex mechanisms

Negative Functional Consequences
- ↓ adaptive response to exercise
- ↑ susceptibility to hypertension, hypotension
- ↑ susceptibility to arrhythmias
- ↓ cerebral blood flow

Risk Factors
- Hypertension, hyperlipidemia
- Inactivity
- Obesity
- Dietary habits
- Tobacco smoking
- Stress, depression
- ↓ social supports

Nursing Interventions
- Teaching about diet, exercise, optimal weight
- If applicable, teaching about smoking cessation
- Teaching about hypertension and dyslipidemia
- Teaching about signs and symptoms of heart disease

Wellness Outcomes
- Improved cardiovascular function
- Prevention of cardiovascular disease
- Normal blood pressure and serum lipids
- Improved longevity and quality of life

Myocardium and Neuroconduction Mechanisms

Age-related changes of the myocardium include amyloid deposits, lipofuscin accumulation, basophilic degeneration, myocardial atrophy or hypertrophy, valvular thickening and stiffening, and increased amounts of connective tissue. The left ventricular wall becomes slightly enlarged in healthy older adults, but any significant myocardial atrophy that occurs is due to pathologic processes. In addition, the left atrium enlarges, even in healthy older adults. Other age-related changes include thickening of the atrial endocardium, thickening of the atrioventricular valves, and calcification of at least part of the mitral annulus of the aortic valve. These changes interfere with the ability of the heart to contract completely. With less effective contractility, more time is required to complete the cycle of diastolic filling and systolic emptying. In addition, the myocardium becomes increasingly irritable and less responsive to the impulses from the sympathetic nervous system.

Age-related changes in cardiac physiology are minimal, and the changes that do occur affect cardiac performance only under conditions of physiologic stress. Even under stressful conditions, the heart in healthy older adults is able to adapt, but the adaptive mechanisms may differ from those of younger adults or be slightly less efficient. The age-related changes that cause functional consequences primarily involve the electrophysiology of the heart (i.e., the neuroconduction system). Age-related changes in the neuroconduction system include a decrease in the number of pacemaker cells; increased irregularity in the shape of pacemaker cells; and increased deposits of fat, collagen, and elastic fibers around the sinoatrial node.

Vasculature

Age-related changes affect two of the three vascular layers, and functional consequences vary, depending on which layer is affected. For example, changes in the tunica intima, the innermost layer, have the most serious functional consequences in the development of **atherosclerosis**, whereas changes in the tunica media, the middle layer, are associated with **hypertension**. The outermost layer (the tunica externa) does not seem to be affected by age-related changes. This layer, composed of loosely meshed adipose and connective tissue, supports nerve fibers and the vasa vasorum, the blood supply for the tunica media.

The tunica intima consists of a single layer of endothelial cells on a thin layer of connective tissue. It controls the entry of lipids and other substances from the blood into the artery wall. Intact endothelial cells allow blood to flow freely without clotting; however, when the endothelial cells are damaged, they function in the clotting process. With increasing age, the tunica intima thickens because of fibrosis, cellular proliferation, and lipid and calcium accumulation. In addition, the endothelial cells become irregular in size and shape. These changes cause the arteries to dilate and elongate. As a result, the arterial walls are more vulnerable to atherosclerosis (discussed in the section on risk factors).

The tunica media is composed of single or multiple layers of smooth muscle cells surrounded by elastin and collagen. The smooth muscle cells are involved in the tissue-forming functions of producing collagen, proteoglycans, and elastic fibers. Because it provides structural support, this layer controls arterial expansion and contraction. Age-related changes that affect the tunica media include an increase in collagen and a thinning and calcification of elastin fibers, resulting in stiffened blood vessels. These changes are particularly pronounced in the aorta, where the diameter of the lumen increases to compensate for the age-related arterial stiffening. Although these changes are viewed as age related, longitudinal and cross-cultural studies are raising questions about the impact of lifestyle variables on arterial stiffness.

Age-related changes in the tunica media cause increased peripheral resistance, impaired baroreceptor function, and diminished ability to increase blood flow to vital organs. Although these changes do not cause serious consequences in healthy older adults, they increase the resistance to blood flow from the heart so that the left ventricle is forced to work harder. Moreover, the baroreceptors in the large arteries become less effective in controlling blood pressure, especially during postural changes. Overall, the increased vascular stiffness causes a slight increase in the systolic blood pressure.

Veins undergo changes similar to those affecting the arteries, but to a lesser degree. Veins become thicker, more dilated, and less elastic with increasing age. Valves of the large leg veins become less efficient in returning blood to the heart. Peripheral circulation is further influenced by an age-related reduction in muscle mass and a concurrent reduction in the demand for oxygen.

Baroreflex Mechanisms

Baroreflex mechanisms are physiologic processes that regulate blood pressure by increasing or decreasing the heart rate and peripheral vascular resistance to compensate for transient decreases or increases in arterial pressure. Age-related changes that alter baroreflex mechanisms include arterial stiffening and reduced cardiovascular responsiveness to adrenergic stimulation. These changes cause a blunting of the compensatory response to both hypertensive and hypotensive stimuli in older adults, so the heart rate does not increase or decrease as efficiently as in younger adults.

 RISK FACTORS THAT AFFECT CARDIOVASCULAR FUNCTION

Many factors affect cardiovascular function by increasing the risk for heart disease, which has been the leading cause of death in the United States for almost a century. Heart disease, or cardiovascular disease, refers to all pathologic processes that affect the heart and circulatory system including specific disease entities, such as coronary heart disease (also called coronary artery disease), arrhythmias, atherosclerosis, heart failure, myocardial infarction, peripheral vascular disease, venous thromboembolism, stroke, and transient ischemic attacks. Although stroke (also called cerebrovascular disease) and transient ischemic attacks are considered cardiovascular conditions because of their underlying pathology, they are considered neurologic conditions in clinical practice because of their effects. (Refer to Chapter 27 for discussion of heart failure; this chapter focuses on conditions that can be addressed through health promotion interventions to reduce all types of cardiovascular disease.)

Researchers, health planners, and health care providers are concerned about risks for cardiovascular disease not only because of its significant prevalence and mortality rate but also because it poses a heavy economic burden. Most importantly from a wellness perspective, there is mounting evidence that most cardiovascular disease is preventable through modification of risk factors (Foody, 2008). Thus, this is a major focus of health promotion efforts, including patient education and motivation for behavior change.

Studies have identified the following risk factors as the most important contributing factors to cardiovascular disease: stress, weight, lipids, diabetes, blood pressure, **physical inactivity**, smoking cessation, inadequate intake of fruit and vegetable, and excessive alcohol consumption (D'Agostino et al., 2008; Dennison & Hughes, 2009; Schenk-Gustofsson, 2009). These conditions can be addressed through medical management and health promotion interventions, as discussed in this chapter and in Chapters 21 (smoking cessation) and 27 (diabetes). Some risk factors, such as age, race, gender, and heredity, cannot be modified, but it is important to consider their influence on a person's overall risk profile. In recent years, there is increasing recognition that race and gender can affect both the risk for developing cardiovascular disease and the chance of having adverse outcomes. For example, there is strong evidence of health disparities associated with increased prevalence and poorer management of heart disease and related risk factors in women and African Americans (e.g., Spertus, Jones, Massoudi, Rumsfeld, & Krumholz, 2009; Taylor et al., 2009; Weiss, 2009). Although age, gender, and race cannot be changed, it is important to recognize variations in manifestation and management of cardiovascular disease that occur in specific groups. Socioeconomic and psychosocial factors also affect the risk profile for heart disease and these factors are pertinent to a holistic approach to care of older adults.

DIVERSITY NOTE

At age 40, lifetime risk for cardiovascular disease in men is 67% and for women it is 50%. By the age of 85 years, the risk is equal in men and women.

DIVERSITY NOTE

The average age of a person having a first major cardiovascular event is 65.8 years in men and 70.4 years in women (Berra, 2008).

Atherosclerosis

Atherosclerosis is a disorder of the medium and small arteries in which patchy deposits of lipids and atherosclerotic **plaques** reduce or obstruct blood flow. It is implicated in 75% of all cardiovascular deaths in the United States (Lewis, 2009). Because atherosclerosis is the underlying pathologic process associated with most cardiovascular disease, the term *atherosclerotic cardiovascular disease* is sometimes used (see discussion on pathologic conditions for details). Several theories about the pathophysiology of atherosclerosis have been proposed since the mid-1970s, and our understanding of atherosclerosis has increased significantly in recent years due to the use of more sophisticated imaging techniques. It is now understood that atherosclerosis is a pathologic condition that begins during childhood with asymptomatic but identifiable changes and progresses through adulthood to the point that it is found in 80% to 90% of adults aged 30 years and older (Lewis, 2009).

Atherosclerosis involves a continuum of changes in the arterial wall that develop in the following sequence (Insull, 2009):

1. *Early fatty streak development during childhood and adolescence:* low-density lipoprotein (LDL) cholesterol particles accumulate in the arterial intima and initiate an inflammatory response.

2. *Early fibroatheroma phase during teens and 20s:* (a) macrophage "foam cells" and other inflammatory cells accumulate, (b) some protective responses are initiated but necrotic debris causes further inflammation, (c) extracellular lipids accumulate and form lipid-rich necrotic cores that occupy 30% to 50% of the arterial wall volume, (d) a fibrous cap, called a plaque, forms over the necrotic core under the endothelium.

3. *Advancing atheroma at 55 years and older:* (a) fibrous cap in a few sites becomes thin and weakened; (b) the thin-capped fibroatheroma is susceptible to rupturing and causing a life-threatening thrombosis; (c) if fibroatheroma does not rupture, it may enlarge and further reduce the arterial lumen; (d) as long as the plaque does not occupy more than 40% of the lumen, the arterial walls can expand to compensate, but if the plaque occupies more arterial space, symptoms result; (e) diseased artery may leak within the arterial wall and provoke further fibrous tissue.

In summary, atherosclerotic changes begin in childhood and can progress to plaque formation. Plaque lesions, which can rupture, remain stable, or continue to grow, are the underlying cause of most cardiovascular disease. Studies have found that multiple asymptomatic cycles of plaque erosion and healing occur in 60% of sudden cardiac deaths before the fatal event (Insull, 2009). Thus, it is important to identify and address risk factors before patients experience symptoms. All the risk factors associated with cardiovascular disease, as described in this section, are risks for the development and progression of atherosclerosis.

Physical Inactivity

Physical inactivity (also called physical deconditioning in reference to cardiovascular function) is a factor that not only increases the risk for cardiovascular disease for all people but also diminishes cardiovascular function in healthy older adults. Thus, even in the absence of pathologic processes, inadequate patterns of physical activity will interfere with the ability of older adults to adapt to age-related cardiovascular changes. According to evidence-based guidelines, the level of physical inactivity that increases the risk for cardiovascular disease is fewer than 30 minutes of moderate physical activity at least 5 days weekly or 20 minutes of vigorous physical activity at least 3 days weekly. National data indicate that 6% and 24% of younger and older adults, respectively, do not achieve adequate levels of physical activity and, therefore, have 1.5 to 2.4 times the relative risk for coronary heart diseases (Lloyd-Jones, 2009). Conditions that often occur in older adults and contribute to physical deconditioning include acute illness, a sedentary lifestyle, mobility limitations, any chronic condition that interferes with physical activity, and psychosocial influences, such as depression or lack of motivation.

Tobacco Smoking

Tobacco smoking is a major avoidable cause of cardiovascular disease, and there is indisputable evidence that all forms of tobacco use (smoking and smokeless or exposure to secondhand smoke) increase the risk for cardiovascular disease and mortality. Research data indicate that cardiovascular disease becomes symptomatic 10 years earlier, and death occurs 13 years earlier in current smokers than in nonsmokers (Surinach et al., 2009). In addition, national data indicate that 35% of smoking-related deaths are due to cardiovascular disease (Lloyd-Jones et al., 2009). Effects of smoking on the cardiovascular system include acceleration of atherosclerotic processes, increased systolic blood pressure, elevated LDL cholesterol level, and decreased high-density lipoprotein (HDL) cholesterol level. Even short exposures to secondhand smoke increase the risk of a heart attack because of immediate adverse effects on the heart, blood, and vascular systems. In addition, nonsmokers who are exposed to secondhand smoke at home or work have 25% to 30% greater risk of developing heart disease (Lloyd-Jones et al., 2009). It should be emphasized that these cardiovascular effects are in addition to the effects of nicotine on respiratory function (see Chapter 21) and other aspects of health (e.g., increased risk for development of many cancers).

Dietary Habits

Randomized controlled trials confirm that dietary habits can increase many risk factors for cardiovascular disease, including weight, blood pressure, glucose levels, and lipoprotein and triglyceride levels. A review of studies summarized the following findings related to dietary habits and cardiovascular health (Lloyd-Jones et al., 2009):

- Total fat intake was less important than type of fat consumed; replacing saturated fat with polyunsaturated fat reduced cardiovascular risk by 24%.
- Each 2% of calories from trans fats were associated with a 23% higher risk of coronary heart disease.
- Intake of 2.5 servings daily of whole grains was associated with a 21% lower risk of cardiovascular disease when compared with 0.2 servings daily.

- When compared with little or no consumption of fish or fish oil, consumption of one to two servings per week of oily fish was associated with a 36% lower risk of cardiovascular mortality.
- Each additional daily serving of fruits or vegetables was associated with a 4% lower risk of coronary heart disease and 5% lower risk of stroke.
- Low-sodium interventions were associated with a 25% lower risk of cardiovascular disease after 10 to 15 years of follow-up.

In addition to studies of specific types of foods, many studies looked at the protective effects of dietary patterns, which are discussed in the section on nursing interventions.

Obesity

Obesity, which is defined by body mass index (BMI) ≥ 30 kg/m^2, is associated with increased risk for many pathologic conditions including stroke, diabetes, **lipid disorders**, atherosclerosis, hypertension, and coronary heart disease. In recent years, increasing attention is being paid to **abdominal obesity** (also called *abdominal adiposity*) as an independent risk factor for cardiovascular disease. Abdominal obesity, defined as a waist circumference more than 102 and 88 cm or waist-to-hip ratio of 0.95 and 0.88 for men and women, respectively, can occur even in people with normal BMI. Significant evidence indicates that abdominal adipose tissue is biologically and metabolically different from subcutaneous fat and, in fact, may have a greater impact on cardiovascular disease than overall obesity (Carr & Tannock, 2009). Analysis of data from the Nurses' Health Study found that higher waist circumference was a strong risk factor for mortality from cardiovascular disease even among normal-weight women (Zhang, Rexrode, Van Dam, Li, & Hu, 2008).

Hypertension

Prevalence for hypertension in American adults aged 65 years and older is 70.8%, with a prevalence of 63.0% and 76.6% for men and women, respectively (McDonald, Hartz, Unger, & Lustik, 2009). Hypertension is defined as blood pressure of 140/90 mm Hg or higher, or a blood pressure that requires treatment with an antihypertensive medication. Hypertension is a disease of the cardiovascular system, and in older adults, it is also an independent risk factor for additional cardiovascular diseases, including coronary artery disease, ischemic stroke, peripheral arterial disease, and congestive heart failure (Aronow, 2008). Since the early 2000s, studies found that blood pressure even at the high end of normal (i.e., 130 to 139/85 to 89 mm Hg) is a risk factor for stroke, myocardial infarction, sudden cardiac death, coronary heart disease, heart failure, renal disease, and all-cause mortality (e.g., Kokubo et al., 2008). Thus, hypertension is both a disease of the cardiovascular system and a risk factor for additional cardiovascular disease.

Until recently, health care practitioners viewed systolic blood pressure as less important than diastolic blood pressure as a criterion for treatment of hypertension. Recent clinical trials, however, support the evidence-based recommendation to treat **systolic hypertension** (also called isolated systolic hypertension) because the risk of cardiovascular disease increases proportionately as systolic pressure increases from 115 mm Hg (Rashidi & Wright, 2009; Williams, Lundholm, & Sever, 2008). This is especially pertinent to older adults because systolic hypertension is the most common type of hypertension in the elderly and is strongly associated with organ damage, and increased risk of cardiovascular disease and mortality (Duprez, 2008).

Risk factors for the development of hypertension include age, ethnicity, genetic factors, overweight, physical inactivity, sleep apnea, psychosocial stressors, and lower education and socioeconomic status. In addition, dietary patterns that increase the risk for hypertension include higher intake of fats and sodium, lower potassium intake, and excessive alcohol consumption (Lloyd-Jones et al., 2009). When dietary patterns of different cultural groups are compared, there is a strong relationship between average daily sodium consumption and prevalence of hypertension (Flegel & Magner, 2009).

The Joint National Committee (JNC) on Detection, Evaluation, and Treatment of High Blood Pressure has published seven reports, with the eighth one planned for publication in late 2011. Because each of these reports revised the classification of hypertension, a blood pressure measurement that was considered normal in 1980 was deemed pathologic in the 2000s. Another consideration is that at one time, the upper normal range for systolic blood pressure was "100 plus your age," so an 84-year-old person could have a systolic blood pressure of 184 and not be diagnosed as having hypertension. This perspective gradually changed and the same standards for determining hypertension apply to adults of all ages. The JNC recommends a classification of hypertension by stages to emphasize the risk of any degree of high blood pressure as a factor in cardiovascular disease (JNC, 2003). To clarify various terms, Table 20-1 defines some of the criteria used regarding blood pressure in older adults.

DIVERSITY NOTE

Significant health disparities are apparent in the control of hypertension, with blacks having a 27% lower chance of adequate control (Lloyd-Jones et al., 2009).

Lipid Disorders

Lipid disorders (also called *dyslipidemias* or *hyperlipidemias*) is a broad term that encompasses all abnormalities of lipopro-

---

TABLE 20-1 Criteria for Normal Blood Pressure and Stages of Hypertension

Adult Blood Pressure	Systolic (mm Hg)		Diastolic (mm Hg)
Normal	<120	And	<80
Prehypertension	120–139	Or	80–89
Hypertension, stage I	140–159	Or	90–99
Hypertension, stage II	≥160	Or	≥100

Source: JNC. (2003). The seventh report of the Joint National Committee on Prevention, Detection, Evaluation, and Treatment of High Blood Pressure. *Journal of the American Medical Association, 289,* 2560–2577.

tein metabolism, including low levels of HDLs (often referred to as "good cholesterol") and elevated levels of total cholesterol, triglycerides, or LDL (often referred to as "bad cholesterol"). Public awareness of the importance of testing for lipid disorders has increased since the early 1980s, when *cholesterol* and *saturated fat* became household words. By the 1990s, numerous studies began confirming a positive association between lipoprotein levels and coronary heart disease, and there was widespread support for cholesterol screening for all adults. During the early 2000s, the National Cholesterol Education Program issued and widely disseminated an updated evidence-based set of guidelines on cholesterol management, called the *Adult Treatment Panel (ATP) III*. These guidelines were updated in 2004 and the updates continue as part of the National Heart, Lung, and Blood Institute plan to develop integrated cardiovascular risk reduction criteria. The ATP III and other evidence-based guidelines emphasize the value of screening for and treating lipid disorders in adults.

Although there is much scientific support for addressing lipid disorders as a risk for cardiovascular disease, questions have been raised about the value of cholesterol screening and treatment for older adults, particularly for those older than 75 years and those who have no cardiovascular disease. According to current evidence-based guidelines, screening for lipid disorders is appropriate for older people who had never been evaluated, but repeated screening is less important for older adults who have normal levels because lipid levels are not likely to change after age 65 (U.S. Preventive Services Task Force, 2008). Current data also indicate that older adults would benefit significantly from lipid-lowering therapy (Ducharme & Radhamma, 2008). Moreover, because older adults have a greater risk for developing coronary heart disease, they are likely to gain more than younger adults from treatment of lipid disorders (U.S. Preventive Services Task Force, 2008). See the Evidence-Based Practice Box 20-1 that summarizes pertinent information about preventing cardiovascular disease.

DIVERSITY NOTE

African Americans and Mexican Americans are less likely than whites to be screened for dyslipidemia (Lloyd-Jones et al., 2009).

Evidence-Based Practice 20-1

Evidence-Based Practice Related to Prevention of Cardiovascular Disease

Statement of the Problem

- Significant advances have been made in preventing and treating cardiovascular disease through medical interventions. However, diet and lifestyle therapies—which are commonly neglected—remain the foundation of clinical intervention for prevention.

Recommendations for Nursing Assessment

- Assess health-related behaviors pertinent to cardiovascular health: dietary patterns, weight, level of physical activity, and smoking.

Recommendations for Nursing Care

- Calculate BMI and discuss with patients.
- Advocate a healthy dietary pattern consistent with American Heart Association recommendations.
- Encourage regular physical activity.
- Discourage smoking among nonsmokers and encourage smoking cessation among patients who do smoke.

Teaching Points for Older Adults and Caregivers

- Consume an overall healthful diet: variety of fruits, vegetables, and grains, especially whole grains; choose fat-free and low-fat dairy products, legumes, poultry, and lean meats; eat fish, preferably oily fish, at least twice weekly; limit intake of saturated and trans fats and cholesterol; limit intake of foods and beverages that have added sugar; select nutrient-dense foods.
- Aim for a healthy BMI of 18.5 to 24.9 kg/m^2.
- Aim for optimal lipid profile: LDL levels <100 mg/dL, HDL >50 mg/dL in women and >40 in men, and triglycerides <150 mg/dL.
- Aim for normal blood pressure: systolic blood pressure <120 mm Hg and diastolic blood pressure <80 mm Hg.
- Adopt dietary modifications that lower blood pressure: reduced salt intake, increased potassium intake, caloric deficit to induce weight loss, moderation of alcohol intake for those who drink.
- Aim for fasting blood glucose level ≤100 mg/dL.
- Be physically active: accumulate ≥30 minutes of physical activity most days of the week and at least 60 minutes most days of the week for people attempting to lose weight or maintain weight loss.
- Avoid use of and exposure to tobacco products.

SOURCES: Diet and lifestyle recommendations revision 2006. A scientific statement from the American Health Association Nutrition Committee.
Lichtenstein AH, Appel LJ, Brands M, Carnethon M, Daniels S, Franch HA, . . . Wylie-Rosett J. (2006). Diet and lifestyle recommendations revision 2006: a scientific statement from the American Heart Association Nutrition Committee. *Circulation 114*(1):82–96.

Metabolic Syndrome

Metabolic syndrome (also called *insulin resistance syndrome*) refers to a group of clinically identifiable conditions, which include lipid disorders, hypertension, and insulin resistance, that increase the risk for developing cardiovascular disease or type 2 diabetes. Each condition is an independent risk for disease, but when they occur together, they disproportionately increase the probability of complication, morbidity, and mortality related to cardiovascular disease or type 2 diabetes (Mazzo, 2008). Criteria for metabolic syndrome have been established by the ATP III guidelines and have also been defined by the International Diabetes Foundation and the World Health Organization. Based on ATP III guidelines, the American Heart Association states that metabolic syndrome is diagnosed when three or more of the following risk factors are present (Lloyd-Jones et al., 2009):

- Central obesity, defined as waist circumference equal to or greater than 40 inches (102 cm) in men or 35 inches (88 cm) in women
- Blood pressure equal to or higher than 130/85 mm Hg
- HDL cholesterol lower than 40 mg/dL in men or equal to or lower than 50 mg/dL in women, or drug treatment for a lipid disorder
- Triglycerides equal to or greater than 150 mg/dL, or specific treatment for hypertriglyceridemia
- Fasting blood glucose level equal to or greater than 100 mg/dL, or drug treatment for increased glucose.

DIVERSITY NOTE

Two studies found that men and whites are more likely to develop metabolic syndrome compared with women and blacks (Lloyd-Jones et al., 2009).

Psychosocial Factors

Psychosocial factors that are associated with increased risk for developing cardiovascular disease include stress, anxiety, depression, social isolation, poor social supports, and personality characteristics, such as higher anger and hostility indices. One focus of current studies is on the relationship between prolonged stress (also called chronic stress) and risk for developing chronic cardiovascular conditions, such as atherosclerosis, hypertension, and lipid disorders. Studies have found the following associations between stress and cardiovascular disease (Larzelere & Jones, 2008; Lee et al., 2010):

- Psychosocial stress was comparable to smoking and hypertension as risk factors for myocardial infarction.
- Chronically stressful situations have been linked to increased risk of coronary artery disease and adverse cardiac events.
- Acute stress has been associated with increased risk for acute cardiovascular events.
- Anger, anxiety, and occupational stress have been found to increase the risk for acute coronary events.
- High levels of emotional distress in patients with congestive heart failure are associated with poorer outcomes.

Studies also indicate that yoga, meditation, and other stress-reduction methods are effective for reducing blood pressure and preventing cardiovascular disease (Sidani & Figueredo, 2009; Sidani & Ziegler, (2008).

Depression has not been identified as a primary risk factor for cardiovascular disease, but it is a risk factor for recurrent coronary events and cardiovascular-related mortality in people who have had a myocardial infarction. Studies also have found that depression accelerates cardiovascular disease in women with diabetes (Evangelista & McLaughlin, 2009). Thus, it is an important consideration with regard to secondary prevention interventions. A recent review of studies that were used for developing evidence-based practice found that prevalence of depression during initial hospitalization for myocardial infarction ranged from 7% to 41% (depending on assessment method), with an average of 20%. This same research review found that up to 60% of patients reported depression 1 month or longer postmyocardial infarction (Green, Dickenson, Nease, & Campos-Outcalt, 2009). Nurses caring for older adults even months after a myocardial infarction need to be aware of this close link so that they can include this dimension in a holistic approach to care.

> **DIVERSITY NOTE**
>
> One study found that African Americans with coronary heart disease were less likely to be treated with antidepressant medications compared with whites despite having similar levels of depression (Waldman et al., 2009).

Heredity and Socioeconomic Factors

Heredity plays a significant role in the risk for developing cardiovascular disease. Large population-based studies show a strong link between reported history of premature parental coronary heart disease and cardiovascular disease, including atherosclerosis and myocardial infarction, in offspring (Lloyd-Jones et al., 2009). Although inherited conditions cannot be changed, people who are aware of having these risk factors may be more motivated to address modifiable risks.

The relationship between socioeconomic status and cardiovascular disease has been a focus of research for several decades. A Centers for Disease Control and Prevention (CDC) survey of adults found that people with less than a high school level of education were twice as likely as college graduates to have multiple-risk factors for cardiovascular disease (Lloyd-Jones et al., 2009). Although income and education are not easily modified, it is important to recognize that these conditions influence not only the risk for cardiovascular disease but also the use of preventive and interventional measures. From a holistic perspective, nurses need to consider these factors when planning health education interventions to address individualized needs of older adults.

Risk for Cardiovascular Disease in Women and Minority Groups

Because cardiovascular disease had long been viewed as a disease of middle-aged men, early research focused primarily, or exclusively, on men. This perspective began changing during the 1990s when studies showed that although the prevalence of cardiovascular disease is lower in younger women than younger men, it increases dramatically after the age of 50 years in women. The following statistics from national databases are indicators of the extent of cardiovascular morbidity and mortality among women in the United States (McSweeney, Cleves, Zhao, Lefler, & Yang, 2010; Weiss, 2009):

- Heart disease and stroke together account for 41.3% of all deaths in women; this is equivalent to a woman dying from cardiovascular disease every minute of every day.
- Cardiovascular disease affects 36.6% of women, with the age-related prevalence increasing from 36.2% for those between the ages of 45 and 54 years to 68.5% for those aged 65 years and older.
- Although many women perceive breast cancer as their greatest threat, cardiovascular disease kills 12 times as many women each year as breast cancer.
- Annual rates of the first major cardiovascular event is similar for men and women, but occurs about 10 years later for women; by the age of 75 years, the lifetime risk for cardiovascular disease is the same in men and women.
- 38% of women versus 25% of men die within 1 year after a first heart attack.
- Women are more likely to have more subtle manifestations of coronary artery disease (e.g., a myocardial infarction), so they are less likely to pursue appropriate evaluation or to be diagnosed accurately.
- Women with cardiovascular disease are less likely than men to be treated according to evidence-based guidelines, and their survival rates are worse.

Along with the growing recognition of unique aspects of cardiovascular disease in women, there has been increasing focus on the disproportionate burden of cardiovascular-related death and disability among minority populations. National data show that African Americans have a higher risk of heart disease and more severe hypertension than whites do. American Indians, Mexican Americans, Native Hawaiians, and some Asian Americans are other groups in which the rate of cardiovascular disease is higher than in whites.

In addition to having more risk factors, African Americans have the highest age-adjusted death rate for cardiovascular disease, and they are more likely than other groups to have risk factors, such as diabetes, obesity, hypertension, and lipid disorders. One study of factors associated with differences in outcomes of black and white patients after a heart attack attributed the disparity in outcomes to black patients having worse risk factors, including diabetes, high cholesterol levels, high blood pressure, and lower socioeconomic status (Spertus et al., 2009).

Another study concluded that there is a clear need for improved methods of identifying and effectively treating dyslipidemia in African Americans (Taylor et al., 2009).

Studies are also focusing on variations of cardiovascular risk factors and interventions in Asian/Pacific Islander Americans. One study found that there may be differences in both therapeutic response and adverse effects of antihypertensive medications between Asian/Pacific Islander Americans and whites (Watson, 2009).

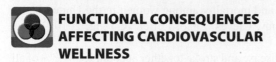

FUNCTIONAL CONSEQUENCES AFFECTING CARDIOVASCULAR WELLNESS

Healthy older adults experience no significant cardiovascular effects when they are resting, but, when they engage in exercise, their cardiovascular function is less efficient. However, older adults who have risk factors for cardiovascular disease are likely to experience negative functional consequences associated with pathologic processes. This section reviews the functional consequences in older adults who have no risk factors, and the sections on nursing assessment and interventions focus on risk factors that can be addressed to prevent pathologic processes that commonly affect cardiovascular function.

Effects on Cardiac Function

Cardiac output, the amount of blood pumped by the heart per minute, is an important measure of cardiac performance because it represents the heart's ability to meet the oxygen requirements of the body. Although reduced cardiac output is common in older adults, it is associated primarily with pathologic, rather than age-related, conditions. With the exception of a slight decrease in cardiac output at rest in older women, healthy older adults do not experience any decline in cardiac output.

Effects on Pulse and Blood Pressure

Normal pulse rate for healthy older adults is slightly lower than that for younger adults, but older adults are likely to have harmless ventricular and supraventricular arrhythmias because of age-related changes that affect cardiac conduction mechanisms. Atrial fibrillation—a more serious arrhythmia— commonly occurs in older adults, but this is associated with pathologic conditions (e.g., hypertension, coronary artery disease) rather than with age-related changes. In most populations across the world, there is an age-related linear increase in systolic blood pressure from age 30 to 40 years, and this change is steeper for women than for men. There also is a progressive decrease in diastolic pressure beginning around age 50 years (Williams et al., 2008).

Effects on the Response to Exercise

A negative functional consequence that affects cardiovascular performance in healthy older adults is a blunted **adaptive response** to physical exercise. Physiologic stress, such as that associated with exercise, increases the demands on the cardiovascular system by four to five times the basal level. The adaptive response involves many aspects of physiologic function, including the respiratory, cardiovascular, musculoskeletal, and autonomic nervous systems. The maximum heart rate achieved during exercise is markedly decreased, and the peak exercise capacity and oxygen consumption decline in older adults. Physical deconditioning and other risk factors account for some of this decline. Similarly, studies confirm that maximum oxygen uptake during exercise decreases with aging but is affected to a greater extent by risk factors, such as prolonged bedrest (McGavock et al., 2009).

Effects on Circulation

Functional consequences also can affect circulation to the brain and the lower extremities. For example, age-related changes in cardiovascular and baroreflex mechanisms can reduce cerebral blood flow to some extent in healthy older adults and to a greater extent in older adults who have diabetes, hypertension, lipid disorders, and heart disease. In addition, increased tortuosity and dilation of the veins, along with decreased efficiency of the valves, lead to impaired venous return from the lower extremities. Consequently, older adults are prone to developing stasis edema of the feet and ankles, and they are more likely to develop venous stasis ulcers.

*M*r. C. is a 64-year-old African American who frequently comes to your Senior Wellness Clinic to have you check his blood pressure. He has been taking hydrochlorothiazide, 25 mg, and verapamil, 120 mg, every morning, and his blood pressures range between 126/80 and 130/84 mm Hg. Mr. C. sees his primary care provider once a year and obtains additional health care through community resources, such as health fairs. Mr. C.'s 86-year-old mother recently died of a cerebrovascular accident, and his father died in his early 50s of a heart attack. Mr. C. has had hypertension since he was 24, and both of his daughters have high blood pressure as well. Neither Mr. C. nor anyone in the household smokes tobacco. He gets very little exercise and weighs 210 pounds, about 30 pounds more than his ideal weight. He reports that he "gets winded easily" when walking up or down a flight of steps or when he has to walk "a long distance" (which he defines as the distance across the parking lot to the senior center). He attributes this to "getting old."

THINKING POINTS

- What age-related changes in cardiovascular function is Mr. C. likely to be experiencing?

- What risk factors are likely to be contributing to Mr. C.'s experience of "getting winded?"
- What risk factors does Mr. C. have for cardiovascular disease?
- What further information would you want to obtain for assessing his risk for cardiovascular disease?

PATHOLOGIC CONDITIONS AFFECTING CARDIOVASCULAR WELLNESS: ORTHOSTATIC AND POSTPRANDIAL HYPOTENSION

Orthostatic and **postprandial hypotension** are conditions that frequently affect cardiovascular function in older adults due to a combination of age-related changes (e.g., decreased baroreflex sensitivity) and risk factors. These cardiovascular conditions are not serious in and of themselves, but they are addressed in this chapter because they can lead to serious consequences. Moreover, they are often overlooked and it clearly is within the realm of nursing to identify hypotension in older adults (see section on Nursing Assessment).

Orthostatic hypotension (also called *postural hypotension*) is defined as a reduction in systolic blood pressure and diastolic blood pressure of at least 20 or 10 mm Hg, respectively, within 1 to 4 minutes of standing after being recumbent for at least 5 minutes. Studies have found that 20% of community-dwelling older adults and 30% to 50% of those in nursing homes have orthostatic hypotension (Mussi et al., 2009). Although orthostatic hypotension can occur in healthy older adults, it is more likely to occur in those who have risk factors, such as the pathologic conditions and adverse medication effects listed in Box 20-1. In addition, the risk can be increased by the total number of medications in regular use and by a combination of conditions, such as Parkinson's disease and anti-Parkinson medications (Hiitola, 2009).

One study found that age, pre-hypertension, hypertension, and diabetes mellitus were important determinants of orthostatic hypotension in a population of community-dwelling adults (Wu, Yang, Lu, Wu, & Chang, 2008). Orthostatic hypotension can be asymptomatic or it can be accompanied by symptoms such as fatigue, lightheadedness, blurred vision, or cognitive difficulties. Although it might seem to be a relatively harmless condition, it can affect the safety and quality of life and lead to serious negative functional consequences. Studies have found that it may cause up to 30% of all syncopal events and is associated with increased overall mortality and increased risk of falls and cardiovascular diseases (Farrell, 2009; van Hensbroek et al., 2009; Verwoert et al., 2008). Moreover, hypotension is one of the few treatable neurologic conditions that is a risk for falls (Arbogast, Alshekhlee, Hussain, McNeeley, & Chelimsky, 2009).

Postprandial hypotension, defined as a systolic blood pressure reduction of 20 mm Hg or more within 2 hours of eating a meal, occurs in 34% to 65% of older adults (Jian & Zhou,

 Box 20-1 Risk Factors for Hypotension

Risks for Orthostatic Hypotension
Pathologic Processes
- Hypertension, including isolated systolic hypertension
- Parkinson's disease
- Cerebrovascular disorders
- Diabetes
- Anemia
- Autonomic dysfunction
- Arrhythmias
- Volume depletion (e.g., dehydration)
- Electrolyte imbalances (e.g., hyponatremia, hypokalemia)

Medications
- Antihypertensives
- Anticholinergics
- Phenothiazines
- Antidepressants
- Anti-Parkinson agents
- Vasodilators
- Diuretics
- Alcohol

Risks for Postprandial Hypotension
Pathologic Processes
- Systolic hypertension
- Diabetes mellitus
- Parkinson's disease
- Multisystem atrophy

Medications
- Diuretics
- Antihypertensive medications ingested before meals

2008). Physiologic changes that can cause postprandial hypotension include impaired baroreflex mechanisms, quicker rate of gastric emptying, the release of vasoactive gastrointestinal hormones, and impaired autonomic regulation of gastrointestinal perfusion. Carbohydrates, and glucose in particular, may contribute to the development of postprandial hypotension. Older adults who have falls, syncope, weakness, or dizziness should be evaluated for postprandial hypotension because it can lead to stroke and coronary heart disease if it is not recognized and treated (Jian & Zhou, 2008).

NURSING ASSESSMENT OF CARDIOVASCULAR FUNCTION

From a wellness perspective, nursing assessment of cardiovascular function focuses on identifying risks for cardiovascular disease and the older adult's knowledge about his or her risk profile because many risks can be addressed through health education interventions. Moreover, when older adults would benefit from improving their health-related behaviors (e.g., diet, exercise), nurses need to assess their readiness for changing behaviors, as discussed in Chapter 5. Assessment of physical aspects of cardiovascular function (e.g., heart rate, blood pressure) is similar in older and younger adults, but nurses also need to assess for hypotension. In addition, nursing assessment needs to consider that older adults may have atypical manifestations of cardiovascular disease (e.g., a heart attack).

◆ Wellness Opportunity

Nurses address body–mind–spirit interconnectedness by identifying stress-related factors that increase the risk for cardiovascular disease and encouraging the use of stress management methods, such as meditation.

Assessing Baseline Cardiovascular Function

Physical assessment indicators of cardiovascular function (e.g., peripheral pulses and heart rhythm and sounds) are the same for all healthy adults. Nurses must keep in mind, however, that older adults are more likely to have chronic conditions that affect cardiovascular function. The following findings are common in older adults, but in the absence of symptoms or other abnormal findings, they usually are not indicative of any serious pathologic process:

- Auscultation of a fourth heart sound
- Auscultation of short systolic ejection murmurs
- Difficulty percussing heart borders
- Diminished or distant-sounding heart sounds
- Electrocardiographic changes such as arrhythmias, left axis deviation, bundle branch blocks, ST-T wave changes, and prolongation of the P-R interval.

If a murmur, arrhythmia, or any other unusual finding is detected, it is important to determine whether it reflects a new development, a preexisting but previously unidentified condition, or a preexisting condition that has already been evaluated. The nurse asks questions to determine the person's awareness of such abnormal findings. Any of the following terms might be used by older adults to describe arrhythmias: fluttering, palpitations, skipped beats, extra beats, or flip-flops. It is advisable to ask the older person about a history of arrhythmias before auscultation, because asking immediately after auscultation could cause undue concern.

Arrhythmias may be caused by cardiac diseases, electrolyte imbalances, physiologic disturbances, or adverse medication effects; alternatively, they may be harmless manifestations of age-related changes. Likewise, murmurs may be caused by age- or disease-related conditions. Therefore, when murmurs or arrhythmias are detected, their significance is assessed in relation to the person's history as well as in relation to the potential underlying causes. It is also important to find out the date of the person's last electrocardiogram because this may provide baseline information regarding the duration of asymptomatic or unrecognized changes.

Assessing Blood Pressure

Although only a few nurses have primary responsibility for medical management of blood pressure, all nurses are responsible for accurate assessment of blood pressure and for deci-

sions regarding the implications of these findings. Thus, all nurses need to be familiar with the most current guidelines for detection of hypertension so that health promotion efforts can be directed toward interventions. Despite mounting medical evidence that the identification and management of hypertension has important health benefits, fewer than 40% of people with hypertension achieve good control in community settings (Banegas et al., 2008). Nurses are in a key position to detect hypertension, provide health education, and refer older adults for further medical evaluation and treatment.

Accurately assessing blood pressure in older adults may be more difficult than in younger adults for several reasons. First, blood pressure in older adults is more variable and has an increased tendency to fluctuate in response to postural changes and other factors. In addition, older adults commonly have **pseudohypertension**, which is the phenomenon of elevated systolic blood pressure readings that result from the inability of the external cuff to compress the arteries in older people with arteriosclerosis. This phenomenon explains the finding of extremely elevated systolic blood pressure readings in people without any evidence of end-organ damage and with normal diastolic blood pressure readings. Another assessment consideration is the common occurrence of **white coat hypertension** (also called *isolated office hypertension*), which is the phenomenon of blood pressure readings being high during office visits to a primary care practitioner but normal when self-assessed at home.

In recent years, **home blood pressure monitoring**, which is the practice of self-measurement of blood pressure, has been endorsed by national and international guidelines including those posted by the American Heart Association and the Preventive Cardiovascular Nurses Association (Pickering et al., 2008). Self-monitoring provides a more accurate assessment base of information, which is particularly important for older adults because they are more susceptible to white coat hypertension and their systolic readings are more variable. Moreover, self-measurement of blood pressure can also be used to detect orthostatic or postprandial hypotension if readings are taken in both sitting and standing positions. In addition, studies suggest that home blood pressure monitoring can lead to better control of hypertension if health care professionals use the information and take appropriate action (Mallick, Kanthety, & Rahman, 2009).

Assessment of blood pressure in older adults is aimed at detecting not only hypertension but also orthostatic and postprandial hypotension. Box 20-2 summarizes guidelines for accurate assessment of blood pressure in older adults, including the technique for assessing for orthostatic and postprandial hypotension.

Identifying Risks for Cardiovascular Disease

The assessment of risks for cardiovascular disease, with emphasis on identifying modifiable risk factors, provides a basis for health promotion interventions. Hypertension, lipid disorders, and smoking cessation (discussed in Chapter 21) are

Box 20-2 Guidelines for Assessing Blood Pressure

For Accurate Blood Pressure Measurement in Older Adults

- Recognize that blood pressure readings are likely to vary, particularly in response to external factors (e.g., meals or postural changes).
- Blood pressure measurements are likely to have diurnal variations, with lowest levels during the night and highest levels after rising in the morning.
- The person should wait 1 hour after eating to have his or her blood pressure checked, except when checking for postprandial hypotension.
- The person should not have ingested caffeine or smoked a cigarette within 30 minutes before having his or her blood pressure checked.
- The person should be seated and resting for 5 minutes before having his or her blood pressure checked.

For Assessment of Orthostatic Hypotension

- Maintain the person's arm in the same position (either parallel or perpendicular to the torso) during supine and standing positions.
- Obtain initial blood pressure reading after the person has been in a sitting or lying position for at least 5 minutes.
- Obtain second blood pressure reading after the person has been standing for 1 to 3 minutes.

For Assessment of Postprandial Hypotension

- Obtain initial blood pressure reading before a meal.
- Obtain second and third reading at 15-minute intervals after the meal is completed.

Method of Assessing Blood Pressure

- The person should be seated with arm bared and feet flat on the floor.
- Support the person's arm as near to the heart level as possible.
- Ask the person to refrain from talking while you check his or her blood pressure.
- Use a sphygmomanometer that has been checked for accuracy.
- Use an appropriate-sized cuff (i.e., the length of the cuff bladder should be at least 80% of the circumference of the arm, and the width should be 20% wider than the diameter of the arm).

- Record the cuff size that is used. (Cuffs that are too small will yield falsely high readings, whereas cuffs that are too large will yield falsely low readings.)
- Fit the deflated cuff firmly around the upper arm, with the center of the cuff bladder over the brachial artery and the bottom of the cuff about 1 to 1½ inches above the bend of the arm.
- Inflate the cuff to 20 or 30 mm Hg above the palpated systolic blood pressure.
- Deflate the cuff at a rate of 2 to 3 mm Hg per second.
- Measure systolic blood pressure at the first sound and diastolic blood pressure at the onset of silence.
- If auscultatory gaps are heard, estimate the systolic blood pressure by applying the cuff, palpating the radial pulse, and inflating the cuff until the pulse is no longer felt.
- Record the magnitude and range of the gap (e.g., 184/82 mm Hg, auscultatory gap 176–148).
- If a very low diastolic blood pressure is heard, record the onset of Korotkoff phases IV and V (e.g., 138/72/10 mm Hg). Also, be sure not to press too hard on the stethoscope.
- Measure blood pressure in both arms the first time it is assessed; then measure it in the arm with the higher reading on subsequent determinations.
- If sounds are difficult to auscultate, support the person's arm above his or her head for 30 seconds. Then inflate the cuff, have the person lower the arm, and measure the blood pressure.
- If it is necessary to recheck the blood pressure in the same arm, deflate the cuff fully before reinflating it and wait at least 2 minutes before taking another measurement.

Normal Findings

- Normal blood pressure is less than 120 mm Hg systolic blood pressure, and less than 80 mm Hg diastolic blood pressure.
- The normal difference between lying/sitting and standing systolic blood pressure is 20 mm Hg or less after standing for 1 minute.
- The normal difference between lying/sitting and standing diastolic blood pressure is 10 mm Hg or less after standing for 1 minute.

---

important remediable conditions for older adults who have these risks. In addition, obesity, physical inactivity, and certain dietary habits are risk factors that can be addressed through improved health-related behaviors. Figure 20-1 is an example of one of the many easy-to-use assessment tools that are available to identify risk factors. Nurses can use Box 20-3 as a guide for nursing assessment of risks.

Wellness Opportunity

Nurses promote personal responsibility and self-awareness by teaching older adults to use self-assessment tools (e.g., Figure 20-1) to identify their risks for heart disease.

Assessing Signs and Symptoms of Heart Disease

Assessment of older adults for heart disease is complicated by the fact that the symptoms often differ from the expected manifestations. Congestive heart failure, for example, often

begins very subtly, and the early manifestations may be mental changes secondary to the physiologic stress. Thus, older adults are likely to be in more advanced stages of heart failure before an accurate diagnosis is made. Likewise, older people with angina and acute myocardial infarctions are likely to have subtle and unusual manifestations, called **atypical presentation**, rather than the classic symptom of chest pain. Between one-fourth and two-thirds of all myocardial infarctions are not clinically recognized as such, with women and older adults having a higher rate of atypical presentation. Studies also indicate that women and older adults are more likely to seek help for atypical symptoms during the months before they experience an acute coronary event (Graham, Westerhout, Kaul, Norris, & Armstrong, 2008). Atypical signs and symptoms include fatigue; nausea; anxiety; headache; cough; visual disturbance; shortness of breath; and pain in the jaw, neck, or throat.

An important nursing assessment consideration is that older adults as well as health care professionals are likely to attribute

What Is Your Risk of Developing Heart Disease or Having a Heart Attack?

In general, the higher your LDL level and the more risk factors you have (other than LDL), the greater your chances of developing heart disease or having a heart attack. Some people are at high risk for a heart attack because they already have heart disease. Other people are at high risk for developing heart disease because they have diabetes (which is a strong risk factor) or a combination of risk factors for heart disease. Follow these steps to find out your risk for developing heart disease.

Step 1 **Check the table below to see how many of the listed risk factors you have; these are the risk factors that affect your LDL goal.**

Major Risk Factors That Affect Your LDL Goal

- O Cigarette smoking
- O High blood pressure (140/90 mmHg or higher or on blood pressure medication)
- O Low HDL cholesterol (less than 40 mg/dL)*
- O Family history of early heart disease (heart disease in father or brother before age 55; heart disease in mother or sister before age 65)
- O Age (men 45 years or older; women 55 years or older)

If your HDL cholesterol is 60 mg/dL or higher, subtract 1 from your total count.

Even though obesity and physical inactivity are not counted in this list, they are conditions that need to be corrected.

Step 2 **How many major risk factors do you have? If you have 2 or more risk factors in the table above, use the risk scoring tables on the opposite page (which include your cholesterol levels) to find your risk score. Risk score refers to the chance of having a heart attack in the next 10 years, given as a percentage.**
(Use the Framingham Point Scores on the opposite page.)

My 10-year risk score is _____%.

Step 3 **Use your medical history, number of risk factors, and risk score to find your risk of developing heart disease or having a heart attack in the table below.**

If You Have	You Are in Category
Heart disease, diabetes, or risk score more than 20%*	I. Highest Risk
2 or more risk factors and risk score 10–20%	II. Next Highest Risk
2 or more risk factors and risk score less than 10%	III. Moderate Risk
0 or 1 risk factor	IV. Low-to-Moderate Risk

Means that more than 20 of 100 people in this category will have a heart attack within 10 years.

My risk category is _____.

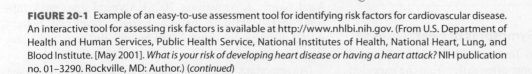

FIGURE 20-1 Example of an easy-to-use assessment tool for identifying risk factors for cardiovascular disease. An interactive tool for assessing risk factors is available at http://www.nhlbi.nih.gov. (From U.S. Department of Health and Human Services, Public Health Service, National Institutes of Health, National Heart, Lung, and Blood Institute. [May 2001]. *What is your risk of developing heart disease or having a heart attack?* NIH publication no. 01–3290. Rockville, MD: Author.) *(continued)*

Men
Estimate of 10-Year Risk for Men

(Framingham Point Scores)

Age	Points
20-34	-9
35-39	-4
40-44	0
45-49	3
50-54	6
55-59	8
60-64	10
65-69	11
70-74	12
75-79	13

Total Cholesterol	Points				
	Age 20-39	Age 40-49	Age 50-59	Age 60-69	Age 70-79
<160	0	0	0	0	0
160-199	4	3	2	1	0
200-239	7	5	3	1	0
240-279	9	6	4	2	1
≥280	11	8	5	3	1

	Points				
	Age 20-39	Age 40-49	Age 50-59	Age 60-69	Age 70-79
Nonsmoker	0	0	0	0	0
Smoker	8	5	3	1	1

HDL (mg/dL)	Points
≥60	-1
50-59	0
40-49	1
<40	2

Systolic BP (mmHg)	If Untreated	If Treated
<120	0	0
120-129	0	1
130-139	1	2
140-159	1	2
≥160	2	3

Point Total	10-Year Risk %
<0	< 1
0	1
1	1
2	1
3	1
4	1
5	2
6	2
7	3
8	4
9	5
10	6
11	8
12	10
13	12
14	16
15	20
16	25
≥17	≥ 30

| 10-Year risk _____% |

Women
Estimate of 10-Year Risk for Women

(Framingham Point Scores)

Age	Points
20-34	-7
35-39	-3
40-44	0
45-49	3
50-54	6
55-59	8
60-64	10
65-69	12
70-74	14
75-79	16

Total Cholesterol	Points				
	Age 20-39	Age 40-49	Age 50-59	Age 60-69	Age 70-79
<160	0	0	0	0	0
160-199	4	3	2	1	1
200-239	8	6	4	2	1
240-279	11	8	5	3	2
≥280	13	10	7	4	2

	Points				
	Age 20-39	Age 40-49	Age 50-59	Age 60-69	Age 70-79
Nonsmoker	0	0	0	0	0
Smoker	9	7	4	2	1

HDL (mg/dL)	Points
≥60	-1
50-59	0
40-49	1
<40	2

Systolic BP (mmHg)	If Untreated	If Treated
<120	0	0
120-129	1	3
130-139	2	4
140-159	3	5
≥160	4	6

Point Total	10-Year Risk %
< 9	< 1
9	1
10	1
11	1
12	1
13	2
14	2
15	3
16	4
17	5
18	6
19	8
20	11
21	14
22	17
23	22
24	27
≥25	≥ 30

| 10-Year risk _____% |

U.S. DEPARTMENT OF HEALTH AND HUMAN SERVICES
Public Health Service
National Institutes of Health
National Heart, Lung, and Blood Institute

NIH Publication No. 01-3290
May 2001

FIGURE 20-1 (continued)

Box 20-3 Guidelines for Assessing Risks for Cardiovascular Disease in Older Adults

Questions to Identify Risk Factors for Cardiovascular Disease

- Do you have, or have you ever had, any heart or circulation problems (e.g., stroke, angina, heart attack, blood clots, or peripheral vascular disease)? *If yes, ask the usual questions about type of therapy, and so on.*
- When was the last time you had an electrocardiogram?
- What is your normal blood pressure? Have you ever been told that you have high blood pressure, or borderline high blood pressure?
- Do you take, or have you ever taken, medications for heart problems or blood pressure? *If yes, ask the usual questions about type, dose, duration of therapy, and the like.*
- Do you smoke, or have you ever smoked? *If yes, ask additional questions, such as those appropriate for assessing respiratory function, Chapter 21.*
- Do you know what your cholesterol levels are? When was the last time you had your cholesterol checked?
- Do you have diabetes? When was the last time you had your blood sugar (glucose) level checked and what was the result?
- What is your usual pattern of exercise?

Additional Considerations Regarding Risk Factors

- Calculate BMI and compare the person's ideal weight to his or her present weight.
- Determine usual dietary habits, paying particular attention to the person's intake of sodium, fiber, and types of fat. (This information is usually obtained during the nutritional assessment.)

atypical symptoms to other conditions, such as arthritis or indigestion, or even to "normal aging." Therefore, nurses need to keep in mind that complaints about fatigue; digestion; respiration; or pain in the arms, shoulders, or upper trunk can be indicators of cardiac disease. Assessment is further complicated by the fact that older adults often have more than one underlying condition that could be responsible for these symptoms. It is not unusual, for example, for an older person to have an esophageal reflux disorder as well as a history of ischemic heart disease. Nurses also need to consider that older adults who have mobility impairments or other functional limitations may not be active enough to experience exertion-related symptoms. Therefore, in addition to focusing the assessment on the usual manifestations of cardiovascular function, the nurse must incorporate information about other systems and overall functioning. In addition, a baseline electrocardiogram is helpful in establishing the possibility of silent or atypical myocardial ischemia.

Assessing Knowledge About Heart Disease

In addition to assessing signs and symptoms, nurses need to assess the older adult's knowledge about manifestations of heart disease. This is particularly important because immediate medical attention is a major factor in determining outcomes of heart attacks, and all people need to be aware of the warning signs so that they can initiate appropriate help-seeking actions. Thus, nurses should ask at least one question to determine the older

adult's knowledge about the signs and symptoms of a heart attack. Nurses also can include a question about what the person would do and whom they would call if they thought they were experiencing a heart attack. Box 20-4 summarizes the guidelines for assessing cardiovascular function and detecting cardiovascular disease in older adults, emphasizes the assessment components that are unique to older adults, and refers to additional assessment components that apply to adults in general.

DIVERSITY NOTE

Knowledge of heart attack and stroke symptoms is lacking among adults in the United States and is lowest among older adults, racial minorities, and other groups who are at highest risk for cardiovascular disease (Bell et al., 2009).

NURSING DIAGNOSIS

If the nursing assessment identifies risks for cardiovascular disease, a nursing diagnosis of Ineffective Health Maintenance may be applicable. This diagnosis is defined as

Box 20-4 Guidelines for Assessing Cardiovascular Function in Older Adults

Questions to Assess for Cardiovascular Disease

- Do you ever have chest pain or tightness in your chest? If yes, ask the usual questions to explore the type, onset, duration, and other characteristics.
- Do you ever have difficulty breathing? If yes, ask the usual questions regarding onset and other characteristics.
- Do you ever feel lightheaded or dizzy? If yes, ask about specific circumstances, medical evaluation, and methods of dealing with symptoms and ensuring safety.
- Do you ever feel like your heart is racing, is irregular, or has extra or skipped beats? If yes, ask about any prior medical evaluation.
- Have you ever been told that you had a heart murmur? If yes, ask about any prior medical evaluation.

Information Obtained During Other Portions of an Assessment that May Be Useful in Assessing Cardiovascular Function

- Do you tire easily or feel that you need more rest than is ordinarily required?
- Do you have any problems with indigestion?
- Do your feet or ankles ever get swollen?
- Do you wake up at night because of difficulty breathing or because of any other discomfort? Have you made any adjustments in your sleeping habits because of difficulty breathing (e.g., do you use more than one pillow or sleep in a chair)?
- Do you have any pain in your upper back or shoulders?

Interview Questions to Assess for Postural Hypotension

- Do you ever feel lightheaded or dizzy, especially when you get up in the morning or after you've been lying down?
- *If yes:* Is this feeling accompanied by any additional symptoms, such as sweating, nausea, or confusion?
- *If yes:* Do any of the risks listed in Box 20-1 apply to you? *If yes, ask about any prior medical evaluation.*

"inability to identify, manage, and/or seek out help to maintain health" (NANDA International, 2009). Related factors common in older adults include lack of physical activity and insufficient knowledge about preventive measures. For older adults with impaired cardiovascular function, applicable nursing diagnoses may include Activity Intolerance, Decreased Cardiac Output, and Ineffective Tissue Perfusion (Cardiopulmonary). The nursing diagnosis of Risk for Injury may be appropriate for older adults with orthostatic or postprandial hypotension, particularly in the presence of additional risk factors for falls and fractures (e.g., osteoporosis, neurologic disorders, and medication side effects).

Wellness Opportunity

Nurses can use the wellness nursing diagnoses, Readiness for Enhanced Nutrition or Readiness for Enhanced Knowledge, for older adults who are interested in developing heart-healthy dietary habits or learning about health-promoting behaviors to prevent heart disease.

PLANNING FOR WELLNESS OUTCOMES

When older adults have risks for cardiovascular disease, nurses can apply any of the following Nursing Outcomes Classification (NOC) terminologies to identify wellness outcomes in their care plans: Health Orientation, Health-Promoting Behavior, Knowledge: Diet, Knowledge: Health Behavior, Risk Control: Cardiovascular Health, Risk Control: Tobacco Use, and Weight Control. Wellness outcomes for older adults with cardiovascular disease include Cardiac Disease Self-Management, Circulation Status, Health Seeking Behavior, Knowledge: Cardiac Disease Management, Tissue Perfusion: Cardiac, and Tissue Perfusion: Peripheral. Additional outcomes include maintaining blood pressure within the normal range and preventing negative consequences of orthostatic or postprandial hypotension (e.g., falls and fractures).

Wellness Opportunity

Nurses address body–mind–spirit interconnectedness by including stress level as an outcome directed toward reducing the risk for cardiovascular disease.

NURSING INTERVENTIONS TO PROMOTE HEALTHY CARDIOVASCULAR FUNCTION

From a wellness perspective, nursing interventions to promote healthy cardiovascular function focus on primary and secondary prevention of cardiovascular disease. These interventions address specific risk factors, such as smoking, hypertension, obesity, and lipid disorders as well as preventive measures, such as optimal levels of physical activity, heart-healthy dietary patterns, and stress-reduction actions. Although pharmacologic and medical interventions are often used to reduce risk factors, teaching about health promotion actions is a nursing intervention that is appropriate in almost all situations. In addition to addressing risks for cardiovascular disease, nurses can address orthostatic or postprandial hypotension and the related functional consequences, such as falls and fractures.

Nurses can use the following Nursing Interventions Classification (NIC) terminologies in care plans to promote cardiovascular wellness: Cardiac Care, Coping Enhancement, Counseling, Exercise Promotion, Health Education, Meditation Facilitation, Nutritional Counseling, Self-Responsibility Enhancement, Simple Guided Imagery, Simple Relaxation Therapy, and Teaching: Individual.

Addressing Risks Through Nutrition and Lifestyle Interventions

Nutrition interventions can be used to address risk factors in all adults and are particularly important for prevention or management of obesity, hypertension, and lipid disorders. Research reviews related to dietary influences on cardiovascular disease support the following evidence-based recommendations (Katcher, Lanford, & Kris-Etherton, 2009; Van Horn et al., 2008):

- 25% to 35% of energy needs should come from dietary fat, with less than 7% coming from saturated fats and trans fats combined, and with less than 200 mg/day of cholesterol
- Although 25 g/day of soy protein is a good substitute for animal protein to decrease saturated fat intake, it does not reduce LDL cholesterol to any significant degree
- Diets should include mushrooms, olive oil, cruciferous vegetable, whole-grain breads, and foods that are high in vitamin B complex
- 2 to 3 g/day of plant sterols and stanols (found in yogurt, margarines, and some cereals) can decrease total cholesterol and LDL cholesterol by as much as 15%; however, sterols/stanols can reduce absorption of carotenoids and fat-soluble vitamins
- Alcoholic beverages in the amount of one drink daily for women and two drinks for men may be beneficial for preventing cardiovascular disease; however, people who do not consume alcohol should not start drinking and it is clearly contraindicated in some conditions (e.g., cardiomyopathy, hypertension, arrhythmias, and risk for alcoholism)
- Current evidence does not support the use of antioxidant supplements, but diets should include fruits and vegetables that are rich in nutrients, including antioxidants.

Many studies have looked at the effects of a **Mediterranean dietary pattern**, which is characterized by higher intakes of fish, poultry, nuts, fruits, legumes, vegetables, and lower intake of red and processed meats. Overall, the Mediterranean dietary pattern results in lower intake of saturated and trans fats and higher intake of monounsaturated and polyunsaturated fats. In addition, complex carbohydrates are the main type of carbohydrates. Research studies have found that this dietary pattern has significant benefits both for primary prevention of coronary heart disease in the general population and for secondary prevention for people who already have pathologic changes (Lloyd-Jones et al., 2009; Sparling & Anderson, 2009).

The **DASH dietary pattern**, which refers to the *Dietary Approaches to Stop Hypertension*, is an evidence-based eating plan that is promoted by many organizations including the National Institutes of Health and the American Heart Association. This dietary pattern is characterized by high intake of fruits, vegetables, and plant proteins from grains, nuts, and legumes; moderate intake of low- or nonfat dairy foods; and low intake of sodium and animal protein and is widely recognized as a primary and secondary preventive intervention for hypertension. Studies have identified the following beneficial effects of DASH-type diets: lowered blood pressure, decreased LDL and triglyceride levels, lower risk of coronary heart disease and stroke, and lower all-cause mortality in people with hypertension (Fung et al., 2008; Lloyd-Jones et al., 2009; Parikh, Lipsitz, & Natarajan, 2009). A longitudinal study of women who developed heart failure found that women who followed the DASH diet had a 37% lower rate after adjusting for other risk factors (Levitan, Wolk, & Mittleman, 2009).

Another focus of nutrition-related research is on the potential benefits of commonly consumed foods and beverages, such as chocolate and tea, that are rich in polyphenols. There is increasing evidence that cocoa and chocolate may improve cardiovascular function and exert antioxidant, anti-inflammatory, antiplatelet, and antihypertensive effects (Frishman, Beravol, & Carosella, 2009). Epidemiologic studies indicate that cocoa and other polyphenols can reduce the risk of cardiovascular disease, but long-term clinical trials are needed before evidence-based recommendations can be determined (Corti, 2009; Grassi, 2009). Similarly, although epidemiologic studies have found an association between green tea intake and reduced risk for cardiovascular disease, clinical trials are not sufficient to support an evidence-based recommendation (Ferguson, 2009; Schneider & Segre, 2009). One study found that highly fermented black tea may be equally potent as green tea in promoting beneficial cardiovascular effects (Lorenz et al., 2009).

Additional lifestyle interventions that are effective for preventing cardiovascular disease include remaining physically active, managing stress, refraining from smoking, and maintaining ideal body weight. Research reviews identify strong evidence supporting the importance of physical exercise as an intervention for preventing cardiovascular disease and improving life expectancy (Katcher et al., 2009). Specific positive effects on cardiovascular function identified in studies include weight loss; reduced blood pressure; improved overall cardiac function; lower rates of cardiovascular disease; improved lipid, glucose, and triglyceride levels; and decreased risk of developing diabetes and cardiovascular disease (Nesto, 2008). Positive effects of exercise on other aspects of health are noted throughout this text, and nurses can incorporate this

information when they teach about the many positive functional consequences of regular physical exercise.

Smoking is a major risk factor for cardiovascular disease, and quitting smoking is beneficial for people at any age. A longitudinal study found that smoking cessation was the most important independent predictor of mortality in patients who had coronary artery bypass graft surgery, with those patients who quit smoking gaining 3 years in life expectancy compared with those who continued to smoke (van Domburg, Reimer, Hoeks, Kappetein, & Rogers, 2008). Benefits of smoking cessation as a secondary prevention intervention begin immediately and are as effective in older adults as they are in younger people. An important nursing responsibility is to provide health education regarding smoking cessation, as discussed in Chapter 21.

Secondary Prevention

When nurses care for older adults who have cardiovascular disease, referrals for secondary prevention programs, such as cardiac rehabilitation, are an important part of care (Figure 20-2). Despite evidence-based guidelines recommending cardiac rehabilitation programs, referral rates are low and one study found that only 14% of Medicare patients with acute myocardial infarctions had enrolled (Mazzini, Stevens, Whalen, Ozonoff, & Balady, 2008). Although referrals need to be initiated by primary care practitioners, nurses have an important responsibility to encourage participation when referrals are

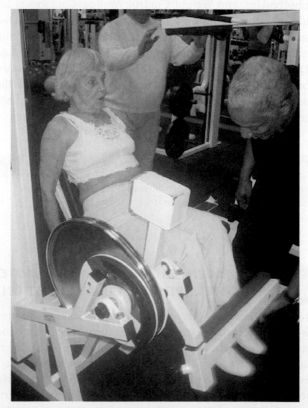

FIGURE 20-2 Exercise is an important preventive intervention. (Courtesy of Monte Unetic.)

made. Nurses also can suggest that patients ask their primary care practitioners about a referral for preventive services such as stress management, cardiac rehabilitation, smoking cessation, or exercise counseling.

DIVERSITY NOTE

Asians, Hispanics, and Native Americans are less likely than white older adults to receive post–acute cardiac rehabilitation services (Dolansky et al., 2010).

Wellness Opportunity

Nurses communicate positive attitudes about aging by talking with older adults about personal responsibility for addressing risks for cardiovascular disease and communicating that it's never too late to incorporate healthy behaviors into daily life.

Addressing Risks Through Pharmacologic Interventions

Before and during the 1990s, hormonal replacement therapy was recommended for menopausal women as an intervention for preventing cardiovascular disease. This recommendation was based on epidemiologic studies, but it was reversed in 2002 when longitudinal and large-scale investigations concluded that risks outweighed the benefits as a preventive intervention. The use of low-dose aspirin is another pharmacologic intervention that has been investigated for the prevention of cardiovascular disease, with emphasis on determining whether the potential benefits outweigh the increased risks for gastrointestinal bleeding and hemorrhagic stroke. In the early 2000s, studies concluded that the balance of benefit and harm is most favorable in people with a high risk for, or a history of, cardiovascular disease. In 2009, the U.S. Preventive Task Force (USPTF, 2009) published updated evidence-based guidelines with the following recommendations:

- Men aged 45 to 79 years and women aged 55 to 79 years: encourage aspirin use when potential cardiovascular benefit outweighs potential harm of gastrointestinal hemorrhage or ischemic strokes
- Men and women aged 80 years and older: no recommendation due to insufficient evidence

Box 20-5 summarizes health education interventions regarding risk for cardiovascular disease in older adults.

Preventing and Managing Hypertension

Although relatively few nurses prescribe medications for hypertension, all nurses need to understand current guidelines and recommendations for management of hypertension because they are responsible for making appropriate decisions related to blood pressure. Nursing interventions for people with hypertension also include evaluating a patient's response to prescribed medications and teaching about interventions for hypertension. In addition, nurses can promote wellness

Box 20-5 Health Promotion Activities to Reduce the Risks for Cardiovascular Disease

Detection of Risks
- Have blood pressure checked annually.
- If the total serum cholesterol level is less than 200 mg/dL, have it rechecked every 5 years. If the total serum cholesterol level is between 200 and 239 mg/dL, follow dietary measures to reduce it and have it rechecked annually. If the total serum cholesterol level is 240 mg/dL or more, obtain a further medical evaluation.

Reduction of Risks
- Give high priority to smoking cessation, if you smoke.
- Avoid passive smoking (i.e., inhaling smoke from other people's cigarettes).
- Maintain weight at a level less than 110% of ideal weight.
- Exercise daily, and engage in aerobic exercise (i.e., exercise that increases the pulse rate) several times weekly for 30 to 45 minutes each time.
- Avoid foods that are high in sodium, and follow dietary measures to reduce serum cholesterol levels.
- Discuss with your primary care provider the use of low-dose aspirin therapy as a preventive measure, particularly if there is any history of coronary artery disease or cerebrovascular events.

by teaching about self-care measures for preventing and treating hypertension. This is particularly important because lifestyle modifications—including diet, weight loss, physical activity, and moderation of alcohol—are an integral component of effective hypertension management (Padiyar, 2009).

The **stepped-care approach** to management of hypertension was introduced in the first JNC report, published in the 1970s, and it has been consistently recommended in subsequent reports. This approach recommends that lifestyle modifications be tried initially, followed by pharmacologic interventions to achieve ideal blood pressure. Lifestyle interventions that have the most significant impact on hypertension are substantial weight loss and a dietary pattern that includes low-sodium and high-potassium foods (Sica, 2008). Dietary guidelines for the United States recommend that daily sodium intake be no more than 2300 mg/day for children aged 2 years and older and that it be no more than 1500 mg/day for those in specific groups, including all blacks, people with hypertension, and all middle-aged and older adults. This recommendation for lower sodium intake applies to 69.2% of U.S. adults; however, national surveys estimate that the average intake of sodium among children aged 2 years and older is more than 3400 mg/day (CDC, 2009). Thus, nurses have important responsibilities with regard to teaching older adults and their caregivers about sodium intake.

Many medications are used for treating hypertension, and selection of the best medication is based on variables such as therapeutic effectiveness and the presence of concomitant conditions. The classes of medications that are used most commonly to manage hypertension are diuretics, beta-blockers, angiotensin-converting enzyme (ACE) inhibitors,

Box 20-6 Guidelines for Nursing Management of Hypertension

Health Promotion Interventions

The following lifestyle modifications are recommended for all people with hypertension:

- Avoidance of tobacco
- Weight reduction when appropriate (i.e., when the person weighs more than 110% of his or her ideal weight)
- 30 to 45 minutes of exercise, such as brisk walking, at least five times weekly
- Limitation of alcohol intake to one drink per day (e.g., 2 ounces of 100-proof whiskey, 8 ounces of wine, or 24 ounces of beer).

The following nutritional interventions are recommended for all people with hypertension:

- Sodium intake limited to 1.5 g daily
- Avoidance of processed foods
- Daily intake of 7 to 8 servings of grains and grain products and 8 to 10 servings of fruits and vegetables

Considerations Regarding the Treatment of Hypertension

- Risks from and definitions of hypertension apply to all age categories (refer to Table 20-1 for criteria).
- A person's blood pressure should be measured at least three times before making any decisions about treatment.
- Home blood pressure monitoring is recommended for initial and on-going assessment.
- The safety of antihypertensive agents is improved by carefully selecting the medication, starting with low doses, and changing the medication regimen gradually, in small increments, if necessary.
- The goals of hypertensive treatment are to control blood pressure by the least intrusive means and to prevent cardiovascular morbidity and mortality.
- Treatment is directed toward achieving and maintaining a systolic blood pressure of <130/80 mm Hg if this can be achieved without compromising cardiovascular function.
- For older adults with isolated systolic hypertension or systolic blood pressure levels of 140 to 160 mm Hg, lifestyle modifications should be the first treatment step.

and calcium channel blockers. Studies have found that all of these classes of antihypertensives are equally effective, but individual patient responses may vary depending on factors such as age and ethnicity. For example, one large study found that a calcium channel blocker was more effective in blacks, an ACE inhibitor was best for young white men, and a beta-blocker worked best in older white men (Sica, 2008). Another research review concluded that the additive effect of antihypertensives from two different classes is approximately five times more effective in lowering blood pressure than increasing the dose of one drug (Wald, Law, Morris, Bestwick, & Wald, 2009).

In recent years, there is increasing emphasis on selecting a drug that not only treats hypertension but also prevents major cardiovascular events and mortality. A review of studies concluded that the type of drug used was less important than the degree to which blood pressure is controlled with regard to reducing the risk of major cardiovascular events (Sica, 2008). Selection of antihypertensives also is based on consideration of potential adverse effects, which is particularly important for older adults (Corrigan & Pallaki, 2009). For example, there is increasing concern about adverse metabolic effects associated with diuretics and beta-blockers in some people (Johnson et al., 2009). One advantage of combining drugs from two classes is that hypertension can be controlled effectively and with fewer adverse effects with lower doses of each drug (Wald et al., 2009). Box 20-6 summarizes guidelines for interventions for hypertension and includes health education information about nutrition and lifestyle interventions. Resources for health education and evidence-based practice for hypertension are listed at the end of this chapter. Figure 20-3 illustrates examples of some of the culturally specific health education materials that are available at the National Institutes of Health.

DIVERSITY NOTE

Asian/Pacific Islander Americans are more likely than whites to experience coughing as an adverse effect of ACE inhibitors (Watson, 2009).

Wellness Opportunity

Nurses promote personal responsibility for managing hypertension by talking with older adults about self-monitoring of blood pressure.

*M*r. C. is now 70 years old and his blood pressure fluctuates between 130/88 and 146/94 mm Hg. He continues to take hydrochlorothiazide, 25 mg, and verapamil, 120 mg, every morning. Mr. C. and his wife live with their daughter and her teenage children. Mr. and Mrs. C. usually do the family grocery shopping, and his wife and daughter prepare the family meals. A diet history reveals that the family usually eats fried fish or chicken about four times a week and pig's feet or ham hocks for the other main meals. Common side dishes are corn, okra, grits, cornbread, sweet potatoes, black-eyed peas, and fried greens. For cooking, the family uses lard, salt pork, or bacon drippings. Their usual beverage is decaffeinated coffee with sugar and cream. The family generally has cereal and toast for breakfast, but they have bacon and eggs on Saturdays and Sundays. Mr. and Mrs. C. eat their noon meal at the senior center 5 days a week. Mr. C.'s weight is still about 30 pounds more than his ideal weight. For the past several years, he has participated in the exercise program at the senior center, but gets little additional exercise and continues to complain of "getting winded" when he walks across the parking lot.

THINKING POINTS

- What additional information would you obtain for further assessment of Mr. C.'s cardiovascular status?
- What nutritional and lifestyle interventions would you discuss with Mr. C. regarding his hypertension?
- What teaching materials would you use for health education with Mr. C.?

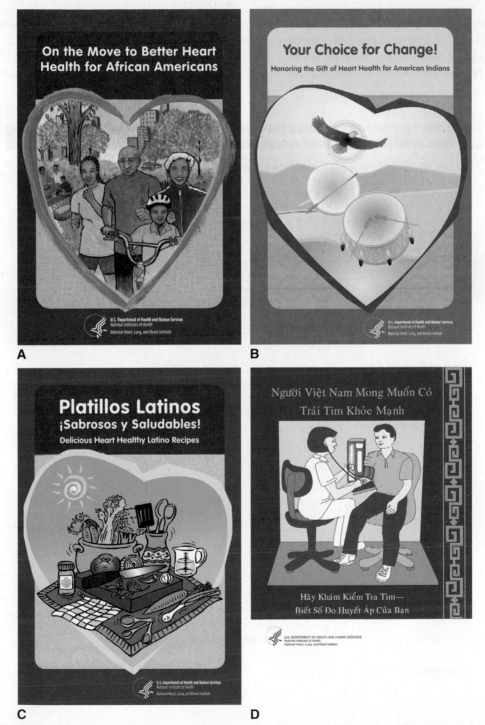

FIGURE 20-3 Examples of culturally specific health education materials that are available from the National Institutes of Health.

Preventing and Managing Lipid Disorders

Although nurses usually do not prescribe medications for treatment of lipid disorders, they are responsible for teaching about preventing and managing lipid disorders. Thus, nurses need to be familiar with lipid disorders treatment guidelines, such as the *ATP III*. This revised report focuses on people aged 50 years and older and encourages health care providers to consider a number of risk factors for people of any age when evaluating the need for interventions. Thus, goals for lipid profiles vary depending on the number of risk factors. For example, the LDL goal for healthy people with no risk factors is less than 160 mg/dL, but the LDL goal for someone with multiple risks is less than 100 mg/dL. Recent evidence indicates that the therapeutic goal for LDL in high-risk patients should be less than

70 mg/dL (Sachdeva et al., 2009). For links to the most up-to-date guidelines visit thePoint at http://thePoint.LWW.com/Miller6e. The updated ATP recommendations (Grundy et al., 2004) lists the following conditions as risk factors:

- Cardiovascular disease (e.g., angina, angioplasty, bypass surgery)
- Cerebrovascular conditions (e.g., ischemic stroke, transient ischemic attacks, symptomatic carotid artery stenosis)
- Peripheral vascular conditions
- Diabetes mellitus.

As with treatment of hypertension, nutrition and lifestyle interventions are the first-line approaches, and medications (e.g., statins) are prescribed if goals are not achieved with non-pharmacologic interventions. Essential nutrition and lifestyle

---

 Box 20-7 Nutritional Interventions for People With High Cholesterol

Dietary Measures to Promote a Healthy Lipid Profile

- Include foods that are high in fiber content in your daily diet (e.g., whole grains).
- Include soy proteins in your daily diet (e.g., tofu, soy milk).
- Eat a minimum of two servings of fatty fish weekly.
- Limit total fat intake to less than 30% of your total daily calorie intake.
- Limit total daily cholesterol intake to 200 mg.
- Use nonfat or low-fat dairy desserts.
- Consumption of butter or margarine should be limited, but margarines that contain stanols are beneficial (e.g., Becanol).
- Use egg whites, omega-3 eggs, or egg substitutes.
- Limit consumption of lean meats to five or fewer 3- to 5-ounce servings per week. Trim fat off meats and the skin off poultry.
- Avoid eating processed meats (e.g., bacon, bologna, sausage, hot dogs).
- Avoid gravies, fried foods, and organ meats.

Guide to Types of Fats

Type of Fat	Sources	Examples	Effect on Lipid Profile
Saturated fatty acids	Animal fats and some vegetable oils (usually solid at room temperatures)	Meat, poultry, butter, and lauric and palm oils	Negative: increases LDL and total cholesterol
Trans fatty acids	Vegetable oils that are processed into margarine or shortening	Dairy products, baked goods, snack foods	Negative: increases LDL cholesterol and lowers HDL cholesterol
Monounsaturated fatty acids	Vegetable oils (usually liquid at room temperatures)	Olive, peanut, and canola oils	Positive: decreases LDL
Polyunsaturated fatty acids	Seafood and vegetable oils (soft or liquid at room temperatures)	Corn, sunflower, safflower, canola, and linoleic oils	Positive: decreases LDL
Omega-3 fatty acids	Fatty fish	Tuna, salmon, herring, mackerel	Positive: decreases LDL cholesterol and triglycerides

LDL, low-density lipoprotein; HDL, high-density lipoprotein.

Box 20-8 Education Regarding Orthostatic and Postprandial Hypotension

Preventing and Managing Orthostatic and Postprandial Hypotension
- Maintain adequate fluid intake (i.e., eight glasses of noncaffeinated beverages daily).
- Eat five or six smaller meals daily, rather than large meals.
- Avoid excessive alcohol consumption.
- Avoid sitting or standing still for prolonged periods, especially after meals.

Health Promotion Measures Specific to Orthostatic Hypotension
- Change your position slowly, especially when moving from a sitting or lying position to a standing position.
- Before standing up, sit at the side of the bed for several minutes after rising from a lying position.
- Maintain good physical fitness, especially good muscle tone, and engage in regular, but not excessive, exercise. (Swimming is an excellent form of exercise because the hydrostatic pressure prevents blood from pooling in the legs.)
- Wear a waist-high elastic support garment or thigh-high elastic stockings during the day, and put them on before getting out of bed in the morning.
- Sleep with the head of the bed elevated on blocks.
- During the day, rest in a recliner chair with your legs elevated.
- Take measures to prevent constipation and avoid straining during bowel movements.

- Avoid medications that increase the risk for orthostatic hypotension, particularly if additional risk factors are present (refer to Box 20-1).
- Avoid sources of intense heat (e.g., direct sun, electric blankets, and hot baths and showers) because these cause peripheral vasodilation.
- If taking nitroglycerin, do not take it while standing.

Health Promotion Measures Specific to Postprandial Hypotension
- Minimize the risk for postprandial hypotension by taking antihypertensive medications (if prescribed) 1 hour after meals rather than before meals.
- Eat small, low-carbohydrate meals.
- Avoid alcohol consumption.
- Avoid strenuous exercise, especially for 2 hours after meals.

Safety Precautions if Hypotension Cannot Be Prevented
- Reduce the potential for falls and other negative functional consequences of postprandial hypotension by remaining seated (or by lying down) after meals.
- Call for assistance if help is needed with walking.
- Adapt the environment to minimize the risk and consequences of falling (e.g., ensure good lighting, install grab bars, keep pathways clear).

interventions for lipid disorders include dietary modifications, maintenance of ideal body weight, and incorporation of regular exercise in one's daily routine. Nutrition interventions focus on dietary fat intake, with emphasis on limiting foods containing saturated fats and trans fatty acids and increasing foods that are high in polyunsaturated and monounsaturated fats. Box 20-7 summarizes health education interventions for prevention and management of lipid disorders in older adults.

Preventing and Managing Orthostatic or Postprandial Hypotension

Interventions aimed at preventing orthostatic and postprandial hypotension can be initiated as health measures for older adults who have any of the risk factors listed in Box 20-1. For older adults with symptomatic orthostatic hypotension, interventions to alleviate the problem are important for maintaining quality of life and preventing serious consequences. In addition, nurses address safety issues by implementing interventions that are directed toward preventing falls and fractures, as discussed in Chapter 22.

For older adults with postprandial hypotension, interventions can be implemented around mealtimes. In institutional or home care settings, registered dietitians may be helpful in developing a plan for addressing postprandial hypotension, but in any setting, nurses assume responsibility for health education about interventions. In older adults with postprandial hypotension, low-carbohydrate meals may be effective in

addressing postprandial hypotension. Also, agents that slow down the rate of gastric emptying, such as xylose and the natural food supplement guar gum, may alleviate postprandial hypotension. One study found that the hypoglycemic agent acarbose is effective and safe for treating postprandial hypotension (Jian & Zhou, 2008). Additional interventions are summarized in Box 20-8, which can be used as a tool for educating older adults about orthostatic and postprandial hypotension.

EVALUATING EFFECTIVENESS OF NURSING INTERVENTIONS

One measure of the effectiveness of health promotion interventions is the extent to which the older adult verbalizes correct information about the risks. Also, the older adult may verbalize intent to change or eliminate the lifestyle factors that increase the risk of impaired cardiovascular function. For example, the older adult may agree to join an exercise program and follow dietary measures to reduce serum cholesterol levels. Effectiveness of interventions can also be measured by determining the actual reduction in risk factors. For example, the person's serum cholesterol level may decrease from 238 to 198 mg/dL after 6 months of regular exercise and dietary modifications. For older adults with impaired cardiovascular function, nurses evaluate the extent to which the signs and symptoms are alleviated and the extent to which older adults verbalize correct information about managing their condition.

*M*r. C. is now 74 years old and continues to come to the Senior Wellness Clinic for monthly blood pressure checks. He reports that his doctor recently started him on a medication for high cholesterol and told him to "watch my diet," but gave no further information or educational materials about what to do about his cholesterol.

NURSING ASSESSMENT

Mr. C. has no knowledge about dietary sources of cholesterol, and is unaware that his diet, which he terms "soul food," is high in cholesterol. Although he says that he has heard a lot about "good and bad cholesterol" in the news, he does not know which foods are good or bad. He tries to buy foods that say "no cholesterol" on the label, but says that the labels are too confusing about the different kinds of fats.

NURSING DIAGNOSIS

Your nursing diagnosis is Altered Health Maintenance related to lack of regular exercise, dietary habits that contribute to hyperlipidemia, and insufficient information about lifestyle factors that increase the risk of cardiovascular disease. Evidence of these risk factors comes from Mr. C.'s inactivity, eating patterns, history of hypertension, and family history of cardiovascular disease. Also, Mr. C. has verbalized insufficient information about the relationship between exercise and cardiovascular function and about dietary measures to control cholesterol.

NURSING CARE PLAN FOR MR. C.

Expected Outcome	Nursing Interventions	Nursing Evaluation
Mr. C.'s knowledge of risk factors for cardiovascular impairment will increase.	• Discuss the risk factors for impaired cardiovascular function, using Figure 20-1 and information from Box 20-3. • Emphasize the risk factors that can be addressed through lifestyle modifications (e.g., exercise, weight loss, and dietary measures to control cholesterol levels).	• Mr. C. will be able to describe his risk factors for cardiovascular disease. • Mr. C. will identify those risk factors that he can address through lifestyle changes.
Mr. C.'s knowledge of the relationship between diet and serum cholesterol levels will increase.	• Use teaching materials obtained from the American Heart Association to illustrate the relationship between diet and serum cholesterol levels. Provide a copy of these pamphlets for Mr. C. to take home. • Suggest that Mr. C. discusses the information in the pamphlets with his wife and daughter. • Ask Mr. C. to bring his wife to the nursing clinic next month so that you can talk with both of them about dietary measures to control cholesterol.	• Mr. C. will accurately describe the relationship between food intake and cholesterol levels. • Mr. C. will identify family eating habits that contribute to his elevated serum cholesterol level.
Mr. C. will modify one dietary habit that contributes to his high cholesterol level.	• Work with Mr. C. to make a list of the foods associated with high cholesterol levels (e.g., fried foods, ham hocks, lard, bacon, and eggs). • Give Mr. C. a copy of Box 20-7 and use it to discuss dietary measures to reduce cholesterol. • Ask Mr. C. to select one change in dietary habits that will have a positive effect on his cholesterol level (e.g., switching from lard to vegetable oil for frying foods).	• Mr. C. will state that he is willing to change one eating habit that contributes to his high cholesterol level. • Next month, Mr. C. will report that he has changed one eating pattern that contributes to high cholesterol levels.

Expected Outcome	Nursing Interventions	Nursing Evaluation
Mr. C. will increase his knowledge about the relationship between exercise and cardiovascular function.	• Use pamphlets from the American Heart Association to teach about the effects of aerobic exercise on cardiovascular function. • Review information about the relationship between exercise and weight.	• Mr. C. will describe the beneficial effects of regular aerobic exercise.
Mr. C. will begin exercising on a regular basis.	• Discuss ways in which Mr. C. can incorporate regular exercise into his daily activities. • Invite Mr. C. and his wife to participate in the daily Eldercise program that is offered following the noon meal at the senior center.	• Mr. C. will verbalize a commitment to perform 30 minutes of exercise 3 days a week.
Mr. C. will eliminate lifestyle factors that increase the risk for cardiovascular disease.	• Ask Mr. C. to invite his wife to your monthly appointments so that she can also receive important health education. • Identify a plan that will enable Mr. and Mrs. C. to gradually incorporate additional dietary measures aimed at reducing cholesterol into the family meal plans. • Identify a plan that will enable Mr. and Mrs. C. to include 30 minutes of exercise 5 times a week. • Discuss weight reduction with Mr. C. and emphasize that dietary modifications and regular exercise are interventions that should facilitate weight loss.	• Mr. C.'s total cholesterol level will be ≤200 mg/dL at the end of 6 months. • Mr. C.'s serum cholesterol level will remain below 200 mg/dL. • Mr. C. will report that he engages in 30 minutes of exercise 5 times weekly. • Mr. C. will report that he follows the dietary measures presented in Box 20-7. • Mr. C.'s weight will be reduced to between 180 and 198 pounds, and he will maintain that weight.

THINKING POINTS

• What factors affect Mr. C.'s ability to manage his cardiovascular condition and address his risk factors, and how would you address these factors in your interventions?

• Explore some of the health education listed at the end of this chapter to find teaching tools that would be appropriate for Mr. C.

Chapter Highlights

Age-Related Changes That Affect Cardiovascular Function
• Degenerative changes of myocardium
• Arterial stiffening
• Thicker, less elastic, more dilated veins
• Increased peripheral resistance
• Altered baroreflex mechanisms

Risk Factors That Affect Cardiovascular Function
• Atherosclerosis
• Physical inactivity
• Tobacco smoking
• Dietary habits
• Obesity, especially abdominal obesity
• Hypertension
• Lipid disorders
• Metabolic syndrome
• Psychosocial factors
• Heredity and socioeconomic factors
• Special considerations for women and minority groups

Functional Consequences Affecting Cardiovascular Wellness
• Effects on cardiac function
• Effects on pulse and blood pressure
• Effects on response to exercise
• Effects on circulation

Pathologic Condition Affecting Cardiovascular Function
• Orthostatic and Postprandial Hypotension

Nursing Assessment of Cardiovascular Function (Figure 20-1; Table 20-1; Boxes 20-2 through 20-4)
• Baseline cardiovascular function (heart rate, sounds, and rhythm)
• Blood pressure, including hypertension and orthostatic or postprandial hypotension
• Risks for cardiovascular disease, with emphasis on modifiable conditions

- Signs and symptoms of heart disease
- Knowledge about heart disease

Nursing Diagnosis
- Ineffective Health Maintenance
- Decreased Cardiac Output
- Ineffective Tissue Perfusion (Cardiopulmonary)

Planning for Wellness Outcomes
- Health-Promoting Behaviors
- Risk Control: Cardiovascular Health
- Risk Control: Tobacco Use
- Cardiac Disease Self-Management

Nursing Interventions to Promote Healthy Cardiovascular Function (Boxes 20-5 through 20-8; Evidence-Based Practice)
- Teaching about nutrition and lifestyle interventions (exercise, heart-healthy diet, optimal body weight, cessation of smoking if applicable)
- Evidence-based practice related to promoting cardiovascular health
- Referrals for secondary prevention programs for older adults who have cardiovascular disease
- Pharmacologic interventions for prevention of cardiovascular disease
- Lifestyle and pharmacologic interventions for hypertension
- Medication, nutrition, and lifestyle interventions for lipid disorders
- Prevention and management of orthostatic and postprandial hypotension

Evaluating Effectiveness of Nursing Interventions
- Verbalization of correct information about risks
- Reported participation in health promotion interventions (e.g., heart-healthy diet, regular exercise, weight reduction, and smoking cessation when applicable)
- Indicators of cardiovascular function within normal range (e.g., blood pressure, serum lipids)
- If applicable, alleviation of signs and symptoms of cardiovascular disease

Critical Thinking Exercises

1. Discuss how each of the following factors influences cardiovascular function, including orthostatic hypotension: lifestyle, medications, age-related changes, and pathologic conditions.
2. Demonstrate how you would teach a home health aide to assess blood pressure and orthostatic hypotension correctly.
3. Describe the questions and considerations that you would include in an assessment of cardiovascular function in an older adult who has no complaints of heart problems, but who has a history of falling twice in the past month and who has not been evaluated by a primary care provider in the past year.

4. You are asked to give a health education talk entitled "Keeping Your Heart Healthy" at a senior center. What information would you include in the presentation? What local resources (i.e., specific contact information for agencies or organizations in your area) would you suggest your audience contact for further information? What audiovisual aids would you use? How would you involve the participants in the discussion?
5. You are working in an assisted-living facility in which several of the residents have orthostatic hypotension. What would you include in your health education regarding management of orthostatic hypotension?

Resources

For links to these resources and additional helpful Internet resources related to this chapter, visit thePoint. at http://thePoint. lww.com/Miller6e.

Clinical Tools

American Heart Association
- Interactive self-assessment tools related to blood pressure and cardiovascular risks
- Interactive quizzes to test heart-health knowledge on topics such as fats, cholesterol, physical activity, and high blood pressure

Hartford Institute for Geriatric Nursing
- *Try This: Best Practices in Nursing Care to Older Adults*
  Issue SP3 (2010), Cardiac Risk Assessment of the Older Cardiovascular Patient; The Framingham Global Risk Assessment Tools
  Issue SP4 (2010), Vascular Risk Assessment of the Older Cardiovascular Patient: The Make-Brachial Index (ABI)

National Heart Lung and Blood Institute
- Health-risk calculators related to blood pressure and heart conditions

Evidence-Based Practice

Mosca, L., Banks, C. L., Benjamin, E. J., Berra, K., Bushnell, C., Dolor, R. J., et al. (2007). Evidence-based guidelines for cardiovascular disease prevention in women: 2007 update. *Circulation, 115,* 1481–1501.

National Heart Lung and Blood Institute
- Cardiovascular Risk Reduction Guidelines in Adults: Cholesterol Guideline Update (ATP IV), Hypertension Guideline Update (JNC 8), Obesity Guideline Update (Obesity 2), Integrated Cardiovascular Risk Reduction Guideline.

National Guideline Clearinghouse
- Diet and lifestyle recommendations for cardiovascular health
- Exercise promotion: walking in elders
- Nutrition practice guideline for hypertension
- Lipid disorders
- Hypertension

Health Education

American Heart Association
- Heart-health information in Spanish, Vietnamese, Simplified Chinese, and Traditional Chinese

American Stroke Association

Centers for Disease Control and Prevention
- WISEWOMAN program to prevent disease among women most in need

- Office of Minority Health: information on cardiovascular disease in racial and ethnic minority populations

DASH diet

Heart and Stroke Foundation of Canada

National Heart, Lung, and Blood Institute
- Publications about heart health for selected audiences, including African Americans, Asian Americans/Pacific Islanders, Latinos, Native Americans/Alaska Natives, and Women
- Online toolkit with resources to address heart disease in women
- Latino Cardiovascular Health Resources: Salud para su Corazon (For the health of your heart)

National Stroke Association

REFERENCES

Lichtenstein, A. H., Appel, L. J., Brands, M., Carnethon, M., Daniels, S., Franch, H. A., . . . Wylie-Rosett, J. (2006). Diet and lifestyle recommendations revision 2006: A scientific statement from the American Heart Association Nutrition Committee. *Circulation, 114*(1), 82–96.

Arbogast, S. D., Alshekhlee, A., Hussain, Z., McNeeley, K., & Chelimsky, T. C. (2009). Hypotension unawareness in profound orthostatic hypotension. *The American Journal of Medicine, 122*, 574–580.

Aronow, W. S. (2008). Hypertension and the older diabetic. *Clinics in Geriatric Medicine, 24*, 489–501.

Banegas, J. R., Segura, J., de la Sierra, A., Gorostidi, M., Rodriguez-Artalejo, F., Sobrinho, J., . . . Spanish Society of Hypertension ABPM Registry Investigators. (2008). Gender differences in office and ambulatory control of hypertension. *The American Journal of Medicine, 121*, 1078–1084.

Bell, M., Lommel, T., Fischer, J. G., Lee, J. S., Reddy, S., & Johnson, M. A. (2009). Improved recognition of heart attack and stroke symptoms after a community-based intervention for older adults, Georgia, 2006–2007. *Preventing Chronic Disease, 6*(2), 1–11.

Berra, K. (2008). Lipid-lowering therapy today. *Journal of Cardiovascular Nursing, 23*(5), 414–421.

Cademartiri, F., LaGrutta, L. L., de Feyter, P. J., & Kresstin, G. P. (2008). Physiopathology of the aging heart. *Radiology Clinics of North America, 46*, 653–662.

Carr, M C., & Tannock, L. L. (2009). Body-fat distribution and mortality risk: Thinking small. *Circulation, 117*, 1627.

Centers for Disease Control and Prevention. (2009). Application of lower sodium intake recommendations to adults: United States, 1999–2006. *MMWR: Morbidity and Mortality Weekly Report, 58*(11), 281–283.

Corrigan, M. V., & Pallaki, M. (2009). General principles of hypertension management in the elderly. *Clinics in Geriatric Medicine, 25*, 207–212.

Corti, R. (2009). Cocoa and cardiovascular health. *Circulation, 119*, 1433–1441.

D'Agostino, R. B., Ramachandran, S. V., Pencina, M. J., Wolf, P. A., Cobain, M., Massaro, J. M., & Kannel, W. B. (2008). General cardiovascular risk profile for use in primary care. *Circulation, 117*, 743–753.

Dennison, C. R., & Hughes, S. (2009). Should we screen for risk factors or disease? A current debate in the prevention of cardiovascular events. *Journal of Cardiovascular Nursing, 24*, 18–20.

Dolansky, M. A., Xu, F., Zullo, M., Shishehbor, M., Moore, S. M., & Rimm, A. A. (2010). Post-acute care services received by older adults following a cardiac event. *Journal of Cardiovascular Nursing, 25*, 342–349.

Ducharme, N., & Radhamma, R. (2008). Hyperlipidemia in the elderly. *Clinics in Geriatric Medicine, 24*, 471–487.

Duprez, D. A. (2008). Systolic hypertension in the elderly: Addressing an unmet need. *The American Journal of Medicine, 121*, 179–184.

Evangelista, O., & McLaughlin, M. A. (2009). Review of cardiovascular risk factors in women. *Gender Medicine, 6*, 17S–36S.

Farrell, T. W. (2009). Orthostatic hypotension. *Ferri's clinical advisor, 2009*. Philadelphia: Mosby Elsevier.

Ferguson, L. R. (2009). Nutrigenomics approaches to functional foods. *Journal of the American Dietetic Association, 109*, 452–458.

Figueredo, V. M. (2009). The time has come for physicians to take notice: The impact of psychosocial stressors on the heart. *The American Journal of Medicine, 122*, 704–712.

Flegel, K., & Magner, P. (2009). Get excess salt out of our diet. *Canadian Medical Association Journal, 181*, 263.

Foody, J. M. (2008). Prevention as the intervention. *Cardiology Clinics, 26*, xiii–xv.

Frishman, W. H., Beravol, P., & Carosella, C. (2009). Alternative and complementary medicine for preventing and treating cardiovascular disease. *Disease of the Month, 55*, 121–192.

Fung, T. T., Chiuve, S. E., McCullough, M. L., Rexrode, K. M., Logroscino, G., & Hu, F. B. (2008). Adherence to a DASH-style diet and risk of coronary heart disease and stroke in women. *Archives of Internal Medicine, 168*, 713–720.

Graham, M. M., Westerhout, C. M., Kaul, P., Norris, C. M., & Armstrong, P. W. (2008). Sex differences in patients seeking medical attention for prodromal symptoms before an acute coronary event. *American Heart Journal, 156*(6), 1210–1216.e1.

Grassi, D. (2009). Flavonids, vascular function, and cardiovascular protection. (2009). *Current Pharmacy Des, 15*(10), 1072–1084.

Green, L. A., Dickenson, W. P., Nease, D. E., & Campos-Outcalt, D. (2009). AAFP guideline for the detection and management of post-myocardial infarction depression. *Annals of Family Medicine, 7*, 71–79.

Grundy, S. M., Cleeman, J. I., Merz, N. B., Brewer, H. B. Jr., Clark, L.T., Hunninghake, D. B., . . . Stone, N. J. (2004). Implications of recent clinical trials for the National Cholesterol Education Program Adult Treatment Panel III Guidelines. *Circulation, 110*, 227–239.

Hiitola, P. (2009). Postural changes in blood pressure and the prevalence of orthostatic hypotension among home-dwelling elderly aged 75 years or older. *Journal of Human Hypertension, 23*, 33–39.

Insull, W. (2009). The pathology of atherosclerosis: Plaque development and plaque responses to medical treatment. *The American Journal of Medicine, 122*, S3–S14.

Jian, Z., & Zhou, B. (2008). Efficacy and safety of acarbose in the treatment of elderly patients with postural hypotension. *Chinese Medical Journal, 121*, 2054–2059.

Johnson, J. A., Boerwinkle, E., Zinch, I., Chapman, A. B., Bailey, K., Cooper-DeHoff, R. M., . . . Turner, S. T. (2009). Pharmacogenomics of antihypertensive drugs: Rationale and design of the Pharmacogenomic Evaluation of Antihypertensive Responses (PEAR) study. *American Heart Journal, 157*, 442–449.

Joint National Committee on Prevention, Detection, Evaluation, and Treatment of High Blood Pressure (JNC). (2003). The Seventh Report of the Joint National Committee on Prevention, Detection, Evaluation, and Treatment of High Blood Pressure. *Journal of the American Medical Association, 289*, 2560–2577.

Katcher, H. I., Lanford, J. L. G., & Kris-Etherton, P. M. (2009). Lifestyle approaches and dietary strategies to lower LDL-cholesterol and triglycerides and raise HDL-cholesterol. *Endocrinology and Metabolic Clinics of North America, 38*, 45–78.

Kokubo, Y., Kamide, K., Okamura, T., Watanabe, M., Higashiyama, A., Kawanishi, K., & Kawano, Y. (2008). Impact of high-normal blood pressure on the risk of cardiovascular disease in a Japanese urban cohort. *Hypertension, 52*, 652–659.

Larzelere, M. M., & Jones, G. N. (2008). Stress and health. *Primary Care Clinical Office Practice, 35*, 839–856.

Lee, K. S., Song, E. K., Lennie, T. A., Frazier, S. K., Chung, M. L., Heo, S., . . . Moser, D. K. (2010). Symptom clusters in men and women with heart failure and their impact on cardiac event-free survival. *Journal of Cardiovascular Nursing, 25*, 263–272.

Levitan, E. B., Wolk, A., & Mittleman, M. A. (2009). Consistency with the DASH diet and incidence of heart failure. *Archives of Internal Medicine, 169*, 851–857.

Lewis, S. J. (2009). Prevention and treatment of atherosclerosis: A practitioner's guide for 2008. *The American Journal of Medicine, 122*, S38–S50.

Lloyd-Jones, D., Adams, R., Carnethon, M., DeSimone, G., Ferguson, B., Flegal, K., . . . American Heart Association Statistics Committee and Stroke Statistics Subcommittee. (2009). Heart disease and stroke statistics–2009 update. *Circulation, 119*, e1–e161.

Lorenz, M., Urban, J., Engelhardt, U., Baumann, G., Stangl, K., & Stangl, V. (2009). Green and black tea are equally potent stimuli of NO production and vasodilation: New insights into tea ingredients involved. *Basic Research in Cardiology, 101*(1), 100–110.

Mallick, S., Kanthety, R., & Rahman, M. (2009). Home blood pressure monitoring in clinical practice: A review. *The American Journal of Medicine, 122*, 803–810.

Mazzini, M. J., Stevens, G. R., Whalen, D., Ozonoff, A., & Balady, G. J. (2008). Effect of an American Heart Association Get with the Guidelines program-based clinical pathway on referral and enrollment into cardiac rehabilitation after acute myocardial infarction. *American Journal of Cardiology, 101*, 1084–1087.

Mazzo, A. D. (2008). Insulin resistance syndrome and glucose dysregulation in the elderly. *Clinics in Geriatric Medicine, 24*, 437–454.

McDonald, M., Hartz, R. P., Unger, A. N., & Lustik, M. B. (2009). Prevalence, awareness, and management of hypertension, dyslipidemia, and diabetes among United States adults aged 65 and older. *Journal of Gerontology: Medical Sciences, 64A*, 256–263.

McGavock, J. M., Hastings, J. L., Snell, P. G., McGuire, D. K., Pacini, E. L., Levine, B. D., & Mitchell, J. H. (2009). A forty-year follow-up of the Dallas bed rest and training study: the effect of age on cardiovascular response to exercise in men. *Journal of Gerontology: Medical Sciences, 64A*, 293–299.

McSweeney, J. C., Cleves, M. A., Zhao, W., Lefler, L. L., & Yang, S. (2010). Cluster analysis of women's prodromal and acute myocardial infarction symptoms by race and other characteristics. *Journal of Cardiovascular Nursing, 25*, 311–322.

Mussi, C., Ungar, A., Salvioli, G., Menozzi, C. Bartoletti, A., Giada, F. . . . For the Evaluation of Guidelines in Syncope Study 2 Group. (2009). Orthostatic hypotension as cause of syncope in patients older than 65 years admitted to emergency departments for transient loss of consciousness. *Journal of Gerontology: Medical Sciences, 64A*, 801–806.

NANDA International. (2009). *Nursing diagnoses: Definitions and classification 2009–2011*. Oxford, UK: Wiley-Blackwell.

Nesto, R. W. (2008). Comprehensive clinical assessment of modifiable cardiometabolic risk factors. *Clinical Cornerstone, 9*, S9–S19.

Padiyar, A. (2009). Nonpharmacologic management of hypertension in the elderly. *Clinics in Geriatric Medicine, 25*, 213–219.

Parikh, A., Lipsitz, S. R., & Natarajan, S. (2009). Association between a DASH-like diet and mortality in adults with hypertension: Findings from a population-based follow-up study. *American Journal of Hypertension, 22*, 409–416.

Pickering, T. G., Miller, N. H., Ogedegbe, G., Krakoff, L. R., Artinian, N. T., & Goff, D. (2008). Call to action on use and reimbursement for home blood pressure monitoring. *Journal of Cardiovascular Nursing, 23*, 299–323.

Rashidi, A., & Wright, J. T. (2009). Drug treatment of hypertension in older hypertensives. *Clinics in Geriatric Medicine, 25*, 235–244.

Sachdeva, A., Cannon, C. P., Deedwania, P. C., Labresh, K. A., Smith, S. C., Dai, D., . . . Fonarow, G. C. (2009). Lipid levels in patients hospitalized with coronary artery disease: An analysis of 136,905 hospitalization in Get With The Guidelines. *American Heart Journal, 157*, 111–117.e2.

Schenk-Gustafsson, K. (2009). Risk factors for cardiovascular disease in women. *Maturitas, 63*, 186–190.

Schneider, C., & Segre, T. (2009). Green tea: Potential health benefits. *American Family Physician, 79*, 591–594.

Sica, D. A. (2008). Management of hypertension in the outpatient setting. *Primary Care: Clinics in Office Practice, 35*, 451–473.

Sidani, M., & Ziegler, C. (2008). Preventing heart disease: Who needs to be concerned and what to do. *Primary Care: Clinics in Office Practice, 35*, 589–607.

Sparling, M. C., & Anderson, J. J. B. (2009). The Mediterranean Diet and cardiovascular disease. *Nutrition Today, 44*(3), 124–133.

Spertus, J. A., Jones, P. G., Massoudi, F. A., Rumsfeld, J. S., & Krumholz, H. M. (2009). Factors associated with racial differences in myocardial infarction outcomes. *Annals of Internal Medicine, 150*, 314–324.

Surinach, J. M., Alvarez, L. R., Coll, R., Carmona, J. A., Sanclemente, C., Aguilar, E., . . . FRENA, Investigators. (2009). Differences in cardiovascular mortality in smokers, past-smokers, and non-smokers: Findings from the FRENA registry. *European Journal of Internal Medicine, 20*, 522–526.

Taylor, H. A., Akylbekova, E. L., Garrison, R. J., Sarpong, D., Joe, J., Walker, E., . . . Steffes, M. W. (2009). Dyslipidemia and the treatment of lipid disorders in African Americans. *The American Journal of Medicine, 122*, 454–463.

U.S. Preventive Services Task Force. (2008). Screening for lipid disorders in adults: Recommendation Statement. Retrieved from http://ahrq.gov/clinic/uspstf08/lipid/lipidrs.htm.

U.S. Preventive Services Task Force. (2009). Aspirin for the prevention of cardiovascular disease: U.S. Preventive Services Task Force Recommendation Statement. *Annals of Internal Medicine, 150*, 396–404.

Van Domburg, R. T., Reimer, W. S., Hoeks, S. E., Kappetein, A. P., & Rogers, A. J. (2008). Three life-years gained from smoking cessation after coronary bypass surgery: A 30 year follow-up study. *American Heart Journal, 156*, 473–476.

Van Hensbroek, P. B., Van Dijk, N., Van Breda, G. F., Scheffer, A. C., Van der Cammen, T. J., Lips, P., . . . Combined Amsterdam and Rotterdam Evaluation of FALLs (CAREFALL) study group (2009). The CAREFALL triage instrument identifying risk factors for recurrent falls in elderly patients. *The American Journal of Emergency Medicine, 27*, 23–36.

Van Horn, L., McCoin, M., Kris-Etherton, P. M., Burke, F., Carson, J. A. S., Champagne, C. M., . . . Sikand, G. (2008). The evidence for dietary prevention and treatment of cardiovascular disease. *Journal of the American Dietetic Association, 108*, 287–331.

Verwoert, G., Mattace-Rasso F., Hofman, A., Heeringa, J., Stricker, B. H. C., Breteler, M. M. B., & Witteman, J. C. M. (2008). Orthostatic hypotension and risk of cardiovascular disease in elderly people: The Rotterdam study. *Journal of the American Geriatrics Society, 56*, 1816–1820.

Wald, D. S., Law, M., Morris, J. K., Bestwick, J. P., & Wald, N. J. (2009). Combination therapy versus monotherapy in reducing blood pressure: Meta-analysis on 11,000 participants from 42 trials. *The American Journal of Medicine, 122*, 290–300.

Waldman, S. V., Blumenthal, J. A., Babyak, M. A., Sherwood, A., Sketch, M., Davidson, J., & Watkins, L. L. (2009). *American Heart Journal, 157*, 77–83.

Watson, J. E. (2009). Hypertension in Asian/Pacific Island Americans. *Journal of Clinical Hypertension, 11*(3), 148–152.

Weiss, A. M. (2009). Cardiovascular disease in women. *Primary Care Clinics: Office Practice, 36*, 73–102.

Williams, B., Lindholm, L. H., & Sever, P. (2008). Systolic pressure is all that matters. *The Lancet, 371*, 2219–2221.

Wu, J. S., Yang, Y. C., Lu, F. H., Wu, C. H., & Chang, C. J. (2008). Population-based study on the prevention and correlates of orthostatic hypotension/hypertension and orthostatic dizziness. *Hypertension Research, 31*, 897–904.

Zhang, C., Rexrode, K. M., Van Dam, R. M., Li, T. Y., & Hu, F. B. (2008). Abdominal obesity and risk of all-cause, cardiovascular, and cancer mortality. *Circulation, 117*, 1658–1667.

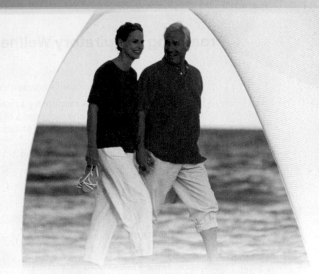

CHAPTER 21

Respiratory Function

LEARNING OBJECTIVES

After reading this chapter, you will be able to:

1. Describe age-related changes that affect respiratory function.
2. Identify risk factors that interfere with respiratory wellness.
3. Discuss the functional consequences that affect respiratory function in older adults.
4. Assess respiratory function, with emphasis on identifying opportunities for health promotion.
5. Identify nursing interventions to improve respiratory function and reduce risk factors that interfere with respiratory wellness.

K E Y   P O I N T S

chronic obstructive pul-
   monary disease (COPD)
ductectasia
elastic recoil
involuntary smoking

kyphosis
lung parenchyma
secondhand smoke
smokeless tobacco

The primary functions of respiration are to supply oxygen to and remove carbon dioxide from the blood. Adequate respiratory performance is essential to life because all body organs and tissues need oxygen. Thus, it is noteworthy that the respiratory system shows less age-related decline than other body systems in healthy, nonsmoking, older adults. The age-related changes that do affect respiratory performance are subtle and gradual, and healthy older adults are able to compensate for these changes. However, when illness, anesthesia, or another complicating factor places extraordinary demands for oxygen on the body, age-related respiratory changes can influence the overall function of the older adult.

 AGE-RELATED CHANGES THAT AFFECT RESPIRATORY FUNCTION

As with other physiologic functions, it is difficult to distinguish the effects of age-related changes from those caused by disease processes and external influences, such as tobacco smoking. Although these influences occur throughout the life span, their cumulative effects become more pronounced in older adults because they interact with age-related changes, such as diminished immune response, or with risk factors, such as diminished mobility.

Upper Respiratory Structures

The nose is often overlooked in discussions of respiratory function, but age-related changes of the upper respiratory structures can influence both comfort and function. For example, age-related connective tissue changes cause the nose to have a retracted columella (the lower edge of the septum) and a poorly supported, downwardly rotated tip. Although these changes are often viewed as having cosmetic, but not functional, effects, they can also cause septal deviations that interfere with the flow of air through the nasal cavity. These changes also can contribute to mouth breathing during sleep, causing snoring and obstructive apnea.

With increasing age, blood flow to the nose diminishes, causing the nasal turbinates to become smaller. Age-related changes also affect the submucosal glands, causing diminished secretions, even in healthy older adults. Because the secretions from the submucosal glands are thin and watery, their function is to dilute the thicker mucus secretions from the goblet cells. With diminished submucosal gland secretions, the mucus in the nasopharynx is thicker and more difficult to remove. This combination of age-related changes in turbinates, blood flow, and submucosal glands results in thicker and dryer secretions and a perception of nasal stuffiness. It also can stimulate the cough reflex and cause a persistent tickle in the throat.

The epiglottis and upper airway structures expel mucus and unwanted material from the lungs and protect the lower airway from harmful substances, ranging in size from microorganisms to large pieces of food. An age-related change

435

Promoting Respiratory Wellness in Older Adults

Nursing Assessment
- Overall respiratory function
- Signs and symptoms of infection
- Tobacco use and attitudes about quitting
- Immunization status

Age-Related Changes
- ↑ stiffness of chest wall
- ↑ anteroposterior diameter
- Enlarged alveoli
- Weaker respiratory muscles
- ↓ response to hypercapnia or hypoxia

Negative Functional Consequences
- ↑ use of accessory muscles
- ↓ cough and gag reflexes
- ↑ energy expenditure for breathing
- ↓ efficiency of gas exchange
- ↑ susceptibility to respiratory infections

Risk Factors
- Tobacco smoking
- Environmental pollutants
- Occupational exposure to respiratory toxins

Nursing Interventions
- Teaching about smoking cessation
- Teaching about flu and pneumonia immunizations
- Teaching about preventing respiratory infections

Wellness Outcomes
- Improved respiratory function
- Decreased risk of respiratory infection
- Improved health from quitting smoking

that affects these structures is calcification of the cartilage, which causes the trachea to stiffen. Another is blunting of the cough and laryngeal reflexes, with a concomitant decrease in coughing in older adults. Age-related reductions in the number of laryngeal nerve endings also have been noted, and these may contribute to diminished efficiency of the gag reflex.

Chest Wall and Musculoskeletal Structures

The chest wall and lungs function like a bellows, with the chest expanding outward in relation to lung expansion. The rib cage and the vertebral musculoskeletal structures are affected by the same kind of age-related changes that affect other musculoskeletal tissue: the ribs and vertebrae become osteoporotic, the costal cartilage calcifies, and the respiratory muscles weaken. Because of these age-related processes, the following structural changes, which can affect respiratory performance, occur: **kyphosis** (i.e., an increased curvature of the spine), shortened thorax, chest wall stiffness, and increased anteroposterior diameter of the chest. As a result of these changes, older adults experience diminished respiratory efficiency and reduced maximal inspiratory and expiratory force. Because older adults compensate for age-related changes by increased use of the diaphragm and other accessory muscles, they are more sensitive to any changes in intra-abdominal pressure. In summary, older adults expend more energy to achieve the same respiratory efficiency as younger adults, but the overall effects on healthy older people are minimal.

Lung Structure and Function

Even in healthy older adults, lungs become smaller and flabbier, and their weight diminishes by approximately 20%. The age-related changes that have the most significant functional consequences are those that occur in the **lung parenchyma**, which is the part of the respiratory system where gas exchange takes place. The affected structures include the terminal bronchioles, alveolar ducts, alveoli, and capillaries. Beginning at around the age of 20 or 30 years, the alveoli progressively enlarge and their walls become thinner. This process of **ductectasia** continues throughout adulthood, causing approximately a 4% loss of alveolar surface area per decade. Because of this loss of alveolar surface, the amount of anatomic dead space increases. Age-related changes cause the pulmonary artery to become wider in diameter with thicker and less extensible walls. The number of capillaries also diminishes, and pulmonary capillary blood volume decreases. Finally, the mucosal bed, where diffusion occurs, thickens.

Elastic recoil is the characteristic that keeps the airway open during inspiration by resisting expansion and maintaining a positive pressure across the lung surface. During expiration, elastic recoil keeps the airways open until the pressure placed on them by the respiratory muscles forces them to collapse. If the airways close prematurely, air is trapped and the lungs cannot expire to their maximum capacity. A combination of age-related changes in the parenchyma and elastic fibers interferes with elastic recoil, which results in early airway closure. This mechanism is responsible for age-related changes in lung volumes and air flow rates.

Specific aspects of lung function, such as air volumes and airflow rates, are measured by pulmonary function tests. In older adults, air volumes are altered because of the age-related changes in the chest wall and in lung elastic recoil. Because various air volumes are interrelated, however, the total lung capacity remains essentially the same because of compensatory mechanisms. Airflow rates are affected to a small degree by age-related changes and to a greater degree by additional variables, such as height, sex, and air volumes. Overall, there is an age-related decline in all airflow rates, but because of the many interacting variables, there is a wide range of normal levels. Table 21-1 summarizes the age-related changes of some lung function parameters.

Because gas exchange is the primary function of the respiratory system, it is the most important functional aspect to consider. Oxygen–carbon dioxide exchange depends on a close match between ventilation (i.e., the amount of air in the lungs) and perfusion (i.e., the amount of blood flowing into the lungs). Because of age-related changes, particularly early airway closure, gas exchange is more likely to be compromised in the lower, rather than the upper, lung regions. Consequently, inspired air is preferentially distributed in the upper regions, and a ventilation-to-perfusion mismatch results. The result of this mismatch is a gradual decrease in arterial oxygen pressure (PaO_2) of approximately 4 mm Hg per decade.

Compensatory changes in respiratory rate are made under conditions of hypercapnia (too much carbon dioxide) or hypoxia (too little oxygen). The response mechanism varies, depending on the stimulus. The response to hypercapnia is initiated by a central chemoreceptor, located in the medulla, whereas the response to hypoxia is initiated by peripheral chemoreceptors, located in the carotid and aortic bodies. When these mechanisms operate efficiently, the respiratory rate and depth increase in response to either low levels of oxygen or high levels of carbon dioxide. Age-related changes cause a 40% to 50% reduction in the ventilatory response to both hypoxia and hypercapnia between the third and eighth decades. Thus, instead of experiencing breathlessness or other

TABLE 21-1 Age-Related Changes in Indicators of Lung Function		
Indicator	**Definition**	**Age-Related Change**
Tidal volume	Amount of air moved in and out during a normal breath	Slight decrease
Residual volume	Amount of air left in the lungs after a forced expiration	Increases by 5%–10% per decade
Forced expiratory volume	Amount of air expelled within 1 second after a maximum inspiration	Decreases 23–32 mL/year in men, 19–26 mL/year in women
Forced inspiratory volume	Maximum volume of air that can be inhaled in addition to tidal volume	Decreases
Forced vital capacity	Maximum volume of air that can be expelled following a maximum inspiration	Decreases 14–30 mL/year in men, 14–24 mL/year in women
Total lung capacity	Amount of air that can be held in the lungs after a maximum inspiratory effort	Unchanged, as a result of compensatory mechanisms
Diffusing capacity	Ability of lungs to transfer gases between the lungs and blood	Declines 2.03 mL/min/mm Hg per decade in men and 1.47 mL/min/mm Hg in women
Arterial oxygen pressure (PaO_2)	Amount of oxygen in arteries	Declines 0.3% per year or 4 mm Hg per decade but remains stable after the age of 75

respiratory symptoms when blood gases are abnormal, older adults are likely to develop mental changes.

RISK FACTORS THAT AFFECT RESPIRATORY WELLNESS

For people of any age, tobacco smoking is the single most important risk factor for lung disease and impaired respiratory function. These risks are both immediate and cumulative. Other risks are mentioned because, particularly for nonsmokers, they can be addressed through health promotion interventions to improve respiratory function. For smokers, however, these other risks are of minimal importance, and attention must be focused on the serious negative consequences of smoking.

Tobacco Use

Tobacco smoking causes detrimental effects through heat and chemical actions on the respiratory system. Burning cigarettes release toxic gases, including carbon monoxide, hydrogen cyanide, and nitrogen dioxide. In addition, burning cigarettes release tobacco tar, which contains nicotine and many other harmful chemicals. Some of the harmful physiologic effects on the respiratory system are bronchoconstriction; early airway closure; inflammation of the mucosa throughout the respiratory tract; and inhibited ciliary action, which leads to increased coughing and mucous secretions and diminished protection from harmful organisms.

> **DIVERSITY NOTE**
>
> Studies suggest that men and women are genetically predisposed to respond differently to tobacco smoke, with men being more likely to develop emphysema-like manifestations and women experiencing more airway affectation (Carrasco-Garrido et al., 2009).

Age-related changes and the cumulative effects of cigarette smoking compound the risks for older adults. Even in otherwise healthy people, smokers have a doubled or tripled rate of decline, compared with nonsmokers, in the forced expiratory volume at 1 second (FEV_1). This reduced FEV_1 is an accelerated and exacerbated age-related change that increases the risk for diseases, such as **chronic obstructive pulmonary disease (COPD)**.

In addition to being associated with detrimental effects on lung functioning, tobacco smoking is strongly associated with increased risk for cancers and other serious diseases of the lungs, cardiovascular system, and many other systems. The following research-based findings substantiate a strong link between tobacco use and disease and mortality in the United States (American Cancer Society, 2008a; American Lung Association, 2008a; Centers for Disease Control and Prevention, 2008a; Shafey, Eriksen, Ross, & Mackay, 2009):

- Tobacco use is associated with at least 15 types of cancers, including lung, stomach, kidney, bladder, pancreas, uterine cervix, and oral cavity.
- Tobacco use accounts for at least 80% of deaths from COPD, 30% of all cancer deaths, and for nearly 20% of deaths from all causes.
- Lung cancer death rate is more than 23 and 13 times higher for current male and female smokers, respectively, than in people who never smoked.
- For smokers aged 65 and older, the risk of dying from a heart attach is 60% higher than for nonsmokers.
- Compared with their nonsmoking counterparts, men and women smokers aged 65 and older are 2 times (men) and 1.5 times (women) as likely to die from a stroke.
- Compared with nonsmokers, cigarette smokers have a far greater chance of developing Alzheimer's disease and other dementias.
- The risk for developing cataracts is two to three times higher in smokers.
- There is strong evidence that smoking cessation even late in life not only adds years to life but also improves quality of life.

> **DIVERSITY NOTE**
>
> Prevalence of cigarette smoking among various groups in the United States is highest for Native Americans/Alaska Natives (37%) and whites (28%), and higher for total of U.S. men (30%) than of women (24%) (Caraballo, Yee, Gfroerer, & Mirza, 2008).

Although pipes and cigars are sometimes viewed as safer than cigarettes, studies indicate that all forms of tobacco are lethal and addictive and have serious health consequences (Shafey et al., 2009). A single large cigar can contain as much tobacco as an entire pack of cigarettes, and although the risk of disease is related to level of inhalation, the only safe option is not smoking cigars at all (American Lung Association, 2008b). Pipe smoking has been associated with an increased risk of death from COPD; cerebrovascular disease; coronary artery disease; and cancers of the lung, larynx, oropharynx, esophagus, colorectum, and pancreas.

Smokeless tobacco (also called nonsmoking tobacco) includes tobacco products that are consumed orally or nasally, without burning or combustion (e.g., snuff, chewing tobacco). These products are associated with increased risk for stroke, cardiovascular disease, periodontal disease, and some cancers (e.g., pancreas).

Another potentially detrimental health effect related to smoking that nurses need to recognize is the potential for altering the effects of medications. Interactions can occur in people who smoke or use nicotine products (including smokeless tobacco) and in people who have recently quit smoking. Interactions can be due directly to the physiologic effects of nicotine or they may be caused by the hydrocarbons in tobacco smoke, which can affect hepatic metabolism of some medications. Additional information and examples of drug–nicotine interactions are discussed in Chapter 8.

Secondhand Smoke and Other Environmental Factors

Secondhand smoke (also called passive smoke or environmental tobacco smoke) is a mixture of smoke that comes primarily from the end of lighted cigarettes, cigars, or pipes (called *sidestream smoke*) and secondarily from smoke that is exhaled by the smoker (called *mainstream smoke*). The Environmental Protection Agency classifies secondhand smoke as a carcinogen because it contains hundreds of carcinogenic chemical compounds.

The terms ***involuntary smoking*** and *passive smoking* refer to the involuntary exposure and breathing in of secondhand smoke. Although negative effects of secondhand smoke were viewed with skepticism when they were first reported in the 1972 Surgeon General's Report, increasing evidence indicates that there is no safe level of exposure to secondhand smoke. The following evidence-based statistics substantiate strong links between secondhand smoke and disease and mortality for adults (American Cancer Society, 2008b; American Lung Association, 2008c; Llewellyn, Lang, Naughton, & Matthews, 2009; Shafey et al., 2009):

- Even brief exposure to secondhand smoke can cause immediate cardiovascular and respiratory damage.
- There is sufficient evidence that nonsmokers exposed to secondhand smoke at home or work increase their risk for lung cancer and coronary artery disease risk by at least 20% to 30%.
- There is suggestive evidence that secondhand smoke increases the risk for stroke, atherosclerosis, breast cancer, nasal sinus cancer, COPD, asthma, chronic respiratory symptoms, and impaired lung function.
- A longitudinal study found that nonsmoking subjects with high salivary cotinine levels from secondhand smoke had increased odds of cognitive impairment.

Another environmental risk factor that can lead to negative functional consequences is the inhalation of air pollutants. Like the effects of cigarette smoking, the effects of air pollution are cumulative over many years and, therefore, have an increased impact on older adults who have been exposed to air pollutants for as many as eight or nine decades.

In addition to being exposed to general air pollutants, older adults who worked in occupations such as mining and firefighting might experience the cumulative and long-term effects of occupational exposure to toxic substances. Because hazards in the workplace were largely unregulated before the

 Box 21-1 Workforces With an Increased Risk for Harmful Respiratory Effects

Firefighters
Miners
Traffic controllers
Shipyard workers
Rubber workers
Aluminum workers
Iron and steel foundry workers
Tunnel and street repair workers
Asbestos workers
Quarry workers
Farmers, agricultural workers, grain handlers
Construction workers
Paper mill workers
Workers exposed to the following: dust, fumes, gases, nickel, arsenic, beryllium, chromium, or radiation

1970s, many older people never benefited from the protections enforced under the Occupational Safety and Health Act. In addition, much of the information now available on the harmful effects of certain chemicals was not widely available when these older adults were working. Even though the exposure to harmful substances may have occurred long ago, the signs and symptoms may not manifest until later adulthood. Box 21-1 lists some job categories that are associated with an increased risk of respiratory disease.

The level of humidity is another environmental condition that can affect respiratory function. For example, dry air can affect the upper airway by further drying the nasal secretions, causing them to be thicker and more difficult to remove. Environmental humidity does not have serious detrimental effects, but it should be considered as a condition that affects overall respiratory wellness.

Additional Risk Factors for Compromised Respiratory Function

A characteristic of respiratory function is that the maximum level reached in the middle and later adulthood is significantly influenced by factors that affected respiratory development in early life. Because respiratory complaints develop when pulmonary function is reduced to half of the maximally attained level, older adults whose peak level was higher during early adulthood can tolerate a greater degree of age-related changes and exposure to risk factors before experiencing respiratory dysfunction. Conversely, older adults who did not attain a high peak level during their 20s will experience the effects of age-related changes and risk factors at an earlier age.

In addition to the age-related changes that involve the respiratory system, age-related changes affecting other systems can also affect respiratory performance. For example, diminished immune response contributes to the increased morbidity and mortality for older adults who have pneumonia and other lower respiratory infections. Conditions that interfere with chest wall expansion also increase the risk for impaired respiratory function. Both kyphosis, which is caused by age-related skeletal changes, and poor posture can interfere with maximum respiratory performance. Other conditions that exacerbate the effects of age-related changes to compromise respiratory function include shallow breathing, activity restrictions, and a recumbent position. Therefore, any older adult who is on bed rest, even for short periods, is at increased risk for impaired respiratory function.

Obesity is another health-related risk factor that can interfere with respiratory function because weight gain and loss are associated with a decline or improvement in lung function. In addition, obesity usually has a negative effect on an individual's overall activity level and this can interfere with optimal respiratory function.

Medications increase the risk for impaired respiratory function in several ways. For example, sedatives and anticholinergic medications can affect upper airway function by drying the mucus. Medications may also influence cough reflexes. Angiotensin-converting enzyme inhibitors, for example, can cause a persistent dry cough.

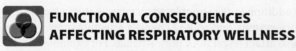

FUNCTIONAL CONSEQUENCES AFFECTING RESPIRATORY WELLNESS

In the absence of smoking and other risk factors, healthy older adults do not experience any significant functional consequences related to respiratory function when performing ordinary activities. Under conditions of physical stress, however, older adults may experience dyspnea and fatigue because their respiratory system is less efficient in gas exchange. Similarly, age-related changes in the respiratory system do not affect exercise capacity, but deconditioning and risk factors can compromise it. Table 21-2 summarizes the functional consequences of age-related changes that affect respiratory wellness. Older adults who smoke or have other risk factors experience the same negative consequences as younger adults, but the effects are cumulative and the consequences are likely to be more serious.

The combination of age-related changes in respiratory function and age-related changes in immunity contributes to an increased risk of acquiring pneumonia and influenza in older adulthood. Older adults are also likely to have multiple risk factors, such as frailty, diminished functional status, or serious illnesses, that further compromise their body's ability to defend against respiratory infections. Studies have identified the following conditions that increase the risk for pneumonia: malnutrition, tobacco use, lung disease, neurologic disease, sedative medications, congestive heart failure, and residence in a long-term care facility (Caterino, 2008).

Aspiration pneumonia is a common and serious respiratory condition in long-term care residents and in older adults with compromised functional status. Factors that increase the risk for aspiration pneumonia include dysphagia, achlorhydria, general debility, tube feeding, malnutrition and dehydration, poor oral hygiene, decreased cough reflex, diminished salivary flow, compromised immune function, and diminished level of consciousness.

In recent years, studies have found an increase in hospitalization admissions for pneumonia in the United States and several European countries (Trotter, Stuart, George, & Miller, 2008). Moreover, there is an age-associated increased risk of complications, including death, from pneumonia and influenza.

TABLE 21-2 Functional Consequences of Age-Related Changes Affecting Respiratory Function

Change	Consequence
Upper airway changes: calcification of cartilage, altered neuromuscular function and reflexes	Snoring, mouth breathing, diminished cough reflex, decreased efficiency of gag reflex
Increased anteroposterior diameter, chest wall stiffness, weakened muscles and diaphragm	Increased use of accessory muscles, increased energy expended for respiratory efficiency
Enlargement of alveoli, thinning of alveolar walls, diminished number of capillaries	Diminished efficiency of gas exchange, decreased arterial oxygen pressure (PaO_2)
Decreased elastic recoil and early airway closure	Changes in lung volumes, slight decrease in overall efficiency
Tidal volume unchanged or slightly diminished, increased residual volume, decreased vital capacity	Total lung capacity unchanged

For example, the death rate from influenza and pneumonia is nearly 130 times higher among people aged 85 and older than among those between ages 45 and 54 (Gorina, Kelly, Lubitz, & Hines, 2008). The higher morbidity and mortality is due in part to the difficulty of diagnosing lower respiratory infections during early stages because the manifestations are subtle and nonspecific (see the section on Nursing Assessment of Respiratory Function).

In addition to being increasingly susceptible to pneumonia and influenza, older adults are susceptible to tuberculosis, particularly as a reactivation of dormant tuberculosis. Risk factors for tuberculosis in older adults include smoking, diabetes, malnutrition, debilitating conditions, or long-term use of corticosteroids. In recent years, the incidence of tuberculosis has been decreasing, but rates remain high for foreign-born people and racial/ethnic minorities. There is wide geographic variation in tuberculosis rates, with four states—California, Florida, New York, Texas—accounting for 49.2% of reported cases in 2008 (Centers for Disease Control and Prevention (CDC), 2009). A higher incidence of tuberculosis in long-term care residents is associated with many risk factors, including the ease with which this disease can spread. Moreover, altered and more subtle disease manifestations interfere with identification and treatment of tuberculosis in older adults.

PATHOLOGIC CONDITION AFFECTING RESPIRATORY FUNCTION: COPD

COPD is a group of diseases, including emphysema, chronic bronchitis, and a subset of asthma, characterized by chronic airflow obstruction that interferes with normal breathing. In addition to tobacco smoking as the primary risk factor, conditions that increase the risk for developing COPD include genetic predisposition, low socioeconomic status, exposure to secondary smoke and other air pollutants, and history of significant childhood respiratory disease.

The most common manifestations of COPD are cough, dyspnea, wheezing, and increased sputum production. The condition is progressive and its cumulative effects become more disabling as the person ages. Functional consequences of COPD for older adults include longer and more frequent

hospitalizations, an increased risk for being discharged to nursing facilities, and impaired health-related quality of life. Moreover, a national survey of more than 1000 patients with COPD found an average of nine comorbid conditions (among them, hypertension, hypercholesterolemia, depression, cataracts, and osteoporosis (Barr et al., 2009). COPD is the fourth leading cause of death in America, with 80% to 90% of the deaths caused by smoking (American Lung Association, 2008d). The Evidence-Based Practice Box 21-1 summarizes recommendations for nursing assessment and care for people with dyspnea, which is called the sixth vital sign in people with COPD (Registered Nurses Association of Ontario, 2005).

NURSING ASSESSMENT OF RESPIRATORY FUNCTION

With the exception of minor differences in physical assessment of the respiratory system, nursing assessment of respiratory function is similar for younger and older adults. However, nurses must be aware of variations in the manifestations of lower respiratory infections when they occur in older adults. Another difference is that nurses assess the different life experiences of older adults with regard to exposure to environmental toxins and attitudes about tobacco use when identifying opportunities for health promotion. From a wellness perspective, nursing assessment of respiratory function focuses on identifying opportunities for health promotion, detecting lower respiratory infections, assessing smoking behaviors, and identifying other risk factors.

Identifying Opportunities for Health Promotion

Nurses interview older adults, or their caregivers, to identify the risk factors that can be addressed through health promotion activities. Because tobacco smoking is the risk factor that has serious detrimental effects on lung health as well as many other aspects of health, nurses assess the potential for influencing all smokers, even older adults, to quit. Health education is based on assessment information about health-related behaviors, such as smoking and avoidance of secondhand smoke, as well as preventive interventions, such as influenza and pneumonia vaccinations. Nurses also assess the attitudes of older adults about these preventive measures, so they can plan appropriate educational approaches. Last, nurses ask older adults about their overall respiratory function to identify respiratory problems that can be addressed in the nursing care

Evidence-Based Practice   21-1
Nursing Care of Dyspnea

Statement of the Problem

- Dyspnea is the sixth vital sign in people with chronic obstructive pulmonary disease (COPD).

Recommendations for Nursing Assessment

- Assess all the following: vital signs, pulse oximetry, lung sounds, chest wall shape and movement, accessory muscle use, productive or nonproductive cough, peripheral edema, ability to complete a full sentence, level of consciousness.
- Assess current level of dyspnea and usual breathing pattern.
- Assess for hypoxemia/hypoxia.
- Identify signs and symptoms of stable and unstable dyspnea and acute respiratory failure.
- Screen for COPD in adults older than 40 years who have a history of smoking by asking each patient these three questions: (1) Do you have progressive activity-related shortness of breath? (2) Do you have a persistent cough and sputum production? (3) Do you experience frequent respiratory tract infections?
- Advocate for spirometry testing for patients who have a history of smoking and are older than 40 years.
- If inhaler is used, assess self-administration technique.

Recommendations for Nursing Interventions

- Acknowledge and accept patient's self-report of dyspnea.
- Administer prescribed oxygen therapy, ventilation modalities, and medications (e.g., bronchodilators, corticosteroids, antibiotics, and psychotropics).
- Implement smoking cessation strategies; consider nicotine replacement and other smoking cessation modalities during hospitalization.
- Remain with patient during episodes of acute respiratory distress.

Recommendations for Teaching Older Adults and Caregivers About Dyspnea

- Prescribed medications, including correct technique for inhaler use.
- Administration of oxygen therapy if prescribed.
- Strategies for secretion clearance, energy conservation, relaxation techniques, nutrition, and breathing retraining.
- Influenza and pneumococcal vaccinations.
- Pulmonary rehabilitation and exercise training as appropriate.
- Smoking cessation strategies if appropriate.
- Disease self-management strategies, including development of action plan and decision-making regarding advanced directives.

SOURCE: Registered Nurses Association of Ontario (RNAO). *Nursing care of dyspnea: The 6th vital sign in individuals with chronic obstructive pulmonary disease.* (March 2005) Toronto, ON: RNAO.

---

plan. Box 21-2 presents an interview format that nurses can use to assess risk factors, overall respiratory function, and opportunities for health education.

✚ Wellness Opportunity

One question a nurse can ask to identify the person's health-promoting behaviors is "What do you do to avoid environmental tobacco smoke?"

Detecting Lower Respiratory Infections

The term *detection* is more accurate than *assessment* with regard to lower respiratory infections because when older adults have pneumonia, they do not always meet the typical assessment criteria. Rather than presenting with a cough, chills, dyspnea, elevated temperature, and elevated white blood cell count, older adults are more likely to have subtler and nonspecific disease manifestations. Even initial chest radiography may not provide accurate diagnostic information. A review of various studies summarized the following ranges for the occurrence of specific manifestations of pneumonia in older adults (Caterino, 2008):

- Fatigue   84%–88%
- Tachypnea   65%–68%
- Cough   63%–84%
- Dyspnea   58%–74%
- History of fever   53%–60%
- Productive sputum   30%–65%
- Tachycardia   37%–40%
- Fever by measurement   12%–32%
- Pleuritic chest pain   8%–32%
- Hemoptysis   3%–13%

This same review found that absence of usual signs and symptoms and presence of altered mental status are especially common in residents of nursing facilities (Caterino, 2008). When assessing older adults, nurses need to recognize that they may not necessarily exhibit the typical manifestations of pneumonia. The most significant finding on physical assessment of the lungs may be a diminished intensity of lung sounds or the presence of rales and rhonchi, which are very nonspecific findings. In addition, a change in mental status or another alteration in functional status, such as falls or incontinence, may be the major clue to pneumonia. Thus, an important nursing responsibility is to detect nonspecific manifestations of pneumonia and collect additional information. This is essential for ensuring a timely diagnosis and preventing complications.

In addition to being aware of the different manifestations of pneumonia in older adults, nurses also must be aware of the varied manifestations of tuberculosis in this population. As with pneumonia, diagnosis and treatment of tuberculosis in older adults are often delayed because of nonspecific assessment findings and the disease may even be overlooked. Studies found that older adults with tuberculosis had a higher frequency of nonspecific symptoms and delayed diagnosis and treatment, which contributes to a higher rate of mortality (Salvado et al., 2010). The common occurrence of false-negative tuberculin skin test reactions in older adults is another reason that tuberculosis may be undetected; however, the two-step Mantoux test with tuberculin purified protein

Box 21-2 Guidelines for Assessing Respiratory Function

Questions to Identify Risk Factors for Respiratory Problems
- Have you had any respiratory problems, such as asthma, chronic lung disease, pneumonia, or other infections?
- Do you have a family history of chronic lung disease?
- Have you ever had tuberculosis?
- Have you ever worked in a job where you were exposed to dust, fumes, smoke, or other air pollutants (e.g., in mining, farming, or any of the occupations listed in Box 21-1)?
- Have you lived in neighborhoods where there was a lot of pollution from traffic or factories?
- Do you smoke now, or have you ever smoked? (If yes, continue with the questions in Box 21-3.)
- Have you been exposed to passive smoke in home, work, or social environments?

Questions to Identify Opportunities for Education About Disease Prevention and Health Promotion
- Have you ever had a pneumonia vaccination? *If yes*, when was the vaccination administered and was a booster ever given?
- Do you get annual influenza vaccinations?

Questions to Assess Overall Respiratory Function
- Do you have any problems with breathing?
- Do you have any wheezing?

- Do you have spells of coughing? *If yes*, When do they occur? How long do they last? What brings them on? Are they dry or productive? Does the phlegm come from your throat or lungs? What does the phlegm look like?
- Do you ever have trouble getting enough air during any particular activities or when you lie down at night?
- Have you stopped doing any particular activities because of problems breathing? For example, have you stopped going up or downstairs, or have you limited the amount of walking you do? (For people with mobility limitations, this question might not be relevant.)
- Do you ever have any chest pain or feelings of heaviness or tightness in your chest?
- Do you use more than one pillow at night, or make any other adjustments, because of trouble with breathing?
- Do you wake up at night because of coughing or difficulty with breathing?
- Do you ever feel as though you can't catch your breath?
- Do you have trouble breathing when the weather is hot, cold, or humid?
- Do you tire easily?

---

derivative (PPD) is the recommended method of assessing for previous exposure to tuberculosis. Because tuberculosis often occurs as a reactivation of dormant disease, nurses must be particularly alert for manifestations of this disease in older adults who have a history of tuberculosis.

Assessing Smoking Behaviors

Although smoking affects all people, regardless of age, some aspects of smoking behaviors differ according to age cohorts. Therefore, an assessment of smoking as a risk factor must address the age-related factors that affect these behaviors. The cohort of people born between 1910 and 1930, for example, is the first age group to be exposed to the social pressures that encouraged smoking without knowing about its detrimental effects. As a result, people who began smoking in the early 1920s, when it became a popular habit for men in the United States, may have smoked for four or five decades before finding out that smoking is harmful. For women in the United States, smoking was not socially acceptable until the mid-1940s. Thus, today's generation of older adults had smoking rates among the highest in American history, with 75% of adult males being current or former smokers in 1960 (American Lung Association, 2008a). Today, the percentage of older adults who smoke (10%) is lower than the rate for other age groups, but older smokers may have an outlook reflected in statements such as, "If I've smoked this long and am still alive, why should I quit now?"

In addition to assessing attitudes about smoking, nurses should assess past and present smoking patterns. Frequency of smoking and type of tobacco smoked are important determinants of the relative risk of smoking. Smokeless tobacco, for example, is not as detrimental to respiratory and cardio-

vascular function as cigarette smoking, but it increases the risk for oral cancer and other types of cancer. Cigarettes vary in the amount of nicotine they contain, and this variable influences the degree of risk associated with a particular type of cigarette. In contrast to younger adults, who began smoking when cigarettes had filters and were lower in nicotine, older adults began smoking when cigarettes had no filters and contained greater amounts of tar and nicotine. Older adults, therefore, are likely to smoke cigarettes that have higher and more harmful nicotine levels. Some older adults, in fact, may still roll their own cigarettes using loose tobacco.

For older adults who smoke, nurses ask questions to determine their readiness to consider quitting smoking as well as their knowledge about the health effects of smoking. This is important because older adult smokers may falsely believe that there are no health benefits to quitting, so they are likely to respond positively to health education about smoking cessation (American Lung Association, 2008a).

Nurses also assess the older adult's perception of smoking as a manifestation of his or her rights and autonomy. For example, nursing home residents may view smoking as the one remaining indicator of their former life and the one pleasurable activity that they can control. As with other health care decisions, adults are entitled to make decisions about their health-related behaviors, but these decisions should be based on full knowledge of the benefits and risks of their choices.

Nurses may need to examine their own attitudes about smoking, especially in relation to older adults. For example, it is important to identify ageist influences that can lead to the view that smoking cessation would not be beneficial for older adults. Similarly, although it is important to respect the rights

Box 21-3 Guidelines for Nursing Assessment of Older Adults Who Smoke

Questions to Assess Smoking Behaviors
- How long have you smoked?
- How much do you smoke?
- What do you smoke?
- Have you smoked other types of tobacco in the past?

Questions to Assess Knowledge of the Risk From Smoking
- Do you think there are any harmful effects of smoking for people in general?
- Do you think you are at risk for any harmful effects from smoking?
- Do you think there are any benefits to quitting smoking?

Questions to Assess Attitudes Toward Smoking
- Have you ever thought about quitting smoking?
- Has any health professional ever talked to you about quitting smoking?
- What do you think about the idea of quitting smoking?
- Have you ever tried to quit? *If yes,* What was your experience with the attempt?
- Would you be interested in finding out information about quitting smoking now?

of older adults who choose to smoke, health care professionals should not exclude older adults from health promotion interventions about smoking simply because they are old. Assessment questions designed to help determine smoking habits and attitudes about smoking are included in Box 21-3.

Wellness Opportunity

To assess smoking behaviors from a whole-person perspective, nurses need to ask questions about the older adults' knowledge of the detrimental effects of smoking as well as their perception of smoking as an expression of autonomy.

Identifying Other Risk Factors

In addition to assessing tobacco use as a risk factor, nurses identify other factors that affect respiratory function in less significant ways. Because maximum respiratory function is attained by early adulthood, nurses assess factors that may have influenced respiratory development in early life. For example, questions about nutrition, respiratory infections, and exposure to cigarette smoke may provide information about the person's vulnerability to the effects of age-related changes and risk factors. For this reason, nurses incorporate questions about exposure to environmental tobacco smoke and harmful air pollutants in their assessments.

Occupational exposure to certain harmful substances is particularly important for smokers because the risk of either one of these factors is compounded when the other factor is present. Nurses also assess the person's level of activity and identify factors that interfere with mobility or routine activities because these conditions can influence the degree to which the person can improve his or her level of activity. If,

for example, people have limited mobility because of arthritis, they may not be able to engage in vigorous physical exercise, but they might benefit greatly from water exercises. Box 21-2 summarizes guidelines for assessing respiratory function in older adults.

Wellness Opportunity

To set the stage for health education about preventive measures, nurses assess the older adult's understanding of influenza and pneumonia vaccinations.

Physical Assessment Findings

Nurses use the usual methods of inspection, palpation, percussion, and auscultation to evaluate respiratory performance in both younger and older adults. Minor differences in assessment findings for healthy older adults include

- Slight increase in the normal respiratory rate, which ranges from 16 to 24 respirations per minute
- Increased anteroposterior diameter
- Forward-leaning posture because of kyphosis
- Increased resonance on percussion
- Diminished intensity of lung sounds
- Increased presence of adventitious sounds in the lower lungs.

Nurses begin the assessment of respiratory function by observing the person's breathing pattern when he or she is walking, changing position, or even sitting. Asking the older adult to sit upright, cough before auscultation, and breathe as deeply as possible with his or her mouth open will facilitate auscultation of breath sounds. When nurses have an opportunity to observe respirations in a sleeping older adult, they may see frequent but brief periods of apnea. This phenomenon is common in older adults and is highly associated with sleep problems, as discussed in Chapter 24, Sleep and Rest. With the exceptions of pneumonia and tuberculosis, the manifestations of most respiratory diseases, such as influenza and COPD, do not differ in older and younger adults.

*M*r. R. is 70 years old and comes with his wife to the senior center where you provide weekly nursing services. Both Mr. and Mrs. R. smoke one to two packs of cigarettes a day. Mr. R. has mild COPD and Mrs. R. has hypertension and coronary artery disease. Every October, the senior center offers flu shots for anyone older than 65 years. As you are preparing to give flu shots, Mr. and Mrs. R. come to you and ask, "Is this the shot that takes care of pneumonia? Our daughter said we should get a pneumonia shot every year, but we don't want a flu shot because our friend says she got the flu from one of those shots and she'll never get a shot again. Can you just give us the pneumonia shot today? We got one from the doctor last year but it's too expensive to get it from him."

THINKING POINTS

- What myths and misunderstandings do Mr. and Mrs. R. express?
- What further assessment questions would you ask?
- What health promotion teaching would you do?

NURSING DIAGNOSIS

The nursing diagnosis of Ineffective Breathing Pattern would be applicable when the nursing assessment identifies factors that may impair the older adult's respiratory function. This diagnosis is defined as "inspiration and/or expiration that does not provide adequate ventilation (NANDA International, 2009). Defining characteristics include bradypnea, dyspnea, orthopnea, tachypnea, altered chest excursion, use of accessory muscles to breathe, and alterations in depth of breathing. If impaired respiratory function interferes with activities of daily living, a nursing diagnosis of Activity Intolerance might be appropriate. Debilitated or chronically ill older adults who live in group settings may be at risk for infections, particularly pneumonia, influenza, and tuberculosis. For example, if a long-term care resident has active tuberculosis, the nursing staff might address the nursing diagnosis of Risk for Infection Transmission for the affected resident and the nursing diagnosis of Risk for Infection for all other residents. Likewise, when influenza affects one or more residents or staff of a long-term care or group living facility, the same nursing diagnoses may be applicable. Ineffective Health Maintenance is a nursing diagnosis that may be used for older adults who have insufficient knowledge about the detrimental effects of active or passive smoking.

Wellness Opportunity

When nurses provide pneumonia or influenza immunizations for older adults, they can use the wellness nursing diagnosis of Readiness for Enhanced Immunization Status.

PLANNING FOR WELLNESS OUTCOMES

When caring for older adults with respiratory problems, nurses identify wellness outcomes as an essential part of the planning process. Nurses can use the following Nursing Outcomes Classification (NOC) terminologies in care plans that address the nursing diagnosis of Ineffective Breathing Pattern: Vital Signs, Respiratory Status: Airway Patency, and Respiratory Status: Ventilation.

For most older adults who have adequate respiratory function, nurses plan for wellness outcomes by addressing their increased vulnerability to pneumonia, influenza, and tuber-

culosis. NOC terminologies pertinent to the nursing diagnosis of Risk for Infection include Immune Status, Immunization Behavior, and Community Risk Control: Communicable Disease.

An appropriate wellness outcome for older adults who lack knowledge about preventing respiratory infections would be Knowledge: Health Behaviors. A specific and easily measured outcome of successful health education might be that older adults obtain immunizations against pneumonia and influenza.

Wellness Opportunity

Nurses promote wellness when their care plans address the immunization status of older adults.

Because tobacco smoking is the most important factor that influences respiratory function, nurses working with older adults who smoke should always consider the possibility of identifying and working toward a goal of reducing or eliminating tobacco use. Thus, for older adults who smoke, NOCs include Risk Control: Tobacco Use and Knowledge: Substance Use Control.

NURSING INTERVENTIONS FOR RESPIRATORY WELLNESS

For all older adults, nursing interventions to promote respiratory wellness focus on protection from secondhand smoke and prevention of respiratory infections. For those who smoke, teaching about smoking cessation is the most important intervention for respiratory wellness. The following Nursing Interventions Classification (NIC) terminologies might be applicable in care plans to promote respiratory wellness: Environmental Risk Protection, Health Education, Immunization/Vaccination Management, Infection Control, Infection Protection, Referral, and Smoking Cessation Assistance.

Promoting Respiratory Wellness

Smoking is the single most important preventable cause of disease and death in the United States and therefore should be a major target of disease prevention activities for all people who smoke tobacco. Because older smokers are likely to have smoking-related functional consequences, smoking cessation will address secondary or tertiary prevention rather than primary prevention. Smoking cessation is widely recognized as a cost-effective health promotion activity that health care professionals should routinely address (United States Preventive Services Task Force, 2009).

For all older adults, disease prevention and health promotion interventions related to respiratory function include pneumonia and influenza vaccinations and education about the importance of avoiding environmental tobacco smoke. These interventions are discussed in the following sections and

Box 21-4 Health Promotion Teaching About Respiratory Problems

Factors That Increase the Risk for Pneumonia and Influenza
- Diabetes or any chronic lung, heart, or kidney disease
- Hospitalization within the past year for heart or lung diseases
- Severe anemia or a debilitating condition
- Confinement to bed or very limited mobility
- Residence in a nursing home or other group living setting
- Immunosuppressive medications

Preventing Respiratory Infection
- Wash your hands frequently with an antibacterial soap or hand sanitizer.
- Avoid hand-to-mouth and hand-to-eye contact.
- Avoid inhaling air that has been contaminated with particles from the cough or sneeze of someone with an infection.
- Avoid crowds during the flu season.
- Be sure that influenza and pneumonia vaccinations are up to date.

Information About Influenza Vaccinations
- New vaccinations are developed every year, based on information about the strains of viruses that are most likely to affect people during the influenza season.
- Vaccines are made from inactivated viruses and, therefore, should have few or no side effects.
- People who are allergic to eggs and egg products should NOT receive influenza immunizations.
- Immunizations do not offer immediate protection because there is a 2- to 3-week delay in developing an antibody response.
- Every year, the manufacturers of the influenza vaccination provide recommendations as to the best time for administering the immunizations for optimal effectiveness. The best time is during the late fall, but the exact time period will vary slightly from year to year.
- Vaccines are not 100% effective, but they are helpful for most older people.
- Influenza immunizations provide protection against the most serious viruses but not against all types of respiratory infections.
- The duration of effectiveness of vaccinations may be shorter than 6 months in some older people; therefore, one vaccination might not protect the person through the entire season.
- Medicare and many other health insurance programs pay for flu shots.

Information About Pneumonia Vaccinations
- Pneumonia vaccinations are recommended for people older than 65 years of age.
- Pneumonia vaccinations were considered one-time-only immunizations, but boosters are now being recommended for older adults who received their initial immunization 5 or more years ago.
- Side effects, if they occur, are not serious and will subside within a few days.
- Common side effects include a slight fever accompanied by pain, redness, or tenderness at the injection site.
- Pneumonia vaccinations are covered by Medicare and other health insurance.

Nutritional Considerations
- Include foods high in zinc and vitamins A, B-complex, C, and E.

summarized in Boxes 21-4 and 21-5. In addition, numerous educational materials are available for use in disease prevention and health promotion interventions, and many of these are available in languages other than English.

 Wellness Opportunity

Nurses promote self-care behaviors by encouraging older adults to use patient teaching materials, which are available from such agencies as American Cancer Society; American Lung Association; Office on Smoking and Health, CDC; and the Lung Association of Canada among others.

Preventing Lower Respiratory Infections

Interventions to prevent pneumonia and influenza are particularly important because more than 85% of deaths due to these diseases were among people aged 65 and older (Gorina et al., 2008). Moreover, pneumonia and influenza are the only diseases of all the leading causes of death in older adults that can be prevented through immunizations and without major investment of time, money, and motivation. Nurses also have important roles in addressing tuberculosis, particularly for medically compromised older adults in long-term and residential care facilities. The following sections discuss the role of the nurse in preventing these types of lower respiratory infections, with emphasis on health education interventions.

The influenza and pneumococcal vaccines are safe and well tolerated in older adults, and studies indicate that these measures reduce morbidity and mortality and decrease hospitalization admission rates for respiratory infections. The CDC recommends both influenza and pneumococcal vaccinations for all people aged 65 and older. Since 1997, the CDC has recommended a one-time booster dose for all people aged 65 or older if they received an initial pneumonia vaccination 5 or more years earlier and if they were younger than 65 years at the time of initial vaccination. Pneumonia vaccinations are also recommended for older adults who are uncertain about their vaccination status.

Although the immunization rate for influenza and pneumococcal vaccinations has been increasing gradually during the past decade, fewer than two-thirds of older adults were immunized during the 2006–2007 influenza season (CDC, 2008c). Many institutional settings have standing orders for influenza and pneumonia vaccinations, and nurses play a primary role in implementing this health promotion intervention in community, residential, and institutional settings. In addition, all health care workers who care for older adults should receive annual influenza vaccinations to prevent transmission, thereby indirectly reducing mortality from influenza in the older population. Box 21-4 summarizes current information about influenza and pneumonia immunizations, along with information about risk factors for these illnesses.

Box 21-5 Health Promotion Teaching About Cigarette Smoking

Attitudes About Smoking

- Stopping smoking at any age is more beneficial than continuing to smoke.
- Many of the harmful effects of smoking are reversed once the smoker quits.
- Although some of the effects of past smoking are irreversible, all of the harmful effects of future smoking can be avoided by quitting now.
- Smoking is a major risk factor for many cancers, including those of the lung, head, stomach, kidney, and pancreas.
- Smoking is a major risk factor for lung and heart disease, including high blood pressure and heart attacks.
- Passive smoking (inhaling smoke from the air) is associated with an increased risk for many diseases.

Type of Tobacco

- The lower the tar and nicotine content of cigarettes, the less harmful the effects. Many cigarettes with lower tar and nicotine levels, however, have additional chemical additives that can be harmful.
- Pipe and cigar smokers are at a higher risk for chronic lung disease than nonsmokers, just as cigarette smokers are.
- The harmful effects of tobacco use on the mouth and upper respiratory tract are equal for all types of tobacco, including smokeless tobacco. All smokers have the same risk for developing cancer of the mouth and upper respiratory tract. Snuff, chewing tobacco, and smokeless tobacco contain nicotine and many other harmful chemicals. The only advantage of smokeless tobacco is that it does not affect other people nearby.

Approaches to Quitting

- Any reduction in present tobacco use is better than maintaining the current level. The negative effects of smoking are directly proportional to the number of cigarettes inhaled.
- Various forms of prescription and over-the-counter nicotine substitutes (e.g., gum, skin patches, and nasal sprays) are available and may be helpful, especially when used in conjunction with counseling and self-help techniques.
- Besides nicotine substitutes, some nonnicotine prescription medications and over-the-counter products may be effective as a component of a smoking cessation program.
- People who are trying to quit smoking should discuss their goals with a health care professional to identify the methods that might be most effective.
- Many self-help programs are available for support and education regarding quitting smoking.
- Information about group programs can be obtained on the Internet or by calling the local office of any of the following organizations: American Lung Association, American Heart Association, or American Cancer Society.

Nonpharmacologic Practices to Help Quit Smoking

- Exercise, music, imagery, massage, meditation, affirmations, deep breathing, stress reduction, social support, or individual or group counseling.

DIVERSITY NOTE

Estimated vaccination rates for people aged 65 and older in 2007 were 70% for non-Hispanic whites, 57% for non-Hispanic blacks, and 54% for Hispanics (CDC, 2008c).

In addition to promoting pneumonia and influenza immunizations, nurses need to promote adequate nutrition and hydration as preventive measures for all older adults. Nurses who care for long-term care residents and older adults with compromised functioning need to implement direct nursing interventions to prevent pneumonia, including aspiration pneumonia. Studies have found that good oral hygiene—including measures to prevent the accumulation of plaque on teeth and dentures—is important for reducing the risk for pneumonia (Bassim, Gibson, Ward, Paphides, & Denucci, 2008; Ishikawa, Yoneyama, Hirota, Miyake, & Miyatake, 2008). Additional nursing interventions for preventing lower respiratory infections include meticulous attention to handwashing and optimal positioning and turning of patients who have limited mobility.

Nurses working in long-term care or other group living facilities are responsible for implementing programs to detect and address tuberculosis. The CDC Web site (www.CDC.gov) provides up-to-date guidelines for screening and diagnostic methods, such as skin testing. It also provides information about interventions for residents with tuberculosis and prevention of the spread of infection among staff and residents.

Any nurse or direct-care staff member working with older adults should undergo periodic skin testing to screen for exposure to tuberculosis.

Eliminating the Risk From Smoking

Educational interventions for older smokers begin by addressing attitudes that influence self-care behaviors. For example, if an older person expresses an "I'm-too-old-to-change" attitude, the initial intervention might be to explore the older adult's understanding of his or her ability to change behavioral patterns. Even though older adults may be long-term smokers, they can successfully quit smoking at rates comparable with their younger counterparts. Nurses can apply information about psychosocial development in older adulthood to encourage older adults to consider the possibility of a behavioral change.

Another commonly expressed belief that nurses can address through health education is "It's too late to do any good." When nurses encounter this type of attitude, they can emphasize that the substantial health benefits derived from quitting smoking are both immediate and long term. Benefits from smoking cessation for people of any age include improved quality of life, decreased susceptibility to smoking-related illnesses (e.g., heart disease and cancer), and a more rapid recovery from illnesses that usually are exacerbated by smoking. Although health benefits of quitting smoking occur at any age, they vary according to the age at which people quit. For example, men and women who quit smoking at the age of 35 increase their life expectancy by 4.5 and 6.1 years, respectively, and those who quit at the age of 65 can expect an increase in life expectancy of 2.0 and 3.7 years, respectively (American Heart Association 2010).

Wellness Opportunity

Nurses support wellness in older adults by communicating that old age is not an inevitable barrier to changing health-related behaviors: It's never too late to quit.

Evidence-based guidelines emphasize the importance of health care providers initiating the topic of tobacco dependence and routinely identifying and intervening with all tobacco users—including light smokers and smokeless tobacco users—at every opportunity (U.S. Department of Health and Human Services, 2008). Additional points of these guidelines are as follows:

- Tobacco dependence is a chronic disease that may require repeated interventions; however, effective treatments can significantly increase rates of long-term abstinence.
- Individual, group, and telephone counseling methods are effective; problem solving and social support as part of treatment are especially effective counseling interventions.
- Nicotine-based medications that reliably increase long-term smoking abstinence are nicotine gum, inhaler, lozenge, patch, and nasal spray.
- Nonnicotine medications that are effective for smoking cessation are sustained-release bupropion (Wellbutrin™) and varenicline (Chantix™); however, in February 2008, the Food and Drug Administration mandated a new warning about neuropsychiatric symptoms that can occur with varenicline.
- Counseling and medication are effective for treating tobacco dependence, but the combination of these methods is more effective than either alone.

Nonpharmacologic interventions that are effective for smoking cessation include exercise, imagery, relaxation, positive self-talk, integration of rewards, and identification of habit breakers for events that trigger smoking (Wynd & Dossey, 2009). Studies have found that for hospitalized patients, advice and support from nursing staff were especially effective for increased success in smoking cessation (Zarling, Burke, Gaines, & Gauvin, 2008).

Nurses can use Box 21-5 as a guide to teaching older adults about quitting smoking. Wynd and Dossey (2009) describe a holistic model that nurses can use to implement smoking cessation care plans with clients. For information about other programs visit thePoint at http://thePoint.lww.com/Miller6e.

*M*r. R. is now 77 years old and attends the senior center with his wife three times a week for meal and social programs. During your weekly senior wellness clinic, he comes to have his blood pressure checked and says that he is thinking about quitting smoking, but that his son just quit and gained a lot of weight and had a lot of trouble sleeping. He's not sure if quitting smoking is worth the effort, especially because his son has been so miserable since he quit. Also, at his age, it probably won't do any good to quit now, he says.

THINKING POINTS

- What further questions would you ask to assess Mr. R.'s readiness to discuss quitting smoking?
- What health promotion teaching would you do?
- What would your response be if you determine that Mr. R. is not ready to consider quitting smoking?

EVALUATING EFFECTIVENESS OF NURSING INTERVENTIONS

Measuring the effectiveness of interventions for the nursing diagnosis of Ineffective Breathing Pattern is based on a reassessment of subjective indicators such as ease of breathing and objective indicators such as lung sounds and respiratory rate and rhythm. An indicator of successful health education interventions for older adults with Ineffective Breathing Pattern is that they can accurately identify factors that can be addressed to improve their respiratory function. Disease prevention interventions for the nursing diagnosis of Risk for Infection could be documented on a record of the person's history of immunizations for pneumonia and influenza. For older adults who smoke and are willing to address this risk factor, effectiveness of interventions would be measured by the person's increased knowledge about the detrimental effects of smoking and by his or her willingness to develop a plan to stop smoking. Long-term effectiveness would be evaluated by the person's successful participation in the smoking cessation program.

*M*r. R. is now 83 years old and recently moved into an assisted living complex where you are employed as the nurse. When he comes in for his flu shot, he asks you how he can get some nicotine gum because he has heard that this is a good way to cut down on cigarettes. Now that he lives in the assisted living complex, he can't smoke in the dining room, and he'd like to chew nicotine gum before and after he eats. He admits that he smokes a pack of cigarettes every day but denies having experienced any bad effects from smoking. Mr. R. sees his doctor for COPD and takes Flovent, two puffs twice a day, and Serevent, two puffs twice a day.

NURSING ASSESSMENT

You begin your nursing assessment by exploring Mr. R.'s attitudes about smoking and ascertaining his knowledge about the harmful effects of cigarette smoking. Mr. R. says he thought about quitting smoking many times but never actually tried to quit because his wife smoked even more than he did until she died a few months ago. He felt it would be too hard to quit as long as she was smoking two packs per day. He also states that he's heard a lot about passive smoking and he figured it wasn't worth trying to quit as long as he was around his wife's cigarette smoke. He states that he's been smoking for 40 years, and if he hasn't gotten lung cancer by now, he's not going to get it at his age. To comply with the rules in the assisted living facility, Mr. R. says he plans to chew nicotine gum when he can't smoke cigarettes, but he sees no reason to quit.

In assessing Mr. R.'s knowledge about the effects of cigarette smoking, you determine that he is aware of some of the harmful effects of passive smoking but has very little information about the detrimental effects of cigarette smoking. He relates that his wife died of lung cancer, but he attributes her death to a history of breast cancer, which she had 10 years before the lung cancer. Mr. R. has no knowledge about cigarette smoking as a risk factor for cardiovascular disease, nor does he realize that his hypertension poses an additional risk. Mr. R. reports that he has experienced no ill effects from cigarette smoking, but when you ask about his history of respiratory infections, he admits he had pneumonia 3 years ago. He says that he received a pneumonia shot 2 years ago, so he doesn't have to worry about getting pneumonia again, and that he has had bronchitis several times, but now that he won't be out shoveling snow, he doesn't worry about getting any lung infections either.

NURSING DIAGNOSIS

Based on the assessment findings, an appropriate nursing diagnosis would be Ineffective Health Maintenance, related to insufficient knowledge about the effects of tobacco use and self-help resources. Some of Mr. R.'s statements reflect a lack of accurate information about the harmful effects of cigarette smoking, particularly regarding risks for respiratory infections and impaired cardiovascular function. Other statements probably reflect an intellectualization of his continued smoking. Your intuition tells you that, with some education and support, he may be willing to quit smoking.

NURSING CARE PLAN FOR MR. R.

Expected Outcome	Nursing Interventions	Nursing Evaluation
Mr. R. will increase his knowledge about the harmful effects of cigarette smoking.	• Give Mr. R. brochures and illustrations provided by the Office on Smoking and Health and use them to discuss the effects of cigarette smoking. • Use brochures from the American Heart Association to discuss the risk factors for cardiovascular disease. • Discuss cigarette smoking as a risk factor for respiratory infections. • Give Mr. R. a copy of Box 21-5 and discuss the immediate and long-term benefits of quitting smoking.	• Mr. R. will verbalize correct information about the risks of cigarette smoking. • Mr. R. will describe the benefits derived from quitting smoking.
Mr. R. will be knowledgeable about techniques for quitting smoking.	• Using information from the American Lung Association, discuss some of the strategies for quitting smoking (e.g., quitting cold turkey, using nicotine substitutes, participating in self-help groups).	• Mr. R. will describe the advantages and disadvantages of the various methods of quitting smoking.
Mr. R. will quit smoking.	• Identify the method Mr. R. prefers for quitting smoking. • Emphasize the importance of nutrition, exercise, and adequate fluid intake. • Agree on realistic goals for smoking cessation. • Discuss supportive resources. Set up weekly appointments at the senior wellness clinic for support and further discussions.	• Mr. R. will report that he has stopped or significantly reduced his smoking.

(case study continues on page 450)

THINKING POINTS

- How would you assess Mr. R.'s readiness and motivation to quit smoking?
- What health education approach would you take with Mr. R.?
- What additional interventions or health education points would you use for Mr. R.?

Chapter Highlights

Age-Related Changes That Affect Respiratory Wellness
(Tables 21-1 and 21-2)
- Upper airway changes (e.g., calcification of cartilage)
- Increased anteroposterior diameter
- Chest wall stiffness, weakened muscles
- Alveoli enlarged and have thinner walls
- Alterations in lung volumes and airflow
- Decreased compensatory response to hypercapnia and hypoxia

Risks Factors That Affect Respiratory Wellness
(Box 21-1)
- Tobacco smoking
- Environmental factors (e.g., pollution, dry air, secondhand smoke)
- Occupational hazards

Functional Consequences Affecting Respiratory Wellness
- Mouth breathing, diminished cough reflex, less efficient gag reflex
- Increased use of accessory muscles, increased energy expended for breathing
- Diminished efficiency of gas exchange, decreased PaO_2 levels
- Decreased vital capacity, slight decrease in overall efficiency
- Increased susceptibility to lower respiratory infections

Pathologic Condition Affecting Respiratory Wellness: COPD
- COPD: a group of diseases, including emphysema, chronic bronchitis, and a subset of asthma, characterized by chronic airflow obstruction

Nursing Assessment of Respiratory Function
(Boxes 21-2 and 21-3)
- Overall respiratory function
- Detection of lower respiratory infections
- Tobacco use and attitudes regarding smoking

Nursing Diagnosis
- Health-Seeking Behaviors
- Ineffective Breathing Pattern
- Risk for Infection

Planning for Wellness Outcomes
- Vital Signs, Respiratory Status: Airway Patency, and Respiratory Status: Ventilation
- Immune Status, Immunization Behavior, and Community Risk Control
- Knowledge: Health Behaviors
- Risk Control: Tobacco Use and Knowledge: Substance Use Control

Nursing Interventions for Respiratory Wellness
(Boxes 21-4 and 21-5)
- Prevention and detection of pneumonia and influenza
- Health education about smoking cessation

Evaluating Effectiveness of Nursing Interventions
- Ease of breathing
- Up-to-date status for pneumonia immunization
- Influenza immunization every year
- For older adults who smoke: active participation in smoking cessation behaviors

Critical Thinking Exercises

1. What will a healthy, nonsmoking, 83-year-old person experience in his or her daily life with regard to respiratory function?
2. What would you include in a health education program, designed for older adults, on the prevention of pneumonia and influenza?
3. How would you address the following statement made by a 71-year-old person: "I've lived this long and don't have lung cancer; why should I start worrying now?"
4. Find the names, addresses, and phone numbers of local agencies that would be appropriate resources for someone interested in quitting smoking. Contact at least one of these organizations to find out specific information about support groups, written materials, and other resources.

Resources

For links to these resources and additional helpful internet resources related to this chapter, visit the Point at http://thePoint.lww.com/Miller6e.

Clinical Tools

Hartford Institute for Geriatric Nursing
- *Try This: Best Practices in Nursing Care to Older Adults* Issue 21 (2007), Immunizations for the Older Adult

Evidence-Based Practice

National Guideline Clearinghouse
- Chronic Obstructive Pulmonary Disease (COPD)
- Nursing Care of Dyspnea
- Tobacco use and dependence

Health Education

American Cancer Society
American Heart Association
American Lung Association
Lung Association of Canada
National Heart, Lung, and Blood Institute Information Center
Office on Smoking and Health, Centers for Disease Control and Prevention

REFERENCES

American Cancer Society. (2008a). *Tobacco & Cancer.* Retrieved from http://www.cancer.org/Cancer/CancerCauses/TobaccoCancer/index.

American Cancer Society. (2008b). *Secondhand smoke.* Retrieved from http://www.cancer.org/Cancer/CancerCauses/TobaccoCancer/secondhand-smoke.

American Heart Association (2010). *American Heart Association Scientific Position on Smoking Cessation.* Retrieved from http://americanheart.org.

American Lung Association. (2008a). *Smoking Among Older Adults Fact Sheet.* Retrieved from http://www.lungusa.org/stop-smoking/facts-figures/smoking-and-older-adults.html.

American Lung Association. (2008b). *Cigar Smoking Fact Sheet.* Retrieved from http://www.lungusa.org/stop-smoking/about-smoking/facts-figures/cigars.html.

American Lung Association. (2008c). *Secondhand Smoke Fact Sheet.* Retrieved from http://lungusa.org/stop-smoking/about-smoking/health-effects/secondhand-smoke.html.

American Lung Association (2008d). *Chronic Obstructive Pulmonary Disease Fact Sheet.* Retrieved from http://www.lungusa.org/lung-disease/copd/resources/facts-figures?COPD-Fact-Sheet.html.

Barr, R. G., Belli, B. R., Mannino, D. M., Petty, T., Rennard, S. I., Sciurba, F. C., . . . Turino, G. M. (2009). Comorbidities, patient knowledge, and disease management in a national sample of patients with COPD. *American Journal of Medicine, 122,* 348–355.

Bassim, C. W., Gibson, B., Ward, T., Paphides, B. M., & Denucci, D. J. (2008). Modification of the risk of mortality from pneumonia with oral hygiene. *Journal of the American Geriatrics Society, 56,* 1601–1607.

Caraballo, R. S., Yee, S. L., Gfroerer, J., & Mirza, S. A. (2008). Adult tobacco use among racial and ethnic groups living in the United States, 2002–2005. *Preventing Chronic Disease, 5*(3), 1–5.

Carrasco-Garrido, P., Miguel-Diez, J., Rejas Gutierrez, J., Martin-Centeno, A., Gobarrt-Vasquez, E., Hernandez-Barrera, V., . . . Jimenez-Garcia, R. (2009). Characteristics of chronic pulmonary disease in Spain from a gender perspective. *BMC Pulmonary Medicine, 9*(2). Retrieved from http://www.biomedcentral.com/1471-2466/9/2.

Caterino, J. M. (2008). Evaluation and management of geriatric infections in the emergency department. *Emergency Medicine Clinics of North America, 26,* 319–343.

Centers for Disease Control and Prevention (2008a). Smoking-attributable mortality, years of potential life lost, and productivity losses—United States, 2000–2004. *MMWR: Morbidity and Mortality Weekly Report, 57*(45), 1226–1228.

Centers for Disease Control and Prevention (2008b). Deaths from chronic obstructive pulmonary disease—United States, 2000–2005. *MMWR: Morbidity and Mortality Weekly Report, 57*(45), 1229–1232.

Centers for Disease Control and Prevention (2008c). Prevention and control of influenza: Recommendations of the Advisory Committee on Immunization Practices, 2008. *MMWR: Morbidity and Mortality Weekly Report, 57*(RR-7), 1–48.

Centers for Disease Control and Prevention (2009). Trends in tuberculosis: United States, 2008. *MMWR: Morbidity and Mortality Weekly Report, 58*(10), 249–253.

Gorina, Y., Kelly, T., Lubitz, J., & Hines, Z. (2008). Trends in influenza and pneumonia among older persons in the United States. *Trends in Health and Aging, 8.* Retrieved from http:/www.cdc.gov/nchs/agingact.htm.

Ishikawa, A., Yoneyama, T., Hirota, K., Miyake, Y., & Miyatake, K. (2008). Professional oral health care reduces the number of oropharyngeal bacteria. *Journal of Dental Research, 87,* 594–598.

Llewellyn, D. J., Lang, I. A., Naughton, F., & Matthews, F. E. (2009). Exposure to secondhand smoke and cognitive impairment in non-smokers: National cross sectional study with cotinine measurement. *British Medical Journal, 338,* 632–634.

NANDA International. (2009). *Nursing diagnoses: Definitions and classification 2009–2011.* Oxford, UK: Wiley-Blackwell.

Registered Nurses Association of Ontario (RNAO). (2005). Nursing care of dyspnea: The 6th vital sign in individuals with chronic obstructive pulmonary disease. Toronto, ON: Author.

Salvado, M., Garcia-Vidal, C., Vazquez, P., Riera, M., Rodriguez-Carballeira, M., . . . Garau, J. (2010). Mortality of tuberculosis in very old people. *Journal of the American Geriatrics Society, 58,* 18–22.

Shafey, O., Eriksen, M., Ross, H., & Mackay, J. (2009). *The tobacco atlas* (3rd ed). Atlanta, GA: American Cancer Society and World Lung Foundation.

Trotter, C. L., Stuart, J. M., George, R., & Miller, E. (2008). Increasing hospital admissions for pneumonia, England. *Emerging Infectious Diseases, 14*(5), 727–733.

United States Preventive Services Task Force (USPSTF). (2009). Counseling and interventions to prevent tobacco use and tobacco-caused disease in adults and pregnant women: U.S. Preventive Services Task Force reaffirmation recommendation statement. *Annals of Internal Medicine, 150*(8), 551–555.

U.S. Department of Health and Human Services, Public Health Service. (2008). *Treating tobacco use and dependence: 2008 Update.* Rockville, MD: USDHHS.

Wynd, C. A., & Dossey, B. M. (2009). Smoking cessation. In B. M. Dossey & L. Keegan (Eds.), *Holistic nursing: A handbook for practice* (5th ed., pp. 443–459). Boston, MA: Jones and Bartlett Publishers.

Zarling, K. K., Burke, M. V., Gaines, K. A., & Gauvin, T. R. (2008). Registered nurse initiation of a tobacco intervention protocol. *Journal of Cardiovascular Nursing, 23,* 443–448.

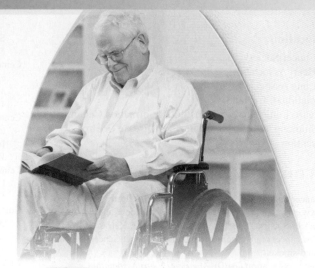

CHAPTER 22

Mobility and Safety

LEARNING OBJECTIVES

After reading this chapter, you will be able to:

1. Delineate age-related changes that affect mobility and safety.

2. Identify risk factors that increase the risk of osteoporosis and influence the safety and mobility of older adults.

3. Discuss the following functional consequences: diminished musculoskeletal function, increased susceptibility to fractures, and increased susceptibility to falls.

4. Discuss the psychosocial and long-term consequences of falls, fractures, and osteoporosis.

5. Conduct a nursing assessment of musculoskeletal performance and risks for falls and osteoporosis.

6. Identify interventions directed toward safe mobility and the elimination of risks for falls and osteoporosis.

K E Y P O I N T S

body sway	osteopenia
bone densitometry	osteoporosis
fall risk assessment	osteoporotic fracture
fear of falling	sarcopenia
osteoarthritis	tai chi

Mobility is one of the most important aspects of physiologic function because it is essential for maintaining independence and because serious consequences occur when independence is lost. For older adults, mobility is influenced by age-related changes to some extent, but risk factors play a much larger role. Because of the many risks that affect mobility, falls and fractures are an unfortunately common occurrence in old age. Older adults, then, have the dual challenge of maintaining mobility skills and avoiding falls and fractures. For these reasons, safety is an integral aspect of mobility.

 AGE-RELATED CHANGES THAT AFFECT MOBILITY AND SAFETY

The bones, joints, and muscles are the body structures most closely associated with mobility, but many additional functional aspects are involved in *safe* mobility. Neurologic function, for example, influences all facets of musculoskeletal performance, and visual function influences the ability to interact safely with the environment. In the musculoskeletal system, **osteoporosis** is the age-related change that has the most significant overall impact, has been studied the most, and is most amenable to interventions aimed at prevention and management.

Bones

Bones provide the framework for the entire musculoskeletal system and work in conjunction with the muscular system to facilitate movement. Additional functions of bone in the human body include storing calcium, producing blood cells, and supporting and protecting body organs and tissues. Bone is composed of a hard outer layer, called cortical or compact bone, and an inner, spongy meshwork, called trabecular or cancellous bone. The proportion of cortical to trabecular components varies according to bone type. Long bones, such as the radius and femur, are composed of as much as 90% cortical cells, whereas flat and vertebral bones are composed primarily of trabecular cells. Both cortical and trabecular bone components are affected by age-related changes, but the rate and impact of age-related changes differ in the two types of bone.

Bone growth reaches maturity in early adulthood, but bone remodeling continues throughout one's lifetime. The following age-related changes affect this remodeling process in all older adults:

- Increased bone resorption (i.e., breakdown of bone that is necessary for remodeling)
- Diminished calcium absorption
- Increased serum parathyroid hormone
- Impaired regulation of osteoblast activity
- Impaired bone formation secondary to reduced osteoblastic production of bone matrix

Promoting Musculoskeletal Wellness in Older Adults

Nursing Assessment
- Usual mobility patterns
- Risks for unsafe mobility
- Risks for osteoporosis
- Health behaviors
- Safety of environment

Age-Related Changes
- ↓ muscle mass
- Degenerative changes of joints
- Slower response of central nervous system
- Osteoporosis

Negative Functional Consequences
- ↓ muscle strength and endurance
- ↑ difficulty performing ADL
- ↑ risk for falls and fractures
- Fear of falling

Risk Factors
- ↓ weight-bearing activity
- ↓ calcium and vitamin D
- Tobacco smoking
- Pathologic conditions
- Adverse medication effects
- Environmental factors
- Gait changes
- ↓ sensory function

Nursing Interventions
- Teaching about exercise
- Teaching about prevention of osteoporosis
- Actions to prevent falls and fall-related injuries
- Addressing fear of falling

Wellness Outcomes
- Safer mobility
- ↓ risk for falls
- Prevention of osteoporosis
- ↓ risk for fractures
- Improved quality of life

- Fewer functional marrow cells due to replacement of marrow with fat cells
- Decreased estrogen in women and testosterone in men.

Muscles

Skeletal muscles, which are controlled by motor neurons, directly affect all activities of daily living (ADLs). Age-related changes that have the greatest impact on muscle function include

- Decreased size and number of muscle fibers
- Loss of motor neurons
- Replacement of muscle tissue by connective tissue and, eventually, by fat tissue
- Deterioration of muscle cell membranes and a subsequent escape of fluid and potassium
- Diminished protein synthesis

The overall effect of these age-related changes is a condition called **sarcopenia**, which is a loss of muscle mass, strength, and endurance.

Joints and Connective Tissue

Numerous age-related changes affect the function of all musculoskeletal joints, including non–weight-bearing joints. In contrast to the bones or muscles, which benefit from exercise, the joints are harmed by continued use and begin to show the effects of wear and tear during early adulthood. In fact, degenerative processes begin to affect the tendons, ligaments, and synovial fluid during early adulthood, even before skeletal maturity is reached.

Some of the most significant age-related joint changes include the following:

- Diminished viscosity of synovial fluid
- Degeneration of collagen and elastin cells
- Fragmentation of fibrous structures in connective tissue
- Outgrowths of cartilaginous clusters because of continuous wear and tear
- Formation of scar tissue and areas of calcification in the joint capsules and connective tissue
- Degenerative changes in the articular cartilage resulting in extensive fraying, cracking, and shredding, in addition to a pitted and thinned surface.

Consequences of these changes include impaired flexion and extension, decreased flexibility of the fibrous structures, diminished protection from forces of movement, erosion of the bones underlying the outgrowths of cartilage, and diminished ability of the connective tissue to transmit the tensile forces that act on it.

Nervous System

Maintenance of balance in an upright position is a complex skill affected by the following age-related changes of the nervous system: altered visual abilities; a decline in the righting reflex; impaired proprioception, particularly in women; and diminished vibratory sensation and joint position sense in the lower extremities. In addition, age-related changes in postural control cause an increase in **body sway**, which is a measure of the motion of the body while standing. Finally, because of the age-related slowing in reaction time, older adults walk more slowly and are less able to respond in a timely manner to environmental stimuli. Researchers have found that older adults can learn to compensate for age-related changes in the central nervous system to avoid falls (Doumas, Rapp, & Krampe, 2009).

Osteopenia and Osteoporosis

Loss of bone mass is an age-related change that affects all adults as they age. The extent to which it occurs, however, is affected by many variables, and emphasis needs to be placed on health promotion interventions that limit the extent and consequences of bone loss (Horan & Timmins, 2009). Because of the widespread availability of simple imaging techniques, called **bone densitometry**, in recent years, bone mass density is now routinely evaluated in adults beginning around their 6th decade. Bone mass density is scored according to standard deviations below that of healthy young adults, called a *T-score*. When a T-score is between 1 and 2.5 standard deviations below this range, the condition is called **osteopenia**; when a T-score is lower than this, the condition is called osteoporosis. Osteoporosis is usually asymptomatic; however, it can cause pain, loss of height, dowager's hump, and increased risk of fractures. In addition to being diagnosed according to bone densitometry scores, osteoporosis is diagnosed when a fracture occurs in the absence of trauma.

Prevalence of osteoporosis increases with age, with 6% at the age of 50 years and 50% after the age of 80 years (Rahmani & Morin, 2009). Although osteoporosis has been recognized as a common condition among postmenopausal women for many decades, only in recent decades has it been recognized as a condition that affects men too. This increase attention is warranted because one-fifth of men and one-half of women aged 50 years and older will have an osteoporotic-related fracture during their lifetime (Khosla, 2010; Rahmani & Morin, 2009).

Gender differences account for the relatively higher rate of osteoporosis among women compared with men. Both men and women reach peak bone mass in their mid-30s, but there are significant differences in patterns of bone loss between men and women. Women have a period of bone mass stability between peak level and the onset of menopause, when declining estrogen levels significantly affect bone mass. During the first decade after the onset of menopause, the annual rate of bone loss may be as great as 7%, but after menopause, it is between 1% and 2%. By contrast, the annual rate of bone loss in men is only about 1% after peak bone mass has been reached. In summary, osteoporosis occurs in both men and women, but women have a much greater percentage of bone loss over their lifetime and experience greater bone loss at an earlier age.

> **DIVERSITY NOTE**
>
> Onset of osteoporosis in men is about one decade later than for women.

 ## RISK FACTORS THAT AFFECT MOBILITY AND SAFETY

The risk factors for safe mobility that are of greatest concern are those that contribute to osteoporosis, fractures, and falls. These risks are of particular importance to nurses because health promotion interventions are appropriate for addressing many of the risk factors. In addition, eliminating or minimizing the risks is likely to prevent the serious functional consequences.

Risk Factors That Affect Overall Musculoskeletal Function

Nutritional deficits and lack of exercise are important risk factors for diminished musculoskeletal performance. Studies have found that low protein intake or the consumption of low-quality protein increases muscle loss in older adults and can lead to sarcopenia (Layman & Rodriquez, 2009). Researchers have also focused on vitamin D deficiency because this vitamin is essential for absorption of calcium and musculoskeletal health. Some studies have found that serum vitamin D levels are correlated strongly with lower extremity function in adults aged 60 years or older and this may explain why vitamin D supplementation at doses of 700 to 1000 IU daily reduces the risk for falls and nonvertebral fractures (Annweiler, Schott, Berrut, Fantino, & Beauchet, 2009; Bischoff-Ferrari et al., 2009; Giovannuci, 2009; Parikh, Avorn, & Solomon, 2009). In addition to being associated with falls and fractures, vitamin D deficiency is associated with reduced handgrip strength, reduced walking distance, less outdoor activity, inability to climb stairs, and impaired leg extension power (Vondracek & Linnebur, 2009).

> **Wellness Opportunity**
>
> Many lifestyle, environmental, and other reversible factors can be addressed for preventing falls and fractures.

Risk Factors for Osteoporosis and Osteoporotic Fractures

Low level of weight-bearing activity, cigarette smoking, excessive alcohol consumption, and inadequate intake of calcium and vitamin D are major lifestyle risk factors that are potentially modifiable. Risk factors that cannot be changed include ethnicity, advanced age, and family history of osteoporosis. Hormonal changes also affect the risk for osteoporosis, particularly with regard to estrogen in women, which has been the focus of research for many decades. In recent decades, researchers are focusing on the role of various sex hormones on the risk for osteoporosis in both men and women. For example, studies have found an association between low bone mineral density (BMD) and low levels of sex hormones in older men, but the exact role of specific hormones has not been determined (Khosla, 2010).

Certain medications and pathologic conditions also increase the risk for osteoporosis. Long-term use of oral or inhaled corticosteroids—a common treatment for asthma, rheumatoid arthritis, and chronic obstructive pulmonary disease—are the medications most frequently associated with secondary osteoporosis. Anticonvulsants, anticoagulants, and

Box 22-1 Risk Factors for Osteoporosis

Factors That Increase the Risk for Osteoporosis and Osteoporotic Fractures
- Female sex
- Age 65 or 70 years or older for women and men, respectively
- Small bones
- Family history of osteoporosis or osteoporotic fracture
- Low calcium intake, both past and current
- Inadequate vitamin D intake
- Lack of weight-bearing activity
- Hormonal deficiency
- Cigarette smoking
- Excessive alcohol intake
- Pathologic conditions (e.g., hypogonadism, hyperparathyroidism, thyrotoxicosis, malabsorption, low gastric acid, pre- or post–solid organ transplant, low gastric acid)
- Medications (e.g., corticosteroids, anticonvulsants, anticoagulants, immunosuppressants, antihormonal agents)

immunosuppressants are other types of drugs that increase the risk for osteoporosis. Recent studies found that selective serotonin reuptake inhibitors were associated with decreased BMD in men (Khosla, 2010).

In addition to identifying risks specifically for osteoporosis, researchers have focused on risks for hip fractures because this type of fracture is so strongly associated with serious and permanent negative consequences. Falls, female sex, low BMD, age 50 to 90 years, tobacco smoking, previous **osteoporotic fractures**, vitamin D deficiency, intake of more than two alcoholic drinks daily, and long-term use of glucocorticoids are major risk factors for hip fractures (Adams & Hewison, 2010; Huntijens et al., 2010; Lawrence, Wenn, Boulton, & Moran, 2010; North American Menopause Society, 2010). Additional risks identified in studies of community-dwelling older people include poor vision, unsteady gait, cognitive impairment, difficulty rising from a chair, excessive caffeine intake, and use of long-acting benzodiazepines or anticonvulsant drugs (Lash, Nicholson, Velez, Van Harrison, & McCort, 2009; Stolee, Poss, Cook, Byrne, & Hirdes, 2009).

Box 22-1 summarizes risks for development of osteoporosis and osteoporotic fractures.

Ms. M. is 55 years old and works as the secretary in the Senior Circle of Care program where you do health screening and educational programs. This program is a "senior wellness program" sponsored by one of the nonprofit hospitals in Minneapolis, Minnesota. Ms. M.'s responsibilities include finding and organizing health education materials under the direction of the nurses. You often go to lunch with her and discuss social and health-related topics.

Ms. M. has always been inquisitive about health-related concerns, and one day she asks your advice about osteoporosis. She says that both she and her mother, who is 83 years old, have been receiving flyers about getting a bone density test, and that her mother asked if she would go with her so that they could both be tested. You know from past conversations that Ms. M.'s mother fractured her wrist a long time ago, but otherwise is relatively healthy. Ms. M. is fairly healthy, although she admits that she "could stand to lose a little weight." You also know from previous discussions that Ms. M. was using hormonal replacement therapy for 3 years but stopped about 4 years ago. In your work as a wellness nurse, you have developed and presented several health education programs about osteoporosis and are fairly familiar with recent literature on osteoporosis.

THINKING POINTS

- Based on what you know about Ms. M., what would you tell her about her risk factors for osteoporosis?
- Based on what you know about Ms. M.'s mother, what additional information would you want to know before advising her about a test for her mother?
- How would you answer Ms. M.'s inquiry?
- What suggestions would you make to help Ms. M. become more knowledgeable about osteoporosis?

Risk Factors for Falls

Falling is unfortunately very common among older adults; it has been the focus of much attention in the United States and many other countries for decades. More than a half century ago, an article titled "On the Natural History of Falls in Old Age" began with the following declaration: "The liability of old people to tumble and often to injure themselves is such a commonplace of experience that it has been tacitly accepted as an inevitable aspect of ageing, and thereby deprived of the exercise of curiosity" (Sheldon, 1960, p. 1685). In recent years, geriatricians and gerontologists have challenged this view that falls are a normal consequence of aging or are accidental or random events. There is now wide agreement that falls and mobility problems result from multiple, diverse, and interacting factors. The current clinical approach is to identify the most likely causes and contributing conditions and to plan interventions to prevent falls. Current emphasis is also on prevention of fractures in people who do fall.

Risk factors for falls can be categorized according to their origin as follows: age-related changes, common pathologic conditions and functional impairments, medication effects, and environmental factors (Box 22-2). Falls are the result of a combination of these factors, rather than one isolated risk factor. Moreover, the risk of falls increases in proportion to the number of fall risk factors. One study found that people with low vision were three times more likely to fall if they were physically inactive compared with those who were active (Lamoureux et al., 2010).

The many studies of reasons for falling in older adults have identified different underlying causes in different age groups. Falls in older adults younger than 75 years are often

---

 Box 22-2 Risk Factors for Falls

Pathologic Conditions and Functional Impairments
- Age-related conditions (e.g., nocturia, osteoporosis, gait changes, postural hypotension, sensory deficits)
- Cardiovascular diseases (e.g., arrhythmias or myocardial infarction)
- Respiratory diseases (e.g., chronic obstructive pulmonary disease [COPD])
- Neurologic disorders (e.g., parkinsonism, cerebrovascular accident [CVA])
- Metabolic disturbances (e.g., dehydration, electrolyte imbalances)
- Musculoskeletal problems (e.g., osteoarthritis)
- Transient ischemic attack (TIA)
- Vision impairments (e.g., cataracts, glaucoma, macular degeneration)
- Cognitive impairments (e.g., dementia, confusion)
- Psychosocial factors (e.g., depression, anxiety, agitation)

Medication Effects and Interactions
- Antiarrhythmics
- Anticholinergics, including ingredients in over-the-counter products (e.g., diphenhydramine)

- Anticonvulsants
- Diuretics
- Benzodiazepines and other hypnotics
- Antipsychotics
- Antidepressants
- Alcohol

Environmental Factors
- Inadequate lighting
- Lack of handrails on stairs
- Slippery floors
- Throw rugs
- Cords or clutter
- Unfamiliar environments
- Highly polished floors
- Improper height of beds, chairs, or toilets
- Physical restraints, including bedrails

associated with trips and slips that are predominantly attributable to a combination of age-related changes and unfavorable environmental conditions. By contrast, falls in people older than 75 years are usually associated with a combination of disease- and medication-related factors.

Pathologic Conditions and Functional Impairment

Nocturia, osteoporosis, sleep problems, gait changes, orthostatic hypotension, decreased muscle strength, hearing and vision impairment, and central nervous system changes are common age-related conditions that can increase the risk of falls in older adults. In general, commonly occurring pathologic conditions are associated with falls in older adults in all of the following ways:

1. Pathologic conditions may be treated with medications that create risks for falling.
2. Illnesses can cause functional impairments, such as vision or mobility limitations.
3. Illnesses may cause metabolic or other physiologic disturbances that create risks for falls.
4. Falls may be one manifestation of an acute illness or a change in a chronic illness.
5. Chronic illnesses interfere with optimal exercise and other health practices that are important in promoting safe mobility.

Functional impairments, regardless of cause, also increase the risk for falls, especially in combination with other risk factors. For example, dementia and depression diminish one's awareness of the environment and can interfere with the ability to process information about environmental stimuli. Older adults with dementia have an annual incidence for falls of around 60%, which is double the rate for older adults without cognitive impairment (Kenny, Rubenstein, & Tinetti, 2010). The following combination of factors is likely to increase the risk for falls in people with dementia: medications, concurrent conditions, decreased level of awareness, diminished ability to cope with environmental surroundings, and associated functional limitations. Older adults who are depressed are at increased risk for falls secondary to gait changes, medication effects, and a diminished ability to concentrate on and respond to environmental factors. Considering all of these possible associations, it is not surprising that most falls resulting in injuries occur in people who have functional impairments and multiple, chronic medical problems.

Medication Effects

Numerous studies have identified hundreds of medications that can contribute to falls, and some studies have looked at the relationship between falls, medications, and diagnoses. Reviews of studies have concluded that diuretics, benzodiazepines, anticonvulsants, antiparkinson agents, antiarrhythmics, sedatives/hypnotics antidepressants, opioid analgesics, nonsteroidal anti-inflammatory agents, and anticholinergic medications are the types of medications that are most consistently and strongly associated with increased risk for falls (Baranzini et al., 2009; Berdot et al., 2009; Carbone et al., 2009; Hanlon et al., 2009; Hegeman, Van Den Bemt, Duysens, & van Limbeek, 2009; Petty et al., 2009; Tsunoda et al., 2010; Woolcott et al., 2009). A recent meta-analysis identified psychotropic medications (i.e., neuroleptics, sedative-hypnotics, anxiolytics, and all types of antidepressants) as the type of medication most consistently identified as a risk for falls (Kenny et al., 2010).

An approach to identifying the relationship between medications and an increased risk for falls is to consider the underlying mechanism of the medication action, as well as the pathologic condition and the potential interactions among various factors. For example, orthostatic hypotension can result from pathologic conditions, age-related changes, or adverse medication effects and can increase the risk for falls. If an 80-year-old person has a pathologic condition (e.g., hypertension) that may cause orthostatic hypotension, and if the person is taking a medication (e.g., a vasodilator) that causes orthostatic hypotension, the risk for falls significantly increases. Therefore, rather than memorizing all of the medications known to increase the risk for falls, nurses can focus their attention on the underlying mechanisms that increase the risk for falls.

The following adverse medication effects can increase the risk for falls: confusion, depression, sedation, arrhythmias, hypovolemia, orthostatic hypotension, delayed reaction time, diminished cognitive function, and changes in gait and balance (e.g., ataxia, decreased proprioception, and increased body sway). Thus, any medication that has one or more of these adverse effects may increase the risk for falls. Other considerations that influence the risk of falls include medication–disease interactions, medication–medication interactions, and medication–alcohol interactions. Also, the dose, half-life, and administration time of the medication can affect the risk for falls. For example, benzodiazepines with long half-lives (e.g., flurazepam) are strongly associated with an increased risk for falls and fall-related injuries. In recent years, zolpidem has become a widely used nonbenzodiazepine sedative-hypnotic for older people because of the high association between benzodiazepines and falls. However, studies have found that zolpidem use is associated with an increased risk of hip fracture in older adults (Rhalimi, Helou, & Jaecker, 2009).

Studies have focused primarily on prescription medications, but over-the-counter medications also can create risks for falls through their adverse effects on psychomotor function. Many over-the-counter preparations for pain, colds, and insomnia contain alcohol or anticholinergics. These ingredients may themselves pose risks or may interact with other medications to increase the risk for falls. The adverse effects of diphenhydramine, a widely used ingredient in over-the-counter products for sleep, colds, and allergies, have received much attention in the media and medical literature. Diphenhydramine has been associated with significant adverse effects on the psychomotor skills necessary for safe driving, and many states include this and other over-the-counter agents in laws pertaining to driving while impaired. Some of the types of medications that are likely to increase the risk for falls are listed in Box 22-2.

Environmental Factors

Some environmental hazards were discussed in Chapter 7, but additional environmental influences must be considered specifically in relation to falls. In institutional settings, for example, falls are most likely to occur in the bedroom and bathroom. In the bedroom, most falls occur while the person is getting in or out of bed, and some falls are related to climbing over side rails or footboards. In the bathroom, falls generally occur while transferring on or off of toilet seats or while hurrying to urinate or defecate. In community settings, most falls occur in the home, particularly in stairways, bedrooms, and living rooms. Environmental hazards that increase the risk of falls in homes include clutter, poor lighting, and lack of handrails on stairs or grab bars in bathrooms.

Physical Restraints

Physical restraints have been used since the 1960s in institutional settings with the intent of protecting impaired people from injury and reducing staff workload. Historically, the belief that using physical restraints protects vulnerable people from falls and shields the institution from liability was widespread. However, questions about using physical restraints and bedrails were first raised during the 1980s and many studies have addressed the safety and effectiveness of these measures. In recent decades, there has been increasing evidence that restraints (including bedrails) increase the risk for falls as well as additional problems, including pressure ulcers, contractures, more serious injury from falls, and increased dependency in ADLs (Castle & Engberg, 2009; Fonad, Emami, Wahlin, Winblad, & Sandmark, 2009). Studies have also found that there is no significant increase in number of falls or use of psychotropic medications after restraint-reduction interventions were implemented (Pellfolk, Gustafson, Bucht, & Karlsson, 2010). Agencies that have recommended using less restrictive devices include the American Nurses Association, the U.S. Food and Drug Administration (FDA), the Centers for Medicare and Medicaid Services (CMS), the Joint Commission (previously known as the Joint Commission on Accreditation of Healthcare Organizations), the American Geriatrics Society, and the British Geriatrics Society.

*M*s. M. is now 67 years old and has retired from her secretarial job. She attends weekly social and lunch gatherings at the local senior center, where you are the wellness nurse. One day she comes to the center with a cast on her left wrist and reports that she fractured her wrist when she slipped and fell on ice in her driveway. You know from prior conversations with her that she stopped taking hormonal therapy several years ago because she had been on it for over 10 years and was concerned about long-term effects. You also know that she takes medications for arthritis, hypertension, and depression and that she self-monitors her blood pressure. In the past 10 years, she has gradually gained "a little weight every year" and her current height/weight is 5'3"/172 pounds. She participates in the weekly "mall walkers" exercise program but does not often exercise independently. She says that "my housework is enough exercise" and that the weekly group exercise activity is "as much as my arthritis will tolerate." She lives in a small one-floor house. Although Ms. M. says she is not really concerned about sustaining any more fractures because she views the recent fall as a "fluke of bad winter luck," she makes an appointment to talk with you. During the appointment, she reports that she is a "little concerned about osteoporosis."

THINKING POINTS

- What risk factors for osteoporosis can you identify from what you already know about Ms. M.?
- What risk factors for falls and fall-related injuries can you identify from what you already know about Ms. M.?
- Can you identify any factors that diminish her risk for falls or fractures?
- What additional information about Ms. M. would be helpful in identifying additional risks for osteoporosis?
- What additional information would be helpful in identifying additional risks for falls and fractures?

PATHOLOGIC CONDITION AFFECTING MUSCULOSKELETAL FUNCTION: OSTEOARTHRITIS

Osteoarthritis is a degenerative inflammatory disease affecting joints and attached muscles, tendons, and ligaments; it is characterized by pain, swelling, and limited movement in joints. Osteoarthritis, a leading cause of disability in the United States, affects older adults disproportionately. Although not all older adults have symptoms of osteoarthritis, the condition is often viewed as an extreme progression of age-related changes. Osteoarthritis is a very complex disease process that results from the interplay of risk factors such as trauma, genetics, obesity, and age-related changes.

DIVERSITY NOTE

Whites and African Americans have similar rates of arthritis, but African Americans have a higher rate of arthritis-related activity limitation.

Because self-care is an important aspect of managing osteoarthritis, nurses focus on health education interventions. Nurses can teach people with osteoarthritis about the following activities for prevention and treatment:

- Participating in a supervised, low-impact exercise program that focuses on improving musculoskeletal strength, balance, and endurance
- Avoiding high-impact activities
- Wearing good shock-absorbing shoes
- Balancing weight-bearing activities with rest periods
- Losing weight if appropriate
- Getting adequate intake of vitamins C and D
- Using walkers and other assistive devices as appropriate to relieve weight-bearing joints, improve balance, or achieve independent functioning
- Using moist heat and analgesics for pain.

Care plans for managing osteoarthritis are most effective when they are based on an interdisciplinary approach that includes medicine, nursing, and physical and occupational therapy. Because there are many medical and surgical interventions for osteoarthritis, nurses emphasize the importance of obtaining regular medical care for ongoing evaluation and treatment as this condition changes. Nurses can also teach older adults about asking for a referral for physical therapy to learn effective muscle strengthening strategies for lower-limb osteoarthritis (Bennell, Hunt, Wrigley, LIm, & Hinman, 2009). Self-care practices that are recommended by evidence-based guidelines include aquatherapy, balance training exercise, land-based exercise, **tai chi**, cold therapy, and weight reduction (if applicable) (Royal Australian College of General Practitioners, 2009; Williams, Brand, Hill, Hunt, & Moran, 2010).

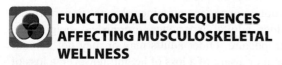

Wellness Opportunity

Older adults with osteoarthritis need to engage in self care activities, including making responsible decisions about promoting optimal comfort and functioning.

FUNCTIONAL CONSEQUENCES AFFECTING MUSCULOSKELETAL WELLNESS

Older adults can partially compensate for age-related changes that affect musculoskeletal function through health promotion interventions, such as good nutrition and physical activity. The functional consequences of osteoporosis, however, are quite serious, as are the functional consequences that result from the many risk factors that contribute to falls and fractures in older adults. As with many other aspects of function in older adulthood, cumulative and interacting effects of risk factors rather than age-related changes most significantly affect function and quality of life.

Effects on Musculoskeletal Function

Muscle strength, endurance, and coordination are affected to some extent by age-related changes, even in the absence of risk factors. Beginning around the age of 40 years, muscle strength declines gradually, resulting in an overall decrease of 30% to 50% by the age of 80 years, with a greater decline in muscle strength in the lower extremities than in the upper extremities. Diminished muscle strength is attributed primarily to age-related loss of muscle mass. In addition, a person's current level of activity and lifelong patterns of exercise can influence muscle strength at any age. Muscle endurance and coordination diminish as a result of age-related changes in the muscles and central nervous system. Because of these changes, older adults experience muscle fatigue after shorter periods of exercise compared with their younger counterparts.

Joint function begins to decline during early adulthood and progresses gradually to cause the following changes in range of motion:

- Decreased range of motion in the upper arms
- Decreased lower back flexion
- Decreased external rotation of the hip
- Decreased hip and knee flexion
- Decreased dorsiflexion of the foot.

These changes result in slowed performance of daily activities, such as writing, eating, grooming, and putting shoes and socks on; difficulty climbing stairs and curbs; and an overall diminished ability to respond to environmental stimuli.

Gait changes, which differ in men and women, are one of the more noticeable functional consequences that occur after the age of 75 years. Women have less muscle control, develop a narrower standing and walking gait, and develop bowlegged-type changes that affect the lower extremities and alter the angle of the hip. Older men develop a wider walking and standing gait, characterized by less arm swing, a shorter stride, decreased steppage height, and a more flexed position of the head and trunk than when they were younger. The overall impact of these changes is that older men and women have a slower walking speed and spend more time in the support phase of gait than in the swing phase. Any significant gait changes that occur are not due to aging alone but are consequences of other conditions, such as osteoarthritis or neurologic disorders (e.g., dementia, Parkinson's disease).

Susceptibility to Falls and Fractures

The combination of age-related changes and multiple interacting risk factors doubly jeopardizes older adults by increasing the probability of both falls and fractures. Fractures are not unique to older adults, but they do differ in many respects from those that occur in younger populations. First, bones of older adults can be fractured with little or no trauma, whereas bones of healthy children and younger adults are usually fractured in response to a forceful impact. Fractures that result from an impact that is no more severe than that which results from falling to the floor from a standing position are classified as osteoporotic fractures (also called *fragility fractures*, or *non-traumatic fractures*). Second, the risk of fractures increases in direct relation to age. Third, it is more likely that fractures in older adults, particularly hip fractures, will have serious consequences affecting independence, quality of life, and morbidity and mortality. Studies show that older adults who have had fractures are at increased risk for functional decline, recurrent falls, permanent admission to a nursing facility, and shortened life expectancy (Ioannidis et al., 2009; Kannegaard, Van Der Mark, Eiken, & Abrahamsen, 2010; Lloyd et al., 2009; Pereira, Puts, Portela, & Sayeg, 2009).

Fear of Falling

Since the early 1980s, gerontologists have recognized a syndrome associated with increased anxiety about falling. The phrase *post-fall syndrome* was initially used to describe a distinct gait pattern adopted by older people who have fallen and been admitted to the hospital for post-fall injuries (Murphy & Isaacs, 1982). In recent years, there has been much research on **fear of falling**, which is the most common reported fear among older adults and has been identified as a public health problem that is of equal importance to falls (Kempen, van Haastreg, McKee, Delbaere, & Zijlstra, 2009). Studies have found that fear of falling is associated with older age, depression, previous falls, use of walking aids, balance impairment, and limitations in ADLs (Sharaf & Ibrahim, 2008; Kempen et al., 2009). Although fear of falling can have a protective effect when it causes older adults to take precautions, studies indicate that excessive concerns about falls leads to activity limitations and alterations in gait that actually decrease walking stability and can increase falls risk (Delbaere, Sturnieks, Crombez, & Lord, 2009). Studies have also found that fear of falling leads to depression, increased anxiety, functional limitations, and decreased quality of life (Boyd & Stevens, 2009; Iglesias, Manca, & Torgerson, 2009; Schmid et al., 2009).

DIVERSITY NOTE

Studies have found that fear of falling is more common in women than men (Filiatrault, Desrosiers, & Trottier, 2009; Kempen et al., 2009).

Family caregivers of older adults may also be quite anxious about potential falls, and they may experience excessive worry about the possibility that the older person might fall. This fear can lead to decisions that restrict an older adult's activities unnecessarily or that result in a move to a setting that provides a greater level of assistance or supervision than the older person desires (Fitzgerald, Hadjistavropoulos, & MacNab, 2009). Although a move to an unfamiliar environment will not necessarily protect the person from falls and may even increase the risk of falls, the caregivers who encourage or make such a decision may derive some peace of mind because they perceive that the older person is safer. It

is now widely recognized that restraints do not prevent falls and are likely to contribute to more serious fall-related injuries; however, some caregivers may falsely believe that restraints and restricted activity are safe and effective fall-prevention interventions.

Wellness Opportunity

Nurses respect older adults' autonomy and involve them in decisions by creatively finding ways to ensure safety while also allowing as much freedom of movement as possible.

NURSING ASSESSMENT OF MUSCULOSKELETAL FUNCTION

Nursing assessment of musculoskeletal function focuses on identifying risks for falls, fractures, and osteoporosis, with particular attention to those factors that can be modified or alleviated through nursing interventions. Nurses can use a **fall risk assessment** tool to identify older adults who might benefit from appropriate preventive interventions.

Assessing Musculoskeletal Performance

Assessment of overall musculoskeletal performance begins with observation of the person's mobility and activities. In addition to watching the person walk, it is especially important to observe the person getting up from a hardback chair without arms. Nurses obtain additional assessment information by asking questions about the person's ability to perform ADLs. When limitations are identified, it is important to find out whether the older adult is using assistive devices to improve mobility, balance, or overall function; safety; and independence. If the person is not using such devices—and may benefit from them—the nurse assesses the person's knowledge about the availability of such devices and his or her attitude about using them because attitudes are likely to influence the acceptability of using recommended aids. Nurses can use the criteria for the functional assessment of all ADLs provided in Chapter 7 together with the assessment information in this chapter.

In addition to experiencing minor changes in performing ADLs, older adults experience diminished height and changes in posture. Older adults may or may not be concerned about or aware of a loss of height; however, a loss of about 2 to 4 cm per decade is normal, owing to osteoporosis and other age-related changes. Including a question about the person's usual height and any noticeable loss of height will give the nurse an opportunity to assess the older adult's awareness of this change. Although the functional consequences of decreased height are minimal, older people who never were very tall may experience increased difficulty performing activities that depend on height. In these situations, they may find that it is safer and more effective to use assistive devices, such as long-handled reachers. They may also

Box 22-3 Guidelines for Assessing Overall Musculoskeletal Function and Risks for Falls and Osteoporosis

Questions to Assess Overall Musculoskeletal Performance
- Do you have any trouble performing your usual activities because of joint limitations?
- Do you have any pain or discomfort in your joints?
- Do you ever feel like you are losing your balance?
- Do you have any trouble walking or getting around?
- Do you use any assistive devices (e.g., a walker, quad cane, or reaching devices) to help you do things?

Questions to Assess Risks for Osteoporosis
Questions to Ask All Older Adults
- Do you know of any blood relatives who have had osteoporosis or who have sustained fractures late in life?
- Have you sustained any fractures during your adult years? (If yes, ask additional questions regarding age at the time, type, location, circumstances, treatment, and so on.)
- Do you take any calcium or vitamin D supplements?
- Have you ever had your bone density measured?
- Have you ever talked with your primary care practitioner about prevention of osteoporosis?
- Do you take any medications for osteoporosis?

Questions to Ask Women
- When did you begin menopause?
- Do you take, or have you ever taken, estrogen or other hormonal therapy? (If yes, ask additional questions regarding type, dose, duration, and so on.)

Questions to Assess Risk for Falls and Fear of Falling
- Have you had any falls in the past few years? (If yes, ask additional questions about the circumstances and ask about pertinent risk factors as summarized in Box 22-2.)
- Are you afraid of falling? (If yes, ask additional questions about specific fears, such as, *What do you think might happen if you were to fall?*)

- Are there any activities you would like to do, but do not do, because of any difficulty moving or getting around? (If yes, ask about specific activities, such as shopping, using public transportation, and so on.)
- Are there any activities you would like to do, but do not do, because you are afraid of falling? (If yes, ask about specific activities, such as going up or down stairs, taking a bath or shower, and so on.)

Observations Regarding Overall Musculoskeletal Performance
- Measure and record the person's present height and stated peak height.
- Observe the individual's walking and gait pattern.
- Observe the person rising from a chair.

Information From the Overall Assessment That Is Also Useful in Assessing Musculoskeletal Function
- Observe and document a functional assessment, as described in Chapter 7.
- How much exercise does the person get on a regular basis? In particular, how much weight-bearing exercise?
- Does the person smoke cigarettes?
- How much alcohol does the person consume?
- What is the person's usual daily intake of calcium and vitamin D?
- Does the person have any medical conditions that are associated with falls or osteoporosis (as summarized in Boxes 22-1 and 22-2)?
- Is the person taking any medications that might create risks for falls (including over-the-counter medications)?
- Does the person have postural hypotension?
- Is the person moderately or seriously visually impaired?
- Does the person have any cognitive impairments or other psychosocial impairments that diminish his or her attention to the environment or interfere with the ability to respond to environmental stimuli?

---

need encouragement to rearrange cupboards so that the most frequently used items are accessible. Another assessment implication of decreased height is that the pants legs of older adults may be too long, especially if the person also has lost weight. Therefore, nurses observe whether the length of clothing increases the risk for falls because this risk can be alleviated through relatively simple interventions. Box 22-3 summarizes guidelines for assessing overall musculoskeletal performance in older adults.

Identifying Risks for Osteoporosis

Nurses assess risks for osteoporosis in all older adults because some health promotion interventions for osteoporosis—such as adequate intake of calcium and vitamin D and participation in regular weight-bearing exercise—are universally applicable. Nurses also identify modifiable risk factors, such as smoking and drinking excessive amounts of alcohol that can be alleviated through lifestyle interventions. If the nursing assessment identifies risk factors that cannot be modified (e.g., long-term use of corticosteroids), this information may

be used to motivate the person to take action to eliminate the risks that can be. Nurses obtain much of the information regarding risks for osteoporosis during an overall assessment or health history, and they consider this information in relation to mobility and safety.

Evidence-based guidelines recommend that people at risk for osteoporotic fractures are best identified through a combination of bone density measurement and an assessment of clinical risk factors (Rahmani & Morin, 2009). Medicare covers the cost of BMD testing every 2 years for people who have risk factors for osteoporosis. Nurses need to be knowledgeable about BMD tests so that they can encourage older adults to talk with their primary care practitioners about these tests. See Box 22-3 for assessment questions and considerations relating to osteoporosis.

Wellness Opportunity

From a holistic perspective, nurses ask older adults to identify enjoyable ways of engaging in weight-bearing activities.

Identifying Risks for Falls and Injury

Identifying fall risks is an essential part of health care for all older adults because it is imperative to initiate preventive interventions. Fall risk assessment is multidimensional and ideally includes observing the person in his or her usual environment. This is important because falls and near falls are caused by multiple interacting conditions that develop over time and require a comprehensive assessment (Zecevic, Salmoni, Lewko, Vandervoort, & Speechley, 2009). Evidence-based guidelines emphasize the effectiveness of a comprehensive fall risk assessment as a basis for interventions that address all the risk factors (Kenny et al., 2010).

The best assessment information is obtained by observing the person in the environment and paying particular attention to the person's awareness of and attention to the environment. Observations are especially helpful in identifying discrepancies between the person's perception of his or her abilities and his or her actual performance. Observations also provide information about adaptive behaviors that otherwise might not be acknowledged. For example, a person might state that he or she has no difficulty with stair climbing, but observations might reveal that the person performs this activity in a highly unsafe manner. Nurses in institutional settings generally do not have opportunities to observe home environments directly, but they can observe the person in the immediate environment and ask the person or caregivers questions about the home setting and their ability to function safely in that setting. They can also consider referrals to home care agencies for home assessment as part of the discharge plan.

Another important aspect of assessing the environment in any setting is identifying the factors that are likely to cause serious injury if a fall does occur. For example, nightstands or any heavy furniture can cause serious injuries, especially if someone hits his or her head while falling. Likewise, furniture with hard or sharp edges can cause serious injuries and bleeding, particularly for people taking anticoagulant drugs. The guidelines summarized in Chapter 7 can be used to assess the safety of any environment and can be applied to all older adults, particularly those who have intrinsic risk factors for falls. Box 22-3 includes assessment questions that are applicable to older adults who are independent or relatively independent.

◆ Wellness Opportunity

Whenever possible, nurses actively involve the older adult and family members in identifying environmental factors that either support or create risks for safe mobility.

Many fall risk assessment tools have been developed and are readily available for use in different settings. The purpose of these tools is to identify people who are at risk for falls so that preventive measures can be implemented. The two types of fall risk assessment tools are functional assessment scales and nursing fall risk tools. Functional assessment scales focus on the person's gait and balance and are used by rehabilitation therapists. Nurses can informally assess gait and balance by asking the person to sit in a firm, straight-backed chair with armrests, stand up from the chair and walk a few steps, then turn around and return to the chair. Nurses also can observe the usual walking pattern of the person, paying particular attention to any gait or balance unsteadiness or unusual patterns. If any abnormalities are noted, nurses can facilitate referrals for further evaluation by a physical therapist. Nursing fall risk assessment tools are widely used in institutional settings as well as home and community-based settings. The Hartford Foundation for Geriatric Nursing recommends the use of the Hendrich II Fall Risk Model (Figure 22-1) in institutional settings as an evidence-based tool for assessing fall risk (Hendrich, 2007). Additional information and a cost-free video demonstrating the application of this tool in a clinical setting is available through collaboration of the Hartford Institute and the *American Journal of Nursing* at http://consultgerirn.org/resources or at www.nursingcenter.com.

Although fall risk assessment tools are useful in identifying people who are at high risk for falls, they do not address the underlying causative factors. When older adults have several risk factors or have already had fall-related injuries, a comprehensive fall assessment should be done in a multidisciplinary setting, such as a geriatric assessment program. A comprehensive fall assessment addresses all the following: cognition, nutrition, environment, medications, pathologic conditions, functional assessment, usual footwear, and a complete physical examination (including visual acuity, musculoskeletal function, and cardiovascular status).

Because fear of falling has negative functional consequences in addition to those associated with actual falls, nurses include at least one question about fear of falling in any assessment of falls and fall risk. If the older person expresses a fear of falling, nurses can ask additional questions in relation to specific activities that may be associated with fears or falls. Assessment questions aimed at identifying fear of falling and related negative functional consequences are included in Box 22-3.

$\mathcal{M}$s. M. is now 75 years old and goes to the senior center three or four times weekly for lunch. You have been the wellness nurse at the center for several years and are quite familiar with Ms. M. because she frequently attends your weekly Healthy Aging class. After your recent class on "Keeping Your Bones Healthy and Moving Well," she made an appointment to see you. She tells you that she has significantly cut down on her exercise because she experienced pain in one knee about a month ago after she took a long walk in the park with her dog. She talked with her doctor about this and was told to start taking ibuprofen, but she has not started taking it because she is not sure how much to take and her knee does not bother her except when she takes a long walk. She used to take her dog for daily walks, but now ties him out so she does not have to go out. Current prescription medications are enalapril, 5 mg twice daily, and hydrochlorothiazide, 25 mg daily. She also takes a multiple vitamin daily and acetaminophen 1000 mg every 6 hours as needed. She continues to live in her one-floor house and is independent in doing all of her household chores. She also is responsible for all year-round outdoor maintenance activities, including mowing the lawn, raking leaves, and shoveling snow.

THINKING POINTS

- What assessment questions from Box 22-3 would you ask Ms. M. at this time?
- Would you use any information from Box 22-1 or Box 22-2 at this time?
- What myths or misunderstandings related to mobility and exercise might be influencing Ms. M.?
- Would you take any steps to assess Ms. M.'s home environment for fall risks?

Hendrich II Fall Risk Model © 2006

Risk Factor	Risk Points	
Confusion/Disorientation/Impulsivity	4	
Symptomatic Depression	2	
Altered Elimination	1	
Dizziness/Vertigo	1	
Gender (Male)	1	
Any Administered Antiepileptics (anticonvulsants): *(Carbamazepine, Divalproex Sodium, Ethotoin, Ethosuximide, Felbamate, Fosphenytoin, Gabapentin, Lamotrigine, Mephenytoin, Methsuximide, Phenobarbital, Phenytoin, Primidone, Topiramate, Trimethadione, Valproic Acid)*	2	
Any Administered Benzodiazepines: *(Alprazolam, Chlordiazepoxide, Clonazepam, Clorazepate Dipotassium, Diazepam, Flurazepam, Halazepam, Lorazepam, Midazolam, Oxazepam, Temazepam, Triazolam)*	1	
Get-up-and-go Test: "Rising from a Chair" *If unable to assess, monitor for change in activity level, assess other risk factors, document both on patient chart with date and time.*		
Ability to rise in single movement-No loss of balance with steps	0	
Pushes up, successful in one attempt	1	
Multiple attempts but successful	3	
Unable to rise without assistance during test *(OR if a medical order states the same and/or complete bed rest is ordered)* *If unable to assess, document this on the patient chart with the date and time*	4	
(A score of 5 or greater = High Risk) **TOTAL SCORE**		

AHI
A VITAL SIGN FOR SAFETY™
Fall Prevention and Risk Management

FIGURE 22-1 The Hendrich II Fall Risk Model, a fall risk assessment tool recommended by the Hartford Institute for Geriatric Nursing. (© Ann Hendrich, Inc.) Used with permission.

NURSING DIAGNOSIS

Impaired Physical Mobility is a nursing diagnosis that is applicable when the assessment identifies limitations in mobility of an older adult. This diagnosis is defined as "limitation in independent, purposeful physical movement of the body or of one or more extremities" (NANDA International, 2009, p. 124). Related factors common in older adults include arthritis, depression, chronic pain, fractured hip, and neurologic disorders (e.g., dementia or Parkinson's disease). If the nursing assessment identifies a history of falls or any risks for falls, the nursing diagnosis of Risk for Falls would be applicable. This diagnosis is defined as "increased susceptibility to falling that may cause physical harm (NANDA International, 2009, p. 312). Related factors common in older adults include all those factors listed in Box 22-2.

In long-term care and rehabilitation settings, nurses frequently address the needs of older adults who have a diagnosis of osteoporosis or a history of fractures. In these situations, as well as in any situation where someone has several risk factors for osteoporosis, a nursing diagnosis of Ineffective Health Maintenance can be used because the focus is on secondary prevention. This diagnosis is defined as the "inability to identify, manage, and/or seek out help to maintain health" (NANDA International, 2009, p. 57).

> **◆ Wellness Opportunity**
>
> Nurses can use the nursing diagnosis Readiness for Enhanced Self Health Management for older adults who are willing to explore opportunities for improving musculoskeletal function and preventing falls and fractures.

PLANNING FOR WELLNESS OUTCOMES

When planning care for older adults who are at risk for osteoporosis, nurses identify wellness outcomes that focus on primary and secondary prevention. In these situations, any of the following Nursing Outcomes Classification (NOC) terms might be pertinent: Health Promoting Behavior, Knowledge: Health Behavior, Risk Control, or Risk Detection.

Nursing goals for an older adult with a nursing diagnosis of Impaired Physical Mobility focus on restoring functional abilities, preventing further loss of function, and preventing falls and injuries. NOC terminology applicable to an older adult with this nursing diagnosis include Balance, Endurance, Mobility, Pain Level, or Activity Tolerance.

Care of older adults with a nursing diagnosis of Risk for Falls focuses on preventing the occurrence of falls and fall-related injuries by implementing fall-prevention programs. The following NOC terminology would be applicable with regard to safety and fall prevention: Risk Control, Risk Detection, Safety Behavior: Fall Prevention, Safety Behavior: Home Physical Environment, Safety Behavior: Personal, Safety Status: Physical Injury, or Safety Status: Falls.

> **◆ Wellness Opportunity**
>
> Wellness outcomes that address the body–mind–spirit interrelatedness for people who are afraid of falling include Coping, Fear Control, Comfort Level, Anxiety Control, and Quality of Life.

 ## NURSING INTERVENTIONS FOR MUSCULOSKELETAL WELLNESS

Nurses have numerous opportunities to promote musculoskeletal wellness because most older adults can benefit from learning about health promotion interventions for improved musculoskeletal function and prevention of osteoporosis, falls, and fractures. Thus, interventions focus not only on direct actions to prevent falls but also on teaching about eliminating or addressing risks. Some Nursing Interventions Classification (NIC) terminologies that would be applicable to the interventions discussed in the following sections include Environmental Management, Exercise Promotion, Fall Prevention, Health Education, Risk Identification, and Teaching: Individual.

Promoting Healthy Musculoskeletal Function and Preventing Falls

Healthy older adults experience only a slight decline in overall musculoskeletal function, but they can compensate for these minor functional consequences by maintaining an active lifestyle. Various types of exercise are beneficial in promoting healthy musculoskeletal function and nurses can encourage older adults to incorporate several exercise strategies into their regular health behavior routines. Positive musculoskeletal effects of exercise include increased bone strength, increased total body calcium, improved coordination, and improved overall body functioning (Treat-Jacobson, Bronas, & Mark, 2010). Flexibility exercises can improve range of motion, and weight-bearing exercise is an essential intervention for osteoporosis. Moderate aerobic exercise can prevent loss of muscle mass in older adults and is especially important for those who are intentionally trying to lose weight (Chomentowski et al., 2009). Studies have also found that resistance exercise improves muscle mass, strength, and function in older adults (Verdijk et al., 2009).

In recent years, there has been increasing attention to holistic types of exercise that address balance, mobility, and the body–mind connection. For example, many studies have found that beneficial effects of tai chi include decreased risk of falls and fractures and improved neuromuscular coordination; postural stability; and muscle strength, endurance, and flexibility (Low, Ang, Goh, & Chew, 2009; Lui, Qin, & Chan, 2008). Tai chi is a traditional Chinese martial art and a mind–body exercise that involves focused attention and a series of fluid and continuous movements. One study found that tai chi was one of the most cost-effective interventions for reducing fall-related hip fractures (Frick, Kung, Parrish, & Narrett, 2010). Much current evidence supports the use of tai chi for older adults in a variety of settings, including community centers, long-term care facilities, and rehabilitation programs in hospitals (Chen, 2010). Studies also support the use of yoga as an effective way of building up BMD after menopause (Fishman, 2009).

The Feldenkrais method is another holistic form of exercise that has been found to improve balance and mobility and to decrease fear of falling in older adults (Ullmann, Williams, Hussey, Durstine, & McClenaghan, 2010). Studies have found that older adults who participated in a series of Feldenkrais method balance classes called Getting Grounded Gracefully improved significantly on several measures of balance and mobility and viewed the intervention positively (Connors, Galea, & Said, 2009; Vrantsidis et al., 2009).

Wellness Opportunity

Walking, dancing, swimming, tai chi, and bicycle riding are examples of wellness intervention that are enjoyable and have positive effects on one's body, mind, and spirit.

Health Education About Osteoporosis

Interventions for prevention and treatment of osteoporosis need to be an integral part of fracture prevention regimens for older adults, particularly in health care settings where a major focus of care is on chronic conditions (e.g., home care and long-term care settings). Although primary care practitioners are responsible for diagnosing and treating osteoporosis, nurses are responsible for health education about osteoporosis interventions and prevention of fractures. Because awareness about osteoporosis in men is just beginning to develop, nurses have a particular responsibility for teaching older men about

A Student's Perspective

This past week, I chose to do the water aerobics with the older adults at the Health and Fitness Centre. I was encouraged by the vitality and general zest for life that these older women showed. I was enlightened by their sense of pride in their health and level of activity. I left with the impression that this group activity was something that each of them attributed her good health to. I also noted that they got more out of this activity than just physical exercise. The social connection that these women had was truly admirable. They were constantly encouraging each other and me during the class. They also used the time just to connect with each other and discuss normal life events.

My take-away lesson from this experience was the importance of having opportunities like this for older adults to exercise their muscles as well as their social personalities. Older adults are often portrayed as socially inferior in today's popular culture, but I felt these older women were living truly balanced lives, maybe more so than me in some respects. I think that often I find myself so busy that I do not take time to invest myself in more meaningful relationships—something that these people are obviously benefiting from.

Clint H.

osteoporosis and fractures. Nurses also need to focus health education on older adults who already have had fractures and on people who have other risk factors, because people who are more vulnerable to the serious consequences of osteoporosis may be more motivated to use preventive interventions. Evidence-based practice for osteoporosis are summarized in Evidence-Based Practice 22-1.

Evidence-Based Practice 22-1
Osteoporosis

Statement of the Problem

- Osteoporosis is underrecognized and undertreated, especially in men and in residents of long-term care facilities.
- Bone mineral density (BMD) is an excellent predictor of fracture risk.
- Nearly half of all white women and about one quarter of men will have an osteoporotic fracture in their lifetime.
- Osteoporotic fractures are a common cause of excess mortality, chronic pain, disability, depression, and deformity

Recommendations for Nursing Assessment

- Assessment of risk factors, especially those that can be addressed through health education (smoking, nutrition, weight-bearing exercise, excessive alcohol intake).
- Early identification of low bone mineral density (BMD) through the use of dual energy x-ray absorptiometry (DXA, DEXA).

Recommendations for Nursing Interventions: Patient Teaching

- Maintain a healthy weight.
- Participate in 30 minutes daily of weight-bearing activities (i.e., walking, aerobics, dancing, resistance training).

- Assure total daily intake of 1200–1500 mg calcium and 800–1000 IU vitamin D in food or supplements.
- Vitamin D supplement is effective for preventing fractures only when used in combination with calcium.
- Implement fall-prevention interventions.
- Have BMD measured at 5-year intervals beginning at the age of 60 years for women with risk factors, at the age of 65 years for those without risks, and at the age of 70 years for men.
- Talk with primary care provider about medications for osteoporosis: bisphosphonates, calcitonin, estrogens, and selective estrogen receptor modulators parathyroid hormone.
- If applicable: quit smoking; limit alcohol to no more than three drinks daily.

SOURCES: Lash et al., 2009; North American Menopause Society, 2010; Rahmani & Morin, 2009; Society of Obstetricians and Gynaecologists of Canada, 2009; Vondracek & Linnebur, 2009.

Health education includes information about risk factors with emphasis on developing a plan to address the modifiable risk factors. Nurses can encourage older adults with risk factors to ask their primary care practitioner about screening tests and interventions. All adults can benefit from lifestyle interventions for osteoporosis, and teaching about these self-care activities is well within the realm of nursing responsibilities. Important self-care interventions for osteoporosis include daily weight-bearing activities, quitting smoking, and limiting alcohol to no more than three drinks daily.

Nurses can also teach older adults and their caregivers about the importance of adequate intake of calcium and vitamin D. A registered dietician, if available, can evaluate a 3-day food history to determine the usual intake of calcium and vitamin D. If intake does not provide at least 1200 mg of calcium and 1000 international units of vitamin D, then health teaching focuses either on increasing dietary intake to the recommended amount or on taking a daily supplement. This is important because a review of studies concluded that vitamin D has the strongest evidence in clinical trials for preventing fractures in older adults (Tinetti & Kumar, 2010). When supplements are used, older adults should be taught that vitamin D may not be effective in preventing fractures unless it is taken

with calcium (DIPART Group, 2010). In long-term care facilities, all care plans should include a review of nutritional interventions for osteoporosis, particularly in relation to preventing fractures. Nurses can take the lead in involving dieticians and primary care providers in developing and implementing appropriate preventive interventions. Box 22-4 summarizes health promotion information that can be used as a guide for teaching older adults about osteoporosis.

Effectiveness of pharmacologic interventions for osteoporosis is measured by their efficacy in increasing bone mass and preventing osteoporotic fractures that are associated with chronic pain, decreased quality of life, and significant morbidity and mortality (Recker, Lewiecki, Miller, & Reiffel, 2009). Hormonal therapies were the first type of intervention for osteoporosis, but since the mid-1990s, the bisphosphonates have become the most commonly used type of medication for preventing osteoporotic fractures. A review of studies concludes that all four approved bisphosphonates reduce relative risk of new vertebral fractures, and three of these drugs (alendronate, risedronate, and zoledronic acid) reduce the relative risk of new nonvertebral fractures, including hip fractures, in postmenopausal women (Bilezikian, 2009). Long-term studies have found that medical treatment of osteoporosis was associated with an 11% reduction in mortality (Bolland, Grey, Gamble, & Reid, 2010; Demontiero & Duque, 2009).

Oral bisphosphonates can cause upper gastrointestinal injury, particularly when taken daily or when there are acidic conditions or preexisting esophageal irritation (Recker et al., 2009). Measures to prevent potential adverse effects on the

Box 22-4 Health Promotion Teaching About Osteoporosis

Health Promotion Interventions for Early Detection and Treatment

- Review risk factors for osteoporosis as summarized in Box 22-1.
- Plan interventions for modifiable risk factors using Box 22-1 and Evidence-Based Practice box 22-1 as guides.
- Encourage discussion with primary care provider about bone mineral density (BMD) tests.
- Encourage discussion with primary care provider about medical interventions for osteoporosis if risk factors are present.
- Encourage discussion with primary care provider about prevention of fractures if osteoporosis is diagnosed.

Lifestyle Interventions

- Implement weight-bearing exercise regimen for 1/2 hour daily.
- Engage in activities such as yoga, swimming, massage, acupressure, and tai chi.
- Wear supportive shoes.
- Discontinue cigarette smoking.
- Maintain ideal body weight.
- Avoid excessive alcohol intake.

Nutritional Interventions

- Calcium supplements often are recommended so that the total intake is 1500 mg per day (average daily calcium intake of older adults is less than 800 mg).

- Foods that are high in calcium include milk, cheese, yogurt, custard, ice cream, raisins, tofu, canned salmon or sardines, and broccoli and other dark green vegetables.
- Provide adequate dietary intake of vitamin D and use 400–800 IU of vitamin D supplement daily; people with osteoporosis may require higher dose.
- Calcium carbonate, which is found in some antacids, is an effective and inexpensive source of elemental calcium; it should be taken with food.
- Limit consumption of beverages containing alcohol, caffeine, or phosphorus.

Special Precautions

- Vitamin D in amounts greater than 400–600 IU per day, and vitamin A in amounts exceeding 5000 IU per day, can have detrimental effects.
- Because calcium may contribute to constipation, measures should be taken to promote bowel function (e.g., regular exercise and adequate fiber and fluid intake).
- Calcium supplements can interact with some medications (e.g., calcium decreases absorption of tetracycline).

gastrointestinal tract include taking the medication in the morning with a full glass of water (not mineral water) at least a half hour before any food. In addition, the person must be in an upright position when taking this medication and avoid lying down for a half hour after the dose. Because of the adverse effects associated with daily oral dosing, newer bisphosphonates have been developed for weekly, monthly, or even annual dosing to increase compliance, and clinical trials of bisphosphonates for up to 10 years have demonstrated the safety and efficacy of these longer-term dosing intervals (Sweet, Sweet, Jeremiah, & Galazka, 2009).

Because most clinical trials of medical interventions for osteoporosis focus primarily on women, much less evidence is available about safe and effective pharmacologic treatments for men with the disease. Bisphosphonates are the most widely studied pharmacologic interventions in men, and by 2002, the FDA had approved alendronate and risedronate for osteoporosis in men. It is likely that when additional bisphosphonates are approved for treatment of osteoporosis, they will be approved for use in both men and women. Calcitonin is another medical intervention that can be used for men with osteoporosis, but its effectiveness in men is still being investigated. Testosterone therapy has been shown to improve BMD and it may, in turn, decrease the risk for fracture in men, but it has been shown to be effective only in men with secondary osteoporosis associated with hypogonadism.

In summary, there is sound evidence that pharmacologic treatment of osteoporosis can improve BMD, reduce the rate of bone loss, and decrease the risk for fracture. Evidence is less clear about pharmacologic interventions for older adults who do not have osteoporosis but have risks for it. Decisions about preventive pharmacologic interventions for people at risk for osteoporosis and fractures must be based on an appraisal of the relative risks and benefits of any particular intervention. Pharmacologic treatment is just one component of a comprehensive management plan that must also include nutritional intake of calcium and vitamin D, physical activity to maintain musculoskeletal function and reduce the risk of falls, and patient education regarding osteoporosis and fall prevention.

*R*ecall that you are the nurse at the wellness program where Ms. M., who is 75 years old, regularly attends your health education programs. Based on additional assessment information, you know that Ms. M. does not take any calcium or vitamin D supplements because she drinks milk twice daily and believes that this should be sufficient. She stopped having menstrual periods when she was 50 years old and began hormonal therapy at that time. She stopped taking estrogen when she was 63 because she began "hearing too many bad things about estrogen." When she fractured her wrist 8 years ago, the orthopedic

surgeon said that her x-rays showed that her "bones were pretty good for her age." She has not had any further x-rays or any BMD tests and says her doctor has never brought up the subject of osteoporosis because "I guess he's too worried about my heart problems to be concerned about my bones." Although she fell once when she was raking leaves last fall and tripped over a small tree stump, she has had no serious fall-related injuries since she fractured her wrist. She does not smoke and drinks alcohol only on major social occasions. When you assessed her blood pressure, you found that her blood pressure while standing was 146/86 mm Hg and while lying was 128/78 mm Hg. Her record of self-monitored blood pressure readings indicates that her usual blood pressure is around 134/82 mm Hg. Her vision is adequate, but she has stopped driving at night and is being monitored by her ophthalmologist for progression of bilateral cataracts. Her eye doctor told her that she is likely to need cataract surgery sometime during the next 2 to 3 years.

THINKING POINTS

- What further assessment information would you want to have?
- What health promotion interventions would you advise for Ms. M.? Specifically, what health teaching would you do with regard to further assessment, lifestyle interventions, nutrition and nutritional supplements, and pharmacologic interventions?
- What educational materials would you use for Ms. M.?
- What follow-up health promotion would you consider for Ms. M.? Specifically, how would you work with Ms. M. to develop long-term health promotion interventions?

Preventing Falls and Fall-Related Injuries

Because falls are multifaceted in their causes, they are best addressed through multidisciplinary fall preventions programs that address conditions in a particular setting and those factors that are unique to each at-risk person. In addition to addressing intrinsic and extrinsic risk factors to reduce the occurrence of falls, comprehensive programs focus on preventing fall-related injuries. Key aspects of fall prevention programs are the identification of people who are at risk for falls and the consistent implementation of preventive actions by all staff. Thus, an important part of these programs is the education of all professional and nonprofessional staff members who have contact with the person who is at risk for falls. Education may involve strategies to heighten staff awareness of the importance of reducing fall risks. For example, posters and brochures may be used initially and periodically as

Box 22-5 A Fall-Prevention Program for Older Adults Being Cared for in Hospitals or Nursing Homes

Identification of Patients/Residents Who Are at Risk for Falling

- Use a nursing judgment and a fall risk assessment tool to identify any risks for falling and fall-related injuries (e.g., medications, osteoporosis, medical conditions, history of falls, impaired cognition, diminished alertness, impaired mobility, age 75 years or older).
- Document the risk factors on the designated fall assessment guide.
- Address any risk factors for falls, osteoporosis, or fall-related injuries that can be modified; this often requires a multidisciplinary approach.
- Reassess the risks for falls and fall-related injuries at predetermined times (e.g., every shift, every day, whenever there is a change in the patient's/resident's functional status).
- Use color-coded items (e.g., brightly colored stickers for the chart, a brightly colored identification band for the person's wrist, and signs near the person's bed and outside the room) to identify those who are included in the fall-prevention program.

Education of the Staff, Patient/Resident, and Family

- Instruct the patient or resident and family about the fall-prevention program and provide written information about preventing falls and obtaining help if falls occur.
- Provide staff education about the fall-prevention program and the risk factors for falls, especially those factors that the staff influences (e.g., use of restraints, selection of footwear).

- Use posters and fliers to heighten staff awareness of the fall-prevention program.

Interventions to Be Implemented for All High-Risk Patients/Residents

- Keep the call light within reach at all times.
- Make sure that ambulatory patients wear sturdy, nonslip footwear when out of bed.
- Offer assistance with activities of daily living (ADLs) and try to anticipate the person's needs before help is needed.
- Encourage the person to call for help when needed.
- Frequently check all people who cannot be relied on to call for help.
- Make sure the bed is in the lowest position possible and the wheels are locked.
- Carefully and frequently assess the environment for factors that increase the risk for either falls or fall-related injuries; address all modifiable risk factors.
- Consider the use of a movement detection device.
- Adhere to institutional policies about use of physical restraints, including bedrails.
- If appropriate, orient the person to person, place, and time every shift and as needed.
- Document fall-prevention interventions on the person's chart.

reminders. Also, some form of patient/resident or chart identification can be used to draw attention to those people who have an increased risk for falls. Box 22-5 describes a fall-prevention program that could be adapted for use in institutional settings.

Addressing Intrinsic Risk Factors

Because any gait and balance impairment increases the risk for falls, interventions that improve mobility are likely to be beneficial in preventing falls. Interventions for improving mobility are implemented primarily by therapists, nurses, and nursing staff, often through an interdisciplinary approach. Teaching about the proper use of mobility aids and other assistive devices is an important part of fall-prevention programs (Figure 22-2). Nurses are responsible for raising questions about whether an older adult may benefit from the use of mobility aids or assistive devices and facilitating a referral to a physical therapist for evaluation and teaching regarding their use. In community settings, nurses can teach older adults and their caregivers about the availability of various mobility aids, transfer assistance devices, and other aids that might improve safety. Nurses can suggest that older adults seek professional help with selecting appropriate mobility aids and assistive devices. Some suppliers of home health care equipment have therapists on staff member who can provide advice and assist with processing claims if the aids are covered by insurance. When mobility aids are prescribed, nurses are responsible for encouraging the person to use the aids and making sure that the aids are accessible.

Nurses are responsible for facilitating referrals for reassessment if questions arise about the safety or effectiveness of mobility aids that are being used.

Because proper footwear is essential to prevent slips and falls, nurses can advise older adults about wearing nonslip footwear for safety. Walking outdoors can be particularly hazardous, especially when winter conditions create a very dangerous environment for older people who have a predisposition for falls. Nurses can emphasize the importance of removing ice and snow from walkways and help older adults explore resources for assistance with this. In addition, a simple gait-stabilizing device, such as the Yaktrax Walker (Figure 22-3), may help prevent outdoor falls when applied and worn properly.

In recent years, fall-prevention literature has emphasized the effectiveness of various exercise routines as an intervention for reducing intrinsic fall risk. An important role for nurses is to identify those older adults who may benefit from gait and balance training programs and to facilitate referrals for physical therapy when appropriate. Nurses are also responsible for encouraging adequate and consistent follow-through with recommended exercise programs. In long-term care settings, nurses generally oversee restorative nursing programs in which nursing assistants help residents with walking and other exercise regimens established by physical therapists. These restorative nursing routines are essential aspects of fall-prevention programs. Group exercise programs are also widely used as fall-prevention interventions that are beneficial to all at-risk people. Many programs incorporate

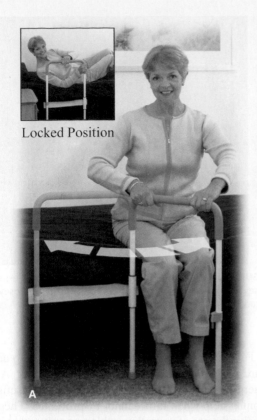

Locked Position

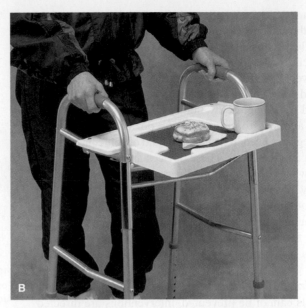

FIGURE 22-2 The use of assistive devices can help reduce the risk of falls. (**A**) Transfer assistive devices are used to facilitate safer transfer in and out of beds. (**B**) Walkers are available in various styles with wheels, brakes, baskets, seats, and other features to improve safety and mobility. (Photographs courtesy of ActiveForever.com.)

exercises aimed specifically at improving gait, balance, ankle strength, or other aspects of fall prevention.

Fall-prevention programs also include multidisciplinary interventions to address medication effects and pathologic conditions that increase the risk for falls. Nurses are responsible for knowing the common adverse effects of medications and raising questions about any effects that increase the risk for falls. Nurses should assess for postural hypotension, for example, as a potential adverse medication effect and as a risk factor for falls. Medication regimens should be reviewed periodically, and nurses can take the lead in suggesting that

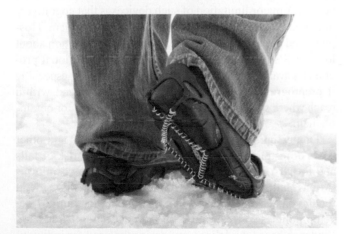

FIGURE 22-3 The Yaktrax Walker is an example of a gait-stabilizing device that can be used to prevent falls on slippery outdoor surfaces. (Photograph courtesy of Yaktrax, LLC.)

pharmacists and prescribing practitioners evaluate medications in relation to fall risks.

Addressing Extrinsic Risk Factors

Interventions for addressing extrinsic risk factors, such as environmental conditions and use of restraints, are applicable for older adults in any setting. Patients who are at risk for falls should receive referrals for environmental home assessments when they are discharged from hospitals. Environmental assessment guidelines provided in Chapter 7 can help with planning interventions that may eliminate or reduce environmental risks. In addition, environmental modifications to improve a person's vision, as discussed in Chapter 17, are applicable to fall prevention.

✦ Wellness Opportunity

Fall-prevention interventions that address the person–environment relationship can be as simple and effective as involving older adults in decisions about removing or replacing slippery throw rugs.

Using Monitoring Devices

Monitoring devices can be very useful in alerting staff to potentially dangerous patient/resident activity, such as getting out of bed or a chair without assistance. Many types of devices are available, but they all transmit a signal to a remote location (e.g., a nursing station) when activated by certain levels of patient/resident movement. Some devices, such as a pad, are applied to the bed or chair, whereas others are attached to the person's clothing. Other devices are programmed specifically for the person's movement in a confined environment, such as his or her room. Most movement-detection devices were originally designed for institutional use, but simplified monitoring and signal systems have now been developed for home use by family caregivers. In home settings, an auditory room-monitoring device may be useful when caregivers need to detect the sound of someone moving around in another room. These devices are widely available in stores where infant care supplies are sold. A major limitation of any movement-detection device is that its effectiveness depends on the timely response of someone who is able to prevent the fall. These devices are not useful for people living alone or for people without responsible and responsive caregivers.

Preventing Fall-Related Injuries and Death

When falls cannot be prevented, interventions are directed toward reducing the risk of fractures and other serious fall-related injuries. Two interventions for preventing fall-related injuries that should be used for all people who are at risk for falls are (1) to implement evidence-based measures for osteoporosis (discussed previously) and (2) to adapt the environment as much as possible to reduce the risk for fall-related injuries. Heavy furniture that is in a pathway where a fall is likely to occur can be moved out of the way or replaced with items that would move easily if the person falls into them. Also, hard edges of furniture and built-in cabinets can be padded. Particular attention should be paid to padding hard edges of bathroom cabinets and either padding or removing swinging shower doors. Using a bed that can be adjusted to a very low position can reduce risk of injury from falling out of bed. Soft mats can be placed near beds and in other locations where people are likely to fall, but caution must be used so that these pads do not become fall risks.

External hip protectors have been available since the 1990s, and many types of hip protectors are now in use in both Europe and North America (Figure 22-4). Hip protectors, which are designed to decrease the impact of a fall, consist of pads with or without hard shells that are placed over the hips and worn under garments. Studies have found that hip protectors represent a "promising strategy" for reducing the risk of hip fracture if they are positioned properly; however, not all studies have demonstrated clinical effectiveness (Cameron et al., 2010; Choi, Hoffer, & Robinovitch, 2010a). Some studies suggest that hip protectors are effective in preventing fractures in people who have low body mass index (BMI) and other risk factors (e.g., previous falls) (Choi, Hoffer, & Robinovitch, 2010b; Koike et al., 2009). Training in martial arts about proper fall technique is another intervention that is being investigated to prevent fall-related injuries and reduce the impact on hips (Groen, Smulders, deKam, Duysens, & Weerdesteyn, 2010).

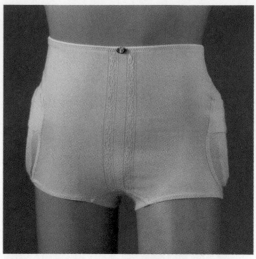

FIGURE 22-4 Hip protectors come in a variety of styles, such as the Posey Community Hipsters (Photograph courtesy of Posey Company, Arcadia, CA).

For people living alone, interventions are also directed toward providing assistance in a timely manner. A personal emergency response system (PERS) can be useful in summoning help when falls cannot be prevented. These devices involve the use of a small portable transmitter that is worn on the person's body or clothing. Examples of such devices are beeper-type devices worn on the belt or pendants worn as necklaces or bracelets. When the person falls, he or she can summon help by using the transmitter to signal a receiver unit attached to the telephone. In turn, a call is automatically made to the PERS provider, who then checks in with the person and calls the local emergency response team or a contact person, such as a neighbor or family member. Some of these devices are set up so that a checkup call is made to the person during any 24-hour period in which the person does not push a reset button or otherwise notify the company that he or she is well. The effectiveness of PERS depends on the ability of the fallen person to signal for help and on the availability of a helping person. A major limitation of such devices is that cognitively impaired people may not be able to learn to use them. Hospitals and home care agencies can provide information about local PERS programs, and information about national programs is available on the Internet. Cordless phones, especially if preprogrammed for emergency help and placed within reach where someone might fall, can also be used for obtaining help.

Finally, nurses need to recognize that bedrails and other types of restraints do not necessarily reduce the risk of falls and are associated with more serious fall-related injuries (Mion, Halliday, & Sandhu, 2008). In recent years, federal regulations have mandated that health care institutions develop policies for restraint reduction or restraint-free care. Evidence-based guidelines emphasize the need for individualized care plans to prevent falls and for education of patients, family members, and all caregiving staff members about the

Statement of the Problem

- About one-third of community-living older adults and more than half of those living in long-term care facilities fall every year; half of those who fall do so more than once.
- Falls are the leading cause of fatal and nonfatal injuries in the United States and a major cause of functional decline, hospital admission, psychological trauma, and institutionalization in older people.
- Fear of falling is consequence of and a risk factor for falls in older adults.

Recommendations for Nursing Assessment

- Multifactorial assessment of fall risks leads to fewer falls and less fear of falling when the assessment is followed by preventive interventions.
- Use good nursing judgment and an evidence-based fall risk assessment tool at the following times: on admission, when patient is transferred to a different unit, when there is a change in the patient's condition, and after a fall has occurred.
- Comprehensive fall assessment of individuals, which should be done following a fall, includes all the following: cognition, nutrition, medications, pathologic conditions, functional assessment, and a complete physical examination (including visual acuity, musculoskeletal function, orthostatic hypotension, and cardiovascular status).
- External factors that should be assessed include lighting, use of assistive devices, usual footwear, lighting, clutter, floor surfaces, presence of grab bars, and hand rails.
- A post-fall assessment should be done immediately and at appropriate intervals after the fall.

Recommendations for Nursing Interventions

- Address medication-related risks: minimize medications, reduce doses or eliminate psychotropic medications.

- Initiate an individually tailored exercise program including balance, strength training, flexibility, tai chi, endurance, cardiovascular, and fitness training.
- Have visual function evaluated as part of an overall fall-prevention program.
- Address postural hypotension and cardiovascular problems.
- Provide vitamin D supplementation in combination with calcium supplements.
- Address foot problems and ensure that the person wears proper nonskid footwear.
- Provide instruction and information to older adults, their caregivers, and health care professionals.
- Establish and implement individualized fall-prevention care plans.
- Teach older adults about fall-prevention interventions, including exercise.
- Facilitate referrals to rehabilitation therapists.

Recommendations for Environmental Interventions

- Modify the home environment to eliminate home fall hazards (e.g., clutter, poor lighting, lack of grab bars, and handrails).
- In institutional settings, implement comprehensive fall-prevention programs that address environmental factors.
- Use visual aids to identify patients/residents who are at risk for falls.
- Use appropriate alerting devices (e.g., personal alarms, pressure sensitive devices) to alert caregivers to potential or actual falls.
- Implement interventions to reduce the risk of harm if falls occur (e.g., hip protectors, low-rise beds, floor mats).

SOURCES: Gray-Miceli, 2008; Hansma, Emmelot-Vonk, & Verhaar, 2010; Kenny et al., 2010; Institute for Clinical Systems Improvement, 2008.

---

concept of restraint-free care as well as fall-prevention measures. Nurses play an extremely important role in decisions about using restraints and in education about their associated risks. Evidence-based practice for prevention of falls are summarized in Evidence-Based Practice 22-2.

Addressing Fear of Falling

Any interventions that reduce the risk of falls are also likely to reduce a person's fear of falling, but some people may need additional interventions to address this problem. The "Falls and Feelings" discussion group is a nursing model that was designed to facilitate discussion of feelings related to falling experiences. The goal for group members was "to enhance self-confidence and life satisfaction, resulting in empowerment of the individual to handle fear of falling" (Gentleman & Malozemoff, 2001, p. 36). Themes of the sessions included risks for falls, prevention of falls, falls and feelings, and fear

as a consequence of falls (Gentleman & Malozemoff, 2001). Nurses can address fear of falling in the same way they address other fears: encourage the expression of feelings and provide education and reassurance about interventions that are being implemented as part of an individualized fall prevention care plan. Family members and caregivers should be included in nursing interventions and health education to address fear of falling. For people living alone, a PERS may be very reassuring and at least alleviate the fear of being helpless if a fall occurs.

EVALUATING EFFECTIVENESS OF NURSING INTERVENTIONS

Nursing care for older adults with impaired musculoskeletal function is evaluated by the degree to which the person achieves and maintains the highest possible level of independence and safe mobility. Nursing care of older adults who are at high risk for osteoporosis is evaluated according to the degree to which the older adult incorporates preventive measures in his or her daily life. For example, older adults might begin a regimen of three half-hour periods of weight-bearing exercise weekly. The nursing care of older adults who are at high risk for falls and fall-related injuries is evaluated according to the extent to which falls and serious injuries are prevented. Nurses cannot, of course, measure the number of falls that do not occur, but they can measure the risk factors that have been addressed in the care plan. Evaluation of these risk factors is facilitated by careful documentation of interventions, such as environmental modifications and fall prevention programs.

Ms. M. is now 89 years old and has been admitted to the hospital for heart failure. Additional medical problems include arthritis, osteoporosis, recurrent depression, early-stage dementia, and history of fractured hip. Current medications include furosemide, 40 mg twice daily; enalapril, 10 mg twice daily; digoxin, 0.125 mg daily; calcitonin nasal spray daily; Os-Cal with D; and sertraline (Zoloft), 50 mg at bedtime. Ms. M. lives alone in an assisted-living facility, where she receives help with her medications and goes to the dining room for meals. You are the nurse on the acute care floor assigned to her care on the day of admission.

NURSING ASSESSMENT

During your initial nursing assessment, Ms. M. is quiet and withdrawn. When you ask about her living situation, she says she moved to the assisted-living facility 2 years ago, after she was hospitalized for treatment of a fractured hip. At the time of the injury, she had been living alone. She had fallen while making her way to the bathroom at night and remained lying on the floor until her daughter came to visit her the next morning. During the past year, Ms. M. reports that she has fallen twice in her room, but that she has been able to call for help and has not had any serious injuries. You determine that Ms. M. will need help in ambulating to the bathroom and that she should be supervised whenever she gets out of bed.

Ms. M. confides that she is worried that she will have to move to the nursing home section of her facility if she falls again. She is very depressed about her lack of energy and her hospitalization for congestive heart failure. A mental status assessment indicates that Ms. M. is alert and oriented but that her short-term memory is impaired. She has a great deal of difficulty with abstract ideas, such as learning to use the call button. You check her vital signs, which are within normal range, with no evidence of postural hypotension.

NURSING DIAGNOSIS

In addition to the nursing diagnoses related to Ms. M.'s medical condition, you identify a nursing diagnosis of Risk for Falls. Related factors include weakness, diuretic and cardiovascular medications, a history of falls, depression, and impaired cognition. You are concerned about preventing falls during her hospitalization.

NURSING CARE PLAN FOR MS. M.

Expected Outcome	Nursing Interventions	Nursing Evaluation
Ms. M. will ambulate safely and avoid falls during her hospitalization.	• Identify Ms. M. as a participant in the fall-prevention program by using an orange wrist bracelet, posting a Fall Alert sign near her bed, and placing an orange Fall Alert sticker on her chart. • Provide Ms. M. with a brochure that explains the fall-prevention program. • Reassess fall risks every shift and document these on the Fall Assessment form included in Ms. M.'s chart. • Talk with Ms. M.'s physician about a referral for physical therapy.	• Ms. M. will receive assistance with ambulation every time she is out of bed. • Ms. M. will not fall during her hospitalization.

Expected Outcome	Nursing Interventions	Nursing Evaluation
	• Keep the call light button within her reach and review instructions for its use every shift.	
	• Assess benefits and risks of using bedrails, and discuss with Ms. M. and her family.	
	• Make sure that the bed is in the lowest possible position with the wheels locked.	
	• Use a movement detection bed pad and explain to Ms. M. that the purpose of the pad is to ensure that the staff knows when she needs to get out of bed.	
	• Every 2 hours, when Ms. M. is awake, the nursing staff will ask her if she needs to go to the bathroom.	

THINKING POINTS

- If you were the nurse on the acute care floor where Ms. M. was a patient, what concerns would you address in a discharge plan? Would you identify any additional nursing diagnoses related to safe mobility and musculoskeletal function? What additional nursing interventions would you plan to supplement the care plan described in this chapter?
- If you were a nurse in the assisted-living facility where Ms. M. lives, what concerns would you have about her care? How would you address these concerns in a care plan?

Chapter Highlights

Age-Related Changes That Affect Mobility and Safety
- Degenerative changes in bones, muscles, joints, and connective tissue
- Central nervous system changes: slowed reactions time, body sway
- Osteopenia and osteoporosis

Risk Factors That Affect Mobility and Safety
- Risk factors for impaired musculoskeletal function: inactivity, inadequate protein and vitamin D intake
- Risk factors for osteoporosis and fractures: inadequate calcium and vitamin D intake, lack of weight-bearing activity, female gender, small bones, increased age, tobacco smoking, excessive alcohol consumption, certain medications (e.g., corticosteroids) (Box 22-1)
- Risk factors for falls: pathologic conditions and functional impairments, medication effects, environmental factors, physical restraints (Box 22-2)

Functional Consequences Affecting Musculoskeletal Wellness
- Diminished muscle strength, endurance, and coordination
- Increased difficulty performing ADLs
- Increased susceptibility to falls
- Increased susceptibility to fall-related injuries, including death
- Fear of falling

Pathologic Condition Affecting Musculoskeletal Wellness
- Osteoarthritis

Nursing Assessment of Musculoskeletal Function
(Box 22-3)
- Assessment of overall musculoskeletal performance
- Risks for osteoporosis (e.g., intake of calcium and vitamin D, history of fractures)
- Identifying risks for falls and injury (Figure 22-1)
- Assessing for safety of the environment

Nursing Diagnosis
- Wellness nursing diagnosis: Readiness for Enhanced Self Health Management
- Related to osteoporosis: Health-Seeking Behaviors, Ineffective Health Maintenance
- Related to fall risks: Impaired Physical Mobility, Risk for Falls
- Additional diagnoses that addresses fear of falling: Fear

Planning for Wellness Outcomes
- Balance, Endurance, Mobility, Activity Tolerance
- Risk Control, Risk Detection
- Safety Behavior: Fall Prevention, Home Physical Environment
- Coping, Fear Control, Comfort Level

Nursing Interventions for Musculoskeletal Wellness
- Teaching about exercise
- Teaching about osteoporosis (e.g., early detection and treatment, lifestyle interventions, nutritional interventions, medications) (Box 22-4, Evidence-Based Practice 22-1)
- Implementing fall prevention programs (e.g., eliminating risks, using monitoring devices, addressing contributing factors) (Box 22-5, Evidence-Based Practice 22-2)

• Preventing fall-related injuries and death (e.g., hip protectors, environmental interventions)
• Addressing fear of falling

Evaluating Effectiveness of Nursing Interventions
• Maintenance of highest level of safe mobility
• Incorporation of preventive measures in daily life to ensure safety and prevent osteoporosis
• Expressed feelings of safety and improved quality of life

Critical Thinking Exercises

1. Identify factors that increase or reduce the risk for osteoporosis.
2. Describe how each of the following age-related changes or risk factors might increase an older person's risk for falls and fractures: nocturia, osteoporosis, medications, altered gait, pathologic conditions, sensory impairments, cognitive impairments, functional impairments, slowed reaction time.
3. Describe the environmental factors that you would assess, in both home and institutional settings, to identify potential risks for falls.
4. Describe how you would design and implement a fall-prevention program in a long-term care facility.
5. How would you deal with a daughter who demanded that restraints be used whenever her 84-year-old mother, who is a patient on your acute care floor, is sitting in a chair?
6. What information would you include in health education about osteoporosis?
7. Use the Internet to find information about fall-prevention products that you might use in clinical practice.

Resources

For links to these resources and additional helpful Internet resources related to this chapter, visit thePoint at http://thePoint.lww.com/Miller6e.

Clinical Tools

American Journal of Nursing and Hartford Institute for Geriatric Nursing
• *How to Try This,* article and video: Hendrich, A. (2007). How to try this: Predicting Patient Falls, article and video. *American Journal of Nursing, 107*(11), 50–58.
Hartford Institute for Geriatric Nursing
• *Try This: Best Practices in Nursing Care to Older Adults* Issue 5 (2007), Fall Risk Assessment for Older Adults: The Hendrich II Fall Risk Model

Evidence-Based Practice

Gray-Miceli, D. (2008). Preventing falls in acute care. In E. Capezuti, D. Zwicker, M. Mezey, & T. Fulmer (Eds.), *Evidence-based geriatric nursing protocols for best practice* (3rd ed., pp. 57–82, 161–198). New York: Springer Publishing Co.
Mion, L. C., Halliday, B. L., & Sandhu, S. K. (2008). Physical restraints and side rails in acute and critical care settings: Legal, ethical, and practice issues. In E. Capezuti, D. Zwicker, M. Mezey, & T. Fulmer (Eds.), *Evidence-based geriatric nursing protocols for best practice* (3rd ed., pp. 503–520). New York: Springer Publishing Co.

National Guideline Clearinghouse
• Prevention of falls in the elderly
• Exercise promotion
• Osteoporosis
• Osteoarthritis

Health Education

American Menopause Foundation, Inc.
Arthritis Foundation
Centers for Disease Control and Prevention
Fall Prevention Center of Excellence
National Arthritis and Musculoskeletal and Skin Diseases Information Clearinghouse
National Osteoporosis Foundation
National Resource Center for Safe Aging

REFERENCES

Adams, J. S., & Hewison, M. (2010). Update in Vitamin D. *Journal of Clinical Endocrinology and Metabolism, 95*(2), 471–478.

Annweiler, C., Schott, A. M., Berrut, G., Fantino, B., & Beauchet, O. (2009). Vitamin D-related changes in physical performance: A systematic review. *Journal of Nutrition, Health and Aging, 13*(10), 893–898.

Baranzini, F., Diurni, M., Ceccon, F., Poloni, N., Cazzamalli, S., Costantini, C., . . . Callegari, C. (2009). Fall-related injuries in a nursing home setting: Is polypharmacy a risk factor? *Bio Medical Central Health Services Research, 9*(228), doi:10.10.1186/1472-6963-9-228.

Bennell, K. L., Hunt, M. A., Wrigley, T. V., Lim, B.-W., & Hinman, R. S. (2009). Muscle and exercise in the prevention and management of knee osteoarthritis: An internal medicine specialist's guide. *Medical Clinics of North America, 93*(1), 161–177.

Berdot, S., Bertrand, M., Dartigues, J. F., Fourrier, A., Tavernier, B., Ritchie, K., & Alpérovitch, A. (2009). Inappropriate medication use and risk of falls-a prospective study in a large community-dwelling elderly cohort. *Bio Med Central Geriatrics, 30,* doi:10.1186/1471-2318-9-30.

Bilezikian, J. P. (2009). Efficacy of bisphosphonates in reducing fracture risk in postmenopausal osteoporosis. *The American Journal of Medicine, 122,* S14–S21.

Bischoff-Ferrari, H. A., Dawson-Hughes, B., Staehelin, H. B., Orav, J. E., Stuck, A. E., Theiler, R., . . . Henschkowski, J. (2009). Fall prevention with supplemental and active forms of vitamin D: A meta-analysis of randomized controlled trials. *BioMed Central, 339,* b3692. doi:10.1136/bmj.b3692.

Bolland, M. J., Grey, A. B., Gamble, G. D., & Reid, I. R. (2010). Effect of osteoporosis treatment on mortality: A meta-analysis. *Journal of Clinical Endocrinology & Metabolism, 95*(3), 1174–1181.

Boyd, R., & Stevens, J. A. (2009). Falls and fear of falling: Burden, beliefs and behaviors. *Age and Ageing, 38*(4), 423–428.

Cameron, I. D., Robinovitch, S., Birge, S., Kannus, P., Khan, K., Lauritzen, J., . . . Kiel, D. P. (2010). Hip protectors: Recommendations for conducting clinical trials—An international consensus statement (part II). *Osteoporosis International, 21*(1), 1–10.

Carbone, L. D., Johnson, K. C., Robbins, J., Larson, J. C., Curb, J. D., Watson, K., . . . Lacroix, A. Z. (2009). Antiepileptic drug use, falls, fractures and BMD in postmenopausal women: Findings from the Women's Health Initiative (WHI). *Journal of Bone & Mineral Research,* doi:10.1359/jbmr.091027.

Castle, N. G., & Engberg, J. (2009). The health consequences of using physical restraints in nursing homes. *Medical Care, 47*(11), 1164–1173.

Chen, K.-M. (2010). Tai chi. In M. Snyder & R. Lindquist (Eds.), *Complementary & alternative therapies in nursing* (6th ed., pp. 373–382.) New York: Springer Publishing Co.

Choi, W. J., Hoffer, J. A., & Robinovitch, S. N. (2010a). The effect of positioning on the biomechanical performance of soft shell hip protectors. *Journal of Biomechanics, 43*(5), 818–825.

Choi, W. J., Hoffer, J. A., & Robinovitch, S. N. (2010b). Effect of hip protectors, falling angle and body mass index on pressure distribution over the hip during simulated falls. *Clinical Biomechanics, 25*(1), 63–69.

Chomentowski, P., Dube, J. J., Amati, F., Stefanovic-Racic, M., Zuh, S., Toledo, F. G. S., & Goodpaster, B. H. (2009). Moderate exercise attenuates the loss of skeletal muscle mass that occurs with intentional caloric restriction—Induced weight loss in older, overweight to obese adults. *Journal of Gerontology Series A: Biological Sciences and Medical Sciences, 64A*(5), 575–580.

Connors, K. A., Galea, M. P., & Said, C. M. (2009). Feldenkrais method balance classes improve balance in older adults: A controlled trial [published online ahead of print June 24, 2009]. *Evidence-Based Complementary and Alternative Medicine*. doi:10.1093/ecam/nep055, 109.

Delbaere, K., Sturnieks, D. L., Crombez, G., & Lord, S. R. (2009). Concern about falls elicits changes in gait parameters in conditions of postural threat in older people. *Journal of Gerontology Series A: Biological Sciences and Medical Sciences, 64A*(2), 237–242.

Demontiero, O., & Duque, G. (2009). Once-yearly zoledronic acid in hip fracture prevention. *Clinical Interventions in Aging, 2009*(4), 153–164.

DIPART Group. (2010). Patient level pooled analysis of 68,500 patients from seven major vitamin D fracture trials in the US and Europe. *British Medical Journal, 340*, b5463. doi:10.1136/bmj.b5463.

Doumas, M., Rapp, M. A., & Krampe, R. T. (2009). Working memory and postural control: Adult age differences in potential for improvement, task priority, and dual tasking. *Journal of Gerontology: Psychological Sciences, 64B*(2), 193–201.

Filiatrault, J., Desrosiers, J., & Trottier, L. (2009). An exploratory study of individual and environmental correlates of fear of falling among community-dwelling seniors. *Journal of Aging & Health, 21*(6), 881–894.

Fishman, L. M. (2009). Yoga for osteoporosis: A pilot study. *Topics in Geriatric Rehabilitation, 25*(3), 244–250.

Fitzgerald, T. G., Hadjistavropoulos, T., & MacNab, Y. C. (2009). Caregiver fear of falling and functional ability among seniors residing in long-term care facilities. *Gerontology, 55*(4), 460–467.

Fonad, E., Emami, A., Wahlin, T. B., Winblad, B., & Sandmark, H. (2009). Falls in somatic and dementia wards at community care units. *Scandinavian Journal of Caring Sciences, 2*(10), 2–10.

Frick, K. D., Kung, J. Y., Parrish, J. M., & Narrett, M. J. (2010). Evaluating the cost-effectiveness of fall prevention programs that reduce fall-related hip fractures in older adults. *Journal of the American Geriatric Society, 58*(1), 136–141.

Gentleman, B., & Malozeimoff, W. (2001). Falls and feelings: Description of a psychosocial group nursing intervention. *Journal of Gerontological Nursing, 27*(10), 35–39.

Giovannucci, E. (2009). Expanding roles of vitamin D. *Journal of Clinical Endocrinology and Metabolism, 94*(2), 418–420.

Gray-Miceli, D. (2008). Preventing falls in acute care. In E. Capezuti, D. Zwicker, M. Mezey, & T. Fulmer (Eds.), *Evidence-based geriatric nursing protocols for best practice* (3rd ed., pp. 57–82, 161–198). New York: Springer Publishing Co.

Groen, B. E., Smulders, E., deKam, D., Duysens, J., & Weerdesteyn, V. (2010). Martial arts fall training to prevent hip fractures in the elderly. *Osteoporosis, International, 21*(2), 215–221.

Hanlon, J. T., Boudreau, R. M., Roumani, Y. F., Newman, A. B., Ruby, C. M., Wright, R. M., . . . for the Health ABC study (2009). Number and dosage of central nervous system medications on recurrent falls in community elders: The health, aging and body composition study. *Journal of Gerontology Series A: Biological Sciences and Medical Sciences, 64A*(4), 492–498.

Hansma, A. H., Emmelot-Vonk, M. H., & Verhaar, H. J. (2010). Reduction in falling after a falls-assessment. *Archives of Gerontology and Geriatrics, 50*(1), 73–76.

Hegeman, J., Van Den Bemt, B. J., Duysens, J., & van Limbeek, J. (2009). NSAIDs and the risk of accidental falls in the elderly: A systematic review. *Drug Safety, 32*(6), 489–498.

Hendrich, A. (2007). How to try this: Predicting patient falls. *American Journal of Nursing, 107*(11), 50–58.

Horan, A., & Timmins, F. (2009). The role of community multidisciplinary teams in osteoporosis treatment and prevention. *Journal of Orthopaedic Nursing, 13*, 85–96.

Huntijens, K. M., Kosar, S., van Geel, T. A., Geusens, P. P., Willems, P., Kessels, A., . . . van Helden, S. (2010). Risk of subsequent fracture and mortality within 5 years after a non-vertebral fracture (published online ahead of print February 17, 2010). *Osteoporosis International*.

Iglesias, C. P., Manca, A., & Torgerson, D. J. (2009). The health-related quality of life and cost implications of falls in elderly women. *Osteoporosis International, 20*(6), 869–878.

Institute for Clinical Systems Improvement. (2008). *Prevention of falls (acute care)*. Bloomington MN: Institute for Clinical Systems Improvement. Retrieved from www.guideline.gov.

Ioannidis, G., Papioannou, A., Hopman, W. M., Akhtar-Danesh, N., Anastassiades, T., Pickard, L., . . . Adachi, J. D. (2009). Relation between fractures and mortality: Results from the Canadian Multicentre Osteoporosis Study. *Canadian Medication Association Journal, 181*(5), 265–269.

Kannegaard, P. N., Van Der Mark, S., Eiken, P., & Abrahamsen, B. (2010). Excess mortality in men compared with women following a hip fracture. National analysis of comedications, comorbidity and survival. *Age and Ageing, 39*(2), 203–209.

Kempen, G. I. J. M., van Haastreg, J. C. M., McKee, K. J., Delbaere, K., & Zijlstra, G. A. R. (2009). Socio-demographic, health-related and psychosocial correlates of fear of falling and avoidance of activity in community-living older persons who avoid activity due to fear of falling. *BioMed Central Public Health, 9*(170), doi:10.1186/1471-2458-9-170.

Kenny, R. A. M., Rubenstein, L. Z., & Tinetti, M. E. (2010). AGS/ABS Clinical Practice Guideline: Prevention of falls in older persons. American Geriatrics Society. Retrieved from www.americangeriatrics.org.

Khosla, S. (2010). Update in male osteoporosis. *Journal of Clinical Endocrinology and Metabolism, 95*(1), 3–10.

Koike, T., Orito, Y., Toyoda, H., Tada, M., Sugama, R., Hosino, M., . . . Takaoka, K. (2009). External hip protectors are effective for the elderly with higher-than-average risk factors for hip fractures. *Osteoporosis International, 20*(9), 1613–1620.

Lamoureux, E., Gadgil, S., Pesudovs, K., Keeffe, J., Fenwick, E., Salonen, S., . . . Rees, G. (2010). The relationship between visual function, duration and main causes of vision loss and falls in older people with low vision (published online ahead of print January 7, 2010) *Graefe's Archives in Clinical and Experimental Ophthalmology*.

Lash, R. W., Nicholson, J. M., Velez, L., Van Harrison, R., McCort, J. (2009). Diagnosis and management of osteoporosis. *Primary Care in Clinical Office Practice, 36*(2009), 181–198.

Lawrence, T. M., Wenn, R., Boulton, C. T., & Moran, C. G. (2010). Age-specific incidence of first and second fractures of the hip. *Journal of Bone Joint Surgery, 92*(2), 258–261.

Layman, D. K., & Rodriguez, N. R. (2009). Egg protein as source of power, strength, and energy. *Nutrition Today, 44*(1), 43–48.

Lloyd, B. D., Williamson, D. A., Singh, N. A., Hansen, R. D., Diamond, T. H., Finnegan, T. P., . . . Singh, M. A. F. (2009). Recurrent and injurious falls in the year following hip fracture: A prospective study of incidence and risk factors from the Sarcopenia and Hip Fracture Study. *Journal of Gerontology Series A: Biological Sciences and Medical Sciences, 64A*(5), 599–609.

Low, S., Ang, L. W., Goh, K. S., & Chew, S. K. (2009). A systematic review of the effectiveness of Tai Chi on fall reduction among the elderly. *Archives of Gerontology and Geriatrics, 48*(3), 325–331.

Lui, P. P. Y., Qin, L., & Chan, K. M. (2008). Tai Chi Chuan exercises in enhancing bone mineral density in active seniors. *Clinics in Sports Medicine, 27*(2008), 75–86.

Mion, L. C., Halliday, B. L., & Sandhu, S. K. (2008). Physical restraints and side rails in acute and critical care settings: Legal, ethical, and practice issues. In E. Capezuti, D. (Ed.), *Evidence-Based Geriatric Nursing Protocols for Best Practice* (3rd ed., pp. 503–520). New York: Springer Publishing Co.

Murphy, J., & Isaacs, B. (1982). The post-fall syndrome. *Gerontology, 28,* 265–270.

NANDA International. (2009). *Nursing diagnoses: Definitions and classification 2009–2011.* Oxford, UK: Wiley-Blackwell.

North American Menopause Society. (2010). Management of osteoporosis in postmenopausal women: 2010 position statement of The North American Menopause Society. *Menopause, 17*(1), 25–54.

Parikh, S., Avorn, J., & Solomon, D. H. (2009). Pharmacological management of osteoporosis in nursing home populations: A systematic review. *Journal of the American Geriatric Society, 57*(2), 327–334.

Pellfolk, T. J., Gustafson, Y., Bucht, G., & Karlsson, S. (2010). Effects of a restraint minimization program on staff knowledge, attitudes, and practice: A cluster randomized trial. *Journal of American Geriatric Society, 58*(1), 62–69.

Pereira, S. R., Puts, M. T. E., Portela, M. C., & Sayeg, M. A. (2009). The impact of hip fracture (HF) on the functional status (FS) of older persons in Rio de Janeiro, Brazil: Results of a prospective cohort study. *Archives of Gerontology and Geriatrics,* doi:10.1016/j.archger. 2009.08.007.

Petty, S. J., Hill, K. D., Haber, N. E., Paton, L. M., Lawrence, K. M., Berkovic, S. F., . . . Wark, J. D. (2009). Balance impairment in chronic antiepileptic drug users: A twin and sibling study. *Epilepsia, 51*(2), 280–288.

Rhalimi M., Helou, R., & Jaecker, P. (2009). Medication use and increased risk of falls in hospitalized elderly patients: A retrospective, case-control study. *Drugs & Aging, 2*(10), 847–852.

Rahmani, P., & Morin, S. (2009). Prevention of osteoporosis-related fractures among postmenopausal women and older men. *Canadian Medical Association Journal, 181*(11), 815–819.

Recker, R. R., Lewiecki, E. M., Miller, P. D., & Reiffel, J. (2009). Safety of bisphosphonates in the treatment of osteoporosis. *The American Journal of Medicine, 122,* S22–S32.

Royal Australian College of General Practitioners. (2009). *Guidelines for the non-surgical management of hip and knee osteoarthritis.* Australian Government: Royal Australian College of General Practitioners.

Schmid, A. A., Acuff, M., Doster, K., Gwaltney-Duiser, A., Damush, T., Williams, L., & Hendrie, H. (2009). Poststroke fear of falling in the hospital setting. *Topics in Stroke Rehabilitation, 16*(5), 357–366.

Sharaf, A. Y., & Ibrahim, H. S. (2008). Physical and psychosocial correlates of fear of falling among older adults in assisted living facilities. *Journal of Gerontological Nursing, 34*(12), 27–35.

Society of Obstetricians and Gynaecologists of Canada. (2009). Menopause and osteoporosis update 2009. *Journal of Obstetrics and Gynaecology Canada, 31,* S1–S3.

Sheldon, J. H. (1960). On the natural history of falls in old age. *British Medical Journal, 2,* 1685–1690.

Stolee, P., Poss, J., Cook, R. J., Byrne, K., & Hirdes, J. P. (2009). Risk factors for hip fracture in older home care clients. *Journal of Gerontology Series A: Biological Sciences and Medical Sciences, 64A*(3), 403–410.

Sweet, M. G., Sweet, J. M., Jeremiah, M. P., & Galazka, S. S. (2009). Diagnosis and treatment of osteoporosis. *American Family Physician, 79*(3), 193–200.

Tinetti, M. E., & Kumar, C. (2010). The patient who falls: "It's always a trade-off". *Journal of the American Medical Association, 303*(3), 258–266.

Treat-Jacobson, D., Bronas, U. G., & Mark, D. L. (2010). Exercise. In M. Snyder & R. Lindquist (Eds.), *Complementary & alternative therapies in nursing* (6th ed., pp. 349–372). New York: Springer Publishing Company.

Tsunoda, K., Uchida, H., Suzuki, T., Watanabe, K., Yamashima, T., & Kashima, H. (2010). Effects of discontinuing benzodiazepine-derivative hypnotics on postural sway and cognitive functions in the elderly. *International Journal of Geriatric Psychiatry,* doi:10.1002.gps.2465.

Ullmann, G., Williams, H. G., Hussey, J., Durstine, J. L., & McClenaghan, B. A. (2010). Effects of Feldenkrais exercises on balance, mobility, balance confidence, and gait performance in community-dwelling adults age 65 and older. *Journal of Alternative and Complementary Medicine, 16*(1), 97–105.

Verdijk, L. B., Gleeson, B. G., Jonkers, R. A. M., Meijer, K., Savelberg, H. H. C. M., Dendale, P., & van Loon, L. J. (2009). Skeletal muscle hypertrophy following resistance training is accompanied by a fiber type-specific increase in satellite cell content I elderly men. *Journal of Gerontology Series A: Biological Sciences and Medical Sciences, 64A*(3), 332–339.

Vondracek, S. F., & Linnebur, S. A. (2009). Diagnosis and management of osteoporosis in the older senior. *Clinical Intervention in Aging, 4,* 121–136.

Vrantsidis, F., Hill, K. D., Moore, K., Webb, R., Hunt, S., & Dowson, L. (2009). Getting grounded gracefully: Effectiveness and acceptability of Feldenkrais in improving balance. *Journal of Aging and Physical Activity, 17*(1), 57–76.

Williams, S. B., Brand, C. A., Hill, K. D., Hunt, S. B., & Moran, H. (2010). Feasibility and outcomes of a home-based exercise program on improving balance and gait stability in women with lower-limb osteoarthritis or rheumatoid arthritis: A pilot study. *Archives of Physical Medicine and Rehabilitation, 91*(1), 106–114.

Woolcott, J. C., Richardson, K. J., Wiens, M. O., Patel, B., Marin, J., Khan, K. M., & Marra, C. A. (2009). Meta-analysis of the impact of 9 medication classes on falls in elderly persons. *Archives of Internal Medicine, 169*(21), 1952–1960.

Zecevic, A. A., Salmoni, A. W., Lewko, J. H., Vandervoort, A. A., & Speechley, M. (2009). Utilization of seniors falls investigation methodology to identify system-wide causes of falls in community-dwelling seniors. *The Gerontologist, 49*(5), 685–696.

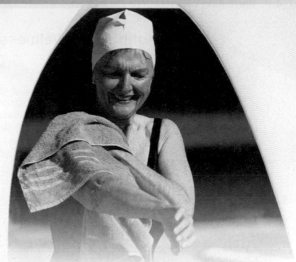

CHAPTER 23

Integument

LEARNING OBJECTIVES

After reading this chapter, you will be able to:

1. Delineate age-related changes that affect the skin, hair, nails, and glands.

2. Describe risk factors that can affect skin wellness for older adults.

3. Discuss the functional consequences of age-related changes and risk factors that affect the skin, hair, nails, and glands.

4. Assess skin in older adults, and recognize normal and pathologic skin changes.

5. Describe the assessment, prevention, and management of pressure ulcers.

6. Implement nursing interventions to address the following aspects of skincare: maintenance of healthy skin, prevention of xerosis, and referrals for the treatment of pathologic skin lesions.

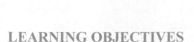

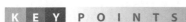	
basal cell carcinoma	photosensitivity
melanoma	pressure ulcer
Mongolian spots	squamous cell carcinoma
photoaging	xerosis

For many people, and particularly for older adults, skin is the most visible indicator of the combined effects of biologic aging, lifestyle, and environment. Thus, the skin, hair, and nails have not only physiologic functions but also many social functions. Physiologically, the skin directly affects all of the following processes:

- Thermoregulation
- Excretion of metabolic wastes
- Protection of underlying structures

- Synthesis of vitamin D
- Maintenance of fluid and electrolyte balance
- Sensation of pain, touch, pressure, temperature, and vibration

The social functions of the skin include facilitating communication and serving as an indicator of race, gender, work status, and other personal characteristics.

Hair serves to protect underlying organs, primarily the skin, from injury and adverse temperatures. In addition, in social contexts, the length and style of one's hair can reflect certain characteristics such as age, gender, and personality. Although hair is one of the most visible manifestations of aging, hair color can easily be altered if gray is viewed as an undesirable indicator of age. Like the skin and hair, nails have both a physiologic and social capacity. Physiologically, nails protect the underlying tissue from injury. In social contexts, nails can reflect personal characteristics such as grooming and occupational activities.

 AGE-RELATED CHANGES THAT AFFECT THE SKIN

The skin is the largest, as well as the most visible, body organ. Structurally, the skin comprises three layers: the epidermis, the dermis, and the subcutaneous tissue. Hair, nails, and sweat glands are also parts of the integumentary system. As with many other aspects of functionality, it is difficult to distinguish between changes that are strictly attributable to aging and those that occur because of risk factors. Genetics, lifestyle, and environmental factors exert a significant effect on skin throughout the lifespan and have a cumulative effect in older adults.

Epidermis

The epidermis is the relatively impermeable outer layer of skin that serves as a barrier, preventing both the loss of body fluids and the entry of substances from the environment. The density of the epidermis varies, depending on the part of the body it covers. The epidermis comprises layers of cells that undergo a continual cycle of regeneration, cornification, and shedding. Epidermal cells develop in the innermost layer of

Promoting Skin Wellness in Older Adults

Nursing Assessment
- Usual activities that affect skin and risk for skin cancer
- Abnormal skin conditions
- Knowledge about risks and protective behaviors
- Risks for pressure ulcers

Age-Related Changes
- ↓ epidermal proliferation
- Thinner dermis, flattened dermal-epidermal junction
- ↓ moisture content
- ↓ sweat and sebaceous glands

Negative Functional Consequences
- Wrinkles, dry skin
- Slower wound healing
- ↓ sweating, shivering, tactile sensitivity
- ↑ susceptibility to skin cancer
- ↑ susceptibility to burns, bruises, and breakdown

Risk Factors
- Exposure to ultraviolet light
- Adverse medication effects
- Personal hygiene practices
- Conditions that ↑ risk for pressure ulcers

Nursing Interventions
- Teaching about self-care for healthy skin
- Teaching about detection and treatment of skin cancer
- Preventing and managing pressure ulcers

Wellness Outcomes
- Improved comfort
- Maintenance of intact and healthy skin
- Elimination of risk for skin cancer
- Absence (or quick healing) of pressure ulcers

the epidermis and continually migrate to the surface of the skin where they are shed. With increasing age, these cells become larger and more variable in shape, and the rate of epidermal turnover gradually decreases.

Melanocytes are epidermal cells that give the skin its color and provide a protective barrier against ultraviolet radiation. Beginning around the age of 25 years, the number of active melanocytes decreases by 10% to 20% each decade. Although this decline occurs in both sun-exposed and sun-protected skin, the density of melanocytes in exposed skin is double or triple that in unexposed skin. With increased age, the number of Langerhans cells, which serve as macrophages, also decreases in both sun-exposed and sun-protected skin; the decrease ranges from 50% to 70% in sun-exposed skin. Another age-related change is a decrease in the moisture content of the outer epidermal layer.

Papillae give the skin its texture and connect the epidermis to the underlying dermis at the dermal–epidermal junction. With increased age, the papillae retract, causing a flattening of the dermal–epidermal junction and diminishing the surface area between the epidermis and dermis. This age-related change slows the transfer of nutrients between the dermis and epidermis. In contrast to other epidermal changes that are more prominent on exposed skin surfaces, this change occurs to some degree on all skin surfaces.

Dermis

The primary functions of the dermis are

- Provision of support for structures within and below this layer
- Nourishment of the epidermis, which has no blood supply of its own
- Coloration
- Sensory perception
- Temperature regulation.

Collagen, which constitutes 80% of the dermis, confers elasticity and tensile strength, which help to prevent tearing and overstretching of the skin. Elastin, which constitutes 5% of the dermis, maintains skin tension and allows for stretching in response to movement. The dermal ground substance, which has a water-binding capacity, determines skin turgor and elastic properties. Blood vessels in the deep plexus play a role in thermoregulation, and those in the superficial plexus supply nutrients to the epidermal layer. Cutaneous nerves in the dermis receive information from the environment regarding pain, pressure, temperature, and deep and light touch.

Beginning in early adulthood, dermal thickness gradually diminishes, with collagen thinning at a rate of 1% per year. Elastin increases in quantity and decreases in quality because of age-related and environmentally induced changes. The dermal vascular bed decreases by approximately one-third with increased age; this contributes to the atrophy and fibrosis of hair bulbs, sweat, and sebaceous glands. Additional age-related changes in the dermis include a decrease in the number of fibroblasts and mast cells.

Subcutaneous Tissue and Cutaneous Nerves

The subcutis is the inner layer of fat tissue that protects the underlying tissues from trauma. Additional functions include the storage of calories, insulation of the body, and regulation of heat loss. With increased age, some areas of subcutaneous tissue atrophy, particularly in the plantar foot surface and in sun-exposed areas of the hands, face, and lower legs. Other areas of subcutaneous tissue hypertrophy, however, with the overall effect being a gradual increase in the proportion of body fat between the third and eighth decades. This increased body fat is more pronounced in women than in men and is most noticeable in the waists of men and the thighs of women. Age-related changes also affect the cutaneous nerves responsible for sensations of pressure, vibration, and light touch.

Sweat and Sebaceous Glands

Eccrine and apocrine sweat glands originate in the dermal layer and are most abundant in the palms of the hands, soles of the feet, and axillae. Eccrine glands, which are important for thermoregulation, open directly onto the skin surface and are most abundant on the palms, soles, and forehead. Apocrine glands are larger than eccrine glands and open into hair follicles, primarily in the axillae and genital area. The sole function of these glands is to produce secretions, which create a distinctive body odor when they decompose. Both eccrine and apocrine glands decrease in number and functional ability with increased age.

Sebaceous glands are present in the dermal skin layer over every part of the body except the palms of the hands and the soles of the feet. These glands continually secrete sebum—a substance that combines with sweat to form an emulsion. Functionally, sebum prevents the loss of water and serves as a mild retardant of bacterial and fungal growth. The secretion of sebum begins to diminish during the third decade, with women having a greater decline than men. In younger adults, sebum production is closely related to the size of the sebaceous glands; however, in older adults, the sebaceous glands increase in size but produce less sebum.

Nails

The rate of nail growth is influenced by many factors including age, climate, state of health, circulation to and around the nails, and activity of the fingers and toes. Nail growth begins to slow in early adulthood, with a gradual decrease of 30% to 50% over the individual's lifespan. Other age-related changes affecting the nails include the development of longitudinal striations and a decrease in lunula size and nail plate thickness. Because of these changes, the nails become increasingly soft, fragile, and brittle and are more prone to splitting. In appearance, the older nail is dull, opaque, longitudinally striated, and yellow or gray.

Hair

Hair color and distribution change to some degree in all older adults, with the most noticeable changes being baldness and gray hair. By the age of 50 years, approximately 50% of people have graying hair and approximately 60% of white men have a noticeable degree of baldness. Graying of the hair results from a decline in melanin production and the gradual replacement of pigmented hairs by nonpigmented ones. Age-related changes also affect hair distribution, with patches of coarse terminal hair developing over the upper lip and lower face in older women and in the ears, nares, and eyebrows of older men. Another age-related change is a progressive loss of body hair, initially in the trunk, then in the pubic area and axillae. In addition, some men are genetically predisposed to baldness, which is attributable to a change in production from coarse terminal hair to fine vellus hair.

DIVERSITY NOTE

White people develop wrinkles and gray hair at an earlier age than other ethnic groups in the United States.

RISK FACTORS THAT AFFECT SKIN WELLNESS

The risk factors that influence the skin and hair of older adults include heredity, lifestyle and environmental factors, and adverse medication effects. Lifestyle and environmental factors have a cumulative effect that manifests more fully during later adulthood, but it is important to identify the risk factors that nurses can address through health education. Risk factors associated with **pressure ulcers** and skin cancer are addressed in the section on Pathologic Conditions Affecting the Skin.

Genetic Influences

Heredity plays an important role in the development of skin and hair changes. People with fair skin, light hair, and light eyes are more sensitive to the effects of ultraviolet radiation than people with dark skin, as evidenced by the fact that skin cancers are common in light-skinned people of northern European ancestry but rare in African Americans.

Lifestyle and Environmental Influences

Smoking, sun exposure, emotional stress, and substance or alcohol abuse are the lifestyle and environmental factors that significantly affect skin wellness. Exposure to ultraviolet radiation is the most significant environmental factor, but adverse climate conditions can also cause negative functional consequences. For example, because the water content of the stratum corneum is influenced by relative humidity, **xerosis** (dry skin) is exacerbated when the relative humidity is below 30%.

Photoaging is the term used to describe skin changes that occur because of exposure to ultraviolet radiation, even at levels that do not cause any detectable sunburn. Although these changes are often viewed as premature aging, they are biologically distinct processes (Habif, 2010). Characteristics of sun-damaged skin include

- Coarse, leathery, and ruddy or yellowed appearance
- Many deep wrinkles, particularly on the face and neck
- Pathologic lesions and seborrheic and actinic keratoses
- Thickened epidermis
- Enlarged sebaceous glands
- Marked loss of elasticity
- Dilated and tortuous blood vessels
- Decreased amounts of mature collagen.

One reason for the common misconception that photoaging is an age-related change is that the cumulative effects of ultraviolet radiation may not be evident until later adulthood.

Cigarette smoking is another factor that has been associated with detrimental skin changes, as well as with hair changes such as balding and gray hair. The skin of people who smoke is likely to have more wrinkles and a grayish discoloration. Smoking also diminishes the skin's ability to protect against ultraviolet radiation damage and increases the risk of skin cancer. Studies of twins consistently identify cigarette smoking and sun exposure as environmental factors that contribute to

skin aging (Guyuron et al., 2009; Martires, Polster, Cooper, & Baron, 2009). A cross-sectional study using a computer analysis of a standardized facial imaging system found that smoking status and topical sun protection were significantly associated with skin condition in older adults (Asakura, 2009).

Cultural factors, societal attitudes, and advertising trends influence hygiene and skincare practices. People in industrialized societies place a high value on frequent bathing and the use of commercial products for hygienic and cosmetic purposes. Although most of the personal practices associated with these values are desirable or harmless in younger adults, they may adversely affect older adults. For example, frequent bathing with harsh deodorant soaps may cause or exacerbate dry skin problems in an older person.

> **Wellness Opportunity**
>
> From a holistic perspective, nurses need to nonjudgmentally consider the influence of cultural and societal attitudes on personal care practices and address any factors that negatively affect self-esteem.

Medication Effects

Common adverse medication effects involving the skin include pruritus, dermatoses, and **photosensitivity** reactions. Less common adverse medication effects on the skin and hair include alopecia and pigmentation changes of the skin or hair. Cytotoxic agents are the type of drug most commonly associated with hair loss, but other drugs that can cause alopecia include anticoagulants, levodopa, indomethacin, propranolol, and drugs that are used for gout and cholesterol (Habif, 2010). In addition, medications can exacerbate age-related skin changes. For example, fluid loss from diuretics can exacerbate xerosis and cause further discomfort or skin problems for the older adult. Another example of the combined effects of aging and medications is that older adults taking anticoagulants are likely to bruise easily and have more extensive bruising.

Dermatoses, or rashes, are the most frequently cited adverse medication effect, and they can be caused by virtually any medication. Medication-related skin eruptions vary widely in their manifestations, including their onset. Drug rashes can occur from 1 day to 4 weeks after initiating or discontinuing the causative medication; the most common type of drug-related skin reaction is maculopapular eruptions. Antibiotics are the type of medication most often associated with skin eruptions; however, any medication can cause skin reactions. Medications that commonly cause dermatitis include allopurinol, ampicillin, bacitracin, erythromycin, gentamicin, miconazole, naproxen, neomycin, penicillin, pseudoephedrine, streptomycin, and inhaled or systemic corticosteroids (Habif, 2010; Nijhawan, Molenda, Airwas, & Jacob, 2009).

Photosensitivity is an adverse medication effect that causes an intensified response to ultraviolet radiation. The inflammatory reaction is initially distributed over sun-exposed areas, but it may spread to nonexposed areas and persist even after the medication is discontinued. Photosensitivity may begin during a seasonal exposure to bright sunlight or during a vacation in an unusually hot climate. Amiodarone, furosemide, naproxen, phenothiazines, sulfonamides, tetracyclines, and thiazides are examples of medications that can cause photosensitivity reactions. Some herbal preparations may also increase the risk of photosensitivity (e.g., St. John's wort) (Habif, 2010).

 ## FUNCTIONAL CONSEQUENCES AFFECTING SKIN WELLNESS

Age-related changes and risk factors negatively affect many functions of the skin including thermoregulation, tactile sensitivity, and response to injury. Age-related changes do not interfere with the protective function of the nails; however, the nails in older persons are brittle and more likely to split. Psychosocial consequences may result when changes in the appearance of the skin and hair are associated with negative attitudes about visible indicators of aging.

Susceptibility to Injury

Progressive degenerative changes of the skin combine with the effects of long-term exposure to the sun and other detrimental environmental conditions to increase the susceptibility of older adults to skin disorders such as skin tears, pressure ulcers, stasis dermatitis, autoimmune skin conditions, and drug reactions (Farage, 2009). In addition, skin lesions often develop, as discussed in the sections on Skin Cancer and Assessment.

Because of the flattened dermal–epidermal junction, older skin is less resistant to shearing forces and is therefore more susceptible to bruises and shear-type injuries. The age-related decrease in dermal thickness compounds the effects of the flattened dermal–epidermal junction, further increasing the susceptibility of older skin to injury and the effects of mechanical stress and ultraviolet radiation. Collagen changes also interfere with the tensile strength of the skin, causing it to be less resilient and more susceptible to damage from abrasive or tearing forces. In addition to advanced age, risk factors associated with skin tears include immobility; polypharmacy; poor nutrition; and sensory, cognitive, or functional impairment (LeBlanc & Baranoski, 2009).

The regeneration of healthy skin takes twice as long for an 80-year-old person as for a 30-year-old person. In perfectly intact skin, this slowed regeneration has no noticeable effects. When skin integrity is compromised, however, this age-related change contributes to delayed wound healing, even for superficial wounds. The consequences of age-related changes that affect the healing of deep wounds include an increased risk for postoperative wound disruption, decreased tensile strength of healing wounds, and increased risk of secondary infections.

DIVERSITY NOTE

Risk factors for skin tears include female sex and white race (LeBlanc & Baranoski, 2009).

Response to Ultraviolet Radiation

The age-related decrease in melanocytes causes older adults to tan less deeply and more slowly when exposed to ultraviolet radiation, and the increased variability in melanocyte density in exposed and unexposed skin may cause a mottled and irregular appearance in the skin's overall pigmentation. A positive functional consequence of age-related melanocyte changes is a decrease in the occurrence of moles beginning around the fourth decade. Aside from these cosmetic effects, a more serious functional consequence of the age-related decrease in melanocytes is the increased incidence of skin cancers in older adults. Other factors that increase the susceptibility of older adults to skin cancers are increased age, decreased number of Langerhans cells, and cumulative exposure to ultraviolet radiation.

Comfort and Sensation

Dry skin is one of the most universal complaints of older adults; indeed, it has been observed in up to 85% of noninstitutionalized older people. Age-related changes, such as diminished output of sebum and eccrine sweat, contribute to a decrease in the moisture content of the skin. Risk factors that may contribute to dry skin include stress, smoking, sun exposure, dry environments, excessive perspiration, adverse medication reactions, excessive use of soap, and certain medical conditions (e.g., hypothyroidism).

Tactile sensitivity begins to decline around the age of 20 years, eventually causing older adults to have a diminished and less intense response to cutaneous sensations. This decline is attributable, at least in part, to age-related changes in Pacinian and Meissner's corpuscles, which are the skin receptors that respond to vibration. Other contributing factors include lower body temperature and functional alterations in the central nervous system. Functionally, older adults are more susceptible to scald burns because of their diminished ability to feel dangerously hot water temperatures.

Thermoregulation is also affected by age-related reductions in eccrine sweat, subcutaneous fat, and dermal blood supply. These age-related changes interfere with sweating, shivering, peripheral vasoconstriction and vasodilation, and insulation against adverse environmental temperatures. Thus, older adults are more at risk for the development of hypothermia and heat-related illnesses, as discussed in Chapter 25.

Cosmetic Effects

The overall cosmetic effect of age-related skin changes is that the skin looks paler, thinner, more translucent, and is irregularly pigmented. Additional indicators of age-related skin changes include sagging, wrinkling, and various growths and lesions. Skin coloration changes are attributable to decreased melanocytes and dermal circulation. Wrinkling and sagging of the skin are caused by age-related changes in the epidermis and dermis, particularly those changes that affect the collagen fibers. Decreased subcutaneous tissue contributes to the sagging of the skin, particularly over the upper arms, by allowing gravity to pull the skin downward.

TABLE 23-1 Functional Consequences Affecting Skin and Appendages

Age-Related Change	Consequence
Decreased rate of epidermal proliferation	Delayed wound healing; increased susceptibility to infection
Flattened dermal–epidermal junction; thinning of dermis and collagen; increased quantity, but decreased quality, of elastin	Decreased resiliency; increased susceptibility to injury, bruising, mechanical stress, ultraviolet radiation, and blister formation
Reductions in dermal blood supply and the number of melanocytes and Langerhans cells	Decreased intensity of tanning; irregular pigmentation; increased susceptibility to skin cancer; diminished dermal clearance, absorption, and immunologic response
Reductions in eccrine sweat, subcutaneous fat, and dermal blood supply	Decreased sweating and shivering; increased susceptibility to hypothermia or hyperthermia
Decreased moisture content	Dry skin; discomfort
Decreased number of Meissner's and Pacinian corpuscles	Diminished tactile sensitivity; increased susceptibility to burns
Slowed nail growth	Increased susceptibility to cracking and injury; delayed healing
Changes in hair color, quantity, and distribution	Negative impact on self-esteem in proportion to negative attitudes

Although these changes in appearance are gradual and do not interfere significantly with physiologic function, the psychosocial consequences of these changes can be significant because of the social value placed on personal appearance and negative attitudes that may be held about growing old. Regardless of age, one's physical appearance has been shown to be an important determinant of self-perception, and modern societies associate attractiveness with young-looking skin.

> **◆ Wellness Opportunity**
>
> Nurses can promote positive attitudes about aging by challenging societal perspectives that associate beauty only with youth.

Because of the high visibility of the face and neck, any signs of increased age that are prominent around the eyes and mouth may be particularly bothersome to the person who wants to avoid visible indications of age. Characteristic signs of advanced age that are evident around the eyes include increased pigmentation, crow's-feet wrinkles, and fat and fluid accumulation in the upper lid and under the eye. Also, because of diminished skin elasticity and the loss and shifting of subcutaneous fat, the neck skin sags, and a double chin may develop. Table 23-1 summarizes the functional consequences resulting from age-related changes of the skin, hair, nails, and glands.

PATHOLOGIC CONDITIONS AFFECTING SKIN: SKIN CANCER AND PRESSURE ULCERS

Skin Cancer

Skin cancer, defined as an abnormal growth of skin cells, is the most common—as well as the most preventable—type of cancer. Older adults are highly vulnerable to the two most common types of skin cancer, primarily because of the cumulative effects of sun exposure. **Basal cell carcinoma**, which is the most common type, occurs most often on the head and neck (Figure 23-1A). If diagnosed and treated during its early stage, the cure rate for basal cell carcinoma is close to 100%; however, if left untreated, it invades the surrounding tissue. **Squamous cell carcinoma**, the second most common type, occurs most commonly on the head, neck, forearms, and dorsal hands. (Figure 23-1B).

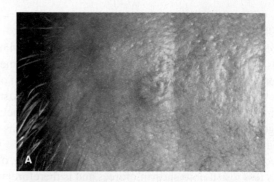
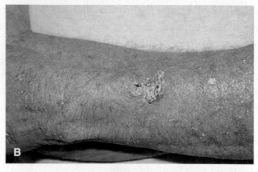
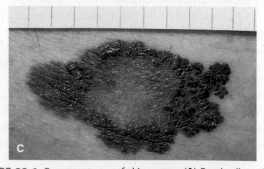

FIGURE 23-1 Common types of skin cancer. (**A**) Basal cell carcinoma. (**B**) Squamous cell carcinoma. (**C**) Melanoma. (**A & B**, Reprinted with permission from Rosenthal, T. C., Williams, M. E., & Naughton, B. J. [2007]. *Office care geriatrics*. Philadelphia: Lippincott Williams & Wilkins; and **C**, from Goodheart, H. P. [2003]. *Goodheart's photoguide of common skin disorders*. Philadelphia: Lippincott Williams & Wilkins.)

Melanoma, which is the most serious type of skin cancer, originates in the melanocytes (see Figure 23-1C). The incidence of melanoma has been gradually increasing in recent decades, with older men accounting disproportionately for the increase (Tucker, 2009). Men aged 60 and 70 years have experienced more than a fourfold and fivefold increase, respectively, in incidence in the United States between 1975 and 2005 (Geller, 2009). Melanoma is the skin cancer most likely to metastasize and cause death, with nearly three-quarters of all melanoma deaths occurring in people aged 55 years and older (Geller, 2009).

DIVERSITY NOTE

The rate of melanoma in African Americans is less than one-twentieth that of whites; however, the 5-year survival rate for minorities is significantly lower than that of whites (72%–81% versus 89.6%) (Geller, 2009).

Early detection and treatment are imperative for improving the outcomes of all types of skin cancer, and nurses have an essential role in assessing and teaching older adults about skin cancer, as discussed in the sections on Nursing Assessment and Nursing Interventions. Nurses also need to be alert to risk factors, so they consider these in their assessments and address them in health promotion. Advanced age increases the risk for all types of skin lesions including skin cancers. Exposure to ultraviolet rays, including those from tanning booths, is a risk factor that is highly associated with skin cancers and that is most amenable to protective measures. Studies indicate that chronic sun exposure, which is the type that one receives during usual daily outdoor activities, is less of a risk for melanoma than intermittent excessive exposure (Berwick &

Erdei, 2009). Additional risk factors for melanoma include a personal or family history of melanoma and fair skin that burns easily and has many large or irregular moles.

Wellness Opportunity

Nurses promote self-care for wellness by teaching older adults to examine their skin for suspicious changes once a month.

Pressure Ulcers

A pressure ulcer is a "localized injury to the skin and/or underlying tissue, usually over a bony prominence, as a result of pressure or pressure in combination with shear and/or friction" (National Pressure Ulcer Advisory Panel, 2007). Although most older adults do not have mobility or activity limitations that are serious enough to increase the risk of skin breakdown, for the small percentage of older people who do, this risk is a major problem with far-reaching negative functional consequences. Because the primary contributing factor in the development of pressure ulcers is persistent pressure, people who lack the ability to move around independently, even for short periods (e.g., during hospitalizations) are most vulnerable (Figure 23-2). Researchers have concluded that prolonged low levels of pressure can be as damaging as short periods of high pressure, particularly in people whose ability to adapt to pressure is impaired (Dealey, 2009).

In recent years, there has been increasing attention to the serious consequences of pressure ulcers, including the high cost, which may be as high as $11 billion annually (Chicano & Drolshagen, 2009). This increased attention is due, at least

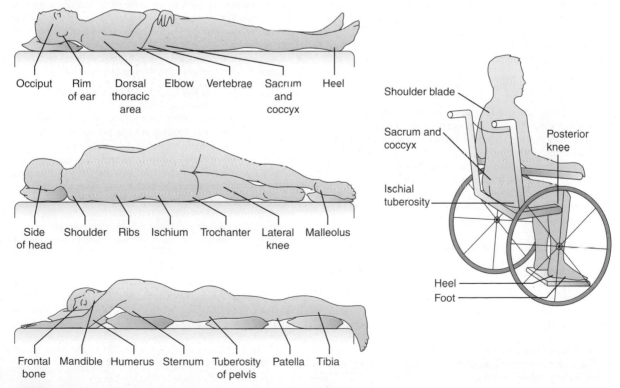

FIGURE 23-2 The risk for the development of pressure ulcers is higher at these points.

in part, to evidence of an almost 80% increase in pressure ulcers in hospitalized patients between 1993 and 2006 (Lyder & Ayello, 2009). Since October 2008, the Centers for Medicare & Medicaid Services has not reimbursed acute care facilities for the care of pressure ulcers that are acquired during the hospitalization because this is considered a preventable condition. Because of this major policy change, healthcare practitioners in acute care settings document the presence of any skin breakdown on admission, and they have increased their efforts to prevent pressure ulcers in all their patients as a major focus of quality improvement programs. This increased attention is warranted, because early preventive interventions are imperative—but greatly underutilized—for hospitalized patients who are at risk for developing pressure ulcers (Rich, Shardell, Margolis, & Baumgarten, 2009). In addition, the Centers for Medicare & Medicaid Services has identified pressure ulcers as a quality indicator for long-term care facilities, so there is increased attention to assessment and prevention in these settings.

Much evidence-based information is available about risk factors, assessment methods, and interventions for preventing and treating pressure ulcers, as summarized in the accompanying Evidence-Based Practice Box 23-1. Nurses can find additional evidence-based information from the organizations listed in the Resources at the end of this chapter. Evidence-based screening tools have been developed for identifying and rating risk factors for pressure ulcer development. In the United States and other countries, the Braden Scale (Figure 23-3) is a commonly used screening tool, and extensive testing supports its validity and reliability (deSouza, Santos, Iri, & Oguri, 2010; Stotts & Gunningberg, 2007). The Hartford Institute for Geriatric Nursing recommends this tool as the best practice for identifying older adults who are at risk for the development of pressure ulcers. Additional information and a cost-free video demonstrating the application of this tool in a clinical setting is available through a collaboration of the Hartford Institute and the *American Journal of Nursing* at http://consultgerirn.org or at www.nursingcenter.com.

Since 1975, healthcare professionals have defined pressure ulcers according to four stages of development. This staging system has been widely used in North America, Europe, and other countries, with leadership coming from the National Pressure Ulcer Advisory Panel (NPUAP). In 2007, the NPUAP added two stages to the system, based on 5 years of work that was reviewed by a consensus conference before final approval. The NPUAP provides many resources including illustrations and quick reference guides in English and other languages (see Resources section). Table 23-2 describes and illustrates the six pressure ulcer stages currently being used in practice settings.

Evidence-Based Practice   23-1
Pressure Ulcers

Statement of the Problem

- Prevalence and incidence rates of pressure ulcers in various settings are as follows: acute care: 10% to 18% prevalence, 0.4% to 38% incidence; long-term care: 2.3% to 28% prevalence, 2.2% to 23.9% incidence; and home healthcare: 0% to 29% prevalence, 0% to 17% incidence
- The heels and sacrum are the two most common sites for the development of pressure; other common sites are the ears, elbows, coccyx, and ischium
- Underlying causative factors are pressure intensity and duration and tissue tolerance
- Important risk factors identified in studies include immobility, surgery, older age, friable skin, urinary and fecal incontinence, compromised nutritional status, cognitive impairment, comorbid conditions, and dependence in activities of daily living, smoking
- Complications of pressure ulcers include sepsis, cellulitis, osteomyelitis, increased length of stay, and financial and emotional cost
- Detection of stage I pressure ulcers is particularly challenging in patients with darkly pigmented skin, and these patients are more likely to die from pressure ulcers

Recommendations for Nursing Assessment

- Identify risk factors using a valid and reliable tool (i.e., Braden or Norton scales)
- Assess skin head to toe on admission to a facility, on discharge, whenever the patient's condition changes, and at appropriate intervals (e.g., daily in acute care, weekly in long-term care during the first month, then periodically according to the patient's condition; on admission and during every visit for home care settings)
- Assess and reassess pressure ulcers according to the 2007 NPUAP Pressure Ulcer Staging System

- During assessments, use natural or halogen lighting rather than under fluorescent lights
- Because patients with darkly pigmented skin may not meet the normal criteria for stage I pressure ulcers, consider additional parameters (e.g., differences in skin over bony prominences compared with surrounding skin, alterations in pain or local sensation, deviations from the usual color for that person)
- If available, use technological devices to improve the detection of stage I pressure ulcers in patients with darkly pigmented skin

Recommendations for Nursing Interventions

- Pressure redistribution interventions: turning and repositioning of patient, use of pressure redistribution surfaces (e.g., alternating pressure mattress, viscoelastic foam cushion and mattress, heel protection boots)
- Nutritional interventions: assessment of nutritional status and appropriate referrals for the services of registered dieticians; provision of adequate calories, nutrients, hydration; appropriate use of supplements
- Skincare: individualize bathing frequency; avoid hot water and excessive rubbing; use moisturizer lotion; protect skin from urine, stool, and other sources of moisture; do not massage bony prominences
- Treatment measures: wound cleansing, moist wound dressings, debridement, pain management, referral to wound care specialists
- Education of professionals, patients, caregivers

SOURCES: Ayello & Sibbald, 2008; Cakmak, Gul, Ozer, Yigit, & Gonu, 2009; Clegg, Kring, Plemmons, & Richbourg, 2009; Dorner, Posthauer, Thomas, & National Pressure Ulcer Advisory Panel, 2009; Institute for Clinical Systems Improvement, 2008; Junkin & Gray, 2009; Lyder, 2009; Lyman, 2009; Shahin, Dassen, & Halfens, 2009; Sprigle, Zhang, & Duckworth, 2009; Wound, Ostomy and Continence Nurses Society, 2009.

BRADEN SCALE FOR PREDICTING PRESSURE SORE RISK

Patient's Name _____ Evaluator's Name _____ Date of Assessment _____

	1	2	3	4				

SENSORY PERCEPTION ability to respond meaningfully to pressure-related discomfort	**1. Completely Limited** Unresponsive (does not moan, flinch, or grasp) to painful stimuli, due to diminished level of consciousness or sedation. OR limited ability to feel pain over most of body.	**2. Very Limited** Responds only to painful stimuli. Cannot communicate discomfort except by moaning or restlessness OR has a sensory impairment which limits the ability to feel pain or discomfort over 1/2 of body.	**3. Slightly Limited** Responds to verbal commands, but cannot always communicate discomfort or the need to be turned. OR has some sensory impairment which limits ability to feel pain or discomfort in 1 or 2 extremities.	**4. No Impairment** Responds to verbal commands. Has no sensory deficit which would limit ability to feel or voice pain or discomfort.
MOISTURE degree to which skin is exposed to moisture	**1. Constantly Moist** Skin is kept moist almost constantly by perspiration, urine, etc. Dampness is detected every time patient is moved or turned.	**2. Very Moist** Skin is often, but not always moist. Linen must be changed at least once a shift.	**3. Occasionally Moist:** Skin is occasionally moist, requiring an extra linen change approximately once a day.	**4. Rarely Moist** Skin is usually dry, linen only requires changing at routine intervals.
ACTIVITY degree of physical activity	**1. Bedfast** Confined to bed.	**2. Chairfast** Ability to walk severely limited or non-existent. Cannot bear own weight and/or must be assisted into chair or wheelchair.	**3. Walks Occasionally** Walks occasionally during day, but for very short distances, with or without assistance. Spends majority of each shift in bed or chair	**4. Walks Frequently** Walks outside room at least twice a day and inside room at least once every two hours during waking hours.
MOBILITY ability to change and control body position	**1. Completely Immobile** Does not make even slight changes in body or extremity position without assistance.	**2. Very Limited** Makes occasional slight changes in body or extremity position but unable to make frequent or significant changes independently.	**3. Slightly Limited** Makes frequent though slight changes in body or extremity position independently.	**4. No Limitation** Makes major and frequent changes in position without assistance.
NUTRITION <u>usual</u> food intake pattern	**1. Very Poor** Never eats a complete meal. Rarely eats more than 1/2 of any food offered. Eats 2 servings or less of protein (meat or dairy products) per day. Takes fluids poorly. Does not take a liquid dietary supplement. OR is NPO and/or maintained on clear liquids or IV's for more than 5 days.	**2. Probably Inadequate** Rarely eats a complete meal and generally eats only about 1/2 of any food offered. Protein intake includes only 3 servings of meat or dairy products per day. Occasionally will take a dietary supplement. OR receives less than optimum amount of liquid diet or tube feeding.	**3. Adequate** Eats over half of most meals. Eats a total of 4 servings of protein (meat, dairy products per day. Occasionally will refuse a meal, but will usually take a supplement when offered. OR is on a tube feeding or TPN regimen which probably meets most of nutritional needs.	**4. Excellent** Eats most of every meal. Never refuses a meal. Usually eats a total of 4 or more servings of meat and dairy products. Occasionally eats between meals. Does not require supplementation.
FRICTION & SHEAR	**1. Problem** Requires moderate to maximum assistance in moving. Complete lifting without sliding against sheets is impossible. Frequently slides down in bed or chair, requiring frequent repositioning with maximum assistance. Spasticity, contractures or agitation leads to almost constant friction.	**2. Potential Problem** Moves feebly or requires minimum assistance. During a move skin probably slides to some extent against sheets, chair, restraints or other devices. Maintains relatively good position in chair or bed most of the time but occasionally slides down.	**3. No Apparent Problem** Moves in bed and in chair independently and has sufficient muscle strength to lift up completely during move. Maintains good position in bed or chair.	
				Total Score _____

FIGURE 23-3 The Braden Scale is a widely used screening tool to identify people at risk for pressure ulcers. Scores = 15–18, at risk; 13–14, moderate risk; 10–12, high risk; <9, very high risk. (From Braden B., & Bergstrom, N. [1988]. Reprinted with permission. Permission to use this tool should be sought at www.bradenscale.com.)

TABLE 23-2 Stages of Pressure Ulcer Development

Stage	Description		
	Normal skin	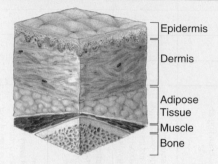	
I	Intact skin with nonblanchable redness of localized area, usually over a bony prominence. Darkly pigmented skin may not have visible blanching, but it may differ in color from the surrounding area.	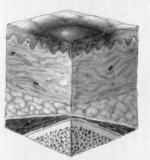	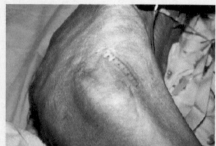
II	Partial thickness loss of dermis presenting as shallow open ulcer with red–pink wound bed, without slough, OR may present as intact or open/ruptured serum-filled blister. This should NOT be applied to skin tears, taper burns, perineal dermatitis, maceration, or excoriation.	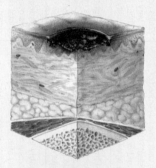	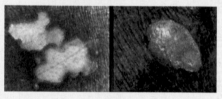
III	Full thickness tissue loss. Subcutaneous fat may be visible, but bone, tendon, or muscle is not exposed. Slough may be present but does not obscure the depth of tissue loss. May include undermining and tunneling. Depth of stage 3 ulcers varies by location, from shallow (e.g., on nose, ear, occiput, malleolus) to very deep where there is significant adiposity.	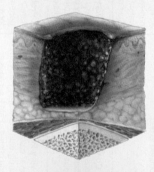	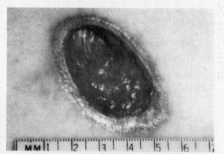
IV	Full thickness tissue loss with exposed bone, tendon, or muscle. Slough or eschar may be present. May include undermining and tunneling. Depth of stage 4 varies by location—from shallow to deep—and may extend into muscle and/or supporting structures, making osteomyelitis possible.	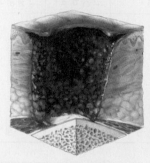	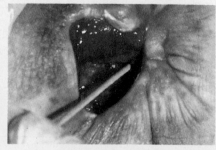

Normal skin labels: Epidermis, Dermis, Adipose Tissue, Muscle, Bone

TABLE 23-2 Stages of Pressure Ulcer Development (*Continued*)

Stage	Description	
Unstageable	Full thickness tissue loss in which the base of the ulcer is covered by slough (yellow, tan, gray, green, or brown) and/or eschar (tan, brown, black) in the wound bed. The true depth cannot be determined until enough slough and/or eschar has been removed to expose the base of the wound. Stable eschar (i.e., dry, adherent, intact without erythema or fluctuance) should not be removed because it is protective.	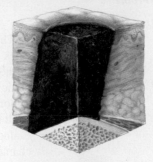
Suspected Deep Tissue Injury	Purple or maroon localized area of discolored intact skin or blood-filled blister due to damage of underlying soft tissue from pressure and/or shear. The area may be preceded by tissue that is painful, firm, mushy, boggy, or warmer or colder than adjacent tissue. May be difficult to detect in individuals with dark skin tones. Evolution may include a thin blister over a dark wound bed.	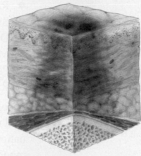

Source: Used with permission from National Pressure Ulcer Advisory Panel (2007). *Updated Staging System.* Available from www.npuap.org.

Once a pressure ulcer develops and is assessed according to the defined stages, it must be reassessed on an ongoing basis. Since 1996, the NPUAP has encouraged the use of a standardized tool for assessing changes in pressure ulcers called the Pressure Ulcer Scale for Healing (PUSH) tool. The PUSH tool scores pressure ulcers according to size, exudates, and tissue type, with changes in the PUSH score over time indicating the progression or regression of the pressure ulcer. This tool and instructions for its use are available at http://www.npuap.org/PDF/push3.pdf.

Although some nurses refer to a "reverse staging" method to document the progression of a later-stage pressure stage to a healed stage, the NPUAP has advised against this practice because it does not accurately reflect the pathophysiologic processes that occur.

 NURSING ASSESSMENT OF SKIN

Because the skin is the largest and most visible organ of the body, it is relatively easy to identify problems that affect it. In addition, the skin may yield clues to other areas of physiologic and psychosocial function such as nutrition, hydration, and personal care. Nurses collect information about the skin, hair, and nails during an assessment interview and through physical examination procedures. Opportunities for direct examination also arise during routine nursing care activities such as assisting with personal care or listening to the lungs and apical heart rate. Noting the characteristics of the skin, hair, and nails can also provide information to validate or raise questions about other areas of function. For example, the observation that an older man has a beard of several days' growth, when combined with assessment information about his overall function, may support conclusions about possible depression or the need for assistance with personal care activities.

Identifying Opportunities for Health Promotion

Assessment questions are aimed at identifying the person's perception of any problems, any risk factors that may contribute to skin problems, and the person's personal care behaviors that influence hair and skin status. Assessing these aspects of skincare can help identify opportunities for health education about risk factors and healthy skincare practices. Older adults may initiate a discussion about age spots or other noticeable skin changes, and they are usually very receptive to information about skin and haircare. Nurses obtain information about medications and other risk factors as part of the overall assessment, and they incorporate this information into the skin assessment. Likewise, other pertinent information obtained during a comprehensive assessment, such as information about fluid intake, nutritional status, and mobility and safety, is applicable to the assessment of the skin. Box 23-1 summarizes assessment questions related to the skin and nails.

Observing Skin, Hair, and Nails

Close inspection of the skin in a warm, private, and well-lit environment is an essential component of skin assessment. Examination of the skin is particularly important because

Box 23-1 Interview Questions for Assessing the Integument

Questions to Assess Risk Factors and Skin Problems
- Do you have any concerns about or trouble with your skin?
- Do you have any problems with rashes, itching, swelling, or dry skin?
- Do you have any sores that will not heal?
- Do you bruise easily?
- Have you been treated for skin cancer or any other skin problems?
- How much time do you spend in the sun?
- Do you spend time in tanning booths?
- Do you do anything to protect yourself from the effects of the sun?

Questions to Assess Personal Care Practices
- How do you manage your bathing?
- How often do you take a bath or shower?
- What temperature water do you use?
- Do you use soap every time you bathe?
- What kind of soap do you use?
- Do you use any kind of skin lotion, creams, or ointments? What kind do you use and how frequently do you use it? Where do you apply it?
- Do you have any problems with your fingernails or toenails?
- Do you get or need any help with nailcare?

DIVERSITY NOTE
Mongolian spots occur in 90% of African Americans, 80% of Asians and Native Americans, and 9% of whites (Andrews, 2008).

The common occurrence of various skin lesions complicates the assessment of skin in older adults. Although most of these changes are harmless, except in terms of their cosmetic consequences, some are cancerous or precancerous. An important aspect of health promotion is to reassure the older adult about the harmless changes and to encourage medical evaluation of the questionable ones. In general, the following characteristics of a skin lesion warrant medical evaluation:

- Redness
- Swelling
- Dark pigmentation
- Moisture or drainage
- Pain or discomfort
- Raised or irregular edges around a flat center.

Also, any lesion that undergoes change, or any sore that does not heal within a reasonable time, should be evaluated further. Evaluation is also indicated when, because of its location, a mole or other skin lesion is subject to frequent rubbing or irritation. When nurses observe a questionable skin lesion, they assess and document all the following characteristics: size, shape, color, location, macular (flat) versus papular (raised), superficial versus penetrating, discrete versus diffuse borders, and the presence or absence of inflammation, redness, or discharge. Terminology related to various skin lesions in older adults is confusing, and many terms are used interchangeably. Table 23-3 describes some of the terms used for skin lesions that are common in older adults; some of these lesions are shown in Figure 23-4.

Nursing assessment of the skin, hair, and nails can provide clues to a broad spectrum of physiologic functioning, particularly when nursing observations are combined with additional assessment information. For example, brown-stained fingertips are an indication of cigarette use, and feces under

older adults may focus on benign conditions, such as xerosis, but not notice more serious conditions such as skin cancer. Nurses observe skin color, turgor, dryness, overall condition, and any growths or pathologic conditions. Nurses also observe and document cultural variations. For example, older adults of Latin, Asian, or African ancestry may have faded **Mongolian spots** (i.e., irregular areas of blue coloration common on the buttocks and lower back and sometimes on the arms, thighs, and abdomen) that might be mistaken for bruises. Also, when assessing for erythema or pressure areas, nurses should keep in mind that early skin changes may be difficult to detect in people with darkly pigmented skin.

TABLE 23-3 Common Skin Lesions in Older Adults

Common Term(s)	Description
Age spots, liver spots, senile lentigines, senile freckles	Pale to dark brown macules, occurring most frequently on exposed areas
Actinic keratosis, solar keratosis	Red, yellow, brown, or flesh-colored papules or plaques; gritty texture; surrounded by erythema; *premalignant*
Senile purpura	Areas of brown or bluish discoloration that look like bruising
Seborrheic keratosis	Brown or black papules or plaques with sharp edges and a waxy or wartlike texture; appearing most frequently on trunk and face
Sebaceous hyperplasia	Yellowish, doughnut-shaped elevations; common on face, particularly in men
Senile angiomas, cherry or ruby angiomas, telangiectasia	Bright, ruby–red, pinpoint, superficial elevations of small blood vessels
Spider angiomas	Tiny, red papules with radiating arms; *may indicate a pathologic condition*
Venous stars	Bluish, irregular, sometimes spider-shaped lesions, appearing mainly on the legs or the chest
Venous lakes, benign venous angiomas	Bluish papules with sharp borders, appearing mainly on the lips or the ears
Acrochordons, skin tags	Flesh-colored, pedunculated, or stalklike lesions
Corns, calluses	Hard masses of keratin caused by repeated pressure or irritation
Xanthelasma	Fatty deposits, usually around the eyes; *may be related to a pathologic condition*, particularly if large or numerous

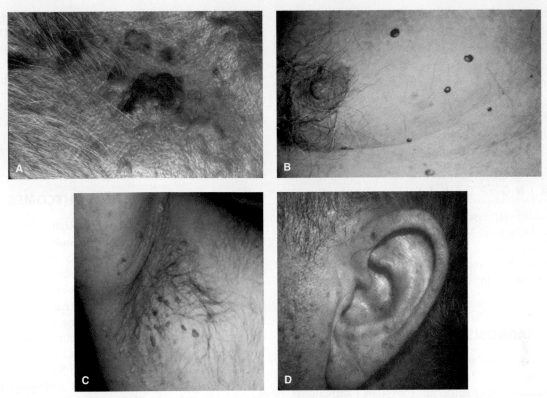

FIGURE 23-4 Common skin lesions in older adults. Seborrheic keratosis (**A**). Cherry angioma (**B**). Skin tag (**C**). Venous lakes or benign venous angiomas (**D**). (**A & D**, Reprinted with permission from Rosenthal, T. C., Williams, M. E., & Naughton, B. J. [2007]. *Office care geriatrics*. Philadelphia: Lippincott Williams & Wilkins; **B**, Reprinted with permission from Weber, J., & Kelley, J. [2002]. *Health assessment in nursing* [2nd ed.]. Philadelphia, PA: Lippincott Williams & Wilkins; **C**, Courtesy of Steifel Laboratories, Inc.)

the fingernails and around the cuticle may be a clue to constipation. In some circumstances, toenails provide clues to mobility difficulties, particularly when extremely long nails curl under the toes. Observations of the skin may provide the only objective evidence of serious functional problems that the older person might not otherwise acknowledge. For example, multiple bruises, particularly in various stages of healing, may be a significant clue to falls, alcoholism, self-neglect, or physical abuse. Observation and documentation of these signs are particularly important when neglect or abuse is suspected but the older adult or caregiver denies any such problems (see Chapter 10 for detailed description of elder abuse).

In assessing the skin for clues to the broader aspects of function, keep in mind that some of the usual manifestations may be altered in older adults. For example, nurses often assess skin turgor on the hands or arms as an indication of hydration status. Because of xerosis and decreased elasticity in the skin of older adults, however, skin turgor is not necessarily a reliable indicator of hydration status. Although the hands or arms may be convenient and socially acceptable sites of inspection, the skin over protected areas, such as the sternum or abdomen, is a more accurate indicator of hydration status in older adults. In nonmedicated older adults, the oral mucous membranes are usually reliable indicators of hydration. However, many medications, including over-the-counter preparations containing anticholinergic ingredients, cause dry mouth.

Another age-related change that complicates the assessment of the skin is delayed wound healing. This change makes it difficult to assess patterns of wound healing using the same standards that are applied to younger adults.

Observations of the hair, skin, and nails provide multiple clues to self-esteem and other aspects of psychosocial function. Physical limitations can interfere with personal grooming, as can psychosocial influences such as lack of motivation or awareness. Thus, evidence of self-neglect in grooming may indicate depression, dementia, or social isolation. The use of hair coloring may reflect the person's attitudes about aging, and unusually deep hues of hair coloring or facial cosmetics may indicate impaired color perception. Nurses can use Box 23-2 as a guide to assessment observations regarding the integumentary system.

*M*s. S. is an 84-year-old white woman who lives in her own home on the coast of Florida. She is quite active and healthy and enjoys golfing and "beach-combing." She attends the local senior center, where you are the wellness nurse. The local chapter of the American Cancer Society is co-sponsoring a skin cancer screening day at the senior center, and you have been asked to prepare a health education program titled "Checking Your Skin for Serious

Changes." You are also assisting the dermatologist with the screening examinations. Ms. S. attends the health education part of your program and says she is not sure if she can stay for the screening. She just has one "age spot," and she knows it is not serious because she has "had a couple skin cancers removed, and this one looks different." You look at the questionable spot, and you assess it as a brown, raised plaque with a gritty texture, about 1 cm in diameter.

THINKING POINTS

- What additional assessment information would you want to obtain from Ms. S.?
- How would you use Table 23-3 and Boxes 23-1 and 23-2 in your assessment?
- What advice would you give to Ms. S. about her skin?

NURSING DIAGNOSIS

When older adults have any skin breakdown nurses can use the nursing diagnosis of Impaired Skin Integrity, defined as "altered epidermis and/or epidermis (NANDA International, 2009, p. 320). When older adults have any risk factors for pressure ulcers, nurses can use the nursing diagnosis of Risk for Impaired Skin Integrity, which is defined as "at risk for skin being adversely altered (NANDA International, 2009, p. 321). Related factors that commonly affect older adults include medications, incontinence, dehydration, limited mobility, nutritional deficits, or a combination of these factors.

If the older adult has any suspect skin lesion, the nursing diagnosis of Ineffective Health Maintenance might be appli-

cable. This is defined as the "inability to identify, manage, and/or seek out help to maintain health" (NANDA International, 2009, p. 57). Nurses could apply this diagnosis to people who do not use protective measures when they are exposed to ultraviolet radiation (from sunlight or tanning booths).

> **Wellness Opportunity**
>
> Nurses can use the wellness nursing diagnosis Readiness for Enhanced Knowledge: Skin Care for older adults who are interested in learning how to address risks for conditions such as dry skin and skin cancer.

PLANNING FOR WELLNESS OUTCOMES

When older adults have conditions that affect skin comfort or integrity, nurses identify wellness outcomes as an essential part of the nursing process. Similarly, when they have risks for conditions that can cause skin problems (e.g., skin cancer or pressure ulcers), nursing goals focus on prevention. For healthy older adults with risk factors (e.g., history of skin cancer) or minor skin problems (e.g., xerosis), applicable Nursing Outcomes Classification (NOC) terminology includes Comfort Level, Tissue Integrity: Skin and Mucous Membranes, Knowledge: Health Behavior, Health Seeking Behavior, Nutritional Status, Risk Control: Cancer, and Symptom Control.

For older adults with pressure ulcers or other types of wounds or skin breakdown, NOC terms include Impaired Skin Integrity, Wound Healing: Primary Intention, and Wound Healing: Secondary Intention. Outcomes are achieved through interventions discussed in the following section.

> **Wellness Opportunity**
>
> Nurses promote wellness when they plan outcomes to address skin comfort and the prevention of skin cancer.

 Box 23-2 Observations Regarding the Integument

Examination of the Skin
- What is the color?
- Are there any areas of irregular pigmentation?
- Are there any areas of sunburn or tan?
- Are there areas that are discolored in any way?
- Are there any indications of poor circulation, particularly in the extremities (e.g., varicosities, or areas of red, blue, or brown discoloration indicative of chronic stasis problems in the lower extremities)?
- What is the skin temperature?
- Is there a marked difference between the temperature of the extremities and that of the rest of the body?
- How does the skin feel in terms of moisture? Is it dry? Clammy? Oily?
- What is the skin's texture? Is it smooth or rough?
- Does the skin look tissue-paper thin?
- What is the turgor of the abdominal skin?
- Are scars present? (If so, describe their location and appearance.) Are there any signs of falling or physical abuse?
- Are any of the lesions described in Table 23-3 present?

Examination of the Hair and Nails
- What are the color, texture, and general condition of the hair?
- What is the distribution pattern of the hair?

- Is there any evidence of dandruff, scaling, or other problems with the hair?
- What are the color, length, cleanliness, and general condition of the toenails and fingernails?
- What are the color and general condition of the nail beds of the toes and fingers?

Personal Care Practices
- What is the person's overall appearance with regard to grooming and attention to personal attractiveness?
- If grooming is poor, does the person express concern about this or provide an explanation?
- Are there any psychosocial factors that influence personal care practices (e.g., is the person socially isolated or overburdened with caregiving responsibilities and, therefore, inattentive to personal care)?
- Are any of the following signs of neglect evident: presence of a body odor; unkempt, uncut, or matted hair; unusually long and unkempt fingernails or toenails; patches of brown crust on the skin; bruises; or any pathologic skin conditions?

NURSING INTERVENTIONS FOR SKIN WELLNESS

Nurses have many opportunities for promoting wellness with regard to comfort, self-esteem, and maintenance of a healthy integumentary system. Nursing interventions for healthy older adults focus on teaching about self-care practices, such as promoting responsibility for identifying and seeking further evaluation for harmful or precancerous lesions. Interventions for physically compromised older adults focus on maintaining intact skin and managing pressure ulcers. Nurses can use the following Nursing Interventions Classification (NIC) terminologies in their care plans: Hair Care, Health Education, Health Screening, Nutrition Therapy, Positioning, Pressure Management, Pressure Ulcer Prevention, Pruritus Management, Risk Identification, Self-Esteem Enhancement, Skin Surveillance, and Wound Care.

Promoting Healthy Skin

Because the condition of the skin depends largely on the overall health of the person, the maintenance of optimal nutrition and hydration is an important intervention in the skincare of older adults. Because environmental conditions and personal care practices also influence the health of the skin, interventions include education of the older adult about these factors. Box 23-3 summarizes teaching points that should be included in the education of older adults, or caregivers of dependent older adults, regarding skin health. Although much of the gerontologic nursing literature advocates limiting baths or showers to one to three times weekly, it is not clear that there is a cause–effect relationship between bathing or showers and dry skin. Other factors, including smoking, dehydration, sun exposure, low environmental humidity, and the use of harsh cleansing products, are likely to contribute to xerosis in older adults.

In recent years, many questions have been raised about whether the common occurrence of vitamin D deficiency is due to the limited sun exposure that is advocated for the prevention of skin cancer. These questions are valid because sunlight is required for vitamin D synthesis in humans, but sunlight is also a well-recognized cause of skin cancer, wrinkles, and photoaging. In addition to preventing vitamin D deficiency, documented health benefits of sunlight include elevated mood and improved energy (Sivamani, Crane, & Dellavalle, 2009). A recent review of evidence related to sunlight and vitamin D concluded that the exposure of arms and legs to sunlight for 5 to 30 minutes between the hours of 10 AM and 3 PM twice a week can prevent vitamin D deficiency without having detrimental effects (Kulie, Groff, Redmer, Hounshell, & Schrager, 2009).

Preventing Skin Wrinkles

The best methods of preventing skin lesions and wrinkles are avoiding too much exposure to sunlight and using a sunscreen with a sun protection factor (SPF) of 15 or higher when exposure to sunlight is unavoidable. Topical products containing

---

 Box 23-3 Health Promotion Teaching About Skin Care for Older Adults

Maintaining Healthy Skin
- Include adequate amounts of fluid in the daily diet.
- Use humidifiers to maintain environmental humidity levels of 40% to 60%.
- Apply moisturizing lotions twice daily or as needed.
- Use moisturizing lotions immediately after bathing, when the skin is still moist.
- Avoid massaging over bony prominences when applying lotions.
- Avoid skincare products that contain perfumes or isopropyl alcohol.
- Avoid multiple-ingredient preparations because unnecessary additives may cause allergic responses.
- Inspect skin monthly for suspicious-looking changes.

Personal Care Practices
- When bathing or showering, use soap sparingly or use a mild, unscented soap (e.g., Dove, Tone, Basis, Aveeno).
- Maintain water temperatures for bathing at about 90°F to 100°F.
- Rinse well after using soap. Whirlpool baths stimulate circulation, but moderate temperatures should be maintained.
- Apply moisturizing products after bathing, rather than using them in the bath water, to minimize the risk for falls on oily surfaces and to maximize the benefits of the emollient.
- Use emollient products containing petrolatum or mineral oil (e.g., Keri, Eucerin, Aquaphor, Vanicream, Vaseline).
- If you use bath oils, take extra safety precautions to prevent slipping.
- If moisturizing products are applied to the feet, wear nonskid slippers or socks before walking.
- Dry your skin thoroughly, particularly between your toes and in other areas where your skin rubs together.
- When drying your skin, use gentle, patting motions rather than harsh, rubbing motions.
- Obtain regular podiatric care.

Avoiding Sun Damage
- Wear wide-brimmed hats, sun visors, sunglasses, and long-sleeved garments when exposed to the sun.
- Wear clothing made of cotton, rather than polyester fabrics, because ultraviolet rays can penetrate polyester.
- Apply sunscreen lotions generously and frequently, beginning 1 hour before sun exposure.
- Use sunscreen lotions with an SPF of 30 or higher. Limit exposure to the sun between 10:00 AM and 3:00 PM to one hour weekly.
- Protect yourself from ultraviolet rays even on cloudy days and when you are in the water.
- Artificial tanning booths use ultraviolet type A rays, which are advertised as harmless, but which have been found to cause damage in high doses.

Preventing Injury From Abrasive Forces
- Do not use starch, bleach, or strong detergents when laundering clothing or linens.
- Use soft terry or cotton washcloths.
- If waterproof pads are necessary, make sure that an adequate amount of soft, absorbent material is placed near the body.

alpha- or beta-hydroxy acids may be beneficial in reversing wrinkles and promoting the regression of solar keratoses. Nurses need to be alert to the possibility that older adults might develop an allergic or sensitivity reaction to some of the ingredients in topical products. Information about the harmful effects of sunlight should be included in health education about the maintenance of healthy skin and prevention of undesirable cosmetic and pathologic skin changes. Also, nurses can encourage people who are concerned about wrinkles and dry skin to discuss medical interventions with their primary care provider.

> **◆ Wellness Opportunity**
>
> Nurses promote wellness by teaching that exposure to ultraviolet light—by sunlight or tanning lights—is a major factor in the occurrence of skin wrinkles, skin cancer, and other skin changes.

Preventing Dry Skin

Petrolatum and other emollients are effective in alleviating dry skin discomfort, because they moisturize and lubricate the skin. The effectiveness of an emollient is based on its ability to prevent water evaporation, so the beneficial effects will be enhanced when it is applied to skin that already has some degree of moisture. Thus, an emollient agent is most effective when it is applied to moist skin immediately after bathing. See Box 23-3 for information on the use of emollients and other interventions designed to prevent or care for dry skin in older adults.

Detecting and Treating Harmful Skin Lesions

Early detection and treatment of cancerous or precancerous skin lesions are key factors in preventing serious functional consequences, because the cure rate for most skin cancers approaches 100% with early excision. The nurse's role is to detect any suspicious-looking lesions and to encourage or facilitate further evaluation. Nurses can encourage all older adults to use the following guide to identify for themselves any skin changes that require further evaluation:

- **A**symmetric shape: irregular or different-looking sides
- **B**order that is irregular: ragged, notched, blurred, irregular
- **C**olor change: different shades, uneven distribution
- **D**iameter: larger than a quarter of an inch (6 mm), increasing.

If the older adult or caregiver has avoided medical evaluation because of fears about cancer, the nurse can provide reassurance about the high cure rate and the minimal chance of long-term problems if early treatment is obtained. Similarly, if they have ignored suspicious changes because they attribute them to "normal aging," nurses can teach about the importance of further evaluation. Box 23-3 includes health promotion information about the prevention and early detection of skin cancer.

> **◆ Wellness Opportunity**
>
> Nurses address the body–mind–spirit interrelationship by allaying unreasonable fears about skin cancer.

*R*ecall that Ms. S. attends the senior center in Florida where you are responsible for presenting a health education program titled "Maintaining Healthy Skin." You plan to emphasize the importance of self-care techniques such as checking for skin changes. Ms. S. is very interested in attending the program and tells you she will be bringing her 80-year-old sister, who also lives in Florida. Ms. S. worries about her sister because she uses a wheelchair and is very frail. You know that several of the participants at the senior program use wheelchairs, and you plan to include health education about the prevention of pressure ulcers.

THINKING POINTS

- Outline your health education points for a half-hour program including specific points about preventing pressure ulcers.
- How would you use Table 23-2 and Box 23-3 in your program?
- Find additional information that you would consider using as educational materials for this program.

EVALUATING EFFECTIVENESS OF NURSING INTERVENTIONS

Nursing care for older adults with dry or itching skin is evaluated by determining the degree to which the interventions alleviate the person's complaints. It may take several weeks for older adults to feel the full effects of skin care interventions because of an age-related delay in dermal response to external stimuli. Also, there is a great deal of individual variation among older adults in their response to interventions. Thus, it may be necessary to evaluate the effects of one type of soap or lotion for several weeks before trying a different brand if the problem does not resolve. Because environmental humidity affects skin comfort, environmental conditions may also influence the evaluation of interventions.

The effectiveness of interventions for older adults at risk for skin breakdown is measured by the absence of pressure ulcers. The effectiveness of interventions for pressure ulcers is determined by the rate of healing and prevention of complications such as osteomyelitis. Because significant cost and quality-of-life issues are associated with pressure ulcers, preventing skin breakdown can have far-reaching positive consequences for older adults who are at risk for developing pressure ulcers.

*M*s. S. is now 92 years old and lives in an assisted-living facility in Florida. She ambulates with a walker and needs assistance with meals, medications, and personal care. Three months ago, her doctor prescribed hydrochlorothiazide 25 mg every morning for isolated systolic hypertension. She has a history of arthritis but does not take any medication for it. Ms. S. attends your monthly nursing clinic for health education and blood pressure monitoring. When she comes to see you in January, she complains of dry skin and discomfort.

NURSING ASSESSMENT

You interview Ms. S. about her personal care practices and find out that she soaks in the tub in lukewarm water three times weekly and enjoys using bath salts and perfumed skin lotions. She spends much of her leisure time outdoors on the patio or in the air-conditioned solarium. She does not use sunscreens because she thinks they are unnecessary and too oily. She states that she has not had sunburn for several years, and that she has built up a good tolerance to the sun. She does not wear sunglasses or sun hats. She reports that she has had three skin cancers removed in the past 10 years, one from her cheek, one from her arm, and one from her ear lobe. She says she does not worry about recurrent skin cancer because she no longer swims outside or sits by the swimming pool. Also, because she does not get sunburned, she believes she is not at risk for skin cancer.

Inspection of Ms. S.'s skin reveals dry, wrinkled skin on her face and arms, and unevenly tanned skin on her face, neck, and extremities. She has many age spots over the exposed skin areas but no suspicious-looking lesions. Ms. S. has blue eyes and fair skin.

NURSING DIAGNOSIS

Your nursing diagnosis is Ineffective Health Maintenance related to excessive sunlight exposure and insufficient knowledge of the effects of ultraviolet light. Evidence for this diagnosis comes from her misconceptions about risk factors for skin cancer and other skin problems. Also, you identify her lack of knowledge about the potential photosensitivity reactions associated with use of hydrochlorothiazide as a factor that contributes to Ineffective Health Maintenance.

NURSING CARE PLAN FOR MS. S.

Expected Outcome	Nursing Interventions	Nursing Evaluation
Ms. S.'s discomfort from dry skin will be alleviated.	• Discuss and describe age-related skin changes. • Discuss risk factors that contribute to skin discomfort (e.g., bath bath salts, perfumed lotions, unprotected exposure to sunlight) • Use Box 23-3 to teach Ms. S. about skincare practices directed toward alleviating dry skin.	• Ms. S. will report that she no longer experiences skin discomfort and dryness.
Ms. S.'s knowledge about risk factors for skin cancer will be increased.	• Discuss the relationship between skin cancer and exposure to ultraviolet rays. • Explain that any exposure to ultraviolet rays is a risk factor for skin cancer. • Emphasize that a history of skin cancer increases the chance of recurrent skin cancer.	• Ms. S. will verbalize an awareness of the risk factors for skin cancer.
The factors that increase Ms. S.'s risk of skin problems and skin cancer will be eliminated.	• Inform Ms. S. that hydrochlorothiazide may increase the risk for photosensitivity, making protective measures increasingly important. • Use Box 23-3 as a guide for discussing measures to avoid sun damage. • Emphasize the importance of using sunscreens and wearing wide-brimmed hats when in the solarium or outside.	• Ms. S. will use measures to reduce the risk for skin cancer and sun damage.

THINKING POINTS

- What risk factors would you address in your care plan?

- How would you promote Ms. S.'s personal responsibility for skincare, including addressing risks for skin cancer?

Chapter Highlights

Age-Related Changes That Affect Skin Wellness
(Table 23-1)
- Decreased rate of epidermal proliferation
- Thinner dermis, flattened dermal–epidermal junction
- Diminished moisture content
- Decreased dermal blood supply
- Fewer sweat and sebaceous glands
- Decreased number of melanocytes and Langerhans cells
- Changes in patterns of hair distribution

Risks Factors That Affect Skin Wellness
- Genetic factors (hair color and distribution, skin cancer)
- Exposure to ultraviolet radiation (sunlight or tanning light)
- Adverse medication effects
- Personal hygiene practices
- Factors that increase the risk for skin breakdown

Functional Consequences Affecting Skin Wellness
(Table 23-1)
- Xerosis (dry skin), discomfort
- Irregular pigmentation and other cosmetic changes
- Increased susceptibility to injury, mechanical stress, and effects of ultraviolet radiation
- Delayed wound healing, increased susceptibility to infection
- Decreased tactile sensitivity, increased susceptibility to burns
- Diminished sweating and shivering, increased susceptibility to hypothermia and heat-related conditions
- Increased risk for skin cancer
- Increased risk for skin breakdown and pressure ulcers

Pathologic Conditions Affecting Skin Wellness
(Figure 23-1, Table 23-2)
- Skin cancer
- Pressure ulcers (Evidence-Based Practice box)

Nursing Assessment of Skin (Table 23-3, Boxes 23-1 and 23-2)
- Abnormal skin conditions
- Personal care practices
- Skin lesions common in older adults (Table 23-3, Figure 23-4)
- Risk for pressure ulcers (Figures 23-2 and 23-3)

Nursing Diagnosis
- Readiness for Enhanced Knowledge: Skin
- Impaired Skin Integrity (or Risk for)
- Ineffective Health Maintenance

Planning for Wellness Outcomes
- Comfort Level
- Tissue Integrity: Skin and Mucous Membranes
- Nutritional Status
- Risk Control: Cancer
- Wound Healing

Nursing Interventions for Skin Wellness (Box 23-3)
- Health promotion teaching about healthy skin
- Preventing skin wrinkles
- Preventing dry skin
- Detecting and treating suspect skin changes
- Preventing and managing pressure ulcers

Evaluating Effectiveness of Nursing Interventions
- Alleviation of complaints (e.g., dryness)
- Evaluation of suspect skin changes
- Absence of pressure ulcers in high-risk older adults
- Wound healing

Critical Thinking Exercises

1. What changes would a healthy 85-year-old person notice with regard to his or her skin, hair, and nails?
2. Describe the questions you would ask and the observations you would make to assess the skin, hair, and nails of an 82-year-old person.
3. Describe at least eight skin lesions that are normal and three skin lesions that require further evaluation.
4. You are asked to give a 20-minute presentation on "Maintaining Healthy Skin" at a senior center. Outline the content of your health education program.
5. What would you teach the family caregivers of a 74-year-old woman who sits in a wheelchair for 14 hours a day with regard to the prevention of pressure ulcers?

Resources

For links to these resources and additional helpful Internet resources related to this chapter, visit thePoint. at http://thePoint.lww.com/Miller6e.

Clinical Tools

American Journal of Nursing and Hartford Institute for Geriatric Nursing
- *How to Try This,* article and video: Stotts, N. A., & Gunningberg, L. (2007). Predicting pressure ulcer risk. *American Journal of Nursing, 107*(11), 40–48.

Hartford Institute for Geriatric Nursing
- *Try This: Best Practices in Nursing Care to Older Adults* Issue 5 (2007), Predicting Pressure Ulcer Risk

Evidence-Based Practice

Ayello, E. A., & Sibbald, R. G. (2008). Preventing pressure ulcers and skin tears. In E. Capezuti, D. Zwicker, M. Mezey, & T. Fulmer (Eds.), *Evidence-Based Geriatric Nursing Protocols for Best Practice* (3rd ed., pp. 403–429). New York: Springer Publishing Co.

National Guideline Clearinghouse
- Pressure ulcer prevention and treatment
- Skin cancer: screening and prevention

Health Education

Agency for Health Care Policy and Research
American Cancer Society
Canadian Cancer Society
National Arthritis and Musculoskeletal and Skin Diseases Information Clearinghouse
National Pressure Ulcer Advisory Panel (NPUAP)

REFERENCES

Andrews, M. M. (2008). Cultural competence in the health history and physical examination. In M. M. Andrews & J. S. Boyle (Eds.), *Transcultural concepts in nursing care* (5th ed., pp. 34–65). Philadelphia, PA: Lippincott, Williams & Wilkins.

Asakura, K. (2009). Lifestyle factors and visible skin aging in a population of Japanese elders. *Journal of Epidemiology/Japan Epidemiological Association, 19*(5), 251–259.

Ayello, E. A., & Sibbald, R. G. (2008). Preventing pressure ulcers and skin tears. In E. Capezuti, D. Zwicker, M. Mezey, & T. Fulmer (Eds.), *Evidence-based geriatric nursing protocols for best practice* (3rd ed., pp. 403–429). New York: Springer Publishing Co.

Berwick, M., & Erdei, E. (2009). Melanoma epidemiology and public health. *Dermatologic Clinic, 27*(2), 205–214.

Cakmak, S. K., Gul, U., Ozer, S., Yigit, Z., & Gonu, M. (2009). Risk factors for pressure ulcers. *Advances in Skin & Wound Care, 22*(9), 412–415.

Chicano, S. G., & Drolshagen, C. (2009). Reducing hospital-acquired pressure ulcers. *Journal of Wound, Ostomy and Continence Nurses Society, 36*(1), 45–50.

Clegg, A., Kring, D., Plemmons, J., & Richbourg, L. (2009). North Carolina nurses examine heel pressure ulcers. *Journal of Wound, Ostomy and Continence Nurses Society, 36*(6), 635–639.

Dealey, C. (2009). Skin care and pressure ulcers. *Advances in Skin and Wound Care, 22*(9), 421–430.

deSouza, D. M., Santos, V. L., Iri, H. K., & Oguri, M. Y. (2010). Predictive validity of the Braden scale for pressure ulcer risk in elderly residents of long-term care facilities. *Geriatric Nursing, 31*, 95–104.

Dorner, B., Posthauer, M. E., Thomas, D., & National Pressure Ulcer Advisory Panel. (2009). The role of nutrition in pressure ulcer prevention and treatment: National Pressure Ulcer Advisory Panel White Paper. *Advances in Skin & Wound Care, 22*(5), 212–220.

Farage, M. A. (2009). Clinical implications of aging skin: Cutaneous disorders in the elderly. *American Journal of Clinical Dermatology, 10*(2), 73–86.

Geller, A. C. (2009). Educational and screening campaigns to reduce deaths from melanoma. *Hematology/Oncology Clinics of North America, 23*(3), 515–527.

Guyuron, B., Rowe, D. J., Weinfeld, A. B., Eshraghi, Y., Fathi, A., & Iamphongsai, S. (2009). Factors contributing to the facial aging of identical twins. *Plastic and Reconstructive Surgery, 123*(4), 1321–1331.

Habif, T. P. (2010). *Clinical dermatology* (5th ed.). St. Louis, MO: Mosby.

Institute for Clinical Systems Improvement. (2008). *Pressure ulcer treatment. Health care protocol.* Bloomington, MN: Institute for Clinical Systems Improvement. Retrieved from www.guideline.gov.

Junkin, J., & Gray, M. (2009). Are pressure redistribution surfaces or heel protection devices effective for preventing heel pressure ulcers? *Journal of Wound, Ostomy and Continence Nurses Society, 36*(6), 602–608.

Kulie, T., Groff, A., Redmer, J., Hounshell, J., & Schrager, S. (2009). Vitamin D: An evidence-based review. *Journal of the American Board of Family Medicine, 22*(6), 698–706.

LeBlanc, K., & Baranoski, S. (2009). Prevention and management of skin tears. *Advances in Skin & Wound Care, 22*(7), 325–332.

Lyder, C. (2009). Closing the skin assessment disparity gap between patients with light and darkly pigmented skin. *Journal of Wound, Ostomy and Continence Nurses Society, 36*(2), 285.

Lyder, C. H., & Ayello, E. A. (2009). Annual checkup: The CMS pressure ulcer present-on-admission indicator. *Advances in Skin and Wound Care, 22*(10), 476–483.

Lyman, V. (2009). Successful heel pressure ulcer prevention program in a long-term care setting. *Journal of Wound, Ostomy and Continence Nurses Society, 36*(6), 616–621.

Martires, K. J., Polster, F. P., Cooper, K. D., & Baron, E. D. (2009). Factors that affect skin aging: A cohort-based survey on twins. *Archives of Dermatology, 145*(12), 1375–1379.

NANDA International. (2009). *Nursing diagnoses: Definitions and classification 2009–2011.* Oxford, UK: Wiley-Blackwell.

National Pressure Ulcer Advisory Panel. (2007). Updated staging system. Retrieved from http://npuap.org.

Nijhawan, R. I., Molenda, M., Airwas, M. J., & Jacob, S. E. (2009). Systemic contact dermatitis. *Dermatology Clinics, 27*, 355–364.

Rich, S. E., Shardell, M., Margolis, D., & Baumgarten, M. (2009). Pressure ulcer preventive device use among elderly patients early in the hospital stay. *Nursing Research, 58*(2), 95–104.

Shahin, E. S. M., Dassen, T., & Halfens, R. J. G. (2009). Incidence, prevention and treatment of pressure ulcers in intensive care patients: A longitudinal study. *International Journal of Nursing Studies, 46*(4), 413–421.

Sivamani, R. K., Crane, L. A., & Dellavalle, R. P. (2009). The benefits and risks of ultraviolet tanning and its alternatives: The role of prudent sun exposure. *Dermatologic Clinics, 27*(2), 149–154.

Sprigle, S., Zhang, L., & Duckworth, M. (2009). Detection of skin erythema in darkly pigmented skin using multispectral images. *Advances in Skin & Wound Care, 22*(4), 172–179.

Stotts, N. A., & Gunningberg, L. (2007). How to try this: Predicting pressure ulcer risk. *American Journal of Nursing, 107*(11), 40–48.

Tucker, M. A. (2009). Melanoma epidemiology. *Hematology/Oncology Clinics of North America, 23*, 383–395.

Wound, Ostomy and Continence Nurses Society. (2009). Wound, Ostomy and Continence Nurses Society position statement on avoidable versus unavoidable pressure ulcers. *Journal of Wound, Ostomy and Continence Nurses Society, 36*(4), 378–381.

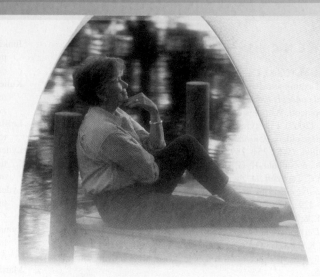

CHAPTER 24

Sleep and Rest

LEARNING OBJECTIVES

After reading this chapter, you will be able to:

1. Delineate age-related changes that affect sleep and rest patterns in older adults.

2. Identify psychosocial, environmental, and physiologic risk factors that influence sleep and rest in older adults.

3. Discuss sleep changes and problems common in older adults.

4. Assess sleep patterns in older adults to identify opportunities for health promotion to improve sleep.

5. Identify nursing interventions to promote optimal sleep and to address risks that interfere with sleep in older adults.

K E Y P O I N T S

advanced sleep phase

circadian rhythm

Epworth Sleepiness
  Scale (ESS)

excessive daytime
  sleepiness

insomnia

obstructive sleep apnea

periodic limb movements
  in sleep (PLMS)

Pittsburgh Sleep Quality
  Index (PSQI)

restless legs syndrome
  (RLS)

sleep latency

Approximately one-third of a person's lifetime is spent in sleep and rest activities, yet little attention is paid to the essential physiologic and psychosocial functions accomplished through these activities. During periods of sleep and rest, many metabolic processes decelerate, production of growth hormone increases, and tissue repair and protein synthesis accelerate. During the deeper stages of sleep, cognitive and emotional information is stored, filtered, and organized. Thus, the quantity and quality of sleep affect many aspects of wellness.

Before the 1930s, research on sleep was nonexistent, and nocturnal sleep was viewed as the absence of daytime activity, rather than as an activity in its own right. In the 1950s, our understanding of sleep patterns improved significantly based on polygraphic measurements that identified sleep cycles. By the 1960s, scientists had identified rapid eye movement (REM), non–rapid eye movement (NREM), and waking stages as three distinct states of consciousness. In the 1970s, sleep disorder centers were established to conduct research on sleep and offer comprehensive evaluation and treatment programs for persons suffering from sleep disorders. By the late 1990s, the American Sleep Disorders Association, a professional organization of primary care providers involved in the diagnosis and treatment of sleep disorders, had more than 2000 members.

In the beginning of the 21st century, print and broadcast media focused public attention on the detrimental effects of sleep deprivation and the large numbers of people affected by inadequate sleep. Numerous Internet sites sprang up, and *sleep apnea syndrome* became part of the common language. Now, health care practitioners are likely to address sleep-related concerns and refer patients for comprehensive sleep studies as a health promotion intervention. Because older adults are as likely as younger adults to benefit from newer information and technology, it is important to understand the specific sleep problems of older adults so that they too can take advantage of the most recent approaches to addressing this important health-related quality-of-life concern.

AGE-RELATED CHANGES THAT AFFECT SLEEP AND REST PATTERNS

Sleep research initially focused on the unique characteristics of each phase of the sleep cycle across the life span, with some attention directed toward sleep changes in older adults. Several decades of research have provided a strong base of information about normal sleep patterns of different age groups, primary sleep disorders (e.g., sleep apnea and **restless legs syndrome [RLS]**), and the complex relationships between sleep and other factors. Studies conclude that "many

Promoting Sleep Wellness in Older Adults

Nursing Assessment
- Usual sleep patterns
- Perception of and satisfaction with sleep
- Pre-bedtime routines
- Risks that interfere with sleep
- Sleep assessment tools

Age-Related Changes
- ↓ time in deep sleep
- ↑ time in light sleep
- ↓ time spent dreaming

Negative Functional Consequences
- ↑ time to fall asleep
- Frequent arousals
- ↑ difficulty returning to sleep
- ↑ time in bed with ↓ sleep
- Poorer quality of sleep

Risk Factors
- Pain, discomfort, nocturia
- Beliefs, attitudes, myths
- Anxiety, depression
- Adverse medication effects
- Pathologic conditions
- Environmental factors

Nursing Interventions
- Teaching about interventions for sleep wellness
- Environmental modifications
- Relaxation and mental imagery
- Teaching about medications and risk factors
- Addressing obstructive sleep apnea

Wellness Outcomes
- Feeling rested and satisfied with sleep
- Improved scores on sleep assessment tools
- Improved quality of life
- Better overall health and functioning

sleep parameters do change with aging, but should not inherently result in fatigue or disrupted daytime functioning" (Gammack, 2008a, p. xi). A wide range of physiologic, environmental, and psychosocial factors interact to affect sleep patterns, and these interrelationships become even more complex with increasing age. Sleep characteristics, which are described according to the quantity of time spent in bed and the depth and quality of sleep, are described in the following sections.

Sleep Quantity

Sleep efficiency, or the percentage of time asleep during the time in bed, influences perceived quality of sleep. Sleep efficiency ranges from 80% to 90% for younger people but diminishes to 50% to 70% for older people (Misra & Malow, 2008). This diminished sleep efficiency is attributed both to prolonged **sleep latency**, which is the time required to fall asleep, and to an increased number of awakenings during the night. Beginning in the fourth decade, the ability to initiate and maintain sleep gradually declines, with an average loss of 28 minutes per decade of life (Espiritu, 2008).

Older adults spend increasing amounts of time in bed, with a decreasing proportion of time in actual sleep. One study found a 28-minute decrease in sleep duration for each decade between the ages of 16 years and 83 years (Van Couter, Spiegel, Tasali, & Leproult, 2008). Other studies indicate that healthy older adults take more daytime naps and spend approximately 1 hour per day napping (Espiritu, 2008). Beneficial effects of daytime naps in older adults include compensation for less nighttime sleep, improved overall functioning, and improved alertness and less daytime sleepiness.

Sleep Quality

Nocturnal sleep patterns are described in terms of sleep cycles and sleep stages. Each sleep cycle, which lasts between 70 and 120 minutes, is a combination of sleep stages. Sleep stages are classified according to the presence or absence of REMs. A typical cycle consists of four NREM stages and one REM stage (also called the dream stage). At the beginning of each cycle, the NREM stages occur sequentially from stage I (lightest sleep) through stage IV (deepest sleep). These stages then occur in reverse order until stage I is reached again and is followed by REM sleep. The cycle repeats during the night, with the length of REM increasing and the length of stages III and IV gradually diminishing (i.e., more time is spent in dream stage and less time in deeper NREM stages as the night progresses). During the NREM stages, muscles gradually relax, body systems function at low levels, and heart and respiratory rates are slower and more regular than during REM or waking periods. Stages III and IV (also known as delta sleep) are the deepest stages, and essential restorative functions and the release of hormones take place during the fourth stage.

Although some dreaming occurs in NREM stages, most active and vivid dreaming occurs during REM sleep. In addition to rapid eye movement, REM sleep is characterized by the following physiologic changes:

- Flaccid muscles
- Fluctuating blood pressure

- Diminished thermoregulatory functions
- Increased gastric acid secretions
- Production of more highly concentrated urine
- An approximately 40% increase in cerebral blood flow
- Irregular and increased rate and rhythm of pulse and respirations
- Clitoral engorgement and increased vaginal blood flow (in women)
- Penile tumescence (in men).

The physiologic alterations that occur during REM may exacerbate some medical problems. For example, increased gastric acid secretion during REM sleep may precipitate gastrointestinal pain for people with peptic ulcer disease. Likewise, people with chronic obstructive pulmonary disease (COPD) may experience dyspnea or even a respiratory crisis because of decreased oxygen saturation during REM periods.

Because the length of stage I sleep increases gradually throughout adulthood, older adults experience longer periods of drowsiness without actual sleep during the early part of the night. In addition, older adults shift more frequently in and out of lighter sleep stages. Between the ages of 20 and 40 years old, the proportion of deep sleep (stages III and IV) decreases gradually until the age of 70 years, when it levels off. In both younger and older adults, stage IV sleep increases significantly during the night after sleep loss. The number of episodes of REM sleep does not change significantly in older adults, but episodes are shorter, resulting in proportionately less time spent in REM. Also, REM sleep stages shift toward the earlier part of the night in older adults. Table 24-1 summarizes the usual adult sleep cycle and typical age-related changes in sleep patterns.

Circadian Rhythm

Sleep patterns are determined, in part, by an individual's **circadian rhythm**, also known as a *biological clock*. Body functions that have a circadian pattern include thermoregulation, sleep–wake cycles, and secretion of many hormones, including cortisol and melatonin. The sleep–wake circadian rhythm generally causes adults to become sleepy between 10 PM and midnight and to awaken feeling rested between 6 AM and

TABLE 24-1 Age-Related Changes in Sleep	
Sleep Characteristics	**Healthy Older Adults (vs. Healthy Younger Adults)**
NREM	
Stages I and II (light sleep)	Gradual increase in quantity, so it accounts for 70% of total sleep time
Stages III and IV (deep sleep)	Proportionate decrease in quantity
REM (dream stage)	Proportionate decrease in quantity
	Begins earlier in the night
	Less intense
Sleep initiation	Longer time to fall asleep
Sleep maintenance	More frequent arousals
Sleep efficiency	Reduced amount of sleep during time in bed, more time in napping to compensate
Sleep schedule	Shift in nocturnal sleep phase to earlier bedtime and wakening

NREM, non–rapid eye movement; REM, rapid eye movement.

8 AM. With increasing age, **advanced sleep phase** occurs, causing older adults to become sleepy earlier in the evening and to awaken earlier in the morning. Age-related alterations in circadian rhythm affect sleep quantity and quality, and these disturbances are likely to be exacerbated by lack of exposure to bright light.

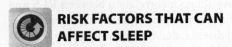

RISK FACTORS THAT CAN AFFECT SLEEP

Although age-related changes affect both the quality and quantity of sleep, they do not necessarily lead to sleep complaints in healthy older adults. For example, in a study of 180 centenarians, 57.4% reported good quality sleep (Tafaro et al., 2007). Rather, the common complaint of sleep problems among older adults is associated with the many psychosocial or physiologic risk factors that frequently affect older adults. In addition, environmental conditions, particularly in institutional settings, can significantly affect the sleep patterns of older adults. Many older adults experience sleep complaints due to several interacting risk factors. One study found that 69% of residents of assisted living facilities reported sleep disturbance, 42% reported primary insomnia, and 35% reported daytime sleepiness, with an association between more functional impairment and sleep complaints (Martin, Alam, Harker, Josephson, & Alessi, 2008).

Psychosocial Factors

Beliefs and attitudes about sleep can have a powerful impact, with many beliefs having a detrimental, anxiety-producing effect. For example, older adults who believe that arousals during the night are abnormal and unhealthy may think they have **insomnia** and seek treatment with medications. Rigid beliefs about the amount of sleep required during the night also can lead to false definitions of insomnia and inappropriate treatment. Likewise, excessive worry about the quantity or quality of sleep can have a negative impact on sleep.

Anxiety, dementia, and depression are psychosocial disorders associated with disrupted sleep. Anxiety and dementia are associated with difficulty falling asleep, frequent arousals during the night, and difficulty returning to sleep. In addition, people with dementia are likely to experience the following sleep alterations: increased time in light sleep stages, very little REM and deep sleep, decreased total sleep time, disrupted sleep–wake cycles, and frequent nighttime arousals and daytime napping. Sleep changes associated with dementia vary according to dementia severity, as discussed in more detail in Chapter 14. Compared with people unaffected by depression, people who are depressed typically take longer to fall asleep, have less deep sleep and more light sleep, awaken more frequently during the night and earlier in the morning, and feel less rested in the morning.

Older adults with few or no interesting activities, work demands, social responsibilities, or environmental stimuli may find it particularly difficult to establish healthy sleeping patterns. Older adults with dementia or depression who are living alone are particularly susceptible to disturbed sleep patterns because of the tendency to stay in bed during the day out of boredom, lack of motivation, difficulty concentrating on interesting activities, or a desire to withdraw from stressful situations. Finally, in any setting, if an older adult spends all of his or her time in the same room, the lack of differentiation between space for waking and sleeping activities may interfere with sleep patterns.

Environmental Factors

Environmental circumstances are another factor that can significantly influence sleep patterns. For people who do not live alone, the actions and demands of other people in the setting, particularly those sharing the same sleeping area, influence sleep patterns. For adults at any age, a change in the sleep environment usually requires a period of adjustment before optimal sleep patterns are established. Thus, older adults may have a particularly difficult time sleeping during the first few nights in a new environment.

In institutional settings, lack of quiet and privacy, conflicting needs of various people, and sleeping in close proximity to others are all factors that can interfere with sleep. Older adults who are accustomed to sleeping alone or with close relations may feel their privacy is being violated in institutional settings where they are required to share a room with people from outside their family. Difficulty falling asleep also may arise if environmental circumstances do not allow the performance of usual prebedtime activities, such as listening to music or reading a book. Schedules of caregivers also may interfere with the sleeping habits of the older adult. For example, in institutional settings, the time for awakening patients/residents is often based on the most efficient use of nursing and dietary time, and patients/residents are expected to adjust their sleep routines accordingly. Likewise, in home settings, dependent older adults may have to adjust their sleep routines to the schedule of their caregivers, who may have work and other responsibilities.

Uncomfortably low or high temperatures, which are often related to inadequate heating or cooling systems, are another environmental factor that can interfere with sleep. Hot and humid conditions can contribute to sleep disturbances in menopausal women by increasing the number of nighttime hot flashes. Noise is another environmental factor that can be more problematic for older adults because around the age of 40 years, people become more sensitive to noise when they are sleeping and can be awakened by less intense auditory stimuli.

Lighting exerts a strong influence on circadian rhythms and can affect sleep patterns in several ways. During the night, excessive light in rooms and hallways, as well as intermittent use of bedside or overhead lighting during care routines, may disrupt sleep. During the day, a lack of sufficient bright light can interfere with nighttime sleep because exposure to bright light is a strong influence on the circadian rhythm. The strong effect of light on sleep is associated with the fact that the body needs light to produce melatonin, a hormone that regulates many physiologic functions, including sleep, body temperature, and the setting of the circadian rhythm. Lack of exposure to bright light is especially problematic in long-term care settings because residents are typically exposed to only a few minutes of bright light daily and daytime light levels tend to be quite low (Martin & Ancoli-Israel, 2008).

In home settings, environmental factors can interfere with the sleep of older adults. For example, older adults who are caregivers may have their sleep interrupted by dependent family members who require care during the night. Conditions such as fear, loneliness, or neighborhood noise are environmental factors that can interfere with sleep in home settings. In any of these situations, a move to an institution may provide the supports and security needed for more peaceful sleeping.

Pathophysiologic Factors

Pathologic processes, physical pain or discomfort, neuromuscular disorders, and adverse effects of chemicals and medications are physiologic factors that can interfere with sleep. Although these risk factors are not unique to older adults, they are increasingly likely to occur in older adults, and are more detrimental in the presence of age-related changes and other risk factors.

Disease processes and physical discomfort interfere with sleep patterns in many ways, with some pathologic conditions being exacerbated during sleep, particularly during the REM sleep stage. Studies have found a correlation between sleep disorders and the following pathophysiologic conditions: malignancies, chronic pain, diabetes mellitus, Parkinson's disease, chronic kidney disease, and COPD (Garcia, 2008). Likewise, cramps in the calf or foot muscles are a nighttime problem for some older adults and may interrupt sleep patterns. Delirium is a condition that is strongly associated with sleep disturbances and, in hospital settings, is one of the most common reasons that nurses request sedatives for their patients (Flaherty, 2008).

✦ Wellness Opportunity

Nurses promote wellness by identifying subtle risk factors, such as chronic pain and discomfort that are often overlooked and that can be addressed through many types of holistic interventions.

Two neuromuscular disorders, RLS and **periodic limb movements in sleep (PLMS)**, have been topics of interest and research in sleep disorder centers since the mid-1970s. RLS is the experience of an almost irresistible urge to move the legs, usually accompanied by unpleasant leg sensations. Symptoms of RLS usually occur in a circadian rhythm, with peak severity between 11 PM and 3 AM, which can interfere

both with initiating and maintaining sleep (Ferri et al., 2008; Spiegelhalder & Hornyak, 2008). In people with dementia, RLS may be a possible cause of motor restlessness and wandering (Martin & Ancoli-Israel, 2008). Studies of RLS prevalence across age groups found a range of 9% to 35% for older age groups (Spiegelhalder & Hornyak, 2008; Wolkove, Elkholy, Baltzan, & Palayew, 2007). In addition to increasing age, researchers have found a correlation between RLS and the following conditions: anemia, depression, fibromyalgia, malignancies, renal disease, diabetes mellitus, anxiety disorders, rheumatoid arthritis, and neurodegenerative diseases. RLS may also be caused or exacerbated by bioactive substances, including caffeine, saccharine, and psychoactive medications (Spiegelhalder & Hornyak, 2008).

PLMS, also known as *nocturnal myoclonus*, is the occurrence of brief muscle contractions, spaced at intervals of about 20 to 40 seconds, that cause leg jerks, or rhythmic movements of muscles in the foot or leg. They occur several times to more than 200 times nightly. Studies indicate that the occurrence of PLMS increases with age, with prevalence rates of 45% among older adults (Wolkove et al., 2007). PLMS can contribute to complaints of insomnia, frequent arousals, and increased daytime sleepiness. In addition to increased age, risk factors for PLMS include caffeine, alcohol, and certain medications (e.g., benzodiazepines and antidepressants). Table 24-2 lists common physiologic processes that commonly occur in older adults and their effects on sleep.

Effects of Bioactive Substances

Adverse effects of medications and chemicals, such as caffeine, alcohol, and nicotine, can interfere with sleep in a number of ways. Caffeine is a central nervous system stimulant that lengthens the sleep latency period and causes awakening during the night. Studies have documented that regular daily caffeine intake is associated with disturbed sleep and increased daytime sleepiness (Roehrs & Roth, 2008). Although low doses of nicotine can have relaxing and sedative effects, higher doses interfere with sleep because of nicotine's stimulant effect as well as its effects on respiration. Alcohol may induce drowsiness as an initial effect, but it suppresses REM sleep and increases the number of awakenings, especially during the latter half of the sleep period. The end result of alcohol consumption is a decrease in total sleep time and an increase in daytime sleepiness. Moreover, people who have consumed alcohol over many years may experience alcohol-related insomnia for a few years after withdrawing from it. If **obstructive sleep apnea** is an underlying causative factor of insomnia, the use of alcohol, hypnotics, or other central nervous system depressants may exacerbate the sleep disorder and lead to increased doses of medication and further detrimental effects. These chemical effects are not unique to older adults; however, adverse effects of medication are more likely to occur in older adults, as discussed in detail in Chapter 8.

Contrary to their primary purpose, some hypnotic medications can cause or contribute to sleep disturbances, especially

TABLE 24-2 Pathophysiologic Factors Affecting Sleep

Risk Factor	Sleep Alteration
Arthritis	Chronic pain and discomfort that interfere with sleep
COPD	Awakening as a result of apnea and respiratory distress
Diabetes mellitus	Awakening secondary to nocturia or poorly controlled blood glucose levels; increased incidence of OSA
Gastrointestinal disorders, ulcers	Nocturnal pain secondary to increased gastric secretions during REM sleep
Hypertension	Early morning awakening
Hyperthyroidism	Increased difficulty falling asleep
Nocturnal angina	Awakening without perception of pain, especially during REM sleep
PLMS, RLS	Awakening caused by recurrent involuntary leg movements
Malignancies	Increased incidence of RLS
Chronic kidney disease	Increase incidence of PLMS, RLS, and OSA
Parkinsonism	Increased time awake; decreased amount of sleep
Dementia	Alterations of all sleep stages
Delirium	Increased somnolence *or* inability to sleep

COPD, chronic obstructive pulmonary disease; OSA, obstructive sleep apnea; PLMS, periodic limb movements in sleep; REM, rapid eye movement; RLS, restless legs syndrome.

when used for more than a few days consecutively because tolerance can develop, sometimes within several days. Also, benzodiazepine hypnotics can have serious adverse effects, especially if the dose is increased to compensate for tolerance. A review of literature concludes that benzodiazepines, when used to treat insomnia, should be avoided because they are associated with unwanted side effects including falls, fractures, mental changes, and diminished daytime alertness and ability to perform everyday tasks (Stone, Ensrud, & Ancoli-Israel, 2008; Tariq & Pulisetty, 2008). Although the nonbenzodiazepine sleep medications, which have been available since 1993, are effective and safer, many older adults continue to use benzodiazepines, which were the most widely prescribed sleep medications after 1970. In addition, older adults often use over-the-counter medications, such as diphenhydramine and other antihistamines, for their sedating effects; however, there is no data to support their effectiveness in improving sleep and they can have serious adverse effects because of their strong anticholinergic actions (Tariq & Pulisetty, 2008).

Other medications that have been associated with disturbed sleep include steroids, antidepressants, aminophylline preparations, thyroid extracts, antiarrhythmic medications, and centrally acting antihypertensives. Table 24-3 summarizes the effects of various medications and chemicals on sleep in older adults.

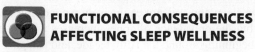 **FUNCTIONAL CONSEQUENCES AFFECTING SLEEP WELLNESS**

The overall functional consequences of age-related sleep changes in sleep (refer to Table 24-1) are insufficient and inefficient sleep and are experienced as poor quality of sleep. In addition, the high prevalence of risk factors that can interfere with sleep increases the vulnerability of older adults to sleep disorders and complaints. Common sleep complaints of older adults include daytime sleepiness, difficulty falling asleep, and frequent arousals during the night. Although estimates of sleep complaints among community dwelling older adults are as high as 80%, most studies indicate that insomnia affects 20% to 50% of the adult population, that it increases with age, and that it affects women more than men (Espiritu, 2008; Garcia, 2008). Studies indicate that poor sleep can lead to additional functional consequences including fatigue, poor cognitive functioning, decreased quality of life, increased depression and anxiety, difficulty with balance and mobility, increased risk for falls, increased potential for a move to an institutional setting, and increased risk for mortality (Benca & Peterson, 2008; Goldman, Ancoli-Israel, & Boudreau, 2008; Misra & Malow, 2008; Walker, 2008).

In the late 1970s, sleep disorders were classified systematically, and standards were established to diagnose these

TABLE 24-3 The Effect of Various Medications and Chemicals on Sleep

Medication or Chemical	Sleep Alteration
Alcohol	Suppression of REM sleep; early morning awakening
Alcohol or hypnotic withdrawal	Sleep disturbances; nightmares
Anticholinergics	Hyperreflexia; overactivity; muscle twitching
Barbiturates	Suppression of REM sleep; nightmares; hallucinations; paradoxical responses
Benzodiazepines	Awakening secondary to apnea
Beta-blockers	Nightmares
Corticosteroids	Restlessness; sleep disturbances
Diuretics	Awakening for nocturia; sleep apnea secondary to alkalosis
Theophylline, levodopa, isoproterenol, phenytoin	Interference with sleep onset and sleep stages
Antidepressants	PLMS; suppression of REM sleep

PLMS, periodic limb movements in sleep; REM, rapid eye movement.

Evidence-Based Practice   24-1
Excessive Sleepiness

Statement of the Problem

- Excessive sleepiness—defined as the inability to maintain alertness, with characteristic hypersomnolence—is common in older adults.
- Causes of excessive sleepiness include medications, environmental and lifestyle factors, age-related changes in chronobiology, chronic health conditions, and medical and psychological disorders (e.g., sleep disorders).
- Healthy older adults experience the following changes in sleep: an increase in transient arousals, longer time until sleep onset and stage 1 sleep, and decrease in quantity and quality of restorative slow-wave sleep.
- Daytime sleepiness is often viewed falsely as normal or unpreventable in older adults; this misperception reduces the likelihood that this condition will be appropriately evaluated and treated.
- Chronic disorders of sleep and wakefulness are among the most common, but overlooked, health problems.
- Consequences of sleepiness and decreased alertness are delayed reaction time and diminished cognitive performance.

Recommendations for Nursing Assessment

- Obtain a sleep history, based on information from both the patient and family members, including information about sleep patterns and sleep-related behaviors.
- Consider using either the Epworth Sleepiness Scale or the Pittsburgh Sleep Quality Scale as a valid and reliable tool for identifying excessive sleepiness.
- Assess for the following causes of excessive daytime sleepiness: obstructive sleep apnea, insomnia, restless legs syndrome, medications, and medical and psychiatric illness.
- When possible, observe patients for snoring, apnea during sleep, excessive leg movements during sleep, and difficulty staying awake during normal daytime activities.

Recommendations for Patient Teaching

Teach older adults and caregivers about the following sleep-promoting measures:
- Use the bed only for sleeping or sex.
- Develop consistent and rest-promoting bedtime routines and maintain the same schedule daily.
- If awakened during the night, avoid looking at the clock.
- Avoid naps or limit to 10–15 minutes.
- Sleep in a cool, quiet environment.
- Avoid the following before bedtime: caffeine, nicotine, alcohol, large meals, exercise, emotionally charged activities.
- If you cannot fall asleep after 15 or 20 minutes, go to another room and engage in a quiet activity until you are sleepy again.

Recommendations for Care

- Work with primary care practitioners to ensure optimal management of medical conditions, psychological disorders, and symptoms that interfere with sleep.
- Teach patients and families about lifestyle measures for improving sleep among all family members.
- Incorporate sleep-hygiene measure and ongoing treatment of existing sleep disorders into the plan of care for older adults in all settings.
- Work with prescribing practitioners to review and, if appropriate, adjust medications that can cause drowsiness or sleep impairment.
- Suggest referral to a sleep specialist for moderate or severe sleepiness or a clinical profile consistent with major sleep disorders.

SOURCE: Adapted from Chasens, E. R., Williams, L. L., & Umlauf, M. G. (2008). Excessive sleepiness. In E. Capezuti, D. Zwicker, M. Mezey, & T. Fulmer (Eds.), *Evidence-based geriatric nursing protocols for best practice* (3rd ed., pp. 459–476). New York: Springer Publishing Co.

---

disorders. Insomnia is classified as a disorder of initiating and maintaining sleep and is one of the most common sleep disorders of older adults. **Excessive daytime sleepiness**, defined as the inability to maintain alertness, is characterized by hypersomnolence (i.e., falling asleep at periodic intervals during a 24-hour period). Excessive daytime sleepiness differs from fatigue, which manifests as difficulty sustaining a high level of functioning. An evidence-based geriatric nursing protocol for best practice states that daytime sleepiness should not be dismissed as an insignificant condition, rather, it should be evaluated by health care providers because it can have significant health effects (Chasens, Williams, & Umlauf, 2008). The protocol is summarized in Evidence-Based Practice Box 24-1.

PATHOLOGIC CONDITION AFFECTING SLEEP: OBSTRUCTIVE SLEEP APNEA

Although medical literature in the late 1880s referred to syndromes in which sleep disorders were associated with brief interruptions in respirations, this phenomenon received little attention until the mid-1970s. In 1988, the U.S. Congress established the National Commission on Sleep Disorders Re-

search to promote prevention, diagnosis, and treatment of obstructive sleep apnea and other sleep disorders. Currently, sleep apnea syndromes have received widespread attention in clinical practice, largely because of research in sleep disorder centers and the increasing availability of evidence-based interventions. Obstructive sleep apnea is the involuntary cessation of airflow for 10 seconds or longer; the occurrence of more than five to eight of these episodes per hour is considered to be pathologic. This condition occurs because the muscles responsible for holding the throat open relax during sleep and block the passage of air. Symptoms of obstructive sleep apnea include daytime fatigue, morning headaches, diminished mental acuity, and loud snoring punctuated by brief periods of silence.

Obstructive sleep apnea is not exclusively a condition of older adults, but the prevalence of apnea increases with advancing age, beginning around the fifth decade, and is higher in men than in women. Prevalence rates for adults older than 60 years range from 37.5% to 62% (Norman & Loredo, 2008). In addition to being associated with increased age, sleep apnea is associated with obesity, dementia, depression, hypertension, hypothyroidism, kyphoscoliosis, deformities of the jaw or nasal structures, and the use of nicotine, alcohol, and medications that depress the respiratory center.

Obstructive sleep apnea has serious consequences because it increases the risk for serious medical conditions and even death. For example, studies confirm that there is a strong independent association between obstructive sleep apnea and all the following conditions: stroke, arrhythmias, hypertension, heart failure, and coronary artery disease (Bradley & Floras, 2009). Moreover, treatment of obstructive sleep apnea results in improved cardiac function, reduced cardiovascular disease, and decrease in mortality rates (Norman & Loredo, 2008). In addition, obstructive sleep apnea interferes with quality of life because it causes excessive daytime sleepiness and other cognitive effects. Adverse cognitive effects include impaired psychomotor vigilance, accuracy, sustained attention, visuospatial learning, executive performance, and motor performance (Norman & Loredo, 2008).

NURSING ASSESSMENT OF SLEEP

Identifying Opportunities for Health Promotion

In recent years, nurses and other health care professionals have focused on the importance of assessing sleep as an essential aspect of wellness and quality of life. Nurses assess sleep patterns to determine the adequacy of the person's usual sleep and rest pattern and to identify factors that either contribute to or interfere with the quality and quantity of sleep. When the assessment identifies health-promoting behaviors that improve sleep, nurses can support these efforts. When nurses identify dysfunctional sleep patterns or risk factors that interfere with sleep, they plan interventions to address the underlying contributing factors. Nurses can address many of the contributing factors through educational interventions when the assessment identifies that misinformation or a lack of knowledge contributes to sleep complaints. Box 24-1 provides guidelines for interviewing independent older adults and caregivers of dependent older adults about sleep and rest patterns.

In addition to obtaining information from older adults and their caregivers, nurses observe behavioral cues of nighttime and daytime rest and activities. This is especially important when objective observations are contrary to subjective complaints. For example, older adults may complain of not sleeping at all, but when observed by caregivers, they may appear to be sleeping during the entire night. By contrast, older adults who deny any problems sleeping may nap frequently and readily fall asleep during daytime activities.

Wellness Opportunity

Nurses can help older adults who are dissatisfied with their sleep identify the risk factors that can be addressed through self-care measures to improve sleep quantity and quality, rather than view this as an inevitable consequence of aging.

Evidence-Based Assessment Tools

Older adults can use evidence-based sleep assessment tools for self-assessment or for self-reporting to health care professionals. Two easy-to-use and readily available tools that

Box 24-1 Guidelines for Assessing Sleep and Rest

Questions to Assess the Perception of Quality and Adequacy of Sleep
- On a scale of 1–10, with 10 as the highest, how would you rate your sleep?
- When you awaken in the morning, do you feel like you are rested?
- Do you feel drowsy or sleepy during the day or early evening?
- Does fatigue interfere with your desired daytime activity level?

Questions to Identify Opportunities for Health Education
- What is your usual time for getting into bed?
- Describe your usual activities during the daytime and evening.
- What are the factors that help you fall asleep (e.g., food or drink, relaxation strategies, environmental influences)?
- What conditions interfere with good sleep (e.g., pain, discomfort, anxiety, depression)?
- Do you take any medicines to help you sleep?
- Do you take medicines to help you stay awake during the day?
- Do you drink alcoholic or caffeinated beverages, or take medicines that contain alcohol or caffeine during the late afternoon or evening? (If yes, how much and what kind?)

- Do you smoke or use nicotine products? (If yes, what kind and how much?)
- Are you aware, or has anyone told you, that you snore or stop breathing during your sleep?
- Do your legs kick or jump involuntarily while you sleep?

Questions to Assess Nighttime Sleep Pattern
- Where do you sleep at night (e.g., bed, couch, recliner chair)?
- How long does it usually take to fall asleep after you get into bed?
- Do you think you lie awake too long before falling asleep?
- After you fall asleep, how many times do you wake up during the night?
- What kinds of things disturb your sleep during the night (e.g., getting up to urinate; activities of roommates or other people in the setting; environmental factors, such as noise or lighting)?
- If changes in living arrangements have occurred in the past few months: Has your sleep pattern changed since . . . (e.g., since you came to this nursing home; since your spouse passed away)?

have been tested for validity and reliability are the **Pittsburgh Sleep Quality Index (PSQI)** and the **Epworth Sleepiness Scale (ESS)**. The PSQI assesses sleep quality and patterns over the past month, and the ESS focuses on daytime sleepiness over the past week. The Hartford Institute for Geriatric Nursing recommends the use of both these tools, and nurses can access the tools and guidelines at http://consultgerirn.org.

---

*M*rs. Z. is 66 years old and recently retired from her job as office manager for a law firm. She considers herself to be in good health, although she has had hypertension for 20 years and osteoarthritis for the past several years. She self-monitors her blood pressure and takes atenolol, 50 mg daily. She occasionally takes an over-the-counter analgesic medication when her arthritis pain bothers her. She just started going to the local senior center once a week for lunch and social and educational activities. During one of your weekly senior wellness clinics, Mrs. Z. comes to talk with you about her difficulty sleeping. She reports that since she has retired, she often wakes up several times during the night and has difficulty returning to sleep. She used to sleep an average of 7 to 8 hours nightly and could easily return to sleep if she woke up during the night. Now she is lucky if she gets 6 hours of sleep because she lies in bed for several hours. She used to go to bed between 10 and 11 PM and get up promptly between 6:30 and 7 AM. Now that she is retired, she goes to bed around 11 PM, but stays in bed until 10 AM if she wakes up during the night and does not get a full night's sleep.

THINKING POINTS

- What age-related changes may be contributing to Mrs. Z.'s dissatisfaction with her sleep?
- What risk factors might be contributing to Mrs. Z.'s dissatisfaction with her sleep?
- What further assessment information would you need to obtain, and how would you obtain it?

NURSING DIAGNOSIS

Nursing diagnoses pertinent to older adults who have sleep problems include Insomnia (i.e., "a disruption in amount and quality of sleep that impairs functioning"); Disturbed Sleep Pattern (i.e., "time-limited interruptions of sleep amount and quality due to external factors"); or Sleep Deprivation (i.e., "prolonged periods of time without sleep") (NANDA International, 2009, pp. 115, 117, 118). When healthy older adults report dissatisfaction with their sleep and express interest in learning self-care activities to improve their sleep pattern,

nurses can use the nursing diagnosis of Readiness for Enhanced Sleep. This wellness nursing diagnosis is defined as "A pattern of natural, periodic suspension of consciousness that provides adequate rest, sustains a desired lifestyle, and can be strengthened (NANDA International, 2009, p. 119).

> **◆ Wellness Opportunity**
>
> Nurses can be alert to opportunities to include the wellness nursing diagnosis of Rreadiness for Enhanced Sleep for older adults in community or long-term care facilities who are willing to explore interventions that improve their sleep patterns.

PLANNING FOR WELLNESS OUTCOMES

When older adults experience sleep disturbances or have risk factors that affect sleep patterns, nurses identify wellness outcomes as an essential part of the nursing process. Nursing Outcomes Classification (NOC) terms that most directly relate to interventions to enhance sleep or address disturbed sleep pattern in older adults are Sleep, Rest, Comfort Level, Personal Well-Being, Anxiety Self-Control, Knowledge: Health Behavior, and Pain: Disruptive Effects.

> **◆ Wellness Opportunity**
>
> Quality of life is a wellness outcome that is achieved through nursing interventions directed toward enhancing sleep.

NURSING INTERVENTIONS FOR SLEEP WELLNESS

Nursing interventions to promote sleep wellness for older adults include health education and direct interventions, such as environmental modifications and comfort and relaxation strategies. As with other aspects of nursing care for older adults, it is essential that nurses individualize the care to address each person's identified needs in various settings. For example, nurses in community settings can focus on teaching older adults and their caregivers about self-care interventions that can improve sleep patterns. In long-term care settings, nurses focus on interventions that can be implemented routinely to improve sleep patterns of residents. In hospital settings, nurses focus primarily on acute medical problems, but sleep disturbances should not be overlooked as an important health concern. Nurses can use the following pertinent Nursing Interventions Classification (NIC) terminologies for documentation of interventions: Sleep Enhancement, Anxiety Reduction, Music Therapy, Risk Identification, Environmental Management, Pain Management, Progressive Muscle Relaxation, and Phototherapy: Mood/Sleep Regulation.

Evidence-Based Interventions

Evidence-based guidelines for interventions to improve sleep and address excessive sleepiness are listed in Resources section at the end of this chapter. All guidelines emphasize initiation of appropriate interventions, including health education about self-care strategies; identification and management of underlying causative conditions; and suitable referrals for further evaluation and treatment. Information in this chapter is based on these guidelines and focuses on interventions that nurses can use in various settings to enhance sleep patterns in older adults.

Self-Care Actions to Promote Healthy Sleep Patterns

Many self-care actions are appropriate for improving sleep, even in people without major sleep complaints. For example, studies confirm that daily moderate physical activity improves sleep for older adults (Guimaraes, deCarvalho, Yanaguibashi, & do Prado, 2008; King et al., 2008). Nurses can use information in Tables 24-1 and 24-2 to teach older adults about normal age-related changes and help them identify risk factors that can affect their sleep. When the assessment identifies contributing factors, nurses can help older adults plan interventions to address these risks. For example, if older adults experience chronic pain or discomfort that interferes with sleep, nurses can help identify appropriate interventions and comfort measures. In addition, nurses can give a copy of Box 24-2 to older adults to teach about actions they can initiate to improve sleep. The box includes brief information about complementary and alternative care practices that are frequently used for sleep problems. Current evidence-based information about complementary and alternative modalities used for sleep is reviewed in the next section to provide a foundation for health education about these practices.

If older adults are not familiar with relaxation techniques for improving sleep, nurses can give them a copy of Box 24-3 and teach them about deep breathing, progressive relaxation, and mental imagery. Cassette tape or CD players with automatic shutoffs can be used to play soothing music or instructions for deep breathing, guided imagery, or relaxation exercises. These products are growing in popularity and can be purchased from many book and music stores or through the Internet.

Complementary and Alternative Care Practices

Commonly used complementary and alternative practices for improving sleep include light therapy, bioactive substances (e.g., melatonin, aromatherapy, herbal products, homeopathic remedies), and body–mind modalities (e.g., yoga, imagery, meditation, tai chi). Evidence-based information about the effectiveness of complementary and alternative practices that older adults are likely to initiate for sleep can be summarized as follows, based on reviews of literature (Gammack, 2008b; Gooneratne, 2008; Joshi, 2008; Ong, Shapiro, & Manber, 2009):

- Melatonin, a sleep-regulating hormone produced by the pineal gland, can be effective in managing circadian sleep disorders, such as those that occur in older adults.

Box 24-2 Health Promotion Teaching About Sleep

Actions to Take
- Establish a bedtime ritual that is effective for you, and try to follow it every night.
- Maintain the same daily schedule for waking, resting, and sleeping.
- Take a warm, relaxing bath in the afternoon or early evening.
- After 1:00 PM, avoid foods, beverages, and medications that contain caffeine or stimulants (e.g., tea, cocoa, coffee, chocolate, sugar, refined carbohydrates, and some over-the-counter pain relievers and cold preparations).
- Prebedtime foods that promote sleep include milk (warm), chamomile tea, and a light snack of complex carbohydrates (e.g., whole grains).
- Use one or more of the following relaxation methods: imagery, meditation, deep breathing, progressive relaxation, soothing music, body or foot massage, rocking in a chair, reading nonstimulating materials, or watching nonstimulating television.
- Perform daily moderate aerobic exercise, preferably before the late afternoon, but avoid vigorous exercise in the evening.
- Assure adequate intake of the following nutrients: zinc, calcium, magnesium, manganese, vitamin C, and vitamin B complex.

Actions to Avoid
- Do not drink alcohol before bedtime because it may cause early morning awakening. If you use alcohol, use only in small amounts.
- Do not smoke cigarettes in the evening because nicotine is a stimulant.

- If your bedtime is temporarily changed, try to keep your waking time as close to the usual time as possible, and avoid staying in bed beyond your usual waking time.
- Do not use your bed for reading or other activities not associated with sleeping.
- If you awaken during the night and cannot return to sleep, get out of bed after 30 minutes and engage in a nonstimulating activity, such as reading, in another room.
- Arise at your usual time, even if you have not slept well.

Complementary and Alternative Care Practices
- Yoga, tai chi, meditation, imagery, aromatherapy, massage, soothing music, relaxation techniques, and a warm bath or warm footbath may be effective in promoting sleep.
- Melatonin, a sleep-regulating hormone, can be effective in improving sleep, but it can interact with other medications and also can cause daytime sleepiness.

Special Precautions
- Although widely promoted as sleep aids, herbs should be used with caution in older adults because of their possible adverse effects.
- Inform your health care professionals about any use of herbs, aromatherapy, or other complementary and alternative care practices.

Box 24-3 Relaxation and Mental Imagery Techniques That Promote Sleep

Deep Breathing
- Focus your attention on your breathing; extend your belly and draw in a deep breath as you count.
- Hold your breath for three or four counts.
- Exhale completely.
- Repeat this pattern, focusing your total attention on breathing.
- Phrases, such as "I am sleepy," or counting may be repeated during each exhalation to help keep your attention focused on breathing.

Progressive Relaxation
- Start by focusing your attention on the muscles in your toes.
- Flex or tense these muscles, and then relax them.
- Repeat two or three times.
- Focus your attention on the muscles in your foot.

- Flex or tense, then relax these muscles, two or three times.
- Repeat this process, progressively focusing on different muscle groups and proceeding from your feet to your head.

Mental Imagery
- Begin with deep breathing exercises to relax yourself.
- Focus your attention on a serene and peaceful scene, visualize the setting, and imagine the sounds (e.g., a beach with waves gently washing ashore).
- Imagine yourself in the setting, lying relaxed, enjoying the environment.
- Keep your attention focused on the scene.
- Imagine repetitive motions, such as waves on the beach or sheep jumping over a fence.

Although a dose range of 0.1 to 10 mg is relatively safe, daytime sleepiness and interference in the effectiveness of calcium channel blockers can be problematic for older adults.

- Valerian has been effective in subjective improvement in sleep in randomized, placebo-controlled trials, and it may increase deep sleep stages.
- Massage therapy has been effective in improving sleep, particularly in people who have conditions that affect sleep, such as stress and fibromyalgia.
- Acupressure, which involves noninvasive stimulation of pressure points, can improve sleep in institutionalized older adults, in patients with end-stage renal disease, and in agitated patients with dementia.
- Relaxation techniques, including imagery and progressive muscle relaxation, are effective for improving sleep in healthy older adults and in those with concomitant conditions, particularly if the technique is practiced twice daily for at least a couple of weeks.
- Meditation techniques, particularly mindfulness meditation, are effective in improving deep sleep and overall sleep, particularly if stress is a contributing factor.
- Tai chi, a Chinese exercise with a meditation component, is effective in improving overall sleep quality and quantity, daytime sleepiness, and general health-related quality of life.
- Listening to soothing music has been shown to improve sleep onset, quality and duration, and daytime function in older people.
- Aromatherapy with lavender essential oil can shorten sleep onset time.

In addition to these modalities, bright light therapy is a modality that can improve sleep in people with seasonal affective disorder (Gammack, 2008b). Studies also indicate that light therapy is effective in reducing agitation and improving sleep and circadian rhythm in people with dementia (Paniagua & Paniagua, 2008). However, there is limited evidence of benefits in healthy older adults or in those with chronic insomnia or nonseasonal depression (Gammack, 2008b).

Wellness Opportunity

Health education about sleep is particularly important in community and long-term care settings because nurses have more opportunities to focus on quality-of-life issues.

Improving Sleep for Older Adults in Institutional Settings

Older adults in acute and long-term care settings have a high prevalence of sleep disturbances, and these disturbances can lead to serious and detrimental health consequences (Flaherty, 2008). For example, lack of sleep in older adults increases their risk for anxiety, delirium, depression, and longer lengths of hospital stay (LaReau, Benson, Watcharotone, & Manguba, 2008). Studies have found that sleep patterns of older adults in long-term care settings are especially fragmented, with residents sleeping for only 58% of the time spent in bed and seldom sleeping for more than 1 hour at a time (Joshi, 2008). Nurses who work evening or night shifts have many opportunities to engage in direct care activities that promote good nighttime sleep, which are in addition to environmental interventions discussed in the next section.

For older adults in any setting, nursing responsibilities include addressing factors that interfere with sleep, ensuring the most comfortable environment possible, and individualizing care plans so that they incorporate personal preferences for optimal sleep conditions. A nursing study of hospitalized older adults identified the following relatively simple nursing actions as interventions to improve sleep (listed in order of patient preferences): assistance with personal hygiene (e.g., toileting, mouth care); awareness of and adherence to usual bedtime; providing a 5-minute head-to-toe massage; straightening bed linens; provision of a bedtime snack; minimizing bedside conversation; and darkening the room (LaReau et al., 2008).

If dementia or depression interferes with sleep onset, the nurse can simply stay with the older person to provide reassurance until the person is able to fall asleep. In addition, relief of pain and anxiety are nursing responsibilities that can influence the sleep of older adults. Older adults who are cognitively impaired may not request analgesics but may give nonverbal cues that pain is interfering with sleep. Nurses should be alert to this possibility and assess for chronic or acute pain. An analgesic taken 30 minutes before bedtime may help induce sleep in people with chronic pain or discomfort.

Because daytime activities influence sleep patterns, care plans in long-term care settings should incorporate appropriate types and amounts of activities in each older adult's daily routine. Also, residents should be exposed to adequate bright lights during the day. Nighttime routines need to be based on a comprehensive assessment of the needs of the older adult and consider any conflicting needs. For example, for some older adults, the need for an uninterrupted night's sleep may outweigh the potential benefits of being awakened for nighttime care tasks. In many situations, the needs can be addressed during the person's usual waking time, rather than performing the tasks on a rigid schedule designed for the convenience of staff.

Modifying the Environment to Promote Sleep

Environmental modifications are among the simplest and most effective interventions to improve sleep, especially in institutional settings. Actions, such as closing bedroom doors and adjusting bedroom lighting, can improve sleep. Elimination of unnecessary staff-initiated noise, especially conversations at the nursing station, is another helpful intervention for patients/residents located near the center of nursing activity. In long-term care settings, nurses can document preferences for bedtime routines that promote sleep on each resident's care plan and assure that these measures are carried out by nursing staff. In long-term care settings where residents share rooms, decisions about room assignments should take into consideration the compatibility of individual needs. Once room assignments have been made, roommate behaviors that interfere with sleep can be addressed by a room change, if necessary.

If a noisy environment contributes to sleeping difficulties, and the noise cannot be controlled or eliminated, the older person may wish to use earplugs. People who live alone, however, should be cautioned about the danger of blocking out protective noises, such as that of a smoke alarm. If environmental noise cannot be eliminated, it can be masked by white noise (e.g., using a fan, air conditioner, soft music, or recordings of white noise). In addition to addressing noise in the environment, interventions address temperature in the sleeping area. The nighttime room temperature should be comfortable, and is usually slightly lower than during the day. In cooler environments, the older adult should wear a nightcap to prevent loss of heat through the head.

Educating Older Adults About Medications and Sleep

Hypnotics may be effective for short-term management of sleep disorders, especially in temporary circumstances, such as in acute care settings; however, the adverse effects of some hypnotics can outweigh their advantages. Guidelines for evidence-based practice encourage the use of behavioral therapies rather than benzodiazepines for treatment of insomnia, particularly in nursing home residents. Studies also confirm that behavioral therapies are effective in improving sleep in hypnotic-dependent older adults (Siebern & Manber, 2010; Soeffing et al., 2008).

Between 1970 and 1993, benzodiazepines (e.g., flurazepam [Dalmane], triazolam [Halcion], temazepam [Restoril]) were the most widely prescribed hypnotics and a major disadvantage was the high incidence of adverse effects that were particularly problematic for frail older adults. Adverse effects associated with benzodiazepines include falls, mental changes, daytime sleepiness, tolerance, dependence, rebound insomnia, suppression of REM sleep, and abuse potential. Because of these adverse effects, benzodiazepines are no longer recommended for older adults. In recent years, the availability of nonbenzodiazepine agents (e.g., zolpidem [Ambien], zaleplon [Sonata], eszopiclone [Lunesta], and ramelteon [Rozerem]) has improved the side effect profile and made it safer for older adults; however, with the exception of eszopiclone, these drugs are not approved for long-term use. As of 2008, eszopiclone was the only hypnotic agent for which a long-term, randomized, double-blind, placebo-controlled study had been performed. Results of the study indicate good safety and effectiveness for improved sleep in older adults (Tariq & Pulisetty, 2008). Despite the improved profile of these newer drugs, however, concerns remain about potential adverse effects including falls, sleep walking, drug interactions, residual sedation, and memory and performance impairment (Sullivan, 2010). Box 24-4 summarizes pertinent teaching points that nurses can use to educate older adults and their caregivers about the effects of alcohol, medications, and certain chemicals on sleep.

> **Wellness Opportunity**
>
> Nurses have important roles in correcting misperceptions about sleep and teaching older adults about nonpharmacologic ways of improving sleep.

Teaching About Management of Sleep Disorders

Evidence-based guidelines emphasize the important role that nurses have in identifying and referring patients for

Box 24-4 Health Promotion Teaching About Medications and Sleep

- Older adults are more susceptible than younger adults to the adverse effects of many prescription sleeping medications, including benzodiazepines (e.g., flurazepam, triazolam, and temazepam).
- Over-the-counter sleeping preparations usually contain diphenhydramine and can have adverse effects, such as confusion, constipation, or blurred vision, either alone or in combination with other medications.
- Sleeping medications, even over-the-counter ones, are likely to have adverse effects that interfere with daytime function and with the quality of nighttime sleep.
- Many hypnotic medications are not effective for long-term use because of increasing tolerance, which may develop within the first week and usually develops after a month of regular use.
- Sleep medications can interfere with the dream stage of sleep and cause a rebound effect, characterized by nightmares and excessive dreaming, after they are discontinued.
- Alcohol is likely to cause nightmares and awakenings during the latter part of the night.
- Medications that can interfere with sleep include steroids, diuretics, theophylline, anticonvulsants, decongestants, and thyroid hormone.
- Combining a sleeping medication with any other medication can be harmful or even fatal.

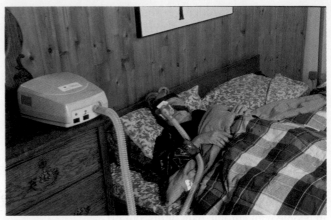

FIGURE 24-1 Illustration of a CPAP machine. (Used with permission from David Weinstein/Custom Medical Stock Photo.)

of the equipment. Figure 24-1 illustrates an older adult using a CPAP machine.

Wellness Opportunity

Nurses promote sleep wellness for older adults who experience sleep problems by teaching about the importance of having any sleep disorder evaluated by a knowledgeable professional.

sleep disorders because they see patients sleep more than any other health care professionals do (Chasens et al., 2008). Thus, when older adults have sleep disturbances that do not respond to health promotion interventions, nurses can teach older adults that there are many safe and effective interventions for addressing sleep disorders. Nurses can also emphasize the importance of addressing sleep disorders as a health issue and encourage older adults to talk with their primary care practitioner about a referral for a comprehensive sleep evaluation.

Teaching about interventions for obstructive sleep apnea is an important nursing responsibility because the disorder affects so many older adults and has serious health consequences, as discussed earlier in this chapter. Many types of interventions are available for treating obstructive sleep apnea, so obtaining a comprehensive evaluation and treatment at a sleep disorders clinic should be considered. The "gold standard" for treating obstructive sleep apnea is continuous positive airway pressure (CPAP) therapy. Studies show that CPAP therapy is effective in decreasing daytime sleepiness, improving some measures of cognitive function, and decreasing the frequency of nocturia in older adults who have obstructive sleep apnea (Norman & Loredo, 2008). People with obstructive sleep apnea are likely to use CPAP equipment, which they have been taught to use independently. However, because older adults with cognitive or functional impairments may need assistance with managing their CPAP machines, nurses need to be able to assist with the use

$\mathcal{M}$rs. Z. returns for further discussion of her sleep problem after filling out the Pittsburgh Sleep Quality Index based on her experiences during the past month. In addition, she has followed your instructions to keep a "sleep log" describing her daily activities, including exercise, and the effect of these activities on her sleep. Per your request, she has documented the types of foods and beverages she consumes regularly. You review the assessment information with her and find out that when she is home, she spends most of her time reading or doing crossword puzzles. She attends the senior center weekly, plays bridge two evenings a week, and goes to lunch with friends a few times every week. She enjoys gardening during the summer but has no other interest in physical activities. She avoids exercise because she is afraid that physical activity "will get the old arthritis all stirred up." On further questioning, she estimates that when she worked, she walked about one half–mile daily. She drinks about "a pot" of coffee daily and has coffee and cookies at bridge games. She enjoys a glass of wine in the evenings. When she wakes up during the night, she usually gets up and goes to the bathroom, then returns to bed and lies there "thinking" until she returns to sleep. Her sleep log reflects that she often stays awake for as long as 2 hours before returning to sleep. She says she's heard that melatonin is good for insomnia and asks your opinion about trying it.

EVALUATING EFFECTIVENESS OF NURSING INTERVENTIONS

The effectiveness of interventions for the nursing diagnosis of Disturbed Sleep Pattern or for the wellness diagnosis of Readiness for Enhanced Sleep can be measured subjectively or objectively. A subjective measurement would be that the older adult reports that he or she feels rested and refreshed upon awakening in the morning. If a sleep assessment tool is used during the initial assessment, it can be used again for a reassessment after interventions have been implemented. An example of an objective measurement would be that the older adult is able to sleep for 6 to 8 hours at night with only brief interruptions, and that the person looks and acts rested during the day.

*M*rs. Z. is now 79 years old and is being admitted to a long-term care facility for skilled care after a total hip replacement. Her diagnoses include osteoarthritis and osteoporosis. After a few weeks in the facility, she plans to return to her ranch-style home where she lives with her husband. Before surgery, she was independent in her activities of daily living, and she expects to regain her independence and walk with a walker. The hospital transfer form has orders for acetaminophen 1000 mg every 8 hours and zolpidem tartrate 5 mg at bedtime as needed.

NURSING ASSESSMENT

During the admission interview, you ask Mrs. Z. about her sleep patterns. She states that for the past few years, she has been awakened frequently at night by her hip pain and other arthritic discomforts. In addition, she reports that she would usually get up three or four times during the night to go to the bathroom. When questioned further, she explains that the pain and discomfort would wake her, and so she would go to the bathroom because she wanted to move around, not because she felt an urge to urinate that often. Although her doctor had prescribed medications for pain, she did not take them regularly because she was concerned about adverse effects. During her 1-week hospitalization, she had taken a sleeping pill several times as well as Tylenol with codeine. Mrs. Z. expresses anxiety about sleeping in the long-term care facility because she says that the noise in the hospital was very disruptive to her sleep. She reports that she feels rested in the morning if she gets at least 6 hours of sleep during the 8 hours she spends in bed. During her hospitalization, she never felt rested in the morning, and was unable to sleep for 6 hours except when she took sleeping pills. Mrs. Z. says that listening to relaxing music helps her to fall asleep.

NURSING DIAGNOSIS

In addition to nursing diagnoses related to Mrs. Z.'s osteoarthritis and hip surgery, you identify a nursing diagnosis of Disturbed Sleep Pattern. Related factors are pain, age-related changes, and environmental conditions. You decide that you will not list nocturia as an associated factor because Mrs. Z. does not feel an urge to void during the night. Rather, she wakes up with pain and then goes to the bathroom. You decide to list age-related changes as a related factor because it is important for Mrs. Z. to understand that, even though she may not awaken with pain, she may awaken because of age-related changes.

NURSING CARE PLAN FOR MRS. Z.

Expected Outcome	Nursing Interventions	Nursing Evaluation
Mrs. Z. will identify factors that influence her sleep pattern.	• Describe age-related changes in sleep patterns. • Discuss the important role of pain-relieving measures in promoting good sleep.	• Mrs. Z. will be able to describe the age-related changes and other conditions that affect her sleeping pattern.

(case study continues on page 510)

Expected Outcome	Nursing Interventions	Nursing Evaluation
Mrs. Z. will consistently obtain 6 hours of sleep nightly without the aid of sleeping medications.	• Administer Tylenol as ordered and evaluate its effectiveness in controlling Mrs. Z.'s pain. • Explain that sleeping medications should be avoided, except for periodic use in short-term situations. • Assign Mrs. Z. to a room that is not close to the nursing station. • Make sure Mrs. Z.'s door is closed at night. • Encourage Mrs. Z. to play quiet music at bedtime. • Give Mrs. Z. a copy of Boxes 24-3 and 24-4 and discuss additional nonpharmacologic methods for promoting sleep.	• Mrs. Z. will report that she is not awakened by pain. • Mrs. Z. will report that she feels rested upon awakening in the morning.

THINKING POINTS

- What additional assessment information pertinent to Mrs. Z.'s sleep patterns would you like to have, and how would you obtain this information?
- What additional nursing interventions would you include in the care plan to address Mrs. Z.'s disturbed sleep pattern? Would you use any of the information in Box 24-2 or give her a copy of it?
- What concerns specifically related to sleep would you have about Mrs. Z. after she is discharged from the skilled nursing facility to her own home? How would you address these concerns in your health promotion interventions?

Chapter Highlights

Age-Related Changes That Affect Sleep and Rest Patterns (Table 24-1)
- Time in bed and total sleep time
- Diminished sleep efficiency
- Alterations in sleep cycles and stages
- Shifts in circadian rhythm

Risks Factors That Affect Sleep Wellness (Tables 24-2 and 24-3)
- Psychosocial factors: beliefs, attitudes, anxiety, depression, boredom
- Environmental factors: noise, light, lack of privacy
- Physiologic factors: pain and discomfort, medication effects, physiologic disorders

Functional Consequences Affecting Sleep Wellness
- Longer time needed to fall asleep
- Frequent arousals during the night
- More time in bed to achieve same quantity of sleep
- Diminished quality of sleep (less dreaming and deep sleep)

Pathologic Condition Affecting Sleep Wellness
- Obstructive sleep apnea

Nursing Assessment of Sleep Patterns (Box 24-1)
- Perception of quantity and quality of sleep
- Factors that affect sleep
- Usual sleep pattern and behaviors that affect it
- Actual sleep pattern (observed in institutional settings)
- Sleep assessment tool

Nursing Diagnosis
- Readiness for Enhanced Sleep
- Disturbed Sleep Pattern

Planning for Wellness Outcomes
- Sleep
- Rest
- Comfort Level
- Personal Well-Being

Nursing Interventions for Sleep Wellness (Boxes 24-2 through 24-4)
- Teaching about interventions to promote healthy sleep patterns
- Modifying the environment
- Individualizing care in institutional settings
- Relaxation and mental imagery techniques
- Teaching about medications that affect sleep
- Addressing obstructive sleep apnea

Evaluating Effectiveness of Nursing Interventions
• Expressed feelings of being rested upon awakening
• Improved score on sleep assessment tool
• Observations that the person is sleeping at night

Critical Thinking Exercises

1. What is an older adult likely to experience with regard to sleep and rest patterns? How would you explain these changes to an older adult?
2. Identify three specific factors in each of the following categories that might interfere with sleep: environmental influences, physiologic disturbances, and psychosocial factors.
3. How would you assess an 82-year-old person who comes to the nursing clinic at the senior wellness center complaining of feeling tired all the time and not getting enough sleep?
4. What would you include in a half-hour presentation on "Tips for Good Sleep" for participants in a senior wellness program at a community-based center?
5. What information about sleep and rest would you include in an in-service program for evening and night shift nursing assistants employed in a long-term care facility?

Resources

For links to these resources and additional helpful Internet resources related to this chapter, visit thePoint at http://thePoint. lww.com/Miller6e.

Clinical Tools

Hartford Institute for Geriatric Nursing
• *Try This: Best Practices in Nursing Care to Older Adults*
  Issue 6.1 (2007), The Pittsburgh Sleep Quality Index (PSQI)
  Issue 6.2 (2007), The Epworth Sleepiness Scale (ESS)

Evidence-Based Practice

Chasens, E. R., Wiliams, L. L., & Umlauf, M. G. (2008). Excessive sleepiness. In E. Capezuti, D. Zwicker, M. Mezey, & T. Fulmer (Eds.), *Evidence-Based Geriatric Nursing Protocols for Best Practice* (3rd ed., pp. 459–476). New York: Springer Publishing Co.
National Guideline Clearinghouse
• Chronic insomnia in adults
• Nonpharmacologic treatment of chronic primary insomnia in the elderly
• Obstructive sleep apnea
• Sleep disorders in long-term care settings

Health Education

American Academy of Sleep Medicine
American Sleep Apnea Association
Better Sleep Council
Better Sleep Council Canada
Canadian Sleep Society
National Center on Sleep Disorders NHLBI Information Center
National Sleep Foundation
Restless Legs Syndrome Foundation

REFERENCES

Benca, R. M., & Peterson, M J. (2008). Insomnia and depression. *Sleep Medicine, 9*(Suppl. 1), S3–S9.

Bradley, T. D., & Floras, J. S. (2009). Obstructive sleep apnoea and its cardiovascular consequences. *Lancet, 373*, 82–93.

Chasens, E. R., Williams, L. L., & Umlauf, M. G. (2008). Excessive sleepiness. In E. Capezuti, D. Zwicker, M. Mezey, & T. Fulmer (Eds.), *Evidence-based geriatric nursing protocols for best practice* (3rd ed., pp. 459–476). New York: Springer Publishing Co.

Espiritu, J. R. D. (2008). Aging-related sleep changes. *Clinics in Geriatric Medicine, 24*, 1–14.

Ferri, R., Manconi, M., Lanuzze, B., Cosentino, F. I., Bruni, O., Ferini-Strambi, L., & Zucconi, M. (2008). Age-related changes in periodic leg movements during sleep in patients with restless legs syndrome. *Sleep Medicine, 9*, 790–798.

Flaherty, J. H. (2008). Insomnia among hospitalized older persons. *Clinics in Geriatric Medicine, 24*, 51–67.

Gammack, J. K. (2008a). Preface. *Clinics in Geriatric Medicine, 24*, xi–xiii.

Gammack, J. K. (2008b). Light therapy for insomnia in older adults. *Clinics in Geriatric Medicine, 24*, 139–149.

Garcia, A. D. (2008). The effect of chronic disorders on sleep in the elderly. *Clinics in Geriatric Medicine, 24*, 27–38.

Goldman, S. E., Ancoli-Israel, S., Boudreau, R. (2008). Sleep problems and associated daytime fatigue in community-dwelling older individuals. *Journal of Gerontology: Medical Sciences, 63A*(10), 1069–1073.

Gooneratne, N. S. (2008). Complementary and alternative medicine for sleep disturbances in older adults. *Clinics in Geriatric Medicine, 24*, 121–138.

Guimaraes, L. H., deCarvalho, L. B. C., Yanaguibashi, G., & do Prado, G. F. (2008). Physically active elderly women sleep more and better than sedentary women. *Sleep Medicine, 9*, 488–493.

Joshi, S. (2008). Nonpharmacologic therapy for insomnia in the elderly. *Clinics in Geriatric Medicine, 24*, 107–119.

King, A. C., Pruitt, L. A., Woo, S., Castro, C. M., Ahn, D. K., Vitiello, M. V., . . . Bliwise, D. L. (2008). Effects of moderate-intensity exercise on polysomnographic and subjective sleep quality in older adults with mild to moderate sleep complaints. *Journal of Gerontology Series A: Biological Sciences and Medical Sciences, 63*, 997–1004.

LaReau, R., Benson, L., Watcharotone, K., & Manguba, G. (2008). Examining the feasibility of implementing specific nursing interventions to promote sleep. *Geriatric Nursing, 29*(3), 197–206.

Lin, C. M., Davidson, T. M., & Ancoli-Israel, S. (2008). Bender differences in obstructive sleep apnea and treatment implications. *Sleep Medicine Reviews, 12*, 481–496.

Martin, J. L., Alam, T., Harker, J. O., Josephson, K. R., & Alessi, C. A. (2008). Sleep in assisted living facility residents versus home-dwelling older adults. *Journal of Gerontology: Medical Sciences, 63A*, 1407–1409.

Martin, J. L., & Ancoli-Israel, S. (2008). Sleep disturbances in long-term care. *Clinics in Geriatric Medicine, 24*, 39 50.

Misra, S., & Malow, B. A. (2008). Evaluation of sleep disturbances in older adults. *Clinics in Geriatric Medicine, 24*, 15–26.

NANDA International. (2009). *Nursing diagnoses: Definitions and classification 2009–2011*. Oxford, UK: Wiley-Blackwell.

Norman, D., & Loredo, J. S. (2008). Obstructive sleep apnea in older adults. *Clinics in Geriatric Medicine, 24*, 151–165.

Ong, J. C., Shapiro, S. L., & Manber, R. (2009). Mindfulness meditation and cognitive behavioral therapy for insomnia: A naturalistic 12-month follow-up. *Explore, 5*(1), 30–36.

Paniagua, M. A., & Paniagua, E. W. (2008). The demented elder with insomnia. *Clinics in Geriatric Medicine, 24*, 69–81.

Roehrs, T., & Roth, T. (2008). Caffeine: Sleep and daytime sleepiness. *Sleep Medicine Reviews, 12*, 153–162.

Siebern, A. T., & Manber, R. (2010). Insomnia and its effective non-pharmacologic treatment. *Medical Clinics of North America, 94*, 581–591.

Spiegelhalder, K., & Hornyak, M. (2008). Restless legs syndrome in older adults. *Clinics in Geriatric Medicine, 24*, 167–180.

Soeffing, J. P., Lichstein, K. L., Nau, S. D., McCrae, C. S., Wilson, N. M., Aquillard, N., . . . Bush, A. J., (2008). Psychological treatment of insomnia in hypnotic-dependent older adults. *Sleep Medicine, 9*, 165–171.

Stone, K. L., Ensrud, K. E., & Ancoli-Israel, S. (2008). Sleep, insomnia and falls in elderly patients. *Sleep Medicine, 9*(Suppl. 1), S18–S22.

Sullivan, S. S. (2010). Insomnia pharmacology. *Medical Clinics of North America, 94*, 563–580.

Tafaro, L., Cicconetti, P., Baratta, A., Brukner, N., Ettorre, E., Marigliano, V., & Cacciafesta, M. (2007). Sleep quality of centenarians: Cognitive and survival implications. *Archives of Gerontology and Geriatrics, 44S*, 385–389.

Tariq, S. H., & Pulisetty, S., (2008). Pharmacotherapy for insomnia. *Clinics in Geriatric Medicine, 24*, 93–105.

Van Couter, E., Spiegel, K., Tasali, S., & Leproult, R. (2008). Metabolic consequences of sleep and sleep loss. *Sleep Medicine, 9*(Suppl. 1), S23–S28.

Walker, M. P. (2008). Cognitive consequences of sleep and sleep loss. *Sleep Medicine, 9*(Suppl. 1), S29–S34.

Wolkove, N., Elkholy, O., Baltzan, M., & Palayew, M. (2007). Sleep and aging: Sleep disorders commonly found in older people. *Canadian Medical Association Journal, 176*(9), 1299–1304.

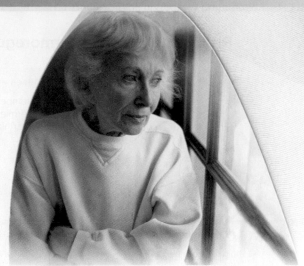

CHAPTER 25

Thermoregulation

LEARNING OBJECTIVES

After reading this chapter, you will be able to:

1. Describe age-related changes that affect an older adult's normal body temperature, febrile response to illness, and response to hot and cold environmental temperatures.

2. Identify risk factors that affect thermoregulation in older adults and increase the potential for hypothermia or hyperthermia.

3. Assess the following aspects of thermoregulation: baseline temperature, risks for altered thermoregulation, hypothermia, hyperthermia, and febrile response to illness.

4. Discuss the functional consequences of altered temperature regulation in older adults.

5. Implement health promotion interventions for preventing hypothermia and hyperthermia in older adults.

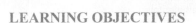

K E Y P O I N T S

accidental hypothermia	heat stroke
acclimatize	hyperthermia
heat exhaustion	hypothermia

The primary function of thermoregulation is to maintain a stable core body temperature in a wide range of environmental temperatures. In the presence of infections, thermoregulation also assists in maintaining homeostasis. Under normal circumstances, the core body temperature is maintained at 97°F (36.1°C) to 99°F (37.2°C) through complex physiologic mechanisms governing heat production and dissipation. Thermoregulation in older adults is affected by age-related changes and is compromised even more by risk factors. Nurses play an important role in promoting healthy thermoregulation and comfort for older adults.

AGE-RELATED CHANGES THAT AFFECT THERMOREGULATION

With increased age, subtle alterations in thermoregulation occur, and these become important considerations in caring for healthy, as well as frail, older adults. Because thermoregulation is a complex process involving many body systems, adaptive responses to environmental temperatures can be altered by many internal and external influences. Internal conditions that affect temperature regulation include metabolic rate; pathologic processes; muscle activity; peripheral blood flow; amount of subcutaneous fat; function of the cutaneous nerves; ingestion of fluid, nutrients, and medications; and the temperature of the blood flowing through the hypothalamus. External influences on thermoregulation include environmental temperature, humidity level, airflow, and the type and amount of clothing and covering used. The following sections address these factors in relation to the ability of older adults to respond to environmental temperatures and in relation to normal body temperature.

Response to Cold Temperatures

In cold environmental temperatures, the body normally initiates physiologic mechanisms to prevent loss of body heat and increase heat production. At the same time, individuals usually initiate protective behaviors to warm the body and protect themselves from adversely cold temperatures. Physiologic mechanisms that prevent heat loss and increase heat production include shivering, muscle contraction, increased heart rate, peripheral vasoconstriction, dilation of the blood vessels in the muscles, insulation of deeper tissues by subcutaneous fat, and release of thyroxine and corticosteroid by the pituitary gland. Protective actions that people commonly initiate in cold temperatures include seeking shelter, ingesting warm fluids, wearing warm clothing or covering, and increasing activity to stimulate circulation.

The following age-related changes, which can affect processes involved with heat loss or production, are likely to

Promoting Healthy Thermoregulation in Older Adults

Nursing Assessment

- Usual baseline temperature
- Risks for hypothermia
- Risks for hyperthermia

Age-Related Changes

- ↓ subcutaneous tissue
- ↓ shivering
- ↓ ability to acclimatize to heat
- ↓ sweating
- ↓ peripheral circulation
- Inefficient vasoconstriction

Negative Functional Consequences

- ↓ ability to respond to adverse temperatures
- ↑ susceptibility to hypothermia or hyperthermia
- ↓ febrile response to illness

Risk Factors

- Age 75 years and older
- Adverse environmental conditions
- Alcohol and medications (e.g., benzodiazepines, phenothiazines)
- Diseases (e.g., cardiovascular, endocrine, or cerebrovascular disorders)

Nursing Interventions

- Maintenance of optimal environmental temperature
- Comfort measures
- Teaching about preventing hypothermia
- Teaching about preventing hyperthermia

Wellness Outcomes

- Decreased risk for hypothermia
- Decreased risk for hyperthermia
- Improved comfort
- Prevention of serious consequences

interfere with an older person's ability to respond to cold temperatures:

- Inefficient vasoconstriction
- Decreased cardiac output
- Decreased muscle mass
- Diminished peripheral circulation

- Decreased subcutaneous tissue
- Delayed and diminished shivering.

These changes begin during the fifth decade, but their impact is not felt until the seventh or eighth decade. The overall effect of these changes is a dulled perception of cold and a concomitant lack of stimulus to initiate protective actions, such as adding more clothing or raising the environmental temperature.

Response to Hot Temperatures

In hot environmental temperatures, or when metabolic heat production is high, the normal mechanisms for heat dissipation are the production of sweat to facilitate evaporation and the dilation of peripheral blood vessels to facilitate heat radiation. When exposed to hot climates or engaged in strenuous activity daily for 7 to 14 days, healthy adults are able to **acclimatize** (i.e., gradually increase their metabolic efficiency to adapt to higher temperatures). The older person's ability to acclimatize and respond to heat stress is altered primarily by age-related changes affecting sweating and cardiovascular function. Older adults have an increased threshold for the onset of sweating, a diminished response when sweating occurs, and a dulled sensation of warm environments. For example, the sweat response to exercise in healthy adults in their mid-60s is about half of that in adults in their mid-20s. Age-related cardiovascular changes interfere with the ability to acclimatize because cardiac output must be sufficient to produce peripheral vasodilation for heat dissipation. Consequently, even healthy older adults are more susceptible to heat stress because they are less able to adapt to hot environments (Platt & Vicario, 2009).

Normal Body Temperature and Febrile Response to Illness

Body temperature is normally maintained at 98.6°F (37°C), plus or minus 1°F, with diurnal variations of 2°F. An elevated temperature, or fever, is the body's protective response to pathologic conditions, such as cancer, infection, dehydration, or connective tissue disease. Although some studies have found that the oral temperature of healthy older adults is lower than that of younger adults, other studies do not support this conclusion (Lu & Dai, 2009). For example, one study of more than 1000 adults in Taiwan during winter and summer seasons concluded that oral temperature of both younger and older adults is lower than 37°C and that environmental temperatures most strongly influence adults aged 85 years and older. A recent nursing review of studies found that mean temperatures ranged from 96°F to 100.7°F (35.6°C to 38.2°C) (Outzen, 2009). Widely accepted definitions of a "fever" include the following: (1) persistent elevation of body temperature of at least 2°F (1.1°C) over baseline values; (2) oral temperatures of 99°F (37.2°C) or greater on repeated measures; and (3) rectal temperatures of 99.5°F (37.5°C) on repeated measurements (Outzen, 2009).

Oral and axillary temperatures are not necessarily an accurate measurement of core temperature in older adults because the difference between their core and skin temperatures is greater and more variable than in younger people. Although rectal temperature has long been viewed as the established standard for measuring body temperature, obtaining it is difficult and very invasive. In recent years, ear thermometry has become the method of choice because it is the least invasive and quickest way of obtaining temperatures, especially in acutely ill patients.

 ## RISK FACTORS THAT AFFECT THERMOREGULATION

Age alone predisposes people to both **hypothermia**, defined as a core body temperature of 95°F (35°C) or lower, and hyperthermia, a body temperature elevated above the person's normal temperature (Holowatz, Thompson-Torgerson, & Kenney, 2010). Because older adults are less able to adapt physiologically to environmental temperatures, even moderately hot or cold environments can be a risk for hypothermia or hyperthermia. In addition, older adults are likely to have pathophysiologic alterations that increase the risk for altered thermoregulation.

Pathophysiologic Conditions That Alter Thermoregulation

The risk for hypothermia is increased by conditions that decrease heat production (e.g., inactivity, malnutrition, endocrine disorders, neuromuscular conditions), increase heat loss (e.g., burns, vasodilation), or affect the normal thermoregulatory process (pathologic conditions of the central nervous system). Major medical conditions associated with hypothermia include cardiovascular disorders, infections, trauma, endocrine disorders, and chronic renal failure (Elbaz et al., 2008). Medications and alcohol can predispose a person to hypothermia by suppressing shivering or inducing vasodilation (e.g., alcohol, psychotropic drugs). For example, official reports of adverse drug reactions cite more than 100 cases of clinically significant hypothermia related to risperidone and other cases due to atypical antipsychotics (e.g., ziprasidone) (Gibbons, Wein, & Paula, 2008). Excessive use of alcohol further increases the risk for hypothermia by dulling sensory perceptions and interfering with cognitive skills necessary for initiating protective behaviors.

The risk for hyperthermia is increased by physiologic alterations that increase internal heat production (e.g., hyperthyroidism, diabetic ketoacidosis) or interfere with the ability to respond to heat stress (e.g., cardiovascular disease, fluid or electrolyte imbalance). Medications can predispose a person to hyperthermia by increasing diuresis (e.g., diuretics), increasing heat production (e.g., salicylate intoxication), or interfering with sweating (e.g., anticholinergics) or peripheral vasodilation (e.g., beta-adrenergic blocking agents). Alcohol increases the risk for hyperthermia by inducing diuresis, and excessive alcohol can increase the risk by increasing heat production.

Environmental and Socioeconomic Influences

Environmental temperatures can increase the vulnerability of older adults, particularly those older than 75 years, to hypothermia or hyperthermia. Although older adults who live in geographic areas with extreme cold or hot seasonal variations are especially vulnerable, studies have found that hypothermia affects older adults even in temperate climates (Elbaz et al., 2008). Other factors interact with environmental conditions to contribute to an increased risk for altered thermoregulation. For example, heat-related illness can be precipitated by even moderate exercise in hot and humid weather, especially if fluid intake is not adequate. If older adults rely solely on their sensation of thirst to signal the need for fluid intake, they can become underhydrated or dehydrated because of the age-related diminished thirst sensation.

In addition to the obvious influence of hot or cold temperatures, substandard living conditions and diets deficient in protein and calories have been associated with hypothermia and hyperthermia. Heat waves are especially hazardous for older adults living in environments with poor ventilation. The detrimental effects are magnified when high temperatures combine with high humidity levels and air pollutants. For older adults living in urban areas with high crime rates, keeping windows closed for safety considerations may restrict ventilation. In Great Britain, the term *urban hypothermia* has been used with reference to older adults living alone in poorly heated dwellings. Likewise, the term *urban hyperthermia* could be applied to older adults living in poorly ventilated houses and apartments, particularly public housing, in cities where heat waves and air pollution are common.

Social isolation is a factor that increases the risk for progression of hyperthermia or hypothermia because people rarely are able to self-report these conditions. Thus, they may not receive help in a timely manner. Older adults who live alone and have dementia may be at increased risk if they do not have the cognitive skills to adjust the thermostat and wear proper clothing or the ability to recognize the symptoms and call for help in a timely manner. Homelessness is another socioeconomic factor that increases the risk for both hypothermia and hyperthermia. Additional risk factors are summarized in Box 25-1.

  Wellness Opportunity

Although the weather cannot be controlled, it is important to identify the environmental factors that affect thermoregulation and that can be addressed through health education about protective actions.

Behaviors Based on Lack of Knowledge

Lack of knowledge about age-related vulnerability to hypothermia and hyperthermia may create risks secondary to inadequate protective measures. For example, when the use of air conditioning or heating is curtailed as a cost-saving measure, younger adults may be able to adjust to the moderately hot or cool temperature, whereas an older adult might become hypothermic or hyperthermic under the same circumstances. If older adults and their caregivers are not aware of the age-related decrease in the perception of environmental

---

 Box 25-1 Risk Factors for Hypothermia or Hyperthermia in Older Adults

Risks for Hypothermia and Hyperthermia
- Age 75+ years
- Adverse environmental temperatures
- Infections or sepsis
- Cardiovascular disorders
- Cerebrovascular disease

Risks for Hypothermia
- Alcohol
- Carcinoma
- Diabetes or hypoglycemia
- Endocrine disorders
- Malnutrition
- Parkinson's disease
- Peripheral neuropathy
- Medications: barbiturates, benzodiazepines, cyclic antidepressants, and phenothiazines

Risks for Hyperthermia
- Alcohol and alcohol withdrawal
- Dehydration
- Diabetic ketoacidosis
- Hyperthyroidism
- Excessive exercise or even moderate exercise in hot environments
- Medications: alpha-adrenergic blocking agents; anticholinergic agents (including antihistamines, phenothiazines, tricyclic antidepressants); benzodiazepines, beta-adrenergic blocking agents, calcium channel blockers, diuretics, and laxatives.

---

temperatures, they may not take appropriate protective measures, such as removing or adding clothing.

In the presence of infection, lack of knowledge about age-related thermoregulatory changes may result in undetected illnesses. For example, caregivers and health care professionals may falsely assume that no infection is present if there is no fever. Similarly, if they believe that the baseline temperature for all adults is 98.6°F (37°C), they may not recognize an elevated temperature in someone whose baseline temperature is lower than this. In addition, lack of knowledge about diurnal temperature variations and age-related changes may contribute to false expectations and undetected illness.

FUNCTIONAL CONSEQUENCES ASSOCIATED WITH THERMOREGULATION IN OLDER ADULTS

A healthy older adult in a comfortable environment will experience few, if any, functional consequences of altered thermoregulation. In the presence of any risk factor, however, hypothermia or hyperthermia may develop in an older adult. Even moderately adverse environmental temperatures can precipitate hypothermia or hyperthermia in an older adult, especially in the presence of additional predisposing factors, such as certain medications or pathologic conditions. For older adults in whom hypothermia or hyperthermia develops, the risk of subsequent morbidity or mortality from this condition is greater than that for their younger counterparts.

In the United States, hypothermia and hyperthermia usually are seasonal hazards that occur during cold spells and heat waves. States with the highest death rates for hypothermia between 1999 and 2002 are Alaska, Montana, Wyoming, New Mexico, and North Dakota. Hypothermia-related deaths also occur in states, such as North and South Carolina, where there are rapid temperature changes, and in states like Arizona with high elevations and colder nighttime temperatures (Falico, Nolte, Siciliano, & Yip, 2005; Murphy et al., 2006). Approximately 10 times as many deaths are reported during heat-wave years in the United States compared to non–heat-wave years (Platt & Vicario, 2009).

Altered Response to Cold Environments

Increased age is associated with an increased vulnerability to hypothermia because most older adults are less aware of a low core body temperature, less efficient in their physiologic response to cold, and less apt to take corrective actions when necessary. A low environmental temperature usually contributes to hypothermia, and the term **accidental hypothermia** is used when low environmental temperature is the primary cause of the condition. Even in normal environmental temperatures, however, the condition can result from serious alterations in homeostasis, such as can occur with anesthesia or endocrine or neurologic disorders. Accidental hypothermia can occur in older adults as a consequence of exposure to moderately cool temperatures, and may affect as many as 10% of older adults living in winter climates (e.g., Great Britain, Canada, and parts of the United States).

In the early stages of hypothermia, the older adult probably will not shiver or complain of feeling cold. In the absence of any protective measures, hypothermia will progress, clouding mental function. The effects of impaired thermoregulation are cumulative, and hypothermia progresses rapidly after the core body temperature falls to 93.2°F (33.9°C). The age-related diminished ability of the kidney to conserve water and the common occurrence of inadequate fluid intake in older adults exacerbate the effects of hypothermia. If the process is not reversed, death from hypothermia will result from the myocardial effects of seriously impaired thermoregulation.

Altered Response to Hot Environments

Functional consequences that affect an older adult's ability to respond to hot environments include delayed and diminished sweating and inaccurate perception of environmental temperatures. Because of these functional consequences, the older adult is more likely to have heat-related illnesses, including **heat exhaustion** and **heat stroke**. Heat exhaustion is a condition that develops gradually from depletion of fluid, sodium, or both. It can occur in active or immobilized older people who are dehydrated or underhydrated and exposed to hot environments. Heat stroke is an even more serious condition that is likely to occur in active older adults because of a combination of age-related thermoregulatory changes and risk factors, such as overexertion and warm environments. Heat stroke can also occur in immobilized older adults in hot environments, either as a progression of untreated heat exhaustion or as a result of a combination of risk factors. The underlying mechanism in heat stroke is an inability to balance the rates of heat production and dissipation. This balance depends primarily on sweating and cardiac output.

In hot environments, the effects of altered thermoregulation are cumulative, and heat-related illnesses progress rapidly after the body temperature reaches 105.8°F (40.6°C). If fluid volume is not adequate to meet the requirements for effective sweating, then hyperthermia will progress even more rapidly. The age-related decrease in thirst sensation can contribute to inadequate fluid intake and diminished thermoregulation. If hyperthermia is not reversed, death will result from respiratory depression.

Altered Thermoregulatory Response to Illness

Age-related changes in the thermoregulatory centers of the hypothalamus diminish the older adult's febrile response to illness and infections. Thus, infections are likely to be undetected until they progress and manifest as a functional decline or change in mental status. Older adults with infections commonly have a normal or even lower than normal temperature, but when their temperature is compared with their baseline temperature, at least a slight elevation is evident. Thus, elevated temperature in older adults can be detected only in relation to their normal baseline temperature.

Altered Perception of Environmental Temperatures

Older adults often report feeling cool or cold, even in very warm environments, and they generally prefer environmental temperatures that are at least 75°F (23.9°C). Inaccurate perceptions of environmental temperatures are associated with pathophysiologic conditions, such as dementia, thyroid disorders, or cardiovascular inefficiency, rather than with age-related changes alone.

Psychosocial Consequences of Altered Thermoregulation

Psychosocial consequences are associated with hypothermia, hyperthermia, or diminished fever response. If hypothermia or hyperthermia is overlooked, or if interventions are not initiated at an early stage, the condition may progress to the point of impairing cognitive function. Likewise, if a diminished or delayed febrile response to an infection is not recognized, a treatable condition may be overlooked and treatment may unintentionally be delayed or denied. Untreated infections are likely to progress in severity and, in older adults, may manifest primarily as a functional decline, such as impaired cognition.

*M*rs. T. is 76 years old and lives alone in a large farmhouse in a rural county in central Ohio. She has lived on this 20-acre farm for 49 years and has been a widow for 2 years. She has four children and eight grandchildren, but they all live in other states. Mrs. T. has been able to manage her farm with a part-time farmhand who comes a couple of times a week to help feed the several dozen chickens and collect eggs. When her farmhand doesn't come, she manages the chores by herself. She has hypertension and type 2 diabetes, and manages reasonably well medically. She adheres to her diabetic diet and takes her medications daily. She sends her farmhand to the city once weekly for groceries and drives to the nearby church on Sundays. Once a month she attends the county senior center, where you are the nurse. It is the middle of July and summer in Ohio this year has been unusually hot and humid. A drought and heat wave are predicted for central Ohio and you are planning to present a health education program called "Hot Tips for Surviving the Summer." You are particularly concerned about Mrs. T. and several other participants who live in isolated areas and have little contact with others.

THINKING POINTS

- What factors increase the risk of Mrs. T. developing a heat-related illness? Which ones would you discuss in your health education program?
- In your health education program, how would you explain heat-related illnesses and the associated signs and symptoms?

NURSING ASSESSMENT OF THERMOREGULATION

Nursing assessment of thermoregulation addresses the older person's baseline body temperature, any risk factors for altered thermoregulation, manifestations of hypothermia or hyperthermia, and febrile response to illness. Nurses use this information for planning health education interventions to prevent hypothermia and hyperthermia. Nurses also use the assessment information to detect hypothermia or heat-related illnesses as quickly as possible so that appropriate interventions can be initiated before serious or irreversible effects occur. Assessment information is also important in detecting infections at an early stage. Nurses obtain much of the pertinent information about risk factors as part of the overall assessment; they also obtain information by observing the environment, measuring the person's body temperature, and

interviewing the older adult and the caregivers of dependent older adults.

Assessing Baseline Temperature

Body temperature measurements show a diurnal fluctuation of 1°F to 2°F, with lower temperatures during sleeping and greater fluctuations during periods of fever-inducing illness. Because older adults normally have a lower body temperature and may have a diminished febrile response to infection, it is especially important to determine the person's usual temperature, as well as to characterize the usual pattern of diurnal variation. Because many types of thermometers are now available (e.g., oral, rectal, tympanic, and bladder probes), it is important to document the method used for assessing temperature. Also, when assessing for hypothermia, it is advisable to use several methods and to make sure that the thermometers are able to detect low body temperatures.

Nurses can encourage older adults in home settings to determine their usual temperature by recording their temperature at different times of the day for several days when they are feeling well. Doing this seasonally by people who live in fluctuating climates and annually by those who live in stable climates provides a baseline for comparison when symptoms of illness or functional decline occur. Nurses can follow this procedure in long-term care settings and record the results as baseline data on the chart. Box 25-2 summarizes the principles underlying nursing assessment of thermoregulation in older adults.

Identifying Risk Factors for Altered Thermoregulation

Anyone older than 75 years is at risk for altered thermoregulation, as are older adults who have one or more of the risk factors listed in Box 25-1. Because so many of the risk factors for altered thermoregulation are modifiable, it is important to identify those that can be addressed through health promotion interventions. Nurses usually identify risk factors involving medications and physiologic disturbances during the overall assessment, and it is important to consider any conditions predisposing the person to hypothermia or hyperthermia. In addition to assessing for risks for hypothermia or heat-related illnesses, nurses must consider a low baseline body temperature as a risk for undetected fever. It is important to document the person's baseline temperature and note this as a risk factor for both hypothermia and undetected febrile conditions if it is below 98°F (36.7°C).

Most nurses do not have the opportunity to observe and assess the older adult's home environment, but they can ask pertinent questions and listen for clues to detect environmental risk factors. For example, older adults who live alone and express concern about keeping the house warm in winter should be considered to be at risk for hypothermia. Likewise, older adults who live in poor housing conditions, or with family members who keep the house at low temperatures during winter months, should be considered to be at risk for

Box 25-2 Guidelines for Assessing Thermoregulation

Principles of Temperature Assessment
- Document the person's baseline body temperature and its diurnal and seasonal variations.
- Assume that even a small elevation above the baseline temperature is a clue to the presence of a pathologic process.
- Document actual temperature and deviations from the baseline, rather than using such terminology as "afebrile."
- Carefully follow all the standard procedures for accurate temperature measurement. Use a thermometer that registers temperatures lower than 95°F (35°C).
- Consider the influence of temperature-altering medications when evaluating a temperature reading (e.g., medications that mask a fever).
- Do not assume that an infection will necessarily be accompanied by an elevated temperature.
- Remember that, in the presence of an infection, a decline in function or change in mental status may be an earlier and more accurate indicator of illness than an alteration in temperature.
- Do not assume that an older adult will initiate compensatory behaviors or complain of discomfort when exposed to adverse environmental temperatures.

Questions to Assess Risk Factors for Hypothermia or Hyperthermia
- Do you have any particular health problems that occur in hot or cold weather?
- Are you able to keep your house or room at a comfortable temperature in both summer and winter months?
- What do you do to cope with hot temperatures in the summer?
- Do you have any difficulty paying your utility bills?
- What forms of protection against the cold do you use in the winter months (e.g., electric blanket, supplemental sources of heat)?

- Have you ever received medical care for exposure to heat or cold?
- Have you ever fallen and not been able to get up or get help?

Observations to Assess Risk Factors for Hypothermia or Hyperthermia
- Does the older person live in a house where the temperature is kept below 70°F (21.1°C) during the winter?
- Does the person drink alcohol or take temperature-altering medications (see Box 25-1)?
- Does the person live alone? If so, what is the frequency of outside contacts?
- Does the person have any pathologic conditions that predispose him or her to hypothermia (e.g., endocrine, neurologic, or cardiovascular disorders)?
- Is the person's fluid and nutritional intake adequate?
- Does the person have postural hypotension? (See Chapter 20, Table 20-2 and Boxes 20-1 and 20-2 for assessment criteria relating to postural hypotension.)
- Is the person immobilized or sedentary? Is the person's judgment impaired because of dementia, depression, or other psychosocial disorders?
- Does the person live in a poorly ventilated dwelling without air-conditioning?
- Are atmospheric conditions very hot, humid, or polluted?
- Does the person engage in active exercise during hot weather?
- Does the person have any chronic illness that predisposes him or her to hyperthermia?
- Is the person at risk for hyponatremia or hypokalemia because of medications or chronic illnesses?

---

hypothermia. Older adults who live in poorly ventilated houses without air conditioning should be considered to be at risk for hyperthermia during heat waves. Interview questions aimed at identifying risk factors for altered thermoregulation are listed in Box 25-2.

Wellness Opportunity

From a holistic perspective, nurses consider that fears about paying utility bills in the winter or about personal safety when windows are open can increase the risk for hypothermia or heat-related conditions

Assessing for Hypothermia

Hypothermia is best detected by measuring core body temperature with a thermometer that registers below 95°F (35°C). Cool skin in unexposed areas, such as the abdomen and buttocks, is a distinguishing characteristic of hypothermia. The environmental temperature may be only moderately cool and the older person will not necessarily shiver or complain of feeling cold. Even in environmental temperatures of 68°F (20°C) or 69°F (20.6°C), an older person may become hypothermic, especially if other risk factors, such as immobility

or hypothermia-inducing medications, are present. Early signs of hypothermia are subtle, and the most objective assessment tool is a comparison of the person's body temperature with their usual baseline temperature. As untreated hypothermia progresses, additional signs may include lethargy, slurred speech, mental changes, impaired gait, puffiness of the face, slowed or irregular pulse, low blood pressure, slowed tendon reflexes, and slow, shallow respirations. Severe stages of hypothermia are characterized by muscular rigidity, diminished urinary function, and a progression of all other manifestations to the point of stupor and coma. The skin will feel very cool, and, contrary to what might be expected, the color of the skin will be pink. Also contrary to what might be expected, a hypothermic person may not shiver, particularly if the body temperature is below 90°F (32.2°C).

Assessing for Hyperthermia

Manifestations of heat-related illnesses range from mild headache to life-threatening respiratory and cardiovascular disturbances. In the early stages of heat-related illness, the person will feel weak and lethargic and may complain of headache, nausea, and loss of appetite. The skin will be warm and dry, and the sweating response may be absent, especially if the person's fluid intake is low. As the heat-related condition progresses, these manifestations will be exacerbated, and the following signs will become evident: dizziness, dyspnea, tachycardia, vomiting, diarrhea, muscle cramps, chest pain, mental impairment, and a wide pulse pressure.

Assessing the Older Adult's Febrile Response to Illness

Because the manifestations of delayed or diminished febrile response to infections are likely to be very subtle, nurses assess for any temperature changes from the person's baseline as well as for additional signs of illness, such as a decline in function or change in mental status. Nurses also should examine assumptions about temperature regulation that may apply to younger adults but not to older adults. For example, the expectation that pneumonia is accompanied by an elevated temperature is not necessarily applicable to older adults, as discussed in Chapter 21. Thus, nurses in long-term care facilities need to be particularly vigilant about subtle temperature changes and other manifestations of fever. A more reliable indicator of elevated temperature in older adults would be an increase of 2°F (1°C) above the person's baseline. See Box 25-2 for a summary of some of these considerations.

> **◆ Wellness Opportunity**
>
> A holistic assessment for febrile conditions requires that nurses identify subtle manifestations, such as behavior changes and slight elevations above the person's baseline temperature, even if the temperature is within the so-called normal range.

NURSING DIAGNOSIS

If the nursing assessment identifies risks for impaired thermoregulation in an older adult, pertinent nursing diagnoses include Hypothermia, Hyperthermia, or Risk for Imbalanced Body Temperature. Hypothermia (and hyperthermia), as Nursing Diagnosis, is defined as body temperature below (above) normal range (NANDA International, 2009). If conditions increase the risk for hypothermia, hyperthermia, and ineffective thermoregulation, the Nursing Diagnosis of Risk for Imbalanced Body Temperature may be appropriate. For example, an 83-year-old woman with diabetes, dementia, and hypertension who is taking a diuretic, an antipsychotic, and an oral hypoglycemic would have many risk factors for both hypothermia and hyperthermia. Related factors that are common in older adults include immobility, advanced age, medication effects, adverse environmental conditions, and acute and chronic illnesses. For older adults living alone, social isolation may be a related factor that increases the risk for experiencing more serious consequences if hypothermia or hyperthermia occurs.

> **◆ Wellness Opportunity**
>
> Nurses can use the nursing diagnosis Readiness for Enhanced Knowledge: Prevention of Hypothermia (or Hyperthermia) for older adults and their caregivers who are interested in learning to address risks for these conditions.

PLANNING FOR WELLNESS OUTCOMES

When caring for older adults with risks for hypothermia or hyperthermia, nurses identify wellness outcomes as an essential component of the nursing process. Nurses can use the following Nursing Outcomes Classification (NOC) terminologies in their care plans addressing risks for altered thermoregulation: Health Promoting Behavior, Hydration, Knowledge: Health Behavior, Knowledge: Personal Safety, Risk Detection, Risk Control, Safe Home Environment, Thermoregulation, and Vital Signs: Body Temperature.

Outcomes vary depending on the setting. In acute care settings, nurses are more likely to focus on outcomes that pertain to the patient's immediate physical condition (e.g., Hydration, Thermoregulation, and Vital Signs: Body Temperature). A focus of nursing care in long-term care settings is early detection of infections. In home and other community settings, nurses might be able to provide group or individual health education for older adults who are at risk for development of hypothermia or heat-related illness, especially during times of extreme weather conditions. In these situations, nurses focus more on teaching about self-care and environmental modifications to prevent hypothermia or hyperthermia.

> **◆ Wellness Opportunity**
>
> Nurses promote wellness when their care plans include health-promoting behaviors to prevent hypothermia and hyperthermia.

 ## NURSING INTERVENTIONS TO PROMOTE HEALTHY THERMOREGULATION

Health promotion interventions to address altered thermoregulation are directed toward primary prevention of hypothermia and heat-related illness. Health promotion interventions also address early detection of altered thermoregulation and prompt initiation of interventions to restore thermal balance and to prevent detrimental effects. Comfort interventions are initiated to promote well-being in older adults. Nurses can use the following Nursing Interventions Classification (NIC) terminologies to document interventions: Environmental Management, Environmental Risk Protection, Health Education, Risk Identification, Surveillance: Safety, Teaching: Individual, and Temperature Regulation.

Addressing Risk Factors

Maintenance of an environmental temperature of around 75°F (23.9°C) is the single most important intervention to prevent hypothermia or hyperthermia. In addition, relative humidity can be altered to minimize the discomfort and detrimental effects associated with extremely warm or cool environments. With comfortable indoor temperatures, the ideal humidity is between 40% and 50%, although an acceptable range is between 20% and 70%. Older adults can be encouraged to humidify the air in their homes during the dry winter months by using humidifiers, either alone or with their heating systems. Simpler measures, such as keeping pans of water on heating vents or using a vaporizer near the bed at night, may be appropriate if a humidifier is unavailable. Older adults living in hot, humid climates may need assistance in applying to elder care community programs that provide window air conditioners, fans, and assistance with summer electric bills.

In many areas of the United States and Canada in which cold winters are the norm, financial assistance for heating bills may be available through government-sponsored programs, such as the Low Income Home Energy Assistance Program's (LIHEAP) Fuel Assistance Program. Other government-sponsored programs provide financial assistance, such as low-interest loans, for home winterization and modernization measures to protect against adverse weather conditions. Older people and their family caregivers should be encouraged to take advantage of these programs, applications for which can be obtained from LIHEAP listed in the Resources section at the end of this chapter.

◆ Wellness Opportunity

Nurses promote wellness for socially isolated older adults by identifying ways of developing a system of social contact, such as a friendly phone call program, that ensures daily contact during periods of adversely hot or cold weather.

Promoting Healthy Thermoregulation

In cool environmental temperatures, interventions to prevent hypothermia include using adequate clothing and covering, especially for the hands, feet, and head because these areas of the body have the heaviest concentration of nerve endings that are sensitive to heat loss. Nurses can encourage older adults to wear caps, thermal socks, and several layers of warm clothing when appropriate. Electric blankets used during the night are a relatively inexpensive form of protection in cool environments, but proper safety precautions must be taken. Space heaters often are used to provide intense heat in a small area, but they can create serious fire and safety hazards. In addition to environmental considerations, special attention must be directed toward ensuring adequate nutrition, including fluid intake, and treating any pathologic conditions.

During heat waves, hyperthermia can affect older adults living in their own homes or in long-term care settings that are not air-conditioned. In long-term care facilities without air-conditioning, nurses need to ensure that all residents have adequate fluid intakes. Nurses also must observe for early signs of hyperthermia, especially in residents who are immo-

bile or who have medical problems, such as endocrine or circulatory disorders, that predispose them to hyperthermia. If only parts of the facility are air-conditioned, nurses can encourage residents to spend time in those areas and can provide assistance for residents who have mobility limitations.

Nurses can teach older adults living in community settings about measures to cool the environment, such as those summarized in Box 25-3. Older adults may be reluctant to use fans or air-conditioners because of a desire to save money on utility bills; however, if they understand the health risks associated with hyperthermia, they may use these appliances judiciously. If the home setting cannot be cooled adequately during heat waves, nurses can encourage older adults to spend time in air-conditioned public places. Additional self-care actions to prevent hyperthermia during heat waves include the provision of adequate fluids and the avoidance of heavy meals and strenuous exercise. Nurses can use Box 25-3, which summarizes interventions for the prevention of hyperthermia, as an educational tool for older adults.

◆ Wellness Opportunity

Nurses can use comfort measures to diminish the sensation of being cold, even if the interventions have no effect on core body temperature.

---

*R*ecall that Mrs. T. is 76 years old and a participant at the county senior center where you will be presenting a health education program.

THINKING POINTS

- How would you incorporate assessment information into your health education program?
- How would you use information from Box 25-3 to teach about preventing heat-related illnesses?
- What specific suggestions would you make about early detection of heat-related illnesses to the participants at this rural senior center?
- How would you find health education materials to use for your program?

EVALUATING EFFECTIVENESS OF NURSING INTERVENTIONS

Nurses evaluate care of older adults diagnosed with Risk for Hypothermia/Hyperthermia or Imbalanced Body Temperature according to the extent to which the risks are eliminated. It is not always possible to know whether risk factors were eliminated, but nurses can evaluate the effectiveness of their teaching by asking for feedback from older adults and their caregivers. Nurses also can suggest referrals for resources and ask the older adult about his or her intent to follow

Box 25-3 Health Promotion Teaching About Hypothermia and Heat-Related Illness

Environmental and Personal Protection Considerations for Preventing Hypothermia

- Maintain a constant room temperature as close to 75°F (23.9°C) as possible, with a minimum temperature of 70°F (21.1°C).
- Use a reliable, clearly marked thermometer to measure room temperature.
- Wear close-knit, but not tight, undergarments to prevent heat loss; wear several layers of clothing.
- Wear a hat and gloves when outdoors; wear a nightcap and socks for sleeping.
- Wear extra clothing in the early morning when your body metabolism is at its lowest point.
- Use flannel bed sheets or sheet blankets.
- Use an electric blanket set on a low temperature.
- Take advantage of programs that offer assistance with utility bills and home weatherization.

Environmental and Personal Protection Action to Prevent Heat-Related Illnesses

- Maintain room temperatures below 85°F (29.4°C).
- If your residence is not air-conditioned, use fans to circulate the air and cool the environment.
- During hot weather, spend time in public air-conditioned settings, such as libraries or shopping malls.
- Drink extra noncaffeinated, nonalcoholic liquids, even if you don't feel thirsty.
- Wear loose-fitting, lightweight, light-colored, cotton clothing.
- Wear a hat or use an umbrella to protect yourself against sun and heat when you are outside.
- Avoid outdoor activities during the hottest time of the day (i.e., between 10:00 AM and 2:00 PM); perform them during the cooler hours of the morning or evening.

- Place an ice pack or cold, wet towels on your body, especially on the head, the groin area, and armpits. Take cool (about 75°F [23.9°C]) baths or showers several times daily during heat waves, but do not use soap every time.

Health Promotion Actions for Maintaining Optimal Body Temperature

- Maintain adequate fluid intake by drinking 8 to 10 glasses of non-caffeinated, nonalcoholic liquid daily.
- Do not rely on your thirst sensation as an indicator of the need for fluid.
- Eat small, frequent meals rather than heavy meals.
- Avoid drinking caffeinated beverages, such as cola and coffee.
- Avoid drinking alcohol.
- In cold weather, engage in moderate physical exercise and indoor activities to increase circulation and heat production.

Nutritional Considerations

- Maintain good nutrition, especially zinc, selenium, and vitamins A, C, and E.

Preventive Measures and Additional Approaches

- Know your normal temperature in the morning and in the evening.
- Know the difference in your temperature in the winter and the summer.
- Obtain pneumonia and influenza immunizations (as discussed in Chapter 21).
- Obtain tetanus and diphtheria vaccinations every 10 years.
- Be aware that melatonin and other bioactive substances (see Box 25-1) might alter temperature regulation; use these substances only under the advice of a health care professional.

---

through. For example, if housing and financial factors increase the risk of hypothermia and heat-related illnesses, nurses can refer the older adult to a program such as LIHEAP and document the person's response to this information.

When nurses teach about preventing hypothermia and heat-related illnesses, effectiveness is evaluated on the basis of the person's ability to describe ways of decreasing the risk factors for hypothermia or heat-related illnesses.

---

*M*rs. T. is now 87 years old and continues to live alone in her own home in a rural area of central Ohio. She has a history of hypertension and diabetic retinopathy, and was recently hospitalized for uncontrolled diabetes. Upon discharge from the hospital in November, she was referred to the Visiting Nurses Association for teaching about insulin administration and monitoring of her diabetic care.

NURSING ASSESSMENT

During your initial visit, you observe that Mrs. T.'s house is poorly maintained and has no insulation or other weatherization. Mrs. T. tells you that she has lived in this house for 60 years and that, in recent years, she has had difficulty keeping up with maintenance because of her poor eyesight and limited income. She has few social contacts, but her daughter visits her every other week and a neighbor visits weekly and brings her groceries. About once a month, friends pick her up and

take her to church. Your assessment reveals that although Mrs. T. has difficulty preparing meals because of her poor eyesight, she is independent in all other activities of daily living.

During your initial visit, you identify several risk factors for hypothermia, so during subsequent visits you follow up with further assessment. You learn that Mrs. T. was taken to the emergency department in January, 2 years ago to be treated for hypothermia. She recalls that her daughter had come for her usual visit and had found her in a very weak and confused state. Her description of the situation is that "they just warmed me up at the hospital and sent me home again. I could have done that myself if my daughter would have just let me be." It is apparent that she did not consider her condition to be of particular concern. In the winter, she keeps her utility bills low by using a small, portable heater in the living room during the day and moving it into the bedroom at night. Mrs. T. keeps her thermostat at 65°F (18.3°C) during the day and 60°F (15.6°C) at night. A neighbor told her that the county office on aging had a program to assist with utility bills, but she is embarrassed to ask her daughter to drive her to the county office to apply for this "welfare help."

NURSING DIAGNOSIS

In addition to addressing the nursing diagnoses related to Mrs. T.'s diabetes, you identify a nursing diagnosis of Risk for Imbalanced Body Temperature, Hypothermia. Related factors include advanced age, diabetes, social isolation, poor housing conditions, low environmental temperatures, and a history of hypothermia.

NURSING CARE PLAN FOR MRS. T.

Expected Outcome	Nursing Interventions	Nursing Evaluation
Mrs. T.'s knowledge about risk factors for hypothermia will be increased.	• Discuss risk factors for hypothermia, with emphasis on Mrs. T.'s diabetes, social isolation, environmental conditions, and history of hypothermia.	• Mrs. T. will be able to state at least four factors that place her at risk for hypothermia.
Mrs. T.'s knowledge about ways of preventing hypothermia will be increased.	• Use Box 25-2 to discuss interventions to prevent hypothermia and to explore waysof applying these interventions to Mrs. T.'s situation.	• Mrs. T. will implement strategies aimed at reducing her risk for hypothermia.
The risk factor of low temperatures in Mrs. T.'s house will be eliminated.	• Inform Mrs. T. about the Low Income Home Energy Assistance Program (LIHEAP) and explain that she may qualify for assistance with utility bills as well as help with weatherization. • Emphasize that LIHEAP is an important health-related program aimed at preventing hypothermia in older adults. • Ask Mrs. T.'s permission to arrange for a home assessment by a LIHEAP staff person.	• Mrs. T. will accept assistance from the LIHEAP program. • Mrs. T. will have her house weatherized. • Mrs. T. will keep her thermostat at 70°F (21.1°C) during the winter.
The risk factor of social isolation will be eliminated.	• Suggest home-delivered meals to Mrs. T. as a means of providing prepared meals and daily contact. • Emphasize that one of the purposes of such programs is to ensure that socially isolated older adults have daily contact with someone who can monitor their well-being. • Ask Mrs. T. for permission to contact her daughter to suggest that she call her mother daily during cold spells to make sure she is okay.	• Mrs. T. will accept home-delivered meals. • Mrs. T.'s daughter will phone daily during cold spells.

THINKING POINTS

• How would you address Mrs. T.'s perception that hypothermia does not have serious health-related implications?

• What additional interventions might you consider to address Mrs. T.'s risk for hypothermia?

Chapter Highlights

Age-Related Changes That Affect Thermoregulation
- Inefficient vasoconstriction
- Decreased cardiac output
- Diminished subcutaneous tissue and muscle mass
- Decreased peripheral circulation
- Delayed and diminished shivering
- Diminished ability to acclimatize to heat.

Risks Factors That Affect Thermoregulation (Box 25-1)
- Environmental factors (e.g., temperatures, humidity)
- Socioeconomic and housing factors (e.g., poor ventilation, inadequate heat, lack of air conditioning)
- Insufficient knowledge about altered thermoregulation
- Medications and alcohol
- Chronic and acute conditions (e.g., infections; cardiovascular, endocrine, and neurologic conditions)
- Inactivity
- Social isolation.

Functional Consequences Affecting Thermoregulation
- Compromised ability to respond to hot or cold environments
- Increased susceptibility to hypothermia and hyperthermia
- Lower baseline temperature
- Diminished febrile response to infections
- Dulled perception of environmental temperatures.

Nursing Assessment of Thermoregulation (Box 25-2)
- Establish baseline temperature, including diurnal variations
- Identify risks for hypothermia or hyperthermia
- Observe for additional manifestations of infections

Nursing Diagnosis
- Readiness for Enhanced Knowledge: Prevention of Hypothermia (or Hyperthermia)
- Risk for Hypothermia
- Risk for Hyperthermia
- Risk for Imbalanced Body Temperature

Planning for Wellness Outcomes
- Health Promoting Behaviors
- Knowledge: Personal Safety
- Risk Detection
- Risk Control
- Safe Home Environment
- Thermoregulation

Nursing Interventions to Promote Healthy Thermoregulation (Box 25-3)
- Maintaining healthy environmental conditions
- Teaching about measures to protect from hypothermia
- Teaching about measures to prevent hyperthermia
- Instituting comfort measures.

Evaluating Effectiveness of Nursing Interventions
- Evidence that risk factors are eliminated

- Feedback about Improved Knowledge Regarding Prevention of Hypothermia and Hyperthermia
- Feedback about Referrals for Community Resources

Critical Thinking Exercises

1. Describe four major functional consequences that an older adult is likely to experience with regard to thermoregulation. How would you explain these changes to an older adult?
2. Explain how each of the following factors might affect an older person's thermoregulation: medications, pathologic conditions, environmental conditions, socioeconomic factors, and lack of knowledge.
3. What would you include in an assessment of thermoregulation in an older adult?
4. What would you teach older adults about hypothermia and its prevention?
5. What would you teach older adults about heat-related illnesses and their prevention?
6. Find appropriate health education materials on the Internet to use in teaching older adults about hypothermia and heat-related illnesses.

Resources

For links to these resources and additional helpful Internet resources related to this chapter, visit thePoint at http://thePoint.lww.com/Miller6e.

Health Education

Health Canada, Canada Health Portal
Low-Income Home Energy Assistance Program (LIHEAP)
National Energy Assistance Referral Hotline
National Institute on Aging (NIA)

REFERENCES

Elbaz, G., Etzion, O., Delgado, J., Porath, A., Talmor, D., & Novack, V. (2008). Hypothermia in a desert climate: Severity score and mortality prediction. *The American Journal of Emergency Medicine, 26*, 683–688.

Fallico, F., Nolte, K., Siciliano, L., & Yip, F. (2005). Hypothermia-related deaths: United States, 2003–2004. *MMWR: Morbidity and Mortality Weekly Report, 54*(7), 173–175.

Gibbons, G. M., Wein, D. A., & Paula, R. (2008). Case Report: Profound hypothermia secondary to normal ziprasidone use. *The American Journal of Emergency Medicine, 26*, 737.e1–737.e2.

Holowatz, L. A., Thompson-Torgerson, C., & Kenney, W. L. (2010). Aging and the control of human skin blood flow. *Frontiers in Bioscience, 1*(15), 718–739.

Lu, S.-H., & Dai, Y.-T. (2009). Normal body temperature and the effects of age, sex, ambient temperature and body mass index on normal oral temperature: A prospective, comparative study. *Science Digest, 46*, 661–668.

Murphy, T., Zumwalt, R., Fallico, F., Sanchez, C., Belson, M., Rubin, C., & Azziz-Baumgartner, E. (2006). Hypothermia-related deaths: United States, 1999–2002 and 2005. *MMWR: Morbidity and Mortality Weekly Report, 55*(10), 282–284.

NANDA International. (2009). *Nursing diagnoses: Definitions and classification 2009–2011*. Oxford, UK: Wiley-Blackwell.

Outzen, M. (2009). Management of fever in older adults. (2009). *Journal of Gerontological Nursing, 35*(5), 17–24.

Platt, M., & Vicario, S. (2009). Heat illness. In J. A. Marx, R. Hockberger, & R. Walls (Eds.), *Rosen's emergency medicine* (7th ed., pp. 1881–1892). St. Louis, MO: Mosby.

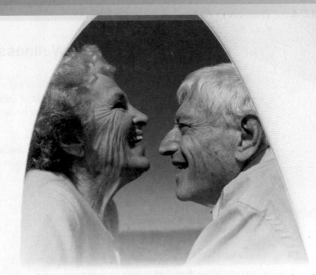

CHAPTER 26

Sexual Function

LEARNING OBJECTIVES

After reading this chapter, you will be able to:

1. Describe age-related changes that affect sexual function in older adults.

2. Discuss risk factors that influence older adults' interest in, opportunities for, and performance of sexual activities.

3. Discuss the functional consequences affecting sexual wellness in older adults.

4. Assess your own attitudes about sexual function in older adults.

5. Apply assessment guidelines in clinical settings when it is appropriate to address sexual wellness.

6. Teach older adults about interventions to promote sexual wellness.

KEY POINTS

andropause

erectile dysfunction

female sexual
   dysfunction

hormonal therapy

hot flashes

human immunodeficiency
   virus (HIV)

menopause

perimenopause

postmenopause

prostatic hyperplasia

urethritis

vaginitis

Because sexual function in older adults encompasses many physiologic and psychosocial aspects of sexuality and intimate relationships, this chapter's perspective is broad. Although sexual function is not a dominant focus of gerontological nursing care in most situations, it is a very important component of quality of life for most older adults. Thus, in long-term care settings and other situations in which quality of life is a focus of care, nurses need to be prepared to assess sexual function and implement nursing interventions that promote sexual wellness.

AGE-RELATED CHANGES THAT AFFECT SEXUAL FUNCTION

A loss of reproductive ability at the onset of **menopause** in women is an age-related change in sexual function that is clearly delineated. **Erectile dysfunction** in older men, often addressed as an age-related change, is more strongly associated with risk factors than with age-related changes and is discussed in the Risk Factors and Pathologic Conditions sections. Other, more subtle age-related changes in sexual function include diminished reproductive abilities in older men and alterations in both male and female responses to sexual stimulation. Older adults generally can compensate for any age-related changes in their response to sexual stimulation; however, when risk factors are present, they may experience additional changes in sexual function.

Changes Affecting Older Women

Hormonally regulated cycles, called *menses*, control female reproductive abilities. With the onset of menses during adolescence, the cyclic release of ova marks the beginning of female reproductive abilities. Reproductive abilities decline around the fifth decade, when the frequency of ovulation diminishes and menstrual cycles become shorter and irregular. Menopause (the cessation of menses), which typically occurs around the age of 49 to 51 years, is a clear indicator that reproduction is no longer possible. **Perimenopause** refers to the several years before menopause when women begin experiencing manifestations of approaching menopause (e.g., changes in menstrual cycles, vasomotor symptoms, vaginal dryness). **Postmenopause** begins 12 months after a woman's last menstrual cycle.

In addition to affecting reproductive ability, menopause influences other aspects of sexual function, predominantly because of the accompanying decline in endogenous estrogen levels. Production of estradiol by the ovaries is the primary

Promoting Sexual Wellness in Older Adults

Nursing Assessment
- Self-assessment of attitudes about sexual functioning and aging
- Cultural influences
- Knowledge about sexual function
- Factors that interfere with sexual function

Age-Related Changes
- Degenerative changes in all reproductive organs
- Diminished levels of hormones
- Cessation of menses (women)

Negative Functional Consequences
- Less intense and slower response to sexual stimulation
- Decreased sexual activity, despite continued interest

Risk Factors
- Societal factors: attitudes, stereotypes, prejudices
- Limited opportunities
- Adverse effects of medications and nicotine
- Functional impairments
- Chronic illnesses

Nursing Interventions
- Teaching about age-related changes
- Addressing risk factors
- Teaching women about hormonal therapy
- Teaching men about interventions for erectile dysfunction

Wellness Outcomes
- Improved quality of life
- Referrals for addressing risk factors
- Increased knowledge and comfort of nursing staff

source of estrogen before menopause, but after menopause, the primary source is estrone, which is converted from androstenedione in skin and fat tissue. Endogenous estrogen levels decline in all postmenopausal women, but the extent and manifestations of estrogen deficiency vary. Factors that affect postmenopausal levels of endogenous estrogen include the interval since the onset of menopause; the production of hormones by the adrenal cortex; changes in the clearance

rates of androgens and estrogens; and body weight, with higher body fat being positively correlated with higher levels of estrogen.

About 70% of all menopausal women experience **hot flashes** (also called *hot flushes*) with one-third of these women requesting treatment for severe symptoms (Ayers, Forshaw, & Hunter, 2010; Luoto, 2009). Hot flashes are a vasomotor symptom that is described as the sudden onset of heat, sweating, and flushing that usually starts in the face, then spreads to the head, neck, chest, torso, and arm; the hot flash typically lasts from 1 to 5 minutes. Sensations of chills, nausea, anxiety, palpitation, and clamminess may also occur. Although the severity of symptoms varies significantly, hot flashes can cause embarrassment, sleep disruptions, significant discomfort, and interruptions in activities, including sexual activities. Hot flashes gradually subside in most women after about 5 years, but 7% experience them for 10 years or longer (Luoto, 2009).

Diminished estrogen levels can directly affect sexual function for older women in several ways. One of the more obvious effects is that breasts become more pendulous and have more fat and less mammary tissue. Vaginal dryness from diminished secretions is another noticeable effect that can affect sexual pleasure unless compensatory interventions, such as a lubricant, are used. Less obvious changes include loss of fullness of the labia, diminished quantity of pubic hair, and atrophy of sexual organs.

In addition to these effects on sexual function and quality of life, estrogen deficiency is associated with increased risk for pathologic conditions, including osteoporosis and cardiovascular disease. Although menopausal hormonal changes have been identified as a risk factor for depression and cognitive decline, studies do not consistently support these conclusions (Weismiller, 2009).

> **DIVERSITY NOTE**
>
> Hot flashes are more prevalent in European and North American women (particularly in African American and Latin American women) and are less common in women who live in India, China, and Japan (Ayers, Forshaw, & Hunter, 2010; Weismiller, 2009).

Changes Affecting Older Men

Male reproductive function depends on the secretion of testosterone and other hormones, the production and release of sperm, and the motility of sperm through the urethra. All organs involved in these processes undergo degenerative changes during later adulthood and gradually diminish the production of viable sperm. Despite these age-related changes, however, some men never lose their reproductive abilities.

The term **andropause** has been used to describe the age-related decline in testosterone in men that begins around the age of 30 years and is analogous to the age-related decline in estrogen in women. Cross-sectional and longitudinal data indicate that a significant percentage of men older than 60 years have serum testosterone levels below the lower limits of young adults (Wang et al., 2009). However, there is significant individual variation among men, with some men maintaining levels that are equal to those of healthy younger men (Orwoll et al, 2006). There is also a significant relationship between low levels of testosterone and cigarette smoking and many chronic illnesses (e.g., hypertension) (Corona & Maggi,

2010; Guay, Seftel, & Traish, 2010). In recent years, the term *late-onset hypogonadism* (also called *testosterone deficiency* or *androgen deficiency*) has been used to describe a syndrome in which serum testosterone level is abnormally low and is associated with symptoms such as low libido, erectile dysfunction, decreased vitality, and depressed mood (Corona, Ferruccio, Morittu, Forti, & Maggi, 2009). Recent studies suggest that low serum testosterone levels are associated not only with diminished sexual function but also with increased risk for pathologic conditions, including cardiovascular disease and type 2 diabetes (Feeley, Saad, Guay, & Traish, 2009).

RISK FACTORS THAT AFFECT SEXUAL FUNCTION

Societal Influences

Because personal attitudes about sexuality are shaped by societal influences, it is important to consider the societal context of attitudes about sexuality, particularly with regard to women and older adults. Strict Victorian standards of morality in Europe and North America strongly influenced many generations, beginning in the 1800s and including those who are older adults today. According to Victorian standards, homosexual activity, public displays of affection, and sex with anyone except a marital partner were totally taboo. During this same time, people viewed menstruation and sexuality as having deleterious effects on women, and medical practitioners removed a woman's sexual organs as a usual treatment. Moreover, masturbation was viewed as an underlying cause of "disasters" that ranged from insomnia and insanity to paralysis, eventual coma, and death (Studd & Schwenkhagen, 2009).

Victorian perspectives were common until 1953 when Kinsey and colleagues published results of their study of *Sexual Behaviours in the Human Female*. This "Kinsey report" brought public attention to previously taboo topics such as orgasm, masturbation, premarital sex, and marital infidelity and was a major turning point in perspectives on female sexuality. In recent decades, attitudes about sexuality changed significantly; however, older adults have been strongly influenced by societal viewpoints of the past. Thus, older adults today may lack accurate information about sexuality and may resist attempts to discuss topics that they consider taboo.

Another factor that influences perspective on sexuality and aging is the strong association in Western societies between sexual attractiveness and physical attractiveness in very gender-specific and stereotypical ways. For example, male sexuality is associated with the image of a tanned, muscular, and youthful man, and female sexuality is associated with the image of a thin, but adequately endowed, young woman. Because these images contrast sharply with typical portrayals of older adults as physically unattractive, they foster a stereotype of "sexless seniors."

These societal influences promote the false perception that older adults have lost the interest in or capacity for sexual activity. This can become a self-fulfilling prophecy if older adults believe this stereotype. Even if older adults do not believe these stereotypes, they may be embarrassed to acknowledge their sexual desires and activities for fear of being considered abnormal.

> **Wellness Opportunity**
>
> Nurses need to avoid reinforcing, or even buying into, the pervasive societal attitudes about "sexless seniors."

Older lesbians, gay men, and bisexuals may be particularly vulnerable to myths and stereotypes about sexuality and aging because they experience an additional layer of misinformation and prejudices related to their sexual orientation. Despite the gradually increasing acceptance of people with diverse sexual orientations in Western societies, older lesbians, gay men, and bisexuals have experienced decades of feeling stigmatized and they are more likely than younger generations to be "closeted" and uncomfortable, or even actively secretive, about their sexual orientation. Some studies have found that older lesbian, gay, and bisexual adults experience more loneliness than heterosexual elders, with higher levels of loneliness being associated with long-term experiences of prejudiced reactions (Fokkema & Kuyper, 2009; Kuyper & Fokkema, 2009). Despite the difficulties inherent in their situation, however, older lesbians, gay men, and bisexuals can enjoy levels of social support and emotional well-being similar to those of older heterosexual people.

> **Wellness Opportunity**
>
> Nurses holistically address sexual wellness by being nonjudgmental about choices of close personal relationships.

Attitudes and Behaviors of Families and Caregivers

In addition to societal influences, the attitudes and behaviors of family members and caregivers who are closest to the older adult can negatively affect the older adult's sexual function. Adult children of older people often find it difficult to deal with the sexuality of their parents because they believe the common stereotype that older adults are asexual. In addition, they may discourage intimate relationships if they fear that a serious relationship would jeopardize their inheritance.

In institutional settings, attitudes of staff members can significantly affect the way in which residents express or repress their sexual needs. Staff members in long-term care facilities are generally unprepared to address issues related to sexuality and aging, and they may hold negative or patronizing attitudes about sexual expression among older adults. In general, nurses tend to ignore the sexual needs of older adults and the only expression of sexual needs by residents of long-term facilities that is considered appropriate is a private, medically approved visit by a spouse. Masturbation and any sexual activities between two unmarried people are usually not tolerated, even when done in private. When the staffs become aware of sexual activities that they consider inappropriate, they often ask family members to intervene, even when the resident is competent. Decisions regarding sexual activity, even between spouses, usually are treated as medical matters. In addition to the prerequisite of medical approval for sexual activity, staff members in long-term care facilities may seek the permission of family members before allowing residents to enjoy sexual activity.

When older adults have dementia, issues related to sexual expression are compounded by questions about competency and the meaning of behaviors. Spouses often are overwhelmed with concerns about caregiving issues that take precedence over sexual relationships and other quality-of-life concerns. Families often question the ability of the person with dementia to make decisions about intimate relationships and sexual expressions, and this is particularly problematic with regard to nonmarital relationships. These decisions are complex and should consider not only the effect on the spouse but also whether the sexual interactions could be beneficial or positive for the person with dementia.

Limited Opportunities for Sexual Activity

The frequency and enjoyment of sexual activities during older adulthood is strongly associated with the importance assigned to sexual activity in the past. As a group, never-married women have the lowest rate of sexual activity compared with other categories of older adults. Although women of all ages are less sexually active than men in their cohort, the difference in their levels of sexual activity widens with increasing age.

Researchers have identified different factors that affect the level of sexual activity for older men and women. For older men, a decline in sexual activity is strongly associated with health problems, whereas for older women, the single most important variable is having a functioning and sexually interested partner (Weismiller, 2009; Wylie & Kenney, 2010). One study found that only 9% of women who were sexually inactive attributed this to personal physical conditions (Huang et al., 2009). A major determinant of having an available sexual partner is the ratio of men to women, which gradually changes with increasing age, from a ratio of 86 men per 100 women between ages 65 and 69 years to a ratio of 41 men per 100 women in the age group of 85 years and older (He, Sengupta, Velkoff, & DeBarros, 2005).

In addition, lack of privacy can limit the older adult's opportunities for sexual activity. Privacy is generally considered a requisite for sexual activity, and adults who live in their own homes are usually able to arrange for this. However, older adults who live in institutions, group settings, or family homes may find it difficult or impossible to arrange for privacy, especially if their sexual needs are ignored or considered abnormal or even morally deviant. Even if some privacy is possible in institutional settings, additional environmental constraints include the inability to lock doors and ensure total privacy and the unavailability of anything larger than a single bed.

Adverse Effects of Medication, Alcohol, and Nicotine

Almost three decades ago, a study published in the *Journal of the American Medical Association* (Slag et al., 1983) identified adverse effects of medication as the single largest cause of erectile dysfunction in men. Slag and colleagues found that 34% of 1180 male patients in a medical clinic were impotent, and 25% of the 188 subjects who subsequently underwent further evaluation were found to have medication-induced erectile dysfunction. In recent years, there has been increasing attention to sexual adverse effects of medications as a major factor that influences quality of life and adherence to prescribed regimens. Although most studies have focused on men, medications are a common cause of sexual dysfunction in both men and women.

Medications adversely affect sexual function through a variety of mechanisms, including their influence on the release of hormones and their actions on the autonomic and central nervous systems. Specific adverse medication effects that interfere with sexual function in men include a decreased or absent libido; difficulty obtaining or maintaining an erection; dry, premature, or retrograde ejaculation; and inability to achieve orgasm. A less common adverse medication effect is priapism, an erection that persists beyond or is unrelated to sexual stimulation, which can lead to permanent erectile dysfunction. Medications that can cause this condition include antipsychotics (e.g., aripiprazole, chlorpromazine, quetiapine, risperidone, and ziprasidone), antidepressants (e.g., trazodone), antihypertensives (e.g., hydralazine, prazosin) and medications used for treating erectile dysfunction (including the over-the-counter preparation of yohimbine) (Anderson, Schmedt, Weinmann, Willich, & Garbe, 2010; Burnett & Bivalacqua, 2007; Myers & Barrueto, 2009). Women may experience the following medication-induced limitations in sexual function: diminished vaginal lubrication, decreased or absent libido, and inability to achieve orgasm. Box 26-1 lists some of the medications that are commonly associated with sexual dysfunction. These effects usually disappear when the medication is discontinued and occasionally the effects will disappear if the dose is decreased.

Because alcohol depresses the central nervous system, it can interfere with sexual function. Although in social settings alcohol can decrease inhibitions and heighten sensual and sexual interest, in excessive amounts, the central nervous system depressant effect of alcohol usually counteracts any

Box 26-1 Medications That Can Interfere With Sexual Function

Ace inhibitors
Alpha-adrenergic blockers or agonists
Antidepressants
Antihistamines
Antiparkinson agents
Antipsychotics
Benzodiazepines
Beta-blockers
Calcium channel blockers
Diuretics
Dopamine agonists
Histamine H_2 antagonists
Monoamine oxidase inhibitors (MAOIs)
Nonsteroidal anti-inflammatory drugs
Alcohol, nicotine, recreational drugs

beneficial effects and interferes with sexual performance. Moderate amounts of alcohol normally do not interfere with sexual performance; however, in combination with other risk factors, such as medications or pathologic conditions, even small amounts of alcohol may be detrimental to the sexual performance of older adults.

Cigarette smoking was first identified as a cause of erectile dysfunction in the mid-1980s, and recent studies have confirmed that smoking increases the risk for sexual dysfunction in both men and women (Kupelian, Araujo, Chiu, Rosen, & McKinlay, 2010; Steinke, Mosack, Wright, Chung, & Moser, 2009). Nicotine interferes with circulation to the sexual organs and accentuates the effects of other risk factors, such as diabetes, hypertension, and vascular disease. Studies also have found that cigarette smoking is associated with earlier onset of menopause and increased the intensity and frequency of hot flashes (Luoto, 2009; Sammel, Freeman, Liu, & Guo, 2009).

Chronic Conditions

Diabetes has consistently been identified as a risk factor for sexual dysfunction, in both men and women. Studies have identified prevalence rates for erectile dysfunction in men with diabetes ranging from 20% to 85%, with higher rates being associated with obesity, older age, and longer duration and poorer control of diabetes (Aslan et al., 2009; Awad, Salem, Gadalla, El Wafa, & Mohamed, 2010; Nehra, 2009; Tamler, 2009). In addition to erectile dysfunction, men with diabetes are likely to experience retrograde ejaculation. Studies indicate that 75% of women with diabetes experience sexual dysfunction, including decreased desire and arousal, orgasmic dysfunction, diminished vaginal lubrication, and pain (Enzlin et al., 2009; Palacios, Castano, & Grazziotin, 2009). Factors that increase the risk for sexual dysfunction in women with diabetes include obesity and hypothyroidism (Veronelli et al., 2009).

Cardiovascular disease is strongly associated with many aspects of sexual dysfunction, including decreased libido, inhibited performance and pleasure, and decreased frequency of sexual activities. Sexual function is affected not only by the physical manifestations of coronary heart disease (e.g., angina and reduced levels of activity) and adverse effects of medications but also by psychological factors that commonly occur in people with cardiovascular disease. For example, even when no physiologic basis exists for abstaining from sexual intercourse after a myocardial infarction, sexual activity is often limited or absent because of fatigue, depression, diminished sexual desire, and fears and anxiety of the person or the sexual partner.

DIVERSITY NOTE

A review of studies concluded that sexual function in women is significantly affected by coronary artery disease and that nurses play a key role in addressing sexual concerns for women with cardiovascular disease (Steinke, 2010).

Gender-Specific Conditions

Prostatic hyperplasia (also called *benign prostatic hypertrophy*) is a pathologic condition in which the prostate gland gradually enlarges and affects the urinary tract and sexual function. This condition affects 20% to 26% of men in their 40s and 80% to 90% of men in their 70s and 80s (Bushman, 2009; Reyes, 2009). Prostatic hypertrophy is highly associated with erectile dysfunction and ejaculatory dysfunction and also is a common cause of urinary incontinence, which can interfere with enjoyment of sexual activities (Rosen et al., 2009).

Sexual function in older women can be affected by their increased susceptibility to **urethritis** and **vaginitis** because of the thinning of the vaginal tissue and the decreased acidity and quantity of vaginal secretions. These conditions can occur after intercourse and cause urinary urgency and burning that persists for several days. They also can interfere with enjoyment of sexual intercourse.

Functional Impairments and Dementia

Functional impairments associated with chronic conditions can interfere with enjoyment of sexual activity in many ways, as in the following examples:

- Chronic obstructive pulmonary disease may cause hypoxia and severe shortness of breath in response to the high physiologic demands of sexual activity.
- Arthritis and other musculoskeletal disorders are likely to be associated with pain, stiffness, muscle spasms, and limited flexibility.
- Urinary incontinence can interfere with satisfying sexual relationships in people of any age, but this condition is more common in older adult.
- Medical conditions and adverse medication effects can have physiologic effects that interfere with all phases of sexual function.

- Dementia, depression, and other conditions that affect psychosocial function can also affect sexual function.

Functional limitations increase with advancing age and are likely to combine with other risk factors to interfere with sexual function. In addition to direct effects, disabilities can indirectly affect sexual function because of the common misperception equating disability with lack of sexual function. This cultural bias, along with other effects of disabilities on self-image, can have a negative impact on sexual function. This is particularly relevant to older adults who live in institutional settings because attitudes of the staff members can affect the residents' expressions of sexuality. A study of factors that influence attitudes about late-life sexuality found that young adults expressed less acceptance of sexual expression and more doubt about ability to consent when older women were described as cognitively impaired (Allen, Petro, & Phillips, 2009).

Sensory impairments can also interfere with sexual function because sensory stimulation is an important part of sexual pleasure and intimate communication. For example, an older adult with impaired hearing may find it difficult or impossible to carry on the intimate conversations that are often a part of sexual interactions. Similarly, hearing impairments can interfere with professional efforts to assess and counsel older adults on this sensitive topic. Likewise, impairments affecting vision, smell, or touch can interfere with some of the usual sensual stimulation associated with sexual activities.

In recent years, gerontologists and clinicians have focused attention on sexual function and intimate relationships in people with dementia. During the later stages of the disease, most people with dementia are indifferent about sex, but issues related to sexual function and intimate relationships often arise during early and middle stages. Loss of sexual desire is the most common effect of dementia on sexual function; however, some people with dementia experience hypersexuality and demand frequent sexual intercourse, particularly men and especially during the middle stages. Some people with dementia exhibit behaviors that are considered sexually inappropriate (e.g., removing clothing or getting into bed with someone); however, these behaviors are caused by cognitive impairments rather than sexual impulses. Sexual expressions of people with dementia in institutional settings include sexual talk, physically intimate touch, and sexual expressions without touching others (Tzeng, Lin, Shyr, & Wen, 2009). Sometimes, the behaviors are normal but they are labeled as problematic because the person is in an institutional setting that is not designed for sexual relationships or because there are questions about the person's ability to make fully informed decisions (Wallace & Safer, 2009).

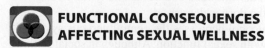

FUNCTIONAL CONSEQUENCES AFFECTING SEXUAL WELLNESS

Sexual function involves reproduction, response to sexual stimulation, and interest and participation in sexual activity. Although reproduction is directly affected by age-related changes, the other two aspects of sexual function are affected more directly by risk factors. In addition, because sexual dysfunctions commonly occur in older men and women as a consequence of risk factors, these are discussed in this section.

Reproductive Ability

For women, loss of reproductive ability is a functional consequence of menopause, caused by the cessation of ova production within 1 year of the last menstrual cycle. Another functional consequence affecting reproduction in women is the increased risk that a fetus will be defective if ova are fertilized during the premenopausal years. The reproductive ability of men, by contrast, gradually declines with age but does not cease completely.

Response to Sexual Stimulation

The Masters and Johnson (1966) investigation has been widely recognized as the landmark study of human physiologic response to sexual stimulation. This study of 694 adults in a laboratory setting identified four phases of physiologic response to sexual stimulation in men and women. An analysis of data on older subjects led to the following conclusions:

- Older adults maintain their ability to respond to sexual stimulation, but their response is slower and less intense.
- Regularly engaging in sexual activity helps older adults respond to sexual stimulation
- Any major changes in response to sexual stimulation are associated with risk factors rather than aging, per se.

Although older adults were greatly underrepresented in this study, the findings of Masters and Johnson have been widely accepted as the knowledge base about age-related changes in physiologic response to sexual stimulation. Normal age-related changes in male and female responses to sexual stimulation and the associated consequences are discussed in the following sections and summarized in Table 26-1.

In recent years, more comprehensive models have been proposed with emphasis on multifactorial factors that influence men and women; however, research on age-related differences is lacking. Current models emphasize the interrelationship between mind and body and conceptualize sexuality in relation to and interaction with variables, such as culture, religion, and social practices (Wylie & Mimoun, 2009).

Sexual Interest and Activity

During the 1940s and 1950s, the Kinsey surveys first brought information about sexual behaviors of older adults to public attention. Since then, other reports confirmed that the frequency of *sexual activity* gradually declines with increasing age; however, *sexual interest and competence* of older adults do not necessarily decline. Despite a reported decline in sexual activity among older adults, a recent survey found that 53% and 25% of adults between the ages of 65 and 74 years and 75 and 85 years, respectively, reported being sexually active (Lindau et al., 2007). In addition, a longitudinal study of four representative samples of 70-year olds in Sweden who were interviewed between 1971 and 2001 reported the following changes in sexual activity and satisfaction: self-reported sexual activity increased, attitudes to sexuality became more positive, the proportion reporting sexual dysfunction decreased, and the proportion reporting a very happy relationship increased as did the proportion reporting a high satisfaction with sexual activity (Beckman, Waern, Gustafson, & Skoog, 2008).

Sexual interest, attitudes, activity, and satisfaction are a continuation of lifelong patterns, and they remain stable in older adulthood unless risk factors interfere with sexual function. Factors that most commonly affect sexual interest and activity in older adults include social circumstances, pathologic conditions, adverse medication effects, and influences of family and caregivers (as discussed in the section on Risk Factors). The sexual needs and interest of older adults,

	Changes in Female Response	**Changes in Male Response**
TABLE 26-1 Functional Consequences for Response to Sexual Stimulation		
Excitement phase	Breasts not as engorged Sexual flush diminished Delayed or diminished vaginal lubrication Decreased expansion of vaginal wall Decreased vasocongestion of labia	Longer time required to attain erection Less firm erection Longer maintenance of erection before ejaculation Increased difficulty regaining an erection if lost Reduced scrotal and testicular vasocongestion
Plateau phase	Decreased areolar engorgement Less intense sexual flush Less intense myotonia Decreased vasocongestion of labia Reduced Bartholin's gland secretions Slower/less marked uterine elevation	Diminished nipple turgidity and sexual flush Less intense muscle tension Slower penile erectile response Delayed and diminished testicular elevation Fewer rectal sphincter contractions Diminution of ejaculatory expulsion force by about 50%
Orgasmic phase	Fewer rectal sphincter contractions Decreased number and intensity of orgasmic contractions	Absent or diminished sense of ejaculatory inevitability Fewer and less intense ejaculatory contractions
Resolution phase	Slower loss of nipple erection Quicker return to pre-excitement stage	Slower loss of nipple erection Longer refractory period Rapid penile detumescence and testicular descent

including residents of long-term care facilities, do not necessarily decrease, but their opportunities for sexual activity are often limited.

In recent decades, studies of sexuality and aging have focused on broader aspects, such as affection, friendships, and intimacy. For older adults, these aspects of sexual function may become more important as the number of acceptable opportunities for sexual activities diminishes. For example, one of the first studies addressing sexual behaviors found that the most common sexual activities in a sample of 202 adults aged 80 to 102 years were touching and caressing without sexual intercourse (Bretschneider & McCoy, 1988). Similarly, Johnson (1996) found that older adults (mean age, 66 years) reported that the sexual activities of kissing, hugging, and hearing loving words were more important than masturbation, oral sex, or sexual conversation. In this study, older women ascribed greater importance to sexual activities of sitting and talking, making oneself more attractive, and saying loving words than did men. By contrast, older men reported greater interest in sexual activities, such as erotic movies and readings, sexual daydreams, and physically intimate activities. More recent studies conclude that older adults in long-term relationships identify factors such as authenticity, communication, intense emotional connection, and a sense of mutual acceptance as characteristics of "great sex" (Kleinplatz & Menard, 2007). In summary, older adults do not lose their interest in or capacity for sexual activity because of age-related changes, but risk factors such as misinformation, social circumstances, pathologic conditions, environmental constraints, and adverse medication effects do commonly interfere with sexual function. A normal consequence of aging, however, is that the response of older men and women to sexual stimulation is slower, less intense, and of shorter duration. As one 79-year-old man was heard to say, "It's like sparklers, not fireworks."

♦ Wellness Opportunity

Nurses need to recognize that many interacting physical and psychosocial factors affect sexual wellness in a unique way for each older adult.

Male Sexual Dysfunction

Erectile dysfunction, defined as the inability to achieve or maintain an erection sufficient for satisfactory sexual function, is the term that has been used since the early 1990s to replace the term *impotence*. The National Institutes of Health proposed this change in terminology to reflect the broader understanding of erectile dysfunction as a complex condition associated with many pathophysiologic conditions and other risk factors. Although erectile dysfunction is not the only type of male sexual dysfunction, it is the one that has been studied the most and has received the most public attention since 1998 because of the availability of medications, such as sildenafil (Viagra), and the widespread publicity about these medications that continues today. Other types of male sexual

dysfunction include problems with ejaculation and diminished desire. Although these problems are associated more strongly with risk factors than with normal aging, the prevalence increases with increasing age.

Studies have found that erectile dysfunction affects 17% to 35% of men between the ages of 40 and 70 years (Laumann, Das, & Waite, 2008; Rosing et al., 2009; Wentzell & Salmeron, 2009). It is currently viewed as a complex disease associated with several interacting factors, the most common physiologic causes being adverse medication effects and pathologic conditions. Medical conditions most strongly associated with erectile dysfunction include hypertension, dyslipidemia, diabetes mellitus, and disorders of the prostate and lower urinary tract (Bianco et al., 2009; Kumar et al., 2009; Nehra, 2009).

Female Sexual Dysfunction

In recent years, health care practitioners and pharmaceutical companies have started addressing **female sexual dysfunction**, similar to the way in which erectile dysfunction has been addressed since the early 1990s. Female sexual dysfunction includes disorders that affect sexual desire (including motivation and physical drive), sexual arousal, orgasm, or pain during sexual activities (i.e., dyspareunia or vaginismus) (Mimoun & Wylie, 2009). Between 40% and 50% of women experience sexual dysfunctions; however, only 12% to 25% of these women associate the sexual problems with personal distress (Clayton & Hamilton, 2009; Palacios et al., 2009).

Many of the same risk factors associated with erectile dysfunction are also associated with female sexual dysfunction: hypertension, hypercholesterolemia, diabetes mellitus, cigarette smoking, pelvic surgeries, and adverse medication effects. In addition, diminished estrogen levels in women who are naturally or surgically menopausal and who are not taking **hormonal therapy** are a major contributing factor (Clayton & Hamilton, 2009). Urinary incontinence, disorders of the pelvic floor (cystocele, vaginal prolapse), and any type of pelvic surgery (e.g., hysterectomy or procedures for urinary incontinence) increase the risk for female sexual dysfunction.

---

*Y*ou are the "wellness nurse" at the senior center where Mr. and Mrs. S. come for the meal program and social interaction. Mr. S. is 73 years old and has hypertension and a history of a heart attack. He takes diltiazem (Cardizem), 300 mg daily; lasix (Furosemide), 20 mg daily; and propranolol (Inderal), 80 mg three times daily. Mrs. S., who is 71 years old, describes herself as generally healthy, but with a history of depression and some arthritis. She takes ibuprofen (Motrin), 400 mg four times daily, and sertraline (Zoloft), 50 mg daily. During your nursing clinics, Mr. S. and several other men have asked you about the drug that is advertised on television for men who have trouble satisfying their partners. The senior center director also has noticed an increased interest in this topic and has asked that you plan a group health information session called "Sexuality and Aging."

THINKING POINTS

- Develop a plan for teaching older adults about the normal changes in sexual function that they are likely to experience.
- What risk factors would you discuss in relation to sexuality and aging?
- What educational materials would you use?
- What teaching would you do about interventions?

PATHOLOGIC CONDITION AFFECTING SEXUAL WELLNESS: HUMAN IMMUNODEFICIENCY VIRUS

Health care practitioners who provide care to older adults are increasingly aware of the need to address **human immunodeficiency virus (HIV)** as a sexually transmitted infection that is becoming more common among older adults. The effectiveness of antiretroviral therapy since the late 1980s has enabled many HIV-infected people to live longer with this condition, which is now considered a chronic disease, before it progresses to acquired immunodeficiency syndrome (AIDS). Because of improved survival as well as the increasing incidence of HIV/AIDS in people aged 50 years, by the years 2015, it is projected that half the people living with this condition will be older adults (Branas et al., 2008). Statistics about HIV/AIDS generally define "older adult" as someone aged 50 years and older based on the Centers for Disease Control and Prevention (CDC) demographic distribution of cases on a bell curve (with an average age of around 30 years). Data from the CDC (2008) indicate that in 2005, people aged 50 years and older accounted for

- 15% of new HIV/AIDS diagnoses
- 24% of people who have HIV/AIDS (increased from 17% in 2001)
- 29% of all people living with AIDS
- 35% of all deaths of persons with AIDS

The CDC also reports significant racial disparity for HIV/AIDS among older adults, with the rate for blacks and Hispanics being 12 and 5 times higher, respectively, than whites. Studies also have found that older women comprise a larger percentage of older adults with HIV, and this disparity is even higher for black women (Martin, Fain, & Klotz, 2008).

Although health-related concerns are associated with HIV/AIDS in anyone, some issues are more strongly associated with HIV/AIDS in older adults, as summarized in Box 26-2. In addition, HIV in older adults can cause neurologic and cognitive changes that can lead to depression and suicidal ideation because of the increased difficulty of coping effectively with the stressors associated with aging and HIV (Vance, Struzick, & Burrage, 2009). Nurses can apply assessment and intervention principles related to preventing suicide in older adults (see Chapter 15) and implement interventions to promote effective coping. Interventions that are appropriate for older adults with HIV include fostering social supports (e.g., support groups, volunteer activities, religious organizations); facilitating referrals to social service agencies (e.g., emergency financial assistance); and encouraging interventions designed to increase hardiness (e.g., cognitive-behavior therapies) (Vance, Childs, Moneyham, & McKie-Bell, 2009).

Risk Factors for HIV

For people of any age, HIV is transmitted through sexual contact, blood contact, needle stick, or perinatally from mother to infant. Among older adults, intravenous drug use and sexual contact between gay men are the primary risk factors associated with HIV infection. However, more than half of HIV infections in older women are attributed to heterosexual transmissions and only about 15% are due to intravenous drug use (Nguyen & Holodniy, 2008). An important consideration with regard to risk factors is that fewer than 10% of older adults who reported at least one risk factor had never had an HIV test performed, and only 15% of this population reported using condoms during sexual activity (Nguyen & Holodniy, 2008).

Box 26-2 Health-Related Concerns Associated With HIV/AIDS in Older Adults

Progression of the Condition
- Older adults are likely to be diagnosed at a later stage, due to lack of screening, poor awareness of risk factors, and failure of health care professionals to recognize and treat HIV/AIDS.
- Older adults have a shorter interval before progression to AIDS, particularly if HIV was diagnosed after the age of 60 years.
- Older adults have a shorter time before death.

Associated Medical Concerns
- HIV/AIDS in older adults increases the risk for diabetes, osteoporosis, parkinsonism, cerebrovascular conditions, cardiovascular conditions, liver disease, and some cancers.
- Dementia occurs more frequently in older HIV patients.
- Drug regimens for HIV/AIDS increase the risk for interactions, particularly with drugs used for anxiety, depression, hyperlipidemia, and erectile dysfunction.

Additional Concerns
- Older adults with HIV/AIDS have higher rates of dementia, depression, and suicidal ideation.
- Older adults are more likely to have less social support due to ageism, living alone, perceived stigma, and nondisclosure of HIV status.

A risk factor specific to older women is that menopausal changes in vaginal mucosa can increase the risk for trauma and sexually transmitted infections during intercourse. Other risk factors that disproportionately affect older women include sexism, physical or sexual abuse, lack of knowledge, lower rates of HIV testing, and more difficulty negotiating safe sex practices (Martin et al., 2008).

Role of Nurses in Assessment and Interventions

Although nurses in gerontological care settings are not expected to be experts in providing care for people with HIV/AIDS, they are expected to holistically assess and address the complex needs of older adults with this condition. Caregivers need to recognize that HIV initially manifests as a nonspecific viral illness with signs and symptoms similar to seasonal flu or mononucleosis (e.g., fever, rash, malaise, myalgia, and pharyngitis). Even without treatment, these manifestations typically subside after about 2 to 3 weeks. HIV antibodies will appear in the blood between 3 and 6 weeks after the initial infection. If treatment is initiated, the latent period can last for 15 years before it progresses to AIDS; without treatment, AIDS will develop and lead to death within 2 to 3 years or sooner (Nguyen & Holodniy, 2008).

Because older adults are not commonly tested for HIV, the infection is likely to be diagnosed at a more advanced stage. Although the current CDC recommendations are for routine, voluntary screening in all people between the ages of 13 and 64 years, some groups recommend at least one-time screening of all sexually active people aged 65 years or older (Nguyen & Holodniy, 2008). One study found that screening of people between the ages of 55 and 75 years is cost-effective for those who have risk factors, including having a sexual partner at risk (Sanders, Bayoumin, Holodniy, & Owens, 2008). Thus, an important role for nurses is to assess for risk factors and encourage testing for older adults who have risk factors.

Treatment of HIV generally includes a combination of antiretroviral agents and other types of medications to control disease progression. The pharmacologic regimen requires close monitoring for therapeutic and adverse effects. Adherence is a common problem for people with HIV/AIDS, for various reasons including cost of medications and adverse effects, making these issues important aspects of assessing older adults with HIV/AIDS.

Nurses have important health promotion responsibilities with regard to wellness for older adults with HIV/AIDS. Their interventions need to be directed toward optimal physical and psychosocial function. Vance and colleagues (2009, 2010) review ways in which gerontological nurses can implement interventions to promote successful aging with HIV. For example, nurses can encourage appropriate levels and types of physical activity to address many of the symptoms associated with HIV.

Teaching about safe sex is a nursing responsibility that is often overlooked when caring for older adults, but it is particularly important with regard to preventing HIV. Older adults need to recognize that safe sex practices are imperative for anyone who has sex with someone other than a long-term partner who is 100% monogamous. Nurses also need to teach about early detection of HIV and other sexually transmitted infections and encourage appropriate testing for anyone with risk factors. Nurses can incorporate information about safe sex in their health education about sexual activity for older adults, as discussed in the section on interventions and summarized in Box 26-5.

NURSING ASSESSMENT OF SEXUAL FUNCTION

Nurses do not necessarily include sexual function in every assessment, but they should assess it whenever they are addressing quality-of-life issues that affect day-to-day function. Thus, assessment of sexual function is especially important in home care and long-term care settings (e.g., nursing facilities, group homes, and assisted living facilities). Sexual function is often neglected in nursing assessments because of the high degree of privacy associated with sexual function and the stereotype of the "sexless senior" that is prevalent in our society. In addition, gender or generational differences between the health professional and the older person may interfere with an assessment of sexual function. Although all of these factors may explain why sexual function in older adults is so often overlooked, they do not justify its exclusion.

Self-Assessment of Attitudes About Sexual Function and Aging

Because of the private nature of sexual function and associated emotional responses and cultural factors, nurses are often uncomfortable discussing it. Additional discomfort occurs because nurses are not confident in dealing with concerns about human sexuality as an integral part of their nursing practice. They are even less comfortable initiating this topic with older adults or with people who are not in a traditional marital relationship. Thus, an assessment of personal attitudes about sexuality and aging is a prerequisite to addressing sexual wellness. Box 26-3 lists some of the questions nurses can use to examine their own attitudes toward the sexual function of older adults. Some questions are specific to adults in long-term care facilities because of the dominant role of nurses in addressing sexual function as a quality-of-life issue for residents.

> ✦ **Wellness Opportunity**
>
> Nurses should take time for self-assessment to increase their comfort with, openness to, and sensitivity about issues related to sexual wellness for older adults.

Significant cultural differences between the nurse and the older adult may increase the difficulty of discussing sexual function. Cultural Considerations 26-1 summarizes some

Box 26-3   Assessing Personal Attitudes Toward Sexuality and Aging

What Do I Believe About Sexuality and Aging?

- Do I hold the misconception that older people, especially unmarried ones, are no longer interested in or capable of sexual activities?
- Do I believe the subtle messages that inaccurately associate sexual activities only with youth and attractiveness?
- Do I hold age-specific standards regarding sexual activity and romantic relationships? (e.g., Do I think it is okay for young adults to kiss or hold hands, but inappropriate or "cute" for older people to do this?)

What Do I Believe About the Nurse's Role With Regard to the Sexual Function of Older Adults?

- Do I base my nursing practice on the misconception that sexual function is strictly a private matter that health professionals should not address?
- Do I view sexual function as an activity of daily living that should be included in a comprehensive assessment of long-term care needs of older adults?
- Do I feel more comfortable discussing sexual function with people who are of the same gender and age range as myself, but very uncomfortable in discussing this matter with people who are old enough to be my parents or grandparents?
- Do I avoid discussion of sexual function with older adults because I believe they are not interested in sexual activity or are uncomfortable discussing this topic?
- Do I avoid discussing sexual function with older adults who are not in traditional marital relationships?

- What beliefs do I hold about the assessment of sexual function based on the age of the person? For example, do I think sexual function should be assessed in sexually active teenagers who are at risk for unwanted pregnancy, but not older people?
- Am I comfortable incorporating health education about safe sex practices with older adults?

What Is My Attitude About Various Expressions of Sexual Activity?

- How do I view sexual activity and romantic relationships between unmarried people, or between people of the same gender?
- How do I view masturbation?
- Do my views about masturbation or sexual activity between unmarried or same-gender people influence my assessment of and interventions for people who engage in these activities?
- Am I tolerant and nonjudgmental toward people whose views and practices are nontraditional or different from mine?

For Nurses in Settings Where Long-Term Needs Are Addressed

- How do I feel about the rights of residents to engage in sexual activity in private, either with themselves or people of their own choosing?
- Do I try to ensure privacy for those residents who desire it?
- If I am aware of the sexual activities of a resident, do I think that I should inform the administrator, a family member, or another " responsible adult?"

---

cultural aspects of sexual function that may be applicable to nursing assessment. Nurses may also be uncomfortable discussing sexual function with older adults who are involved in same-sex or other nontraditional relationships. Thus, an important aspect of self-assessment is to identify attitudes toward nontraditional sexual activities because these attitudes

CULTURAL CONSIDERATIONS 26 - 1

Cultural Aspects of Sexual Function

Expressions of Sexuality and Intimacy

- In some cultures, direct eye contact, especially between a man and woman, is interpreted as an expression of intimacy.
- In some cultures, it is taboo for a man to be alone with a woman other than his wife.
- Touching another person (particularly of the opposite sex) is considered taboo in many cultures.
- In some cultures, heterosexual men and women commonly hold hands with another person of the same gender.
- Only a few cultures value sexual equality between men and women.
- Homosexuality is accepted in some cultures but is considered taboo or is kept secret among family members in others.

Assessment Considerations

- In some cultures, it is considered taboo for postmenopausal women to have their breasts or vagina examined, even by a health care provider.
- Menopausal manifestations may vary in different cultural groups (e.g., most Japanese women do not experience hot flashes).

can influence the assessment and care of people who do not conform to the nurse's expectations. When assessing sexual function, it is important that nurses establish a trusting relationship, have an awareness of gay and lesbian culture and other nontraditional sexual relationships, and communicate a nonjudgmental attitude by using gender-neutral terminology. For example, the word *partner* includes a spouse as well as a same-sex relationship and asking about someone who is a *confidant* is broader than asking about marital status.

Assessing Sexual Function in Older Adults

The goals in assessing sexual function in older adults include providing an opportunity for the older adult to address any issues related to sexual function and identifying risk factors, including lack of information, that can interfere with the older person's sexual function and quality of life. Although the extent of the assessment varies according to individual circumstances, it should include, at a minimum, questions about the gynecologic aspects of female sexual function and the genitourinary aspects of male sexual function. Nurses can easily incorporate these questions into a routine assessment of overall function. If these questions are followed by an open-ended question about sexual interest and activities, the nurse can then respond to the individual needs of the older adult. If problems or risk factors are identified, the nurse is not expected to conduct an in-depth assessment of all aspects of sexual function but should obtain enough information to suggest appropriate

Box 26-4 Guidelines for Assessing Sexual Function in Older Adults

Interview Atmosphere and Communication Techniques
- Ensure both privacy and comfort.
- Be nonjudgmental and matter-of-fact in verbal and nonverbal communication.
- If feasible, sit face-to-face in chairs, rather than conducting the interview while the person being interviewed is in bed.
- If feasible, allow the person being interviewed to wear usual daytime clothing, rather than a hospital gown.

Initiation and Discussion of the Topic
- Begin by acknowledging feelings of discomfort and by stating the reason for discussing this topic. (e.g., "I know that sexuality is a private matter and people are often uncomfortable discussing this topic. However, as a nurse, I consider sexuality to be an aspect of health and well-being, and it may have a significant bearing on your overall care.")
- Include statements that address stereotypes and require a response from the older adult. (e.g., "Our society tends to view old people as being uninterested in sex, but for most older people, this is not true. Many older people are less sexually active than when they were younger, but this is not because of age-related changes. Have you experienced any changes in your sexual activities in the past few years?")
- Initiate the topic near the end of a comprehensive assessment interview, and begin with questions about the physiologic aspects of male or female function, such as those that follow.
- Incorporate at least one question to assess the appropriateness of including information about safe sex practices in your health teaching. (e.g., "If you have sex with partners other than someone who is in a long-term monogamous relationship with you, what precautions do you take?")

Interview Questions to Assess Male Sexual Function
- Have you ever had prostate problems or related surgery? Have you ever been told that you have or had an enlarged prostate?
- How often do you undergo a complete medical examination? When was your last complete physical examination done?
- Do you ever experience dribbling of urine or have problems holding your water?
- Do you have any trouble initiating the stream of urine?
- After you have urinated (passed water), do you still feel like you haven't emptied your bladder completely?
- Do you have to get up during the night to empty your bladder? If so, how many times?
- Have you ever noticed any blood in your urine?
- Do you ever have any discharge from your penis?
- Do you have any sores, lumps, ulcers, irritations, or areas of inflammation on your penis or scrotum?
- Do you have any trouble with erection or ejaculation?

Interview Questions to Assess Female Sexual Function
- How many children, if any, have you had? How many pregnancies?
- At what ages did your menstrual periods begin and end?
- Have you ever had a Pap (Papanicolaou) test? When was your most recent Pap test and gynecologic examination?
- Have you ever had a mammogram? When was the most recent one?
- Have you ever been taught to examine your breasts for lumps?
- Do you examine your breasts for lumps? How often?
- Have you noticed any changes in your breasts? Do you ever have any discharge from your nipples?
- Do you have any burning, itching, or irritation in the vaginal area?
- Do you ever have any vaginal discharge or bleeding?
- Do you have any difficulties with sexual intercourse?

Principles for Assessing Sexual Interest and Activities
- If the older adult makes a clear statement that this topic is irrelevant, do not insist on further questions. If the older adult responds to questions, however, do not discontinue the interview because of your own discomfort.
- Do not assume that an assessment of sexual function is irrelevant to unmarried people.
- For both married and unmarried older adults, use open-ended questions to elicit information about intimate relationships (e.g., "Is there anything you would like to ask or discuss about intimate relationships?").
- For a married person, open-ended questions may be asked about the partner's influence on sexual activities (e.g., "Has your husband experienced any changes in his health that have affected your sexual activities?").
- Listen for statements that reflect myths, a negative self-image, or self-fulfilling prophecies, such as "Of course I stopped being interested in sex after menopause," or "I can't have an erection because I have prostate trouble."
- If risk factors, such as certain medications or pathologic conditions, have been identified earlier in the interview, ask additional questions, such as "Have you had any difficulties with sexual activities since your heart attack?" or "Do you have any questions about the possible effects of diabetes on sexual activity?"
- Emphasize the clinical reason for the questions. ("Sometimes certain illnesses or medications interfere with sexual function, and we want to identify any problems you might be having in this area.")
- Use open-ended questions that allow for either closure of the topic or a further discussion of issues. ("Is there anything you would like to discuss with regard to your sexual relationships?")

resources for further evaluation. Box 26-4 summarizes guidelines for assessing sexual function in older adults.

The Hartford Institute for Geriatric Nursing recommends that nurses use the PLISSIT assessment model as a routine nursing assessment for older adults (Wallace, 2008). The four components of this model are as follows:

- Obtaining **Permission** from the client to initiate sexual discussion
- Providing **Limited Information** about sexual function

- Giving **Specific Suggestions** for the individual to proceed with sexual relations
- Providing **Intensive Therapy** surrounding the issues of sexuality for the client

Additional information and a cost-free video demonstrating the application of this tool in a clinical setting is available through collaboration of the Hartford Institute and the *American Journal of Nursing* at http://consultgerirn. org/resources or at www.nursingcenter.com. Nurses have effectively applied this model to assess and address sexual issues of patients who have stomas or cardiovascular disease (Ayaz & Kubily, 2009; Jaarsma, Steinke, & Gianottem, 2010).

NURSING DIAGNOSIS

When nurses identify risks that interfere with sexual function, or when older adults express an interest in discussing sexual function, the appropriate nursing diagnosis is Ineffective Sexuality Pattern, defined as "expressions of concern regarding own sexuality" (NANDA International, 2009). Related factors commonly identified in older adults include medication effects; endocrine diseases (e.g., diabetes); cardiovascular diseases; genitourinary conditions; functional impairments secondary to chronic conditions (e.g., limited range of motion as a result of arthritis); psychosocial circumstances (e.g., lack of a partner); and myths and misunderstandings about age-related changes. The case example at the end of this chapter addresses this nursing diagnosis.

> **Wellness Opportunity**
>
> The nursing diagnosis of Readiness for Enhanced Knowledge: Sexual Functioning would be applicable to older adults who express an interest in learning about the effects of aging or risk factors on sexual wellness.

PLANNING FOR WELLNESS OUTCOMES

Increased knowledge about sexual function is an expected outcome for older adults who lack accurate information about age-related changes and risk factors. An outcome for residents of long-term care facilities would be Client Satisfaction: Protection of Rights. For a long-term care resident who is gay, lesbian, or bisexual, an applicable outcome would be Client Satisfaction: Cultural Needs Fulfillment. Nurses can use the following additional Nursing Outcomes Classification (NOC) terminologies in care plans to promote sexual wellness for older adults: Body Image, Health Beliefs, Knowledge: Sexual Functioning, Personal Well-Being, Self-Esteem, and Sexual Functioning.

> **Wellness Opportunity**
>
> Quality of Life is a wellness outcome for older adults who achieve more satisfying relationships through a variety of expressions of intimacy.

 ## NURSING INTERVENTIONS TO PROMOTE HEALTHY SEXUAL FUNCTION

Nurses have many opportunities to teach older adults about healthy sexual function as an important aspect of quality of life, particularly in home and long-term care settings. Nurses have an important teaching role because many older adults, as well as family and caregivers, hold stereotypes or have little accurate information about sexuality and aging. Nurses can use the following Nursing Interventions Classification (NIC) terminologies in their care plans: Body Image Enhancement, Energy Management, Health Education, Patient Rights Protection, Risk Identification, Role Enhancement, Self-Awareness Enhancement, Self-Esteem Enhancement, and Teaching: Sexuality.

Teaching Older Adults About Sexual Wellness

Unlike sex therapists or primary health care providers, nurses are not expected to provide sex education or direct interventions; however, nurses are expected to address sexual function as a quality-of-life concern. Nursing responsibilities also include teaching about safe sex practices for older adults who are sexually active with anyone other than their long-term monogamous partner. Health education about sexual wellness for older adults includes the following information:

- Acknowledgment that sexual function is within the usual realm of health promotion for older adults, especially in long-term care settings
- Effects of age-related changes on sexual function
- Risk factors that cause or contribute to problems with sexual function
- Resources for addressing identified problems and risk factors
- Protection from sexually transmitted infections

In addition, nurses in long-term care settings often need to address attitudes of the staff members, families, and residents by providing accurate information and role modeling nonjudgmental behaviors.

In some situations, it is appropriate for nurses to teach older adults, as well as their caregivers, about age-related changes and risk factors that affect sexual function. However, the privacy of this topic requires that nurses use excellent communication skills when teaching about sexual wellness. It is important to be open, respectful, and nonjudgmental, and to avoid the use of medical terminology when discussing sexuality with older adults. Nurses can use printed information written in nontechnical terms, such as the teaching tool in Box 26-5, as a basis of discussion about sexual function for older adults. Nurses can emphasize that any major changes in sexual function are not due to age-related changes alone, and they can use Table 26-1 for further discussion of sexual function in healthy older adults. Many excellent resources for professionals and lay people are available in bookstores and on the Internet.

> **Wellness Opportunity**
>
> Nurses promote personal responsibility for sexual wellness by suggesting sources of accurate information that older adults can use.

Addressing Risk Factors

If an older adult with significant changes in sexual function also has a pathologic condition, takes a medication, or uses any substance that might be a contributing factor, nurses can teach

Box 26-5 Health Education About Sexual Activity for Older People

- Older people remain fully capable of enjoying orgasm, but their response to sexual stimulation usually is slower, less intense, and of shorter duration. Increasing the amount and diversity of sexual stimulation and experimenting with different positions can compensate for these changes and increase sexual enjoyment.
- The "use it or lose it" principle applies to sexual activity.
- Sexual problems in older people occur for the same reasons they occur in younger people. That is, they may be related to illness or disability, medications or alcohol, or psychological and relationship factors. A cause of sexual problems that is unique to older people is the self-fulfilling prophecy of the "sexless senior" stereotype.
- The following habits enhance sexual enjoyment: exercising regularly, avoiding or limiting consumption of alcohol, maintaining optimal health and nutrition, using hearing aids and corrective lenses as needed, and engaging in sexual activities when you are relaxed and your energy level is at its peak.
- If you experience problems with sexual function, seek advice from a professional who is skilled in working with older people. Medical help can be obtained from a urologist, gynecologist, or other medical specialist. If there is no medical basis for the problem, a sex therapist or marriage counselor might be helpful.
- If you engage in sexual activity with anyone other than your long-term monogamous partner, protect yourself from sexually transmitted infections and talk with your health care practitioner about being tested periodically.

Facts Specific to Older Men
- Periodic difficulties with erection and ejaculation do not necessarily indicate that you are impotent.
- After you've reached orgasm, it may be 1 or 2 days before you are able to reach full orgasm again.
- Many new treatment options are available for treating erectile dysfunction (impotence). If your health care provider cannot provide up-to-date information about these options, ask for a referral for an appropriate evaluation and discussion of various options.

Facts Specific to Older Women
- Using a water-soluble lubricant will compensate for decreased vaginal lubrication. Do *not* use petroleum jelly because it is not a very effective lubricant for this purpose and can predispose you to infection.
- Estrogen is beneficial in preventing some problems with sexual function, but the relative risks and benefits of such therapy should be considered and discussed thoroughly with your primary care provider.
- You may have vaginal irritation or urinary tract infections, especially after sexual intercourse, because of age-related thinning of the vaginal wall. Such problems may be avoided by the following interventions:
  - Drink plenty of fluids.
  - Use an estrogen cream or vaginal lubricant.
  - Maintain good hygiene in the vaginal area.
  - If you have a male partner, have him thrust his penis downward, toward the back of your vagina.
  - Empty your bladder before and after intercourse.

about the potential influence of these risk factors. This is particularly important when nurses identify pertinent risk factors, but the older adult attributes sexual problems to old age. For example, an older man may attribute a problem with attaining an erection to age-related changes, when, in fact, he has diabetes and takes an antihypertensive medication that is associated with erectile dysfunction. Nurses can use Box 26-1 to identify some of the medications that can interfere with sexual function. When nurses identify a potential relationship between a risk factor and sexual problems, it is appropriate to suggest that the older adult seek professional advice. A complete medical evaluation by a primary care provider who is knowledgeable about the sexual problems of older adults is usually the best starting point. If medications are causing or contributing to sexual dysfunction, the primary care provider should consider alternative medications or reduced doses if medically feasible. For example, people with hypertension are less likely to have sexual dysfunction when treated with calcium channel blockers, angiotensin-converting enzyme inhibitors, or peripheral alpha-adrenergic receptor blockers. After medical problems are addressed, a mental health professional may be an appropriate resource if problems with sexual function persist.

Arthritis is one of the most common pathologic conditions affecting older adults, and it is often self-managed with little or no medical supervision. Often, the symptoms are not severe enough to motivate the older adult to seek medical evaluation and treatment, but they may interfere with sexual activities. In such cases, nurses can use Box 26-6 to teach about self-care

interventions that may be effective in improving the quality of sexual activities for the older adult with arthritis. Nurses can also suggest that older adults who have arthritis obtain pamphlets from local chapters of the Arthritis Foundation.

Box 26-6 Health Education About Sexual Activity for People With Arthritis

The pain, fatigue, and joint limitations of arthritis may interfere with, but do not have to curtail, your enjoyment of sexual activity. In fact, sexual activity can be beneficial to you because it stimulates the release of cortisone, adrenalin, and other chemicals that are natural pain relievers. The following actions may enhance your sexual enjoyment and minimize the effects of arthritis:
- Engage in sexual activity when you feel least fatigued and most relaxed.
- Use analgesic medications and other methods of pain relief before engaging in sexual activity.
- Use relaxation techniques before engaging in sexual activity. Relaxation techniques that may be helpful for arthritis include warm baths or showers and the application of hot packs to the affected joints.
- Maintain optimal health through good nutrition and a proper balance of rest and activity.
- Experiment with different sexual positions and use pillows for comfort and support.
- Increase the time spent in foreplay.
- Use a vibrator if your ability to massage is limited by arthritis.
- Use a water-soluble jelly for vaginal lubrication.

Another pathologic condition often associated with sexual dysfunction is coronary artery disease, particularly in those who have had myocardial infarctions or who have undergone coronary artery bypass surgery. Studies consistently identify a need for health care professionals to provide information about sexual concerns for patients and their partners not only immediately after a myocardial infarction but for a prolonged period after initial recovery (Mosack & Steinke, 2009). Nurses can encourage older adults to discuss these concerns with their primary care practitioner and can provide health education using the general guidelines outlined in Box 26-7.

Promoting Sexual Wellness in Long-Term Care Settings

Responsibilities of nurses in long-term care settings to address sexual needs differ from those responsibilities of nurses in acute care or home settings in the following ways:

- Intense medical needs of patients in acute care settings take precedence over sexual needs.
- The short duration of stay in acute care settings is not conducive to addressing long-term sexual needs of patients.
- Because of the high degree of privacy and autonomy for people in their own homes, home care nurses are not routinely concerned about sexual needs.

Residents in long-term care facilities, however, usually are not acutely ill, are planning to stay in the facility for a long time, and do depend on the nursing staff to ensure the privacy necessary to meet their personal needs. Thus, the nurse in long-term care facilities must address the sexual needs of residents as an integral part of the overall care plan.

> ### Box 26-7 Health Education About Sexual Activity for People With Cardiovascular Disease
>
> - Participation in a medically supervised exercise program can reduce oxygen requirements during sexual activity and improve the quality of your sex life.
> - The typical energy expenditure for sexual intercourse is equivalent to that used for climbing two flights of steps.
> - Do not engage in sexual activity in extremely hot and humid environments.
> - Wait 3 hours after consuming alcohol or a large meal before initiating sexual activity.
> - Engage in sexual activity when your energy is at its peak and you are feeling rested and relaxed.
> - Avoid sexual activity during times of intense emotional stress.
> - Avoid engaging in sexual activity with a partner with whom you are uncomfortable (e.g., an extramarital partner).
> - Experiment with different positions to find one that is least demanding of your energy.
> - Consider using nitroglycerin, if ordered by your primary care provider, as needed before sexual activity.
> - Know that many types of oral medications for erectile dysfunction can cause serious (even fatal) interactions with nitrates.
> - Consult your primary care provider if you experience chest pain during or after sexual activity, or breathlessness or heart palpitations persisting for 15 minutes after orgasm.

Staff education is an important part of addressing the sexual needs of older adults in long-term care facilities because staff members need to know about all aspects of sexuality and aging, including the lifelong interest in and need for sexual activity and intimate relationships. Audiovisual materials can be used to stimulate discussion about the unique aspects of meeting sexual needs in institutional settings and about the responsibilities and limitations of staff members. Nurses generally participate in such in-services as part of the interdisciplinary team, which also includes social service and administrative staff. Presenters and discussion leaders should be nonjudgmental and matter-of-fact so that they role model the most effective approach for addressing this sensitive topic.

When the ability of a cognitively impaired resident to give informed consent is questionable, an interdisciplinary team can assess competence to participate in an intimate relationship. Emphasis should be placed on the Residents' Rights bill, as defined by the federal government in the 1987 Nursing Home Reform Law. Sexual needs of residents of long-term care facilities are protected through the rights to

- Self-determination
- Participation in their own care
- Independence in making personal decisions
- Reasonable accommodation of their needs and preferences
- Privacy and unrestricted communication with any person of their choice
- Immediate access by their relatives and others, subject to reasonable restriction with the resident's permission

In addition to educating staff members about the sexual needs and rights of residents, nurses are responsible for ensuring privacy for those residents who desire it. If a resident does not have a private room, staff members try to provide privacy, while still respecting the rights of any roommates. Sometimes, the role of the nurse will be that of a negotiator, assisting residents in reaching mutually acceptable agreements about privacy and shared space.

> **Wellness Opportunity**
>
> Nurses respect autonomy by working with other staff members to assess the ability of someone with dementia to make decisions about expressions of sexuality.

Teaching Women About Interventions

Hormonal therapy refers to the use of estrogen alone or with progestogen for symptoms of natural or surgically induced menopause. The relative risks and benefits of hormonal therapy have been hotly debated since the 1940s, and numerous studies have been published with controversial results, particularly since 2002. Studies are ongoing and the debate continues today, but there is consistent emphasis on basing decisions on individualized goals. Thus, an important role for nurses is to encourage women to discuss their personal risks and benefits with a knowledgeable health care practitioner.

The most recent position statement of the North American Menopause Society (2008) summarizes the following conclusions based on a comprehensive review of studies:

- Hormonal therapy is widely recognized as the most effective treatment for vasomotor symptoms (i.e., hot flashes and night sweats) and their potential consequences (e.g., disturbed sleep and diminished quality of life).
- Studies support the initiation of hormonal therapy around the time of menopause to treat menopause-related symptoms; to treat or reduce the risk of certain disorders (e.g., osteoporosis or fractures) in select postmenopausal women; or both.
- The benefit–risk ratio for menopausal hormonal therapy is favorable close to menopause but decreases with aging and with the time since menopause in previously untreated women.
- Vaginal hormonal therapy is recommended for vaginal atrophy.
- Vaginal hormonal therapy may benefit some women with urge incontinence if this is associated with vaginal atrophy, but it is unclear whether hormonal therapy is effective in treating overactive bladder or pure stress incontinence.
- Systemic hormonal therapy may worsen or provoke stress incontinence.
- Vaginal hormonal therapy may reduce the risk of recurrent urinary tract infection.

Because of the controversy surrounding the prescription of hormonal therapy, there is an increasing need for evidence-based recommendations regarding nonhormonal therapies for menopausal symptoms. In addition, women—particularly those who are Asian, Hispanic, and African American—have reported that they need information about management of menopausal symptoms from health care professionals (Im, Lee, Chee, Dormire, & Brown, 2010). Unfortunately, evidence-based information about interventions for menopausal symptoms is currently very limited but is evolving. Nurses can keep up to date on evidence-based information by checking the resources listed at the end of this chapter, and they can encourage women to check these resources. Interventions that are highly recommended and without controversy are those that emphasize a healthy lifestyle (e.g., regular exercise, relaxation techniques, nutritious food, healthy weight). Lifestyle interventions for hot flashes include keeping environmental temperatures cool, avoiding spicy foods, and wearing lightweight clothing. Women can be encouraged to use water-soluble lubricants or prescription estrogen cream for vaginal dryness.

Teaching Men About Interventions

Interventions for erectile dysfunction have been available for several decades, but until recently, these interventions were not widely used, in part, because men did not seek help for this condition. Since 1998, extensive publicity about oral agents that are safe and easy-to-use interventions has brought much attention to this topic and it now commonly recognized as a treatable condition. Sildenafil (Viagra) is the most commonly used drug of this type, called oral phosphodiesterase-5 inhibitors, and the two additional drugs in this class are vardenafil (Levitra) and tadalafil (Cialis). Many recent, large-scale studies have evaluated these drugs and concluded that they are safe and effective as first-line therapies for erectile dysfunction in older adults (Morales, Mirone, Dean, & Costa, 2009; Tsertsvadze et al., 2009). Common adverse effects of these drugs include nausea, headache, flushing, indigestion, and nasal congestion. Some recent studies are finding "emerging evidence" that these drugs are associated with hearing and vision impairments (Snodgrass et al., 2010). These drugs are contraindicated for men taking nitrate medications because they can cause serious and even fatal adverse effects. Apomorphine, which is a dopamine receptor agonist, is another first-line therapy with a safety and efficacy profile similar to the phosphodiesterase-5 inhibitors, but this drug can be used concomitantly with nitrates (Eardley et al., 2010). Apomorphine is administered sublingually.

Testosterone therapy has gained increasing attention in recent years; however, a recent research review concluded that studies do not consistently support the safety and effectiveness of this intervention for improving erections or increasing the frequency of sexual intercourse (Tsertsvadze et al., 2009). Because detrimental effects of testosterone therapy, including prostatic hyperplasia and increased risks of prostate cancer, may outweigh the benefits, it is not widely recommended for management of andropause or sexual dysfunction and is contraindicated in men with breast cancer or prostate cancer. Some herbal preparations (e.g., yohimbine) are promoted for enhancing sexual function in men; however, evidence-based information is unavailable to support these so-called interventions.

In addition to the oral agents that are widely publicized, several types of penile prosthesis implants have been shown to be safe, reliable, effective, and "life-changing" in recent studies (Bettocchi et al., 2009; Eid, 2009). Some of these devices require a surgical procedure, but some can be self-administered. Another pharmacologic approach is the administration of a vasoactive drug, such as alprostadil, as either an intracavernosal injection or a transurethral suppository. Nurses do not need to be familiar with the details of these procedures, but they need to know enough about interventions to suggest that men discuss their options with a physician.

Nurses also need to identify and implement interventions to address risk factors that cause or contribute to sexual dysfunction. For example, teaching about smoking cessation and raising questions about sexual adverse effects of prescribed medications are health promotion interventions that nurses can initiate. Nurses can also teach men to seek medical care for optimal control of chronic conditions that increase the risk for erectile dysfunction (e.g., diabetes, hypertension, hyperlipidemia) (Gratzke et al., 2010). Psychotherapy and behavioral therapy may be used as primary or adjunctive treatment options to address the psychosocial issues that may be contributing to erectile dysfunction. Pelvic muscle exercises, commonly performed as a treatment for urinary incontinence, may also be useful in treating erectile dysfunction. The technique for performing these exercises is described in Chapter 19. Decisions about appropriate treatment options must be based on a comprehensive evaluation by a urologist or a primary care provider who is knowledgeable about erectile dysfunction. The primary responsibility of nurses is to keep up to date on the types of interventions that are available and to teach about the importance of seeking help for erectile dysfunction.

EVALUATING EFFECTIVENESS OF NURSING INTERVENTIONS

Nursing care for older adults with the diagnosis of Altered Sexuality Patterns is evaluated by the degree to which risk factors are eliminated, particularly through the provision of accurate information. For example, older adults may verbalize an improved understanding of the age-related changes that affect their response to sexual stimulation. In turn, this information can alleviate anxiety about sexual performance and improve quality of life. Interventions to alleviate risk factors, such as medical conditions or adverse medication/chemical effects, would be considered successful if the older adult follows through with a referral to an appropriate resource. One measure of successful intervention in long-term care settings would be that staff members increase their understanding of the sexual needs of older adults and are more comfortable allowing appropriate sexual expressions by the residents.

*M*r. and Mrs. S. are now 75 and 73 years old, respectively, and they have moved to an assisted-living facility where you are the nurse. Their health conditions have not changed significantly in the past 2 years, with the exception of Mrs. S. having more difficulty walking because of her arthritis. Mr. and Mrs. S. recently moved to the facility because they needed help with transportation and wanted to live in a place where they had fewer responsibilities and more time to enjoy life. During one of their appointments, Mrs. S. becomes tearful and says she has been disappointed in their move from their own home. She says, "Now we have the time to enjoy our life together, but we seem to be in each other's way all the time. When we lived in our own home, we were so busy with the yard and the housekeeping and all the daily chores, we never had time to think about what we enjoy together. Now I don't have to cook meals and worry about getting to the grocery store, but we aren't enjoying the time we have together."

NURSING ASSESSMENT

On further discussion, Mrs. S. acknowledges that she has talked with her husband about having more "intimate time and resuming sexual activities that have petered out in the past few years because we were always so tired and never seemed to have much time." In reply, Mr. S. has stated that "We're probably too old to do those things, and old people shouldn't expect to have the fun in bed that we used to have." Mrs. S. says she used to believe that, but recently she's been talking with some of the other women in the assisted-living facility who seem to be enjoying sexual activities. Mr. and Mrs. S. relate that they had a good sexual relationship until Mr. S.'s heart attack 5 years ago. After that, he lost interest in sexual activities, even though he was told he could resume all his usual activities except for very strenuous activity, such as shoveling snow. Mrs. S. says she masturbates occasionally, but she doesn't find that very satisfying. Mrs. S. expresses concern about being comfortable in the sexual position they used previously because her arthritis has gotten worse in the past few years.

NURSING DIAGNOSIS

You address Ineffective Sexuality Patterns as your nursing diagnosis for Mr. and Mrs. S. Related factors include myths and lack of information about the age-related changes and risk factors that influence sexual function. Potential risk factors that you identify are Mr. S.'s medications and his lack of information about sexual function after a heart attack.

NURSING CARE PLAN FOR MR. AND MRS. S.

Expected Outcome	Nursing Interventions	Nursing Evaluation
Mr. and Mrs. S.'s knowledge about age-related changes and risk factors that affect sexual function will be increased.	• Use Box 26-5 as a basis for discussion of sexual function in later adulthood.	• Mr. and Mrs. S. will verbalize correct information about sexual function in older adulthood.

(case study continues on page 542)

Expected Outcome	Nursing Interventions	Nursing Evaluation
The risk factors associated with Mr. S.'s heart attack and medication regimen will be addressed.	• Explain that many medications for heart problems and high blood pressure are associated with problems with sexual function. • Use Box 26-7 as a basis for discussing sexual activity as it relates to people with heart problems. • Encourage Mr. S. to talk with his primary care provider about his medication regimen and about his heart condition. Suggest that he inquire whether a different medication would effectively treat his high blood pressure without interfering with sexual function.	• Mr. S. will agree to talk with his primary care provider about the potential relationship between his medications and heart condition and his lack of sexual activity.
The risk factors associated with Mrs. S.'s arthritis will be addressed.	• Use Box 26-6 to discuss sexual activity as it relates to people with arthritis.	• Mrs. S. will identify ways to increase her comfort during sexual activities.

THINKING POINTS

- What risk factors are likely to influence Mrs. S.'s enjoyment of sexual activity?
- What risk factors are likely to affect Mr. S.'s enjoyment of sexual activity?
- What health education would you provide for Mrs. S., and what would you use for patient teaching tools?
- What health education would you provide for Mr. S., and what would you use for patient teaching tools?

Chapter Highlights

Age-Related Changes That Affect Sexual Wellness
- Diminished levels of hormones
- Degenerative changes of reproductive organs
- Cessation of menses and onset of menopause for women

Risk Factors That Affect Sexual Wellness
- Societal influences, especially on attitudes, stereotypes, and prejudices
- Effects of attitudes and behaviors of families and caregivers, especially on dependent older adults
- Limited opportunities for sexual activity (lower ratio of men to women, health conditions)
- Adverse effects of medication, alcohol, and nicotine (Box 26-1)
- Chronic conditions
- Gender-specific conditions
- Functional impairments and dementia

Functional Consequences Affecting Sexual Wellness
- Reproductive ability: ceases in women, diminishes in men
- Response to sexual stimulation: slower and less intense (Table 26-1)
- Sexual interest and activity: maintenance of interest and capacity in most older adults, but diminished sexual activity due to risk factors
- Male and female sexual dysfunction

Pathologic Condition Affecting Sexual Wellness: Human Immunodeficiency Virus
- Increasing numbers of adults aged 50 years and older have HIV/AIDS
- Health-related concerns associated with HIV/AIDS in older adults (Box 26-2)
- Risk factors differ for older adults (less likely to be tested or to practice safe sex)
- Nurses have important roles in identifying new cases of HIV, assessing risks for sexually transmitted infections, and assessing treatment issues (i.e., adverse effects, drug interactions).
- Nurses need to teach about safe sex practices.

Nursing Assessment of Sexual Function
- Self-assessment of attitudes about sexual function and aging (Box 26-3)
- Assessment of cultural influences (Cultural Considerations 26-1)

- General principles of and specific interview questions for nursing assessment (Box 26-4)
- Using the PLISSIT assessment model (Clinical Tools)

Nursing Diagnosis
- Readiness for Enhanced Knowledge: Sexual Functioning
- Ineffective Sexuality Pattern

Planning for Wellness Outcomes
- For residents in long-term care facilities: Client Satisfaction, Protection of Rights; Cultural Needs Fulfillment
- Body Image
- Personal Well-Being
- Self-Esteem
- Sexual Functioning

Nursing Interventions to Promote Sexual Wellness
(Boxes 26-5 through 26-7)
- Teaching older adults about sexual wellness: age-related changes and risk factors
- Addressing risk factors: teaching about sexual activity for people with arthritis or cardiovascular disease
- Promoting sexual wellness in long-term care facilities: staff education, protection of rights, ensuring privacy
- Teaching women about interventions for menopause and men about interventions for erectile dysfunction

Evaluating Effectiveness of Nursing Interventions
- Provision of accurate information to dispel myths and misconceptions
- Improved quality of life
- Referrals to health care professionals for addressing risk factors
- Increased knowledge and comfort of staff in long-term care facilities

Critical Thinking Exercises

1. Describe the attitudinal risk factors on the parts of society, older adults, and health care providers that can interfere with healthy sexual function in older adults.
2. Summarize the functional consequences that are likely to affect sexual function in healthy older men and women.
3. What are the responsibilities of nurses in each of the following settings related to assessment of sexual function in older adults: community setting, acute care facility, and long-term care facility?
4. Describe the assessment and health education approaches you might use for a 73-year-old married man who confides that he has difficulty making his wife "happy in bed."
5. Spend a few minutes answering all the questions included in Box 26-3, Assessing Personal Attitudes Toward Sexuality and Aging. What did you learn about yourself?

Resources

For links to these resources and additional helpful Internet resources related to this chapter, visit thePoint at http://thePoint.lww.com/Miller6e.

Clinical Tools

American Journal of Nursing and Hartford Institute for Geriatric Nursing
- *How to Try This,* article and video: Wallace, M. A. (2008). Assessment of sexual health in older adults: Using the PLISSIT model to talk about sex, *American Journal of Nursing, 108*(7), 52–60.
- *Try this: Best Practices in Nursing Care to Older Adults* Issue 10 (2007), Sexuality Assessment for Older Adults

Evidence-Based Practice

Arena, J. M., & Wallace, M. (2008). Issues regarding sexuality. In E. Capezuti, D. Zwicker, M. Mezey, & T. Fulmer (Eds.), *Evidence-based geriatric nursing protocols for best practice* (3rd ed., pp. 629–647). New York: Springer Publishing Co.
National Guideline Clearinghouse
- Hormonal therapy in menopausal women
- Medical care for menopausal and older women with HIV infection

Health Education

American Association of Sex Educators, Counselors and Therapists
American Menopause Foundation, Inc.
Foundation for Health in Aging
HIV Wisdom for Older Women
New England Association on HIV Over Fifty
North American Menopause Society
Senior Action in a Gay Environment (SAGE)
Sexuality Information and Education Council of the United States

REFERENCES

Allen, R. S., Petro, K. N., & Phillips, L. L. (2009). Factors influencing young adults' attitudes and knowledge of late-life sexuality among older women. *Aging and Mental Health, 13*(2), 238–245.

Anderson, F., Schmedt, N., Weinmann, S., Willich, S. N., & Garbe, E. (2010). Priapism associated with antipsychotics: Role of alpha1 adrenoceptor affinity. *Journal of Clinical Psychopharmacology, 30*(1), 68–71.

Aslan, Y., Sezgin, T., Tuncel, A., Tekdogan, U. Y., Guler, S., & Atan, A. (2009). Is type 2 diabetes mellitus a cause of severe erectile dysfunction in patients with metabolic syndrome? *Urology, 74*(3), 564–565.

Awad, H., Salem, A., Gadalla, A., El Wafa, N. A., & Mohamed, O. A. (2010). Erectile function in men with diabetes type 2: Correlation with glycemic control. *International Journal of Impotence Research, 22*(1), 36–39.

Ayaz, S., & Kubilay, G. (2009). Effectiveness of the PLISSIT model for solving the sexual problems of patients with stoma. *Journal of Clinical Nursing, 18*(1), 154–156.

Ayers, B., Forshaw, M., & Hunter, M. S. (2010). The impact of attitudes towards the menopause on women's symptom experience: A Systemic review. *Maturitas, 65,* 28–36.

Beckman, N., Waern, M., Gustafson, D., & Skoog, I. (2008). Secular trends in self reported sexual activity and satisfaction in Swedish 70 year olds: Cross sectional survey of four populations, 1971–2001. *British Medical Journal, 337,* a279, doi:10.1136/bmj.a279.

Bettocchi, C., Palumbo, F., Spilotros, M., Lucarelli, G., Ricapito, V. D., Palazzo, S., . . . Ditonnob, P. (2009). Penile prosthesis implant: When, what and how. *Journal of Men and Health, 6*(4), 299–306.

Bianco, F. J., McHone, B. R., Wagner, K., King, A., Burgess, J., Patierno, S., & Jarrett, T. W. (2009). Prevalence of erectile dysfunction in men screened for prostate cancer. *Journal of Urology, 74*(1), 89–92.

Branas, F., Berenguer, J., Sanchez-Conde, M., Lopez-Bernaldo de Quiros, J. C., Miralles, P., Cosin, J., & Serra, J. A. (2008). The eldest of older adults living with HIV: Response and adherence highly active antiretroviral therapy. *The American Journal of Medicine, 121*(9), 820–824.

Bretschneider, J. G., & McCoy, N. L. (1988). Sexual interest and behavior in healthy 80- to 102-year-olds. *Archives of Sexual Behavior, 17*, 109–129.

Burnett, A. L., & Bivalacqua, T. J. (2007). Priapism: Current principles and practice. *Urologic Clinics of North America, 34*, 631–632.

Bushman, W. (2009). Etiology, epidemiology, and natural history. *Urologic Clinics of North America, 36*, 403–415.

Centers for Disease Control (CDC). (February, 2008). HIV/AIDS among persons aged 50 and older. http://www.cdc.gov/hiv/topics/older.

Clayton, A. H., & Hamilton, D. V. (2009). Female sexual dysfunction. *Obstetrics and Gynecological Clinics of North America, 36*(209), 861–876.

Corona, G., Ferruccio, N., Morittu, S., Forti, G., & Maggi, M. (2009). Recognising late-onset hypogonadism: A difficult task for sexual health care. *Journal of Men's Health, 6*(3), 210–218.

Corona, G., & Maggi, M. (2010). The role of testosterone in erectile dysfunction. *Nature Reviews Urology, 7*(1), 46–56.

Eardley, I., Donatucci, C., Corbin, J., El-Meliegy, A., Hatzimouratidis, K., McVary, K., . . . Lee S.-W. (2010). Pharmacotherapy for erectile dysfunction. *Journal of Sexual Medicine, 7*(1, Pt 2), 524–540.

Eid, J. R. (2009). What is new for inflatable penile prostheses? *Current Opinion in Urology, 19*(6), 582–588.

Enzlin, P., Rosen, R., Wiegel, M., Brown, J., Wessells, H., Gatcomb, P., . . . the DCCT/EDIC Research Group. (2009). Sexual dysfunction in women with type 1 diabetes: Long-term findings from the DCCT/EDIC study cohort. *Diabetes Care, 32*(5), 780–785.

Feeley, R. J., Saad, F., Guay, A., & Traish, A. M. (2009). Testosterone in men's health: A new role for an old hormone. *Journal of Men's Health, 6*(3), 169–176.

Fokkema, T., & Kuyper, L. (2009). The relation between social embeddedness and loneliness among older lesbian, gay, and bisexual adults in the Netherlands. *Archives of Sexual Behavior, 38*(2), 264–275.

Gratzke, C., Angulo, J., Chitaley, K., Dai, Y. T., Kim, N. N., Paick, J. S., . . . Christian G. Stief. (2010). Anatomy, physiology, and pathophysiology of erectile dysfunction. *Journal of Sexual Medicine, 7*(1, Pt 2), 445–475.

Guay, A., Seftel, A. D., & Traish, A. (2010). Hypogonadism in men with erectile dysfunction may be related to a host of chronic illnesses. *International Journal of Impotence Research, 22*(1), 9–19.

He, W., Sengupta, M., Velkoff, V. A., & DeBarros, K. A. (2005). *65 = in the United States: 2005*. Current Population Reports: Special Studies, P23–209. U.S. Department of Health and Human Services, National Institute on Aging, and U.S. Department of Commerce, U.S. Census Bureau. Available at: www.census.gov/prod/2006pubs/p23–209.pdf.

Huang, A. J., Subak, L. L., Thom, D. H., Van Den Eeden, S. K., Ragins, A. I., Kuppermann, M., . . . Brown, J. S. (2009). Sexual function and aging in racially and ethnically diverse women. *Journal of American Geriatric Society, 57*(8), 1362–1368.

Im, E.-O., Lee, B., Chee, W., Dormire, S., & Brown, A. (2010). A national multiethnic online forum study on menopausal symptom experience. *Nursing Research, 59*(1), 26–32.

Jaarsma, T., Steinke, E. E., & Gianotten, W. L. (2010). Sexual problems in cardiac patients: How to assess, when to refer. *Journal of Cardiovascular Nursing, 25*, 159–164.

Johnson, B. K. (1996). Older adults and sexuality: A multidimensional perspective. *Journal of Gerontological Nursing, 22*(2), 6–15.

Kleinplatz, P. J., & Menard, A. D. (2007). Building blocks toward optimal sexuality: Constructing a conceptual model. *The Family Journal, 15*(1), 72–78.

Kumar, R., Nehra, A., Jacobson, D. J., McGree, M. E., Gades, N. M., Lieber, M. M., . . . St sauver, J. L. (2009). Alpha-blocker use is associated with decreased risk of sexual dysfunction. *Urology, 74*, 82–88.

Kupelian, V., Araujo, A. B., Chiu, G. R., Rosen, R. C., & McKinlay, J. B. (2010). Relative contributions of modifiable risk factors to erectile dysfunction: Results from the Boston Area Community Health (BACH) Survey. *Preventive Medicine, 50*(1–2), 19–25.

Kuyper, L., & Fokkema, T. (2009). Loneliness among older lesbian, gay, and bisexual adults: The role of minority stress. *Archives of Sexual Behavior, 39*(5), 1170–1180.

Laumann, E. O., Das, A., & Waite, L. J. (2008). Sexual dysfunction among older adults: Prevalence and risk factors from a nationally representative U.S. probability sample of men and women 57–85 years of age. *Journal of Sexual Medicine, 5*(10), 2300–2311.

Lindau, S. T., Schumm, L. P., Laumann, E. O., Levinson, W., O'Mircheartaigh, C. A., & Waite, L. J. (2007). A study of sexuality and health among older adults in the United States. *New England Journal of Medicine, 357*(8), 762–774.

Luoto, R. (2009). Hot flushes and quality of life during menopause. *BMC Women's Health, 9*, 13, doi:10.1186/1472–6878-9–13.

Martin, C. P., Fain, M. J., & Klotz, S. A. (2008). The older HIV-positive adult: A critical review of the medical literature. *The American Journal of Medicine, 121*, 1032–1037.

Masters, W. H., & Johnson, V. E. (1966). *Human sexual response*. Boston, MA: Little Brown.

Mimoun, S., & Wylie, K. (2009). Female sexual dysfunctions: Definitions and classification. *Maturitas, 63*, 116–118.

Morales, A. M., Mirone, V., Dean, J., & Costa, P. (2009). Vardenafil for the treatment of erectile dysfunction: An overview of the clinical evidence. *Clinical Interventions in Aging, 4*, 463–472.

Mosack, V., & Steinke, E. (2009). Trends in sexual concerns after myocardial infarction. *Journal of Cardiovascular Nursing, 24*(2), 162–170.

Myers, A., & Barrueto, F. (2009). Refractory priapism associated with ingestion of yohimbe extract. *Journal of Medical Toxicology, 5*(4), 223–225.

NANDA International. (2009). *Nursing diagnoses: Definitions and classification 2009–2011*. Oxford, UK: Wiley-Blackwell.

Nehra, A. (2009). Erectile dysfunction and cardiovascular disease: Efficacy and safety of phosphodiesterase type 5 inhibitors in men with both conditions. *Mayo Clinic Proceedings, 84*(2), 139–148.

Nguyen, N., & Holodniy, M. (2008). HIV infection in the elderly. *Clinical Interventions in Aging, 3*(3), 453–472.

North American Menopause Society. (2008). Position Statement: Estrogen and progestogen use in postmenopausal women: July 2008 position statement of The North American Menopause Society. *Menopause: The Journal of the North American Menopause Society, 15*(4), 584–603.

Orwoll, E., Lambert, L. C., Marshall, L. M., Blank, J., Barrett-Connor, E., Cauley, J., . . . Steve Cummings for the Osteoporotic Fractures in Men Study Group. (2006). Testosterone and estradiol among older men. *Journal of Clinical Endocrinology and Metabolism, 91*, 1336–1344.

Palacios, S., Castano, R., & Grazziotin, A. (2009). Epidemiology of female sexual dysfunction. *Maturitas, 63*, 119–123.

Reyes, J. A. (2009). Lower urinary tract symptoms and sexual function: A current concern for Asian men's health. *Journal of Men's Health, 6*(1), 14–19.

Rosen, R. C., Wei, J. T., Althof, S. E., Seftel, A. D., Miner, M., & Perelman, M. A. (2009). Association of sexual dysfunction with lower urinary tract symptoms of BPH and BPH medical therapies: Results from the BPH registry. *Urology, 73*, 562–566.

Rosing, D., Klebingat, K-J., Berberich, H. J., Bosinski, H. A. G., Loewit, K., & Beier, K. M. (2009). Male sexual dysfunction. *Deutsches Arzteblatt International, 106*(50), 821–828. doi:10.3238/arztebl.2009.0821.

Sammel, M. D., Freeman, E. W., Liu, Z., & Guo, W. (2009). Factors that influence entry into stages of the menopausal transition. *Menopause, 16*(6), 1218–1227.

Sanders, G. D., Bayoumin, A. M., Holodniy, M., & Owens, D. K. (2008). Cost-effectiveness of HIV screening in patients older than 55 years of age. *Annuals of Internal Medicine, 148*(12), 889–903.

Slag, M., Morley, J. E., Elson, M. K., Trence, D. L., Nelson, C. J., Nelson, A. E., . . . Shafer, R. B. (1983). Impotence in medical clinic patients. *Journal of the American Medical Association, 249*, 1736–1740.

Snodgrass, A. J., Campbell, H. M., Mace, D. L., Faria, V. L., Swanson, K. M., & Holodniy, M. (2010). Sudden sensorineural hearing loss associated with vardenafil. *Pharmacotherapy, 30*(1), 112.

Steinke, E. E. (2010). Sexual dysfunction in women with cardiovascular disease: What do we know? *Journal of Cardiovascular Nursing, 25*(2), 151–158.

Steinke, E. E., Mosack, V., Wright, D. W., Chung, M. L., & Moser, D. K. (2009). Risk factors as predictors of sexual activity in heart failure. *Dimensions in Critical Care Nursing, 28*(3), 123–131.

Studd, J., & Schwenkhagen, A. (2009). The historical response to female sexuality. *Maturitas, 63*, 107–111.

Tamler, R. (2009). Diabetes, obesity, and erectile dysfunction. *Gender Medicine, 6*(Suppl 1), 4–16.

Tsertsvadze, A., Fink, H. A., Yazdi, F., MacDonald, R., Bella, A. J., Ansari, M. T., . . . Wilt, T. J. (2009). Oral phosphodiesterase-5 inhibitors and hormonal treatments for erectile dysfunction: A systematic review and meta-analysis. *Annals of Internal Medicine, 151*(9), 650–661.

Tzeng, Y. L., Lin, L. C., Shyr, Y. I., & Wen, J. K. (2009). Sexual behavior of institutionalized residents with dementia–A qualitative study. *Journal of Clinical Nursing, 18*(7), 991–1001.

Vance, D. E. (2010). Aging with HIV: Clinical considerations for an emerging population. *American Journal of Nursing, 110*(3), 42–47.

Vance, D. E., Childs, G., Moneyham, L., & McKie-Bell, P. (2009). Successful aging with HIV: A brief overview for nursing. *Journal of Gerontological Nursing, 35*(9), 19–25.

Vance, D. E., Struzick, T., & Burrage, J. (2009). Suicidal ideation, hardiness, and successful aging with HIV. *Journal of Gerontological Nursing, 35*(5), 27–32.

Veronelli, A., Mauri, C., Zecchini, B., Peca, M. G., Turri, O, Valitutti, M. T., . . . Pontiroli, A. E. (2009). Sexual dysfunction is frequent in premenopausal women with diabetes, obesity, and hypothyroidism, and correlates with markers of increased cardiovascular risk. A preliminary report. *The Journal of Sexual Medicine 6*(6), 1561–1568.

Wallace, M. A. (2008) Assessment of sexual health in older adults: Using the PLISSIT model to talk about sex, *How to Try This,* article and video: *American Journal of Nursing, 108*(7), 52–60.

Wallace, M., & Safer, M. (2009). Hypersexuality among cognitively impaired older adults. *Geriatric Nursing, 30*(4), 230–236.

Wang, C., Nieschlag, E., Swerdloff, R., Behre, H. M., Hellstrom, W. J., Gooren, L. J., . . . Wu, F. C. W. (2009). Investigation, treatment, and monitoring of late-onset hypogonadism in males. *Journal of Andrology, 30*(1), 1–6.

Weismiller, D. G. (2009). Menopause. *Primary Care Clinics in Office Practice, 36*, 199–226.

Wentzell, E., & Salmeron, J. (2009). Prevalence of erectile dysfunction and its treatment in a Mexican population: Distinguishing between erectile function and change and dysfunction. *Journal of Mental Health, 6*(1), 56–62.

Wylie, K., & Kenney, G. (2010). Sexual dysfunction and the ageing male. *Maturitas, 65*, 23–27.

Wylie, K., & Mimoun, S. (2009). Sexual response models in women. *Maturitas, 63*, 112–115.

PART 5

Promoting Wellness in All Stages of Health and Illness

CHAPTER 27

Caring for Older Adults During Illness

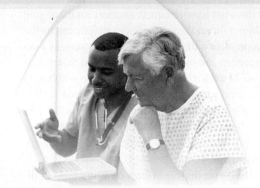

LEARNING OBJECTIVES

After reading this chapter, you will be able to:

1. Describe characteristics of illness in older adults.

2. Discuss the role of nurses in promoting wellness in older adults who are ill.

3. Describe the palliative care model for addressing the needs of older adults during illness.

4. Apply wellness concepts to nursing care of older adults who have cancer, diabetes, or heart failure.

5. Describe the role of nurses in holistically addressing needs of families and caregivers.

KEY POINTS

caregiver burden

caregiver well-being

palliative care

Several factors differentiate care of older adults from that of other populations and add to the challenge of promoting wellness. Foremost among these is the reality that most older adults—and all of those whom nurses care for in acute and long-term care settings—are coping with several or even many pathologic conditions that threaten their wellness. Despite pathologic conditions, however, nurses can identify numerous opportunities to promote wellness, especially by addressing the whole person instead of focusing only on physiologic processes. This chapter discusses a philosophy of holistic care that is applicable for older adults who have chronic or progressively declining conditions. Concepts are applied to nursing care for older adults who have cancer, diabetes, and heart failure.

CHARACTERISTICS OF ILLNESS IN OLDER ADULTS

Older adults commonly have one or more chronic conditions that gradually accumulate and affect their daily functioning and quality of life. Consequently, they typically receive health care on a continuing basis for chronic conditions and periodically for acute episodes. Even when acute conditions are the focus of care, interplay between chronic conditions and one or more acute conditions is likely to affect care. Thus, the health of older adults often fluctuates unpredictably and is usually affected by multiple interacting conditions. When nurses care for older adults who are experiencing illness, then, they address not only the acute conditions but also the interaction among acute and chronic conditions.

In addition to having more chronic conditions, older adults are more likely than their younger counterparts to have serious pathologic conditions (e.g., cancer) and neurodegenerative conditions (e.g., dementia) that seriously compromise their health. The conditions most prevalent among older adults are musculoskeletal conditions, stroke, hypertension, cardiovascular disease, cancer, dementia, diabetes, lung conditions, and hearing and vision impairments. They are also more likely to experience adverse effects from the medications they take for these conditions, as discussed in Chapter 8.

Consequences of illness in older adults may be far reaching and likely to affect both functioning and quality of life.

For example, older adults with heart failure are typically hospitalized when their condition becomes unstable and they are likely to be discharged to skilled care facilities for ongoing care before returning to independent living. These intermittent periods of care in institutional settings are likely to interfere with the person's ability to function independently. Eventually, they can lead to long-term placement in an assisted living or other type of nursing facility, particularly if the older adult does not have adequate support for managing the condition at home. In addition, an illness that threatens the older adult's independence in this way may have serious psychosocial consequences. For example, in the United States, fear of being "put away" in a nursing home is a common—although often unfounded—worry among older people. Because of this anxiety, older people may deny symptoms of illness for fear that the solution will result in a loss of independence; they also may avoid the health care system and experience unnecessary anxiety about minor or treatable illnesses.

The combined and cumulative effects of aging (which diminish physiologic reserves) and disease (which place additional physiologic demands on the person) make it more difficult for older adults to adapt to acute and chronic illnesses. The cumulative effects of all these intermittent and interacting forces can lead to a "yo-yoing" effect: the person experiences a cycle of ups and downs in health, with the "yo-yo" failing to return to the height of its previous cycle. With diminishing resiliency during subsequent cycles, the yo-yo eventually loses its ability to bounce back. Promoting wellness involves holistically addressing the changing needs of older adults as they progress through these cycles of ups and downs. Thus, when nurses care for older adults, they typically address several nursing diagnoses simultaneously, reassessing the situation frequently so that they can modify their goals accordingly. When nurses care for older adults holistically, they should be able to identify at least one wellness outcome in every situation.

✚ Wellness Opportunity

By attending to the body–mind–spirit interconnectedness of older adults, nurses can identify opportunities to provide physical comfort and support emotional and spiritual growth even in situations involving inevitable physical decline.

CONNECTING THE CONCEPTS OF WELLNESS, AGING, AND ILLNESS

Although the concepts of wellness and aging may seem almost contradictory, it is relatively easy to apply wellness to older adults who are healthy, functional, and satisfied with their lives. The greater challenge is to apply the concept of wellness to the nursing care of people who not only are in their 80s, 90s, or even older but are seriously ill or dying. It is necessary in these circumstances to emphasize that wellness applies to the broader context of the body–mind–spirit interrelationship

A Student's Perspective

I learned a lot from my interview this past week. The woman I spoke with has gone through a lot of hardships in her life—and is still going through hardships—but she continues to move forward despite setbacks. She is suffering from physical ailments, but her faith in God keeps her head above water. This woman was open to questioning and insightful with her answers. For being a quiet woman, she has a lot of inner strength she pulls on.

For a while after she was diagnosed with multiple sclerosis, she suffered depression and lost five dress sizes unintentionally. She also became fatigued and withdrawn. This was in line with how it has been shown that physical ailments can cause stress in a person, and that this in turn can cause other physical ailments. She was fortunate (if it can be called so) to be able to lose the amount of weight that she did and not have severe consequences. If this were to happen to someone of lesser weight, the results may have been more serious. This is a first-hand experience of how depression can cause more than just sad feelings as effects. Once she accepted her fate, she gained back two dress sizes and is holding there, which she is content with.

Her daughter has also been diagnosed with multiple sclerosis, which is a blessing and burden at the same time. Her daughter has been diagnosed at a much younger age and has more serious problems with it, causing her to be periodically hospitalized. It is difficult for a mother to watch her daughter go through this, but it's a blessing that she has someone to share the experience with.

As stated earlier, her faith in God keeps her head above water. She still has her bouts with frustration, but she believes that God only gives what we can handle and that He is always there for her. Her strength is encouraging to the people around her. I know it has given me strength.

Anita M.

as well as one's relationships with self, others, and all that is sacred to the individual. When caring for older adults who are ill, nurses have unique opportunities to promote wellness by addressing needs related not only to physical comfort, health, and function but also to emotional comfort and spiritual well-being. For example, nurses can promote wellness during illness through nursing actions such as the following:

- Helping older adults identify personal strengths that are not dependent on their physical health and functioning (e.g., emotional, interpersonal, and spiritual qualities), then identifying strategies that build on or improve these personal characteristics
- Supporting and promoting interpersonal relationships, including the development of new relationships and support resources, that can improve the older adult's health, functioning, and quality of life
- Helping older adults identify realistic goals for quality of life, which can be identified in any situation when wellness is conceptualized in the context of the body–mind–spirit interrelationship
- Facilitating the use of new resources and strengthening the support resources that already are in place for older adults, their families, and caregivers

- Identifying ways of supporting wellness for families and caregivers of dependent older adults.

Personal responsibility for health is an important aspect of wellness for older adults because self-care is essential for achieving optimal health in people who have chronic illnesses. Nurses can help older adults identify ways to assume personal responsibility for their health, even when they are dependent on others for their care. Recent studies emphasize the importance of addressing the decision-making process—as it is influenced by the patient's experiences, values, culture, and other factors—as an integral component of self-care (Song, 2010). Because personal responsibility for health—with regard to both general wellness and specific chronic conditions—often requires that a person address health-related behaviors, nurses can apply principles of behavior change as discussed in Chapter 5. Health promotion programs based on positive approaches, such as motivational interviewing or gain framing, may be particularly effective for older adults with diabetes or heart failure (Mayer et al., 2010; Miller, 2010; Paradis et al., 2010). An important outcome of educational interventions is improved self-efficacy, which is strongly associated with improved self-care health behaviors (Yehle & Plake, 2010).

Health promotion is an important aspect of wellness that should not be overlooked in the care of older adults suffering from illness. Unfortunately, ageist attitudes of health professionals, older adults, and family members can create barriers to health promotion. For example, ageist attitudes contribute to the low rate of cancer screening and other age-based disparities in cancer care for older adults (Kagan, 2008). Although health care professionals may believe that there is little or no benefit from improving health behaviors in later life, studies have debunked many of the myths that influence these ageist attitudes (Ferraro, 2006). Nurses and other health care professionals must be careful not to be influenced by ageist attitudes that would suggest that older adults are too old to learn or change behaviors or too old to benefit from improved health behaviors.

Even when illnesses compromise the health, functioning, and quality of life of older adults, nurses can usually identify wellness-oriented outcomes and interventions if they use a holistic perspective. For example, older adults who have difficulty engaging in the usual "land-based" types of exercise may be able to participate in aquatic exercise programs, which are increasingly available as out-patient therapies (Norton & Jamison, 2010). Studies found that aqua therapy programs improve health outcomes and quality of life for people with osteoarthritis, cardiopulmonary conditions, balance dysfunction, and lymphedema related to breast cancer (Ambroza & Geigle, 2010; Gulick, 2010; Morris, 2010; Tilden, Reicherter, & Reicherter, 2010). Table 27-1 lists examples of Nursing Outcomes Classification (NOC) and Nursing Interventions Classification (NIC) labels that are applicable to addressing psychosocial, comfort, health promotion, and spiritual needs. Nurses can incorporate these outcomes and interventions into care plans in conjunction with addressing the needs that are directly related to the primary health conditions.

HOLISTICALLY CARING FOR OLDER ADULTS WHO ARE ILL: FOCUSING ON CARING AND COMFORTING

Care and comfort are core components of all nursing, but they become even more important when a cure is not feasible. Equating aging with inability to cure is not only inaccurate but also a great disservice to older adults. However, it also is

TABLE 27-1 Nursing Outcomes and Nursing Interventions Classifications for Promoting Wellness in Older Adults During Illness

Type of Needs	Nursing Outcomes Classification (NOC)	Nursing Interventions Classification (NIC)
Psychosocial needs	Anxiety Level, Coping, Decision Making, Fear Level, Participation in Health Care Decisions, Personal Autonomy, Personal Well-Being, Self-Direction of Care, Self-Esteem, Social Involvement, Stress Level, Suffering Severity	Anxiety Reduction, Counseling, Coping Enhancement, Decision-Making Support, Emotional Support, Patient Rights Protection, Resiliency Promotion, Support Group, Simple Guided Imagery, Touch
Comfort needs	Comfort Level, Pain Control, Pain: Disruptive Effects, Sleep, Symptom Control, Thermoregulation	Pain Management, Positioning, Simple Massage, Temperature Regulation, Therapeutic Touch
Health promotion needs	Fall Prevention Behavior; Health Promoting Behavior; Immunization Behavior; Knowledge: Diet, Disease Process, Health Behavior, Health Resources, Illness Care, Medication; Nutritional Status; Physical Fitness; Risk Control; Risk Detection; Self-Care Status; Safe Home Environment	Anticipatory Guidance, Environmental Management: Comfort/Safety, Exercise Promotion, Fall Prevention, Health Education, Immunization Management, Nutrition Management, Risk Identification, Self-Responsibility Facilitation, Simple Relaxation Therapy, Skin Surveillance, Sleep Enhancement, Surveillance: Safety
Spiritual needs	Hope, Spiritual Health	Active Listening, Forgiveness Facilitation, Guilt Work Facilitation, Hope Instillation, Presence, Reminiscence Therapy, Religious Ritual Enhancement, Self-Awareness Enhancement, Spiritual Growth Facilitation, Spiritual Support
Quality-of-life needs	Leisure Participation, Personal Well-Being, Quality of Life	Animal-Assisted Therapy, Aromatherapy, Family Involvement Promotion, Humor, Music Therapy

a disservice to older adults to focus only on curing disease when they reach the point at which treatments are more detrimental than the underlying conditions. Moreover, because of the complexity of illness in older adults, the "turning point" when the focus changes from cure to care is rarely clearly defined. Thus, geriatricians, gerontologists, ethicists, and gerontological nurses increasingly are trying to identify ways to improve quality of life for people whose quantity of life is limited.

The emergence of **palliative care** programs in recent years provides a framework for promoting wellness during serious illness, and this model is increasingly used to address the complex and cumulative effects of conditions for which there is no cure. The World Health Organization (2002) and the National Consensus Project for Quality Palliative Care (2009) describe the following aspects of palliative care:

- Recipients of care are patients and their families facing problems associated with a broad range of persistent, life-threatening, or recurring conditions that adversely affect their daily functioning or will predictably reduce life expectancy.
- Goals are to prevent and relieve suffering, enhance quality of life, optimize function, assist with decision making, and provide opportunities for personal growth.
- Palliative care is applicable early in the course of an illness and should be offered as needs develop and before they become unmanageable.
- Palliative care can be provided concurrently with life-prolonging therapies or as a main focus of care.
- Palliative care is both a philosophy of care and an organized system for delivering comprehensive care.

Hospice services (discussed in Chapter 29) include palliative care, but the programs differ in that entry into hospice requires that the patient be in a terminal state, whereas palliative care services can be provided at any point during the course of a chronic declining condition. Palliative care can be provided in any setting, including acute-care, long-term care, and home settings.

Palliative care models are particularly applicable to holistically addressing the needs of older adults because of the emphasis on quality of life during serious illness. These models promote wellness for older adults by focusing on respect for the individual, sharing caring moments, allowing older adults to direct their own care, and honoring the intrinsic worth and uniqueness of each person (Mahler, 2010). For example, early in the process of providing palliative care for people with dementia, information about the individual's physical, psychological, social, and spiritual background is compiled in a biosketch and incorporated into the care plan so that care can be individualized (Long, 2009).

Some characteristics of palliative care programs that are particularly pertinent to promoting wellness in older adults include the following:

- A primary focus on ensuring comfort and psychosocial and spiritual well-being

- Comprehensive management of distressing symptoms
- Education and support of families and all support people (e.g., friends, volunteers, significant others)
- Consultation, education, and support of professional caregivers (e.g., nurses, nursing assistants, primary care providers)

A study of palliative care for patients in intensive care units found that two key components were assurance of comfort and attention to dignity and personhood (Nelson et al., 2010).

Nurses have an important responsibility to recognize the appropriateness of a referral for palliative care and to initiate discussion of this option with older adults and their families. Studies indicate that lack of knowledge by patients and health care providers is a major barrier to obtaining palliative care services (Melvin, 2010; Melvin & Oldham, 2010). When discussing palliative care services with older adults or their families, nurses can emphasize that although these services are usually provided with hospice programs, palliative care focuses on managing symptoms rather than on care of dying. Information about appropriate referrals and palliative care services is available from the National Hospice and Palliative Care Organization and other organizations listed in the Resources section at the end of this chapter.

APPLYING WELLNESS CONCEPTS IN SPECIFIC PATHOLOGIC OR CHRONIC CONDITIONS

All clinically oriented chapters in this text identify opportunities for nurses to promote wellness in relation to usual aspects of functioning and some common chronic conditions of older adults. Although it is beyond the scope of this book to address pathophysiologic conditions in depth, the next sections highlight some considerations that are more specific to promoting wellness in older adults who have cancer, diabetes, or heart failure. These three conditions are selected as examples and are discussed within the framework of the Functional Consequences Theory to illustrate the application of wellness concepts to care of older adults who are ill.

Promoting Wellness for Older Adults With Cancer

Because cancer is a condition that requires the passage of time before it reaches the stage of being a diagnosable disease, an increased risk of cancer is an unavoidable consequence of aging (White & Cohen, 2008). Thus, the risk of cancer in older adults is about 10 times that of younger adults and about 60% of all newly diagnosed cancers and 70% of all cancer diagnoses occur in people 65 years of age and older (Bond, 2010; Rottenberg et al., 2009). Breast, colon, and prostate cancers occur with increased incidence in older adults (White & Cohen, 2008). Compared with younger adults, those 65 years of age and older are less likely to be screened for cancer and are diagnosed at a later stage (Oncology Nursing Society and Geriatric Oncology Consortium,

2007). Despite the fact that increasing age is a major risk factor for breast cancer, older patients are less likely to be screened and are more likely to present with larger and more advanced tumors and greater lymph node involvement (Petrakis & Paraskakis, 2009).

Cancer is an important focus of health promotion efforts because approximately two-thirds of cancer deaths are from potentially preventable causes (Molokhia & Perkins, 2008). In addition, cancer is one of the most correctable sources of disparities among minority elders who have excess morbidity and mortality in all phases (i.e., screening or diagnostic, treatment, and postcancer survival) (DeLancey, Thun, Jemal, & Ward, 2008). Thus, nurses have important health promotion roles particularly in teaching about cancer prevention and early detection.

Although cancer is highly prevalent among older adults, research, education, treatment, and public policy are limited, so there is a scarcity of evidence-based data specific to the older adult population (Oncology Nursing Society and Geriatric Oncology Consortium, 2007). This lack of data may be the result of ageist beliefs that older adults will not respond to treatment or health education. In addition, older adults themselves are likely to be influenced by their own misperceptions based on outdated beliefs. For example, they may have anxieties and fears based on inaccurate or outdated perceptions of a diagnosis of cancer being a "death sentence." Myths and ageist attitudes also can interfere with symptom management, especially with pain management (see Chapter 28).

Care of older adults with cancer is complicated not only by the pathologic processes of cancer itself but also by the many interacting conditions that can complicate their responses to treatments. Thus, decisions about screening and treatment of cancer are more complex and need to be based not on chronologic age alone but on a multidimensional assessment that considers all the following: effects of normal age-related changes, physical and psychosocial health and functioning, effects of accumulated chronic conditions, life expectancy, potential benefits versus harms, and the individual's values and preferences (White & Cohen, 2008).

Decisions about screening and treatment of cancer in older adults can be complicated for several reasons. When older adults have pathophysiologic conditions that compromise cognitive abilities, these decisions must be made by health care proxies. Although this holds true for many situations with older adults, it is particularly problematic when older adults have cancer because evidence-based guidelines for screening or treatment are often lacking. Treatment-related decisions are also complicated by medical conditions that affect the older adult's ability to tolerate treatments. In addition, older adults are less likely to have family and caregiver supports to assist with complex treatment regimens (e.g., transportation for radiation, assistance with dealing with chemotherapy treatments and effects), and this may affect treatment decisions.

Nursing Assessment

From a health promotion perspective, nurses assess older adults to identify their knowledge and attitudes about screening for the types of cancer most likely to develop. For example, skin cancer is one of the most commonly occurring types, and it can be readily detected through self-examination. Thus, nurses can assess whether older adults understand how important it is to check for skin cancer and what they need to look for (as discussed in Chapter 23). Nurses also assess level of knowledge about prevention of cancer because this provides a base for identifying health promotion goals. When caring for an older adult who has cancer, nurses holistically assess psychosocial aspects such as the meaning of cancer for the individual, coping strengths and supports, and the person's ability to participate in decisions about screening and care.

Wellness Nursing Diagnoses and Wellness Outcomes

Readiness for Enhanced Knowledge is a wellness nursing diagnosis applicable for older adults who are interested in learning about screening and prevention of cancer. This diagnosis would also be applicable if the person is interested in learning more about holistically oriented resources such as hospice services (discussed in Chapter 29). The wellness nursing diagnosis of Readiness for Enhanced Self-Care would be applicable for increasing personal responsibility for older adults who have cancer. For example, this would be particularly applicable with regard to complex decision making regarding cancer treatment.

Two outcomes applicable to prevention and early detection of cancer are Health Promoting Behavior and Knowledge: Health Behavior. Outcomes that are pertinent to holistically caring for older adults with cancer include Comfort, Coping, and Quality of Life.

Nursing Interventions

Health promotion interventions focus on teaching older adults about primary prevention and early detection of cancer through screening, as summarized in Box 27-1. Nurses can encourage older adults and surrogate decision makers to discuss cancer detection and treatment options with their primary care providers with an emphasis on quality of life.

For older adults already diagnosed with cancer, nurses address all aspects of pain and comfort (see Chapter 28). Also, because people with cancer commonly use complementary and alternative therapies, nurses can teach them to obtain information from reliable sources (e.g., the National Cancer Institute and the National Center for Complementary and Alternative Medicine).

In addition, nurses can use evidence-based information to teach about self-care practices that may be effective in alleviating some of the symptoms and discomforts associated with cancer and cancer treatments. For example, studies show that guided imagery—one of the most commonly

Box 27-1 Health Promotion Interventions Related to Cancer and Older Adults

Teaching About Primary Prevention
- Stop smoking (if applicable)
- Avoid secondhand smoke
- Maintain ideal body weight
- Consume at least five servings of fresh fruit and vegetables and 25–30 g of fiber daily
- Limit intake of fats, red meats, and fried foods
- Avoid excessive exposure to sunlight
- Avoid excessive alcohol consumption

Screening Recommendations of the American Cancer Society for Older Adults
- Annual fecal occult blood test
- Flexible sigmoidoscopy and double contrast barium enema every 5 years, OR colonoscopy every 10 years
- Annual prostate-specific antigen and digital rectal examination for men
- Annual mammogram, and Pap test every 2–3 years for women
- Annual checkup by primary care practitioner to examine skin, thyroid, oral cavity, breasts, ovaries, and testicles

recommended integrative therapies for people with cancer— is most effective for psychosocial and quality-of-life indicators, such as anxiety and depression (Fitzgerald & Langevin, 2010). Studies also support the benefits of yoga and meditation for people with cancer (Cameron, 2010; Kreitzer & Reilly-Spong, 2010).

Nurses also need to address the need for information about the disease and treatments. Health education for older cancer patients needs be tailored to the identified and individualized needs. Exploring personal treatment goals is important because older cancer patients may be less willing than younger ones to trade increased survival for their quality of life when considering chemotherapy (Posma, van Weert, Jansen, & Bensing, 2009). Additional wellness-oriented nursing interventions include offering hope, support, and encouragement and considering referrals for hospice and palliative care. Nurses can find additional information about cancer in older adults through the Oncology Nursing Society and Geriatric Consortium and the Hospice and Palliative Care Nurses Association.

Wellness Opportunity

Nurses can promote personal responsibility for wellness by teaching older adults about screening and preventive actions they can take.

Promoting Wellness for Older Adults With Diabetes Mellitus

Diabetes mellitus is one of the most common chronic conditions in older adults, and it affects almost 25% of people aged 60 years and older (Centers for Disease Control and Prevention,

2008). Age-related changes that increase the risk for development of diabetes include declining beta cell function and increased insulin resistance (glucose intolerance). In addition to age-related changes, risk factors for diabetes include obesity, hypertension, family history, physical inactivity, high levels of triglycerides, and low levels of high-density lipoproteins.

DIVERSITY NOTE

Age-adjusted rates of diagnosed diabetes by race: Native American and Alaskan Natives, 16.5%; blacks, 11.8%; Hispanics, 10.4%; Asian Americans, 7.5%; and whites, 6.6% (Centers for Disease Control and Prevention, 2008).

Disease management and nursing care related to diabetes are complicated by the common occurrence of concomitant conditions in older adults. For example, infections can affect the optimal doses of insulin and hypoglycemic agents, and chronic arthritis or periodic flare-ups of gout are likely to affect the older adult's level of activity. Another complicating factor is that older adults are likely to be taking medications that can lead to disease instability. For example, older adults are likely to have acute or chronic conditions that require treatment with prednisone, which, in turn, affects control of blood glucose. Conditions that occur more commonly in older adults such as dementia, depression, and functional limitations can interfere with self-management of diabetes, as can dependence on others who interfere with meals or financial constraints that affect ability to purchase medications and appropriate foods. Diabetes is a well-recognized risk factor for renal failure, retinopathy, neuropathy, and cardiovascular diseases (including stroke, hypertension, myocardial infarction, and coronary artery disease). These conditions contribute to the significantly increased morbidity associated with diabetes (Grady, Entin, Entin, & Brunye, 2009). In addition, studies indicate that diabetes is a risk factor for cognitive decline, impaired myocardial function, depression, and lumbar spinal stenosis (Andersson et al., 2010; Anekstein et al., 2010; Lin et al., 2009; Maggi et al., 2009).

Nursing Assessment

Although nurses are not expected to diagnose diabetes, they are expected to know about variations in diagnostic indicators that are specific to older adults. For example, the renal threshold for glucose increases in older adults, so glycosuria may not be an accurate indicator. The American Diabetes Association (2010) states that any one of the following four conditions is diagnostic indicator for diabetes:

- Glycosylated hemoglobin (HbA$_{1c}$) $\geq$6.5%
- Fasting blood glucose $\geq$126/dl (8-hour fast)
- Symptoms of hyperglycemia (e.g., polyuria, polydipsia, weight loss) and a random (i.e., anytime during the day) blood glucose $\geq$200 mg/dl
- 2-hour blood glucose value during oral glucose tolerance test $\geq$200 mg/dL with glucose load of 75 g

Box 27-2 Assessment Guidelines for Older Adults With Diabetes

Considerations About the Meaning of Diabetes
- What terminology is appropriate for discussing the condition (e.g., older adults may refer to diabetes as "sugar")?
- What is the person's understanding of diabetes?

Considerations for Disease Management
- What is the person's understanding of personal responsibility for managing diabetes?
- Socioeconomic influences: Who does grocery shopping and meal preparation? What foods are included in the usual meal pattern? What is the usual "budget" for food? Where does the person eat meals?
- What cultural factors affect health beliefs, disease management, food preparation, eating patterns, and health-related behaviors, such as exercise?
- What concomitant conditions affect the older adult's self-care abilities?

Considerations Regarding the Influence of Ageist Attitudes
- Do ageist attitudes (of the older adult, caregiver, or health care professionals) interfere with setting wellness-oriented goals? (e.g., "I've been eating donuts for breakfast all my life, why should I worry about that now at my age?")
- Does the older adult (or do others) inaccurately associate a sense of hopelessness with his or her condition because of advanced age? (e.g., "At my age, I can't do anything about my sugar levels.")

The HbA$_{1c}$ is routinely used to monitor glucose control in people with diabetes over the previous months, with the target goal being a level less than 7% to reduce microvascular and neuropathic complications.

In addition to the usual nursing assessment parameters for diabetes, a holistic nursing approach for older adults addresses issues, such as the meaning of the condition to the person, identification of ageist attitudes that may affect management, and socioeconomic and cultural influences. Box 27-2 summarizes some questions that are more specific to assessment of diabetes in older adults from a wellness perspective.

Wellness Nursing Diagnoses and Wellness Outcomes

Readiness for Enhanced Knowledge is a wellness nursing diagnosis applicable for older adults who are interested in learning about diabetes, particularly with regard to improved understanding of how this condition affects their health. Nurses can use the wellness nursing diagnosis of Readiness for Enhanced Self-Care when they care for older adults who are interested in improving personal responsibility for management of their condition, including preventing complications.

Outcomes that would be pertinent to promoting wellness in older adults with diabetes include Diabetes Self-Management, Blood Glucose Level, Health Promoting Behavior, Knowledge: Diabetes Management, and Self-Care Status.

Nursing Interventions

Care plans for older adult with diabetes include all the usual interventions that apply to all adults with diabetes (e.g., teaching about nutrition, exercise, medications, glucose monitoring, and other aspects of self-care). Teaching about self-management with a focus on lifestyle—diet, physical activity, weight management, and smoking cessation—is widely recognized as the cornerstone of diabetes care and prevention of complications. Research indicates that improved health behavior for middle-aged and older adults was associated with a decrease in HbA$_{1c}$ levels of 0.6% to 1% (Chiu & Wray, 2010; Ripsin, Kang, & Urban, 2009). In addition to teaching about lifestyle interventions, nurses should emphasize the importance of ophthalmologic care, podiatric care, prevention of injury, and observations of wound healing. Health education interventions need to address the needs of specific cultural groups because studies found that culturally relevant lifestyle interventions can improve diabetes-related behaviors and clinical outcomes (Castro et al., 2009). Nurses can use the resources listed in Chapter 5 to find culturally appropriate health education programs that are pertinent to older adults with diabetes.

Nurses may need to address factors that are more common among older adults, such as involving and teaching caregivers, compensating for memory deficits, and identifying the most cost-effective ways of obtaining medications and glucometer supplies. Older adults with diabetes may benefit from referrals for community-based services, including home-delivered meals, assistance with grocery shopping or meal preparation, participation in group meal programs, transportation to appointments, and assistance with medication management or glucose monitoring. Providing such services for an older adult with diabetes is often an essential element in ensuring optimal control and supporting the person's ability to remain in his or her own home.

Nurses also may need to address fear and anxiety in older adults and caregivers and to encourage discussion of feelings about diabetes and the impact of this chronic condition on the person's health and lifestyle. Nurses can help older adults identify safe and enjoyable ways of engaging in physical activity, especially if they have concomitant conditions that affect their ability to exercise. For example, swimming or aquatherapy classes may be more appropriate than walking for an older adult who has arthritis or problems with balance.

Wellness Opportunity

Nurses can teach all older adults about actions they can take to prevent diabetes by using resources, such as the tools adapted from the Diabetes Prevention Program, which are available from the National Diabetes Education Program at www.ndep.nih.gov.

Promoting Wellness for Older Adults With Heart Failure

Heart failure has the distinction of being the most common admission and readmission diagnosis for hospitalization in older adults in the United States and the most expensive medical condition (Hernandez et al., 2010). Moreover, as many as 57% of admissions are potentially preventable with adequate self-care, including medication adherence and monitoring of symptoms (Jurgens, Hoke, Byrnes, & Riegel, 2009). In addition to recurrent hospitalizations, other common consequences of heart failure in older adults include the following:

- Increased likelihood for developing arrhythmias, which can threaten life or cause syncopal episodes
- Increased risk for hypotension and falls because of compromised cardiovascular function and adverse medication effects
- Increased risk for hospital-acquired iatrogenic conditions, such as *Clostridium difficile* infection
- Increased risk for drug interactions and adverse medication effects, especially if the older adult has concomitant conditions and requires several types of medications
- High incidence of sleep disorders
- Shorter life expectancy

Because of consequences such as these—which make it a major source of chronic disability, increased mortality, and impaired quality of life—heart failure in older adults has emerged as a major focus of health promotion interventions.

DIVERSITY NOTE

Data analyses indicate that the percentage of risk associated with modifiable conditions—which could prevent heart failure—is 49% for whites and 68% for blacks (Kalogeropoulos et al., 2009).

Nursing Assessment

Nurses assess for signs and symptoms of heart failure in older adults using the same assessment techniques that apply to adults of any age. However, older adults are more likely to have concomitant conditions that can affect the assessment. For example, because older adults with mobility limitations may not exert themselves enough to experience dyspnea, nurses need to consider other limiting factors when they assess the effects of heart failure on respirations. Nurses need to ask very direct assessment questions about signs and symptoms because older adults have poor symptom recognition and are likely to attribute early symptoms, such as fatigue and shortness of breath, to normal aging (Riegel et al., 2010; Jurgens et al., 2009).

Another assessment consideration is that older adults with heart failure are likely to have some degree of chronic renal failure, which often fluctuates within an abnormal range. Thus, nurses need to identify and document the older adult's usual indicators of renal function (i.e., ranges of blood urea nitrogen and creatinine that are typical for that individual). Because older adults with heart failure and renal failure are at increased risk for electrolyte imbalance and adverse medication effects, nurses need to assess for these and other consequences. For example, hyperkalemia, which can be life-threatening in people with heart failure, can be caused by cardiovascular medications such as angiotensin-converting enzyme (ACE) inhibitors, angiotensin II receptor blockers, and aldosterone antagonists (Poggio, Grancelli, & Miriuka, 2010).

In addition to assessing signs and symptoms of heart failure, nurses assess risk factors, paying particular attention to those that can be addressed through health promotion interventions. Factors that increase the risk for heart failure include hypertension, coronary artery disease, myocardial infarction, family history of heart failure, hyperthyroidism, diabetes, smoking, and obesity. Even though older adults may have long-term patterns of behavior that affect disease management (e.g., smoking, inadequate physical activity, or high-sodium diets), nurses need to assess attitudes about changing these behaviors so that they can address this in health promotion teaching. Additional wellness-focused assessment considerations that are important for older adults who have heart failure are outlined in Box 27-3.

Wellness Nursing Diagnoses and Wellness Outcomes

Nurses can use the wellness nursing diagnosis of Readiness for Enhanced Therapeutic Regimen Management to promote increased personal responsibility for management of heart failure and prevention of hospitalizations and other complications. The wellness nursing diagnosis of Readiness for Enhanced Fluid Balance might be applicable when older adults with heart failure are interested in learning about actions they can take to improve and maintain fluid and electrolyte balance.

 Box 27-3 Assessment Guidelines for Older Adults With Heart Failure

Considerations About the Meaning of Heart Failure
- What is the older adult's understanding of heart failure?
- What terminology is appropriate for discussing the condition? Does the term *failure* cause anxiety or fear?
- What personal experiences or those of significant others are influencing the older adult's response to cardiovascular disease? (e.g., How life-threatening does the person perceive this to be?)

Considerations Regarding the Influence of Ageist Attitudes
- Do ageist attitudes interfere with health promotion interventions? (e.g., Do health care providers avoid teaching about smoking cessation because they think the person is too old to quit or to benefit from quitting?)

Considerations Regarding Disease Management
- Does the older adult have questions or fears about engaging in therapeutic or enjoyable activities (e.g., exercise, swimming, sexual relationships)? If so, would he or she benefit from health education about this?
- Do socioeconomic factors affect disease management (e.g., limited income that interferes with ability to purchase needed medications or healthy foods)?

Outcomes that are pertinent to promoting wellness in older adults with heart failure include Cardiac Disease Self-Management, Energy Conservation, Health Promoting Behavior, and Knowledge: Cardiac Disease Management.

Nursing Interventions

Wellness-oriented care plans for older adults with heart failure focus on teaching about actions the person can take to achieve the best possible level of functioning and quality of life despite the chronic condition. For example, nurses can teach older adults about planning appropriate rest and "energy management" techniques to achieve optimum quality of life with limited energy. A systematic review found that health education interventions provided by nurses were beneficial for secondary prevention in heart failure, with regard to lipids, blood pressure, weight loss, physical activity, dietary intake, cigarette smoking, psychosocial measures, quality of life, and mortality (Allen & Dennison, 2010). Teaching about symptom recognition is an important aspect of self-care because older adults may not associate signs and symptoms with heart failure. One study found that teaching older adults to keep a symptom diary, including documentation of daily body weights, can be helpful for symptom recognition and self-care (White, Howie-Esquivel, & Caldwell, 2010). From a holistic perspective, nurses also need to address psychosocial consequences associated with heart failure, such as fear, anxiety, loneliness, and depression (discussed in Chapters 12, 13, and 15).

In addition to providing the usual patient teaching about medications, nurses caring for older adults with heart failure must monitor for digoxin toxicity (because there is a very narrow therapeutic range) and provide patient education about drug interactions and the effect of drugs and other concomitant conditions. For example, nonsteroidal anti-inflammatory drugs, including over-the-counter ones, are associated with development of heart failure and can interfere with antihypertensives and ACE inhibitors. One study found that use of nonsteroidal anti-inflammatory agents is common among elderly heart failure patients and may lead to hospitalizations (Muzzarelli et al., 2009).

> **Wellness Opportunity**
>
> Because stress-reduction activities are especially important when older adults have chronic conditions, such as heart failure, nurses can suggest relaxation and health promotion activities such as deep breathing, meditation, and guided imagery.

ADDRESSING NEEDS OF FAMILIES AND CAREGIVERS

During periods of illness—whether acute, chronic, or declining—the importance of relationships increases in proportion to the need not only for physical care but also for emotional and spiritual care. Thus, when nurses care for older adults during illness, families and caregivers are an integral focus of care. Even with the increasing availability of formal services for older adults in the United States, families and friends continue to provide 80% to 90% of the care given to dependent older adults in the community. For older adults who have dementia or other conditions that cause progressive declines in functioning, the role of caregiver usually evolves gradually and can last for years. Even in situations in which older adults do not have progressively declining conditions, families of older adults frequently deal with intermittent and cumulative conditions that require intense medical care or rehabilitative services. It is not uncommon for families of older adults to take on roles of care managers and find themselves negotiating health care services for at least one and sometimes several parents, grandparents, aunts, uncles, and other relatives and "significant others."

The term **caregiver burden** is commonly used to describe the financial, physical, and psychosocial problems that family members experience when caring for older adults who are impaired or suffering from illness. Specific functional consequences associated with caregiver burden include depression; disturbed sleep; social isolation; family discord; career interruptions; financial difficulties; lack of time for self; poor physical health; psychological/emotional/mental strain; and feelings of anger, guilt, grief, anxiety, hopelessness, and helplessness. Some of the stressors that contribute to caregiver burden are multiple demands on the caregiver, lack of control over the situation, loss of social support, impairment of the care recipient, duration and intensity of care, dependency in activities of daily living, unpredictability and recurrence of illness, and problem behaviors of the care recipient (Coon & Evans, 2009; Tamayo, Broxson, Munsell, & Cohen, 2010).

Although most studies have focused on the burdens of caregiving, there is increasing recognition that **caregiver well-being** can be a positive consequence of caring for a dependent loved one. Positive outcomes identified in studies include personal growth, strengthening of relationships, feelings of satisfaction, and increased self-esteem (Winter, Bouldin, & Andresen, 2010). Caregivers are more likely to experience positive effects when they have more choice about the situation or when they perceive themselves as interdependent with the care receiver (e.g., as a spouse) (Poulin et al., 2010; Winter et al., 2010). One study found that a high proportion of caregivers of family members with dementia or stroke found satisfaction from promoting the care recipient's well-being and from experiencing a sense of fulfillment or personal achievement (Mayor, Ribeiro, & Paul, 2009). Cultural factors also significantly affect the experience of being a caregiver, as discussed in Chapter 1, especially with regard to societal perceptions of family roles and responsibilities. (see Cultural Considerations Box 1-1 in Chapter 1.)

Nurses address teaching needs of older adults' families, partners, and significant others as an essential nursing responsibility related to continuity of care for patients in all health care settings. Consistent with this responsibility,

TABLE 27-2 Nursing Outcomes and Nursing Interventions Classifications for Promoting Wellness in Caregivers

Type of Needs	Nursing Outcomes Classification (NOC)	Nursing Interventions Classification (NIC)
Needs related to caregiver role	Caregiver Adaptation to Patient Institutionalization, Caregiver Emotional Health, Caregiver Endurance Potential, Caregiver Home Care Readiness, Caregiver Lifestyle Disruption, Caregiver–Patient Relationship, Caregiver Performance: Direct/Indirect Care, Caregiver Physical Health, Caregiver Stressors, Caregiver Well-Being	Caregiver Support, Case Management, Counseling, Energy Management, Family Support, Family Integrity Promotion, Resiliency Promotion, Role Enhancement, Self-Awareness Enhancement, Support Group
Needs related to using resources and managing care	Information Processing, Knowledge: Health Resources, Participation in Health Care Decisions, Role Performance	Decision-Making Support, Health Education, Health System Guidance, Referral, Respite Care, Support System Enhancement, Teaching: Individual, Telephone Consultation
Psychosocial needs	Anxiety Level, Coping, Decision Making, Depression Level, Family Coping, Family Resiliency, Fear Level, Grief Resolution, Loneliness Severity, Self-Esteem, Stress Level	Active Listening, Anticipatory Guidance, Anxiety Reduction, Cognitive Restructuring, Coping Enhancement, Emotional Support, Grief Work Facilitation, Mood Management, Presence, Simple Guided Imagery
Spiritual and quality-of-life needs	Hope, Leisure Participation, Quality of Life, Sleep, Social Involvement, Social Support, Spiritual Health	Forgiveness Facilitation, Guilt Work Facilitation, Hope Instillation, Humor, Sleep Enhancement, Spiritual Support

nurses follow standards of care and document the teaching they provide regarding caregiving instructions, but they do not necessarily address the broader needs of caregivers because of barriers, such as time constraints and perception of this as a nonessential aspect of care. However, when nurses care for dependent older adults, it is important to recognize that even the basic needs of the older adult cannot be met without a strong support system. Thus, nurses need to identify outcomes and interventions to prevent caregiver burnout and enhance the ability of families and other caregivers to provide the necessary care. For example, studies found that skill-training interventions improved caregiver health and

quality of life (Coon & Evans, 2009; Elliott, Burgio, & DeCoster, 2010).

Interventions also need to focus on improving the function and well-being of the care recipient. A study found that the burden experienced by family caregivers of depressed older adults was alleviated after the care recipient was treated with antidepressants (Martire et al., 2010). As with all aspects of caring for older adults, there is great individual variation among families, caregivers, and care recipients, so there are many varied interventions to address caregiver issues. The Evidence-Based Practice Box 27-1 summarizes research findings related to interventions for family caregivers, and Table 27-2

Evidence-Based Practice 27-1

Family Caregiving

Statement of the Problem

- More than 80% of the care for dependent older adults is provided by family.
- Caregiving activities include assistance with daily activities, illness-related care (medication management, assessing and addressing symptoms, carrying out treatments), and care management activities (advocacy, accessing and coordinating services, navigating health care and social service systems).
- Caregivers typically experience higher levels of stress and depression and lower levels of physical health and subjective well-being.
- Increased caregiver strain is associated with lack of preparedness for the role, caring for someone with dementia, and poor quality relationships between care giver and care recipient.

Recommendations for Nursing Assessment

- Parameters of assessment: (1) caregiving context (e.g., roles and responsibilities, duration of caregiving, physical environment, financial status, potential resources, cultural factors); (2) caregiver's perception of health and functional status of care recipient (functional and cognitive limitations); (3) caregiver preparedness (skills, knowledge); (4) quality of relationship between caregiver and care recipient; (5) indicators of problems with care (unhealthy environment, inappropriate financial management); (6) caregiver's health status (self-rated health, physical and mental health, rewards of caregiving)

- Assessment tool: Caregiver Strain Index (Hartford Foundation for Geriatric Nursing)

Recommendations for Interventions

- Identify caregiver needs and address them through health education or referrals
- Assist in identifying strengths in the caregiving situation
- Help caregivers identify and manage their physical and emotional responses
- Psychoeducational skill building: education related to care recipient behavior management, management of caregiver depression and feelings (e.g., anger, frustration), problem solving, relaxation, "Coping with Caregiving" classes, support groups
- Psychotherapeutic counseling: cognitive behavioral therapy
- Multicomponent skill building: family therapy, individualized counseling and support

SOURCES: Messecar, D. C. (2008). Family caregiving. In E. Capezuti, D. Zwicker, M. Mezey, & T. Fulmer (Eds.), *Evidence-based geriatric nursing protocols for best practice* (3rd ed., pp. 127–160). New York: Springer Publishing Co.; Coon, D. W., & Evans, B. E. (2009). Empirically based treatments for family caregiver distress: What works and where do we go from here? *Geriatric Nursing, 30*, 426–436.

lists NOC and NIC terms that are applicable to promoting wellness for families and caregivers who are involved with care of ill or dependent older adults.

Chapter Highlights

Characteristics of Illness in Older Adults
- Presence of many interacting conditions and factors (e.g., acute illness, chronic conditions, psychosocial factors, environmental conditions, age-related changes, medication effects)
- Complexity of interpreting signs and symptoms (e.g., vague or atypical manifestations)
- Far-reaching consequences (e.g., loss of independence due to fractured hip)
- Cumulative effects of aging and illness making adaptation difficult
- Older adults likely experiencing a "yo-yoing" pattern of health, with gradually diminishing resiliency.

Connecting the Concepts of Wellness, Aging, and Illness
- A holistic perspective enables nurses to identify ways of promoting wellness by addressing needs related to physical health and functioning and emotional and spiritual well-being.
- An important aspect of wellness is promoting personal responsibility for health through self-care measures and management of chronic conditions.
- Nurses challenge ageist attitudes and provide health education to foster behavior change when appropriate.
- Many NIC and NOC terms are applicable in care plans that address psychosocial, comfort, health promotion, and spiritual needs (Table 27-1).

Holistically Caring for Older Adults Who Are Ill: Focusing on Caring and Comforting
- Palliative care is a holistic approach to caring for patients with advanced progressive illnesses through prevention, assessment, and treatment of pain and other physical, psychosocial, and spiritual problems.
- Nurses have important roles in suggesting referrals for palliative care and talking with older adults and their families about the scope of these services.

Promoting Wellness for Older Adults With Cancer
- Older adults are disproportionately affected by cancer, they are less likely to be screened for cancer, and they are diagnosed at a later stage.
- From a health promotion perspective, nurses assess older adults to identify their knowledge and attitudes about screening for the types of cancer that they are most likely to develop.
- Nurses holistically address the needs of older adults already diagnosed with cancer.
- Nurses can teach older adults about primary prevention interventions and about screening recommendations (Box 27-1).

Promoting Wellness for Older Adults With Diabetes
- Diabetes is common among older adults, with the highest prevalence among Native American and Alaskan Natives, blacks, and Hispanics.
- Disease management and nursing care related to diabetes are complicated by the common occurrence of concomitant conditions and by the increased vulnerability of older adults to complications.
- In addition to usual assessment parameters, nurses identify ageist attitudes and the meaning of diabetes (Box 27-2).
- Care plans for older adults with diabetes include all the usual interventions and additional teaching points (e.g., teaching caregivers, referring for community-based services, and appropriate ways of engaging in physical activity).

Promoting Wellness for Older Adults With Heart Failure
- Heart failure is the leading cause of hospitalizations and readmissions among older adults in the United States and as many as 57% of admission are potentially preventable with adequate self-care.
- In addition to assessing all the usual signs and symptoms of heart failure, nurses assess effects of other conditions, risk factors that can be addressed through health promotion, and other aspects that are specific to older adults (e.g., the effects of ageist attitudes).
- In addition to all the usual teaching points, wellness-oriented care plans focus on teaching about actions the person can take to achieve the best possible level of functioning and quality of life, despite the effects of heart failure.

Addressing Needs of Families and Caregivers
- Nurses promote caregiver well-being by identifying and addressing issues related to caregiver burden (Evidence-Based Practice Box 27-1).
- Many NIC and NOC terms are applicable in care plans that address caregivers with regard to role performance; use of resources and management of care; and psychosocial, spiritual, and quality-of-life needs (Table 27-2).

Critical Thinking Exercises

1. Identify an older person (in your personal life or clinical experience) who has recently been hospitalized and address the following in relation to that person:
   - How many different conditions (e.g., acute and chronic illness, functional limitations, support resources, psychosocial factors, or environmental factors) affected how the person was able to adapt to the hospitalization?
   - How did these factors affect the outcome for the person (e.g., longer hospitalization, increased dependency on others, discharge plans)?
   - Select two NOC and NIC terms from Table 27-1 that you could apply to a care plan to promote wellness for this person.

2. Think about your expectations for older adults who are affected by multiple interacting conditions and identify any ageist attitudes or assumptions that are likely to affect your care.

3. Find information about local resources for palliative care and prepare yourself to teach older adults and their families about this service.

4. Identify a situation in your personal life or clinical experience that requires caregiving assistance from a family member at least once weekly and address the following in relation to this situation:
   - What benefits (rewards) and stresses is the caregiver likely to experience?
   - Select two NOC and NIC terms from Table 27-2 that you could apply to a care plan to address the needs of this caregiver.

Resources

For links to these resources and additional helpful Internet resources related to this chapter, visit thePoint at http://thePoint. lww.com/Miller6e.

Clinical Tools

American Journal of Nursing and Hartford Institute for Geriatric Nursing
   - *How to Try This,* article and video: Onega, L. L. (2008). *American Journal of Nursing, 108*(9), 62–69.
   - *Try this: Best Practices in Nursing Care to Older Adults* Issue Number 13 (Revised 2007), Caregiver Strain Index (CSI)

Evidence-Based Practice

Balas, M. C., Casey, C. M., & Happ, M. B. (2008). Comprehensive assessment and management of the critically ill. In E. Capezuti, D. Zwicker, M. Mezey, & T. Fulmer (Eds.), *Evidence-based geriatric nursing protocols for best practice* (3rd ed., pp. 565–593). New York: Springer Publishing Co.

Coon, D. W., & Evans, B. E. (2009). Empirically based treatments for family caregiver distress: What works and where do we go from here? *Geriatric Nursing, 30,* 426–436.

Coviello, J., & Chyun, D. A. (2008). Fluid overload: identifying and managing heart failure patients at risk for hospital readmission. In E. Capezuti, D. Zwicker, M. Mezey, & T. Fulmer (Eds.), *Evidence-based geriatric nursing protocols for best practice* (3rd ed., pp. 595–614). New York: Springer Publishing Co.

Messecar, D. C. (2008). Family caregiving. In E. Capezuti, D. Zwicker, M. Mezey, & T. Fulmer (Eds.), *Evidence-based geriatric nursing protocols for best practice* (3rd ed., pp. 127–160). New York: Springer Publishing Co.

Overcash, J. (2008). Cancer assessment and intervention strategies. In E. Capezuti, D. Zwicker, M. Mezey, & T. Fulmer (Eds.), *Evidence-based geriatric nursing protocols for best practice* (3rd ed., pp. 615–628). New York: Springer Publishing Co.

Health Education

American Cancer Society
Hospice and Palliative Nurses Association
National Diabetes Education Program
National Hospice and Palliative Care Organization
Oncology Nursing Society

REFERENCES

Allen, J. K., & Dennison, C. R. (2010). Randomized trials of nursing interventions for secondary prevention in patients with coronary artery disease and heart failure. *Journal of Cardiovascular Nursing, 25*(3), 207–220.

Ambroza, C., & Geigle, P. R. (2010). Aquatic exercise as a management tool for breast cancer-related lymphedema. *Topics in Geriatric Rehabilitation, 26*(2), 120–127.

American Diabetes Association. (2010). Executive summary: Standards of medical care of diabetes-2010. *Diabetes Care, 33*(S1), S4–S10.

Andersson, C., Gislason, G. H., Weeke, P., Hoffmann, S., Hansen, P. R., Torp-Pedersen, C., & Søgaard, P. (2010). Diabetes is associated with impaired myocardial performance in patients without significant coronary artery disease. *Cardiovascular Diabetology Journal, 9*(3), 1–6.

Anekstein, Y., Smorgick, Y., Lotan, R., Agar, G., Shalmon, E., Floman, Y., & Mirovsky, Y. (2010). Diabetes mellitus as a risk factor for the development of lumbar spinal stenosis. *Israel Medical Association Journal, 12*(1), 16–20.

Bond, S. M. (2010). Physiological aging in older adults with cancer, implications for treatment decision making and toxicity management. *Journal of Gerontological Nursing, 36*(2), 24–38.

Cameron, M. E. (2010). Yoga. In M. Snyder & R. Lindquist (Eds.), *Complementary & alternative therapies in nursing* (6th ed., pp. 123–133) New York: Springer Publishing Co.

Castro, S., O'Toole, M., Brownson, C., Plessel, K., & Schauben, L. (2009). A diabetes self-management program designed for urban American Indians. *Preventing Chronic Disease, 6*(4), 1–5.

Centers for Disease Control and Prevention. (2008). *Estimates of diagnosed diabetes now available for all U.S. counties.* Retrieved from www.cdc.gov/media/pressrel/2008/r4080624.htm.

Chiu, C.-J., & Wray, L. A. (2010). Factors predicting glycemic control in middle-aged and older adults with type 2 diabetes. *Preventing Chronic Disease, 7*(1), 1–5.

Coon, D. W., & Evans, B. (2009). Empirically based treatments for family caregiver distress: What works and where do we go from here? *Geriatric Nursing, 30*(6), 426–436.

DeLancey, J. O. L., Thun, M. J., Jemal, A., & Ward, E. M. (2008). Recent trends in black-white disparities in cancer mortality. *Cancer Epidemiology Biomarkers & Prevention, 17*(11), 2908–2912.

Elliott, A. F., Burgio, L. D., & DeCoster, J. (2010). Enhancing caregiver health: Findings from the resources for enhancing Alzheimer's Caregiver Health II Intervention. *Journal of the American Geriatrics Society, 58*(1), 30–37.

Ferraro. K. F. (2006). Health and aging. In R. H. Binstock & L. K. George (Eds.), *Handbook of aging and the social sciences* (6th ed., pp. 238–256). San Diego, CA: Academic Press.

Fitzgerald, M., & Langevin, M. (2010). Imagery. In M. Snyder & R. Lindquist (Eds.), *Complementary & alternative therapies in nursing* (6th ed., pp. 663–89) New York: Springer Publishing Co.

Grady, J. L., Entin, E. B., Entin, E. E., & Brunye, T. T. (2009). Using message framing to achieve long-term behavioral changes in persons with diabetes. *Applied Nursing Research,* doi:10.1016/j.apnr.2009.03.007.

Gulick, D. T. (2010). Effects of aquatic intervention on the cardiopulmonary system in the geriatric population. *Topics in Geriatric Rehabilitation, 26*(2), 93–103.

Hernandez, A. F., Hammill, B. G., Peterson, E. D., Yancy, C. W., Schulman, K. A., Curtis, L. H., & Fonarow, G. C. (2010). Relationships between emerging measures of heart failure processes of care and clinical outcomes. *American Heart Journal, 159*(3), 406–413.

Jurgens, C. Y., Hoke, L., Byrnes, J., & Riegel, B. (2009). Why do elders delay responding to heart failure symptoms? *Nursing Research, 58*(4), 274–282.

Kagan, S. H. (2008). Ageism in cancer care. *Seminars in Oncology Nursing, 24*(4), 246–253.

Kalogeropoulos, A., Georgiopoulou, V., Kritchevsky, S. B., Psaty, B., Smith, N. L., Newman, A. B., . . . Butler, J. (2009). Epidemiology of incident heart failure in a contemporary elderly cohort, the health, aging, and body composition study. *Archives of Internal Medicine, 169*(7), 708–715.

Kreitzer, M. J., & Reilly-Spong, M. (2010). Meditation. In M. Snyder & R. Lindquist (Eds.), *Complementary & alternative therapies in nursing* (6th ed., pp. 149–167) New York: Springer Publishing Co.

Lin, E. H. B., Heckbert, S. R., Rutter, C. M., Katon, W. J., Ciechanowski, P., Ludman, E. J., . . . Von Korff, M., (2009). Depression and increased mortality in diabetes: Unexpected causes of death. *Annals of Family Medicine, 7*(5), 414–420.

Long, C. O. (2009). Palliative care for advanced dementia. *Journal of Gerontological Nursing, 35*(11), 19–25.

Maggi, S., Limongi, F., Noale, M., Romanato, G., Tonin, P., Rozzini, R., . . . for the ILSA Study Group. (2009). Diabetes as a risk factor of cognitive decline in older patients. *Dementia and Geriatric Cognitive Disorders, 27*(1), 24–33.

Mahler, A. (2010). The clinical nurse specialist role in developing a geropalliative model of care. *Clinical Nurse Specialist, 24*(1), 18–23.

Martire, L. M., Schultz, R., Reynolds, C. F. III., Karp, J. F., Gildengers, A. G., & Whyte, E. M. (2010). Treatment of late-life depression alleviates caregiver burden. *Journal of the American Geriatrics Society, 58*(1), 23–29.

Mayer, C., Williams, B., Wagner, E. H., LoGerfo, J. P., Cheadle, A., & Phelan, E. A. (2010). Health care costs and participation in a community-based health promotion program for older adults. *Preventing Chronic Disease, 7*(2), 1–6.

Mayor, M. S., Ribeiro, O., & Paul, C. (2009). Satisfaction in dementia and stroke caregivers: A comparative study. *Rev Latino-Americana de Enfermagem, 17*(5), 620–624.

Melvin, C. S. (2010). Patients' and families' misperceptions about hospice and palliative care, listen as they speak. *Journal of Hospice and Palliative Nursing, 12*(2), 107–115.

Melvin, C. S., & Oldham, L. (2009). When to refer patients to palliative care, triggers, traps, and timely referrals. *Journal of Hospice and Palliative Nursing, 11*(5), 291–301.

Messecar, D. C. (2008). Family caregiving. In E. Capezuti, D. Zwicker, M. Mezey, & T. Fulmer (Eds.), *Evidence-based geriatric nursing protocols for best practice* (3rd ed., pp. 127–160). New York: Springer Publishing Co.

Miller, N. H. (2010). Motivational interviewing as a prelude to coaching in healthcare settings. *Journal of Cardiovascular Nursing, 25*(3), 247–251.

Molokhia, E. A., & Perkins, A. (2008). Preventing cancer. *Primary Care Clinics in Office Practice, 35*, 609–623.

Morris, D. M. (2010). Aquatic therapy to improve balance dysfunction in older adults. *Topics in Geriatric Rehabilitation, 26*(2), 104–119.

Muzzarelli, S., Tobler, D., Leibundgut, G., Schindler, R., Buser, P., Pfisterer, M. E., & Brunner-La Rocca, H. P. (2009). Detection of intake of nonsteroidal anti-inflammatory drugs in elderly patients with heart failure. How to ask the patient? *Swiss Medicine Weekly, 139*(33–34), 481–485.

National Consensus Project for Quality Care. (2009). *Clinical practice guidelines for quality palliative care.* Retrieved from www.nationalconsensusproject.org.

Nelson, J. E., Puntillo, K. A., Pronovost, P. J., Walker, A. S., McAdam, J. L., Ilaoa, D., & Penrod, J. (2010). In their own words: Patients and families define high-quality palliative care in the intensive care unit. *Critical Care Medicine, 38*(3), 808–816.

Norton, C., & Jamison, L. (2010). Spectrum of aquatic exercise programming for elderly individuals. *Topics in Geriatric Rehabilitation, 26*(2), 140–147.

Oncology Nursing Society and Geriatric Oncology Consortium Joint Position on Cancer care for older adults (2007). *Oncology Nursing Forum, 34*, 623–624.

Paradis, V., Cossette, S., Frasure-Smith, N., Heppell, S., & Guertin, M.-C. (2010). The efficacy of a motivational nursing intervention based on the stages of change on self-care in heart failure patients. *Journal of Cardiovascular Nursing, 25*(2), 130–141.

Petrakis, I. E., & Paraskakis, S. (2009). Breast cancer in the elderly. *Archives of Gerontology and Geriatrics, 50*, 179–184.

Poggio, R., Grancelli, H. O., & Miriuka, S. G. (2010). Understanding the risk of hyperkalaemia in heart failure: Role of aldosterone antagonism. *Postgraduate Medical Journal, 86*(1013), 136–142.

Posma, E. R., van Weert, J. C. M., Jansen, J., & Bensing, J. M. (2009). Older cancer patients' information and support needs surrounding treatment: An evaluation through the eyes of patients, relatives and professionals. *BioMed Central Nursing, 8*(1), doi:10.1186/1472-6955-8-1.

Poulin, M. J., Brown, S. L., Ubel, P. A., Smith, D. M., Jankovic, A., & Langa, K. M. (2010). Does a helping hand mean a heavy heart? Helping behavior and well-being among spouse caregivers. *Psychology and Aging, 25*(1), 108–117.

Riegel, B., Dickson, V. V., Cameron, J., Johnson, J. C., Bunker, S., Page, K., & Worrall-Carter, L. (2010). Symptom recognition in elders with heart failure. *Journal of Nursing Scholarship, 42*(1), 92–100.

Ripsin, C. M., Kang, H., & Urban, R. J. (2009). Management of blood glucose in type 2 diabetes mellitus. *American Family Physician, 79*(1), 29–36.

Rottenberg, Y., Barchana, M., Liphshitz, I., & Peretz, T. (2009). The changing face of cancer in the elderly: Only a demographic change? *Archives of Gerontology and Geriatrics,* doi:10.1016/j.archger.2009.05.011.

Song, M. K. (2010). Diabetes mellitus and the importance of self-care. *Journal of Cardiovascular Nursing, 25*(2), 93–98.

Tamayo, G. J., Broxson, A., Munsell, M., & Cohen, M. Z. (2010). Caring for the caregiver. *Oncology Nursing Forum, 37*(1), E50–E57.

Tilden, H. M., Reicherter, E. A., & Reicherter, F. (2010). Use of an aquatics program for older adults with osteoarthritis, from clinic to the community. *Topics in Geriatric Rehabilitation, 26*(2), 128–139.

White, H. K., & Cohen, H. J. (2008). The older cancer patient. *Nursing Clinics of North America, 43*, 307–322.

White, M. M., Howie-Esquivel, J., & Caldwell, M. A. (2010). Improving heart failure symptom recognition, a diary analysis. *Journal of Cardiovascular Nursing, 25*(1), 7–12.

Winter, K. H., Bouldin, E. D., & Andresen, E. M. (2010). Lack of choice in caregiving decision and caregiver risk of stress, North Carolina, 2005. *Preventing Chronic Disease, 7*(2), 1–5,

World Health Organization. (2002). *National cancer control programmes: Policies and managerial guidelines* (2nd ed.). New York: World Health Organization.

Yehle, K. S., & Plake, K. S. (2010). Self-efficacy and educational interventions in heart failure: A review of the literature. *Journal of Cardiovascular Nursing, 25*(3), 175–188.

CHAPTER 28

Caring for Older Adults Experiencing Pain

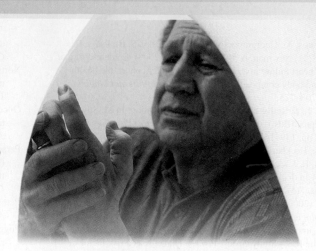

LEARNING OBJECTIVES

After reading this chapter, you will be able to:

1. Define acute versus persistent pain and identify the scope of the problem of pain, including barriers to effective pain management in older adults.

2. Explain the physiology of pain and identify treatment options.

3. Examine and dispel commonly held myths and beliefs about persistent pain in older adults.

4. Provide age-appropriate assessment techniques for effective pain management and patient advocacy for pain management issues.

5. Describe principles of analgesic medication use in older adults.

6. Apply principles of wellness to nursing care of older adults experiencing pain.

7. Discuss cultural aspects of pain.

KEY POINTS

acute pain	pain
addiction	pain intensity
adjuvant analgesics	pain receptors
dependence	perception
nociception	persistent pain
nonopioid analgesics	tolerance
opioid analgesics	

The experience of **pain** is not unique to older adults, but the higher rate of chronic conditions in this patient population places them at increased risk for pain. Nurses who care for older adults have an important responsibility to assess pain to plan appropriate pain management interventions. In addition, nurses need to be able to address common misconceptions about pain in older adults and implement effective pain management plans. This chapter provides a base of information about common types of pain and discusses assessment and management interventions that are important for addressing pain in older adults.

ACUTE VERSUS PERSISTENT PAIN

Pain is an unpleasant sensory and emotional experience associated with actual or potential tissue damage (Gordon et al., 2005). McCaffrey (1968) presented the most commonly used definition of pain as being whatever the experiencing person says it is, existing whenever she or he says it does.

Acute pain is sharp, immediate pain from an injury to tissue, but it is also triggered by physiologic malfunction or severe illness. It is a warning signal of possible or actual tissue damage, and is the normal, predicted physiologic response to an adverse chemical, thermal, or mechanical stimulus. Acute pain is generally time limited and is responsive to anti-inflammatory and opioid medications as well as other approaches. Acute pain may be due to trauma or an acute medical or orthopedic problem. Additional types of acute pain are postoperative pain; acute exacerbations of pain associated with chronic medical problems, such as cancer or postherpetic neuralgia; and pain associated with medical procedures.

The importance of effectively treating acute pain and providing greater comfort with the use of new medications and techniques must be emphasized, both for the individual's quality of life and for the broader health care effects. Failure to effectively treat acute pain can lead to prolonged hospital stays and delayed recovery. Uncontrolled postoperative pain is reported by approximately 50% of patients, and it is the most common cause for unexpected hospital readmissions (Polomano, Dunwoody, Krenzischek, & Rathmell, 2008). Specifically important for older adults is the potential for acute pain to develop into **persistent pain** (Shipton & Tait, 2005).

Clinical practice guidelines, established by professional groups including the American Pain Society (APS), the International Association for the Study of Pain (IASP), and the American Geriatric Society (AGS), define persistent pain as

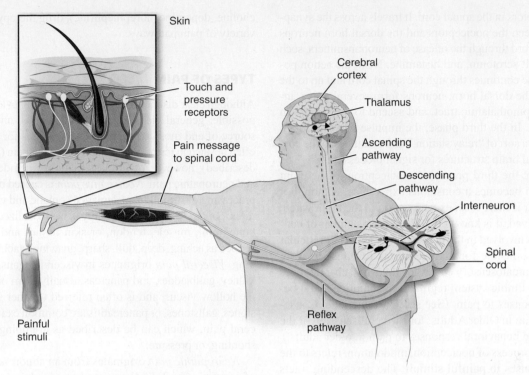

FIGURE 28-1 Processes involved in the physiology of pain.

a multidimensional phenomenon characterized by unpleasant sensory and emotional experiences. Persistent pain is a state in which pain persists beyond the usual course of an acute disease or healing of an injury, and it is associated with actual or potential tissue damage that continues for a prolonged period of time that may or may not be associated with a recognizable disease process (American Geriatric Society, 2002; Gordon et al., 2005). The APS uses a time period of 6 months to designate persistent pain (Gordon et al., 2005). Although the terms *persistent* and *chronic* are often used interchangeably, for many older adults, chronic pain has become a label associated with negative images and stereotypes. These negative connotations are often associated with psychiatric problems, ineffective treatment options, apathetic attitudes toward pain management, or drug-seeking behavior. The term *persistent pain* depicts more positive attitudes by patients and professionals (American Geriatric Society, 2002).

ANATOMY AND PHYSIOLOGY OF PAIN

Pain, which is a subjective experience, involves both an emotional quality and a physiologic sensation. **Nociception** is the physiologic occurrence of a measurable pain signal involving the transmission of information to the spinal cord and brain about inflammation or tissue damage. Despite the unpleasant feeling of pain, nociception is a critical component of the body's defense mechanism, rapidly warning the central nervous system to initiate motor neurons to minimize the detected potential for harm. Four basic processes occur with nociception: (1) transduction, (2) transmission, (3) **perception**, and (4) modulation (Figure 28-1).

Transduction is the conversion of one energy form to another. A noxious stimulus of a mechanical, thermal, or chemical nature causes tissue damage, resulting in a release of substances that activate nociceptors and lead to the generation of an impulse known as an *action potential*. Primary afferent nociceptors are classified according to their diameter, degree of myelination, and conduction velocity. The largest-diameter fibers, A-beta fibers, respond maximally to light touch or moving stimuli. They are present primarily in nerves that innervate the skin. In healthy individuals, the activity of these fibers does not produce pain. There are two other classes of primary afferents: the small-diameter myelinated Λ-delta (Λ fibers) and the unmyelinated (C fiber) axons. These fibers, known as primary afferent nociceptors or **pain receptors**, are present in nerves to the skin and to deep somatic and visceral structures. Most A and C afferents respond maximally only to intense or pain-inducing stimuli and produce the subjective experience of pain when they are electrically stimulated. This stimulation occurs when damaged cells release sensitizing substances, such as substance P, histamine, and prostaglandins, which trigger changes in the neuron cell membrane that permit an influx of sodium ions as well as other ion transfers. The resulting change in electrical charge generates an action potential, and the signal is transmitted to the central nervous system.

Transmission is the continuation of the action potential from the site of damage to the spinal cord and then to the brain. Transmission occurs in three phases. First, the action potential generated at the site of damage travels to the termination site of the nociceptors in the spinal cord. It travels across the synaptic cleft between the nociceptors and the dorsal horn neurons of the spinal cord through the release of neurotransmitters, such as substance P, serotonin, and histamine. Next, the action potential impulse continues through the spinal cord and up to the brain. From the dorsal horn, neurons form several tracts, including the spinothalamic tract, and ascend to the brainstem and thalamus. In the third phase, the impulse moves through the thalamus, a sort of "relay station," and continues to the cortex and central brain structures for signal processing.

Perception, the third process of nociception, is the point at which pain becomes a conscious experience. Although it is still unclear if there is an exact location in the brain where pain is perceived, it is known that there are a number of central structures involved in the perception of pain. The reticular system is responsible for the autonomic response to pain, whereas the somatosensory cortex localizes and characterizes pain, and the limbic system regulates the emotional and behavioral responses to pain. (See section Functional Consequences of Pain in Older Adults, for further discussion of the emotional and behavioral responses to pain in older adults.)

The final process of nociception, modulation, refers to the body's responses to painful stimuli. The descending tracts from the brain to the periphery follow the same pathway down the spinal cord to the dorsal horn. The descending tract neurons release substances, such as endogenous opioids, serotonin, and norepinephrine, which are capable of inhibiting the transmission phase of the noxious impulse, resulting in analgesia. These modulatory systems explain the action of tricyclic antidepressants for pain management.

The physiology of pain perception as described is the "normal" process by which acute pain is experienced. Although persistent pain follows the same basic principles, there are several key differences between the physiology of acute pain and persistent pain. Persistent pain is multifactorial in origin and can be affected by age, sex, ethnicity, and previous experiences with pain. Persistent pain often cannot be explained by objective clinical measures alone; its cause may be idiopathic and influenced by the patient's psychological makeup. Thus, recognition of the potential combination of physiologic and psychological processes at work in persistent pain may assist in guiding the development of appropriate pain management regimens.

The etiology of persistent pain is not well understood; it can occur in the absence of apparent illness or after incomplete healing from injury. With persistent pain, the central nervous system continues to process pain signals as though new injuries were occurring. The perception of persistent pain is associated with the upregulation of genes for sensory neuron–specific channels in which regulating proteins for signaling pain contain genetic components that, when continuously exposed to pain signals, can predispose certain persons to persistent pain. Because physiologic changes that occur during pain signal processing involve many neurotransmitters (e.g., substance P, serotonin, prostaglandins, bradykinin, leukotrienes, histamine, norepinephrine) and receptors (e.g., opioid, serotonin, acetyl-choline, dopamine, norepinephrine), drug therapy can target a variety of pain pathways.

TYPES OF PAIN

Although clear distinctions between types of pain are not always possible, general classifications help nurses understand the source of and most appropriate interventions for pain. Pain is often defined in terms of acute and persistent pain (as previously described); however, other classifications include nociceptive and neuropathic pain. *Nociceptive pain* is caused by the normal processing of stimuli from damaged somatic and visceral structures. *Somatic pain*, which usually is well localized, arises from bone, joint, muscle, tendon, or skin tissues and is often described as aching, deep, dull, sharp, gnawing, stabbing, or throbbing. *Visceral pain* originates in visceral organs, such as the kidney, gallbladder, and pancreas, usually from obstruction of the hollow viscus, and is often referred to other sites. Kidney stones, gallstones, or pancreatitis are common examples of visceral pain, which can be described as cramping, squeezing, shooting, or pressure.

Neuropathic pain originates from an abnormal processing of sensory stimuli by the central or peripheral nervous system. Centrally generated pain is caused by either injury to the nervous system (e.g., phantom pain from an amputation) or dysregulation of the autonomic nervous system (e.g., burning pain below the level of a spinal cord lesion). Peripherally generated pain has two causes: mononeuropathies or polyneuropathies. Mononeuropathy results in pain along a known peripheral nerve pathway (e.g., nerve root compression or trigeminal neuralgia), and polyneuropathy occurs along the distribution of many peripheral nerves (e.g., diabetic neuropathy or Guillain-Barré syndrome). Neuropathic pain is described as burning, numbness, radiating, shooting, stabbing, tingling, or hypersensitivity to touch.

One final classification of pain that is often used is that of cancer pain. Although *cancer pain* is not a physiologic classification, it has distinct characteristics. Cancer pain is a complex phenomenon in which pain can be acute, persistent, nociceptive, or neuropathic. Cancer pain can be caused by tumor progression, treatments and medications administered for the cancer, or even treatments for the side effects of the cancer treatments.

CAUSES OF PAIN IN OLDER ADULTS

Pain is a widespread problem for older adults, affecting 25% to 50% of community-dwelling older adults and 50% to 75% of residents in long-term care facilities (Dumas & Ramadurai, 2009; Planton & Edlund, 2010). In addition, 80% to 85% of persons older than 65 years experience at some point in time a significant health problem that predisposes them to pain (Rustoen et al., 2005; Tsai & Means, 2005). Causes of acute pain in older adults include injury or trauma and surgical procedures, both planned and emergency. Although acute pain is a predictable consequence of surgical procedures, approximately 50% of surgical patients report inadequate pain relief, resulting in unnecessary moderate-to-severe pain (Polomano Rathnell, Kenzischek, & Dunworthy, 2008). Pain-related hospital readmissions are more common than all other postoperative reasons, including surgical conditions and bleeding.

People older than 65 years have an increased rate of chronic conditions that are associated with persistent pain and pain-associated declining physical function. Common causes of persistent pain in older adults include arthritis, osteoporosis, postherpetic neuralgia, and diabetic peripheral neuropathy.

AGE-RELATED CHANGES THAT AFFECT PAIN

Although age-related changes in pain perception are not well understood, the process is altered by underlying neurochemical, neuroanatomic, and neurophysiologic mechanisms. Moreover, pain management is affected by age-related changes in the pharmacokinetics and pharmacodynamics of analgesic medications. Some age-related changes that can affect the pharmacologic treatment of pain include decreased renal function, decreased lean body weight, decreased liver mass and hepatic blood flow, decreased serum protein concentrations, and decreased pulmonary function. These physiologic changes can alter the absorption, distribution, metabolism, elimination, and side effects of analgesic medications in older adults. However, little is known about changes in the perception of pain due to the aging process. The misconception that older adults are not able to feel pain as intensely as younger adults should not reduce the aggressiveness of pain management in this population. The undertreatment of pain is a much greater concern.

The typical pain symptoms manifested in younger adults may not always be present in older adults. Older adults may be less likely to report pain because they do not want to "complain," or they believe that it is a part of the natural aging process. In older adults, pain is likely to manifest as mental changes, restlessness, aggression, fatigue, or agitation. The lack of "expected" symptoms might lead to a misdiagnosis or delay in treatment, especially if the older adult is reluctant to admit to having pain.

BARRIERS TO PAIN MANAGEMENT

Despite the progress in understanding the physiology of pain and the advances in its assessment and treatment, there are many barriers nationwide to the appropriate recognition and management of pain. These obstacles exist at many levels, from health care systems to insurance providers, and from health care providers to patients and family members. Nurses need to recognize these barriers so they can not only assess and manage pain but also advocate for the needs of patients. Table 28-1 lists some of the barriers to pain management, along with problems and possible solutions that nurses can address.

FUNCTIONAL CONSEQUENCES OF PAIN IN OLDER ADULTS

Functional consequences of pain in older adults include diminished physical function and higher levels of disability. In particular, persistent pain is associated with significant loss of lower extremity function (Eggermont, Bean, Guralnik, & Leveille, 2009). Psychosocial consequences include fatigue, anxiety, depression, sleep disturbances, and loss of independence. Consequences associated with the undertreatment of pain include decreased quality of life, social isolation and negative effects on relationships, impaired function, physical deconditioning, sleep disturbances, fatigue, depression, and anxiety. These consequences are not unique to older adults; however, their effects can be particularly devastating in this population, causing unnecessary suffering and compounding the inherent toll of persistent pain.

An essential aspect of optimal pain management is recognizing the unique way in which each individual experiences pain. Pain is interpreted differently by each person and is influenced by many factors. Past pain experiences can influence one's current perception of pain by triggering "memories" in the pain pathways. In addition, age, sex, beliefs, values, and culture can influence the meaning and interpretation of pain for each individual. Moreover, expectations of what the pain means and attitudes about the pain can affect the degree to which patients tolerate it. Box 28-1 lists specific factors that can worsen or improve pain for older adults.

CULTURAL ASPECTS OF PAIN ASSESSMENT AND MANAGEMENT

Cultural background can significantly influence the way pain is experienced and how it is managed. These cultural variations

---

Box 28-1 Factors Affecting the Experience of Pain

Factors That Worsen Pain
- Insomnia/fatigue
- Anxiety
- Fear
- Isolation
- Boredom
- Anger
- Sadness
- Depression

Factors That Improve Pain
- Nonpharmacologic approaches
- Medications
- Sleep/rest
- Understanding/validation
- Companionship
- Diversional activity
- Reduction in anxiety
- Elevation of mood

Copyright 2005, Casey Shillam. Used with permission.

TABLE 28-1 Barriers to Effective Pain Management

Source of the Barrier	Problems Contributing to the Barrier	Possible Solutions to Overcoming the Barrier

Patients and families	• Attitude that pain cannot be effectively managed and is a normal part of aging
	• Family burnout (families are often involved in educating, goal setting, and primary caregiving)
	• Belief that pain is an atonement for past actions that must be endured
	• Belief that pain is inevitable
	• Belief that "complaining" equals "burden," or results in retribution
	• Belief that health care providers are "always right"; self-advocacy is not appropriate
	• Belief that morphine is used only at the end of life
	• Fear of addiction to medication
	• Stigma of opiate use
	• Side effects, which may be difficult to manage or impossible to treat
	• Fear of the underlying meaning of the pain (e.g., that it indicates worsening of the disease process)
		• Provide education about the treatments for side effects
		• Explain the mechanism of action of morphine and its appropriate use for pain management
		• Explain the differences between "addiction" and "tolerance"
		• Present nonpharmacologic alternatives:
		  ▪ Physical therapy
		  ▪ Massage
		  ▪ Body/energy work
		  ▪ Acupuncture
		  ▪ Chiropractic or naturopathic care
		  ▪ Behavioral or mental health therapies
		  ▪ Biofeedback
		  ▪ Pilates, yoga

Health care providers	• Belief that older adults have a higher pain tolerance • Belief that patients with dementia do not experience pain • Belief that older adults cannot tolerate potent opioid analgesic medication • Fear of being investigated for excessive prescribing of opioids • Fear of the consequences of hospital policies for aggressive pain treatment • Lack of resources in rural/outlying areas • Insufficient communication between members of the health care team • Inadequate knowledge about pain and how best to manage it	• Complete continuing education in pain management (as for licensure renewal) • Attend educational seminars provided to health care workers by hospitals on prescription regulations with strategies for providing safe, structured pain management • Participate in a pain management clinic or team for referral of complex pain management cases

Health care system/institution	• Cultural and political climate resistant to change in the standards of care
	• Systems do not encourage a multidisciplinary approach to pain management
	• Lack of a shared language among disciplines for communicating about pain
	• Lack of motivation to improve pain management standards (belief that the problem is already being adequately addressed)
	• Lack of health care provider accountability for effective pain relief
		• Encourage institutions to:
		  ▪ Identify key players among upper management and clinicians to include in discussions for change to standards of care
		  ▪ Select a system-wide pain rating system, using clear, concise terminology for routine pain assessment and documentation
		  ▪ Offer education from a policy perspective on the implications of unrelieved pain (e.g., increased length of stay and health care costs)
		  ▪ Implement measures to hold individual providers responsible for appropriate pain assessment and treatment

Insurance companies/ payment plans	• Lack of reimbursement for opioid treatment • Lack of reimbursement for multidisciplinary pain centers • Lack of reimbursement for nonpharmacologic interventions	• Advocate for patients by contacting insurance companies that refuse to pay for treatment • Advocate for policy-level changes to reimbursement formularies • Assume a leadership or consultation position in an insurance company

can influence nursing assessment and interventions in many ways. For example, people from cultures that are stoical in their approach may be reluctant to acknowledge pain, may not accept analgesics, and may want to bear their pain alone and silently. In contrast, people from cultural groups that are more expressive about pain may believe that verbal expressions and outbursts are effective coping mechanisms and they may want

caregivers to attend to their needs (Narayan, 2010). As with other aspects of culturally appropriate care, nurses need to be aware of different expressions of pain commonly used by cultural groups, while at the same time avoiding stereotypes. Cultural Considerations Box 28-1 provides examples of ways in which cultural groups may express pain and suggests nursing implications related to these cultural variations.

CULTURAL CONSIDERATIONS 28-1

Expressions of Pain Associated with Selected Cultural Groups

Group	Pain Expression	Nursing Implications
Haitians	Pain is described as *doule,* but Haitians may be vague about the location because they believe that the whole body is affected. Injections are the preferred method for medication administration, followed by elixirs, tablets, and capsules.	Acknowledge that the whole *body* is affected, but ask the person to identify specific points. Consider cultural preferences regarding medication administration.
Japanese	Bearing pain is considered a virtue and a matter of family honor. *Itami* is the word for pain. Because addiction is a strong taboo, patients may be reluctant to accept pain medication.	Encourage the expression of pain as an important component of accurate assessment. Consider the use of regularly scheduled medications rather than a patient-controlled approach.
Jews	Verbalization of pain is acceptable and common. Individuals want to know the cause of the pain, which is just as important as obtaining relief.	Talk with patients about causes of pain.
Navajo Indians	Pain is viewed as something to be endured and patients may not request pain medication but may be using herbal medicines.	Use nonjudgmental approach to ask about herbal medicines. Consult with pharmacist to determine if herbal approaches can be incorporated into treatment plan. Offer pain medication and explain that it will promote healing.
Puerto Ricans	May be outspoken in expressing pain (e.g., *Ay!* is a verbal moaning of *dolor).* May prefer oral or intravenous analgesics rather than injections or rectal medications. May use heat, herbal teas, and prayer for pain management.	Use appropriate pain assessment tools; do not judge pain expression as an exaggeration.
Somalians	May express pain as being one half of the body. Pain may be an expression of sadness or social and psychological discomfort.	Assess whether pain is an expression of physical or emotional symptoms.
Turks	Pain may be expressed through emotional outbursts or verbal complaints.	Recognize a wide range of pain expressions.

Source: Purnell, L. D. (2009). *Culturally competent health care.* Philadelphia, PA: F.A. Davis.

Nurses can apply the following guidelines for pain management when caring for patients from various cultural backgrounds (Al-Atiyyat, 2009):

- Use culturally appropriate assessment tools.
- Recognize variations in expressions of pain across cultures.
- Be sensitive to different styles of communicating pain.
- Recognize that expressions of pain may not be acceptable within a culture.
- Appreciate that the meaning of pain varies across cultures.
- Develop personal awareness of values and beliefs that may affect responses to pain.

Nurses can find additional resources related to cultural aspects of pain in older adults at http://thePoint.lww.com/Miller6e.

NURSING ASSESSMENT OF PAIN IN OLDER ADULTS

A basic pain assessment is a simple task to perform; however, a comprehensive pain assessment is one of the most complex, and important, nursing responsibilities. Unrelieved pain and unnecessary suffering for older adults result from an incomplete or inaccurate pain assessment, or from failure to perform one at all. The major mistakes associated with a pain assess-

ment include failure to assess pain, failure to accept a patient's report of pain, and failure to act on the patient's report of pain. A pain assessment *is* asking and believing the patient, assessing the critical components of the pain experience, assessing the cause of the pain, and communicating the findings of the pain assessment to the health care team. Pain assessment *is not* relying only on changes in vital signs; deciding that the patient does not "look in pain"; basing pain assessment only on how much the nurse believes a procedure or disease "should" hurt; assuming sleeping patients do not have pain; and assuming a patient will tell the nurse when he or she is in pain. Box 28-2 summarizes assumptions that should and should not be made when assessing pain in older adults.

Several organizations have proposed guidelines for the assessment of pain in older adults, including the Hartford Institute for Geriatric Nursing, the National Gerontological Nursing Association, and the AGS (see the Resource section at end of chapter for more information).

Collecting Pertinent Information

An essential first step in assessing pain is recognizing that many older adults refer to pain by using words, such as *burning, discomfort, aching, soreness,* or *hurting.* The nurse should also observe for physical indicators of pain, which include grimacing, muscle tension, rubbing or protecting body parts, rapid or excessive eye blinking, or a sad or frightened

Box 28-2 Assumptions Made by Nurses Regarding Pain Assessment

Assumptions That Should be Made in All Situations
- Self-report is the gold standard for pain assessment.
- Pain assessment must be regular, systematic, and documented in order accurately to evaluate treatment effectiveness.
- Both patients and health care providers have personal beliefs, prior experiences, insufficient knowledge, and mistaken beliefs about pain and pain management that
  - Influence the pain management process
  - Must be acknowledged and addressed before optimal pain relief can be achieved.

Assumptions That Should be Made in Specific Situations
- The majority of hospitalized older adults suffer from both acute and chronic pain.
- People with dementia have the same physiologic experience of pain as those who do not have any cognitive impairment.

- People with cognitive impairment experience pain but are often unable to verbalize it; however, there may be nonverbal indicators.
- People with dementia have pain if they have conditions or are in situations that typically cause pain; therefore, medicate for pain even if they are unable to report it.

Assumptions That Should Not be Made
- All older adults complain about pain.
- Older adults cannot or will not comply with complex or alternative therapies.
- Older adults are unreliable historians and will not accurately report their pain.
- Older adults will under-report their pain because they believe that pain is an inevitable aspect of aging.

Sources: National Gerontological Nursing Association. (2002). Innovations in clinical practice: Chronic pain management in older adults. Available at www.ngna.org/pdfs/Chronic%20Pain%20ICP.pdf; The Hartford Institute for Geriatric Nursing. (2000). Assessing pain in older adults. *Try This: Best Practices in Nursing Care to Older Adults, 7;* and The Hartford Institute for Geriatric Nursing. (2003). Assessing pain in persons with dementia. *Try This: Best Practices in Nursing Care for Older Adults With Dementia, 1*(2), both available at http://consultgerirn.org.

facial expression (see section Assessment in Cognitively Impaired Older Adults, for further discussion of the nonverbal indicators of pain). Verbalizations and vocalizations can also indicate the presence of pain and can include sighing or moaning, chanting or calling out "Help," noisy breathing, yelling "Ow" or "Ouch," swearing or cursing, or stop commands like "Stop" or "Don't do that."

If nurses are not familiar with the older adult, they need to elicit a history of recent changes in function from the patient, family members, or caregivers because these changes can be indicators of pain. Information about the usual activities of daily living (ADLs) and baseline measures of functioning are useful in assessing changes that are indicative of pain. It is also important to recognize the relationship between pain and the person's mood and psychological function. For example, nurses can use age-specific and cognitive-appropriate scales such as the Geriatric Depression Scale (see Chapter 15) and the tools recommended by the Hartford Institute for Geriatric Nursing listed in the Clinical Tools at the end of this chapter. Finally, the nurse must recognize that medication effects and chronic medical conditions can influence both the experience of pain and the treatment of that pain. Nurses can use the questions in Box 28-3 as a guide for collecting pertinent information throughout the pain assessment.

Assessment of Pain Components

Nurses assess the following components of the pain experience: intensity, impact on ADLs, quality, location, physical findings, temporal characteristics, aggravating and alleviating factors, analgesic history, patient goals and expectations, and the meaning of pain and the patient's attitudes. **Pain intensity** is the state of being unpleasant, or the subjective determina-

tion of the strength, concentration, or force of the symptom of pain. The subjective report of the intensity is the component most often addressed in pain assessment because it is the most easily identified indicator of improvement or worsening. Intensity is the component that is often considered the "fifth vital sign" and it is assessed by using a rating scale, such as the Numerical Rating Scale (NRS) to document the patient's report on a scale of 0 to 10. The Verbal Descriptor Scale (VDS) rates pain on a continuum with verbal cues ranging from no pain to mild pain, moderate pain, severe pain, very severe pain, to the worst pain possible. Often this scale

Box 28-3 Sample Questions for Pain Assessment in Older Adults

- How strong is your pain right now?
- What was the worst/average pain over the past week?
- How many days over the past week have you been unable to do what you would like to do because of your pain?
- How often do you participate in pleasurable activities such as hobbies, socializing with friends, travel? Over the past week, how often has pain interfered with these activities?
- How often do you exercise? Over the past week, how often has pain interfered with your ability to exercise?
- How often does pain interfere with your ability to think clearly?
- How often does pain interfere with your appetite? Have you lost weight as a result?
- How often does pain interfere with your sleep? How often over the past week has this scenario occurred?
- Has pain interfered with your energy, mood, personality, or relationships with other people?
- Over the past week, how often have you taken pain medication?
- How would you rate your health at the present time?

Pain intensity scales

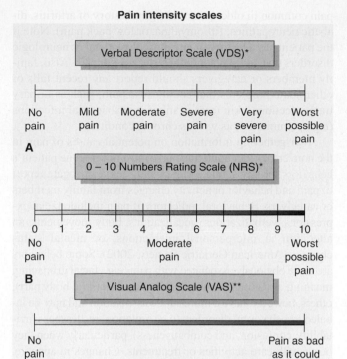

* If used as a graphic rating scale, a 10-cm baseline is recommended.

** A 10-cm baseline is recommended for VAS scales.

FIGURE 28-2 Examples of pain rating scales: (**A**) Verbal Descriptor Scale, (**B**) Numerical Rating Scale, and (**C**) Visual Analog Scale.

is used in conjunction with the NRS. Figure 28-2 illustrates three commonly used pain intensity scales. It is important to document the patient's self-report of his or her pain rating, not your personal impression of what you think the rating "should" be. In addition to consistently using the same tool each time, nurses should document additional assessment comments in the chart when appropriate.

Assessing the effects of pain on ADLs not only provides additional information for the nurse but also may help older adults recognize subtle ways in which pain interferes with their lives. Thus, nurses should ask how often in the past week the pain or discomfort has interfered with self-care or the usual ability to perform activities, such as bathing, eating, dressing, and going to the toilet. Limiting the time frame to the past week helps the patient to focus attention on the present, rather than recalling how pain has fluctuated over the course of months or years. Nurses should also ask about the effects of pain states on complex activities, such as driving, paying bills, preparing meals, shopping for groceries, and taking care of home-related chores.

Assessing the quality of the pain based on specific descriptors used by older adults is helpful in determining the underlying pain mechanism as somatic, visceral, or neuropathic, as discussed in section Types of Pain. Nurses should document the location of the pain on a figure drawing in the patient's

chart. Location can be identified simply by asking the patient to mark the location on a figure drawing, or by having the patient point to the location on his or her own body. If there is more than one site, letters may be used for distinguishing the different sites for documentation, (e.g., A, B, C, and so forth). This step of assessment is critical for delineating different areas of pain because they may be different types of pain. Each location may require an individual approach to management.

Physical findings may also aid in assessing the location of the pain. Although pain assessment cannot rely only on physical findings, the nurse must observe the site of pain; note any changes in skin color, warmth, irritation, or integrity; and review any pertinent physical assessment data.

Temporal characteristics describe the course of the pain experience using the following parameters: onset, duration of episodes, frequency (i.e., constant or intermittent), and variations with time of day or certain activities. It is logical to assess aggravating and alleviating factors in conjunction with temporal characteristics. This goal is accomplished by inquiring about what makes the pain better or worse, if the pain is affected by movement or changing position, and if any non-pharmacologic methods help to alleviate the pain.

Analgesic history can also be taken at this time and should include information on the patient's current medication use, the onset and duration of maximal analgesia with medication use, and the number of medications that are being taken on a set schedule versus those taken only as needed (p.r.n.). The nurse must also thoroughly assess and document analgesic use within the previous 24 hours because a patient can have very different pain ratings depending on whether analgesics have been taken on the day of the assessment. This is also the time to inquire about problems the patient has had with side effects of medications as well as any fears of potential side effects or **addiction** to pain medication.

When assessing pain, nurses must evaluate the patient's goals and expectations, as well as the meaning he or she associates with the pain. Some older adults may fear the onset of pain as an indicator of a progressive terminal illness or disease process, and others may view pain as a positive sign that they are still alive for another day. Nurses assess the meaning and context of the pain in relation to actual and potential effects on functional and psychosocial activities, such as sleep, physical activities, recreational activities, personal relationships, and work. These areas can influence older adults' perception of the severity of the pain and their willingness to participate in a pain management regimen. This time is also the point at which to gain an understanding of the patient's short- and long-term goals of treatment. Does the patient expect to return to baseline functioning, or is he or she expecting to continue to experience some pain? Another important issue to determine is the patient's acceptable level of pain and to incorporate this acceptable level as a goal of the pain management regimen. Is a pain level of 5 on the 0 to 10 NRS acceptable to the patient, or is 3 the target pain level?

A crucial step that is often overlooked is the reassessment of pain frequently and regularly. In acute care settings, nurses should assess the effectiveness of the treatment shortly after the administration of pain medication (30 to 60 minutes) and whenever pain management interventions are changed. Nurses also need to reassess whenever patients experience changes in any of the critical components of pain. This reassessment includes questions regarding pain severity and length of time the pain was relieved with the previous intervention.

Assessment in Cognitively Impaired Older Adults

Even though damage to the central nervous system can affect cognitive skills necessary for communicating the experience of pain, people with dementia still experience pain sensations to a degree similar to that of cognitively intact older adults (Schuler, Njoo, Hestermann, Oster, & Hauer, 2004). Despite the known similarity in the prevalence of pain between cognitively impaired and cognitively intact older adults, nursing home documentation indicates that only 50% of residents with severe cognitive impairment receive pain medications compared with 80% of their cognitively intact counterparts (Reynolds, Hanson, DeVellis, Henderson, & Steinhauser, 2008). This discrepancy indicates a significant undertreatment of pain in those with cognitive impairments.

Pain assessment in cognitively impaired older adults, which is necessary for appropriate pain management, can be a difficult task for nurses. The disease processes associated with dementia and cognitive impairments interfere with the patient's ability to interpret the pain stimulus through the step of perception in the pain pathway. The affective response to the pain sensation that occurs in both the perception and modulation phases is affected by this central nervous system damage (Scherder et al., 2005). Although difficult, it is possible to attain a comprehensive pain assessment in older adults with cognitive impairment with the right information and the right tools.

According to the hierarchy of pain assessment principles, self-report is the gold standard for pain assessment, and all attempts should be made to obtain this self-report from the patient (McCaffery & Pasero, 1999). Patients with mild-to-moderate cognitive impairment often are able to provide an accurate self-report of pain. However, in advanced stages of cognitive disease, the ability to self-report decreases, and eventually self-reporting is no longer possible. When nurses cannot obtain a self-report, as with nonverbal older adults or those with cognitive impairments, they should take the following steps:

- Look for clues to the potential causes of pain.
- Observe the patient's behaviors.
- Obtain pertinent information about pain and behaviors from family members or caregivers.
- Attempt an analgesic trial.

If the nurse is not familiar with the cognitively impaired patient, information should be obtained from someone who does know him or her, such as a family member or caregiver. Always ask the patient to rate his or her pain (Table 28-2). The nurse must also search for potential causes of pain or discomfort. A thorough medical history should be gathered, with particular attention paid to conditions associated with chronic pain common in older persons (e.g., a history of arthritis, diabetic neuropathies, fibromyalgia, or low back pain). Note if the patient has a history of any musculoskeletal or neurologic disorders that could potentially be a cause of pain. Also, family members or caregivers should report any recent falls or other acute problems that could cause pain, such as urinary tract infections, skin tears or injuries, or bacterial infections (e.g., pneumonia), as well as chronic conditions.

After gathering information on potential causes of pain in the nonverbal older adult, the nurse must observe the patient's behaviors for any subtle changes and seek a surrogate report of pain and behavior or activity changes from family members or caregivers. Behavioral indicators of pain include facial expressions, verbalizations, vocalizations, body movements, an alteration in interpersonal interactions, or mental status changes (American Geriatric Society, 2002). Some behaviors are more obviously associated with pain (e.g., facial grimacing, moaning, groaning, or rubbing a suspected painful body part); others, however, have a more subtle association and may be labeled as behavioral disorders (e.g., agitation, restlessness, irritability, confusion, and combativeness), particularly when they occur with care activities or treatments. Changes in appetite, functional level, or usual activities also can be clues to pain. Thus, nurses need to document behaviors as well as changes in patterns that may be indicative of pain exacerbation.

Many pain assessment tools have been developed specifically for nonverbal older adults with dementia. A recent review of 14 tools recommended the Pain Assessment in Advanced Dementia (PAINAD) for daily assessments and the Pain Assessment Checklist for Seniors with Limited Ability to Communicate (PACSLAC) for baseline and follow-up assessments in long-term care settings (Herr, Bursch, Ersek, Miller, & Swafford, 2010). Nurses can find up-to-date information about pain assessment tools for nonverbal older adults at http://thePoint.lww.com/Miller6e.

Finally, nurses should attempt an analgesic trial to investigate any changes in behavior or activity that are thought to result from pain. Using data collected during a comprehensive pain assessment, the nurse estimates the intensity of pain and selects an appropriate analgesic based on the principles of analgesic medication discussed in the following section. For example, acetaminophen 500 to 1000 mg every 8 hours may be an appropriate first step when mild-to-moderate pain is suspected in a patient with a history of mild osteoarthritis. If behaviors continue to indicate potential pain, it may be appropriate to begin low-dose opioids and titrate upward (increase the dose) as indicated, because these medications are effective in decreasing pain-related agitation (Manfredi et al., 2003).

PRINCIPLES OF ANALGESIC MEDICATION

The rapid pace of change in the world of analgesic development makes it difficult to maintain proficiency in pain management medications unless one specializes in this field. However, if nurses have a basic understanding of the principles

TABLE 28-2 Principles of Pain Assessment in Older Adults With Cognitive Impairment

Principle	Steps to Achieve in Pain Assessment
Know the person	• Develop a relationship with the patient • Include family members or caregivers in obtaining history of the patient's painful conditions and behavior or activity changes
Ask the person	• Always assume the person can communicate with you and understand a rating scale • If at first you don't succeed, try, try again • Use the same words they use: "hurting," "uncomfortable," "sore," "tender," "achy," etc. • Try asking, "Are you comfortable?" • Gently touch the suspected painful area and ask again about the specific site • Document and communicate with the health care team what works and what language is used by the person
Use multiple resources	• Review the chart for a current or past history of painful diagnoses • Talk with direct caregivers • Talk with family and close friends • Communicate with other nurses, pharmacists, and physical and occupational therapists
Individualize pain care plans	Include the following: • Pain-related diagnoses • Pain-related medication use and bowel care • Unique expressions of pain • Unique expressions of comfort • Individualized strategies for promoting comfort and reducing pain
Promote comfort	Take the following steps during pain assessment: • Ask for assistance from caregivers • Use warm supplies • Keep the person warm and covered • Provide timely warnings • Maximize the person's control • Respond to evidence of pain with sincere apology and reassurance
Prevent discomfort	Ensure the following during pain assessment: • Toileting and personal hygiene needs are met • Clothing is slightly oversized and not restrictive, and shoes fit well (not rubbing on toes) • Movement and seating are conducted with great care to avoid any sudden or jarring movements that could initiate pain

Copyright 2005, Casey Shillam. Used with permission.

of analgesic medication administration, and learn a few medications well, they will know where to go to find more specific information about developing complex pain management regimens. This section presents the basic information needed for understanding the administration of analgesics, covers medication cautions specific to older adults, discusses the issues surrounding fear of addiction and side effects, and provides some disease-specific treatment recommendations.

Classifications of Analgesics

Analgesics are divided into three different groups: nonopioids, opioids, and adjuvants. The term *narcotic* has become obsolete and should not be used in clinical practice because the media and general population apply the term to substances that have the potential for abuse, such as cocaine, that

actually have no analgesic properties. The terms **nonopioid** and **opioid** **analgesics** should be used in place of *nonnarcotic* and *narcotic*.

Nonopioid analgesics include acetaminophen; nonaspirin, nonsteroidal anti-inflammatory drugs (NSAIDs); and aspirin. Nonopioids act at the site of the injury to decrease pain; NSAIDs, for example, inhibit the release of prostaglandin from damaged cells. Opioid analgesics are natural, semisynthetic, or synthetic drugs that relieve pain by binding to multiple types of opioid receptors in the central nervous system. As a result of this action, the release of neurotransmitters is blocked and the pain impulse cannot cross the synapse into the dorsal horn during the transmission phase of the pain pathway. Examples of opioids are codeine, morphine, tramadol, fentanyl, and methadone. **Adjuvant analgesics** are medications that have a primary indication other than the treatment of pain, such as an antidepressants or anticonvulsants, but relieve pain in some conditions. Adjuvants most often act on the modulation phase of the pain pathway by interfering with the reuptake of serotonin and norepinephrine, which inhibit the transmission of nociceptive impulses. All three groups are effective in the perception phase, acting in different ways to decrease the conscious experience of pain perception.

The World Health Organization's Three-Step Pain Relief Ladder for Pain Management

The AGS has endorsed the use of the World Health Organization's (WHO) pain relief ladder as a guide for the treatment of persistent pain in older adults (American Geriatric Society, 2002). Nurses can apply this approach for selecting analgesics on the basis of the intensity of the pain, using analgesics from each of the three different classifications, and building on previously effective treatments. The three steps of the WHO's pain relief ladder (Figure 28-3) address different levels of pain intensity, and also allow for the fact that not all people experience pain in the same way along the same trajectory. Therefore, tailoring therapeutic regimens to individual needs is considered the gold standard of pain management for older adults (American Geriatric Society, 2002). Based on this AGS guideline, treatment does not necessarily begin at Step 1 and progress sequentially. For example, it may be appropriate to begin at Step 3 or titrate more rapidly for an older adult who is experiencing excruciating pain.

Step 1 of the WHO pain relief ladder addresses mild pain (i.e., ranging from 1 to 3 out of 10 on an NRS) by recommending the use of nonopioid analgesics initially, with the addition of an adjuvant if it is deemed appropriate. Although

nonopioids are generally viewed as having fewer risks of side effects than opioids, this misconception is a dangerous one. The use of NSAIDs poses many serious side effects for older adults because they can cause significant end-organ toxicity. Thousands of hospitalizations occur annually as a result of gastric bleeding caused by these drugs. Excessive use of NSAIDs can also result in renal insufficiency, decreased platelet aggregations, and even death. Acetaminophen is often considered a "safe" alternative to NSAIDs because it is a very effective analgesic with few side effects and does not cause problems with the stomach, kidneys, or platelets. However, the most common side effect associated with the overuse of acetaminophen is a deadly one: hepatotoxicity. It is important to recognize that the recommended ceiling dose for acetaminophen (i.e., 4 g daily) is for *healthy individuals* with no previous liver or metabolic complications. *Extreme caution* must be taken with older adults using any nonopioid medication. Levels of acetaminophen must also be carefully monitored if an older adult is using a combination medication (an opioid plus acetaminophen) for breakthrough pain because levels greater than the safe maximum can easily be reached. This principle is critically important for patient teaching because older adults may not realize that many over-the-counter products (e.g., arthritis pain relievers, Tylenol PM) contain acetaminophen that must be factored into the daily maximum dose.

If the pain continues to be in the mild-to-moderate range (e.g., it worsens from a 3 to a 5 of 10 on an NRS), and is not adequately relieved by the use of a nonopioid, then Step 2 suggests adding a weak opioid, or opioid combination, to the regimen. This step *builds on* the previous one; it does not replace the use of the Step 1 nonopioid analgesics. Step 2 should also include a method of providing around-the-clock analgesia by using a breakthrough medication. For example, a patient would take acetaminophen 500 mg every 6 hours and use one tablet of Percocet (i.e., 5 mg oxycodone plus 325 mg acetaminophen) every 4 hours as needed for breakthrough pain. This combination of acetaminophen and Percocet contains only half the maximum recommended dose of acetaminophen for older adults.

If the pain persists or worsens (i.e., ranging from 7 to 10 on an NRS), the interventions in Step 3 should be considered. Although both Steps 2 and 3 include the use of an opioid, different types of opioids are used in each step. Because Step 2 opioid drugs (e.g., Lortab 5/500, Tylenol #3, or Percocet) include fixed doses of acetaminophen, the extent to which these opioids can be used is limited by the recommended maximum daily dose of acetaminophen for older adults. Thus, the use of stronger opioids is the appropriate next step. Step 3 builds on Steps 1 and 2, with the continued use of nonopioids and adjuvants. Opioid use in Step 3 must be scheduled around the clock and still include some type of breakthrough pain medication. Opioids prescribed for breakthrough pain should also have a short half-life so that they can be rapidly titrated for severe pain episodes. Opioids for around-the-clock administration should be delivered in a controlled-release formula, ensuring that the administration rate remains constant.

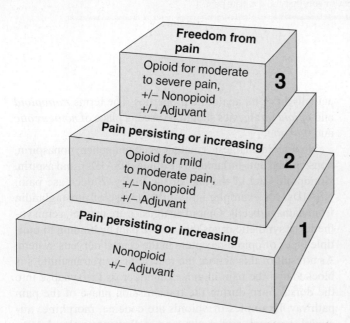

FIGURE 28-3 World Health Organization pain relief ladder. (Copyright 2005, World Health Organization. Redrawn with permission.)

Management of Side Effects and Risks of Tolerance, Dependence, and Addiction

Because the fear of side effects and addiction is one of the greatest barriers to effective pain management in older adults, nurses may need to address this fear appropriately when developing a pain management regimen. In addition, side effects, especially constipation, are often limiting and potentially quite dangerous. All potential side effects of medications must be addressed in the plan, and the patient must be reassured that most side effects can be managed safely. When nurses care for patients who are taking opioid analgesics, they must incorporate a regimen for maintaining bowel function in the care plan because constipation is an expected side effect that should be dealt with proactively. Constipation, which occurs in up to 95% of patients treated with opioids, is caused by a slowing down of peristalsis and a decreased urge to defecate (Lentz & McMillan, 2010). Although medication **tolerance** can be considered a physiologic protective mechanism that helps the body become accustomed to the medication so that adverse effects gradually diminish, this mechanism does not extend to constipation. Therefore, the risk will not diminish, and in fact can increase. Box 28-4 summarizes a recommended regimen for maintaining bowel function in people taking opioid analgesics.

Nurses need to teach patients and their families about the differences between tolerance, **dependence**, and addiction to help them understand that the risk of addiction is minimal and the effective management of pain can improve quality of life and decrease the negative sequelae of unmanaged pain. Many older adults fear addiction to opioids, and many of their family members may stigmatize the use of opioids. Tolerance to and dependence on opioids are not the same as addiction to opi-

> **Box 28-4 Recommendations for Maintaining Bowel Function in Patients Taking Opioid Medications**
>
> **Points to Remember**
> - *Tolerance* is your ally with regard to all side effects except constipation.
> - The hand that writes the opioid order should also write the bowel regimen order.
> - Constipation is an expected adverse effect that should be dealt with from the start.
>
> **Before Requesting a Laxative**
> - Rule out other causes of constipation.
> - Do not give laxatives if abdominal pain is present.
> - Reassess daily for responses.
>
> **A Bowel Program Can Include**
> - Senna = docusate tablets (Senokot-S)
> - Lactulose
> - Bisacodyl (Dulcolax)
> - Magnesium hydroxide (milk of magnesia)
> - Nonpharmacologic remedy: daily administration of a fruit paste (including such ingredients as senna tea leaves, prunes, raisins, or figs)

> **A Student's Perspective**
>
> *My aging client complains periodically about pain in her shoulder. She has stated that she does not want to take anything besides aspirin when she has pain and that aspirin seems to take care of her pain. She does not take the aspirin every day. She's afraid of taking pain medications because she does not want to rely on strong medications and she is afraid of becoming addicted. I explained to her the consequences of untreated pain and also tried to ease her fears of pain medication. She assured me that she will see her physician if the pain becomes severe when aspirin does not help her.*
>
> *Thelma M.*

oids, but the three terms are often confused. The APS defines tolerance as a pharmacodynamic response at the neurophysiologic level due to chronic drug administration (Gordon et al., 2005). Tolerance is manifested by a decrease in one or more therapeutic effects of the medication (e.g., less analgesia) or its side effects (e.g., sedation, respiratory depression, or nausea). Tolerance should be viewed as a descriptive term that refers to a change in the relationship between the therapeutic effect and the dose, not as a negative label implying addictive behavior. Dependence is defined as a physiologic phenomenon manifested by the development of withdrawal symptoms on sudden discontinuation of the medication. The best approach to withdrawal symptoms is to reduce the dose gradually, rather than abruptly discontinuing the drug. Again, physical dependence does not indicate the presence of addiction; rather, it means that the patient depends on the treatment to live, much as a person with hypothyroidism is physically dependent on thyroid replacement to survive, but is not addicted to thyroid replacement. This distinction should be made very clear to the patient and the family.

In contrast to dependence and tolerance, addiction is a *psychological* dependence on the medication (Gordon et al., 2005). Addiction is no longer narrowly defined in relation to the symptoms of withdrawal; instead, it is described according to the following three behavioral characteristics:
- Compulsive use of the drug
- Loss of control over the use of the drug
- Use of the drug in spite of harm.

Based on this definition, it is clear that the continued use of opioids for pain relief does not indicate addiction, regardless of the dose or length of time the person has been using the medication.

Developing a Wellness-Focused Pain Management Plan

Although the management of pain in older adults is complex, principles of wellness focus on developing a comprehensive and individualized pain management care plan based on the assessment. Nursing interventions for managing pain depend on the nature of the pain (acute vs. persistent) as well as on the patient's personal experiences and preferences. Incorporating wellness approaches to the care of this population includes the patient as a partner in decision making and planning.

Principles for wellness when responding to acute pain include consideration of preemptive analgesia before surgical procedures, use of multimodal analgesic therapies by combining analgesics with different mechanisms of action to decrease overall doses of individual medications and reduce adverse events, and administering analgesics by alternate routes such as by transdermal mechanisms instead of oral, intramuscular, or intravenous routes (Polomano, 2008). Nonpharmacologic approaches are also effective for managing acute pain. Meditation, acupuncture, and therapeutic touch have all shown positive effects in acute pain management (Morone, Lynch, Greco, Tindle, & Weiner, 2008; Monroe, 2009; Madsen, Gotzsche, & Hrobjartsson, 2009).

These principles of wellness can also be applied to the older adult with persistent pain. Meditation, acupuncture, and therapeutic touch are effective not only for managing acute pain but also for persistent pain (Morone et al., 2008; Monroe, 2009; Madsen et al., 2009). A review of studies found that energy-healing modalities (i.e., Reiki, therapeutic touch, and healing touch) are effective as an adjunct to traditional treatment approaches to decrease the amount of pain medicine required or increase the time between dosages of narcotic analgesics (Fazzino, Griffin, McNulty, & FitzPatrick, 2010). In addition, the use of nature-related visual distraction (pictures and videos of nature) and audio stimuli (nature sounds or music) has demonstrated reduction in pain (Kline, 2009).

Self-care strategies are an important aspect of wellness-oriented care for older adults with chronic pain. One exemplary program for improving pain management in long-term care, called the Campaign Against Pain, empowers residents by teaching them about self-management interventions to help with pain management (Long et al., 2010). Another program found that older adults could learn mind–body interventions for self-care pain management by using online modules (Berman, Iris, Bode, & Drengenberg, 2009).

When adding analgesic medication into the wellness approach to pain management, nurses need to communicate with other members of the health care team to formulate a plan that clearly establishes and addresses the patient's pain goals, anticipated side effects, and proposed interventions for those side effects. Patients and designated family members are included as members of the decision-making team. Key points include working closely with all members of the interdisciplinary team; recognizing that prescribers, such as nurses, have their own values, beliefs, and potential biases about pain; approaching the prescriber as a colleague with mutual goals for the patient; and documenting objectively and frequently to establish evidence and validate requests. Also, proposed interventions should be based on evidence-based guidelines (i.e., the WHO pain relief ladder) and should include nonpharmacologic interventions, when appropriate. Although nurses cannot be expected to know

TABLE 28-3 Managing Pain in Older Adults With Common Chronic Conditions			
Type of Pain	**Characteristics of Pain**	**Nonpharmacologic Treatments**	**Pharmacologic Treatments**
Persistent back pain	• Difficult to manage • Up to 85% of back pain has no obvious etiology • Often more than one etiology	• Cognitive–behavioral therapy • Physical therapy • Yoga	• NSAIDs with caution for GI bleeds • Opioids in conjunction with nonpharmacologic methods • Adjuvant analgesics, such as tricyclic antidepressants in patients also diagnosed with depression
Osteoporosis pain	• Intensifies with sitting or standing and is relieved by bed rest • Exacerbated by sudden movements • May be an indirect consequence of multiple vertebral compression fractures	• Instructed stretching • Bed rest and bracing (for acute pain) • Rehabilitative physical therapy • Supportive pillows • Ice massage • Patient education • Social support	• NSAIDs with caution for GI bleeding • Opioid–nonopioid combination with short-acting opioids, or controlled-release opioids, with caution because sedation can increase risk of falls and fractures • Opioid-induced constipation can lead to straining, thereby increasing risk of osteoporotic fractures; carefully titrate dosage and prescribe a laxative
Osteoarthritis pain	• Characterized as deep, aching, poorly localized • Usual sites of involvement are the interphalangeal joints, lumbar and cervical spine, and weight-bearing joints	• Exercise • Weight control • Rest • Joint care	• Acetaminophen has been shown to relieve pain as effectively as NSAIDs for many patients with osteoarthritis. • NSAIDs with caution for GI bleeding (although all NSAIDs work similarly, each has a different chemical compound with slightly different side effects) • Celecoxib (Celebrex), a COX-2 inhibitor, is still being prescribed although other COX-2 inhibitors have been taken off the market. • Topical pain-relieving creams, rubs, and sprays (e.g., capsaicin cream) • Corticosteroids

GI, gastrointestinal; NSAID, nonsteroidal anti-inflammatory drug.

all the implications of all analgesics, they can become experts on frequently used drugs and keep references handy for the rest. Finally, nurses can develop expertise in nonpharmacologic interventions, which can often be the most effective and comforting interventions for patients. For specific recommendations for managing pain in some common chronic conditions, see Table 28-3.

Chapter Highlights

Acute Versus Persistent Pain

- Two commonly accepted definitions of pain are (1) an unpleasant sensory and emotional experience associated with actual or potential tissue damage and (2) whatever the person experiencing it says it is existing whenever she or he says it does.
- Acute pain is time-limited and responsive to analgesics, whereas persistent pain continues for a prolonged period and may or may not be associated with a recognizable disease process.

Anatomy and Physiology of Pain

- Nociception, which is the physiologic occurrence of a measurable pain signal, involves the four processes of transduction, transmission, perception, and modulation (Figure 28-1).

Types of Pain

- Pain can be classified as nociceptive or neuropathic pain; nociceptive pain is further classified as either somatic or visceral pain.
- Cancer pain is a complex phenomenon in which pain can be acute, persistent, nociceptive, or neuropathic.

Causes of Pain in Older Adults

- For 80% to 85% of people aged 65 years and older, a significant health problem is associated with pain.

Age-Related Changes That Affect Pain

- Age-related changes can affect pain perception and pain management, and pain symptoms may present differently in older and younger adults.

Barriers to Pain Management

- Nurses need to identify and address problems that create barriers to effective pain management in older adults (Table 28-1).

Functional Consequences of Pain in Older Adults

- The functional consequences of pain in older adults include diminished physical function, loss of mobility, higher levels of disability, and decreased quality of life.
- Untreated pain can lead to anxiety, depression, or even suicide.

Nursing Assessment of Pain in Older Adults

- Nurses need to assess factors that can worsen or improve pain for older adults (Box 28-1).

- Nurses can base their assessment of pain in older a... on certain assumptions (Box 28-2).
- Box 28-3 summarizes sample questions for pain assessment.
- Nurses need to apply specific principles of pain assessment for older adults who are cognitively impaired (Table 28-2).
- Figure 28-2 illustrates some of the commonly used pain scales that are applicable to assessing pain in older adults.

Principles of Analgesic Medication

- Principles of analgesic administration are outlined in the World Health Organization's pain relief ladder (Figure 28-3) and applied to some common chronic conditions in Table 28-3.
- Nurses need to address adverse effects of analgesics, with particular attention to maintaining bowel function (Box 28-4).
- Nurses need to teach patients and their families about the differences between tolerance, dependence, and addiction.

Critical Thinking Exercises

1. Identify an older person in your recent clinical experience who has talked with you about persistent pain and address the following in relation to that person:
   - What factors listed in Box 28-1 affect the person's experience of pain?
   - What assumptions from Box 28-2 are applicable to assessment of pain in that person?
2. Review the barriers to effective pain management related to patients and families (Table 28-1) and identify ways in which you could overcome these barriers when you care for older adults in clinical practice.
3. Review the information about tolerance, dependence, and addiction and write a sentence for each of these concepts in terms that you could use for teaching older adults and their caregivers.

Resources

For links to these resources and additional helpful Internet resources related to this chapter, visit thePoint at http://thePoint. lww.com/Miller6e.

Clinical Tools

American Journal of Nursing and Hartford Institute for Geriatric Nursing
- *How to Try This,* article and video: Flaherty, E. (2008). Using pain-rating scales with older adults. *American Journal of Nursing, 108*(6), 40–47.
- *How to Try This,* article and video: Horgas, A., & Miller, L. (2008). Pain assessment in people with dementia. *American Journal of Nursing, 108*(7), 62–70.

City of Hope, Pain Resource Center
Hartford Institute for Geriatric Nursing
- *Try This: Best Practices in Nursing Care to Older Adults* Issue 7 (2007), Pain Assessment for Older Adults Issue D2 (2007), Assessing Pain in Persons With Dementia Issue SP1 (2010), Assessment of Nociceptive Versus Neuropathic Pain in Older Adults

Evidence-Based Practice

National Guideline Clearinghouse

Health Education

American Pain Foundation
American Society for Pain Management Nursing
Foundation for Health in Aging
Partners Against Pain

REFERENCES

Al-Atiyyat, N. M. H. (2009). Cultural diversity and cancer pain. *Journal of Hospice and Palliative Nursing, 11*, 154–164.

American Geriatric Society. (2002). The management of persistent pain in older persons. *Journal of the American Geriatrics Society, 50*(6, Suppl.), S205–S224.

Berman, R. L. H., Iris, M. A., Bode, R., & Drengenberg, C. (2009). The effectiveness of an online mind-body intervention for older adults with chronic pain. *The Journal of Pain, 10*, 68–79.

Dumas, L. G., & Ramadurai, M. (2009). Pain management in the nursing home. *Nurse Clinicians of North America, 44*, 197–208.

Eggermont, L. H., Bean, J. F., Guralnik, J. M., & Leveille, S. G. (2009). Comparing pain severity versus pain location in the MOBILIZE Boston study. *Journal Gerontology: Biological Sciences and Medical Sciences, 64*, 763–770.

Fazzino, D., Griffin, M. T. Q., McNulty, S. R., & FitzPatrick, J. J. (2010). Energy healing and pain. *Holistic Nursing Practice, 24*, 79–88.

Gordon, D. B., Dahl, J. L., Miaskowski, C., McCarberg, B., Todd, K. H., Paice, J. A., . . . Carr, D. B., (2005). American pain society recommendations for improving the quality of acute and cancer pain management: American Pain Society Quality of Care Task Force. *Archives of Internal Medicine, 165*(14), 1574–1580.

Herr, K., Bursch, J., Ersek, M., Miller, L. L., & Swafford, K. (2010). Use of pain-behavioral assessment tools in the nursing home: Expert consensus recommendations for practice. *Journal of Gerontological Nursing, 36*(3), 18–29.

Kline, G. A. (2009). Does a view of nature promote relief from acute pain? *Journal of Holistic Nursing, 27*(3), 159–166.

Lentz, J., & McMillan, S. C. (2010). The impact of opioid-induced constipation in patients near the end of life. *Journal of Hospice and Palliative Nursing, 12*, 29–38.

Long, C. O., Morgan, B. M., Alonzo, T. R., Mitchell, K. M., Bonnell, D. K., & Beardsleay, M. E. (2010). Improving pain management in long-term care. *Journal of Hospice and Palliative Nursing, 12*, 148–155.

Madsen, M. V., Gotzsche, P. C., & Hrobjartsson, A. (2009). Acupuncture treatment for pain: Systematic review of randomized clinical trials with acupuncture, placebo acupuncture, and no acupuncture groups. *British Medical Journal, 338*, 330–338. doi:10.1136/bmj.a3115.

Manfredi, P., Breuer, B., Wallenstein, S., Stegmann, M., Bottomley, G., & Libow, L. (2003). Opioid treatment for agitation in patients with advanced dementia. *International Journal of Geriatric Psychiatry, 18*(8), 700–705.

McCaffery, M., & Pasero, C. (1999). Assessment. Underlying complexities, misconceptions, and practical tools. In M. McCaffery & C. Pasero (Eds.), *Pain: clinical manual* (2nd ed., pp. 35–102). St. Louis, MO: Mosby.

McCaffrey, M. (1968). *Nursing practice theories related to cognition, bodily pain and man-environmental interactions.* Los Angeles, CA: UCLA Students Store.

Monroe, C. M. (2009). The effects of therapeutic touch on pain. *Journal of Holistic Nursing, 27*(2), 85–92.

Morone, N. E., Lynch, C. S., Greco, C. M., Tindle, H. A., & Weiner, D. K. (2008). "I felt like a new person." The effects of mindfulness meditation on older adults with chronic pain: Qualitative narrative analysis of diary entries. *The Journal of Pain, 9*(9), 841–848.

Narayan, M. C. (2010). Culture's effects on pain assessment and management. *American Journal of Nursing, 110*(4), 38–47.

Planton, J., & Edlund, B. J. (2010). Regulatory components for treating persistent pain in long-term care. *Journal of Gerontological Nursing, 36*(4), 49–56.

Polomano, R. C., Dunwoody, C. J., Krenzischek, D. A., & Rathmell, J. P. (2008). Perspective on pain management in the 21st century. *Pain Management Nursing, 9*(1), S3–S10.

Polomano, R. C., Rathmell, J. P., Krenzischek, D. A., & Dunwoody, C. J. (2008). Emerging trends and new approaches to acute pain management. *Pain Management Nursing, 9*(1), S33–S41.

Reynolds, K. S., Hanson, L. C., DeVellis, R. F., Henderson, M., & Steinhauser, K. E. (2008). Disparities in pain management between cognitively intact and cognitively impaired nursing home residents. *Journal of Pain and Symptom Management, 35*(4), 388–396.

Rustoen, T., Wahl, A. K., Hanestad, B. R., Lerdal, A., Paul, S., & Miaskowski, C. (2005). Age and the experience of chronic pain: Differences in health and quality of life among younger, middle-aged, and older adults. *Clinical Journal of Pain, 21*(6), 513–523.

Scherder, E., Oosterman, J., Swaab, D., Herr, K., Ooms, M., Ribbe, M., . . . Benedetti, F. (2005). Recent developments in pain in dementia. *British Medical Journal, 330*, 461–464.

Schuler, M., Njoo, N., Hestermann, M., Oster, P., & Hauer, K. (2004). Acute and chronic pain in geriatrics: Clinical characteristics of pain and the influence of cognition. *Pain Medicine, 5*(3), 253–262.

Shipton, E. A., & Tait, B. (2005). Flagging the pain: Preventing the burden of chronic pain by identifying and treating risk factors in acute pain. *European Journal of Anaesthesiology, 22*(6), 405–412.

Tsai, P., & Means, K. M. (2005). Osteoarthritic knee or hip pain: Possible indicators in elderly adults with cognitive impairment. *Journal of Gerontological Nursing, 31*(8), 39–45.

CHAPTER 29

Caring for Older Adults at the End of Life

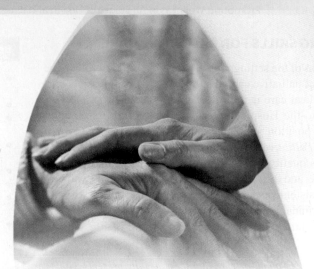

LEARNING OBJECTIVES

After reading this chapter, you will be able to:

1. Identify factors that influence attitudes toward death.
2. Describe cultural and historical approaches to end-of-life care.
3. Explain the nurse's role in end-of-life care.
4. Identify the common characteristics of "quality of life" and a "good death."
5. Describe palliative care and hospice nursing.
6. Assess physical, psychological, social, and spiritual care needs for older adults at the end of life.
7. Identify appropriate nursing interventions to address symptoms commonly experienced by older adults at the end of life.

KEY POINTS

death
death with dignity
dying
end of life
hospice

medicalization
palliation
rehumanizing
spiritual well-being

Because of the dramatic increases in life expectancy and the trend toward living longer with chronic conditions, there has been increasing interest in and emphasis on end-of-life care. Advances in medical knowledge and technology have shifted the focus of care to prolonging and sustaining life because many illnesses that once were fatal (e.g., cancer, cardiovascular disease) are now chronic conditions. Because of these changes, health care providers focus not only on preventing and curing disease but also on managing chronic illness and promoting quality of life. For people in the terminal stages of an illness, the focus of health care is on optimal comfort and quality of life for people who are dying and for their families. In older adults, **death** is usually associated with the cumulative effects of chronic illness and many interacting conditions, rather than a single cause.

THE DYING PROCESS AND DEATH

Although life and death appear to be clear concepts, the lack of an exact definition of the terms *life*, **dying**, and *death* can at times cloud the goals of care. According to the American Geriatrics Society's (AGS's) position statement on *The Care of Dying Patients* (AGS, 2002), birth and death give definition to life as the period of time in between. Death is an irreversible lifeless state in which the physiologic functions of life are absent. Dying is regarded as a less specific, individualized process in which an organism's life comes to an end (i.e., the final portion of the life cycle). When does the dying process begin? People are considered to be dying when they are ill with a progressive condition that is expected to end in death and for which there is no treatment that can substantially alter the outcome (AGS, 2002). The length of the dying process varies and depends on the individual's holistic situation. Its duration may be a matter of minutes, hours, weeks, or months.

The **end of life** is the period for patients when "there is little likelihood of cure for their disease(s); further aggressive therapy is judged to be futile; and comfort is the primary goal" (Wilke & TNEEL Investigators, 2003, p. 9). This period can last from hours to months, and it encompasses the time during which a person is actively dying. **Palliation** is defined as "the relief of suffering when cure is impossible" (Wilke & TNEEL Investigators, 2003, p. 41). Palliative care is an evolving professional specialization, defined by the Robert Wood Johnson Foundation Last Acts Task Force (2002) as the "comprehensive management of the physical, psychological, social, spiritual, and existential needs of patients, particularly those with incurable, progressive illness. The goal of palliative care is to help patients achieve the best possible quality of life through minimizing suffering, controlling symptoms, and restoring functional capacity, while remaining sensitive to personal, cultural, and religious values, beliefs, and practices."

NURSING SKILLS FOR PALLIATIVE CARE

Regardless of the setting, nurses take on a primary role in the delivery of palliative care at a time in which aggressive, curative medical care is no longer feasible or appropriate. According to the Hospice and Palliative Nurses Association (HPNA) position statement on the *Value of Professional Nurse in Palliative Care*, nurses have long advocated for attention to quality of life throughout the lifespan, including end of life, and they are the healthcare professionals who provide consistent presence to patients and families who are facing terminal illness (HPNA, 2008). The position statement describes nursing skills for effective end-of-life care as follows:

> *Advanced terminal or chronic illness usually presents with not one, but multiple and often complex symptoms that affect the body, mind, and spirit of the patient. These symptoms require the professional nurse to employ highly trained skills and provide holistic care that is consistent with the goals of the patient and family . . . . Competent, patient-centered nursing practice for palliative care includes expert assessment skills, critical thinking, comprehensive pain and symptom management of the whole patient, effective communication skills, and a professional knowledge base to support ethical decision making. These are the skills that patients and families value highly as death approaches. HPNA (2008, p.1)*

PERSPECTIVES ON DEATH AND DYING

During the last hundred years, society witnessed significant change in the perception and management of death. Before the 20th century, death was more readily accepted as an inevitable and normal part of life. Illness and death were family centered, with care provided by family members in their homes. As health care became more sophisticated, a shift occurred. Hospital-based care provided by physicians, nurses, and other professionals replaced the family caregiving model. This **medicalization** of end-of-life care has had a major impact on the dying experience in the last three to four decades: end-of-life experiences in formal health care facilities are often technologically driven and dehumanized (Saunderson & Brener, 2007).

Nursing is a leading force in the palliative care movement—a natural fit given the holistic tradition of the profession. In the past two to three decades, as **hospice** has grown, so has a realization that the end of life can be positively affected by returning to basics. Goals are slowly refocusing on comfort, companionship, and caring, with nurses in a pivotal role. This **rehumanizing** of death and dying recognizes and respects the process as an important and meaningful stage of the continuum of human life. Box 29-1 presents strategies for rehumanizing death.

Sites of Death and Dying

Since the beginning of the 20th century, when most people died in their homes, the place of death gradually shifted, so

---

Box 29-1 Strategies for Rehumanizing Death

- Reintroduce a peaceful sense of harmony between dying people and the process of dying.
- Provide the support of community participation in dying rituals.
- Support the harmonious acceptance of death as ordinary and natural, not a social evil.
- Emphasize the comforting roles of fellowship, ritual, and ceremony.
- Facilitate, even mandate, the notion that dying should be a culturally shared community experience.
- Culturally legitimize the pain and suffering that often accompanies dying.
- Provide a common base of participation and sense of belonging; attach the dying person to the community of living.

Source: Saunderson, C. A., & Brener, T. H. (Eds.). (2007). *End of life: A nurse's guide to compassionate care* (p. 281). Philadelphia, PA: Lippincott Williams & Wilkins.

---

that by the 1990s, only 20% of people died at home or in noninstitutional settings. However, that trend is reversing, and in 1999, 25% of deaths occurred in private homes (Wilke & TNEEL Investigators, 2003). According to the report by the Robert Wood Johnson Foundation Last Acts Task Force (2002), a national coalition to improve care and caring near the end of life, 50% of Americans aged 65 years and older die in hospitals, although more than 70% state their desire to die at home. The deaths are often preceded by multiple physician visits and expensive life-prolonging treatments.

Studies indicate that between 24% and 30% of deaths among older Americans occur in long-term care facilities (Munn et al., 2008; Menec, Nowicki, Blandford, & Veselyuk, 2009). A national nursing home survey found that the number of hospice patients receiving care in nursing homes has been increasing significantly in recent years (Bercovitz, Decker, Jones, & Remsburg, 2008). Concerns have been raised about end-of-life care in nursing facilities. For example, Menec et al. (2009) found that unnecessary and inappropriate hospitalizations of long-term care residents close to the end of life are common and have a particularly negative impact.

Views of Death and Dying in Western Culture

As a result of many interacting factors, Western culture has tended to deny or ignore the universality of death. During the last several decades, responsibility for the dying experience has been informally and more exclusively delegated to clinicians, with a majority of deaths occurring in hospitals. In health care settings, physicians are usually the major decision makers because of their medical expertise. Many older adults revere physician suggestions and recommendations for treatment, even though they do not always fully understand the issues, options, or potential consequences. Older adults are often reluctant to question physicians, and they may set aside their personal values, ideas, and wishes to follow the advice of their doctor. Consequently, they may not explore their options of dying in places other than hospitals or institutional settings.

In studies of social gerontology, Markson (2003) identified the following four contemporary societal values or beliefs that shape the general outlook on aging and death:

1. Work and activity are intertwined with self-worth, and chronic illness or disability is associated with the end of productivity and loss of purpose. Consequently, people may not acknowledge illness and aging because they are viewed as predecessors to death.

2. Through self-determination and individual responsibility, anyone can do anything if he or she tries hard enough. Because human life has inherent limitations, this false mentality is a major underpinning to the denial of aging and death in the 21st century.

3. Medical advances of the last several decades foster the belief that aging, illness, and even death can be manipulated, managed, and controlled.

4. Authority over and responsibility for death has subtly transferred from religious leaders to physicians. Consequently, the ability to cure illness and prolong life has imbued life and death with qualities that are more humanistic and less spiritual.

In some ways, society is more accepting of an older adult's death compared with that of a younger person. The rationale for this attitude is that older people have had an opportunity to "live their lives." Sometimes, death is viewed as a blessing, taking an older adult out of a situation of suffering and reduced capacity. Caregivers often express relief when death occurs, stating that "he wouldn't have wanted to live like this."

Despite these prevalent attitudes and beliefs, in the past 20 to 30 years, society in general has begun to culturally acknowledge and integrate an increasing acceptance of life's end. This change has been largely provoked by the baby boom generation facing its own aging process while simultaneously dealing with their parents' aging and health issues. Ethical questions and challenges have surfaced as a result of problems in care and rising associated costs. For example, in the midst of the assisted suicide debate, society has begun asking a second layer of questions: "What value is there in the last phase of life? Can there be any meaning and value in the process of dying? Can there be value in grieving? Can there be value in caring for people as they die?" (Byock, 2006). The changing demographics and increase in the numbers of older adults dying will be an impetus for continued discussion and changes in social policies.

Older Adults' Perspective on Death and Dying

How do older adults view death when mortality becomes imminent? Common stereotypes about old age contribute to the myth that older adults are ready to die because their lives have lost their value. These beliefs have been proven to be ageist. On the contrary, although studies have suggested that death anxiety decreases with advancing age, older adults' feelings about death vary according to individual social circumstances and life experiences (Markson, 2003). In spite of their chronologic years, many older adults have life goals they expect to fulfill; consequently, they are not ready to die.

> ### A Student's Perspective
>
> *This week, I learned that it is okay to accept that an elderly patient is ready to die and that is his/her wish. I had a patient who requested that we not perform any measures—just give him his beer with lunch, wine with dinner, and some pain medicine to make him comfortable. He stated that he has led a good life and is ready to go see God. That is really hard for me because it's my job to help people and save lives. The other aspect of that is helping people die a dignified death—it's just a really TOUGH aspect!!!*
>
> *Sarah E.*

Although younger generations may feel a sense of entitlement to a long life, many older adults hold the opposite view. They may be more accepting of the possibility of imminent death, viewing long life as a privilege. Young people tend to place life and death on opposite ends of the spectrum, and feel threatened and cheated by death because of the opportunity for living that is lost. From their vantage point, older adults more frequently view death as a natural part of life's continuum, and the process of dying as a period of self-actualization. Even though physical decline is a main theme of aging and dying, for many older adults, this time of life is one of growth and fulfillment. From this holistic perspective on death and dying, old age can be turned into an opportunity for development and death into an ultimate accomplishment.

Health Care Professionals' Perspective on Death and Dying

Health care facilities have been institutionally designed to be centers for disease care and disease cure. Given this orientation, practitioners and health care professionals often view death as something to be avoided because it symbolizes professional and personal incompetence or failure. Prolonging life, even at the expense of quality, was thought to be the ultimate accomplishment: a symbol of success for patients, families, and the health care teams involved.

In recent decades, palliative and end-of-life care have become part of the medical mainstream, and health care professionals realize they can find meaning and satisfaction in caring for people who are dying and their loved ones. As experts, professionals in the disciplines of hospice and palliative care play a key role in promoting awareness and understanding in this process of social, cultural, and professional maturation. Standards of care define and guide health professionals' practice to include clear communication, ethical decision making, technical competence, and intensive management of symptoms, respecting the dying individual's autonomy. The issue of quality of life versus quantity of life at all costs has redefined the professional perspective.

To provide effective end-of-life care, nurses need to examine their own feelings and attitudes, which may affect the care they provide. Personal beliefs about death are shaped by experiences from the time of birth, with the family as the primary influence. Religious affiliations, popular media and culture, and ethnic background contribute to one's reactions to death and dying. Whether death is discussed as part of normal life or whether it is seen as "the enemy" influences care. Nurses need to learn about clinical aspects of end-of-life care, and they must also take time to process their own feelings and concerns. Some questions to ponder for self-awareness and insight include the following (Ohio State University Health Sciences Center, 2003):

- When you hear the word "death," what comes to your mind? What do you personally fear the most? What are you most curious about?
- How old were you the first time someone close to you died? How was grief handled in your family? What do you believe happens to you when you die?
- Have you ever seen anyone die? What was that like for you?
- How do your own attitudes and previous experiences affect the way you work with dying patients now?

Because of the nature of their work as care providers, nurses are in an ideal position to serve primary roles in achieving quality end-of-life experiences for older adults.

Culturally Diverse Perspectives on Death and Dying

Nurses providing holistic care to older adults at the end of life need to recognize the effects of culture on the dying experience because cultural beliefs and practices are particularly influential with regard to end-of-life care (Hampton et al., 2010; Salman & Zoucha, 2010). Cultural factors can affect all the following aspects of end-of-life nursing care:

- Perceptions of a good death
- Acceptance of hospice and palliative care services
- Lines of communication about pending death and end-of-life decisions
- Expectations about medical interventions (e.g., decisions about resuscitation)
- Place where death occurs
- Practices and rituals near the end of death and immediately following death
- Decisions about autopsy or organ donations.

Because the experience of death and dying is very personal, nurses should incorporate cultural considerations into individualized assessments and be aware of diverse beliefs and attitudes associated with the experience of death and dying. Cultural Considerations Box 29-1 provides information about death rituals that are commonly associated with specific groups. It also suggests interventions that nurses can apply in different situations. As with other aspects of culturally appropriate care, nurses need to be aware of different practices that may be associated with particular groups; at the same time, they need to avoid stereotypes.

A Student's Perspective

I found myself in a situation today in which I quickly recognized the importance of the lesson on cultural sensitivity in nursing. My aging client unfortunately had a significant change over the weekend, and her husband requested for her to be transported to the hospice inpatient unit. As she and I sat on her bed, she verbalized her acceptance that her disease is terminal. She wept as she voiced her heartache in telling her family of her "disappointment." Even though she is Catholic, because of her Chinese heritage and her family's Buddhist belief in "saving face," she worries that she has let her family down. While she expressed her thoughts, I listened and provided emotional support, which seemed to ease some of her grief. We transported her to the hospice unit, and I assisted in making her comfortable with the new environment. When I went out to the nurses' station to give my report, the receiving nurse's first comment to me was, "I see she is Asian and you have her religious preference documented as Catholic. Are you sure that is correct?" Because of our recent discussions and reading on cultural sensitivity, I quickly realized how we as nurses can make incorrect assumptions in categorizing individuals based on their ethnicity. I reported about my client's childhood history, her parents' belief in Buddhism, the Catholicism she was taught in school, and her long and strong Catholic faith. I found myself really understanding the importance of educating ourselves as nurses about different cultures and the effect of cultural belief systems on individualized health care. As difficult as it was for me to leave my client in a strange environment, I felt that the information I had learned and shared would enable the staff to be respectful of her beliefs, which in turn would be a positive experience for my client during her stay.

Deborah L.

QUALITY OF CARE AT THE END OF LIFE

During the 1990s and early 2000s, reports from several major institutions—including the Institute of Medicine and the Robert Woods Johnson Foundation—identified serious problems with end-of-life care in the United States. These reports found that many people experienced discomfort and suffering from end-of-life symptoms because health care professionals did not possess the skills and knowledge required to meet the needs of a dying person. To address some of the problems, the Nathan Cummings Foundation and the Robert Wood Johnson Foundation developed the Toolkit of Instruments for Measuring End-of-life Care (TIME) to help health care professionals identify opportunities for improving care. The End of Life Nursing Education Consortium (ELNEC) is a major initiative to improve nursing care for people who are near the end of life. A recent study concluded that the ELNEC project has been tremendously successful in improving nursing knowledge at end of life during the past decade (Whitehead, Anderson, Redican, & Stratton, 2010). Information about these and other educational programs is listed in the Resources at the end of this chapter.

CULTURAL CONSIDERATIONS 29 - 1

Death Rituals Commonly Associated With Specific Groups

Group	Death Ritual	Intervention
African Americans	May respond to news of death of a loved one by *falling out* (i.e., sudden collapse, paralysis, and inability to see or speak).	Recognize that this is a culturally based response and not an emergency medical condition; provide support.
Amish Appalachians	Provide a wake-like "sitting up" during the night for seriously ill and dying family members.	Arrange for privacy and accommodate family members staying overnight.
Cubans, Filipinos, Mexicans	A large gathering of relatives and friends may attend the dying person and place religious artifacts around the person; candles are lit after death to illuminate the path of the spirit to the afterlife.	Arrange for a gathering place close to the dying person; find electric candles if open flames are not allowed; summon clergy for religious rituals; do not move religious items.
Europeans	Believe that the dying person should not be left alone.	Make accommodations for family members to be present at all times.
Haitians	Family members gather and pray when death is imminent and may cry uncontrollably; all family members try to be at the person's bedside at the time of death.	Make accommodations for privacy, encourage family to bring in religious objects, allow families to participate in postmortem care if they desire to do so.
Hindus, Indians	Priest and eldest son may perform death rites, with all male relatives assisting; women may respond with loud wailing.	Provide a supportive and private environment; offer understanding of death rituals and grief behaviors.
Japanese	Family members gather at the bedside at the time of death, with the eldest son having particular responsibilities at the time.	Notify eldest son of pending death, identify lines of communication if eldest son is not available.
Jews	Dying person should not be left alone; death rituals vary and some are not performed on the Sabbath or holy days.	Ask the closest relative specifically about postmortem practices.
Koreans	Family members are expected to stay with the person who is dying and assist with care.	Support family in caring for the person.
Mexicans	Some, especially women, may have an *ataque de nervios* (i.e., the person exhibits hyperkinetic and seizure-like activity to release strong emotions) on hearing of the death of a loved one.	Recognize that this is a culture-bound syndrome and treatment is usually not necessary; remain with the person, provide support, and involve family with assistance if possible.
Muslim groups	The bed should be turned to face the holy city of Mecca, family recites prayers from the Qur'an.	Facilitate positioning of the bed whenever possible, provide privacy for prayers.
Navajo Indians	It is taboo to talk about a fatal disease or dying; the issue needs to be discussed in the third person, as if it is occurring in someone else.	Avoid suggesting that someone is dying because this may be interpreted as a wish that the person be dead.
Puerto Ricans	Death is perceived as a time of crisis; the head of the family (i.e., usually the oldest daughter or son) is responsible for receiving the news of death.	Allow time for family to view, touch, and stay with the body before it is removed; ask if the family wants a clergy member called.
Vietnamese	Flowers are avoided during illness because they are usually reserved for rites of the dead.	Ask permission from the patient or family before placing flowers in a room.

Source: Purnell, L. D. (2009). *Culturally competent health care.* Philadelphia, PA: F. A. Davis.

Promoting Wellness at the End of Life

Wellness at the end of life is closely connected to the concept of a "good death," which has been described by Western societies as a **death with dignity**. A death with dignity is specifically characterized by a dying experience in which (Wilke & TNEEL Investigators, 2003):

- The patient's and family's wishes are respected.
- The patient and family feel a sense of control over the situation.
- The patient is physically comfortable.
- The patient is psychologically comfortable.
- The patient has spiritual support available according to her or his wishes.

These characteristics are in accord with the "Dying Patient's Bill of Rights," a document created at a workshop on "The Terminally Ill Patient and the Helping Person" by Linda Austin (1975) to identify concretely the dignified care that dying people deserve (Box 29-2). This document continues to be helpful as a fundamental guide for defining goals and interventions for individualized end-of-life care.

Box 29-2 The Dying Person's Bill of Rights

I have the right to be treated as a living human being until I die.

I have the right to maintain a sense of hopefulness, however, changing its focus may be.

I have the right to express my feelings and emotions about my approaching death in my own way.

I have the right to participate in decisions concerning my care.

I have the right to expect continuing medical and nursing attention even though cure goals must be changed to comfort goals.

I have the right not to die alone.

I have the right to be free from pain.

I have the right to have my questions answered honestly.

I have the right not to be deceived.

I have the right to have help from and for my family in accepting my death.

I have the right to die in peace and with dignity.

I have the right to retain my individuality and not be judged for my decisions, which may be contrary to the beliefs of others.

I have the right to be cared for by caring, sensitive, knowledgeable people who will attempt to understand my needs and will be able to gain some satisfaction in helping me face my death.

I have the right to be cared for by those who can maintain a sense of hopefulness, however, changing this might be.

I have the right to expect that the sanctity of the human body will be respected after death.

I have the right to discuss and enlarge my religious and/or spiritual experiences, whatever these may mean to others.

Source: Austin, L. (1975). *Dying patient's bill of rights.* Created at The Terminally Ill Patient and the Helping Person Workshops. Sponsored by the Southwest Michigan Inservice Education Council in Lansing, MI.

DIVERSITY NOTE

A study of 284 Muslims of 14 nationalities identified the following priorities as important components of a "good death": dignity, privacy, spiritual and emotional support, access to hospice care, ability to issue advance directives, and time to say goodbye (Tayeb, Al-Zamel, Fareed, & Aboueillail, 2010).

For many older adults, a "good death" is part of the process of "aging well," but both processes are very individualized and strongly influenced by cultural and spiritual factors. In the continuum of life, the experiences of aging, the end of life, and death are opportunities for self-actualization. Defining a "good death" for older adults is extremely personal and often dependent on the effects of aging and illness on the person's level of function and independence. The goal of nursing is to support this stage of life and help patients maintain optimal personal dignity.

Patient comfort, which has always been a core nursing responsibility, is an essential component of death with dignity. The word "patient" is derived from the Latin word *patiens*, which means "one who endures" or "one who suffers." The word "comfort" comes from the Latin *confortare*, which means "to strengthen." Literally, then, nurses who provide comfort to patients are strengthening those who suffer. This definition is particularly appropriate for nurses who provide care for patients at the end of life that is built on the following beliefs (Wilke & TNEEL Investigators, 2003):

- The dying are not people for whom "nothing can be done."
- Patients deserve to be assured that *everything* will be done to prevent them from dying in pain, without dignity.
- Patients will not die alone, isolated from those they love and who love them.

Hospice Care

Hospice refers to a philosophy of care that seeks to support dignified dying or a good death experience for those with terminal illnesses. Hospice care involves a core interdisciplinary team of professionals and volunteers who provide medical, psychological, and spiritual support as well as support for the patient's family. These services are provided by public and private agencies in home- or facility-based care settings, or in freestanding, short-term residential facilities.

The term *hospice* (from the same linguistic root as "hospitality") was first applied to specialized care for dying patients in the 1960s by physician and nurse Dame Cicely Saunders, who founded the first modern hospice—St. Christopher's—in a residential suburb of London. During a guest lecture for medical students, nurses, social workers, and chaplains at Yale University, Saunders introduced the idea of hospice care and emphasized holistic services and symptom control. This lecture sparked interest, which led to the development of hospice care as it is known today.

In 1969, psychiatrist Elisabeth Kübler-Ross published *On Death and Dying*. This book, based on interviews with dying patients, identified five stages through which many terminally ill patients progress: denial, anger, bargaining, depression, and acceptance (Kübler-Ross, 1969). The book was well received by all disciplines and drew attention to the needs of dying people. In 1972, Kübler-Ross testified at the first national hearings conducted by the U.S. Senate Special Committee on Aging, on the subject of death with dignity. In her testimony she stated,

A Student's Perspective

When I left the nursing home today I felt better about working with people facing the certain end of their lives. Mr. F. had a really positive attitude about his inoperable brain tumor and it made me understand that I am the one who feels uncomfortable with death. He expressed that his life has meaning and that he is here for a reason. He told me about some of his goals in life: he plans to get out of the nursing home so that he can travel around the country in an RV with his wife. He seemed to imply that even if that goal never occurred, it was OK, that it was mostly something to look forward to. All of the communication with Mr. F. had a huge impact on me. It gave me a whole new perspective on how people view their lives. This man is suffering from this terrible disease, yet he still finds hope and has goals in life.

Erin H.

We live in a very particular death-denying society. We isolate both the dying and the old, and it serves a purpose. They are reminders of our own mortality. We should not institutionalize people. We can give families more help with home care and visiting nurses, giving the families and the patients the spiritual, emotional, and financial help in order to facilitate the final care at home. National Hospice and Palliative Care Organization (NHPCO) (n.d.)

In 1982, Congress created a Medicare hospice benefit, which provided federal financial support to people dying of a terminal illness. Hospice benefits have become increasingly available and are now supported by many health insurance plans. Advantages of these services include the following:

- Hospice treats the person, not the disease; focuses on the family, not the individual; and emphasizes the quality of life, not the duration.
- Hospice care relies on the combined knowledge and skill of an interdisciplinary team of professionals, including physicians, nurses, home care aides, social workers, counselors, and volunteers.
- Hospice care is a cost-effective alternative to the high costs associated with hospitals and traditional institutional care.

Hospice eligibility criteria, which are defined by Medicare, require a physician referral, including a statement that a patient is terminally ill and has a life expectancy of 6 months or less. This requirement is problematic because it is difficult to predict the length of time before death. As a result, many patients have missed opportunities for services and had their benefits delayed until the last few weeks of life. Despite the substantial increase in the use of hospice services in recent years, the mean length of service has decreased from 25 days in 1998 to 20 days in 2007 (Connor, 2009).

An important role of nurses is to advocate for referrals to engage hospice support earlier for the benefit of older adult patients and their families. Hospice programs offer the following services:

- Physician and nursing care
- Home health aide
- Therapies such as music, art, and other supportive services
- Social work and counseling services
- Spiritual care
- Volunteer support
- Bereavement counseling, including support programs for 1 year after death
- Medical equipment and supplies
- Drugs related to the disease
- Inpatient care for symptom management, caregiver respite, or both.

 NURSING INTERVENTIONS IN END-OF-LIFE CARE

To assist patients and their families in attaining death with dignity in a caring manner, the nurse must possess the following skills: interpersonal communication abilities; expertise in the assessment and treatment of the physical, psychosocial, and spiritual dimensions of dying; the ability to relate prognoses to patients and families; and knowledge of resources. Nurses assist patients and families with end-of-life tasks, such as identifying sources of support (e.g., hospice), managing symptoms, supporting life-closure processes, and planning for rites and rituals at the time of death and after. Nurses have primary roles not only in assisting with these tasks but also in teaching families about the signs of imminent death and management of the dying processes.

McSteen and Peden-McAlpine (2006) discuss the primary role of nurses as advocates serving as guides, liaisons, and supporters during the dying experience. Guiding activities include providing and clarifying information and options in a manner that supports the decision making of the dying individual and his or her family. In addition, the nurse advocate serves as a liaison between the family and members of the health care team. Including family members in their loved ones' dying process ultimately has a positive impact on the experience. Finally, the nurse advocate acts to support the choices and decision making of patients and families, setting aside his or her own perspective as a health care professional.

Nurses will gain personal and professional satisfaction from serving as care providers, coordinators, and advocates for older adults at the end of life. Fulfillment can be obtained from knowing that patients die in comfort, with their dignity intact and their wishes and values respected.

Promoting Communication

The National Institutes of Health consensus statement on improving end-of-life care (National Institutes of Health Consensus Development Program, 2004) identified numerous transitions that people face at the end of life, including physical, emotional, spiritual, and financial. Nurses have many opportunities to intervene in each of these realms by using communication strategies and interpersonal skills. These interventions include presence, compassion, touch, recognition of an individual's autonomy, and honesty (Box 29-3).

Communication is the cornerstone of interpersonal relationship building. When caring for people who are dying, communication is critically important to all involved, and its importance is magnified by the unpredictability of the situation. Nurses can help dying patients express their needs by using open, honest, direct, and empathetic communication, even when they may be uncertain about what to say. (See Box 29-4 for examples of what to say as well as what not to say.) Dying patients value the ability to express themselves; in particular, older adults value the opportunity to achieve closure and say good-bye.

Offering Spiritual Support

Spiritual support provided by nurses is widely recognized as an important component of end-of-life care because it contributes to the dying person's quality of life (Murray, 2010; Wallace & O'Shea, 2007). **Spiritual well-being** at the end of

Box 29-3 Supportive Interventions for Relationship Building

Presence	A core nursing intervention, presence can be described as a "gift of self" in which the nurse is available and open to the situation.
	Presence can be demonstrated through verbal communication, valuing what the patient says, accepting the patient's meaning for things, and remembering or reflecting.
Compassion	The nurse strives to be totally and compassionately *with* the patient and family, allowing the most positive experience.
Touch	A powerful therapeutic intervention, touch communicates an offer of unconditional acceptance. It can be both healing and life affirming, a means of communicating genuine care and compassion.
Recognition of autonomy	The nurse realizes and respects the individual's right to make all end-of-life decisions.
Honesty	The nurse is often in a front-line position to communicate/explain what can be expected. Compassionate honesty builds trust with the older adult facing death and his or her family.
Expert communication	At any given moment, nurses need to be able to assess the patient and family, implement a plan to comfort them, and communicate clearly and supportively throughout.
Assisting in transcendence	At the highest level of care, nurses provide emotional support that facilitates the experience of self-transcendence and a sense of triumph over death.

Source: Saunderson, C. A., & Brener, T. H. (Eds.). (2007). *End of life: A nurse's guide to compassionate care* (p. 6). Philadelphia, PA: Lippincott Williams & Wilkins.

life includes meaningful existence, the ability to find meaning in daily experience, and the ability to transcend physical discomfort and prepare for death (Ferrell & Coyle, 2006). Nurses assess spiritual needs both initially and on an ongoing basis because these needs are likely to change during the end-of-life process. Nurses can apply information from Chapter 13 to assess spirituality in older adults.

Nursing diagnoses pertinent to spiritual care during the end of life are Risk for Spiritual Distress, Spiritual Distress, and Readiness for Enhanced Spiritual Well-being. The following nursing interventions relevant to spiritual care at the end of life are as follows: Active Listening, Coping Enhancement, Emotional Support, Guilt Work Facilitation, Hope Instillation,

Presence, Religious Ritual Enhancement, Spiritual Support, and Touch. Nurses also make referrals for pastoral care, hospital chaplains, parish nurses, or other spiritual support resources when appropriate. Hospice programs provide spiritual support and can provide resources to assist nurses in addressing spiritual needs of patients and families.

Managing Symptoms

Although the end-of-life period and dying are very individualized and unpredictable processes, some symptoms occur commonly and require expert and timely nursing care, particularly for older adults who may experience more symptoms

Box 29-4 Communicating With Dying Patients and Their Families

What to Say
- What do you need me to do for you?
- Is there anyone I can call for you?
- I'm here to listen.
- No need to rush. Take your time.
- It's okay to cry. Let me get you a tissue.
- Would you like to be left alone?
- Would you like to share some memories?

What Not to Say
- She's in a better place now.
- He lived a full life.
- She's out of her pain.
- It'll be all right.
- Don't cry.
- Be strong.
- He'd want you to get on with your life.

Source: Saunderson, C. A., & Brener, T. H. (Eds.). (2007). *End of life: A nurse's guide to compassionate care* (p. 18). Philadelphia, PA: Lippincott Williams & Wilkins.

A Student's Perspective

I had a special experience with a man at the nursing and rehab center. "Mort" and I had great conversations, and he quickly became a friend. Mort was suffering from cardiovascular failure, and I knew he did not have long to live. I interviewed Mort and then wrote a paper about his life. I wrote the paper early so that I could read it to Mort before his health declined any more. I read my paper to Mort one morning, and he listened with a seeming sense of sacredness about the words being read. This was his life, and I could tell that it meant a lot to him that I wrote it all down. When I finished, Mort simply said, "I thank you . . . I thank you." He asked me to put the paper in a safe place so it would not get ruined. Mort and I had a special connection; he was a hero to me. The following week, I went to the clinic and found out that Mort had passed away. I am grateful that I had the opportunity to know Mort and to grow and learn from his good life. I am glad that I could serve him at this final time and help him reflect on his life.

Amy C.

(Ogle & Hopper, 2005). Symptoms, which can occur at any time, include fatigue and weakness, constipation, dyspnea, nausea and vomiting, dehydration, decreased appetite, and pain. Because these symptoms usually occur in combination, management is challenging and it is not always possible to control every symptom completely. Although not every patient will have a peaceful passing, nurses and other health care professionals must make every effort to manage symptoms and alleviate distress to the extent possible.

Nurses can use information in Table 29-1 and the following sections as a guide to nursing assessment and interventions for some of the commonly occurring symptoms. In addition, nurses can use information in Chapter 28 to address pain, which is a symptom that occurs frequently at the end of life and is one of the most feared symptoms associated with death. This chapter addresses the symptoms only in relation to the end of life; other pertinent topics are discussed more comprehensively in other chapters: confusion or delirium (Chapter 14), depression (Chapter 15), constipation (Chapter 18), and sleep problems (Chapter 24).

Fatigue (Asthenia)

Fatigue is one of the most commonly reported symptoms at the end of life. Fatigue is often described as tiredness, or lack of physical strength and endurance, or decreased mental concentration. Older adults may have reduced energy or activity tolerance caused by usual aging changes, so it is important for the nurse to establish a baseline for comparison and meaningful interpretation. Fatigue is generally a symptom with underlying causes related to disease processes or conditions, such as anemia, malnutrition, infection, drug therapy, or depression. Other concurrent end-of-life symptoms, such as pain and dyspnea, may exacerbate fatigue.

Constipation

Constipation, a reduced frequency of bowel movements, can include passing hard stools, straining to pass a stool, or impaction (hard stool that is blocked). Constipation may be accompanied by pain, abdominal fullness, and reduced bowel sounds. In general, older adults are at increased risk for constipation because of medications, dietary patterns, and decreased physical activity. Factors that increase the risk for constipation at the end of life include pain medications (discussed in Chapter 28), dehydration, kidney failure, elevated calcium levels, and disease effects (e.g., ascites, spinal cord damage, colon or pelvic cancers). One study found that constipation was the most common and frustrating adverse effect of opioids in patients near the end of life (Lentz & McMillan, 2010).

Dyspnea

Dyspnea is a sensation of shortness of breath or breathlessness. It has been described as a sensation of suffocation or being smothered that can generate fear that death is occurring. A study of almost 6000 patients receiving hospice care found a high prevalence of breathlessness during the 3 months leading to death, with increasing prevalence and severity closer to the time of death (Currow et al., 2010). Dyspnea may result from abnormalities or imbalanced states in the pulmonary, cardiac, neuromuscular, or metabolic systems, as well as arising from psychological causes.

Nausea and Vomiting

Nausea and vomiting are common symptoms associated with terminal illness. Causes of nausea and vomiting at the end of life include the following:

- Irritation/obstruction of gastrointestinal tract (bowel obstruction, constipation, cancer tumor, delayed emptying of stomach from ascites, tumor pressure [often called *squashed stomach syndrome*])
- Medication side effect (particularly opioids such as morphine)
- Ear infection or labyrinthitis
- Electrolyte imbalance, sepsis
- Kidney failure, liver failure
- Increased intracranial pressure (brain tumor, cerebral edema, intracranial bleeding, metastasis)
- Foul odors
- Anxiety, fear.

Dehydration

Because older adults normally have an age-related decrease in body water, they become dehydrated more easily. Causes of dehydration at the end of life include reduced or inadequate oral intake, medications such as diuretics, vomiting, diarrhea, and fever. Symptoms of dehydration can interfere with comfort by causing dry mouth, constipation, confusion, and skin impairment.

Anorexia and Cachexia

Additional symptoms include anorexia, a lack of appetite that progresses to the inability to eat, and cachexia, which is a general state of malnutrition in which there is loss of fat, muscle, and bone mineral content. People with cachexia usually do not respond to increased intake or nutritional supplements (Ferrell & Coyle, 2006). Even before the terminal illness, older adults often have less lean tissue, so there is less reserve and malnutrition can progress quickly. Factors that contribute to anorexia and cachexia include nausea and vomiting, constipation, dehydration, weakness, depression, pain, oral candidiasis or dry mouth, gastritis, and medication side effects.

Symptoms During the Active Dying Process

When it becomes apparent that a dying person has only a few days to live, it is especially important that the nurse work closely with the individual and his or her family to help them understand the dying process and anticipate changes. Guidance about what to expect helps reduce fear and anxiety (Ogle & Hopper, 2005). Characteristic physical signs indicate the "active dying" process. In most situations, the individual has

TABLE 29-1 Guide to Nursing Assessment and Interventions for Common Symptoms at the End of Life

Symptom	Nursing Assessment	Nursing Interventions	Pharmacologic Interventions
Fatigue (asthenia)	Assess for associated conditions, including infection, fever, pain, depression, insomnia, anxiety, dehydration, hypoxia, medication effects.	Inform older adult and family of the normality of fatigue at end of life. Pace activities and care according to tolerance. Exercise if tolerated. Promote optimal sleep, with regular times of rest, sleep, and waking.	Corticosteroids, although generally contraindicated in older adults, may decrease fatigue in patients with cancer. Treat associated conditions (e.g., with antibiotics, antidepressants).
Constipation	Identify risks (e.g., chronic laxative users, medications). Perform abdominal assessment, including palpation for distention, tenderness, or masses and auscultation of bowel sounds and pitch. Assess patients taking pain medications daily. Monitor the character of the bowel movements. Check the rectum if the older adult has not had a bowel movement in more than 3 days or is leaking liquid stool (which can occur with an impaction).	Anticipate and prevent constipation with emphasis on fiber, fluid intake, and activity, but recognize that patients may have difficulty tolerating the optimal interventions. Promote regular routine. Strongest propulsive contractions occur after breakfast; provide patient privacy at this time.	Individualize laxative regimen based on the cause(s) of constipation, history, and preferences. Use bulk-forming and stool-softening agents for patients with normal peristalsis. A laxative regimen (with stimulant laxative) may be ordered for patients taking a pain medication known to cause constipation. Stimulant laxatives are the most appropriate for opioid-induced constipation.
Dyspnea	*Respiratory:* Assess vital signs, including oxygen saturation, breathing pattern, and use of accessory muscles. Auscultate breath sounds. Assess cough (type, if present). Check for tachypnea and cyanosis. *General:* Assess for restlessness, anxiety, and activity tolerance.	Pace activities and rest. Provide oxygen, usually at 2–4 L per cannula (avoid using face mask because of discomfort and sensation of smothering). Provide calm reassurance. Use a fan to circulate air and help reduce the feeling of breathlessness. Position for optimal respiratory function (e.g., leaning forward over a table with a pillow on top is helpful for COPD; on the side with head slightly elevated for unresponsive patient). Teach patient to use pursed-lip breathing, and encourage relaxation techniques to reduce muscle tightness and associated sensation of breathlessness.	Treat causes. Treat symptoms with morphine or hydromorphone, which relieves the breathless sensation in almost all cases. Use antianxiety agents or antidepressants if appropriate (and if perception of breathlessness is exaggerated because of anxiety or depression). Corticosteroids can be used for their anti-inflammatory effects in certain conditions (e.g., COPD, radiation pneumonitis).
Nausea and vomiting	Assess for potential cause (e.g., constipation, bowel obstruction). Palpate abdomen and check for distention. Assess vomitus for fecal odor. Assess heartburn and nausea, which may occur after meals in squashed stomach syndrome. Assess pain (e.g., pain on swallowing may indicate oral thrush; pain on standing may be caused by mesenteric traction). Hiccups occur with uremia.	Offer frequent, small meals; serve foods cold or at room temperature. Apply damp, cool cloth to face when nauseated. Provide oral care after vomiting.	Medications need to be specific to the cause: • Squashed stomach syndrome, gastritis, and functional bowel obstruction: metoclopramide (contraindicated in full bowel obstruction) • Chemical causes, such as morphine, hypercalcemia, or renal failure: haloperidol • If caused by dysfunction of vomiting center (e.g., associated with mechanical bowel obstruction, increased intracranial pressure, motion sickness): meclizine or diphenhydramine
Dehydration	Assess for clinical signs of hydration (e.g., skin turgor over the upper chest or forehead). Assess buccal membranes for moistness. Assess vital signs: pulse, orthostatic blood pressure.	Encourage fluids as tolerated; offer ice chips and popsicles if swallowing. Provide frequent oral care; use swabs or moistened toothettes.	Give intravenous fluids or administer clysis per advance directives. Discuss continued diuretic use with physician.
Anorexia and cachexia	Assess for weight loss. Assess for levels of weakness and fatigue. Conduct physical examination for decreased fat, muscle wasting, decreased strength. Assess mental status, including depression.	Remove unpleasant odors. Provide frequent oral care. Treat pain optimally. Provide frequent, small meals. Provide companionship. Serve meals in a place that is separate from the bed area. Involve patient with meal planning. Collaborate with dietician for nutritional analysis and meal planning. Encourage culturally appropriate foods. Consider using an alcoholic beverage before meals.	Medications that are used to stimulate appetite, promote weight gain, and provide a sense of well-being: megestrol acetate, corticosteroids, and mirtazapine. Metoclopramide is used to improve gastric motility and appetite.

COPD, chronic obstructive pulmonary disease.

become totally dependent on others for all aspects of care, with less wakeful or alert time. Levels of consciousness may change or fluctuate. The person has little or no interest in the oral intake of food or fluids. Physiologic changes occur in breathing patterns, circulation slows down, sensory awareness decreases, and muscle weakness occurs as a result of decreased tone. In addition to these physiologic manifestations, up to 85% of patients experience delirium during the last weeks of life, with agitation being a common manifestation (Clary & Lawson, 2009). Table 29-2 summarizes some signs and symptoms that occur within days of death. Nurses should describe plans for care to give reassurance that comfort needs will be met. The overall focus of nursing care at this point is to continue to promote physiologic and psychological comfort, while assisting the older adult in achieving a peaceful, dignified death. The Dying Person's Bill of Rights (Box 29-2) continues to provide guidance for care in the final hours of life.

When death does not occur suddenly, the older adult may have opportunities for final closure. Reminiscence and life review can promote self-actualization during this time. Participation in decisions concerning the person's death, as well as those concerning the continuation of life for loved ones, can assist in bringing inner peace. Older adults often reach a point of readiness and anticipation of death, and they may communicate that they are ready to make the transition from life to death. Nurses can use therapeutic communication techniques to acknowledge their expressions in a genuine and supportive manner. Final good-byes to family members and friends are also difficult for those being left behind. Nurses can offer and coordinate grief support through the hospice or palliative care team, or through chaplains or other meaningful religious and spiritual resources.

TABLE 29-2 Signs and Symptoms of Death Within Days

Physiologic Change	Signs and Symptoms
Altered breathing patterns	• Breathing initially becomes more shallow • Cheyne-Stokes respirations • Noisy breathing (death rattle)
Changing circulation	• Limbs, ears, and nose become cold to touch or mottled in appearance • Decreased blood pressure • Pulse may weaken and become irregular • Diaphoresis • Possible increase in dependent edema • No urine output or small amount of very dark urine (anuria or oliguria)
Decreased muscle tone	• Relaxed facial muscles, lower jaw drops, mouth open • Decreased/loss of gag reflex • Difficulty swallowing • Abdominal distention due to decreased gastrointestinal activity • Possible urinary and fecal incontinence due to relaxation of sphincter muscles
Decreased senses	• Reduced level of consciousness • Blurred or distorted vision • Decreased taste and smell (probable continued sense of hearing)

Source: Saunderson, C. A., & Brener, T. H. (Eds.). (2007). *End of life: A nurse's guide to compassionate care.* Philadelphia, PA: Lippincott Williams & Wilkins.

*P*art I: Mr. Bauer is a 91-year-old man with medical diagnoses including hypertension, type 2 diabetes mellitus, history of cerebrovascular accident, and benign prostatic hyperplasia. He was taking the following medications, lisinopril (Prinivil), 20 mg daily; aspirin, 81 mg daily; furosemide (Lasix), 40 mg daily; potassium, 20 mEq daily; and acetaminophen (Tylenol) as needed for arthritis pain. He has lived at home by himself for the last 15 years since the death of his wife. He has three adult children, all living out of state, who visit on average once monthly. He is very well known in his neighborhood as the older man who helps everyone. He loves his home and spends his days "keeping house." His favorite chores include mowing the grass in the summer and blowing the snow in the winter. He owns and drives a car to the local supermarket and barber and to the cemetery to visit his wife's grave. In late summer, he had an accident with his lawn mower that drew his family's attention to the fact that he was losing his strength. While mowing his grass, he fell over the lawn mower, scraping his face on the cement. He required emergency department (ED) evaluation and treatment, including stitches for facial lacerations. He later admitted that, before his fall, he had been experiencing dizziness, especially when getting out of his easy chair.

Three weeks after his ED evaluation, Mr. Bauer's daughter came to visit. She was shocked to see her father looking so "thin and gaunt." Mr. Bauer admitted that he had lost a few pounds over the summer and still didn't have much energy. He stated that he wasn't sleeping well at night, with his sleep disrupted every 30 to 45 minutes because of the need to urinate. To control his urination, he had decided to limit his drinking fluids to less than 8 oz daily. Mr. Bauer's daughter noticed that in spite of his weight loss, his abdomen was very large and distended. "Do you have any aches?" she asked her father. He nodded yes and grabbed his lower abdomen.

THINKING POINTS

- Based on symptoms and history, what points would you address in your nursing assessment?
- What nursing problems would you address in Mr. Bauer's nursing care plan?
- What are some probable causes of Mr. Bauer's abdominal discomfort?
- What would the appropriate nursing interventions be?
- What health teaching would you provide?

*P*art II: Mr. Bauer and his daughter have a follow-up office visit with his primary care physician. On arrival, his vital signs are as follows: temperature, 98° PO; apical pulse, 82 beats per minute and irregularly irregular; respirations, 24 per minute; and blood pressure sitting, 98/50. When standing to walk to the scale for his weight measurement, he swayed a bit, grabbed the wall, and then steadied himself. "I just got a little dizzy," he admitted. As the office nurse, you immediately grabbed the blood pressure cuff and took his blood pressure in the standing position. It was 70/40. Mr. Bauer's pulse at that time was 90 and irregular. Noting the vital sign changes, the physician ordered some laboratory tests. Blood samples for testing were drawn in the office. With results pending, no changes were made in his medical care at that time.

THINKING POINTS

- What are your immediate nursing concerns for Mr. Bauer based on information about his decline during the past 6 months?
- What risk factors are likely to be contributing to Mr. Bauer's dizziness?
- What patient teaching is indicated at this time?

*P*art III: Mr. Bauer's blood test results come back the next day, confirming dehydration and malnutrition:

- Sodium: 150
- Potassium: 3.7
- Serum albumin: 3.0
- Prealbumin: 14
- Blood urea nitrogen: 35
- Serum creatinine: 1.7

The physician discontinued Mr. Bauer's furosemide and lisinopril and suggested a follow-up visit in 2 weeks. Two days before his next appointment, Mr. Bauer's daughter called the office to relay that her father had fallen and was taken to the hospital for evaluation. A workup revealed that he had a transient ischemic attack and was now too weak to eat and he was experiencing difficulty swallowing. The family declined a feeding tube and a hospice referral was made.

THINKING POINTS

- Identify two priority nursing diagnoses appropriate for Mr. Bauer at this time.

- For each diagnosis, list two to three nursing interventions.

Mr. Bauer died in the hospital 1 week after his fall, on the day he was scheduled for discharge.

Chapter Highlights

End-of-Life Transitions
- The end of life is the period in which there is little likelihood of cure, and comfort is the primary goal.

Cultural and Historical Perspectives on Death and Dying
- There is a gradual trend toward dying at home, which is where most people say they want to die, and where most people did die during the early part of the 20th century.
- American society is moving beyond the culture of denial of death and finding ways to address death as an integral part of life (Box 29-1).
- Cultural factors significantly affect attitudes toward death and dying (Cultural Considerations Box 29-1).

Quality of Care at the End of Life
- Nurses and other health care professionals have strong roles in supporting death with dignity (Box 29-2).
- Hospice is a philosophy of care whose goal is to support dignified dying and a good death experience for people who are terminally ill.

Nursing Interventions in End-of-Life Care
- Nurses use many interventions, including verbal and nonverbal communication (Boxes 29-3 and 29-4), to address the complex needs of patients who are dying and their families.
- Nurses assess and address common symptoms that occur during the end of life, including fatigue, constipation, dyspnea, nausea and vomiting, dehydration, and anorexia (Table 29-1).
- Nurses holistically address needs of patients and families during the immediate end-of-life process (Table 29-2).

Critical Thinking Exercises

1. Review the section on Health Care Professionals' Perspective on Death and Dying and spend a few minutes answering the questions for self-reflection.
2. Review Cultural Considerations 29-1 and think about how each of the points listed applies to your personal perspectives on death and dying.
3. From a nursing perspective, identify the ways in which caring for patients at the end of life differs from caring for patients with acute care needs.
4. From a nursing perspective, identify the ways in which caring for patients at the end of life differs from caring for patients who have chronic illnesses.

Resources

For links to these resources and additional helpful Internet resources related to this chapter, visit thePoint at http://thePoint.lww.com/Miller6e.

Clinical Tools

Center to Advance Palliative Care
Promoting Excellence in End-of-Life Care
TIME: Toolkit of Instruments for Measuring End-of-life Care

Evidence-Based Practice

National Guideline Clearinghouse
- End-of-life care
- Quality palliative care
- Interventions to improve palliative care of pain, dyspnea, and depression at the end of life
- Family preparedness and end-of-life support before death of a nursing home resident

Health Education

American Association of Colleges of Nursing, End-of-Life Care (ELNEC)
Dying Well
Growth House: Guide to Death, Dying, Grief, Bereavement, and End of Life Resources
Hospice and Palliative Nurses Association
National Association for Home Care & Hospice

REFERENCES

American Geriatrics Society (AGS). (2002, November). *Position statement: The care of dying patients*. Retrieved from www.americangeriatrics.org/products/positionpapers/careofd.shtml.

Austin, L. (1975). *Dying patient's bill of rights*. Created at The Terminally Ill Patient and the Helping Person Workshops. Sponsored by the Southwest Michigan Inservice Education Council in Lansing, MI.

Bercovitz, A., Decker, F. H., Jones, A., & Remsburg, R. E. (2008). End-of-life care in nursing homes: 2004 National Nursing Home Study. *National Health Statistics Reports* (9), 1–5.

Byock, I. (2006). Where do we go from here? A palliative care perspective. *Critical Care Medicine, 34*, S416–S420.

Clary, P. L., & Lawson, P. (2009). Pharmacologic pearls for end-of-life care. *American Family Physician, 79*(12), 1059–1065.

Connor, S. R. (2009). U.S. hospice benefits. *Journal of Pain and Symptom Management, 38*, 105–109.

Currow, D. C., Smith, J., Davidson, P. M., Newton, P. J., Agar, M. R., & Abernethy, A. P. (2010). Do the trajectories of dyspnea differ in prevalence and intensity by diagnosis at the end of life? *Journal of Pain and Symptom Management, 39*, 680–690.

Ferrell, B. R., & Coyle, N. (2006). *Textbook of palliative nursing* (2nd ed.). New York: Oxford University Press.

Hampton, M., Baydata, A., Bourassa, C., McKay-McNabb, K., Goodwill, K., McNabb, P., & Boekelder, R. (2010). Completing the circle: Elders speak about end-of-life care with aboriginal families in Canada. *Journal of Palliative Care, 26*(1), 6–14.

Hospice and Palliative Nurses Association (HPNA). (2008, October). *Position statement: Value of the professional nurse in palliative care*. Retrieved from www.hpna.org.

Kübler-Ross, E. (1969). *On death and dying*. New York: Macmillan.

Lentz, J., & McMillan, S. C. (2010). The impact of opioid-induced constipation on patients near the end of life. *Journal of Hospice and Palliative Nursing, 12*(1), 29–38.

Markson, E. (2003). *Social gerontology today*. Los Angeles, CA: Roxbury.

McSteen, K., & Peden-McAlpine, C. (2006). The role of the nurse as advocate in ethically difficult care situations with dying patients. *Journal of Hospice and Palliative Nursing, 8*, 259–269.

Menec, V. H., Nowicki, S., Blandford, A., & Veselyuk, D. (2009). Hospitalizations at the end of life among long-term care residents. *Journal of Gerontology: Medical Sciences, 64A*, 395–402.

Munn, J. C., Dobbs, D., Meier, A., Williamsn, C. S., Biola, H., & Zimmerman, S. (2008). The end-of-life experience in long-term care: Five themes identified from focus groups with residents, family members, and staff. *The Gerontologist, 48*, 485–494.

Murray, R. P. (2010). Spiritual care beliefs and practices of special care and oncology RNs at patients' end of life. *Journal of Hospice and Palliative Care, 12*, 51–58.

National Hospice and Palliative Care Organization (NHPCO). (n.d.). *The history of hospice care*. Retrieved from http://www.nhpco.org.

National Institutes of Health Consensus Development Program. (2004, December 6–8). *National Institutes of Health state-of-the-science conference statement on improving end-of-life care*. Retrieved from http://consensus.nih.gov/2004/2004EndOfLifeCareSOS024html.htm.

Ogle, K., & Hopper, K. (2005). End of life care for older adults. *Primary Care: Clinics in Office Practice, 32*, 811–828.

Ohio State University Health Sciences Center, Office of Geriatrics & Gerontology. (2003). Series to understand, nurture and support end-of-life transitions (SUNSET). Retrieved from http://sunset.osu.edu.

Purnell, L. D. (2009). *Culturally competent health care*. Philadelphia, PA: F.A. Davis.

Robert Wood Johnson Foundation Last Acts Task Force. (2002, November). *Means to a better end: A report on dying in America today*. Retrieved from www.rwjf.org/files/publications/other/meansbetterend.pdf.

Salman, K., & Zhoucha, R. (2010). Considering faith within culture when caring for the terminally ill Muslim patient and family. *Journal of Hospice and Palliative Nursing, 12*, 156–163.

Saunderson, C. A., & Brener, T. H. (Eds.). (2007). *End of life: A nurse's guide to compassionate care*. Philadelphia, PA: Lippincott Williams & Wilkins.

Tayeb, M. A., Al-Zamel, E., Fareed, M. M., & Aboueillail, H. A. (2010). A "good death": Perspectives of Muslim patients and health care providers. *Annals of Saudi Medicine, 30*, 215–221.

Wallace, M., & O'Shea, E. (2007). Perceptions of spirituality and spiritual care among older nursing home residents at the end of life. *Holistic Nursing Practice, 21*, 285–289.

Whitehead, P. B., Anderson, E. S., Redican, K. J., & Stratton, R. (2010). Studying the effects of the end-of-life nursing education consortium at the institutional level. *Journal of Hospice and Palliative Nursing, 12*, 184–193.

Wilke, D., & TNEEL Investigators. (2003). *Toolkit for nurturing excellence at end-of-life transition (TNEEL)*. University of Washington School of Nursing. Retrieved from www.tneel.uic.edu/tneel.asp.

Index

Index

Note: Page numbers followed by the letter *b* denoted boxes, those followed by *f* denote figures, and those followed by *t* denote tables.

A

abdominal obesity, 412
abstract thinking, 239
accidental hypothermia, 517
acclimatize, 515
accommodation, 335
acetaminophen, 121
  usage of, 570
A Core Curriculum in Ethnogeriatrics, 22
acquired immunodeficiency syndrome (AIDS), 533
active life expectancy, 47–48
activities of daily living (ADLs), 47, 95, 387, 453, 566
  assessment of, 99–101, 100*b*
  and dementia, 266, 277*b*
activity theory, of aging, 52
acuity, 335
acupressure, in sleep improvement, 506
acute care for elders (ACE) units, 77
acute care settings, 77–78
  for dementia, 274–275
    hospital-at-home model, 77–78
    role of nurses, 78
    specialized geriatric acute care units, 77
    subacute care units, 77
    transitional care models, 78
acute glaucoma, 344
acute organic brain syndrome. *See* delirium
acute pain, 560
adaptive response, 416
addiction, 567
adjuvant analgesics, 569–570
adult day centers, 84–85
adult protective services, 179–181
  principles of, 181*b*
Adult Treatment Panel (ATP) III, 413
advance directives, 151–153
  do not resuscitate order, 152
  durable power of attorney for health care, 152–153
  Five Wishes document, 151
  living wills, 152
Advanced Practice Registered Nurse (APRN), 61
advanced sleep phase, 499
Advancing Excellence in America's Nursing Homes, 80
adverse medication effects, 122, 129–130
affective function, assessment, 240–244
  anxiety, 241–242
  depression, 243
  guidelines, 240–241, 244*b*
  happiness/well-being, 243–244
  mood, 241
  self-esteem, 242–243
African Americans
  caregiving relationships of, 7
  death rituals and intervention in, 579

health disparities in, 27
heart disease risk, 415
overview of, 26–27
age attribution, 7
age identity, 3
ageism, 5–8
  Ageism Survey, 6, 6*f*
  attitudes of nurses on, addressing of, 8
  cultural perspectives and, 6, 7
  definition of, 5
  effects of, 6–8
  manifestations of, 5–6
age-related changes, 36, 39–40, 39*b*
  on cardiovascular function, 408–410
  on digestion and eating patterns, 358–362
  on hearing, 311–314
  on mobility and safety, 452–454
  on pain, 563
  on respiratory function, 435–438
  and risk factors, difference between, 39
  on sexual function, 525–527
  on skin, 477–479
  on sleep and rest, 496–499
  on thermoregulation, 513–515
  on urinary function, 383–386
  on vision, 333–338
age-related macular degeneration (AMD), 339, 342*t*, 343
  dry type, 343
  wet type, 343
age stratification theory, of aging, 52–53
aging
  attitude towards
    ageism, 5–8
    shifting trends, 5
  and death, relationship between, 48
  definitions of, 3–4
  demographics of, 9–11, 10*t*
  and disease, relationship between, 48
  global, 16, 17*b*
  images of, 1–2
  myths/realities about, 8–14, 9*t*, 36
  successful, 4–5
  and wellness, relationship between, 2
aging anxiety, 7
aging in place, 76*b*
aging successfully, concept of, 4
aging, theories of
  biologic theories, 49–51
  holistic perspective, on aging, 56–57
  psychological theories, of aging, 54–56
  sociocultural theories, of aging, 51–53
akathisia, 242
alcohol
  adverse effects of, 529 (*See also* sexual function)
  and medications interactions, 128, 128*t*
  sleep disorder, 500

alcoholics anonymous (AA), 297
alertness level, assessment of, 236
alpha-adrenergic blocking agents, usage of, 400
Alzheimer's disease, 258
  assessments for
    CSADL, 101
    GDS/FAST, 265, 266*t*
  cigarette smoking and, 438
  distinguishing features, 261*t*
  familial, 262
  pathologic changes associated with, 261–262, 262*f*
  preclinical, 263, 263*f*
  prevalence, 261
  risks for, 262–263
  vision impairments in, 339
American Academy of Anti-Aging Medicine, 8
American Academy of Ophthalmology, 350
American Association of Retired Persons (AARP), 52
American Diabetes Association, 552
American Geriatrics Society (AGS), 21, 59, 60, 458, 560, 575
American Heart Association and the Preventive Cardiovascular Nurses Association, 418
American Indians/Alaskan Natives, caregiving relationships of, 7
American Journal of Nursing, 371, 462, 484, 536
American Lung Association, 443
American Nurses Association (ANA), 60, 458
American Nurses Credentialing Center (AACN), 60
American Occupational Therapy Association, 109
American Optometric Association, 350
American Pain Society (APS), 560
American Sleep Disorders Association, 496
amyloid precursor protein, 261
analgesics, classifications of, 569–570
anatomy, of pain, 561–562
androgen deficiency. *See* late onset hypogonadism
andropause, 527
angiotensin-converting enzyme (ACE), 425, 554
anorexia, at the end of life, 583
anosognosia, 266
anti-aging interventions, 8
anti-aging movement, 8
anticholinergics, 122–123, 388
  adverse effects, 130
antidepressant medications
  commonly used, 300*t*
  nursing responsibility for, 300–301, 301*b*
  types of, 299–300
antidiuretic hormone (ADH), 385
antimuscarinic agents, adverse effects of, 400
antipsychotic medications, 123
  and people with dementia, 131

anxiety, 241–242
aphasia, 238
apocrine sweat glands, 479
apomorphine, 540
apoptosis theory, of aging, 50
Appalachian people, 32
aqueous humor, 343. *See also* glaucoma
arcus senilis, 333
arrhythmias, 418
Artifacts of Culture Change Tool, 80
artificial nutrition and hydration, and ethical
    issues, 154–155
artificial urinary sphincter, usage of, 401
Asian Americans
    cardiovascular disease in, 415
    eating patterns in, 366
Asians and Pacific Islanders, 29–30
    cultural overview, 29–30
        Asian Indians, 29
        Chinese, 29
        Filipinos, 29
        Japanese, 30
        Koreans, 30
        Vietnamese, 29–30
aspirin, 425
assessments. *See also* functional assessment;
        psychosocial assessment
    of ADLs, 99–101, 100*b*
    for Alzheimer's disease, 101, 265
    of bioactive substances, 131–136
    of cardiovascular function, 417–422
    of cognitive function, 193–194
    of dementia, 269–270
    of digestion and nutrition, 369–371, 372*b*,
        373*f*
    of driving safety, 108–110
    of elder abuse and neglect, 168–174
    of end of life transition, 584*t*
    of environmental safety, 106–107, 107*b*
    geriatric, 106
    by gerontologists
        active life expectancy, 47–48
        activities of daily living, 47
        life span/life expectancy, 46
        mortality rates, 46–47
    of health and functioning, 94–110
    of hearing, 318–321
    of IADLs, 101, 101*b*
    of insight, 239
    of musculoskeletal function, 460–462
    of pain, 565–568
    of psychosocial function, 212
    of respiratory function, 441–445
    of sexual function, 534–537
    of skin, 487–489
    of sleep and rest, 503–504
    of spiritual needs, 253*b*
    of thermoregulation, 517–520
    of urinary function, 391–393
    of vision, 345–348
    of wheelchair fit, 106, 106*t*
assisted-living facilities, 14, 15*b*, 81–82
assistive device
    behavioral cues, 321*b*
    for falls reduction, 469*f*
    listening, 323–325
    for mobility and safety, 459
    for urinary function, 393
atherosclerosis, 410
    and cardiovascular disease, 411
attitudes, towards aging
    effects of ageism, 6–8
    historical attitude, 5
    of nurses, 8

atypical presentation, 419
auditory nervous system, 314
auditory room-monitoring device, usage of, 470
automatic and effortful processing theory, 190
autonomy, definition of, 149

B
baby boomers, 9
Balanced Budget Act of 1997, 82
barbiturates, 123
baroreflex mechanisms, 410
basal cell carcinoma, 482, 482*f*
Beers prescription criteria, 122–123
behavioral and psychological symptoms of
        dementia (BPSD), 268
behavioral cues and hearing loss, 320, 321*b*
benign prostatic hyperplasia, 387
benign prostatic hypertrophy. *See* prostatic
        hyperplasia
benzodiazepines, 123
    adverse effects of, 507
    hypnotics and sleep disorder, 501
Best Practices in Care for Older Adults, 39
beta-amyloid, 261
bile, in digestion, 360
bioactive substances, 113–118
    age-related influences on, 118–120
    assessment of use and effects, 131–136
    diagnosis, 136
    effects of, 500–501 (*See also* sleep and rest)
    functional consequences, 129–131
        adverse effects potential, 129–130
        altered mental status, 130–131
        altered therapeutic effects, 129
        anticholinergic toxicity, 130
        antipsychotic medication effects, 131
        drug-induced parkinsonism, 131
        tardive dyskinesia, 131
    herbs, 115–116, 117*t*–118*t*
    homeopathy, 116, 118
    medication (*See* medications)
    medication interactions, 125–129
        with alcohol, 128, 128*t*
        with caffeine, 128, 128*t*
        with herbs, 126–127
        with medication, 125–126, 127*t*
        with nicotine, 128–129, 129*t*
        with nutrients, 127–128, 127*t*
    metabolic pathways of, 119, 120*t*
    risk factors, 120–125
        adverse effects nonrecognition, 125
        communication barriers, 122
        financial considerations, 124–125
        inappropriate prescribing practices,
                122–123
        lack of information, 122
        medication nonadherence, 124
        myths and misunderstandings, 121–122
        pathologic processes and functional
                impairments, 121
        polypharmacy, 124
biodemography, 47
biofeedback and stimulation devices, in urinary
        function, 397–398
biogerontology, 48
biologic aging, definition of, 49
biological clock. *See* circadian rhythm
biologic theories, of aging, 49–51
    apoptosis theory, 50
    caloric restriction theory, 50
    conclusions about, 50
    cross-linkage theory, 49
    free radical theory, 49

    genetic theory, 50
    immunity theory, 49–50
    neuroendocrine theory, 49
    relevant to nurses/nursing, 50–51
    wear-and-tear theory, 49
bipolar disorder, 290
bisphosphonates and osteoporotic fractures
        prevention, 466–467
bladder, urinary
    suspension surgery, goal of, 401
    and urinary tract, 385
bladder diary, 393, 394*f*
bladder record. *See* bladder diary
blepharochalasis, 333
blood pressure
    assessment of, 418, 419*b*
    cardiovascular wellness and, 416
    criteria for normal, 413*t*
    diastolic, 413
    measurement in older adults, 419*b*
    self-measurement of, 418
    and sleep disorder, 498
    smoking and, 412
    systolic, 413
board-and-care home, 15*b*
body mass index (BMI), 368, 412, 470
body sway, 454
bone
    age-related changes in, 452–453
    densitometry, 454
    function of, 452
    mass density, 454
bone mineral density (BMD), 455
bowel function
    constipation and, 374
    in patients taking opioid medications,
        571*b*
Braden Scale, usage of, 484, 485*f*
Brain Health Initiative, 65
brain imaging techniques, 260
bright-light therapy, 302
British Geriatrics Society, 458
bupropion, 448
Bureau of Health Professions Health Resources
        and Services Administration, 22

C
cachexia, at the end of life, 583
caffeine, 128
caffeine intake and sleep disorder, 500
calcitonin and osteoporosis prevention, 467
calcium intake and osteoporosis prevention, 466
caloric restriction theory, of aging, 50
calories, 361
campaign against pain, 572
cancellous bone, 452
cancer pain, 562
cancer patients, 550–552
    assessments, 551
    diagnosis and wellness outcomes, 551
    interventions for, 551–552, 552*b*
carbohydrates, role and requirements of, 361
cardiovascular disease, 408
    and sexual dysfunction, 530
cardiovascular function
    age-related changes, 408
        baroreflex mechanisms, 410
        myocardium and neuroconduction
                mechanisms, 409–410
        vasculature, 410
    assessment of, 417–418
        baseline cardiovascular function, 418
        blood pressure, 418

easy-to-use assessment tools, 420*f*–421*f*
guidelines for, 422*b*
heart disease, signs and symptoms of, 419–422
identifying risks for, 418–419
knowledge about heart disease, 422
diagnosis, 422–423
functional consequences
cardiac function, effects on, 416
circulation, effects on, 416
pulse and blood pressure, effects on, 416
response to exercise, effects on, 416
interventions
effectiveness evaluation of, 429
health education, 425*b*
hypertension, 425–426
lipid disorders, 428–429, 428*b*
nutrition and lifestyle interventions, 423–424
orthostatic hypotension, 429
pharmacologic, 425
secondary prevention, 424–425, 424*f*
pathologic conditions, 417
risk factors, 410–411
atherosclerosis, 411
dietary habits, 412
heredity and socioeconomic factors, 415
hypertension, 412–413, 413*t*
lipid disorders, 413
metabolic syndrome, 414
obesity, 412
physical inactivity, 411–412
psychosocial factors, 414–415
tobacco smoking, 412
in women and minority groups, 415–416
wellness outcomes, 423
caregiver burden, 16, 555
caregiver well-being, 555
care management services, 87
case management services, 87–89
cataracts, 338, 339, 341–343
causes of, 341
cortical, 341–342
nuclear, 342
posterior subcapsular, 342
catastrophic reaction, 269
centenarians, studies of, 48–49
Centers for Disease Control and Prevention (CDC), 64, 65, 415, 441, 533
Centers for Medicare and Medicaid Services (CMS), 399, 458, 484
cerumen, 311
chest wall and musculoskeletal structures, 436–437
Chinese, caregiving relationships of, 7
chlorhexidine, 375
cholelithiasis, 360
choroidal neovascularization, 343
Chronic Care: A Call to Action for Health Reform, 64
chronic care models, 87
chronic confusion, 270
chronic glaucoma, 344
chronic obstructive pulmonary disease (COPD), 364, 388, 438
and dyspnea, 498
functional consequences of, 441
risk factor of, 441
chronic organic brain syndrome (COBS), 258
chronic pain, 561
chronologic age, 3
cigarette smoking
adverse effects of, 438
and cataracts, 339
erectile dysfunction and, 529

health promotion teaching about, 447*b*
and skin changes, 480
and testosterone levels, 527
ciliary body, 335. *See also* eye
cimetidine (Tagamet), 126
circadian rhythm, 498–499
circumstantiality, 235
Civil Rights Act of 1964, 23
clearance rate, drug, 114–115
Cleveland Scale for Activities of Daily Living (CSADL), 101, 102*f*–105*f*, 105
clopidogrel (Plavix), 126
closed-captioned television, usage of, 324
Cochrane Review, 61
cognitive function, 187–199
age-related changes, 187–191
adult psychological development, 190–191
central nervous system, 188–189
fluid and crystallized intelligence, 189
memory, 189–190
assessments of, 193–194
cultural factors and, 193
diagnosis, 194
functional consequences, 193, 194*b*
interventions, 194–198
adaptations of health education materials, 197–198, 197*b*
education and training, 195, 196*b*
effectiveness evaluation, 198
improving concentration and attention, 195
participation in mentally stimulating activities, 195, 197
risk factors, 191–193
medication effects, 192
personal/social/attitudinal influences, 191
physical/mental health factors, 192
smoking/environmental factors, 192–193
stage theories, 190–191
wellness outcomes, 194
cognitive reserve, 189, 264–265
cohousing communities, 15*b*
color perception, 335
Comfort Care DNR, 152
communication
with adults with dementia, 276
during end of life transition, 581
and hearing, 316–317
nonverbal, cultural factors of, 231
for psychosocial assessment, 229–233
creating environment for, 231–233
enhancement of, 230–231, 234*b*
identifying barriers, 229–230
community-based services, 84–86
adult day centers, 84–85
health promotion programs, 85
parish nursing programs, 85
respite services, 85
role of nurses, 85–86
community resources for older adults, 84*b*
community settings
for dementia care, 275
compact bone, 452
competency, 150
complementary and alternative medicine (CAM), 115
for healthy sleep, 505–506
Comprehensive Geriatric Education Program (CGEP), 60
compression of morbidity, 47
conductive hearing losses, 316
confabulation, 235
Confusion Assessment Method (CAM), 257
congregate housing, 15*b*

constipation, 369
at the end of life, 583
health education regarding, 375*b*
contextual theories, memory, 190
continence training, 397
goal of, 399, 399*b*
continuous positive airway pressure (CPAP), 508, 508*f*
continuum of care, for older adults, 75, 76*b*.
See also settings, for health care
development of, 75–76, 76*f*
coordination of care, models of, 86–88
care management services, 87
case management services, 87–88
chronic care models, 87
comprehensive models, 86–87
cornea, 335
corneal arcus. *See* arcus senilis
cortical bone. *See* compact bone
cortical cataracts, 341–342
corticosteroids, 455
cosmetic effects, of age-related skin changes, 481–482
critical flicker fusion, 338
cross-linkage theory, of aging, 49
crystallized intelligence, 189
cultural and socioeconomic factors, in eating patterns, 365–366
cultural aspects, of pain management, 563–565
cultural competence, and transcultural nursing, 21–23
cultural self-assessment, 21–22, 22*b*
linguistic competence, 23
sources of information on, 22–23
use of interpreters, 23, 24*b*
cultural diversity/groups, of U.S. older adults, 20–21, 26–31
African Americans, 26–27
American Indian and Alaska Native, 30–31
Asians and Pacific Islanders, 29–30
Hispanics/Latinos, 27–29
cultural factors
of death/dying, 578, 579
of digestion and nutrition, 365–366
of eating patterns, 365–366
cultural self-assessment, 21–22, 22*b*
culture-bound syndromes, 209, 210*t*
culture change movement, 80–81
Culture & Clinical Care, 22
cycles per second (cps), 311
cytochrome P-450 system, 119

D

daily food intake in older adults, guidelines for, 377*b*
darifenacin, 400
dark adaptation, 337
DASH dietary pattern, 424
dazzling glare, 337
death/dying. *See also* end of life transition
caregivers response, 577
death with dignity, 579
definition of, 575
demographics of, 577
Dying Person's Bill of Rights, 580*b*
nursing skills for palliative care, 576
perspectives on, 576*b*
culturally diverse, 578, 579
health care professionals', 577–578
older adults', 577
sites of, 576
in western culture, 576–577

death/dying (*Continued*)
  process, 575
  promoting communication, 581
  signs and symptoms of, 585*t*
decibels (dB), 311
decisional autonomy, 151
decision-making capacity, 150–151
dehydration and bladder irritability, 387
dehydration, at the end of life, 583
delirium, 255–259, 500
  assessment, 256–257
  diagnosis, 257
  functional consequences, 256
  hyperactive, 255
  hypoactive, 255
  interventions, 257–259, 258*f*
  prevalence rates, 256
  research findings related to, 254*t*
  risk factors, 256
  types, 255
delirium, medication-induced, 130–131
delusions
  definition of, 244
  delirium associated, 245
  dementia associated, 246
  depression associated, 246–247
  distinguishing features of, 245*t*
  paranoid disorder associated, 247
  physiologic causes, 245*t*
dementia, 259–280
  assessment of, 269–270, 270*b*
    initial, 269
    interference with, 269
    ongoing, 269–270
  associated factors, 264–265
  coping and daily living with, 271*b*
  diagnosis, 260, 270–271
  distinguishing features, 261*t*
  distinguishing features of, 294*t*
  functional consequences, 265–267
    behavioral and psychological symptoms,
      268–270
    personal experiences, 266–268, 267*b*
    self-awareness, 266, 267*b*
    stages of dementia, 265–266
  and functional impairments, 530
  interventions, 271–279
    communication facilitation, 276, 277*b*
    in different settings, 273–275
    effectiveness evaluation, 279
    environmental modifications, 275–276, 277*b*
    pharmacologic, 276, 278–279
    promoting wellness, 273, 273*b*
    studies of, 270*t*
    theoretical frameworks, 273
  strategies to prevent cognitive decline, 265*t*
  terminology descriptions, 259
  theories about, 259–260
  types of, 260, 261*t*
    Alzheimer's disease, 261–263
    frontotemporal dementia, 264
    Lewy body dementia, 264
    vascular dementia, 263–264
  and urinary incontinence, 388
  wellness outcomes, 271
demographic trends, in United States, 9–11,
    10*b*, 10*f*
dependence, 571
depression, 287
  assessment of, 243
  assessments of, 294
    cultural factors, 295
    screening tools, 295
    unique manifestations, 294–295

and cardiovascular disease, 415
classification of, 290
diagnosis, 296
distinguishing features of, 294*t*
functional consequences, 293*b*
  physical health and functioning,
    292–293
  psychosocial/quality of life, 293–294
interventions, 296–302
  antidepressant medications, 299–300, 300*t*,
    301*b*
  complementary and alternative therapies,
    302, 302*b*
  ECT education, 301
  education/counseling, 298–299
  effectiveness evaluation, 302
  exercise/nutrition, 297–298
  psychosocial function, 297
  referrals for therapy, 299
  risk factors alleviation, 297
late-life, 287
risk factors
  demographic/psychosocial, 290–291
  functional impairments, 291–292
  medical conditions, 291–292, 291*b*
  medications/alcohol, 292, 292*b*
and sleep disorder, 499
and suicide, 302–305
theories
  biologic theories, 289
  cognitive triad theory, 289
  dementia, 289
  genetic theories, 289
  learned helplessness theory, 288
  psychosocial theories, 287–288
  vascular depression, 289–290
wellness outcomes, 296
younger *vs.* older adults, 294*t*
depression in Alzheimer's disease, 290
depth perception, 337–338
dermatitis, cause of, 480
dermatoses, 480
dermis
  collagen in, 479
  elastin in, 479
  functions of, 479
desvenlafaxine, 300
detrusor, 385
developmental intelligence, 191
diabetes, 552–553
  assessments, 552–553
  and cataracts, 339
  diagnosis and wellness outcomes, 553
  guidelines for assessment of, 553*b*
  interventions, 553
  and sexual dysfunction, 529
diagnosis
  of bioactive substances, 136
  of cardiovascular function, 422–423
  of cognitive function, 194
  of delirium, 257
  of dementia, 260
  of depression, 296
  of digestion and nutrition, 372–374
  of elder abuse and neglect, 174
  of hearing, 321–322
  of mobility and safety, 464
  of psychosocial function, 212–213
  of respiratory function, 445
  of sexual function, 537
  of skin, 490
  of sleep and rest, 504
  of suicide, 305
  of thermoregulation, 520

of urinary function, 395
of vision, 348
*Diagnostic and Statistical Manual of Mental
    Disorders, 4th Edition, Text Revision
    (DSM-IV-TR)*, 290
dietary approaches to stop hypertension, 424
dietary fiber, 361
dietary habits and cardiovascular disease,
    412
dietary reference intakes (DRIs), 361
digestion and nutrition
  age-related changes
    esophagus and stomach, 360
    intestinal tract, 360
    liver, pancreas, and gallbladder, 360
    oral cavity, 359–360
    smell and taste, 358
  assessment of
    behavioral cues to, 371*b*
    interviewing, 369–370, 370*b*
    MNA-SF, 373*f*
    observing cues to, 370
    physical assessment and laboratory
      information, 370–371, 372*b*
    using assessment tools, 371
  constipation, 369
  diagnosis, 372–374
  functional consequences
    ability to procure, prepare, and enjoy
      food, 367
    nutritional status and weight changes, 368,
      368*f*
    oral function, changes in, 367–368
    quality of life, 368–369
  interventions
    daily food intake, guidelines for, 377*b*
    evaluating effectiveness of, 377
    food guide pyramid for, 378*f*
    promoting optimal nutrition and preventing
      disease, 376–377
    promoting oral and dental health, 375–376,
      376*b*
    risk factors, 374–375, 375*f*
  nutritional requirements, age-related changes
      in, 360–361
    calories, 361
    carbohydrates and fiber, 361
    fats, 361
    water, 361–362
  risk factors, 362, 362*t*
    cultural and socioeconomic factors,
      365–366
    environmental factors, 366–367
    functional impairments and disease
      processes, 363–364
    lifestyle factors, 364–365
    medication effects, 364, 365*t*
    myths and misunderstandings, behaviors
      based on, 367
    oral care, conditions related to, 363, 363*b*
    psychosocial factors, 365
  wellness outcomes, 374
digital hearing aids, 326
diminished speech discrimination, 317
diphenhydramine, adverse effects of, 457
disengagement theory, of aging, 52
do not resuscitate (DNR) order, 152
"donut hole" period, 125
driving cessation, 204
driving rehabilitation programs, 109
driving safety assessment, 108–110
  addressing risk factors, 109
  referring to community resources,
    109–110

risk identification, 108–109
working with caregivers, 110
driving skills and vision changes, 340
drug-induced parkinsonism, 125, 131
drusen, 343
dry eyes
  causes of, 338
  comfort measures for, 350
dry skin
  prevention of, 491*b*, 492
  risk factors of, 481
ductectasia, 437
durable power of attorney for health care, 152–153
dying, 575
Dying Person's Bill of Rights, 580*b*
dyslipidemias. *See* lipid disorders
dysphagia, 363, 364
dyspnea
  at the end of life, 583
  nursing care of, 442

E

earwax. *See* cerumen
eccrine glands, role of, 479
ectropion, 333
Eden Alternative, 81
education/health promotion
  about constipation, 375*b*
  about fall prevention, 468*b*
  about hearing, 319*b*
  about oral and dental care, 376*b*
  about orthostatic and postprandial
      hypotension, 429*b*
  about osteoporosis, 465–467
  about respiratory function, 441, 443*b*
  about sexual function, 538*b*, 539*b*
  about skin care, 491*b*
  about sleep and rest, 503*b*
  about urinary wellness, 396*b*
  about vision, 346*b*
  during illness, 553, 555
elastic recoil, 437
elder abuse and neglect
  assessments, 168–174
    activities of daily living, 171
    cultural aspects, 173–174
    degree of frailty, 171
    environmental influences, 172–173
    injuries/bruises/physical harm, 169–171
    nutrition and hydration, 169
    pathologic conditions, 171
    physical health, 169–171
    psychosocial function, 171–172
    support resources, 172
    threats to life, 173
    unique aspects of, 168–169
  characteristics, 162–163
  cultural considerations, 164–165
  definition of, 162
  diagnosis, 174
  forms of, 167
  functional consequences, 167–168
  increase in reports of, 163
  interventions, 175–177, 178*f*
    in community settings, 176
    effectiveness evaluation, 182
    in institutional settings, 175
    in multidisciplinary teams, 176–177
    nursing protocol, 180*b*
    prevention/treatment, 177
    referrals, 176–177
  legal interventions, 178–182
    adult protective services, 179

assessment, 179–180
consultation services, 180
ethical issues, 181–182, 182*t*
providing care, 180–181
reporting/collaborating, 179
testifying in court, 180
in nursing homes, 166–167
overview of, 162–165
prevalence and causes, 163–164
profiles, 164*b*
risk factors, 165–166
  caregiver factors, 165
  invisibility, 165
  psychosocial factors, 165
  vulnerability, 165
sites of accidental bruises, 170*f*
as social problem, 163
types of services needed in, 177, 178*f*
wellness outcomes, 175
elderspeak, 214
electroconvulsive therapy (ECT), 301
elimination half-time, drug, 114
empowering model, of phases of mature
    aging, 191
end of life, definition of, 575
End of Life Nursing Education Consortium
    (ELNEC), 578
end of life transition
  assessment and interventions, 584*t*
  cultural perspectives of, 578
  dying process/death, 575
  interventions
    active dying process symptoms in, 583–585
    anorexia and cachexia, 583
    constipation, 583
    dehydration, 583
    dyspnea, 583
    fatigue, 583
    managing symptoms, 582–585
    nausea and vomiting, 583
    promoting communication, 581, 582*b*
    spiritual support, 581–582
  quality of care for, 578
    hospice care, 580–581
    promoting wellness, 579–580
enophthalmos, 333
entropion, 333
environmental circumstances and sleep disorder,
    499–500
environmental factors
  and urinary function, 388–389, 389*b*
  in eating patterns, 366–367
environmental modifications
  for preventing incontinence, 399–400, 400*b*
    (*See also* urinary function)
  for sleep improvement, 507
  and visual wellness, 350, 350*b*, 351*b*
environmental modifications, as health
    promotion interventions, 68
Environmental Protection Agency, 439
environmental tobacco smoke. *See* secondhand
    smoke
environment, concept of, in Functional
    Consequences Theory, 39*b*, 42
epidermis, 477–479
  role of, 477
Epworth Sleepiness Scale (ESS), 504
erectile dysfunction, 525, 532
  and cigarette smoking, 529
esophagus and stomach, in digestion, 360
estradiol, production of, 525
estrogen levels and sexual function, 527
eszopiclone, 507
ethnogeriatrics, 21, 22

Evercare model, 86–87
everyday competence, 106
evidence-based practice, 61, 68, 72 (see page
    xxix in the front matter of this text for a
    complete list of evidence-based
    practice features)
excessive daytime sleepiness, 502
executional autonomy, 151
executive dysfunction, 239–240
exercise and healthy musculoskeletal function, 464
Exploritas, 197
external ear, 311–312
eye, 335–336, 335*f*
  appearance and tear ducts, 333–335

F

falls
  and fall-related injuries, prevention of, 467–471
    addressing extrinsic risk factors, 469
    addressing fear of falling, 471
    addressing intrinsic risk factors, 468–469, 469*f*
    fall prevention programs, 468*b*
    monitoring devices, usage of, 469–470
    preventing fall-related injuries and death,
        470–471
    Yaktrax Walker, 468, 469*f*
  fear of falling, 460
  and fractures, susceptibility to, 459–460
  and injury, identifying risks for, 462
  risk assessment, 460
    tools, usage of, 462
  risk factors for, 456–458, 456*b* (*See also*
      mobility and safety)
    environmental factors, 458
    medication effects, 457–458
    pathologic conditions and functional
        impairment, 457
    physical restraints, 458
fatigue, at the end of life, 583
fats
  function of, 361
  saturated, 361
  unsaturated, 361
fecal impaction and urinary incontinence, 388
Federal Interagency Forum on Aging-Related
    Statistics, 376
Feldenkrais method, 465
female sexual dysfunction, 532
fesoterodine, 400
fever, definition of, 515
fiber, role and requirements of, 361
Filipinos, caregiving relationships of, 7
Five Wishes document, 151, 155
fluid and crystallized intelligence theory, 189
fluid intelligence, 189
food guide pyramid, for older adult, 378*f*
footwear and fall prevention, 468
forced expiratory volume at 1 second (FEV$_1$), 438
foster care, 15*b*
fovea, 336
fragility fractures, 460
free radical theory, of aging, 49
frontotemporal dementia, 264
  distinguishing features of, 261*t*
functional age, 4
functional assessment, 95–106
  of ADLs, 99–101, 100*b*
  of cognitive ability, 101–105
  form for, 97, 98*f*–99*f*
  of IADLs, 101, 101*b*
  tools for, 95, 97–99, 97*f*
  for use of adaptive/assistive devices, 105–106
  wheelchair, fit assessment, 106, 106*t*

functional assessment scales, usage of, 462.
     See also musculoskeletal function
functional consequences, 37–39, 39*b*
     of cardiovascular function, 416
     of digestion, 367–369, 368*f*
     of hearing, 316–318
     of musculoskeletal function, 459–460
     negative, 37–38
     of pain, 563
     positive, 38–39
     of respiratory function, 440–441, 440*t*
     of sexual function, 530–532
     of skin, 481–482
     of sleep and rest, 501–502
     of thermoregulation, 516–517
     of urinary function, 389–390
     of vision, 339–340
functional disability, 47–48
functional impairments, affect urinary
     function, 387
Functional Consequences Theory for
     Promoting Wellness in Older
     Adults, 36–43, 38*f*
     application for wellness promotion, 42–43
     basic premises, 37
     concepts underlying, 37–42, 39*b*
          age-related changes and risk factors,
               39–40
          environment, 42
          functional consequences, 37–39
          health, 41–42
          nursing, 41
          person, 40–41
     vs. functional assessment, 39

G
gallbladder, in digestion, 360
gastrointestinal tract and urinary incontinence,
     388
generalized anxiety disorder (GAD), 241
generic drugs, 140–141
genetic influences and skin wellness, 480
genetic theory, of aging, 50
genitourinary tract, conditions of
     benign prostatic hyperplasia, 387
     pelvic floor dysfunction, 387
Geriatric Depression Scale-Short Form
     (GDS-SF), 295, 296*f*
geriatric medicine, 59
Geriatric Resource Nurse (GRN) model, 78
geriatrics, 59
Geriatrics journal, 59
Germans, caregiving relationships of, 7
gerontological advanced practice nurse
     (GAPN), 61
gerontological nursing, 60–63
     development timelines, 62*f*
     education for, 60–61
     evidence-based practice for, 61, 63
     history and development of, 60
     roles of advanced practice nurses in, 61
     standards of performance, 60*b*
Gerontological Society of America, 59
gerontologists
     assessments by
          active life expectancy, 47–48
          activities of daily living, 47
          life span/life expectancy, 46
          mortality rates, 46–47
     biogerontology subspecialty, 48
gerontology, 59
gerotranscendence theory, of
     aging, 55

glare, 337
     dazzling, 337
     scotomatic, 337
     veiling, 337
glaucoma, 343–345
     acute, 344
     and cataracts, 339
     chronic, 344
     normal-tension, 341*f*, 344
Global Deterioration Scale/Functional
     Assessment staging (GDS/FAST),
     Alzheimer's disease, 265, 266*t*
glomerular filtrate, definition of, 383
glomerular filtration rate (GFR), 383–384
Greeks, caregiving relationships of, 7
Green House Project, 81
Growing Old: The Process of Disengagement, 52
guardianship, 150
Guided Care model, 87
Guided Care Program for Families and
     Friends, 87
Guide to Culturally Competent Health Care, 22

H
hair color, age-related changes affect, 479
Haitians, caregiving relationships of, 7
hallucinations
     definition of, 244
     delirium associated, 247–248
     dementia associated, 248
     depression associated, 248
     distinguishing features of, 245*t*
     paranoid disorder associated, 248–249
Hartford Foundation for Geriatric Nursing, 462
Hartford Institute for Geriatric Nursing, 22, 122,
     484, 504, 536, 565
health
     concept of, in Functional Consequences
          Theory, 39*b*, 41–42
     defined, 63
health belief systems, 24
health care services, payment for, 88–90.
     See also payments, for health care
          services
health care workforce, diversity in, 20–21
health disparities, 24–25
     causes of, 25
     definition of, 25
     for diabetes and heart disease, 25*f*
     in older adults, 25
health education
     for health promotion, 68
     for oral and dental care, 376*b*
     for osteoporosis, 465–467, 466*b*
     for sexual wellness, 537, 538*b*
     for urinary wellness, 396*b*
     for visual wellness, 348–350, 349*b*
Health Empowerment Theory, 63
health promotion, 63–71
     concept of, 63
     initiatives, 64–65, 65*b*
     interventions for
          environmental modifications, 68
          guidelines for, 67*b*
          health education, 68
          physical activity, promotion of, 68, 69*t*
          risk-reduction interventions, 67–68
          screening programs, 65–66
          types and examples of, 65–68, 66t
     for older adults, 64
     role of nurses in, 63
     transtheoretical model of, 69–70, 71*t*
health-related quality of life, concept of, 64

healthy aging, 59
     studies of, 48–49
Healthy Aging and Depression program, 65
Healthy Aging Phenotype, 46
Healthy People 2010, 25
Healthy People 2020, 64–65
hearing
     age-related changes, 313*f*
          auditory nervous system, 314
          external ear, 311–312
          functional consequences of, 313*t*
          inner ear, 313–314
          middle ear, 312–313
     assessments of
          interviewing about hearing changes,
               318–320, 319*b*
          observing behavioral cues, 320
          using hearing assessment tools, 320–321
     diagnosis, 321–322
     functional consequences
          communication, effects on, 316–317
          hearing loss, effects of, 317–318
     interventions
          communicating with hearing-impaired older
               adults, 328
          compensating for hearing deficits,
               323–327
          effectiveness evaluation, 329
          preventing and alleviating impacted
               cerumen, 323
          promoting hearing wellness, 322–323
     pathologic condition affecting, 318
     risk factors
          disease processes, 316
          impacted cerumen, 315
          lifestyle and environmental factors, 314–315
          medication effects, 315–316
     wellness outcomes, 322
hearing aid, 325–327
     use and care of, 327
Hearing handicap inventory for the elderly
     (HHIE-S), 319
hearing-impaired people, communication
     techniques, 328*b*
heart disease, signs and symptoms of, 419–422
heart failure, 553–555
     assessments, 554, 554*b*
     consequences of, 554
     diagnosis and wellness outcomes, 554–555
     interventions, 555
heat exhaustion, 517
heat stroke, 517
Hendrich II Fall Risk Model, usage of,
     462, 463*f*
herbs (botanicals), 115–116
     commonly used, 117, 117*t*–118*t*
     and medications, with similar bioactivity, 115*t*
     potential adverse effects, 116, 116*t*
     tips for usage of, 139*b*
heredity and cardiovascular disease, 415
heredity factors and skin wellness, 480
hertz (Hz), 311
high-density lipoprotein (HDL), 412
high-level wellness, 2
hip protectors, usage of, 470, 470*f*
Hispanic Americans
     cultural overview, 27–29
          Cubans, 28
          Mexicans, 28
          Puerto Ricans, 28
Holistic Nursing Scope and Standards of
     Practice, on cultural competence, 21
holistic perspective, on aging, 56–57
home blood pressure monitoring, 418

home care services
    long-term home care, 83
    skilled home care, 83
    sources for, 83–84
    trends in, 82–83
homecare suite, 15b
homeless older adults, 32
homeopathic remedies, 116, 118
homeostasis, effects on, 389. *See also* Urinary
        function
hormonal level and osteoporosis, 455
hormonal therapy, 532
    for vasomotor symptoms treatment, 540
hospice, 576
Hospice and Palliative Nurses Association
        (HPNA), 552, 576
    on withdrawing life-sustaining therapies, 155,
        156b
hospice care, 580–581. *See also* end of life
        transition
Hospital Admission Risk Profile (HARP)
        screening tool, 77
hospital-at-home models, 77–78
Hospital Elder Life Program (HELP), 77
    for delirium management, 257, 258f
hot flashes, 526–527
Human Genome Project, 50
human immunodeficiency virus (HIV)
    health-related concerns, 533b
    risk factors for, 533–534
    role of nurses, 534
    treatment of, 534
human needs theory, of aging, 54
humidity level and respiratory function, 439
hydration, assessment of, 169
hyperlipidemias. *See* Lipid disorders
hypertension, 410
    and cardiovascular disease, 412–413
    nursing management of, 426b
    prevention and management of, 425–426, 427f
    stages of, 413t
hyperthermia
    assessment for, 519–520
    risk factors for, 516b
hypnotics, in sleep disorders management, 507
hypotension, risk factors for, 417b
hypothermia, 515
    assessing for, 519
    definition of, 520
    health promotion teaching, 522b
    risk factors for, 516b

I
illness
    characteristics of, 547–548
    concepts of wellness, and aging, 548–549
    families and caregivers, addressing needs of,
        555–557, 556t
    holistic care, 549–550
    NOC and NIC in, 549t
    palliative care programs, 550
    pathologic conditions
        cancer, 550–552
        diabetes mellitus, 552–553
        heart failure, 553–555
illusions. *See also* hallucinations
    definition of, 244
    distinguishing features of, 245t
Immigration Act, 1965, 20
immunity theory, of aging, 49–50
immunosenescence, 49–50
impacted cerumen, 315
impaired hearing, risk factors for, 314b

impotence, 532
Improving the Lives of LGBT Older Adults, 33
incompetent person, 150
Independence at Home model, 87
indwelling catheters
    and urinary tract infections, 387
    usage of, 387
infantilization, 214
informal caregivers, 15
inner ear, 313–314
insight, 239
    assessment of, 239
insomnia, 499, 502
Institutes for Learning in Retirement (ILR), 197
instrumental activities of daily living
        (IADLs), 97
    assessment of, 101, 101b
insulin resistance syndrome. *See* metabolic
        syndrome
intermediate nursing home care, 79
intermittent clean catheterization, 399
International Association for the Study of Pain
        (IASP), 560
International Diabetes Foundation, 414
Interpreter Facilitation for Individuals with
        Limited English Proficiency, 23
interpreters, use of, 23, 24b
interventions. *See also* Nursing Interventions
        Classification (NIC)
    for cardiovascular function, 423–429
    for digestion and nutrition, 374–377, 375f,
        376b, 377b, 378f
    for end of life transition, 581–585
    for hearing wellness, 322–328, 322b
    for musculoskeletal function, 464–472
    for respiratory function, 445–448
    for sexual function, 537–541
    for skin, 491–492
    for sleep and rest, 504–509
    for thermoregulation, 520–521
    for urinary function, 395–403, 396b, 402b
    for visual wellness, 348–353, 349b–352b
intestinal tract, digestion in, 360
Into Aging, 8
involuntary smoking, 439
iris, 335. *See also* Eye
isolated office hypertension. *See* white coat
        hypertension

J
Japanese, caregiving relationships of, 7
Joanna Briggs Institute, 61
John A. Hartford Foundation, 61
Joint Commission, 458
Joint National Committee (JNC), 413
joints and connective tissue, age-related changes
        in, 454
Journal of Gerontology, 59
Journal of the American Geriatrics Society, 60
Journal of the American Medical Association, 529

K
Kayser-Jones Brief Oral Health Status
        Examination, 370
kidneys and urinary excretion, 383–385
Koreans, caregiving relationships of, 7
kyphosis, 436

L
laboratory information, in urinary elimination
        assessment, 393
Langerhans cells, 478

late-life anxiety, detection and assessment of,
        242
late-life depression, 287. *See also* depression
late-onset hypogonadism, 527
Latinos. *See* Hispanic Americans
learned helplessness, 212
learned helplessness theory, 288
legal and ethical issues, 149–159
    advance directives, 151–153
        do not resuscitate order, 151
        durable power of attorney for health care,
            152–153
        living wills, 151
    autonomy and rights, 149–151
        competency, 149–150
        decision-making capacity, 150–151
    cultural aspects of, 155–156
    ethical issues
        in artificial nutrition and hydration, 154–155
        in everyday care of older adults, 153–154
    long-term care settings and, 153, 154
    role of nurses, 156–159, 158b
lens, 335. *See also* eye
lesbian, gay, bisexual, and transgender (LGBT)
        older adults, 32–33
Lewy body dementia, 264
    distinguishing features of, 261t
life-course theory, of aging, 54–55
life events, affecting daily life, 202–206
life expectancy, 46, 46f
life review, 216
life span, 46
lifestyle and environmental factors
    for hearing wellness, 314–315
    in skin wellness, 480
lifestyle interventions and hypertension, 425
lighting and sleep disorder, 499–500
linguistic competence, 23
lipid disorders, 412
    and cardiovascular disease, 413
    prevention and management of, 428–429, 428b
lipofuscin, 49, 360
liver, in digestion, 360
*Live Well, Live Long: Health Promotion and
        Disease Prevention for Older Adults*
        program, 65
living wills, 152
long-term care, 76b
long-term care insurance, 90
long-term care settings
    for dementia care, 273–274, 274b
low-density lipoprotein (LDL), 411
lower respiratory infections
    detection of, 442–443
    prevention of, 446–447
Low Income Home Energy Assistance
        Program's (LIHEAP), 521, 522
low-vision aids, for improving visual
        performance, 350–351, 352b
lung parenchyma, 437
lung structure and function, 437–438, 437t

M
MacArthur Research Network on Successful
        Aging, 4, 11
magnetic resonance imaging (MRI), 323
mainstream smoke, 439
male sexual dysfunction, 532
management
    of hypertension, 426b
    pain, 563–565, 571
    of sleep disorders, 507–508
    of vision, 342t

Mantoux test, 442
massage therapy, in sleep improvement, 506
mechanical presbycusis, 314
Medicaid, 89–90
medicalization, 576
Medicare, 88
  insurance plans, 89*b*
Medicare Part D prescription drug program,
  125
Medicare Select policy, 89
medication reconciliation, 137
medications
  absorption of oral medications, 113–114
  adverse effects of, 529, 529*b* (*See also* sexual
    function)
  age-related decreased clearance rate, 119*b*
  assessments, 132–133
    and cultural factors, 134
    guidelines for, 133*b*
  Beers criteria for, 122–123
  considerations regarding use of, 113–115
  devices for adherence, 140*f*
  effects and risk for falls, 457–458 (*See also*
    mobility and safety)
  effects in hearing wellness, 315–316
  effects in skin, 480–481
  effects in urinary function, 388, 388*t*
  guidelines for assessment of, 133*b*
  and herbs, with similar bioactivity, 115*t*
  inappropriate, 124
  interactions, 125–129
    with alcohol, 128, 128*t*
    with caffeine, 128, 128*t*
    with herbs, 126–127
    with medication, 125–126, 127*t*
    with nicotine, 128–129, 129*t*
    with nutrients, 127–128, 127*t*
  interventions for healthy-taking of,
    136–142
    adherence factors, 139–141
    decreasing medications number, 141–142
    education, 137–139
    evaluation of, 142
    evidence-based interventions, 136–137
  nonadherence to, 124
  polypharmacy, 124
  prescribing cascade, 125
  safe and effective use of, tips on, 138*b*
  in treating urinary incontinence, 400, 400*t*
  unrecognized adverse effects, 125, 126*t*
meditation techniques, in sleep improvement,
  506
mediterranean dietary pattern, 423
melanocytes, 478
melanoma, 482*f*, 483
melatonin, role of, 505–506
memory
  assessment of, 236–237
  in older adults, theories on, 190
  primary, 189
  recognition, 189
  secondary, 189
Ménière disease, 316
menopause, 525
menses, 525
metabolic presbycusis, 314
metabolic syndrome, 414
  risk factors of, 414
metamemory, 190
Mexican Americans, caregiving relationships
  of, 7
middle ear, 312–313
mild cognitive impairment (MCI), 263
mindfulness, 195

Mini-Cog, for cognitive impairment, 234
Mini-Mental State Examination (MMSE), 231
Minimum Data Set (MDS), 106, 153
mini nutritional assessment (MNA), 371
mini nutritional assessment-short form
  (MNA-SF), 373
mixed hearing loss, 316
mixed urinary incontinence, 390
mobility and safety
  age-related changes
    bones, 452–453
    joints and connective tissue, 454
    muscles, 453–454
    nervous system, 454
    osteopenia and osteoporosis, 454
  diagnosis, 464
  musculoskeletal function, pathologic
    condition, 458–459
  risk factors, 454–455
    falling, 456–458, 456*b*
    musculoskeletal function, 455
    osteoporosis and osteoporotic fractures, 455
  wellness outcomes, 464
Mongolian spots, 488
monoamine oxidase inhibitors (MAOIs), 299
movement-detection devices, usage of, 470
muscles, 453–454
  age-related changes in, 453–454
musculoskeletal function
  assessment of
    guidelines for, 461*b*
    identifying fall risks, 462
    musculoskeletal performance, 460–461
    osteoporosis, risks for, 461
  functional consequences
    effects on, 459
    falls and fractures, susceptibility to, 459–460
    fear of falling, 460
  interventions for
    evaluating effectiveness of, 471–472
    fall prevention programs, 468*b*
    health education, 465–467
    healthy musculoskeletal function and
      preventing falls, 464–465
    preventing falls and fall-related injuries,
      467–471
  pathologic condition, 458–459
  risk factors, 455
myocardium and neuroconduction mechanisms,
  409–410
myths and misunderstandings, 8, 9*t*
  in eating patterns, 367
  urinary function and, 386–387

N

nail growth, factors affecting, 479
narcotic, 569
Nathan Cummings Foundation, 578
National Association for the Visually
  Handicapped (NAVH), 350
National Association of Chronic Disease
  Directors (NACDD), 65
National Association of Insurance
  Commissioners, 89
National Center for Chronic Disease Prevention
  and Health Promotion, 64
National Center on Elder Abuse, 162
National Cholesterol Education Program, 413
National Commission on Sleep Disorders
  Research, 502
National Consensus Project for Quality Palliative
  Care, 550
National Council on Aging (NCOA), 65

National Family Caregiver Support Program,
  90
National Gerontological Nursing Association,
  565
National Hospice and Palliative Care
  Organization, 550
National Institute for Occupational Safety and
  Health, 315
National Institute of Nursing Research (NINR),
  63
National Institutes of Health (NIH), 139, 532
National Long-Term Care Ombudsman program,
  153
National Long-Term Care Survey, 48
National Pressure Ulcer Advisory Panel
  (NPUAP), 484, 487
National Senior Service Corps, 297
*National Standards for Culturally and
  Linguistically Appropriate Services*
  (CLAS standards), 23
nausea and vomiting, at the end of life, 583
neglect. *See* elder abuse and neglect
nervous system, 454
neural presbycusis, 314
neuroendocrine theory, of aging, 49
neuropathic pain, 562
neuroplasticity, 189
neurostimulator, 398
nicotine, 128–129
  adverse effects of, 529 (*See also* sexual
    function)
  intake and sleep disorder, 500
nociception, 561
  modulation, 562
  perception, 562
  transduction, 561
  transmission, 561–562
nociceptive pain, 562
nocturia, 387
  causes of, 390
  functional consequences of, 390
nocturnal myoclonus. *See* periodic limb
  movements in sleep (PLMS)
noise and sleep disorder, 499
noise-induced hearing loss (NIHL), 315
nonopioid analgesics, 569
non-rapid eye movement (NREM), 496, 498
nonsteroidal anti-inflammatory drugs (NSAIDs),
  569
  usage of, 570
non traumatic fractures. *See* fragility fractures
normal-tension glaucoma, 341*f*, 344
North American Menopause Society, 540
nose, age-related connective tissue changes in,
  435
nuclear cataracts, 342
numerical rating scale (NRS), 566, 567, 567*f*
Nurse Reinvestment Act of 2002, 60
nurses
  addressing attitudes of, 8
  cultural self-assessment for, 21–22, 22*b*
  gerontological nursing education, 60–61
  in lower respiratory infections prevention,
    446–447
  role in legal and ethical issues, 156–159
  use of health promotion interventions by, 63
Nurses Improving Care to the Hospitalized
  Elderly (NICHE), 61, 77
nursing
  concept of, in Functional Consequences
    Theory, 39*b*, 41
  gerontological (*See* gerontological nursing)
nursing fall risk assessment tools, usage of, 462
nursing home, 78

nursing home care
  intermediate nursing home care, 79
  levels of, 78–79
  long-term care, admission to, 79, 79f
  new models of
    assisted-living facilities, 81–82
    and culture change movement, 80–81
    Pioneer Network, 81
    roles for nurses in, 82
  restorative care, 79
  role of nurses, 80
  skilled nursing home care, 78–79
  special care units, 79–80
  trends in, 79
Nursing Home Diversion program, 90
Nursing Home Reform Law, 539
Nursing Home Residents' Bill of Rights, 153, 154b
nursing interventions classification (NIC)
  for bioactive substances, 136
  for cardiovascular disease, 423
  for cognitive wellness, 195
  for delirium, 257
  for dementia, 272
  for depression, 296
  for digestion, 374
  for elder abuse, 175
  for hearing, 322
  for illness, 549, 549t, 556t
  for mobility and safety, 464
  for psychosocial wellness, 195
  for respiratory function, 445
  for sexual function, 537
  for skin, 491
  for sleep and rest, 504
  for thermoregulation, 520
  for vision, 348
Nursing Knowledge International, 63
nursing outcomes classification (NOC)
  for abused older adult, 175
  for bioactive substances, 136
  for cardiovascular disease, 423
  for cognitive wellness, 194
  for delirium, 257
  for dementia, 271
  for depression, 296
  for digestion, 374
  for hearing, 322
  for illness, 549, 549t, 556t
  for mobility and safety, 464
  for respiratory function, 445
  for sexual function, 537
  for skin, 490
  for sleep and rest, 504
  for thermoregulation, 520
  for vision, 348
nutritional status and weight changes, in older adults, 368, 368f
nutrition and lifestyle interventions, in cardiovascular disease, 423–424
nutrition assessment tools, usage of, 371

O
obesity
  and cardiovascular disease, 412
  and respiratory function, 440
obstructive sleep apnea, 500, 502–503
  symptoms of, 502
Occupational Safety and Health Act, 439
older adults, 4
  age-related variations in laboratory values in, 96t
  caregiving needs of, 14–15

cultural groups of, 26–31
depression in, 303 (See also depression)
digestive and nutritional wellness in, 359
diversity of, 20–33
educational levels by race/Hispanic origin, 12f
in families, 14–16
Functional Consequences Theory perspective on, 39b, 40–41
grandchildren caregiving by, 16
health characteristics of, 11, 11b
health disparities affecting, 25
homeless, 32
housing options for, 15b
illness in, 547–548
LGBT elders, 32–33
living arrangements of, 11–14, 14f
marital status by sex/age, 13f
population projections, 21f
poverty level by race/Hispanic origin, 12f
promoting urinary wellness in, 384
as recipients and givers of care, 15–16
in rural areas, 32
socioeconomic characteristics of, 11–13, 13b
U.S. cultural diversity of, 20–21
in world, 16, 17b
Older Americans Act (OAA), 3, 82, 90, 374
olfaction, 358
Omnibus Budget Reconciliation Act (OBRA), 106, 153
Oncology Nursing Society and Geriatric Consortium, 552
On Death and Dying, 580
On Lok Senior Services program, 86
opioid analgesics, 569
oral and dental health, promoting, 375–376, 376b
oral cavity, 359–360
oral function, changes in, 367–368
oral health, conditions in, 363, 363b. See also Digestion and nutrition
oral mucosa, age-related changes of, 360
organic brain syndrome (OBS), 259
orientation, assessment of, 235–236
orthostatic hypotension, 417
  prevention and management of, 429, 429b
osteoarthritis, 458–459
  prevention and treatment of, 459
osteopenia, 454
osteoporosis, 452, 454
  health education for, 465–467, 466b
  prevalence of, 454
  risk factors for, 455, 455b
  risk identification for, 461
osteoporotic fractures, 455
otosclerosis, 316
otoscope
  guidelines for, 321b
  usage of, 320
Outing Age 2010, 33
overactive bladder (OAB), 390
  risk factor of, 390
over-the-counter drugs, 121
oxybutynin, 400

P
PACE programs, 86
pain
  acute, 560
  acute vs. persistent, 560–561
  age-related changes affect, 563

assessments, 565, 566b
  cognitively impaired older adults, 568, 569t
  collecting pertinent information, 565–566
  pain components, 566–568
  sample questions, 566b
cancer, 562
causes of, 562–563
chronic, 561
cultural aspects of, 563–565
factors affecting, 563b
functional consequences, 563
management, barriers in, 563, 564t
neuropathic, 562
nociceptive, 562
persistent, 560, 561
principles of analgesic medication, 568–569
  classifications of, 569–570
  pain management plan, 571–573, 572t
  side effects management, 571, 571b
  WHO's pain relief ladder, 570, 570f
rating scales, 567f
somatic, 562
types of, 562
visceral, 562
Pain Assessment Checklist for Seniors with Limited Ability to Communicate (PACSLAC), 568
Pain Assessment in Advanced Dementia (PAINAD), 568
pain intensity, 566
pain receptors, 561
palliation, 575
palliative care, 550
pancreas, in digestion, 360
papillae, 478
paradox of wellbeing, 191
paranoia, 244–245
parish nurse programs, 85
Partnership for Prescription Assistance, 141
passive smoke. See secondhand smoke
pathologic conditions
  cardiovascular function, 417
  falls in older adults, 457
  respiratory function, 441
  sexual function, 533–534
  of skin, 482–487
  sleep and rest, 502–503
Patient Health Questionnaire (PHQ-2), 295
Patient Self-Determination Act (PSDA), 151
payments, for health care services
  long-term care insurance, 90
  Medicaid, 89–90
  Medicare, 88, 89b
  medigap insurance, 88–89
  OAA funds, 90
  out-of-pocket spending, 88, 88f
pelvic floor dysfunction, 387
pelvic floor electrical stimulation, 398
pelvic floor muscle training (PFMT), 396, 397, 397b
  goal of, 397
  in pubococcygeal muscle identification, 397
perceived age, 3
perception, 561
percutaneous endoscopic gastrostomy (PEG) tube, 155
perimenopause, 525
periodic limb movements in sleep (PLMS), 500
periurethral injections, usage of, 401
persistent pain, 560, 561
  treatment of, 570
personal emergency response system (PERS), 470
personal listening system, 323

Person-Environment Fit Theory, 42
pessaries, usage of, 398
phacoemulsification, 342
pharmacodynamics, 113
pharmacokinetics, 113
pharmacologic interventions, for cardiovascular
    disease prevention, 425
phonemes, 317
phosphodiesterase-5 inhibitors, 540
photoaging, 480
photosensitivity, 480
physical activity, as health promotion
    intervention, 68, 69*t*
physical inactivity, 411
    and cardiovascular disease, 411–412
physiology, of pain, 561–562, 561*f*
Pioneer Network, 81
Pittsburgh Sleep Quality Index (PSQI), 504
plaques, 411
pneumococcal vaccines, 446
pneumonia, in older adults, 440
polypharmacy, 124
posterior subcapsular cataracts, 342
post-fall syndrome, 460
postmenopause, 525
postprandial hypotension, 417
    prevention and management of, 429, 429*b*
postural hypotension. *See* orthostatic
    hypotension
potentially inappropriate medications (PIMs),
    122
    prevalence of, 123*t*
presbycusis, 314, 317
presbyopia, 337
presbyphagia, 360
prescription assistance programs, 141
pressure ulcer, 480, 483–487
    risk for development of, 483, 483*f*
    stages of, 486*t*–487*t*
pressure ulcer scale for healing (PUSH),
    487
prevention
    of dry skin, 491*b*, 492
    of falls and fall-related injuries, 467–471
    of hypertension, 425–426, 427*f*
    of lipid disorders, 428–429, 428*b*
    of lower respiratory infections, 446–447
    of orthostatic hypotension, 429, 429*b*
    of osteoarthritis, 459
    of osteoporotic fractures, 466–467
    of postprandial hypotension, 429, 429*b*
    of skin wrinkles, 491–492
Prevention Research Centers on Healthy Aging
    Research Network (PRC-HAN), 4
Program of All-inclusive Care for the Elderly
    (PACE) mode, 85
program theory of aging, 50
*Promoting Exercise and Behavior Change in
    Older Adults,* 69
prompted voiding, 395
prostatic hyperplasia, 530
protein, 361
protein-calorie malnutrition. *See* protein-energy
    malnutrition
protein-energy malnutrition, 368
pseudodementia, 259
pseudohypertension, 418
psychological theories, of aging, 54–56
    gender and aging theory, 55
    gerotranscendence theory, 55
    human needs theory, 54
    life-course and personality development
        theories, 54–55
    relevance to nurses/nursing, 55–56

psychosocial assessment, 226–253
    affective function, 240–244
        anxiety, 241–242
        depression, 243
        guidelines, 240–241, 244*b*
        happiness/well-being, 243–244
        mood, 241
        self-esteem, 242–243
    communication skills for, 229–233
        creating environment for, 231–233
        enhancement of, 230–231, 234*b*
        identifying barriers, 229–230
    contact with reality, 244–249
        delusions, 244–247
        guidelines for, 249*b*
        hallucinations and illusions, 247–249
        special considerations, 249
    decision-making capacity, 238–239
    executive function, 239–240
    mental status assessment, 233–238, 236*b*,
        238*b*
        alertness/attention, 236
        higher language skills, 238, 238*b*
        memory, 236–237
        motor function/psychomotor behaviors,
            234–235
        orientation, 235–236
        physical appearance, 234
        response to interview, 235
        social skills, 235
        speech and language characteristics,
            237–238, 238*b*
    overview of, 226–229
    procedure for, 227–228
    purposes of, 227
    religion/spirituality, 251–253, 253*b*
    scope of, 228–229
    social supports, 249–251, 251*b*
        barriers to, 251
        economic resources, 251
        social network, 250–251
psychosocial factors
    and cardiovascular disease, 414–415
    in eating patterns, 365 (*See also* digestion and
        nutrition)
    and sleep disorder, 499 (*See also* sleep and
        rest)
psychosocial function, 202–221
    assessment, 212
    diagnosis, 212–213
    functional consequences, 212
    influential factors
        cultural considerations, 209–211
        religion/spirituality, 208–209
    interventions, 213–219, 218*b*
        addressing role loss, 216
        addressing spiritual needs, 217–218
        coping strategies, 221*t*
        decision-making involvement, 215–216
        encouraging life review/reminiscence,
            216
        fostering social supports, 217
        healthy aging classes, 218–219
        self-esteem enhancement, 214, 215*b*
        sense of control promotion, 215
    life events and, 202–206, 203*f*
        ageist attitudes, 205–206
        chronic illness, 204
        death of friends and family, 205
        driving vehicle, 204–205
        functional impairments, 204
        relocation, 204
        retirement, 203–204
        widowhood, 205

    risk factors, 211–212
    theories about, 206–208
        coping, 207–208
        emotional development, 206
        stress, 206–207
    wellness outcomes, 213
Puerto Ricans, caregiving relationships of, 7
pulsed magnetic therapy, 398
purified protein derivative (PPD), 442–443

Q

quality of care
    at the end of life transition, 578
        hospice care, 580–581
        promoting wellness, 579–580

R

rapid eye movement (REM), 496, 498
    sleep, characteristics of, 498
Recommended Dietary Allowances
    (RDAs), 360
Re-engineered Hospital Discharge (RED)
    program, 78
reminiscence, 216
renal tubules and urine concentration, 385
Resident Assessment Instrument (RAI), 153
resident-centered care, 80
residents, 78
Residents' Rights bill, 539
respiratory function
    age-related changes
        chest wall and musculoskeletal structures,
            436–437
        lung structure and function, 437–438, 437*t*
        upper respiratory structures, 435–436
    assessments of
        guidelines for, 443*b*
        health promotion, identifying opportunities
            for, 441–442
        lower respiratory infections, detecting,
            442–443
        older adults who smoke, 444*b*
        physical assessment findings, 444–445
        smoking behaviors, assessment of, 443–444
    COPD, 441
    diagnosis, 445
    functional consequences, 440–441, 440*t*
    interventions
        eliminating the risk from smoking, 447–448
        evaluating effectiveness of, 448
        health promotion teaching, 446*b*
        lower respiratory infections, 446–447
        promoting respiratory wellness, 445–446
    risk factors
        compromised respiratory function, 439–440
        secondhand smoke, 439
        tobacco use, 438–439
        workforces, 439*b*
    wellness outcomes, 445
respite services, 85
restless legs syndrome (RLS), 496
    and sleep disorder, 500
restorative care, 79
retained awareness, 266
retina, 335
retinal–neural pathway, 336
retirement community, 15*b*
Retooling for an Aging America, 64
risk factors, 36, 39*b*, 40
    for cardiovascular function, 410–416
    for digestion and nutrition, 362–367, 362*t*,
        363*b*, 365*t*

for hearing, 314–316
for mobility and safety, 454–458
for respiratory function, 438–440
for sexual function, 527–530
for skin, 480–481
for sleep and rest, 499–501
for thermoregulation, 515–516
for urinary function, 386–389, 388*t*, 389*b*
for vision, 338–339
risk-reduction interventions, for older adults,
67–68
Roadwise Review, 109
Robert Wood Johnson Foundation Last Acts Task
Force, 575
Roy's Adaptation Model, 63
rural older adults, 32
Russians, caregiving relationships of, 7

S

sacral nerve stimulation therapy, 398
saliva, in food digestion, 359–360
sandwich generation, 14
sarcopenia, 454
saturated fats, 361
scaffolding theory of aging and cognition,
189
scotomatic glare, 337
screening programs, for older adults, 65–66
secondhand smoke, 439
Selective Optimization With Compensation
theory, 63, 206
selective serotonin reuptake inhibitors (SSRIs),
299–300
self-care actions, for sleep improvement, 505
self-esteem, 203, 214, 215*b*
senescence, 48
senility, 259
sensorineural hearing losses, 316
sensory presbycusis, 314
serotonin and norepinephrine reuptake inhibitors
(SNRIs), 299
Services and Advocacy for Gay, Lesbian,
Bisexual, and Transgender Elders
(SAGE), 33
settings, for health care
acute care, 77–78
community-based services, 84–86
home care services, 82–84
new nursing home care models, 80–82
nursing home, 78–80
Sexual Behaviours in the Human Female, 527
sexual function
age-related changes
older men, 527
older women, 525–527
assessments of, 535–537, 536*b*
self-assessment, 534–535, 535*b*
cultural aspects of, 535
diagnosis, 537
functional consequences, 530–531
female sexual dysfunction, 532
male sexual dysfunction, 532
reproductive ability, 531
response to sexual stimulation, 531
sexual interest and activity, 531–532
interventions
addressing risk factors, 537–539
evaluating effectiveness of, 541
health education for, 538*b*
long-term care settings, 539, 539*b*
teaching about sexual wellness, 537
teaching men, 540–541
teaching women, 539–540

pathologic condition
health-related concerns, 533*b*
HIV, risk factors for, 533–534
nurses, role of, 534
risk factors
chronic conditions, 529–530
families and caregivers, attitudes and
behaviors of, 528
functional impairments and dementia, 530
gender-specific conditions, 530
medication, alcohol, and nicotine, adverse
effects of, 529
sexual activity, limited opportunities for,
528–529
societal influences, 527–528
wellness outcomes, 537
sexual stimulation
functional consequences for, 531*t*
response to, 531
shared housing, 15*b*
"SHOW ME" functional assessment tool, 95
sidestream smoke, 439
sildenafil, 540
skilled nursing home care, 78–79
skin
age-related changes
dermis, 479
epidermis, 477–479
hair, 479
nails, 479
subcutaneous tissue and cutaneous nerves,
479
sweat and sebaceous glands, 479
assessments of
health promotion, identifying opportunities
for, 487
interview questions for, 488*b*
observing skin, hair, and nails, 487–489,
490*b*
skin lesions, 488*t*
diagnosis, 490
functional consequences, 482*t*
comfort and sensation, 481
cosmetic effects, 481–482
susceptibility to injury, 481
ultraviolet radiation, response to, 481
interventions
detecting and treating harmful skin lesions,
492
evaluating effectiveness of, 492
preventing dry skin, 492
preventing skin wrinkles, 491–492
promoting healthy skin, 491, 491*b*
pathologic conditions affecting skin,
482–487
risk factors
genetic influences, 480
lifestyle and environmental influences,
480
medication effects, 480–481
social functions of, 477
wellness outcomes, 490
skin cancer, 482–483
skin lesions, 488*t*, 489*f*
characteristics of, 488
detection and treatment of, 491*b*, 492
occurrence of, 488
skin wrinkles, prevention of, 491–492
skipped-generation households, 16
sleep and rest
age-related changes, 496–497, 498*t*
circadian rhythm, 498–499
sleep quality, 498
sleep quantity, 497–498

assessments of
evidence-based assessment tools, 503–504
health promotion, identifying opportunities
for, 503, 503*b*
diagnosis, 504
functional consequences, 501–502
health promotion teaching, 508*b*
interventions for
complementary and alternative care
practices, 505–506
educating older adults, 507
environmental modifications to promote
sleep, 507
evaluating effectiveness of, 509
evidence-based interventions, 504–505
health promotion teaching, 505*b*
institutional settings, improving sleep in,
506–507
self-care actions, 505
sleep disorders, teaching about management
of, 507–508
medications effect on, 501*t*
pathologic condition affecting, 502–503
relaxation and mental imagery techniques, 506*b*
risk factors
bioactive substances, effects of, 500–501
environmental factors, 499–500
pathophysiologic factors, 500, 501*t*
psychosocial factors, 499
wellness outcomes, 504
sleep apnea syndrome, 496
sleep latency, 497
sleep–wake circadian rhythm, causes of, 498
small-house nursing home, 81
smell and taste, 358. *See also* digestion and
nutrition
smokeless tobacco, 438
smoking
behaviors, assessment of, 443–444 (*See also*
respiratory function)
and cardiovascular disease, 424
cessation, 445
and respiratory disease, 445
risk elimination, 447–448
Snellen chart, usage of, 347, 347*b*
social isolation, 213
and hyperthermia, 516
social network, 250–251
Social Readjustment Rating Scale (SRRS), 207
social skills, assessment of, 235
societal influences, and sexual function, 527–528
sociocultural theories, of aging, 51–53
activity theory, 52
age stratification theory, 52–53
disengagement theory, 52
emerging theories, 53
person–environment fit theory, 53
relevance to nurses/nursing, 53
subculture theory, 52
socioemotional selectivity theory, 191, 206
solifenacin, 400
somatic pain, 562
sound amplification, 323
special care units (SCUs), 79–80
spiritual well-being, 581
squamous cell carcinoma, 482, 482*f*
stage theories, of adult cognitive development,
190–191
*Standards of Professional Gerontological
Nursing Performance,* 60*b*, 61
Stephen Ministries, 252
stepped-care approach, 425
stereopsis, 338
St. John's wort, 302

Stokes/Gordon Stress Scale (SGSS), 207, 207*t*
stress, 206
stressors theory, 206–207
stress urinary incontinence, 390
subacute care units, 77
subculture theory, of aging, 52
subcutaneous tissue and cutaneous nerves, 479
subjective age, 3
successful aging, 4–5
suicide, 292, 302–305
    assessment of risk for, 303–305, 304*b*
    diagnosis, 305
    interventions for, 305, 305*b*
    rates by race/ethnicity, 303*f*
sun-damaged skin, characteristics of, 480
sun protection factor (SPF), 491
Supercentenarian Research Foundation, 48
surgical and minimally invasive procedures, in treating urinary incontinence, 401
survivorship curve, 46–47
    rectangularization of curve, 47
sweat and sebaceous glands, 479
systolic hypertension, 413

T

tacrine (Cognex), 276
tactile sensitivity, 481. *See also* skin
tadalafil, 540
tai chi, 459, 464
    in sleep improvement, 506
tardive dyskinesia, 123, 131
telehealth, 86
terazosin, 388
testosterone
    levels and cigarette smoking, 527
    therapy and osteoporosis prevention, 467
testosterone deficiency. *See* late-onset hypogonadism
The Care of Dying Patients, 575
thermoregulation
    age-related changes
        normal body temperature, 515
        response to cold temperatures, 513–515
        response to hot temperatures, 515
    assessment of
        baseline temperature, 517
        febrile response to illness, 520
        hyperthermia, 519–520
        hypothermia, 519
        risk factors for, 517–519
    diagnosis of, 520
    functional consequences, 516–517
        altered perception of environmental temperatures, 517
        altered response to hot environments, 517
        altered thermoregulatory response to illness, 517
        cold environments, altered response to, 517
        psychosocial consequences, 517
    guidelines for assessing, 519*b*
    interventions
        addressing risk factors, 520–521
        evaluating effectiveness of, 521–522
        promoting healthy thermoregulation, 521
    primary function of, 513
    risk factors
        environmental and socioeconomic influences, 515–516
        lack of knowledge, 516
        pathophysiologic conditions, 515
    wellness outcomes, 520

thirst perception and urinary function, 386
tinnitus, 318
tobacco
    smoking and cardiovascular disease, 412
    use and respiratory disease, 438–439, 441
tolerance, 571
    definition of, 571
tolterodine, 400
Toolkit of Instruments for Measuring End-of-life Care (TIME), 578
trabecular bone. *See* cancellous bone
transcultural nursing, 21
transitional care, 78
Transitional Care Model (TCM): Hospital Discharge Screening Criteria for High Risk Older Adults, 78
Transtheoretical model (TTM), of health promotion, 69–70, 71*t*
    action stage, 70
    contemplation stage, 69–70
    maintenance stage, 70
    precontemplation stage, 69
    preparation stage, 70
tricyclic antidepressants, 123
Try This: Best Practices in Nursing Care to Older Adults, 95, 180
t-score, 454
tuberculin skin test, 442
tuberculosis, in older adults, 441
tunica intima
    age-related changes in, 410
    composition of, 410
    role of, 410

U

ultraviolet radiation and skin wellness, 481
unit-dose medication systems, 139
United States Pharmacopoeia (USP) mark, 116, 116*f*
unsaturated fats, 361
upper respiratory structures, 435–436
urban hyperthermia, 516
urban hypothermia, 516
urethritis, 530
urge urinary incontinence, 390
urinalysis, 371
urinary control devices, usage of, 398–399, 398*f*
urinary elimination, patterns of, 394*f*
urinary function
    age-related changes
        bladder and urinary tract, 385
        control mechanisms, 385–386
        control over urination, 386
        kidneys, 383–385
    assessment of
        health promotion, identifying opportunities for, 392–393, 393*b*
        laboratory information, 393
        talking about urinary function, 391–392
        urinary elimination, 392*b*
    diagnosis, 395
    functional consequences
        homeostasis, effects on, 389
        voiding patterns, effects on, 389–390
    interventions
        evaluating effectiveness, 402–403
        health education, 396*b*
        managing incontinence, 401, 402*b*
        promoting continence and alleviating incontinence, 396–401
        urinary wellness, teaching about, 395–396

pathologic condition affecting, 390–391
    risk factors
        environmental factors, 388–389, 389*b*
        functional impairments, 387
        medication effects, 388, 388*t*
        myths and misunderstandings, 386–387
        pathologic conditions, 387–388
    wellness outcomes, 395
urinary incontinence, 383, 390–391
    cause of, 388
    mixed, 390
    prevalence of, 390
    signs and symptoms of, 390
    stress, 390
    urge, 390
U.S. Department of Health and Human Services, 448
U.S. Food and Drug Administration (FDA), 458
U.S. Preventive Services Task Force (USPSTF), 295
U.S. Senate Special Committee on Aging, 580

V

vaginal hormonal therapy, 540
vaginitis, 530
valerian, in sleep improvement, 506
values clarification, 154
vardenafil, 540
varenicline, 448
vascular dementia, 263–264
    distinguishing features of, 261*t*
vascular depression, 289–290
veiling glare, 337
verbal descriptor scale (VDS), 566, 567*f*
Vietnamese, caregiving relationships of, 7
the village, 15*b*
visceral pain, 562
vision
    age-related changes, 336–337
        altered color vision, 338
        delayed dark and light adaptation, 337
        diminished acuity, 337
        diminished critical flicker fusion, 338
        diminished depth perception, 337–338
        eye, 335–336
        increased glare sensitivity, 337
        loss of accommodation, 337
        reduced visual field, 337
        retinal–neural pathway, 336
        slower visual information processing, 338, 338*t*
        tear ducts and eye appearance, 333–335
    assessment of
        identifying opportunities for health promotion, 345–346
        interviewing about changes, 345, 346*b*
        observing cues to visual function, 346, 347*b*
        standard vision tests, 347–348, 347*b*
    diagnosis, 348
    disease conditions affecting, 342*t*
    functional consequences
        driving, effects on, 340
        quality of life, effects on, 340
        safety and function, effects on, 339–340
    guidelines for using magnifying aids, 353*b*
    interventions
        dry eyes, comfort measures for, 350
        environmental modifications, 350, 350*b*, 351*b*
        evaluating effectiveness of, 353
        eye care practitioners, 349*b*

health promotion interventions, 348–350, 349b
    low-vision aids, 350–351, 352b
    quality of life, maintaining and improving, 351–353
pathologic conditions affecting
    AMD, 343
    cataracts, 341–343
    glaucoma, 343–345
    risk factors, 338–339
    wellness outcomes, 348
visual acuity, 337
visual field, 337
visual impairment, 336
vitamin D
    deficiency and musculoskeletal health, 455
    intake and osteoporosis prevention, 466
    and skin cancer, 491
vitamin D deficiency, screening for, 66
voiding patterns and urinary incontinence, 389–390. *See also* urinary function

W
warfarin (Coumadin), 126
wear-and-tear theory, of aging, 49
wellness
    cultural perspectives on, 23–24
    defined, 63
    and nursing care of older adults, 2–3
    and older adults, 2
wellness outcomes, 37
    for cardiovascular function, 423
    for cognitive function, 194
    for dementia, 271
    for depression, 296
    for digestion and nutrition, 374
    for elder abuse and neglect, 175
    for hearing, 322
    for mobility and safety, 464
    for psychosocial function, 213
    for respiratory function, 445
    for sexual function, 537
    for skin, 490
    for sleep and rest, 504

    for thermoregulation, 520
    for urinary function, 395
    for vision, 348
wheelchairs, fit assessment, 106, 106t
white coat hypertension, 418
widowhood, 205
women and minority groups, cardiovascular disease in, 415–416
World Health Organization (WHO), 550
    pain relief ladder, 570, 570f

X
xerosis, 480
xerostomia, 360

Y
yaktrax walker, 468, 469f

Z
zolpidem, 457